www.harcourt-international.com

Bringing you products from all Harcourt Health Sciences companies including Baillière Tindall, Churchill Livingstone, Mosby and W.B. Saunders

- **Browse** for latest information on new books, journals and electronic products
- **Search** for information on over 20 000 published titles with full product information including tables of contents and sample chapters
- **Keep up to date** with our extensive publishing programme in your field by registering with eAlert or requesting postal updates
- **Secure online ordering** with prompt delivery, as well as full contact details to order by phone, fax or post
- **News** of special features and promotions

If you are based in the following countries, please visit the country-specific site to receive full details of product availability and local ordering information

USA: www.harcourthealth.com

Canada: www.harcourtcanada.com

Australia: www.harcourt.com.au

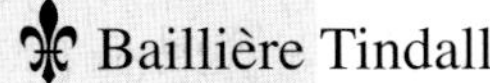

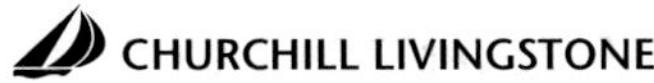

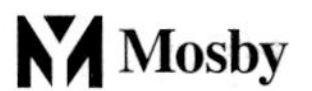

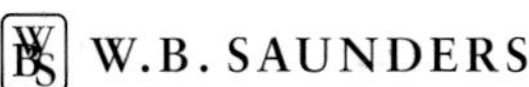

SIXTH EDITION

IMMUNOLOGY

Ivan Roitt

MA DSc(Oxon)Hon FRCP(Lond) FRCPath FRS
Emeritus Professor of Immunology
Royal Free and University College Medical School
University College London, UK

Jonathan Brostoff

MA DM(Oxon) DSc(Med) FRCP(Lond) FRCPath
Senior Research Fellow
Professor Emeritus of Allergy and Environmental Health
Division of Life Sciences
King's College London
London, UK

David Male

MA PhD
Professor of Biology, Department of Biological Sciences
The Open University
Milton Keynes, UK

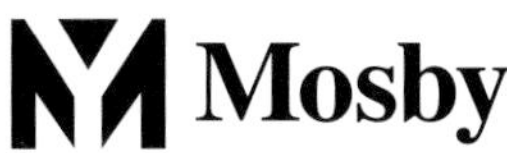

EDINBURGH LONDON NEW YORK PHILADELPHIA ST LOUIS SYDNEY TORONTO 2001

MOSBY
An imprint of Elsevier Science Limited

First published by Gower Medical Publishing Ltd, 1985 ISBN 0-906923-35-2
Second edition published by Gower Medical Publishing Ltd, 1989
ISBN 0-3974-4573-3
Third edition published by Mosby-Year Book Europe Ltd, 1993
ISBN 0-397-44765-5
Fourth edition published by Mosby, an imprint of Times Mirror International Publishers Ltd, 1996 ISBN 0-7234-2178-1
Fifth edition published by Mosby, an imprint of Mosby International Ltd
1998 ISBN 0 7234 29189

Sixth edition 2001
Reprinted 2002

ISBN 0 7234 31892
International Student Edition ISBN 0 7234 32422
Reprinted 2002

British Library Cataloguing in Publication Data
A catalogue record for this book is available from the British Library

Library of Congress Cataloging in Publication Data
A catalog record for this book is available from the Library of Congress

Note
Medical knowledge is constantly changing. As new information becomes available, changes in treatment, procedures, equipment and the use of drugs become necessary. The authors, contributors and the publishers have taken care to ensure that the information given in this text is accurate and up to date. However, readers are strongly advised to confirm that the information, especially with regard to drug usage, complies with the latest legislation and standards of practice.

Commissioning Editor: Louise Crowe, Richard Furn
Project Development Manager: Janice Urquhart
Project Manager: Frances Affleck
Design direction: Judith Wright
Illustration Manager: Bruce Hogarth
New illustrations by: Sandie Hill
Illustrations by: Richie Prime, Lynda Rosemary Payne

The publisher's policy is to use **paper manufactured from sustainable forests**

Printed in Spain

Preface

As we started to plan the 6th edition of Immunology, it soon became clear that the steady progress in the subject during the last few years has lead to a new way of understanding immune responses. So we have completely reorganised the first half of the book which covers basic immunology. In addition, all sections have been thoroughly revised and updated to reflect the continuing rapid progress in both basic and clinical immunology.

The opening chapters describe the building blocks of the immune system – cells, organs and the major receptor molecules, including antibodies, T cell receptors and MHC molecules. Information on the development of the leucocyte populations and antigen receptors has now been placed alongside the text describing their functions.

The following chapters deal with the initiation of the immune response, leading from antigen presentation and co-stimulation through cell activation pathways to the actions of cytokines. Finally three chapters discuss the principle effector arms of the immune response, TH2 responses with antibody production, TH1 responses and mononuclear phagocytes, and cytotoxicity, including Tc cells and NK cells. The chapter on immunoregulation has been revised to reflect this way of thinking, while the chapter on tolerance has been extensively rewritten to provide a bridge to the understanding of autoimmunity.

Our aim in this revision has been to provide readers with a sound understanding of the immune responses which underlie clinically important areas, namely defence against infection, hypersensitivity states and allergy, immunopathology, tumour immunotherapy and transplantation. We have maintained what we believe to be an important feature of the book, namely a clear description of the scientific principles of clinical immunology, integrated with histology, pathology, and clinical examples.

A new feature of the book is the use of problem-based learning for basic immunology and clinical case studies as appropriate. A set of solutions to the problems is also included, although some of the questions are open ended and would form a good basis for class discussion or tutorials.

A great strength of this book is the interlinked products which enhance learning and provide different ways of approaching the subject. Free with this book is a disk containing three sample animations taken from the highly successful Immunology Interactive CD-ROM (Male, Brostoff, Gray, Roitt) and a link to a supporting website:

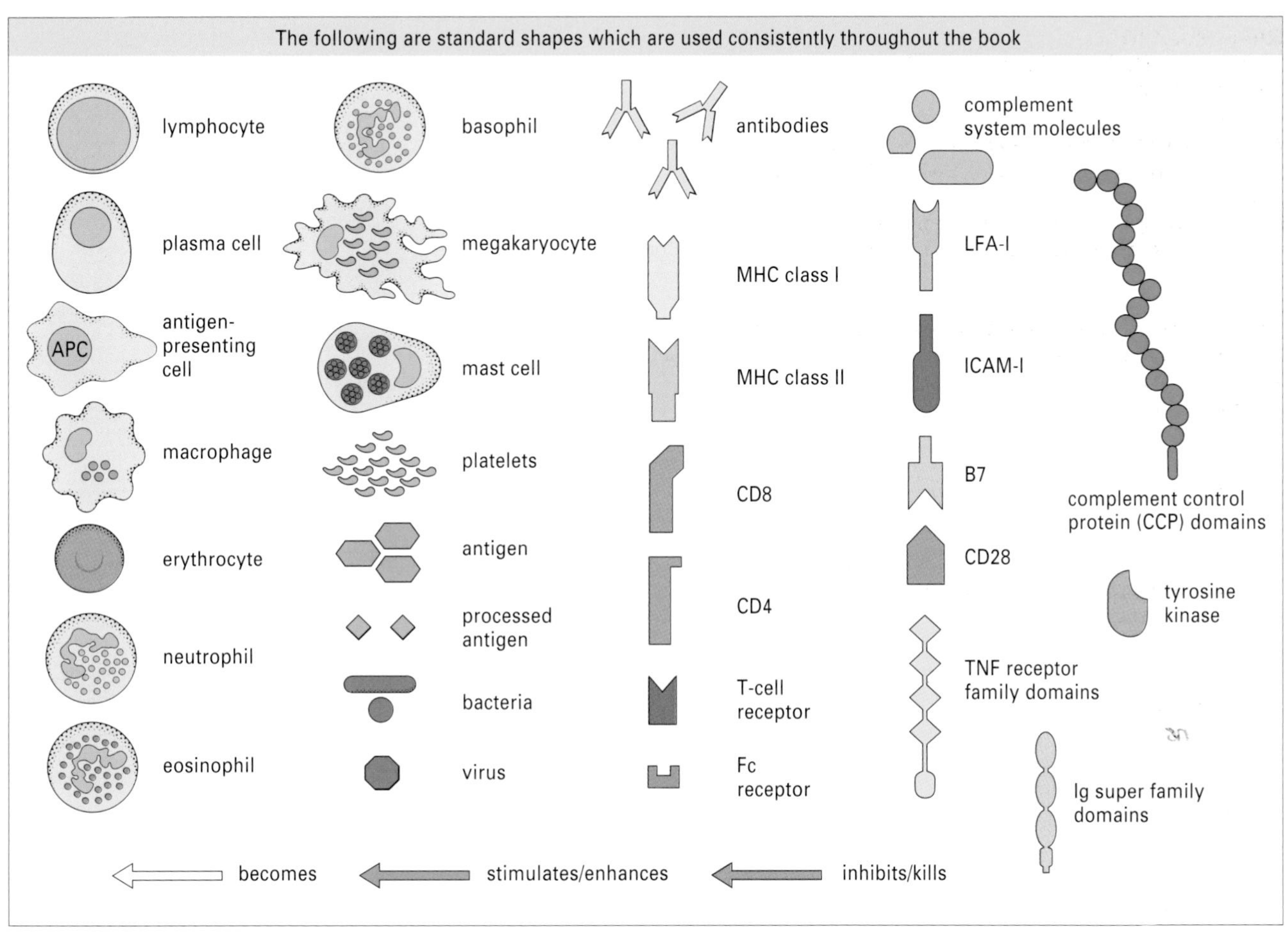

www.fleshandbones.com/immunology/roitt. This website hosts the illustrations from the book in downloadable format. Also available separately is *Immunology: An Illustrated Outline*, Third edition (Male).

We wish our readers well in their study of immunology, a subject which continues to excite and surprise us, and which underpins many other areas of biology and biomedical sciences.

Ivan Roitt
Jonathan Brostoff
David Male

Contents

11. Regulation of the immune response

Anne Cooke

12. Immunological tolerance

David Wraith

13. Evolution of immunity

John Horton, Norman A. Ratcliffe

14. Immunity to viruses

Tony Nash

15. Immunity to bacteria and fungi

Graham A. W. Rook

16. Immunity to protozoa and worms

Janette E. Bradley

17. Vaccination

Peter Beverley

18. Tumour immunology

Peter Beverley

19. Primary immunodeficiency

Fred S. Rosen

20. Secondary immunodeficiency

Ian Weller

21. Hypersensitivity – Type I

Tom Platts-Mills

22. Hypersensitivity – Type II

David Male

23. Hypersensitivity – Type III

Frank Hay, Olwyn M. R. Westwood

24. Hypersensitivity – Type IV

Warwick Britton

25. Transplantation and rejection

Ian Hutchinson

26. Autoimmunity and autoimmune disease

Ivan Roitt

27. Immunological techniques

Michael Steward

Appendices

Contributors

Professor Frances Balkwill
Translational Oncology Laboratory
St Bartholomew's and Royal London School of Medicine and Dentistry
London, UK

Professor Peter Beverley
Edward Jenner Institute for Vaccine Research
Compton, Berkshire, UK

Professor Janette E. Bradley
Chair of Immunoparasitology
School of Biological Sciences
University of Nottingham
Nottingham, UK

Professor Warwick Britton
Centenary Institute for Cancer Medicine and Cell Biology, and Department of Medicine
University of Sydney, Sydney, Australia

Professor Jonathan Brostoff
Senior Research Fellow,
Professor Emeritus of Allergy and Environmental Health
King's College London
London, UK

Professor Anne Cooke
Professor of Immunology
Department of Pathology
University of Cambridge, Cambridge, UK

Professor Marc Feldman
Head of Cytokine and Immunology Research Section
Kennedy Institute of Rheumatology
Professor of Cellular Immunology
Department of Rheumatology
Imperial College of Medicine
London, UK

Professor Siamon Gordon
Sir William Dunn School of Pathology
University of Oxford, Oxford, UK

Professor Carlo E. Grossi
Department of Experimental Medicine
University of Genova, Italy

Professor Frank Hay
Professor of Immunology and Society of Apothecaries
Lecturer in the History of Medicine
Department of Biochemistry and Immunology
St George's Hospital Medical School
London, UK

Dr John Horton
Reader in Immunology
Department of Biological Sciences
University of Durham
Durham, UK

Professor Ian Hutchinson
Professor of Immunology
School of Biological Sciences and Faculty of Medicine
University of Manchester
Manchester, UK

Professor Peter M. Lydyard
Professor of Immunology
Royal Free and Middlesex Hospital Medical School
London, UK

Professor David Male
Professor, Department of Biological Sciences
The Open University
Milton Keynes, UK

Dr Joseph C. Marini
Cellular and Cytokine Immunology
Kennedy Institute of Rheumatology
London, UK

Professor Tom Platts-Mills
Head of Asthma and Allergic Disease Center
University of Virginia
Charlottesville, USA

Professor Tony Nash
Department of Veterinary Pathology
University of Edinburgh, Edinburgh, UK

Professor Norman A. Ratcliffe
Biomedical and Physiological Research
School of Biological Sciences
University of Wales, Swansea, Wales, UK

Professor Ivan Roitt
Emeritus Professor of Immunology
Director of The Institute of Biomedical Science
University College London Medical School
London, UK

Professor Graham A. W. Rook
Professor of Medical Microbiology
Royal Free and University College London Medical School, Windeyer Institute of Medical Sciences
London, UK

Professor Fred S. Rosen
James L. Gamble Professor of Pediatrics
Harvard Medical School
President
Center for Blood Research
Senior Physician
Children's Hospital, Boston, USA

Professor Michael Steward
Professor of Immunology
Department of Infectious and Tropical Diseases
London School of Hygiene and Tropical Medicine
London, UK

Professor John Trowsdale
Immunology Division
Department of Pathology
University of Cambridge
Cambridge, UK

Professor Malcolm Turner
Immunobiology Unit
Institute of Child Health
University College London
London, UK

Professor Ian Weller
Professor of Sexually Transmitted Diseases
Royal Free and University College Medical School
University College London
London, UK

Dr Olwyn M. R. Westwood
MSc Programme Co-ordinator
School of Life Sciences
University of Surrey Roehampton
London, UK

Professor David Wraith
Professor of Experimental Pathology
Department of Pathology and Microbiology
University of Bristol
Bristol, UK

1 Introduction to the immune system

- **The immune system has evolved to protect us from pathogens.** Some, such as viruses, infect individual cells; others, including many bacteria, divide extracellularly within tissues or the body cavities.
- **The cells which mediate immunity include lymphocytes and phagocytes.** Lymphocytes recognize antigens on pathogens. Phagocytes internalize pathogens and degrade them.
- **An immune response consists of two phases.** In the first phase, antigen activates specific lymphocytes that recognize it; in the effector phase, these lymphocytes coordinate an immune response that eliminates the source of the antigens.
- **Specificity and memory** are two essential features of adaptive immune responses. The immune system mounts a more effective response on second and subsequent encounters with a particular antigen.
- **Lymphocytes have specialized functions.** B cells make antibodies; cytotoxic T cells kill virally infected cells; helper T cells coordinate the immune response by direct cell–cell interactions and the release of cytokines, which help B cells to make antibody.
- **Antigens are molecules which are recognized by receptors on lymphocytes.** B lymphocytes usually recognize intact antigen molecules, while T lymphocytes recognize antigen fragments on the surface of other cells.
- **Clonal selection involves recognition of antigen by a particular lymphocyte;** this leads to clonal expansion and differentiation to effector and memory cells.
- **The immune system may break down.** This can lead to immunodeficiency or hypersensitivity diseases or to autoimmune diseases.

Our environment contains a great variety of infectious microbes – viruses, bacteria, fungi, protozoa and multicellular parasites. These can cause disease, and if they multiply unchecked they will eventually kill their host. Most infections in normal individuals are short-lived and leave little permanent damage. This is due to the immune system, which combats infectious agents.

Because microorganisms come in many different forms, a wide variety of immune responses are required to deal with each type of infection. In the first instance, the exterior defences of the body present an effective barrier to most organisms, and very few infectious agents can penetrate intact skin (*Fig. 1.1*). However, many gain access across the epithelia of the gastrointestinal or urogenital tracts. Others can infect the nasopharynx and lung. A small number, such as malaria and hepatitis B, can only infect the body if they enter the blood directly.

The site of the infection and the type of pathogen largely determine which immune responses will be effective. The most important distinction is between pathogens which invade the host's cells and those which do not. All viruses, some bacteria and some protozoan parasites replicate inside host cells, and to clear an infection the immune system must recognize and destroy these infected cells. Many bacteria and larger parasites live in tissues, body fluids or other extracellular spaces, and the responses to these pathogens are quite different. During the course of an infection, however, even intracellular pathogens must reach their target cells by moving through the blood and tissue fluid. At this time they are susceptible to elements of the immune system, which normally counter extracellular pathogens (*Fig. 1.2*).

This chapter introduces the basic elements of the immune system and of immune responses, which are detailed in Chapters 2–18. There are various ways in which the immune system can fail, leading to immunopathological reactions, and these are outlined in the second half of the book. However, it is important to stress that the primary function of the immune system is to eliminate infectious agents and to minimize the damage they cause.

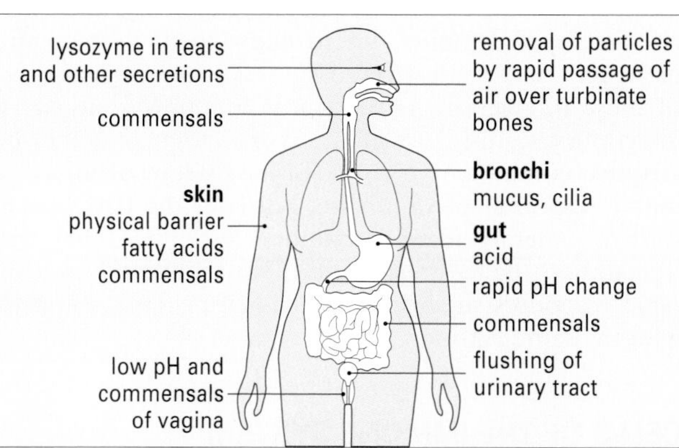

Fig. 1.1 Most of the infectious agents that an individual encounters do not penetrate the body surface, but are prevented from entering by a variety of biochemical and physical barriers. The body tolerates a number of commensal organisms, which compete effectively with many potential pathogens.

ADAPTIVE AND INNATE IMMUNITY

Any immune response involves, firstly, recognition of the pathogen or other foreign material, and secondly a reaction to eliminate it. Broadly, the different types of immune response fall into two categories: innate (or non-adaptive) immune responses and adaptive immune responses. The important difference between these is that an adaptive

Intracellular and extracellular pathogens

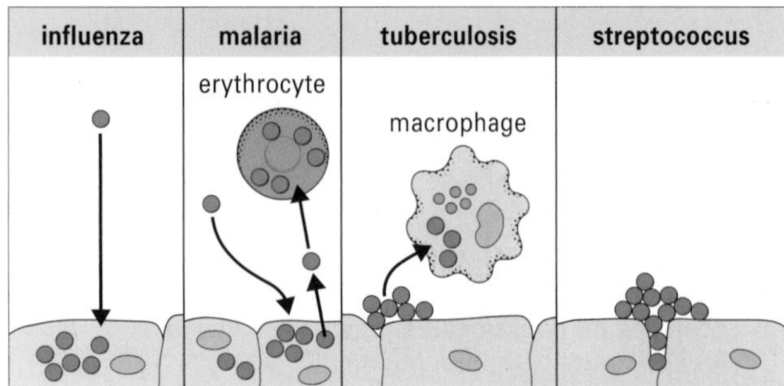

Fig. 1.2 All infectious agents spread to infect new cells by passing through the body fluids or tissues, but many pathogens must infect cells of the body to divide. For example, viruses such as influenza must invade cells to reproduce, while *Plasmodium* spp. (malaria) have two separate phases of division, either in cells of the liver or in erythrocytes. The mycobacteria which cause tuberculosis can divide extracellularly or within macrophages. Some bacteria such as the streptococci, which produce sore throats and wound infections, generally divide outside cells.

Interaction between lymphocytes and phagocytes

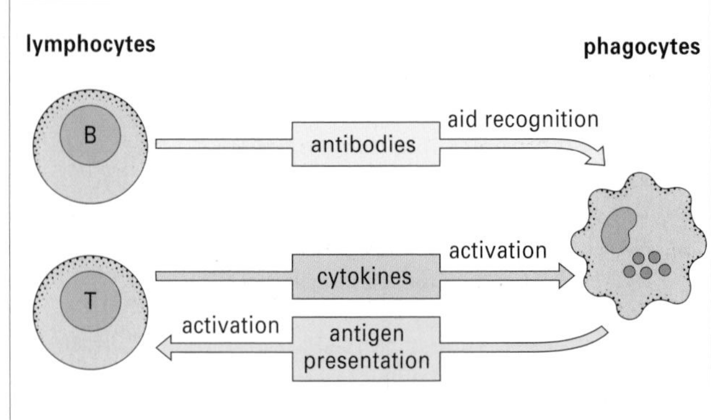

Fig. 1.3 B lymphocytes release antibodies, which bind to pathogens and their products and so aid recognition by phagocytes. Cytokines released by T cells activate the phagocytes to destroy the material they have taken up. In turn, mononuclear phagocytes can present antigen to T cells, thereby activating them.

immune response is highly specific for a particular pathogen. Moreover, although the innate response does not alter on repeated exposure to a given infectious agent, the adaptive response improves with each successive encounter with the same pathogen: in effect the adaptive immune system 'remembers' the infectious agent and can prevent it from causing disease later. For example, diseases such as measles and diphtheria induce adaptive immune responses which generate a life-long immunity following an infection. The two key features of the adaptive immune response are thus specificity and memory.

Immune responses are produced primarily by leucocytes, of which there are several different types.

Phagocytes and innate immune responses – One important group of leucocytes is the phagocytic cells, such as the monocytes, macrophages and polymorphonuclear neutrophils. These cells bind to microorganisms, internalize them and then kill them. Because they use primitive non-specific recognition systems which allow them to bind to a variety of microbial products, they mediate innate immune responses. In effect they act as a first line of defence against infection.

Lymphocytes and adaptive immune responses – Another important set of leucocytes is the lymphocytes. These cells are central to all adaptive immune responses, because they specifically recognize individual pathogens, whether they are inside host cells or outside in the tissue fluids or blood. In fact there are several different types of lymphocyte, but they fall into two basic categories, T lymphocytes (or T cells) and B lymphocytes (or B cells). B cells combat extracellular pathogens and their products by releasing antibody, a molecule which specifically recognizes and binds to a particular target molecule, called the antigen. The antigen may be a molecule on the surface of a pathogen, or a toxin which it produces. T lymphocytes have a wider range of activities. Some are involved in the control of B lymphocyte development and antibody production. Another group of T lymphocytes interacts with phagocytic cells to help them destroy pathogens they have taken up. A third set of T lymphocytes recognizes cells infected by virus and destroys them.

Interaction between lymphocytes and phagocytes – In practice there is considerable interaction between the lymphocytes and phagocytes. For example, some phagocytes can take up antigens and show them to T lymphocytes in a form they can recognize, a process which is called antigen presentation. In turn, the T lymphocytes release soluble factors (cytokines), which activate the phagocytes and cause them to destroy the pathogens they have internalized. In another interaction, phagocytes use antibodies released by B lymphocytes to allow them to recognize pathogens more effectively (*Fig. 1.3*). One consequence of these interactions is that most immune responses to infectious organisms are made up of a variety of innate and adaptive components. In the earliest stages of infection, innate responses predominate, but later the lymphocytes start to generate adaptive immune responses. They then 'remember' the pathogen, and mount more effective and rapid responses should the individual become reinfected with the same pathogen at a later date.

CELLS OF THE IMMUNE SYSTEM

Immune responses are mediated by a variety of cells, and by the soluble molecules which they secrete. Although the leucocytes are central to all immune responses, other cells in the tissues also participate, by signalling to the lymphocytes and responding to the cytokines released by

Components of the immune system

cell	leucocytes: lymphocytes			leucocytes: phagocytes			leucocytes: auxiliary cells			other
	B cell	T cell	large granular lymphocyte	mononuclear phagocyte	neutrophil	eosinophil	basophil	mast cell	platelets	tissue cells
soluble mediators	antibodies	cytokines		complement			inflammatory mediators			interferons cytokines

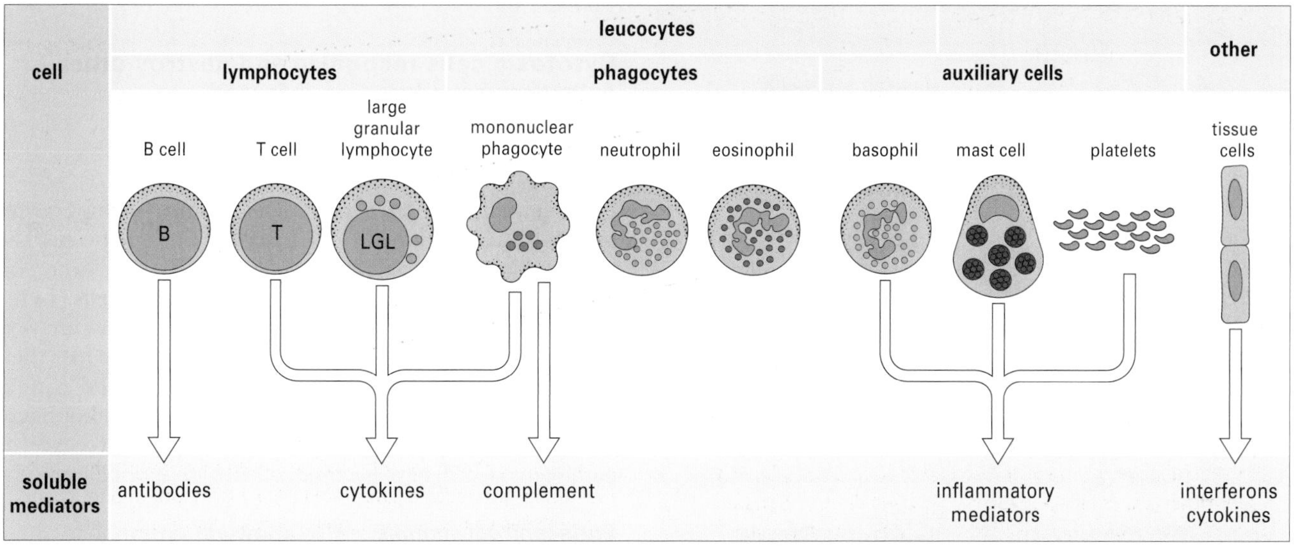

Fig. 1.4 The principal components of the immune system are shown, indicating which cells produce which soluble mediators. Complement is made primarily by the liver, although there is some synthesis by mononuclear phagocytes. Note that each cell produces and secretes only a particular set of cytokines or inflammatory mediators.

T lymphocytes and macrophages. *Figure 1.4* lists the main cells and molecules involved in immune reactions.

Phagocytes internalize antigens and pathogenic microorganisms and degrade them

Mononuclear phagocytes – The most important group of long-lived phagocytic cells belongs to the mononuclear phagocyte lineage. These cells are all derived from bone marrow stem cells, and their function is to engulf particles, including infectious agents, internalize them and destroy them. For this purpose they are strategically placed where they will encounter such particles. For example, the Kupffer cells of the liver line the sinusoids along which blood flows, while the synovial A cells line the synovial cavity (*Fig. 1.5*). Blood cells belonging to this lineage are called monocytes. In time, these migrate from the blood into the tissues, where they develop into tissue macrophages. These cells are very effective at presenting antigens to T lymphocytes (see Chapter 2).

Polymorphonuclear neutrophils – Polymorphonuclear neutrophils, often just called neutrophils or PMN, are another important group of phagocytes. Neutrophils constitute the majority of the blood leucocytes and develop from the same early precursors as monocytes and macrophages. Like monocytes, they migrate into tissues, particularly at sites of inflammation, but neutrophils are short-lived cells, which engulf material, destroy it and then die.

Lymphocytes occur as two major types, B cells and T cells, which are responsible for specific recognition of antigens

Lymphocytes are wholly responsible for the specific immune recognition of pathogens, so they initiate adaptive immune responses. All lymphocytes are derived from bone-marrow stem cells, but T lymphocytes then develop in the thymus, while B lymphocytes develop in the bone marrow (in adult mammals).

B cells – Each B cell is genetically programmed to encode a surface receptor specific for a particular antigen. Having recognized its specific antigen, the B cells multiply and differentiate into plasma cells, which produce large amounts of the receptor molecule in a soluble form that can be secreted. This is known as antibody. These antibody molecules are large glycoproteins found in the blood and tissue fluids: because they are virtually identical to the original receptor molecule, they bind to the antigen that initially activated the B cells.

T cells – There are several different types of T cells, and they have a variety of functions. One group interacts with mononuclear phagocytes and helps them destroy intracellular pathogens; they are called type-1 T-helper cells or TH1 cells. Another group interacts with B cells and helps them to divide, differentiate and make antibody: these are the TH2 cells. A third group of T cells is responsible for the destruction of host cells which have become infected by viruses or other intracellular pathogens – this kind of action is called cytotoxicity and these T cells are hence called T-cytotoxic (TC) cells. In every case, the T cells recognize antigens, but only when they are presented on the surface of the other cell by so-called major histocompatibity complex (MHC) molecules. They use a specific receptor to do this, termed the T-cell antigen receptor (TCR). This is related, both in function and structure, to the surface antibody which B cells use as their antigen receptors. T cells generate their effects, either by releasing soluble proteins, called cytokines,

Cells of the mononuclear phagocyte lineage

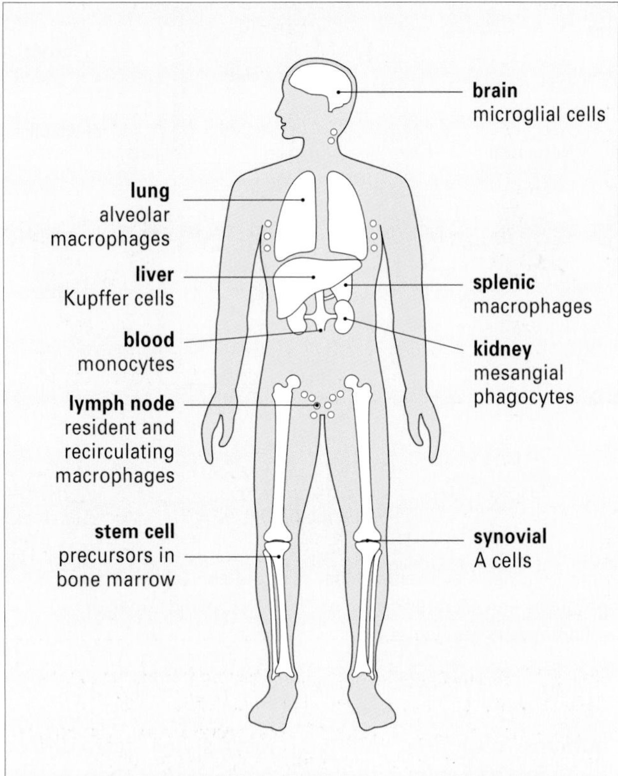

Fig. 1.5 Many organs contain phagocytic cells derived from blood monocytes which are manufactured in the bone marrow. Monocytes pass out of the blood vessel and become macrophages in the tissues. Resident phagocytic cells of different tissues were previously referred to as the reticuloendothelial system, but they too appear to belong to the monocyte lineage.

which signal to other cells, or by direct cell–cell interactions. The principal functions of lymphocytes are summarized in *Figure 1.6*.

Cytotoxic cells recognize and destroy other cells that have become infected

Several cell types have the capacity to kill other cells, of which the Tc cell is especially important.

Large granular lymphocytes – The group of lymphocytes known as large granular lymphocytes (LGLs) also has the capacity to recognize the surface changes that occur on a variety of tumour cells and virally infected cells. LGLs damage these target cells, but unlike Tc cells, they are very effective at recognizing cells which lack, or have lost their MHC molecules. This action is sometimes called natural killer (NK) cell activity. Additionally, both macrophages and LGLs recognize and destroy some target cells (or pathogens) which have become coated with specific antibody.

Eosinophil polymorphs – Also known as eosinophils, these are a specialized group of leucocytes which have the ability to engage and damage large extracellular parasites, such as schistosomes.

All of these cell types damage their different targets by releasing the contents of their intracellular granules close to them. Other molecules secreted by the cytotoxic cells, but not stored in granules, contribute to the damage.

Auxiliary cells control inflammation

A number of other cells mediate inflammation, the main purpose of which (see below) is to attract leucocytes and the soluble mediators of immunity towards a site of infection.

Basophils and mast cells – These have granules containing a variety of mediators that produce inflammation in surrounding tissues. These mediators are released when the cells are triggered. They can also synthesize and secrete a number of mediators which control the development of immune reactions. Mast cells lie close to blood vessels

Functions of lymphocytes

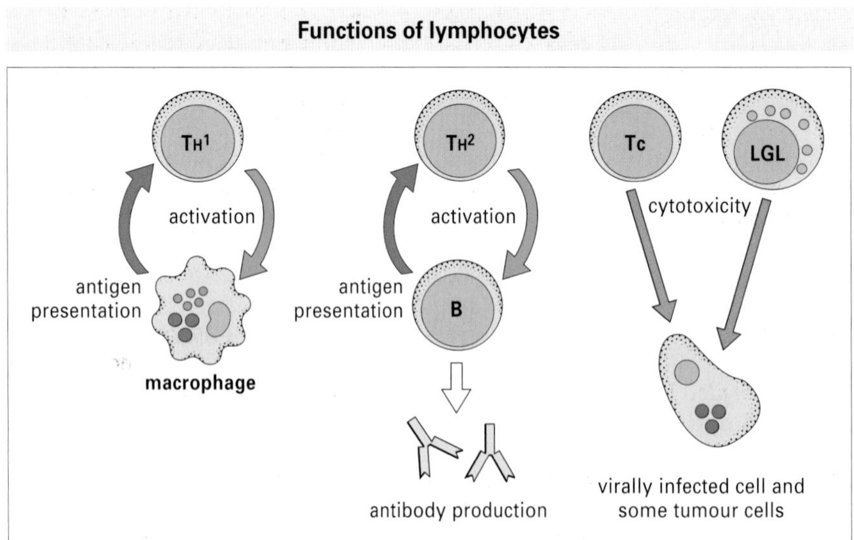

Fig. 1.6 Macrophages present antigen to type-1 T helper cells (TH1) which release cytokines that activate the macrophages to destroy microorganisms they have phagocytosed. B cells present antigen to TH2 cells, which release cytokines which activate them, causing them to divide and differentiate. Cytotoxic T cells (Tc) and large granular lymphocytes (LGL) recognize and destroy virally infected cells.

in all tissues, and some of their mediators act on cells in the vessel walls. Basophils are functionally similar to mast cells but are mobile, circulating cells.

Platelets – These can also release inflammatory mediators when activated during thrombogenesis or by means of antigen–antibody complexes.

SOLUBLE MEDIATORS OF IMMUNITY

A wide variety of molecules are involved in the development of immune responses. These include antibodies and cytokines, produced by lymphocytes, and a variety of other molecules that are normally present in serum. The serum concentration of a number of these proteins increases rapidly during infection and they are therefore called acute phase proteins. One example is C-reactive protein (CRP), so called because of its ability to bind to the C-molecule of pneumococci. This promotes their uptake by phagocytes, a process known as opsonization (see *Fig. 1.10*). Molecules such as antibody, complement and C-reactive protein that promote phagocytosis are said to act as opsonins.

Complement proteins mediate phagocytosis, control inflammation and interact with antibodies in immune defence

The complement system is a group of about 20 serum proteins whose overall function is the control of inflammation. The components interact with each other, and with other elements of the immune system. For example, a number of microorganisms spontaneously activate the complement system, via the so-called alternative pathway, which is an innate, non-specific reaction. This results in the microorganism being coated by complement molecules, leading to its uptake by phagocytes. The complement system can also be activated by antibodies bound to the pathogen surface (via the 'classical pathway'), when it co-mediates a specific, adaptive response.

Complement activation is a cascade reaction, with each component sequentially acting on others, in a similar way to the blood-clotting system. Activation by either the classical or the alternative pathway generates protein molecules or peptide fragments which have the following effects:

- Opsonization of microorganisms for uptake by phagocytes and eventual intracellular killing.
- Attraction of phagocytes to sites of infection (chemotaxis).
- Increased blood flow to the site of activation and increased permeability of capillaries to plasma molecules.
- Damage to plasma membranes on cells, Gram-negative bacteria, enveloped viruses or other organisms which have induced the activation. This in turn can produce lysis of the cell or virus and reduce the infection.
- Release of further inflammatory mediators from mast cells.

These functions are outlined in *Figure 1.7* and detailed in Chapter 3.

Complement functions

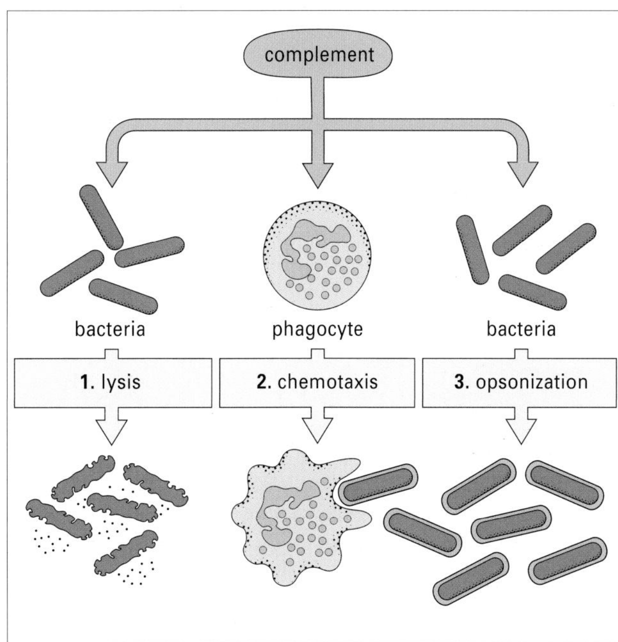

Fig. 1.7 (**1**) The complement system has an intrinsic ability to lyse the cell membranes of many bacterial species. (**2**) Complement products released in this reaction attract phagocytes to the site of the reaction – chemotaxis. (**3**) Complement components coat the bacterial surface – opsonization – allowing the phagocytes to recognize the bacteria and engulf them. These reactions may be triggered by the intrinsic ability of the complement system to recognize microbial components or by antibodies bound to the microorganism.

Cytokines signal between lymphocytes, phagocytes and other cells of the body

Cytokine is the general term for a large group of molecules involved in signalling between cells during immune responses. All cytokines are proteins, some with sugar molecules attached (glycoproteins). The different cytokines fall into a number of categories, and those produced by lymphocytes may be called lymphokines. The principal sets of cytokines are outlined below.

Interferons (IFNs) – These are particularly important in limiting the spread of certain viral infections. One group of interferons (IFNα and IFNβ) is produced by cells which have become virally infected; another type, IFNγ, is released by certain activated T cells. IFNs induce a state of antiviral resistance in uninfected tissue cells (*Fig. 1.8*). They are produced very early in infection and are the first line of resistance to a great many viruses.

Interleukins (ILs) – These are a large group of cytokines (IL-1 to IL-22) produced mainly by T cells, although some are also produced by mononuclear phagocytes, or by tissue cells. They have a variety of functions, but most of them are involved in directing other cells to divide and differentiate.

Colony-stimulating factors (CSFs) – These are primarily involved in directing the division and differentiation of bone-marrow stem cells, and the precursors of blood

Interferons (IFNs)

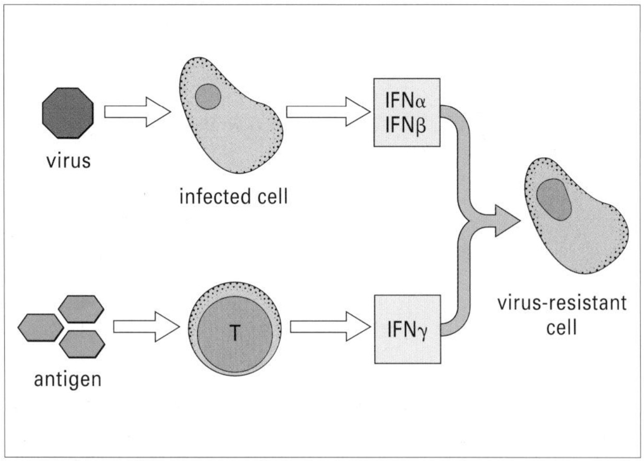

Fig. 1.8 When host cells become infected by virus, they may produce interferon. Different cell types produce interferon-α (IFNα) or interferon-β (IFNβ); interferon-γ (IFNγ) is produced by some types of lymphocyte (T) after activation by antigen. Interferons act on other host cells to induce a state of resistance to viral infection. IFNγ has many other effects as well.

leucocytes. The balance of different CSFs is partially responsible for the proportions of different cell types that will be produced. Some CSFs also promote further differentiation of cells outside the bone marrow. For example, macrophage-CSF (M-CSF) promotes the development of monocytes in bone marrow and macrophages in tissues.

Chemokines – This large group of chemotactic cytokines direct movement of cells around the body, from the blood stream into tissues and to the appropriate location within each tissue. Some of the chemokines also activate cells to carry out particular functions.

Other cytokines – Of these, the tumour necrosis factors, TNFα and TNFβ and transforming growth factor-β (TGFβ), have a variety of functions, but are particularly important in mediating inflammation and cytotoxic reactions.

Each set of cells releases a particular blend of cytokines, depending on the type of cell and whether it has been activated. For example, the TH1 cells release one set of cytokines which promote their interactions with mononuclear phagocytes, while the TH2 cells release a different set which allow them to activate B cells. Some cytokines may be produced by all T cells, and some just by a specific subset. Equally important is the expression of cytokine receptors. Only a cell which has the appropriate receptors can respond to a particular cytokine. For example the receptors for interferons, mentioned above, are present on all nucleated cells in the body, but other cytokines are much more restricted in their distribution. In general, cytokine receptors are specific for their own individual cytokine, but this is not always so. In particular many of the chemokine receptors respond to several different chemokines. This is discussed in more detail in Chapters 3 and 7.

Antibody specifically binds to antigen and then mediates secondary effects

Antibodies (Ab), also called immunoglobulins (Ig), are a group of serum molecules produced by B lymphocytes. In fact, as explained earlier, they are the soluble form of the B cells' surface antigen receptor. All antibodies have the same basic structure, but they differ in the region that binds to the antigen. In general, each antibody can bind specifically to just one antigen.

While one part of an antibody molecule (the Fab portion) binds to antigen, other parts interact with other elements of the immune system, such as phagocytes, or one of the complement molecules. In effect, antibodies act as flexible adaptors, allowing various elements of the immune system to recognize specific pathogens and their products (*Fig. 1.9*).

The part of the antibody molecule that interacts with cells of the immune system, is termed the Fc portion. Neutrophils, macrophages and other mononuclear phagocytes have Fc receptors on their surface. Consequently, if antibody binds to a pathogen, it can link to a phagocyte via the Fc portion. This allows the pathogen to be ingested and destroyed by the phagocyte (phagocytosed) – the antibody acts as an opsonin. Phagocytes can recognize

Antibody – a flexible adaptor

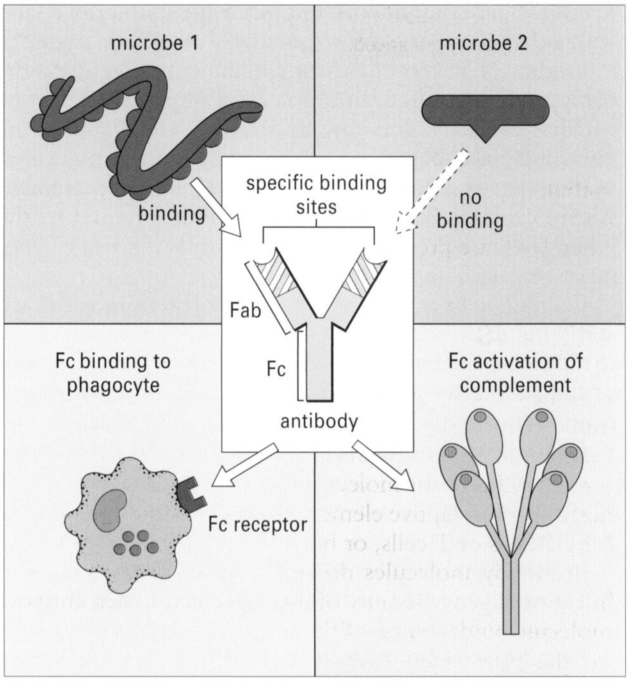

Fig. 1.9 When a microorganism lacks the inherent ability to activate complement or bind to phagocytes, the body provides antibodies as flexible adaptor molecules. The body can make several million different antibodies able to recognize a wide variety of infectious agents. Thus the antibody illustrated binds microbe 1, but not microbe 2, by its 'antigen-binding portion' (Fab). The Fc portion may activate complement or bind to Fc receptors on host cells, particularly phagocytes.

Opsonization

phagocyte	opsonin	binding
1	–	±
2	complement C3b	+ +
3	antibody	+ +
4	antibody and complement C3b	+ + + +

Fig. 1.10 (**1**) Phagocytes have some intrinsic ability to bind directly to bacteria and other microorganisms. (**2**) This is much enhanced if the bacteria have activated complement. They will then have bound C3b so that the cells can bind the bacteria via C3b receptors. (**3**) Organisms which do not activate complement well, if at all, are opsonized by antibody (Ab), which can bind to the Fc receptor on the phagocyte. (**4**) Antibody can also activate complement and if both antibody and C3b opsonize the microbe, binding is greatly enhanced.

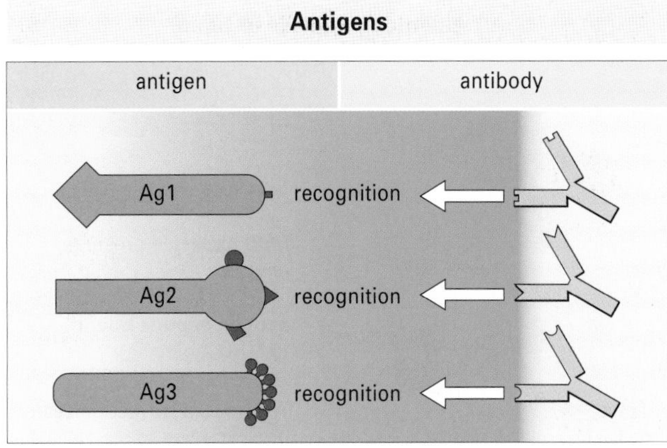

Fig. 1.11 Molecules that generate antibodies are called antigens. Antigen molecules each have a set of antigenic determinants, also called epitopes. The epitopes on one antigen (Ag1) are usually different from those on another (Ag2). Some antigens (Ag3) have repeated epitopes. Epitopes are molecular shapes recognized by antibodies of the adaptive immune system. Each antibody recognizes one epitope rather than the whole antigen. Even simple microorganisms have many different antigens which may be protein, lipid or carbohydrate.

material using either activated complement (C3b) or antibody as the opsonin, but phagocytosis is most effective when both are present (*Fig. 1.10*).

ANTIGENS

Originally the term antigen was used for any molecule that induced B cells to produce a specific antibody (*anti*body *gen*erator). Now however the term is much more widely used to indicate any molecule that can be specifically recognized by the adaptive elements of the immune system, that is by B cells or T cells, or both.

Antibody molecules do not bind to the whole of an infectious agent. Because of their specificity, each antibody molecule binds to one of the many molecules – antigens – on the microorganism's surface. There may be several different antibodies for a given pathogen, each binding to a different antigen on that pathogen's surface. Each antibody binds to a restricted part of the antigen called an epitope. A particular antigen can have several different epitopes or repeated epitopes (*Fig. 1.11*). Antibodies are specific for the epitopes rather than the whole antigen molecule.

The way in which a sufficient diversity of antibody molecules is generated to bind to all the different antigens encountered in a lifetime is explained in Chapter 4.

Antigen recognition is the foundation of all adaptive immune responses

T cells also recognize antigens, but they recognize antigens originating from within cells that are presented at the surface of the host cell as small polypeptide fragments. For example, a host cell that has been infected with a virus will express small fragments of viral proteins on its surface, thus making it instantly recognizable by cytotoxic T cells. The antigen fragments are presented on the surface of the cell by a specialized group of molecules. These are encoded in a set of genes known as the major histocompatibility complex (MHC), and are consequently called MHC molecules. The T cells use their antigen-specific receptors (TCRs) to recognize the antigenic peptides bound to these MHC molecules (*Fig. 1.12*).

The essential point to remember about antigen, is that it is the initiator and driving force for all adaptive immune responses. The immune system has evolved to recognize antigens, destroy them and eliminate the source of their production – bacteria, virally infected cells, etc. When antigen is eliminated, immune responses switch off.

IMMUNE RESPONSES

You will recall that there are two major phases of any immune response:

- Recognition of the antigen.
- A reaction to eradicate it.

In adaptive immune responses, lymphocytes are responsible for immune recognition, and this is achieved by clonal selection.

T-cell recognition of antigen

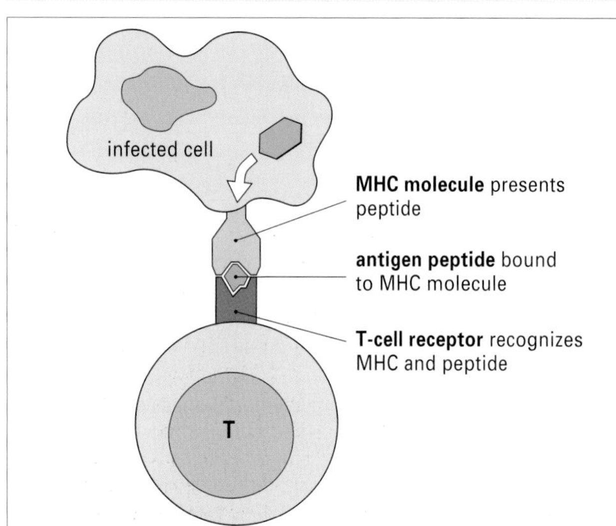

Fig. 1.12 T cells recognize antigens that originate within other cells, such as viral peptides from infected cells. They do this by binding specifically to antigenic peptides presented on the surface of the infected cells by molecules encoded by the major histocompatibility complex (MHC molecules). The T cells use their specific receptors (TCRs) to recognize the unique combination of MHC molecule plus antigenic peptide. Unlike B cells, which recognize just a portion of the antigen, a T cell recognizes residues from both the MHC molecule and the antigen peptide.

B-cell clonal selection

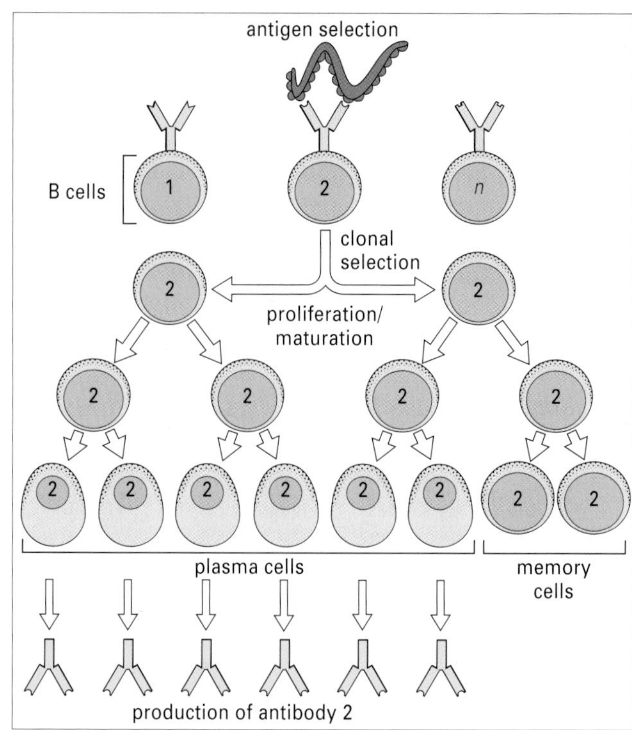

Fig. 1.13 Each antibody-producing cell (B cell) is programmed to make just one antibody, which is placed on its surface as an antigen receptor. Antigen binds to only those B cells with the appropriate surface receptor – B cell 2 in this example. In this way these cells are stimulated to proliferate and mature into antibody-producing cells, and the longer-lived memory cells, all having the same antigen-binding specificity.

Clonal selection involves proliferation of cells that recognize a specific antigen

Each lymphocyte (whether a B cell or T cell) is genetically programmed to be capable of recognizing essentially only one particular antigen. The immune system as a whole can specifically recognize many thousands of antigens, so the lymphocytes recognizing any particular antigen must represent only a minute proportion of the total. How then is an adequate immune response to an infectious agent generated? The answer is that when an antigen binds to the few cells that can recognize it, they are induced to proliferate rapidly. Within a few days there are a sufficient number to mount an adequate immune response. In other words, the antigen selects for and generates the specific clones of its own antigen-binding cells (*Fig. 1.13*), a process called clonal selection. This operates for both B cells and T cells.

One might wonder how the immune system can 'know' which specific antibodies will be needed during an individual's lifetime. In fact, it does not. The immune system generates antibodies that can recognize an enormous range of antigens even before it encounters them. Many of these will never be called upon to protect the individual against infection. However, there are a tremendous number of infectious organisms, and many of them have the capacity to change their antigens through mutation. As examples, new strains of influenza arise every year, while the virus which causes AIDS mutates many times even within one individual. This makes it necessary for many different antibodies to be available, just in case they are ever needed.

Lymphocytes that have been stimulated, by binding to their specific antigen, take the first steps towards cell division. They express new receptors which allow them to respond to cytokines from other cells, which signal proliferation. The lymphocytes may also start to secrete cytokines themselves. They will usually go through a number of cycles of division, before differentiating into mature cells, again under the influence of cytokines. For example, proliferating B cells eventually mature into antibody-producing plasma cells. Even when the infection has been overcome, some of the newly produced lymphocytes remain, available for restimulation if the antigen is ever encountered again. These cells are called memory cells, since they retain the immunological memory of particular antigens. It is memory cells that confer the lasting immunity to a particular pathogen.

Different immune effector mechanisms are available for handling the vast range of diverse pathogens

There are numerous ways in which the immune system can destroy pathogens, each way being suited to a given

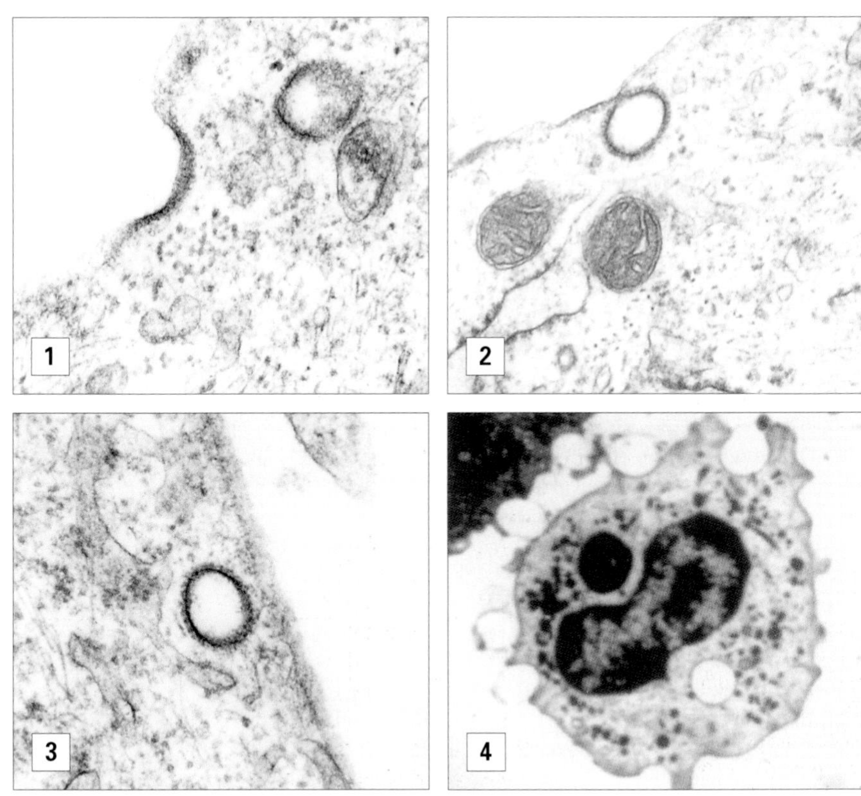

Fig. 1.14 Electronmicrograph studies of endocytosis and phagocytosis. These micrographs show stages of invagination, leading to endocytosis of material from the extracellular environment. Molecules or small particles bound to cell surface receptors cluster towards pits in the membrane (1). The cell extends processes around the developing endosome which is then pinched off (2) and internalised (3). Phagocytosis is a similar process which occurs on a larger scale. Micrograph 4, shows a human phagocyte engulfing latex beads, bound to the cell membrane. (Panels 1–3 courtesy of Dr A. Stevens and Professor J. Lowe. Panel 4 courtesy of Professor C.H.W. Horne.)

type of infection at a particular stage of its life cycle. These defence mechanisms are often referred to as effector systems.

Neutralization – In one of the simplest effector systems, antibodies can combat certain pathogens just by binding to them. For example, antibody to the outer coat proteins of some rhinoviruses (which cause colds) can prevent the viral particles from binding to and infecting host cells.

Phagocytosis – More often antibody is important in activating complement, or acting as an opsonin to promote ingestion by phagocytes. Phagocytic cells, which have bound to an opsonized microbe, engulf it by extending pseudopodia around it. These fuse and the microorganism is internalized in a phagosome (*Fig. 1.14*). The phagocytes have several ways of dealing with this material. For example, macrophages convert molecular oxygen to form microbicidal reactive oxygen intermediates (ROIs) and NO•, which are secreted into the phagosome. Neutrophils contain lactoferrin, which chelates iron and prevents some bacteria from obtaining that vital nutrient. Finally, granules and lysosomes fuse with the phagosome, pouring enzymes into the phagolysosome, which digest the contents (*Fig. 1.15*). The mechanisms involved are described fully in Chapters 9 and 15.

Cytotoxic reactions – Cytotoxic reactions are effector systems directed against whole cells that are in general too large for phagocytosis. The target cell may be recognized either by specific antibody bound to the cell surface, or by T cells using their specific TCRs. In cytotoxic reactions the

Phagocytosis

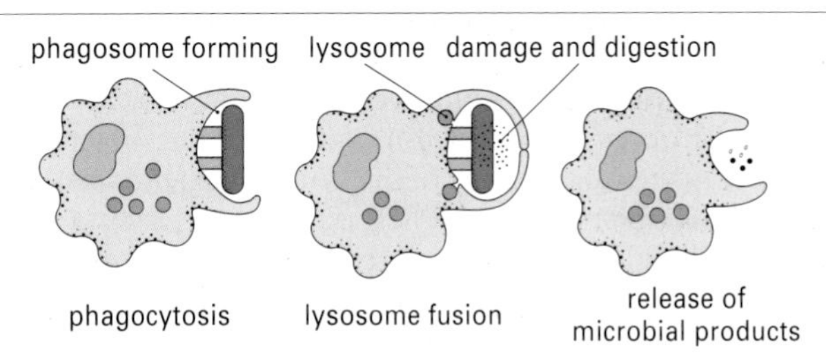

Fig. 1.15 Phagocytes arrive at a site of inflammation by chemotaxis. They may then attach to microorganisms by way of their non-specific cell surface receptors. Alternatively, if the organism is opsonized with a fragment of the third complement component (C3b) and/or antibody, attachment will be through the phagocyte's receptors for C3b and/or Fc (see *Fig. 1.10*). If the phagocyte membrane now becomes activated, microbicidal oxygen metabolites are formed and the infectious agent is taken into a phagosome by pseudopodia extending around it. Once inside, lysosomes fuse with the phagosome to form a phagolysosome and the infectious agent is killed. Undigested microbial products may be released to the outside.

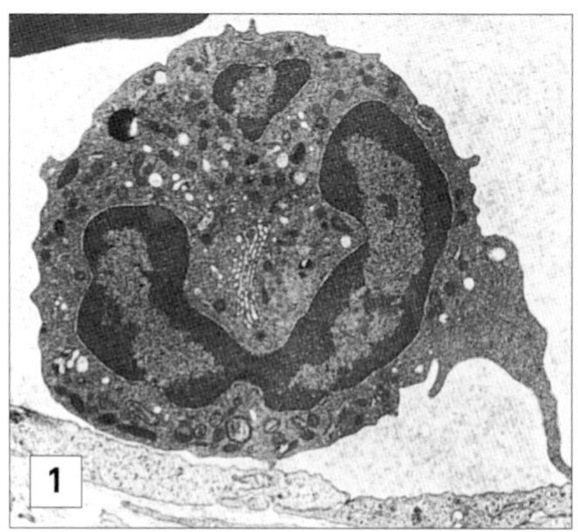

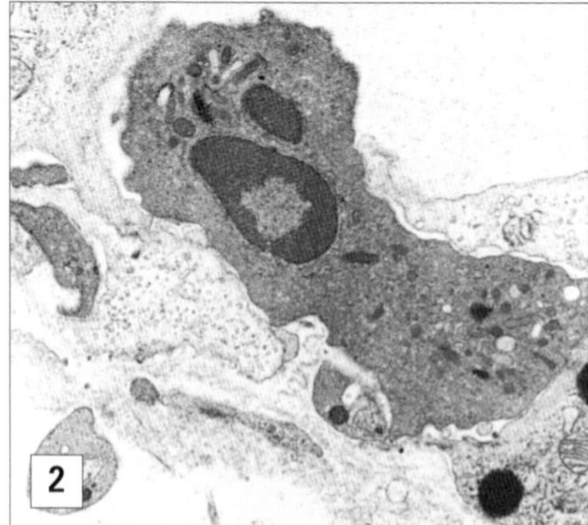

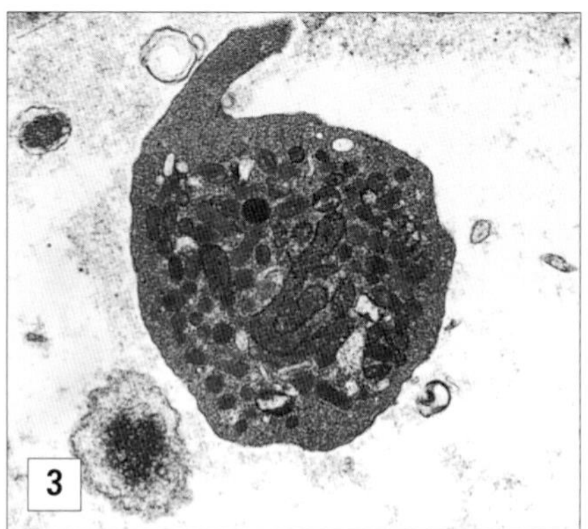

Fig. 1.16 Three phases of neutrophil migration across endothelium. (**1**) A neutrophil adheres to endothelium in a venule. (**2**) The cell extends its pseudopodia between the endothelial cells and migrates towards the basement membrane. (**3**) A neutrophil which has traversed the endothelium. The entire process is sometimes referred to as diapedesis. ×4000. (Courtesy of Dr I. Jovis).

attacking cells direct their granules towards the target cell, in contrast to phagocytosis where the contents are directed into the phagosome. The granules of cytotoxic T cells contain molecules called perforins which can punch holes in the outer membrane of the target. (In a similar way, antibody bound to the surface of a target cell can direct complement to make holes in its plasma membrane.) Some cytotoxic cells can also signal to the target cell to embark upon a programme of self-destruction – a process called apoptosis.

INFLAMMATION

The cells of the immune system are widely distributed throughout the body, but if an infection occurs it is necessary to concentrate them and their products at the site of infection. The process by which this occurs is inflammation. Three major events occur during this response:

- Blood supply to the infected area is increased.
- Capillary permeability is increased due to retraction of the endothelial cells. This permits larger molecules than usual to escape from the capillaries, and thus allows the soluble mediators of immunity to reach the site of infection.
- Leucocytes migrate out of the venules into the surrounding tissues. In the earliest stages of inflammation, neutrophils are particularly prevalent, but in later stages monocytes and lymphocytes also migrate towards the site of infection.

Chemotaxis and cell migration – The process of cell migration is controlled by chemokines on the surface of venular endothelium in inflamed tissues. Chemokines activate the circulating cells causing them to bind to the endothelium and initiating leucocyte migration across the endothelium (*Fig. 1.16*). Once in the tissues, cells migrate towards the site of infection by a process of chemical attraction known as chemotaxis. For example, phagocytes will actively migrate up concentration gradients of certain (chemotactic) molecules. Particularly active is C5a, a fragment of one of the complement components (*Fig. 1.17*), which attracts both neutrophils and monocytes. When purified C5a is applied

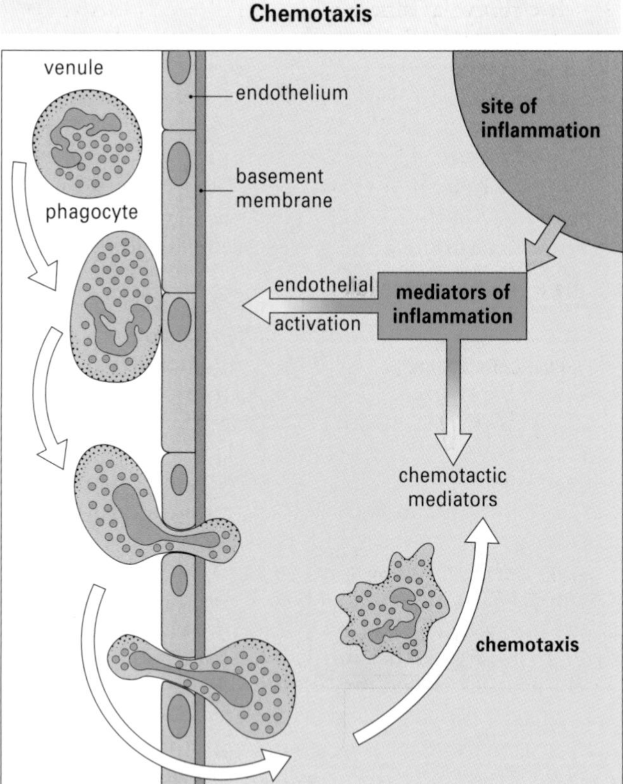

Fig. 1.17 At a site of inflammation, tissue damage and complement activation by the infectious agent cause the release of mediators of inflammation (e.g. C5a, a fragment of complement and one of the most important chemotactic peptides). These mediators diffuse to the adjoining venules, causing passing phagocytes to adhere to the endothelium. The phagocytes insert pseudopodia between the endothelial cells and dissolve the basement membrane. They then pass out of the blood vessels and move up the concentration gradient of the chemotactic mediators in the direction of the site of inflammation (chemotaxis).

to the base of a blister *in vivo*; neutrophils can be seen sticking to the endothelium of nearby venules shortly afterwards. The cells then squeeze between the endothelial cells and move through the basement membrane of the microvessels to reach the tissues. This process is described more fully in Chapter 3.

DEFENCES AGAINST EXTRACELLULAR AND INTRACELLULAR PATHOGENS

It will be clear that there is a fundamental difference between immune responses to extracellular and intracellular pathogens. In dealing with extracellular pathogens, the immune system aims to destroy the pathogen itself and neutralize its products. In response to intracellular pathogens, there are two options. Either the T cells can destroy the infected cell – cytotoxicity – or they can activate the cell to deal with the pathogen for itself. This occurs, for example, when helper T cells release cytokines which activate macrophages to destroy organisms they have taken up.

Because many pathogens have both intracellular and extracellular phases of infection, different mechanisms are usually effective at different times. For example, the polio virus travels from the gut, through the blood stream to infect nerve cells in the spinal cord. Antibody is particularly effective at blocking this early phase of infection. However, to clear an established infection, Tc cells or natural killer (NK) cells must kill any cell that has become infected. Consequently, antibody is important in limiting the spread of infection, and preventing reinfection with the same virus, while cytotoxic cells are essential to deal with infected cells (*Fig. 1.18*). These considerations play an important part in the development of effective vaccines.

VACCINATION

One area in which immunological studies have had most immediate and successful application is in the field of vaccination. The principle of vaccination is based on two key elements of adaptive immunity, namely specificity and memory. Memory cells allow the immune system to mount a much stronger response on a second encounter with antigen. This secondary response is both faster to appear and more effective than the primary response.

The aim in vaccine development is to alter a pathogen or its toxins in such a way that they become innocuous without losing antigenicity. This is possible because antibodies and T cells recognize particular parts of antigens, the epitopes, and not the whole organism or toxin. Take, for example, vaccination against tetanus. The tetanus bacterium produces a toxin which acts on receptors to cause tetanic contractions of muscle. The toxin can be modified by formalin treatment so that it retains its epitopes but loses its toxicity; the resulting toxoid is used as a vaccine (*Fig. 1.19*). Whole infectious agents, such as the polio virus, can be attenuated so they retain their antigenicity but lose their pathogenicity.

Vaccination is discussed in more detail in Chapter 17.

Reaction to extracellular and intracellular pathogens

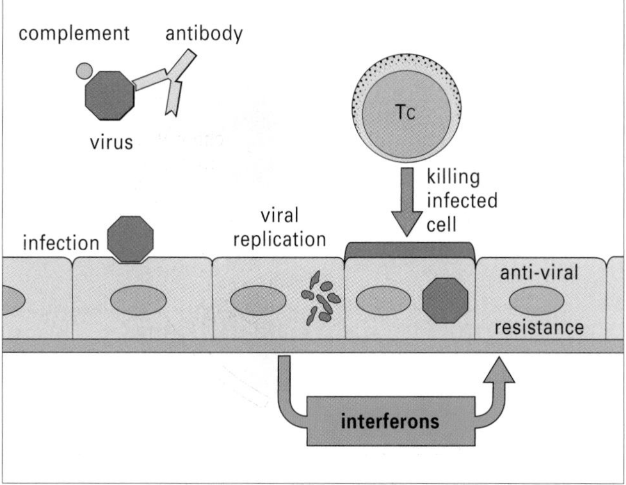

Fig. 1.18 Different immunological systems are effective against different types of infection, here illustrated as a virus infection. Antibodies and complement can block the extracellular phase of the life cycle, and promote phagocytosis of the virus. IFNs produced by infected cells can signal to uninfected cells, and induce a state of antiviral resistance in them. Viruses can only multiply within living cells; Tc cells are effective at recognizing and destroying the infected cells before significant replication has occurred.

Principle of vaccination

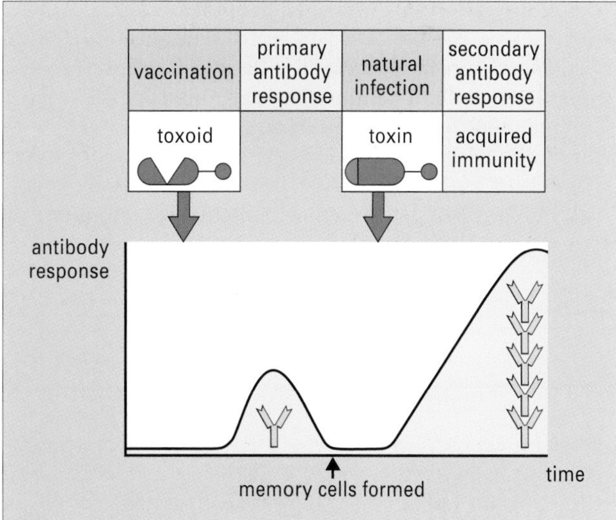

Fig. 1.19 The principle of vaccination is illustrated by immunization with tetanus toxoid. Chemical modification of tetanus toxin produces a toxoid which has lost toxicity but retains its epitopes. Thus, a primary antibody response to these epitopes is produced following vaccination with toxoid. In a natural infection the toxin re-stimulates B memory cells, which produce the faster and more intense secondary antibody response to the epitope, so neutralizing the toxin.

IMMUNOPATHOLOGY

Up to this point, the immune system has been presented as an unimpeachable asset. It is certainly true that deficiencies in any part of the system leave the individual exposed to a greater risk of infection, although other parts of the system may partly compensate for such deficiencies. Clearly, strong evolutionary pressure from infectious microbes has lead to the development of the immune system in its present form. However, there are occasions when the immune system is itself a cause of disease or other undesirable consequences (*Fig. 1.20*).

In essence the system can fail in one of three ways.

Inappropriate reaction to self antigens: autoimmunity – Normally the immune system recognizes all foreign antiens and reacts against them, while recognizing the body's own tissues as 'self' and making no reaction against them. The mechanisms by which this discrimination between 'self' and 'non-self' is established, are described in Chapter 12. If the system should react against self components, autoimmune disease occurs. Examples of autoimmune disease are rheumatoid arthritis and pernicious anaemia (see Chapter 26).

Ineffective immune response: immunodeficiency – If any elements of the immune system are defective, the individual may not be able to fight infections adequately. These conditions are termed immunodeficiency. Some are hereditary deficiencies, which start to manifest themselves shortly after birth, while others, such as acquired immunodeficiency syndrome (AIDS), develop later (see Chapters 19 and 20).

Overactive immune response: hypersensitivity – Sometimes immune reactions are out of all proportion to the damage that may be caused by a pathogen. The immune system may also mount a reaction to a harmless antigen, such as a food molecule. The immune reactions may cause more damage than the pathogen, or antigen, and in this case we speak of hypersensitivity (see Chapters 21–24). For example, molecules on the surface of pollen grains are recognized as antigens by particular individuals, generating the symptoms of hayfever or asthma.

Failure of the immune system

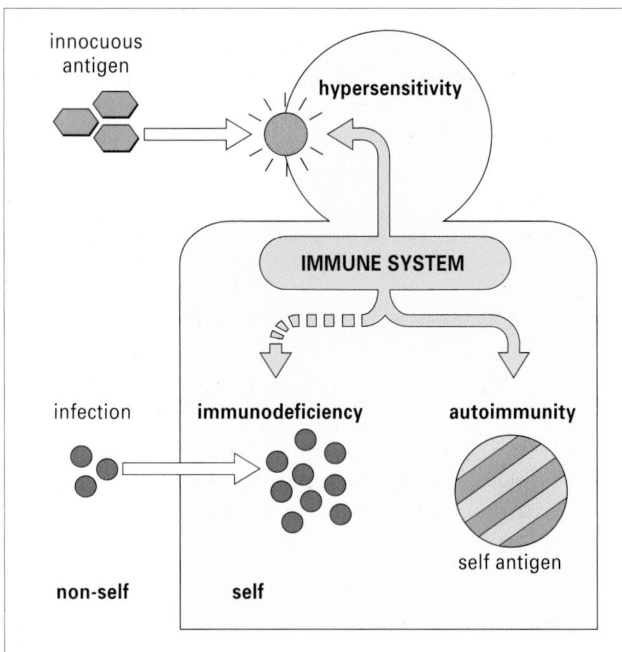

Fig. 1.20 There are three principal ways in which the immune system can fail – hypersensitivity, immunodeficiency and autoimmunity. The first two are due to an inappropriately large or small immune response, respectively. Autoimmunity is caused by a failure of self/non-self discrimination in immune recognition.

Finally, there are occasions when the immune system acts normally, but the immune responses it produces are inconvenient in the context of modern medicine. The most important examples of this are in blood transfusion and graft rejection. In these cases it is necessary to match carefully the donor and recipient tissues so the immune system of the recipient does not attack the donated blood or graft tissue. These problems are, however, a small price to pay for an essential system of the body, which is absolutely vital to protect individuals against infection.

CRITICAL THINKING • Specificity and memory in immune responses (Explanations on p. 453)

The recommended schedules for vaccination against different diseases are strikingly different. Two examples are given below. For tetanus, the vaccine is a modified form of the toxin released by the tetanus bacterium. The vaccine for influenza is either an attenuated non-pathogenic variant of the virus, which is given intranasally, or a killed preparation of virus given intradermally. Both of the vaccines induce antibodies which are specific for the inducing antigen.

Pathogen	Type of vaccine	Recommended for:	Vaccination	Effectiveness
Tetanus	Toxoid	Everyone	Every 10 years	100%
Influenza A	Attenuated virus	Health workers and older people	Annually	Variable 0–90%

1.1 Why is it only necessary to vaccinate against tetanus every 10 years, while antibodies against the toxoid disappear from the circulation within a year?

1.2 Why is the vaccine against tetanus always effective, whereas the vaccine against influenza protects on some occasions but not others?

1.3 Why is tetanus recommended for everyone and influenza for only a restricted group of 'at-risk' individuals, even though influenza is a much more common disease than tetanus?

DISCUSSION POINT

If we could immunize every person in the world against influenza-A in one year, do you think that this would lead to the total eradication of the disease?

2 Cells, tissues and organs of the immune system

- **Most cells of the immune system** derive from haemopoietic stem cells.
- **Development and differentiation of different cell lineages** depend on cell interactions and cytokines.
- **Each cell type expresses characteristic surface molecules (markers)** which identify them.
- **Phagocytic cells** are found in the circulation (monocytes and granulocytes) and reside in tissues (e.g. Kupffer cells in the liver).
- **Eosinophils, basophils, mast cells and platelets participate in the inflammatory response.**
- **Antigen-presenting cells** are required by T cells to enable them to respond to antigens.
- **B and T lymphocytes express antigen receptors**, which are required for the antigen recognition.
- **There are two major subpopulations of T lymphocytes** which have helper and cytotoxic activities.
- **B cells** can differentiate into antibody-secreting plasma cells, following activation.
- **Lymphoid organs and tissues** are either primary (central) or secondary (peripheral).
- **Lymphoid stem cells develop and mature within the primary lymphoid organs** – the thymus and bone marrow; this process is called lymphopoiesis.
- **T lymphocytes developing in the thymus are subject to positive and negative selection processes.**
- **The diverse antigen repertoires found in mature animals** are generated during lymphopoiesis, by recombination of gene segments encoding the TCR and Ig.
- **Mammalian B cells develop mainly in the fetal liver and from birth onwards in the bone marrow.** This process continues throughout life. B cells also undergo a selection process at the site of B-cell generation.
- **Lymphocytes** migrate to, and function in, the secondary lymphoid organs and tissues.
- **The systemic lymphoid organs** include the spleen and lymph nodes.
- **The mucosa-associated lymphoid tissue (MALT)** includes all the lymphoid tissues associated with mucosae.
- **Peyer's patches** are a major site of lymphocyte priming to antigens crossing mucosal surfaces of the small intestine.
- **Lymphoid organs** protect different body sites; the spleen responds to blood-borne antigens; the lymph nodes respond to lymph-borne antigens and the MALT protects the mucosal surface.
- **Most lymphocytes recirculate around the body;** there is continuous lymphocyte traffic from the blood stream into lymphoid tissues and back again into the blood via the thoracic duct and right lymphatic duct.

In Chapter 1, we encountered the two major groups of cells, lymphocytes and phagocytes, which comprise the immune system. These and other specialized cells that provide protection against invading organisms are found throughout the body within the blood stream, in specialized organs – the lymph nodes and spleen and beneath the epithelial tissues lining the respiratory, gastrointestinal and genitourinary sytems. These cells derive mainly from undifferentiated 'self-renewing' haemopoietic stem cells (HSCs) through a process of differentiation (*Fig. 2.1*). This is mediated by microenvironmental factors including cell-to-cell interactions and the presence of soluble or membrane-bound cytokines. In addition to their different appearances, cells can be distinguished by their surface markers, which have been collated into the 'CD system', described below and in Appendix 2.

Totipotent HSCs are found in the yolk sac, liver, spleen, bone marrow and in some mesenchymal areas of the embryonic and fetal mammal. After birth and throughout adult life they are normally found only in the bone marrow, where they give rise to four major cell lineages: erythroid (erythrocytes), megakaryocytic (platelets), myeloid (granulocytes and mononuclear phagocytes) and lymphoid (lymphocytes), the latter two being the most important in terms of protection against exogenous pathogens. Antigen-presenting cells are largely, but not exclusively, derived from myeloid precursors. The myeloid and lymphoid lineages are both critical to the functioning of the immune system.

CELLS OF THE INNATE IMMUNE SYSTEM

Phagocytes

Phagocytes belong to two major lineages – monocytes/macrophages and polymorphonuclear granulocytes. The latter have a lobed, irregularly shaped (polymorphic) nucleus. They are classified into neutrophils, basophils and eosinophils, on the basis of how their cytoplasmic granules stain with acidic and basic dyes. The three types of cells have distinct effector functions. Most numerous are the neutrophils, also called PMNs (polymorphonuclear neutrophils), which constitute the majority of leucocytes (white blood cells) in the blood stream (around 60–70% in adults). The other family of phagocytes consists of circulating cells, the monocytes and of cells that reside within the interstitium of various organs (e.g. spleen, liver, lungs) where they display distinctive morphological features and perform diverse functions.

Mononuclear phagocytes are widely distributed throughout the body

The mononuclear phagocyte system has two main functions, which result from the activities of two different types of bone marrow-derived cells:

- 'Professional' phagocytic macrophages, whose main role is to remove particulate antigens.
- Antigen-presenting cells (APCs), whose role is to take up, process and present antigenic peptides to T cells.

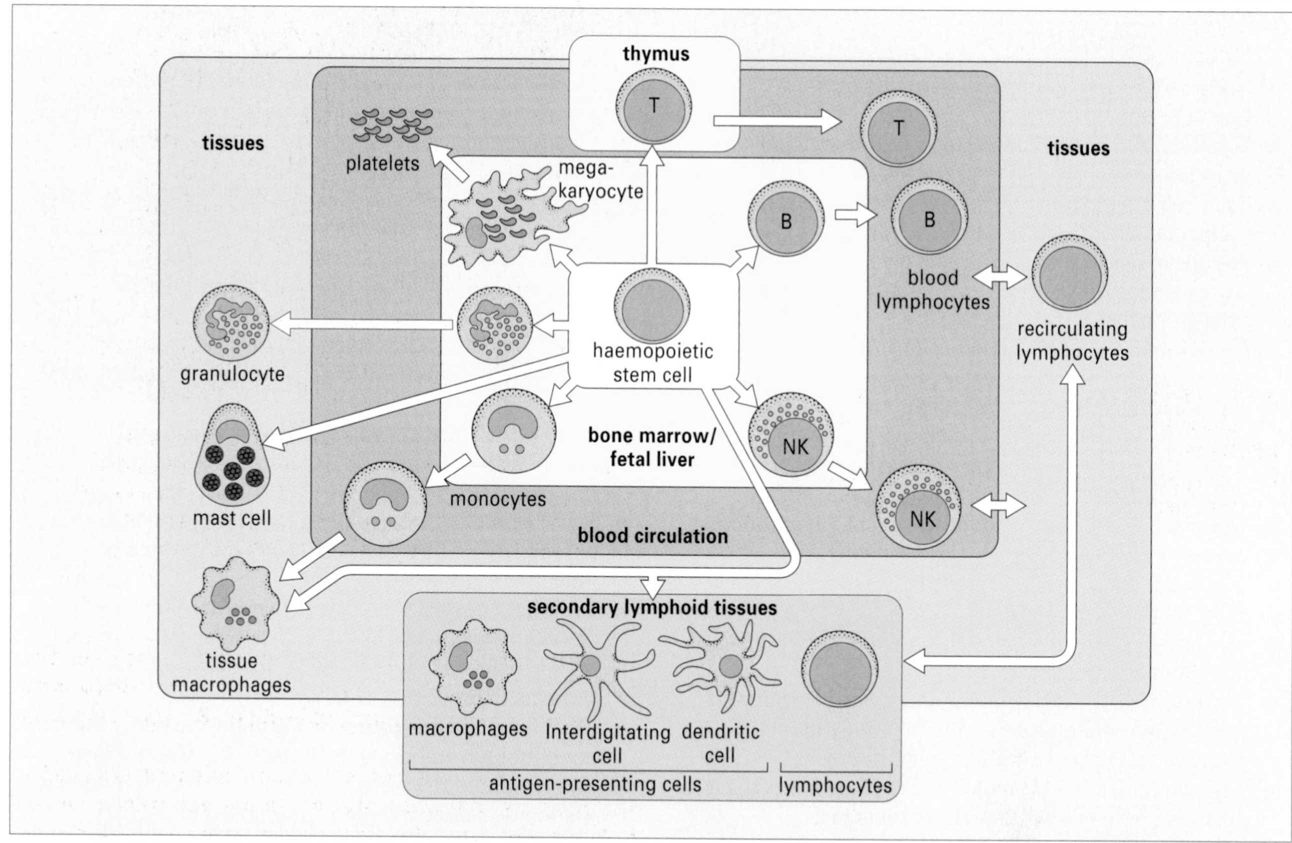

Fig. 2.1 All the cells shown arise from the haemopoietic stem cell. Platelets produced by megakaryocytes are released into the circulation. Granulocytes and monocytes pass from the circulation into the tissues. Mast cells are identifiable in all tissues. B cells mature in the fetal liver and bone marrow in mammals, whereas T cells mature in the thymus. The origin of the large granular lymphocytes with NK activity is probably the bone marrow. Lymphocytes recirculate through secondary lymphoid tissues. Interdigitating cells and dendritic cells act as antigen-presenting cells in secondary lymphoid tissues.

APCs will be considered together with the cells that are responsible for the adaptive T-cell-mediated immune response. Phagocytic macrophages are found in many organs (see *Fig. 1.5*). Examples of these are Kupffer cells in the liver (*Fig. 2.2*) and microglial cells in the brain (*Fig. 2.3*).

Myeloid progenitors in the bone marrow differentiate into promonocytes and then into circulating monocytes which migrate through the blood vessel walls into the various organs to become macrophages. The human blood monocyte is large (10–18 μm diameter) relative to the lymphocyte. It has a horseshoe-shaped nucleus and contains azurophilic granules (*Fig. 2.4*). Ultrastructurally, the monocyte possesses ruffled membranes, a well-developed Golgi complex and many intracytoplasmic lysosomes (*Fig. 2.5*). These lysosomes contain peroxidase and several acid hydrolases which are important for intracellular killing of microorganisms.

Monocytes/macrophages actively phagocytose organisms or even tumour cells *in vitro*. Microbial adherence,

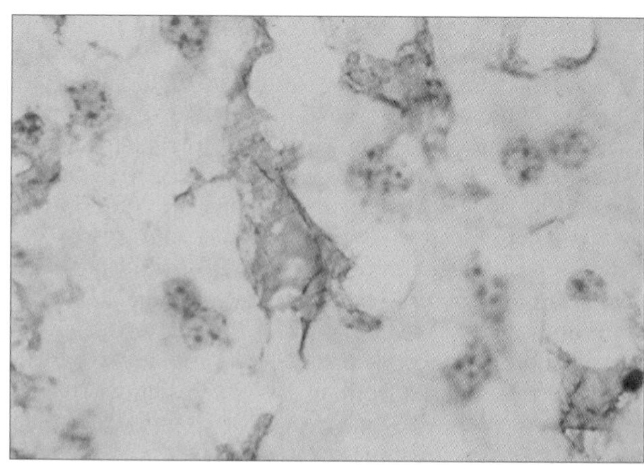

Fig. 2.2 Kupffer cells. Kupffer cells in the normal mouse liver stain strongly positive with antibody to F4/80. Sinusoidal endothelial cells and hepatocytes are F4/80 negative. (Courtesy of Professor S. Gordon and Dr D. A. Hume.)

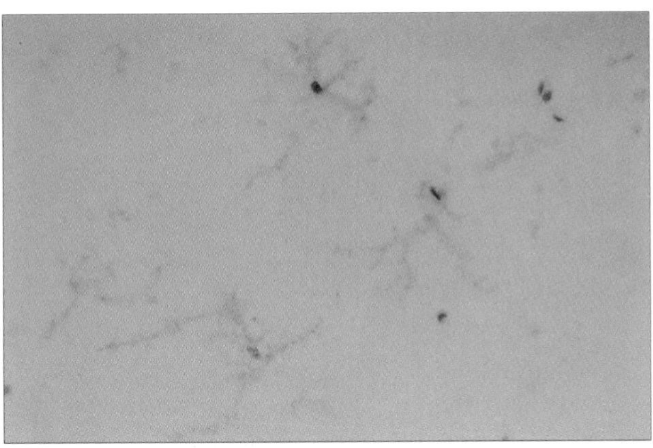

Fig. 2.3 Microglial cells. The highly arborized mature resident macrophage within adult mouse brain is stained with antibody to F4/80. Resting microglia appear to occupy distinct non-overlapping fields within the adult CNS. (Courtesy of Professor V. H. Perry and Professor S. Gordon.)

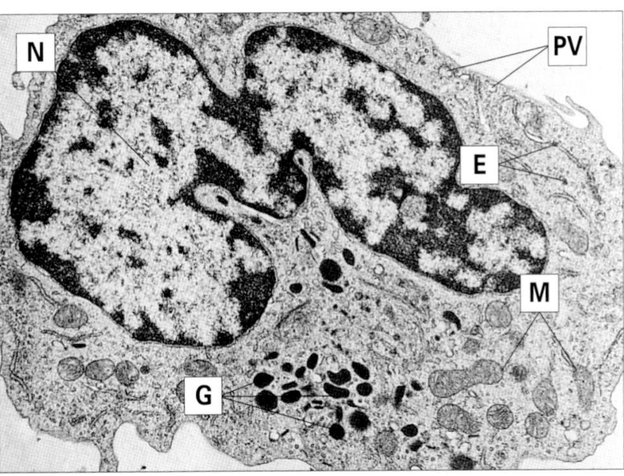

Fig. 2.5 Ultrastructure of the monocyte. This shows the horseshoe-shaped nucleus (N), the pinocytotic vesicles (PV), lysosomal granules (G), mitochondria (M) and isolated rough endoplasmic reticulum cisternae (E). ×8000. (Courtesy of Dr B. Nichols, from *J Cell Biol* 1971;**50**:498, with permission.)

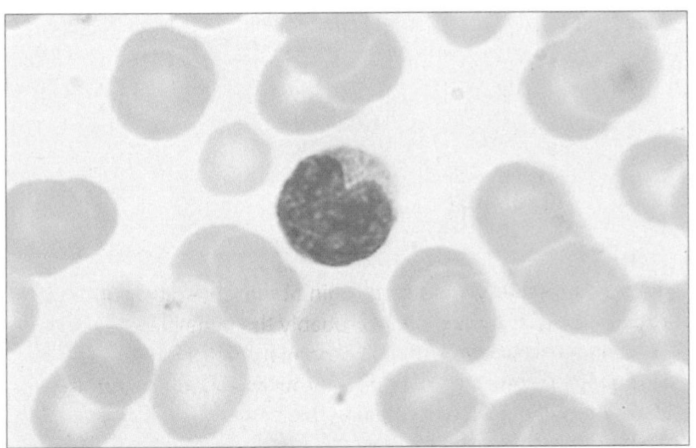

Fig. 2.4 Morphology of the monocyte. Blood monocytes have a characteristic horseshoe-shaped nucleus and are larger than most circulating lymphocytes. Giemsa stain. ×1200.

followed by ingestion, occurs through specialized receptors. These receptors mainly attach to sugars or lipids on the microbial surface and include scavenger receptors, toll receptors and mannose receptors. Monocytes/macrophages also have receptors for IgG and complement with which the microorganism may become coated.

Polymorphs are produced in three different types

Polymorphonuclear granulocytes (often referred to as polymorphs or granulocytes) mainly consist of neutrophils and are released from the bone marrow at a rate of around 7 million per minute. They are short-lived (2–3 days) relative to monocytes/macrophages, which may live for months or years. Like monocytes, PMNs adhere to endothelial cells lining the blood vessels (marginate) and extravasate by squeezing between the endothelial cells to leave the circulation (see *Fig. 1.16*). This process is known as diapedesis. Adhesion is mediated by receptors on the granulocytes and ligands on the endothelial cells, and is promoted by chemoattractants (chemokines) such as interleukin-8 (IL-8) (see Chapter 3 and Appendix 4).

Granulocytes do not show any inherent specificity for antigens, but they play an important role in acute inflammation (usually synergizing with antibodies and complement) in protection against microorganisms. Their predominant role is phagocytosis and destruction of pathogens. The importance of these cells is shown in individuals with reduced white cell numbers, or with rare genetic defects which prevent polymorph extravasation in response to chemotactic stimuli. Both defects markedly increase susceptibility to infection.

Neutrophils are short-lived phagocytic cells

Neutrophils comprise over 95% of the circulating granulocytes. They have a characteristic multilobed nucleus and are 10–20 μm in diameter (*Fig. 2.6*).

Chemotactic agents for neutrophils include protein fragments released when complement is activated (e.g. C5a), factors derived from the fibrinolytic and kinin systems, the products of other leucocytes and platelets, and the products of certain bacteria. Chemotactic stimuli result in neutrophil margination (adhesion to endothelial cells) and diapedesis.

Neutrophils have a large arsenal of antibiotic proteins stored in two main types of granules. The primary (azurophilic) granules are lysosomes containing acid hydrolases, myeloperoxidase and muramidase (lysozyme). The secondary (specific) granules contain lactoferrin and lysozyme. In addition to these enzymes and to lactoferrin, the granules also contain the antibiotic proteins – defensins, seprocidins, cathelicidins and bacterial permeability inducing (BPI) protein. Ingested organisms are contained within vacuoles termed phagosomes, which fuse with the lysosomes to form phagolysosomes.

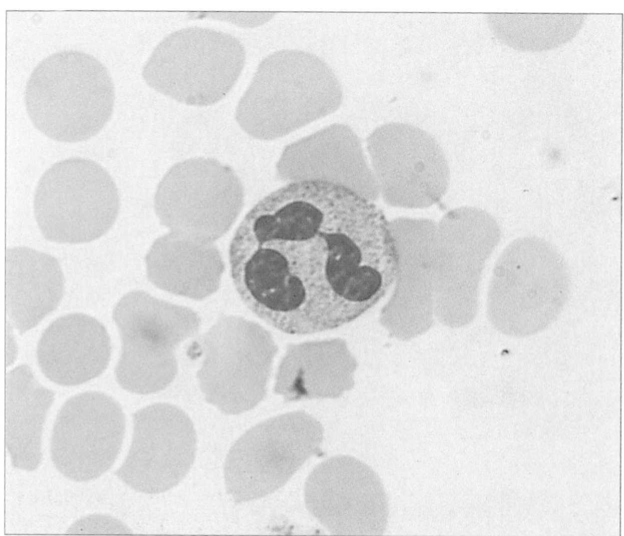

Fig. 2.6 Morphology of the neutrophil. One mature neutrophil in a blood smear showing multilobed nuclei. Giemsa stain. ×1500. (Adapted from Zucker-Franklin D, Greaves MF, Grossi CE, *et al. Atlas of Blood Cells: Function and Pathology*. Vol II. 2nd edn. Milan: EE Ermes, Philadelphia: Lea and Febiger, 1988.)

Extracellular release of granules and cytotoxic substances by neutrophils can also occur when they are activated by immune complexes through their Fcγ receptors. This may be an important pathogenetic mechanism in immune-complex diseases (type III hypersensitivity, see Chapter 23).

Development of phagocytes

Myelopoiesis (development of myeloid cells) commences in the liver of the human fetus at about 6 weeks of gestation. Studies in which colonies have been grown *in vitro* from individual stem cells have shown that the first progenitor cell derived from the haemopoietic stem cells (HSCs) is the colony-forming unit (CFU), which can give rise to granulocytes, erythrocytes, monocytes and megakaryocytes (CFU–GEMM). Maturation of these cells occurs under the influence of colony-stimulating factors (CSFs) and of several interleukins, including IL-1, IL-3, IL-4, IL-5, IL-6 and IL-7. These factors, which are important in the positive regulation of haemopoiesis, are derived mainly from stromal cells in the bone marrow, but are also produced by mature forms of differentiated myeloid and lymphoid cells. Other cytokines (e.g. transforming growth factor-β, TGFβ) may downregulate haemopoiesis. The development of phagocytes is set out in *Figure 2.7*. The further differentiation of monocytes into macrophages, myeloid dendritic cells and osteoclasts is described fully in Chapter 9 (see *Fig. 9.1*).

Monocytes and neutrophils develop from a common precursor cell

Monocyte development

CFU–GMs taking the monocyte pathway give rise initially to proliferating monoblasts. These cells differentiate into

Development of granulocytes and monocytes

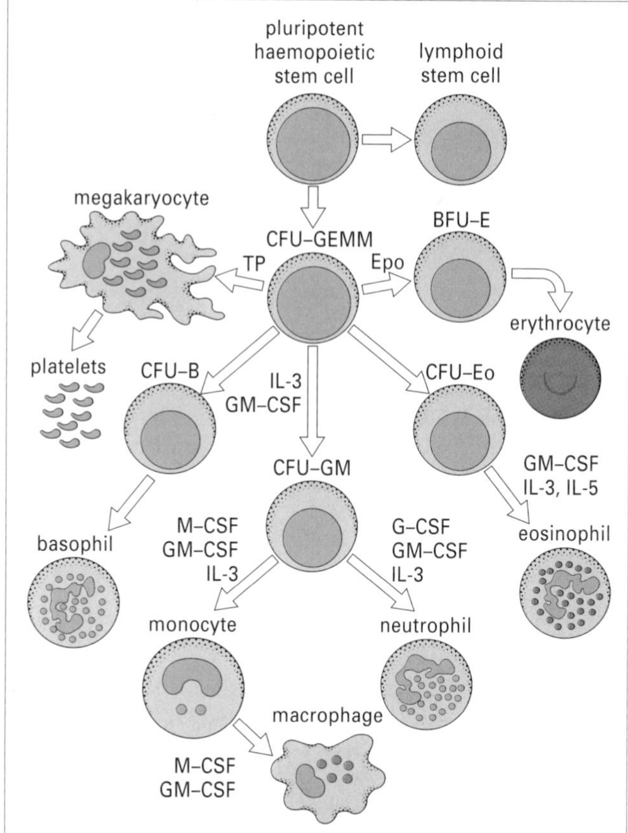

Fig. 2.7 Pluripotent haemopoietic stem cells generate colony-forming units (CFU). CFU–GEMMs have the potential to give rise to all blood cells except lymphocytes. IL-3 and granulocyte–macrophage colony-stimulating factor (GM–CSF) are required to induce this stem cell to enter one of five pathways (i.e. to give rise to megakaryocytes, erythrocytes via burst-forming units, basophils, neutrophils or eosinophils) and are also required during further differentiation of the granulocytes and monocytes. Eosinophil (Eo) differentiation from CFU–Eo is promoted by IL-5. Neutrophils and monocytes are derived from the CFU–GM through the effects of G–CSF and M–CSF, respectively. Both GM–CSF and M–CSF, and other cytokines (including IL-1, IL-4 and IL-6), promote the differentiation of monocytes into macrophages. Thrombopoietin (TP) promotes the growth of megakaryocytes. B = basophil; BFU–E = erythrocytic burst-forming unit; Epo = erythropoietin; G = granulocyte; M = monocyte.

promonocytes and finally into mature circulating monocytes. Circulating monocytes are thought to be a replacement pool for tissue-resident macrophages, e.g. lung macrophages. The different types of macrophages form the mononuclear phagocyte system.

CD34, like other early maturation markers, is lost in mature neutrophils and monocytes/macrophages. However, monocytes, unlike neutrophils, continue to express significant levels of MHC class II molecules. These molecules are important for the presentation of antigen to T cells. Monocytes also acquire many of the same surface molecules as mature neutrophils (*Fig. 2.8*). Studies of

Main markers of monocytes, macrophages, granulocytes, mast cells and platelets

marker	monocyte	macrophages	granulocytes	mast cells	platelets
CD11a	+	+	+	+	–
CD11b	+	–	+	+	–
CD13	+	–	+	–	–
CD14	+	–	–	–	–
CD15	–	–	–	–	+
CD16(FcγRIII)	–	+(ss)	+	–	–
CD23(FcεRII)	+	+	+(e)	+	+
CD32(FcγRII)	+	+	+	+	+
CD33	+	–	–	–	–
CD35(CR1)	+	–	–	–	–
CD41	–	–	–	–	+
CD42	–	–	–	–	+
CD64(FcγR1)	+	+	+(a)	–	–
CD68	–	+	–	–	–
FcεR1	+(a?)	+(a?)	+(b)	+	–

Fig. 2.8 Descriptions of the Fc receptors can be found in *Figures 4.22* and *4.23*. ss = subset, a = activated, b = basophils, e = eosinophils

myeloid cell lines *in vitro* (believed to represent distinct stages of monocyte differentiation) indicate that both phagocytic efficiency and Fc receptor-mediated cytotoxicity are optimal only in mature macrophages whereas generation of the cytokine IL-1 by monocytes is equally good at birth and in adults.

Neutrophil development

The colony-forming unit–granulocyte macrophage (CFU–GM) cell is the precursor of both neutrophils and mononuclear phagocytes. As the CFU–GM differentiates along the neutrophil pathway, several distinct morphological stages are distinguished. Myeloblasts develop into promyelocytes and myelocytes, which mature and are released into the circulation as neutrophils. The one-way differentiation of cells from the CFU–GM into mature neutrophils is the result of acquiring specific receptors for growth and differentiation factors at successive stages of development.

Surface differentiation markers disappear or are expressed on the cells as they develop into granulocytes. For example, MHC class II molecules and CD38 are expressed on the CFU–GM, but not on mature neutrophils. Other surface molecules acquired during the differentiation process include CD13, CD14 at low density, CD15 (the Lewis X blood group hapten), the β_1-integrin chain (CD29), VLA-4 (CD49d, α chain), the leucocyte integrins CD11a, b, c and d associated with CD18 β_2-chains, complement receptors and CD16 Fcγ receptors (see Appendix 2 for a list of additional markers).

It is difficult to assess the functional activity of different developmental stages of granulocytes, but it seems likely that the full functional potential is realized only when the cells are mature. There is some evidence that neutrophil activity, as measured by phagocytosis or chemotaxis, is lower in fetal than in adult life. However, this may be due, in part, to the lower levels of opsonins present in the fetal serum, rather than to a characteristic of the cells themselves. To become active in the presence of opsonins, neutrophils must interact directly with microorganisms and/or with cytokines generated by a response to antigen. This limitation could reduce neutrophil activity in early life. Activation of neutrophils by cytokines and chemokines is also a prerequisite for their migration into tissues.

Eosinophils

Human blood eosinophils usually have a bilobed nucleus and many cytoplasmic granules that stain with acidic dyes,

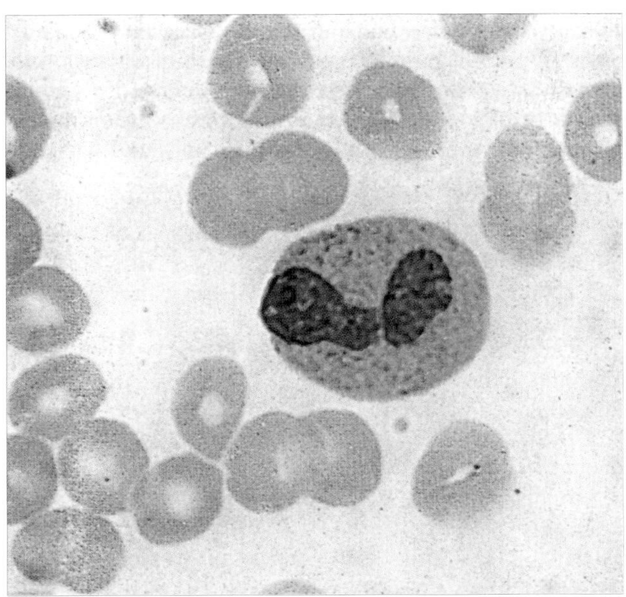

Fig. 2.9 Morphology of the eosinophil. The bilobed nucleus and eosinophilic granules in the cytoplasm are of note. Giemsa stain. ×1000. (Adapted from Zucker-Franklin D, Greaves MF, Grossi CE, *et al. Atlas of Blood Cells: Function and Pathology.* Vol II. 2nd edn. Milan: EE Ermes, Philadelphia: Lea and Febiger, 1988.)

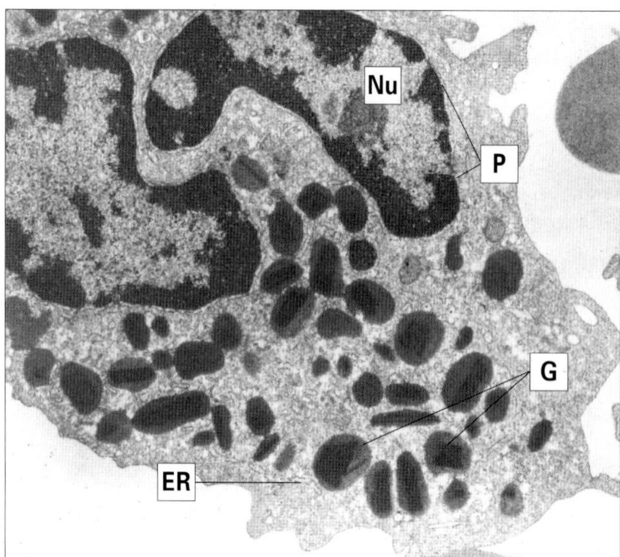

Fig. 2.10 Ultrastructure of a human eosinophil. The mature eosinophil contains granules (G) with central crystalloids. Nu = nucleus; ER = endoplasmic reticulum; P = nuclear pores. ×17 500. (Adapted from Zucker-Franklin D, Greaves MF, Grossi CE, *et al. Atlas of Blood Cells: Function and Pathology.* Vol II. 2nd edn. Milan: EE Ermes, Philadelphia: Lea and Febiger, 1988.)

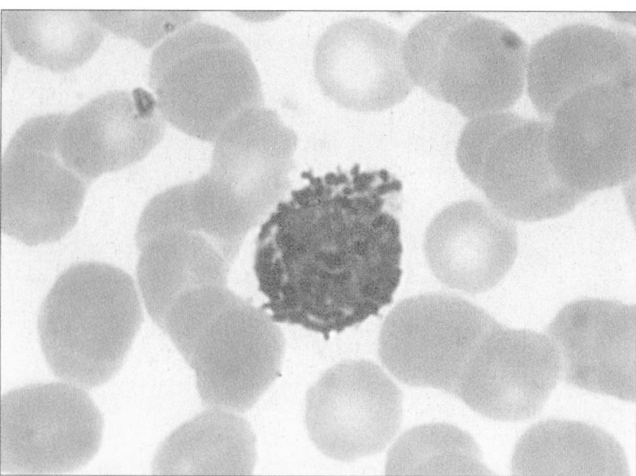

Fig. 2.11 Morphology of the basophil. This blood smear shows a typical basophil with its deep violet-blue granules. Wright's stain. ×1000.

e.g. eosin (*Fig. 2.9*). They comprise 2–5% of blood leucocytes in healthy, non-allergic individuals. Although not their primary function, they appear to be capable of phagocytosing and killing ingested microorganisms. The granules in mature eosinophils are membrane-bound organelles with crystalloid cores that differ in electron density from the surrounding matrix (*Fig. 2.10*).

Certain stimuli will cause eosinophils to degranulate. Degranulation involves fusion of the intracellular granules with the plasma membrane and release of the granule contents into the extracellular environment. This type of reaction is the only way that these cells can use their granule armament against large pathogens (e.g. shistosomula), which cannot be phagocytosed. Eosinophils are thought to play a specialized role in immunity to parasitic worms using this mechanism (see Chapter 18). Eosinophils also release histaminase and aryl sulphatase, which inactivate the mast cell products, histamine and some of the leukotrienes. The effect of the eosinophil factors is thus to dampen down the inflammatory response and reduce granulocyte migration into the site of invasion.

Basophils and mast cells

Basophils are found in very small numbers in the circulation, accounting for less than 0.2% of leucocytes (*Fig. 2.11*). The mast cell, which is not found in the circulation, is indistinguishable from the basophil in a number of its properties, although it displays distinctive morphological features.

There are two different kinds of mast cells; the mucosal mast cell (MMC) associated with mucosae, and the connective tissue mast cell (CTMC). MMCs appear to depend on T cells for their proliferation, while the CTMCs do not. Both types of mast cells can be seen under light microscopy using basic dyes (*Fig. 2.12*). Mature blood basophils have randomly distributed granules surrounded by membranes (*Fig. 2.13*). The granules in both basophils and mast cells contain heparin, leukotrienes, histamine and eosinophil chemotactic factor of anaphylaxis (ECF-A).

The stimulus for mast cell or basophil degranulation is often an allergen (an antigen causing allergic reaction). To be effective, an allergen must cross-link IgE molecules bound to the surface of the mast cell or basophil via its high-affinity Fc receptors for IgE (FcεRI). Degranulation of a basophil or mast cell results in all the contents of the granules being released very rapidly. This occurs by intracytoplasmic fusion of the granules, followed by discharge of their contents (*Fig. 2.14*). Mediators such as histamine, released by degranulation, cause the adverse symptoms

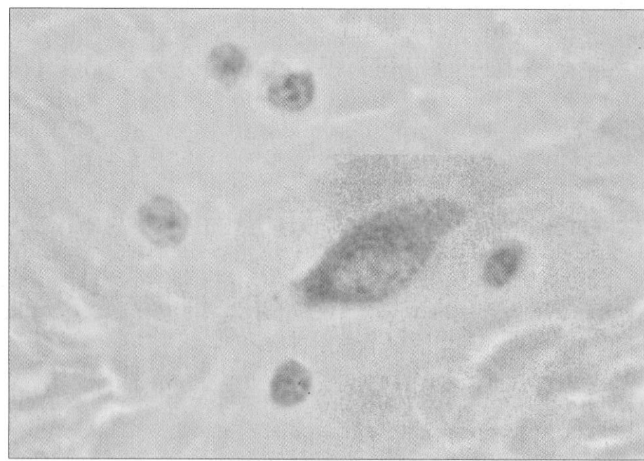

Fig. 2.12 Histological appearance of human connective tissue mast cells. This micrograph shows dark blue cytoplasm with purple granules. Alcian blue and safranin stain. ×600. (Courtesy of Dr T. S. Orr.)

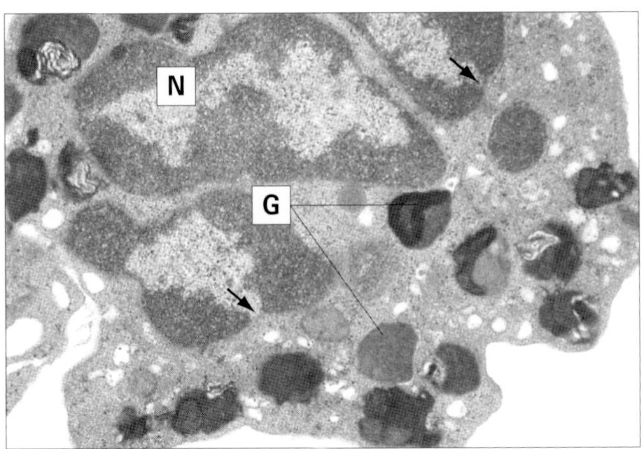

Fig. 2.13 Ultrastructure of the basophil. Note the segmented nucleus (N) and the large cytoplasmic granules (G). ×11 000. (Adapted from Zucker-Franklin D, Greaves MF, Grossi CE, *et al. Atlas of Blood Cells: Function and Pathology.* Vol II. 2nd edn. Milan: EE Ermes, Philadelphia: Lea and Febiger, 1988.)

of allergy but, on the positive side, they also play a role in immunity against parasites by enhancing inflammation. Mast cell functional markers are summarized in *Figure 2.8.*

Platelets

Blood platelets, in addition to their role in blood clotting, are involved in immune responses and especially in inflammation. They are derived from megakaryocytes in the bone marrow and contain granules (*Fig. 2.15*). The adult human produces 10^{11} platelets each day. On average, 30% of them are sequestered in the spleen. Platelets express class I MHC products, receptors for IgG (CD32; FcγRII), and low-affinity receptors for IgE (FcεRII; CD23). In addition, megakaryocytes and platelets carry receptors for factor VIII and other molecules important for their function, such as the GpIIb/IIIa complex (CD41) and the GpIb/GpIx complex (CD42: see *Fig. 2.8*). The GpIIb/IIIa complex is a cytoadhesin, and is responsible for binding to fibrinogen, fibronectin and vitronectin. In addition, both this complex and the GpIb/GpIx complex are receptors for von Willebrand factor. There is an additional vitronectin receptor, CD51. Both receptors and adhesion molecules are important in the activation of platelets. Following injury to endothelial cells, platelets adhere to, and aggregate at, the endothelial surface of damaged vascular tissue. They release substances contained within two types of granules which include serotonin and fibrinogen. This results in an increased capillary permeability, activation of complement and hence attraction of leucocytes.

Natural killer (NK) cells

Natural killer (NK) cells account for up to 15% of blood lymphocytes and express neither T-cell nor B-cell antigen receptors.

Most surface antigens detectable on NK cells by monoclonal antibodies are shared with T cells or monocytes/macrophages. Monoclonal antibodies to CD16 (FcγRIII) are commonly used to identify NK cells in purified lymphocyte populations. CD16 is involved in one of the activation pathways of NK cells, and is also expressed by neutrophils, some macrophages and some γδ T cells.

On granulocytes, CD16 is linked to the surface membrane by a phosphatidylinositol glycan (PIG) linkage, whereas NK cells, macrophages and γδ T cells express the transmembrane form of the molecule. The CD56 molecule, a homophilic adhesion molecule of the Ig superfamily (N-CAM), is another important marker of NK cells. The absence of CD3, but the presence of CD56 and/or CD16, is currently the most reliable marker for NK cells in man, although both markers can also be found on a minority of T cells (mostly with $CD3^+/CD8^+$ phenotype). Markers of NK cells are shown in *Figure 2.16* and in more detail in Appendix 2. Resting NK cells also express the β chain of the IL-2 receptor, an intermediate affinity receptor of 70 kDa, and the signal transducing common γ chain of the IL-2 and of other cytokine receptors. Therefore, direct stimulation with IL-2 results in activation of NK cells. Interestingly, this 70 kDa receptor is also expressed on all of the T cells that display large granular lymphocyte (LGL) morphology, namely <5% of $CD4^+$ T cells and 30–50% of $CD8^+$ T cells. All of these cells respond to IL-2 by acquiring non-specific cytotoxic functions and are known

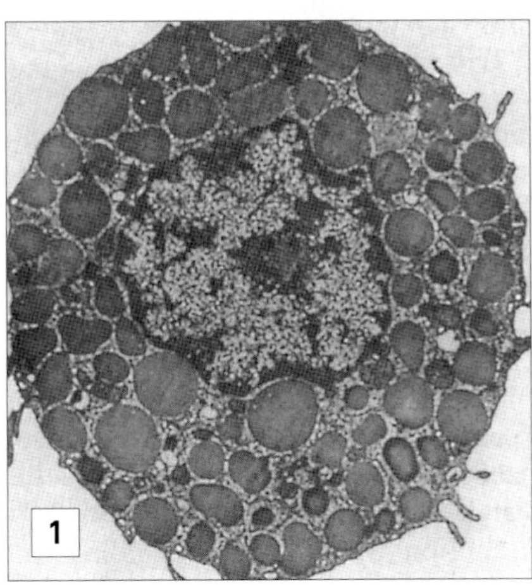

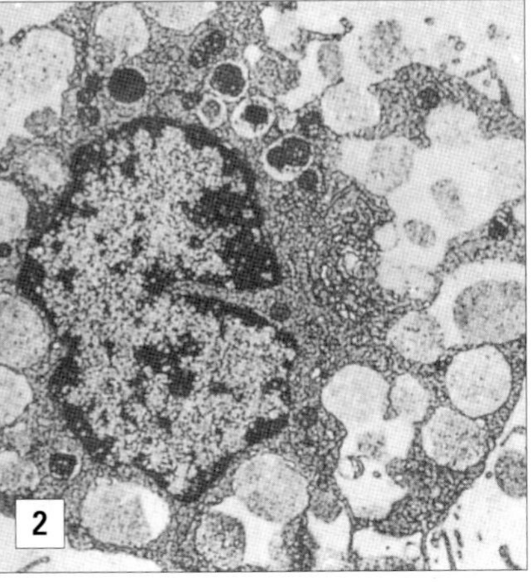

Fig. 2.14 Electron micrograph study of rat mast cells. Rat peritoneal mast cells show electron-dense granules (**1**). Following incubation with anti-IgE, vacuolation with exocytosis of the granule contents has occurred (**2**). Transmission electron micrographs, ×2700. (Courtesy of Dr D. Lawson.)

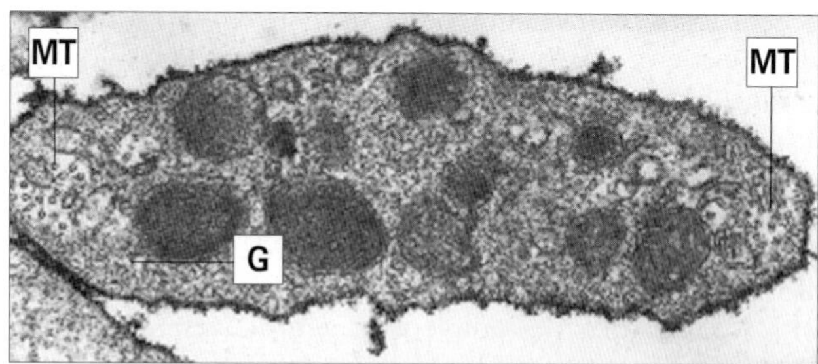

Fig. 2.15 Ultrastructure of a platelet. Cross-section of a platelet showing two types of granules (G) and bundles of microtubules at either end (MT). ×42 000. (Adapted from Zucker-Franklin D, Greaves MF, Grossi CE, *et al. Atlas of Blood Cells: Function and Pathology*. Vol II. 2nd edn. Milan: EE Ermes, Philadelphia: Lea and Febiger, 1988.)

Surface markers of human NK cells

marker	also present on
CD16 (FcγRIII)	minority of T cells granulocytes, some macrophages
CD56	minority of T cells
CD57	some T cells
IL-2R (β chain)	resting and activated T cells
CD94, CD158 (killer inhibitory receptors)	some T cells

Fig. 2.16 Several of the characteristic markers of NK cells also occur on other minor populations of leucocytes. Note that the killer inhibitory receptors (KIRs) may also occur as activating receptors (KARs), depending on which type of intracytoplasmic segment is linked to the extracellular portion (see Chapter 10).

collectively as lymphokine activated killer (LAK) cells. LAK cells kill fresh tumour cells and a broader spectrum of neoplastic targets in comparison to those lysed by resting NK cells.

The function of NK cells is to recognize and kill virus-infected cells and certain tumour cells (*Fig. 2.17*). The mechanism of recognition is not fully understood but involves both activating and inhibitory receptors, described in Chapter 10. Cells of the body expressing MHC molecules are protected against cytotoxicity mediated by NK cells; thus K562, the cells commonly used to measure NK cell function do not express HLA molecules. Down-regulation or modification of MHC molecules in virus-infected cells and some tumours makes them susceptible to NK cell-mediated killing.

NK cells are also able to kill targets coated with IgG antibodies via their receptor for IgG (FcγRIII: CD16). This property is referred to as antibody-dependent cellular cytotoxicity (ADCC). NK cells release interferon-γ (IFNγ) and other cytokines (e.g. IL-1 and GM–CSF) when activated, which may be important in the regulation of haemopoiesis and immune responses.

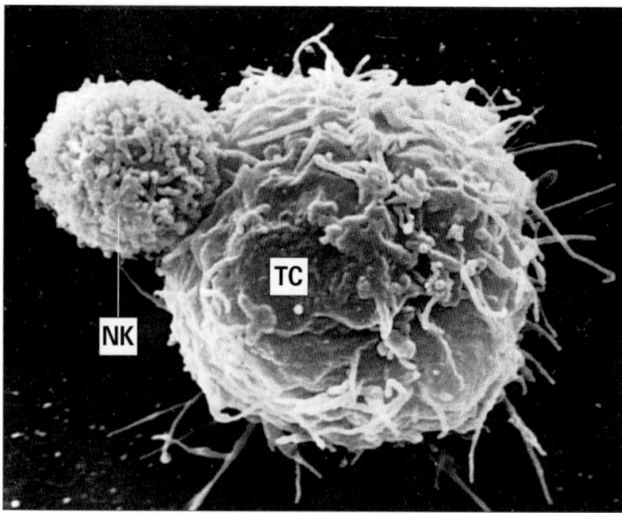

Fig. 2.17 An NK cell (NK) attached to a target cell (TC). ×4500. (Courtesy of Dr G. Arancia and W. Malorni, Rome.)

CELLS OF THE ADAPTIVE IMMUNE SYSTEM

Antigen-presenting cells (APCs)

APCs are a heterogeneous population of leucocytes with very efficient immunostimulatory capacity. Some have a pivotal role in the induction of functional activity of T-helper (TH) cells and, in this regard, are seen as the interface between the innate and adaptive immune systems; some communicate with other leucocytes.

APCs are found primarily in the skin, lymph nodes, spleen, within or underneath most mucosal epithelia and in the thymus (*Fig. 2.18*). Langerhans' cells in the skin and in other squamous epithelia migrate as 'veiled cells', via the afferent lymphatics into the paracortex of the draining lymph nodes. Here, these cells interact with T cells and are termed interdigitating cells (IDC: *Fig. 2.19*). This migration provides an efficient mechanism for carrying antigen from the skin and mucosa to the TH cells located in the lymph nodes. These APCs are rich in class II MHC molecules, which are important for presenting antigen to TH cells.

The follicular dendritic cells (FDC) are found in the primary and secondary follicles of the B-cell areas of the lymph nodes, spleen and MALT and present antigen to B cells (see below). They are a non-migratory population of cells which form a stable network by establishing strong intercellular connections via desmosomes (*Fig. 2.20*). They lack class II MHC molecules but bind antigen via complement receptors (CD21 and CD35), which attach to complement associated with immune complexes (iccosomes). They also express Fc receptors. Another kind of APC has recently been described within the germinal centre (GC) of secondary B-cell follicles, the MHC class II positive germinal centre dendritic cell (GCDC). In contrast to FDC, they are migrating cells which on arrival in the GC interact with T cells.

APCs present in the thymus, are also called IDCs, and

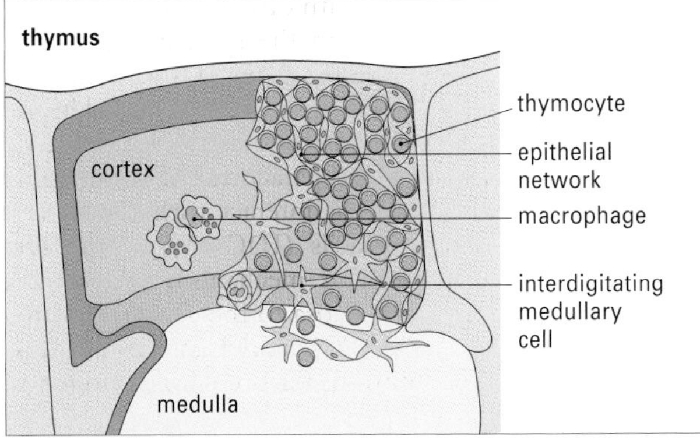

Fig. 2.18 Bone-marrow-derived antigen-presenting cells (APCs) are found especially in lymphoid tissues, in the skin and in mucosa. APCs in the form of Langerhans' cells are found in the epidermis and are characterized by special granules (the tennis-racquet-shaped Birbeck granules). These cells, rich in MHC class II, carry processed antigens and migrate via the afferent lymphatics (where they appear as 'veiled' cells) into the paracortex of the draining lymph nodes. Here they make contact with T cells. These 'interdigitating cells', localized in the T-cell-dependent cells areas of the lymph node, present antigen to T-helper cells. Exposure of antigen to B cells occurs on the follicular dendritic cells (FDCs) in the germinal centres of B-cell follicles. Some macrophages located in the outer cortex and marginal sinus may also act as APCs. In the thymus, APCs occur as interdigitating cells in the medulla.

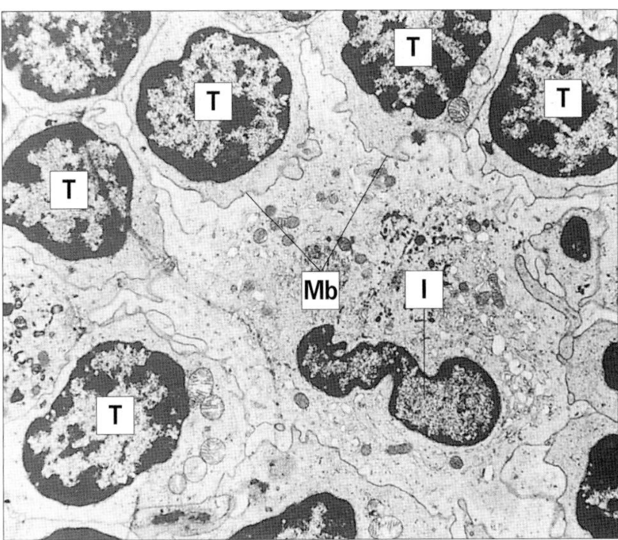

Fig. 2.19 Ultrastructure of an interdigitating dendritic cell (IDC) in the T-cell area of a rat lymph node. Intimate contacts are made with the membranes of the surrounding T cells. The cytoplasm contains a well-developed endosomal system and does not show the Birbeck granules characteristic of skin Langerhans' cells. I = IDC nucleus; Mb = IDC membrane; T = T-cell nucleus. ×2000. (Courtesy of Dr B. H. Balfour.)

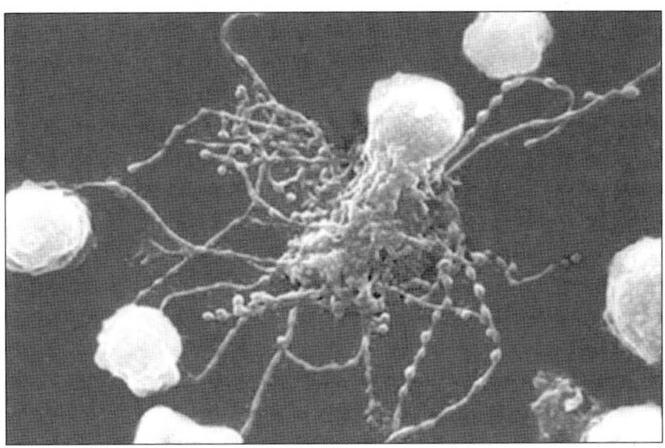

Fig. 2.20 Follicular dendritic cell. An isolated follicular dendritic cell from the lymph node of an immunized mouse 24 hours after injection of antigen. The FDC is of intermediate maturity with smooth filiform dendrites typical of young FDCs, and beaded dendrites which participate in the formation of iccosomes of mature FDCs. The adjacent small white cells are lymphocytes. (Electron micrograph kindly provided by Dr Andras Szakal; reproduced by permission of the *Journal of Immunology*.)

are especially abundant in the medulla. The thymus is of crucial importance in the development and maturation of T cells, and it appears that the IDCs play a role in deleting T cells that react against self antigen. This process is referred to as 'negative selection' (see Chapter 12).

The majority of APCs are bone marrow derived although their haemopoietic progenitor cell remains undefined. For example, within 100 days of bone-marrow transplantation, all epidermal Langerhans cells of the recipient have been replaced with cells of donor origin. Following stimulation *in vitro* with GM–CSF and IL-4, monocytes lose their phagocytic capacity and transform into efficient class II MHC-expressing APCs with dendritic morphology. The FDCs of the primary and secondary lymphoid follicles are not bone marrow derived, but are of mesenchymal origin.

Dendritic cells interacting with T cells are not the only APCs with this property since both macrophages and classical B cells are rich in class II MHC membrane molecules, especially after activation, and are thus able to process and present specific antigens to (activated) T cells (see Chapter 6). Distinguishing markers found on different kinds of APCs are shown in *Figure 2.21.*

Somatic cells other than immune cells do not normally express class II MHC molecules, but cytokines such as IFNγ and TNFα can induce the expression of class II molecules on some cell types, and thus allow them to present antigen, e.g. skin and thyroid epithelium, endothelia. This induction of 'inappropriate' class II expression might contribute to the pathogenesis of autoimmune diseases and to prolonged inflammation.

Lymphocytes

Large numbers of lymphocytes are produced daily in the primary or central lymphoid organs (thymus and postnatal bone marrow). Some of these cells migrate via the circulation into the secondary lymphoid tissues (spleen, lymph nodes and mucosa-associated lymphoid tissues). The average human adult has about 2×10^{12} lymphoid cells and the lymphoid tissue as a whole represents about 2% of total body weight. Lymphoid cells account for about 20% of the leucocytes in the adult circulation. Many mature lymphoid cells are long-lived, and persist as memory cells for many years.

Lymphocytes are morphologically heterogeneous

In a conventional blood smear, lymphocytes vary in both size (6–10 μm in diameter) and morphology. Differences are seen in the nuclear to cytoplasmic (N : C) ratio, the nuclear shape, and the presence or absence of azurophilic granules.

Two distinct morphological types are seen in the circulation as determined by light microscopy and a haematological stain such as Giemsa. The first type is relatively small, is typically agranular and has a high N : C ratio. The second type is larger, has a lower N : C ratio, contains cytoplasmic azurophilic granules and is known as the large granular lymphocyte (LGL). LGL should not be confused with granulocytes, monocytes or their precursors, which also contain azurophilic granules (*Fig. 2.22*).

Resting blood T cells – The majority of these express αβ T-cell receptors (see 'T cells' below) and can show either of the above morphological patterns. The majority (≈95%) of TH cells and a proportion (≈50%) of T cytotoxic (TC) cells are of the smaller type (non-granular with a high N : C ratio). They also carry a cytoplasmic structure termed the 'Gall body', which consists of a cluster of primary lysosomes associated with a lipid droplet. The Gall body is

Markers on antigen-presenting cells

cell markers	Langerhans' cells	interdigitating cells	follicular dendritic cells	GCDC	B cells	macrophages
MHC II	+	+	–	+	+	±
FcγRII (CD32) FcγRI (CD64)	+ ±	– –	+ –	+ –	+ –	+ +
CD35 (CR1)	+	–	+	+	+	+
CD21	–	–	High	Low	+	+
CD2	–	–	–	+	–	–
CD4	+	–	–	+	–	+
CD1a	+	–	–	–	–	–
CD40	?	High	+	Low	High	+
NSE	–	–	–	–	–	+
Phagocytosis	–	–	–	–	–	+

Fig. 2.21 Langerhans' cells (LC), interdigitating dendritic cells (IDC), germinal centre dendritic cells (GCDC) and B cells are rich in MHC class II for communicating with CD4⁺ T cells. CD4 expressed by only some APCs may allow their infection with HIV. Macrophages (M) possess low levels of MHC class II for antigen presentation and are mainly phagocytic cells. Follicular dendritic cells (FDC) located within the primary and secondary follicles do not express class II MHC, but have high levels of FcγR, CR1 and CR2 to enable them to trap immune complexes (iccosomes) for presentation to B cells. NSE = non-specific esterase.

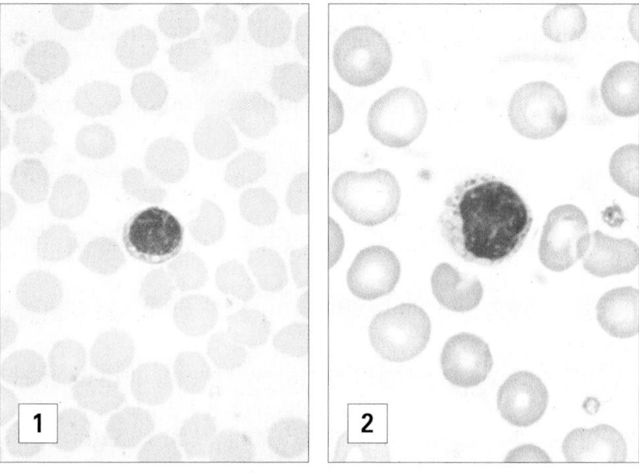

Fig. 2.22 Morphological heterogeneity of lymphocytes. (**1**) The small lymphocyte has no granules, a round nucleus and a high N : C ratio. (**2**) The large granular lymphocyte has a lower N : C ratio, indented nucleus and azurophilic granules in the cytoplasm. Giemsa stain. (Courtesy of Dr A. Stevens and Professor J. Lowe.)

easily identified by lysosomal enzyme cytochemistry and electron microscopy (*Fig. 2.23*). The other morphological pattern is shown by <5% of TH cells and by about 30–50% of TC cells. These display LGL morphology, with primary lysosomes dispersed in the cytoplasm and a well-developed Golgi apparatus (*Fig. 2.24*). Interestingly, TC cells with LGL morphology are not detected in mice.

The γδ T-cell population (γδT) is another subset which displays LGL characteristics. These cells have a dendritic morphology in lymphoid tissues (*Fig. 2.25*); when cultured *in vitro* they may adhere to surfaces, showing a variety of morphological features (*Fig. 2.26*).

Resting blood B cells – These cells do not have Gall bodies or LGL morphology and their cytoplasm is predominantly occupied by scattered monoribosomes (*Fig. 2.27*). Activated B cells with developing rough endoplasmic reticulum are occasionally seen in the circulation (*Fig. 2.28*).

Lymphocytes express characteristic surface markers

Lymphocytes (and other leucocytes) express a large number of different molecules on their surfaces, which can be used to distinguish ('mark') cell subsets. Many of these cell markers can now be identified by specific monoclonal

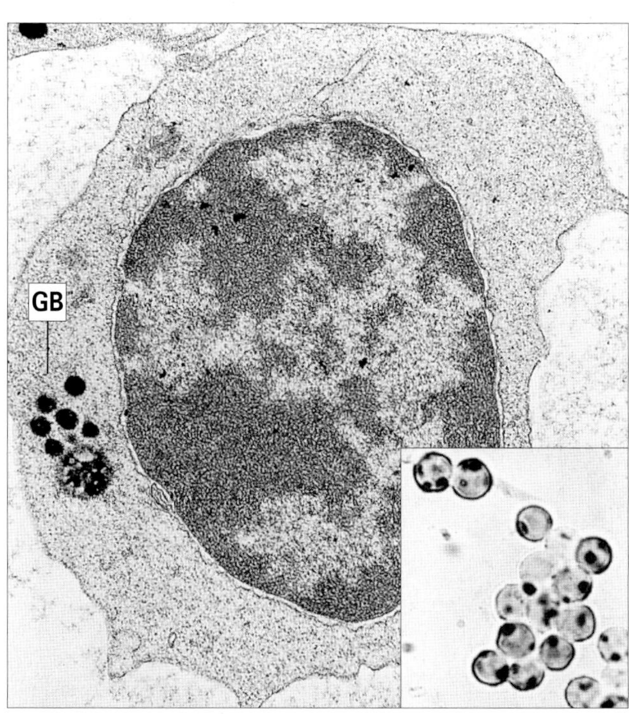

Fig. 2.23 Ultrastructure of a non-granular T cell. This electron micrograph shows the Gall body (GB) that is characteristic of the majority of resting T cells. It consists of primary lysosomes and a lipid droplet (arrow). ×10 500. Inset: This structure is also seen as a single 'spot' after staining for non-specific esterases in light microscopy. ×400. (Adapted from Zucker-Franklin D, Greaves MF, Grossi CE, *et al. Atlas of Blood Cells: Function and Pathology.* Vol II. 2nd edn. Milan: EE Ermes, Philadelphia: Lea and Febiger, 1988.)

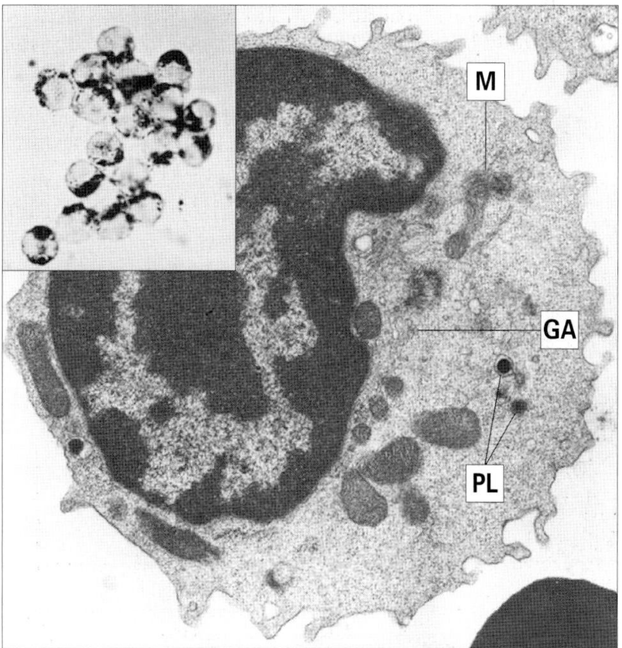

Fig. 2.24 Ultrastructure of T cells with granular morphology. These cells characteristically have electron-dense peroxidase-negative granules (primary lysosomes, PL), scattered throughout the cytoplasm, with some close to the Golgi apparatus (GA). There are many mitochondria (M) present. ×10 000. Inset: Cytochemical staining for acid phosphatase shows a granular pattern of staining under light microscopy. ×400. (Adapted from Zucker-Franklin D, Greaves MF, Grossi CE, *et al. Atlas of Blood Cells: Function and Pathology.* Vol II. 2nd edn. Milan: EE Ermes, Philadelphia: Lea and Febiger, 1988.)

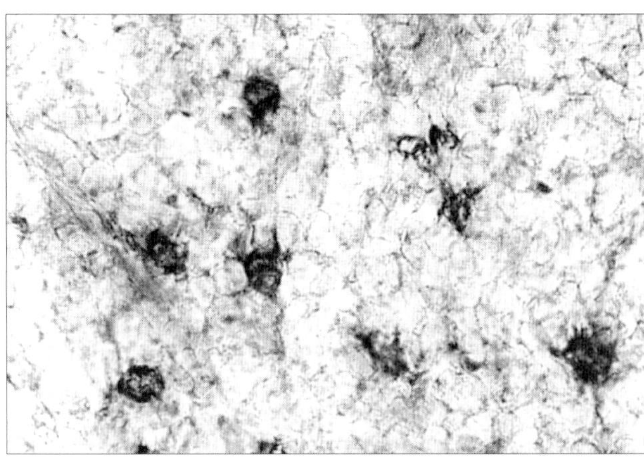

Fig. 2.25 Dendritic morphology of γδ T cells in the tonsil. This T-cell population is predominantly localized in the interfollicular T-cell-dependent zones. Note the dendritic morphology of the cells. Anti-γδ T cell mAb and immunoperoxidase. ×900. (Courtesy of Dr A. Favre, from *Eur J Immunol* 1991;**21**:173, with permission.)

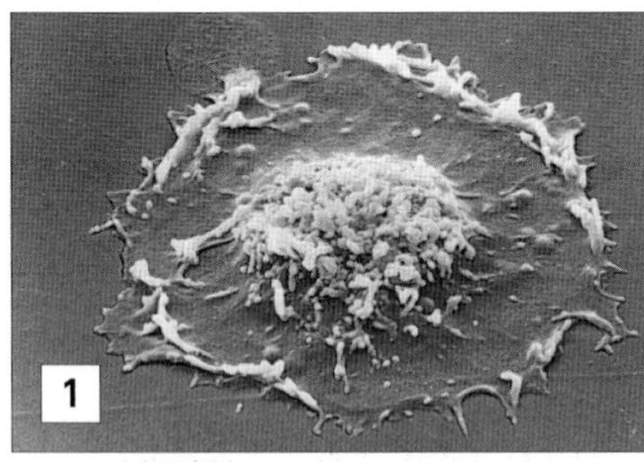

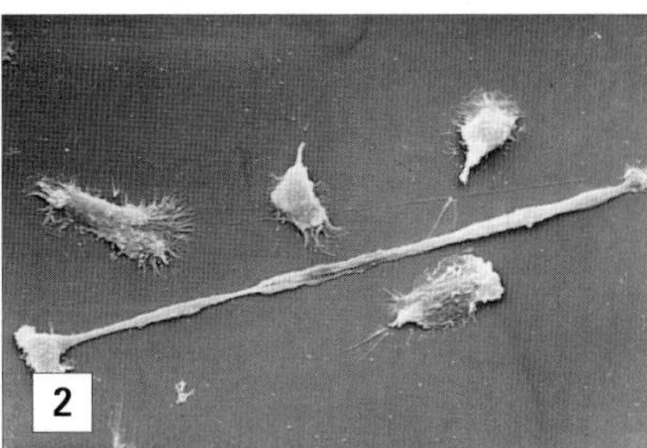

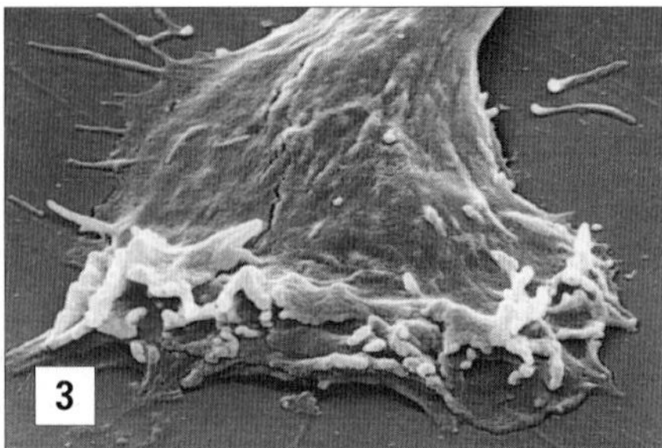

Fig. 2.26 Morphological changes in cloned γδ T cells *in vitro*. Cells adhere to the substrate in a similar way to macrophages. ×6000. (**2**) The cells become elongated with uropod formation, extending two polar filopodia. ×2000. (**3**) Adhesion plaques are formed at the terminal ends of the filopodia. ×20 000. (Courtesy of Dr G. Arancia and Dr W. Malorni, from *Eur J Immunol* 1991;**21**:173, with permission.)

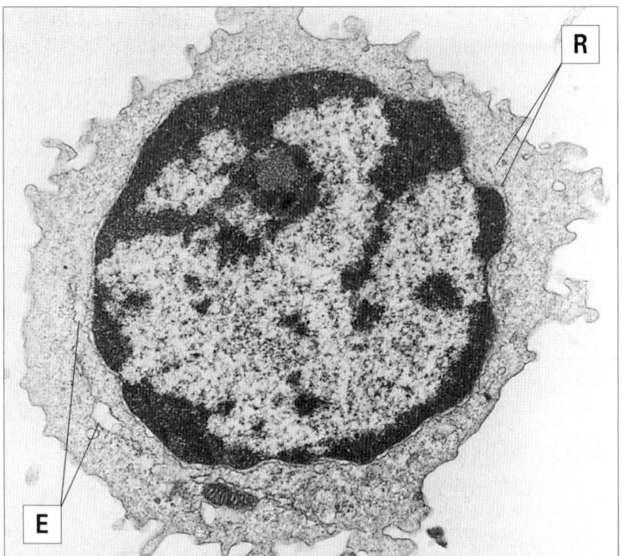

Fig. 2.27 Ultrastructure of resting B cells. These cells have no Gall body or granules. Scattered ribosomes (R) and isolated strands of rough endoplasmic reticulum (E) are seen in the cytoplasm. Development of the Golgi-lysosomal system in the B cell occurs on activation. ×11 500.

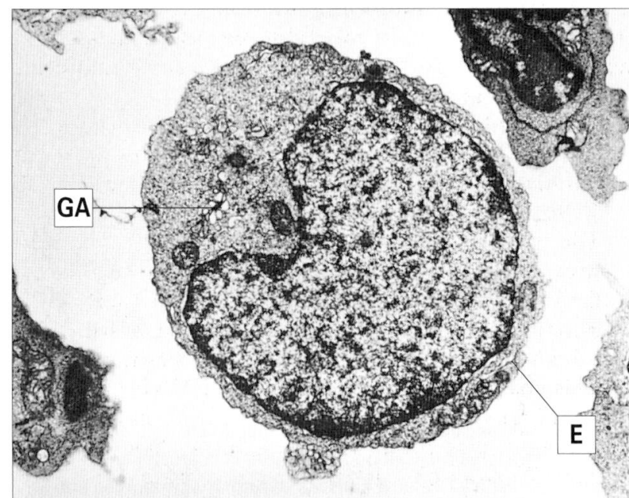

Fig. 2.28 Ultrastructure of B-cell blasts. The main feature of activated B cells is the development of the machinery for immunoglobulin synthesis. This includes rough endoplasmic reticulum (E), free polyribosomes and the Golgi apparatus (GA), which is involved in glycosylation of the immunoglobulins. ×7500.

antibodies (mAb). A systematic nomenclature has been developed, in which the term CD (Cluster Designation) refers to groups (clusters) of mAb, each cluster binding specifically to a particular molecule. The CD system derives from analysis of mAb against human leucocyte antigens, produced mainly in mice. The work is carried out in many laboratories worldwide, and a series of International Workshops determine the patterns of mAb binding to different leucocyte populations, and the molecular weight of the markers. Monoclonal antibodies with similar characteristics, defined by these criteria, are grouped together and given a CD number. However, it is now customary to use the CD marker to indicate the molecule recognized by each group of monoclonal antibodies (a list of CD markers is given in Appendix 2).

Molecular markers are further defined according to the information they offer about the cell. For example:

- Lineage markers identify a specific lineage, for example CD3, found only on T cells.
- Maturation markers are transiently expressed during differentiation, for example CD1 present on developing thymocytes but not on mature T cells.
- Activation markers, for example the low-affinity T-cell growth factor (IL-2) receptor (CD25) is only expressed when cells are stimulated by antigens or mitogens.

Although it is sometimes useful to define markers in this way, it is not always possible to do so. A maturation marker for one lineage is sometimes an activation marker for the same lineage. For example, CD10 present on immature B cells is lost on mature B cells but reappears on activation. Furthermore, 'activation' markers may already be present at low density on cells, but increase following activation. An example of this is provided by MHC class II molecules that show increased expression on monocytes following their activation by IFNγ.

There are families of cell markers

Cell surface molecules belong to different families which have probably evolved from a few ancestral genes. These families are distinguished by their molecular structure and include the following major groups:

- The *immunoglobulin superfamily* comprises molecules with structural characteristics similar to those of the immunoglobulins. This family includes CD2, CD3, CD4, CD8, CD28, MHC class I and II and many more.
- The *integrin* family consists of heterodimeric molecules with α and β chains. There are several integrin subfamilies; all members of a particular subfamily share a common β chain, but each has a unique α chain. One subfamily (the β_2-integrins) uses CD18 as the β chain. This chain can be associated with CD11a, CD11b or CD11c or αd – these combinations make up the lymphocyte function antigens LFA-1, Mac-1 (CR3), p150,95 and $\alpha d\beta_2$ surface molecules respectively – and are commonly found on leucocytes. A second subfamily (the β_1-integrins) has CD29 as the β chain, again associated with various other peptides and includes the VLA (very late activation) markers.
- *Selectins* (CD62, E, L and P), expressed on leucocytes (L) or activated endothelial cells and platelets (E and P). They have lectin-like specificity for a variety of sugars expressed on heavily glycosylated membrane glycoproteins, for example CD43.
- *Proteoglycans,* typically CD44, have a number of glycosaminoglycans (GAG) binding sites (e.g. for chondroitin sulphate), and bind to extracellular matrix components (typically, hyaluronic acid).

Other families include the tumour necrosis factor (TNF) and nerve growth factor (NGF) receptor superfamily, the C-type lectin superfamily, the family of receptors with seven transmembrane segments (tm7) and the superfamily with four membrane-spanning segments (tm4, e.g. CD20).

It should be emphasized that markers expressed by lymphocytes can often be detected on cells of other lineages, for example CD44 (commonly expressed by epithelial cells). Surface molecules can be demonstrated using fluorescent antibodies as probes (*Fig. 2.29*). This is exploited by the technique of flow cytometry, which can enumerate and separate cells on the basis of their size and fluorescent staining (see *Fig. 27.9*), and which has allowed a detailed dissection of lymphoid cell populations.

The major functions of the above families of marker molecules is to allow the lymphocytes to communicate with their environment. They are extremely important in cell trafficking, adhesion and activation.

T cells

T cells can be distinguished by their different antigen receptors

The definitive T-cell lineage marker is the T-cell antigen receptor (TCR). There are two defined types of TCR: one is a heterodimer of two disulphide-linked polypeptides (α and β); the other is structurally similar but consists of γ and δ polypeptides. Both receptors are associated with a set of five polypeptides, the CD3 complex, and together form the T-cell receptor complex (TCR–CD3 complex; see Chapter 5). Approximately 90–95% of blood T cells are αβ T cells and the remaining 5–10% are γδ T cells.

Immunofluorescent demonstration of T-cell markers

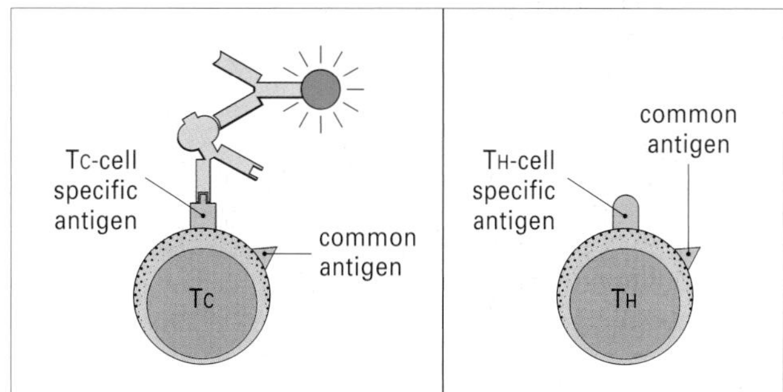

Fig. 2.29 Mouse monoclonal antibodies directed towards a T-cell subset-specific antigen on a T-cytotoxic (Tc) cell, will bind to such cells, but not to T-helper (TH) cells (e.g. CD8). The bound antibody is detected using antibodies to mouse immunoglobulin coupled to a fluorescent molecule. This provides a method for identifying and enumerating T-cell subsets.

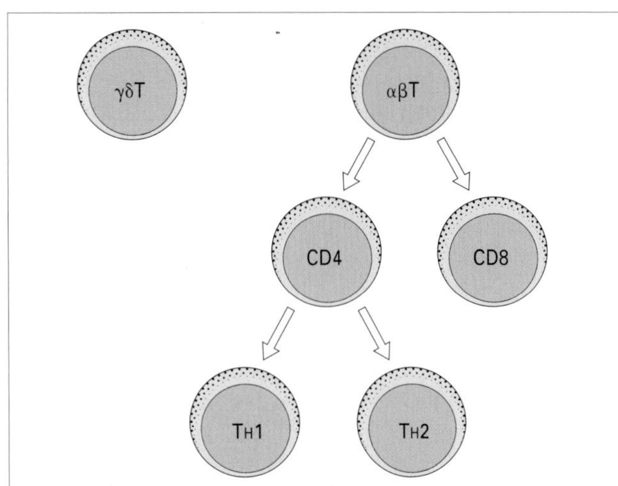

Fig. 2.30 T cells express either γδ or αβ TCR. T cells are divided into CD4 and CD8 subsets which determine whether they see antigen (peptides) with MHC class II or I, respectively. $CD4^+$ T cells can be further subdivided into TH1 and TH2 on the basis of their cytokine profiles.

αβ T cells are further distinguished by their expression of CD4 or CD8

αβ T cells are subdivided into two distinct non-overlapping populations; a subset which carries the CD4 marker and mainly 'helps' or 'induces' immune responses (TH), and a subset which carries the CD8 marker and is predominantly cytotoxic (TC). $CD4^+$ T cells recognize their specific antigens in association with major histocompatibility complex (MHC) class II molecules, whereas $CD8^+$ T cells recognize antigens in association with MHC class I molecules (see Chapter 6). Thus, the presence of CD4 or CD8 limits (restricts) the type of cell with which the T cell can interact (*Fig. 2.30*). A small proportion of αβ T cells express neither CD4 nor CD8 and these 'double negative' T cells might have a regulatory function. Similarly, most circulating γδ cells are 'double negative', although a few of them are $CD8^+$. By contrast, most γδ T cells in tissues express CD8.

There are functional subsets of αβ$CD4^+$ and $CD8^+$ T cells

These populations can be further subdivided into functional subsets based on the phenotypic expression of CD28 and CTLA-4 (CD152). Expression of CD28 by $CD4^+$ T cells allows the delivery of a costimulatory signal on recognition of antigen by αβ T cells (and prevents anergy which would follow engagement of TCR with antigen alone). These cells also express CTLA-4 following binding of CD28 to its ligands B7-1 (CD80) and B7-2 (CD86) found on APCs. Interaction of CTLA-4 with these same ligands now induces downregulation of T-cell functions. In addition, αβ T cells express different isoforms of the leucocyte common antigen, CD45. It is believed that CD45RO rather than CD45RA is related to cell activation and is a marker of memory cells. Other criteria have been used to subdivide αβ T-cell subsets. For example, 5–10% of circulating T cells express NK cell markers (CD56, CD57 and CD11b/CD18). These cells do not produce IL-2 and proliferate weakly in response to antigens and mitogens.

αβ T lymphocytes can also be classified on the basis of cytokine production

Functional diversity of T cells has also been demonstrated by analysis of TH clones for cytokine secretion patterns. In mice and in men, two groups of $CD4^+$ T-cell clones have been identified. The TH1 subset secretes IL-2 and IFNγ, and the TH2 subset produces IL-4, IL-5, IL-6 and IL-10 (see *Fig. 7.12*). TH1 cells mediate several functions associated with cytotoxicity and local inflammatory reactions. Consequently, these cells are important for combating intracellular pathogens including viruses, bacteria and parasites. TH2 cells are more effective at stimulating B cells to proliferate and produce antibodies, and therefore function primarily to protect against free-living microorganisms (humoral immunity).

γδ T cells are common in mucosal surfaces and in murine epidermis

γδ T cells are relatively frequent in mucosal epithelia but form only a minor subpopulation of circulating T cells (around 5%). The majority of intraepithelial lymphocytes (IELs) are γδ T cells and express CD8, a marker not found on most circulating γδ T cells. It has been shown that $CD8^+$ γδ T cells have a specific repertoire of T-cell receptors biased towards certain bacterial/viral antigens (superantigens), and current opinion is that these cells may play an important role in protecting the mucosal surfaces of the body. Some γδ T cells may recognize antigens directly, i.e. with no need for APCs.

T cells share some markers with other cell lineages

So far, we have described the cell markers and antigen-specific receptors which define T-cell subsets. There are also a number of other surface molecules, expressed on all T cells (pan T-cell markers), which are found on cells of other lineages. The receptors for sheep erythrocytes (CD2) are a good example. Under normal circumstances, the CD2 molecule, together with the TCR–CD3 complex and other membrane-bound glycoproteins, is involved in activating T cells when it binds to the appropriate ligands. CD2 is also found on about 75% of $CD3^-$ NK cells. Another molecule involved in T-cell activation, CD5, is expressed on all T cells and on a subpopulation of B cells. Although CD5 can bind to CD72, it is debatable whether or not this is the physiological ligand in B cells. CD7 is present on the majority of NK cells and T cells. Murine T cells express markers similar to those detected on human T cells. A summary of the main markers that distinguish T cells from B cells – the other main lymphocyte population, – is shown in *Figure 2.31.*

Suppressor T cells

Although there is clear evidence for the existence of antigen-specific suppressor T cells (Ts), it is unlikely that they represent a functionally separate T-cell subset. There is also evidence that both $CD4^+$ and $CD8^+$ T cells can

Main distinguishing markers of T and B cells

CD number	T cells	B cells
Antigen receptor	TCR ($\alpha\beta$ or $\gamma\delta$)	Ig
CD1	–	+
CD2	+	–
CD3	+ (*)	–
CD4	+ (ss)	–
CD5	+	+ (ss)
CD8	+ (ss)	–
CD16	+ (ss$)	–
CD19	–	+
CD20	–	+
CD21	+ (ss)	+
CD22	–	+ (ss)
CD23	+ (ss)	+
CD28	+	?
CD32	–	+
CD40	–	+
CD79a	–	+ (**)
CD79b	–	+ (**)

Fig. 2.31 *Part of the T-cell receptor complex: ss, subset; ss$, subset of $\gamma\delta$ T cells: **part of the B-cell receptor complex.

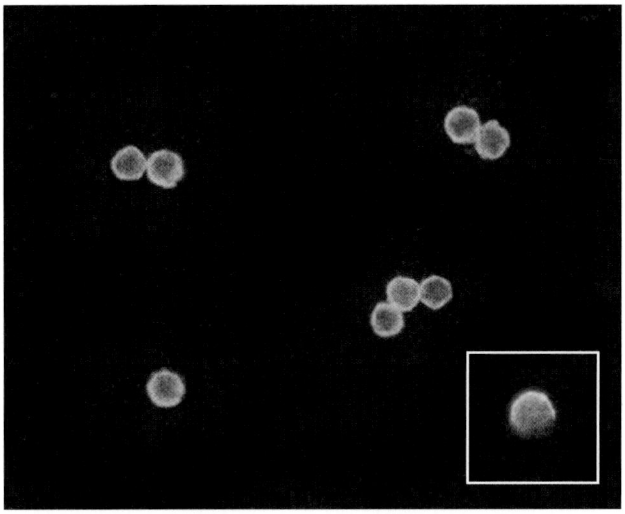

Fig. 2.32 B cells stained for surface immunoglobulin. B cells stained with fluorescent anti-IgM in the cold show a surface ring-like pattern under UV light. A polar redistribution (capping) is seen when the cells are incubated at 37°C in the presence of the antibody (inset). ×300. (Adapted from Zucker-Franklin D, Greaves MF, Grossi CE, *et al. Atlas of Blood Cells: Function and Pathology.* Vol II. 2nd edn. Milan: EE Ermes, Philadelphia: Lea and Febiger, 1988.)

suppress immune responses and this might operate through direct killing of APCs, through 'suppressive' cytokines, for example TGFβ, negative regulation of signal transduction (CTLA-4 interaction with its ligands; see above) or via the idiotype network (see Chapter 11).

B cells

About 5–15% of the circulating lymphoid pool are B cells defined by the presence of surface immunoglobulin. These are constitutively produced and are inserted into the cell surface membrane where they act as specific antigen receptors. These receptors can be detected on the cell surface using fluorochrome-labelled antibodies specific for immunoglobulin. Immunofluorescence staining shows a 'ring-like' pattern over the B cell (*Fig. 2.32*). Divalent antibodies to surface immunoglobulin bind to and cross-link the surface receptors, producing 'patches' of immunoglobulin on the cell surface. On warming up, most of these complexes are actively swept along the cell surface and are seen as a 'cap' over one pole of the cell (see *Fig. 2.32 inset*). Capping is followed by internalization and degradation of the Ig. Capping may also be seen with other surface glycoproteins and is not exclusive to B cells.

Cell surface immunoglobulin and signalling molecules form the 'B-cell receptor' complex

The majority of human B cells in peripheral blood express two immunoglobulin isotypes on their surface, IgM and IgD (see Chapter 4). On any B cell, the antigen-binding sites of these isotypes are identical. Fewer than 10% of the B cells in the circulation express IgG, IgA or IgE, although these are present in larger numbers in specific locations of the body, for example, IgA-bearing cells in the intestinal mucosa. Immunoglobulin associated with other molecules on the B-cell surface forms the 'B-cell antigen receptor complex' (BCR). These 'accessory' molecules consist of disulphide-bonded heterodimers of Igα (CD79a) and Igβ (CD79b). The heterodimers interact with the transmembrane segments of the immunoglobulin receptor, and like the separate molecular components of the TCR/CD3 complex, are involved in cellular activation (see *Fig. 4.1* and *5.2*).

Other B-cell markers and subsets

The majority of B cells carry MHC class II antigens, which are important for cooperative (cognate) interactions with T cells. These class II molecules consist of I–A or I–E in the mouse and HLA-DP, DQ and DR antigens in man. Complement receptors for C3b (CD35) and C3d (CD21) are commonly found on B cells and are associated with activation and, possibly, 'homing' of the cells. CD19/CD21 interactions with complement associated with antigen plays a role in antigen-induced B-cell activation via the antigen-binding antibody receptor. Fc receptors for exogenous IgG (FcγRII, CD32) are also present and play a role in negative signalling to the B cell (see Chapter 11).

CD19, CD20 and CD22 are the main markers currently used to identify human B cells. Other human B cell markers are CD72 to CD78. The CD72 molecule has also been described for murine B cells (Lyb-2) together with B220, a high molecular weight (220 kDa) isoform of CD45 (Lyb-5). CD40 is an important molecule on B cells which is involved in cognate interactions between T and B cells (see *Fig. 8.10*).

CD5⁺ B lymphocytes are a distinctive cell subset

Many of the first B cells that appear during ontogeny express CD5, a marker originally found on T cells. These cells (termed B-1 cells) are found predominantly in the peritoneal cavity in mice and there is some evidence for a separate differentiation pathway from 'conventional' B cells (B-2 cells). They express their immunoglobulins from unmutated or minimally mutated germline genes. $CD5^+$ B cells produce mostly IgM, but also some IgG and IgA. These so-called natural antibodies are of low avidity but, unusually, they are polyreactive and are found at high concentration in the adult serum. $CD5^+$ cells may respond well to TI (T-independent) antigens. They may also be involved in antigen processing and antigen presentation to T cells, and probably play a role in both tolerance and antibody responses. Functions proposed for natural antibodies include the following: the first line of defence against microorganisms; clearance of damaged self components; and 'idiotype network' interactions within the immune system. Characteristically, these antibodies also react against autoantigens including DNA, Fc of IgG, phospholipids and cytoskeletal components. Since CD5 has been shown to be expressed by B2 cells when they are activated appropriately, there is still some controversy as to whether CD5 represents an activation antigen on B cells. The current theories therefore support the notion for there being two different kinds of $CD5^+$ B cells. Although the function of CD5 is unknown on human B cells, it is associated with the BCR and may be involved in the regulation of B-cell activation.

B-cell differentiation leads to the formation of plasma cells and memory cells

Following B-cell activation, many B-cell blasts mature into AFCs, which progress *in vivo* to terminally differentiated plasma cells. Some B blasts do not develop rough endoplasmic reticulum cisternae. These cells are found in germinal centres and are named follicle centre cells or centrocytes. Under light microscopy, the cytoplasm of the plasma cells is basophilic; this is due to the large amount of RNA being utilized for antibody synthesis in the rough endoplasmic reticulum. At the ultrastructural level, the rough endoplasmic reticulum can often be seen in parallel arrays (*Fig. 2.33*). Plasma cells are infrequent in the blood, comprising less than 0.1% of circulating lymphocytes. They are normally restricted to the secondary lymphoid organs and tissues but are also abundant in the bone marrow. Antibodies produced by a single plasma cell are of one specificity and immunoglobulin class. Immunoglobulins can be visualized in the plasma cell cytoplasm by staining with fluorochrome-labelled specific antibodies (*Fig. 2.34*). Many plasma cells have a short lifespan, surviving for a few days and dying by apoptosis (*Fig. 2.35*), whereas a subset of plasma cells with a long lifespan (months) has been recently described in the bone marrow. See *Figure 2.31* for a comparison of B-cell markers with those of T cells.

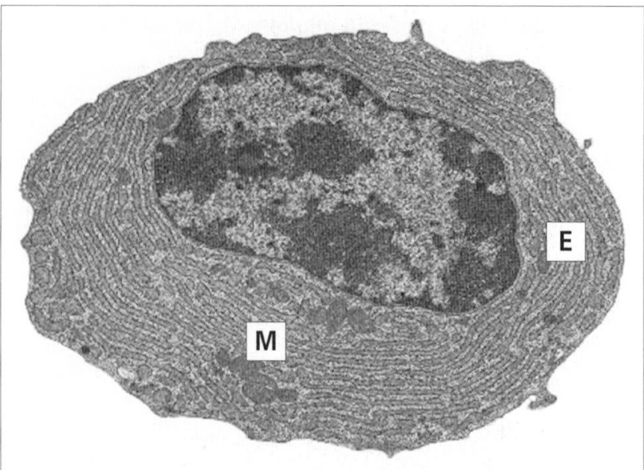

Fig. 2.33 Ultrastructure of the plasma cell. The plasma cell is characterized by parallel arrays of rough endoplasmic reticulum (E). In mature cells, these cisternae become dilated with immunoglobulins. Mitochondria (M) are also seen. ×5000. (Adapted from Zucker-Franklin D, Greaves MF, Grossi CE, *et al. Atlas of Blood Cells: Function and Pathology.* Vol II. 2nd edn. Milan: EE Ermes, Philadelphia: Lea and Febiger, 1988.)

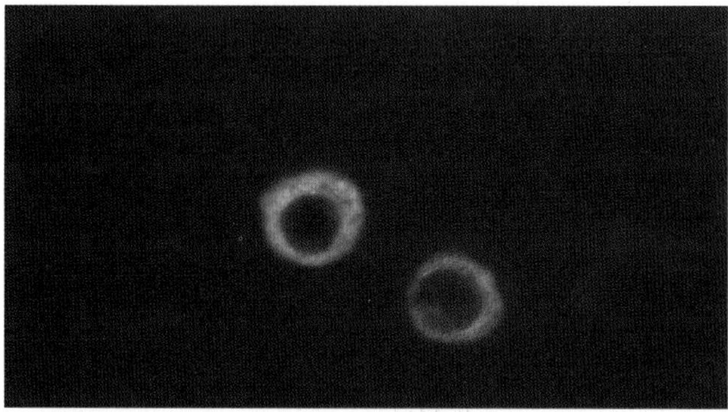

Fig. 2.34 Immunofluorescent staining of intracytoplasmic immunoglobulin in plasma cells. Fixed human plasma cells, treated with fluoresceinated anti-human-IgM (green) and rhodaminated anti-human-IgG (red), show extensive intracytoplasmic staining. As the distinct staining of the two cells shows, plasma cells normally only produce one class or subclass (isotype) of antibody. ×1500. (Adapted from Zucker-Franklin D, Greaves MF, Grossi CE, *et al. Atlas of Blood Cells: Function and Pathology.* Vol II. 2nd edn. Milan: EE Ermes, Philadelphia: Lea and Febiger, 1988.

LYMPHOID TISSUES

The cells involved in the immune response are organized into tissues and organs in order to perform their functions most effectively. These structures are collectively referred to as the lymphoid system. The lymphoid system comprises lymphocytes, accessory cells (macrophages and APCs) and, in some tissues, epithelial cells. It is arranged into either discretely encapsulated organs or accumulations of diffuse lymphoid tissue. The major lymphoid organs and tissues are classified into either primary (central) or secondary (peripheral; *Fig. 2.36*). In essence, lymphocytes are produced in the primary lymphoid organs and function within the secondary lymphoid organs and tissues.

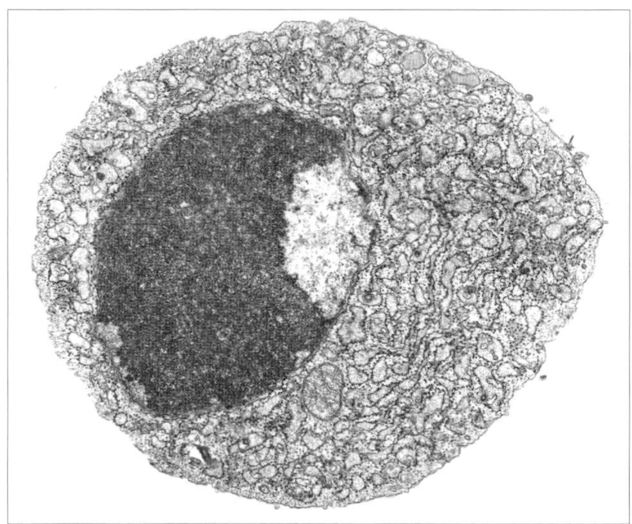

Fig. 2.35 Plasma cell death by apoptosis. Plasma cells are shortlived and die by apoptosis (cell suicide). Note the nuclear chromatin changes, which are characteristic of apoptosis. ×5000.

Primary lymphoid organs

Primary lymphoid organs are the major sites of lymphocyte development. Here, lymphocytes differentiate from lymphoid stem cells, proliferate and mature into functional cells. In mammals, T cells mature in the thymus, B lymphocytes in the fetal liver and bone marrow (see Chapter 8). Birds have a specialized site of B-cell generation, the bursa of Fabricius. It is in the primary lymphoid organs that lymphocytes acquire their repertoire of specific antigen receptors in order to cope with antigenic challenges that individuals receive during their lifespan. In these primary lymphoid organs the cells with receptors for autoantigens are mostly eliminated, whilst in the thymus T cells also 'learn' to recognize self-MHC molecules. There is evidence that some lymphocyte development occurs outside the primary lymphoid organs.

The thymus is the site of T-cell development

The thymus in mammals is a bilobed organ, located in the thoracic cavity, overlying the heart and major blood vessels. Each lobe is organized into lobules separated from each other by connective tissue trabeculae. Within each lobule, the lymphoid cells (thymocytes) are arranged into an outer cortex and an inner medulla (*Fig. 2.37*). The tightly packed cortex contains the majority of relatively immature proliferating thymocytes; more mature cells are found in the medulla, implying a differentiation gradient from cortex to medulla. Mature thymocytes in the medulla express CD44, which is not detected in cortical thymocytes. This receptor, which binds to hyaluronate and other extracellular matrix components, is found on all trafficking cells and is not expressed on sessile lymphocytes. There is a network of epithelial cells throughout the lobules which plays a role in the differentiation process from bone marrow-derived prethymic cells to mature T lymphocytes.

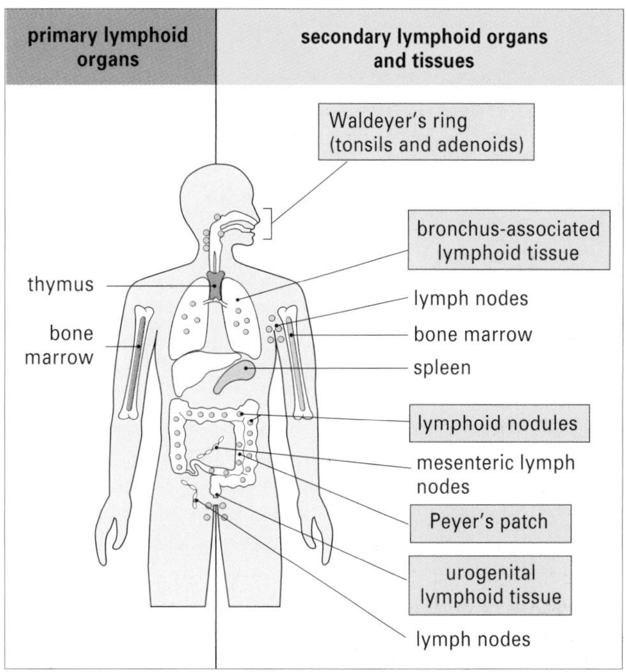

Fig. 2.36 Thymus and bone marrow are primary lymphoid organs. They are sites of maturation for T and B cells respectively. Cellular and humoral immune responses occur in the secondary (peripheral) lymphoid organs and tissues. Secondary lymphoid organs can be classified according to the body regions which they defend. The spleen responds predominantly to blood-borne antigens. Lymph nodes mount immune responses to antigens circulating in the lymph, entering through the skin (subcutaneous lymph nodes) or through mucosal surfaces (visceral lymph nodes). Tonsils, Peyer's patches and other mucosa-associated lymphoid tissues (blue boxes) react to antigens which have entered via the surface mucosal barriers. Note that the bone marrow is both a primary and a secondary lymphoid organ.

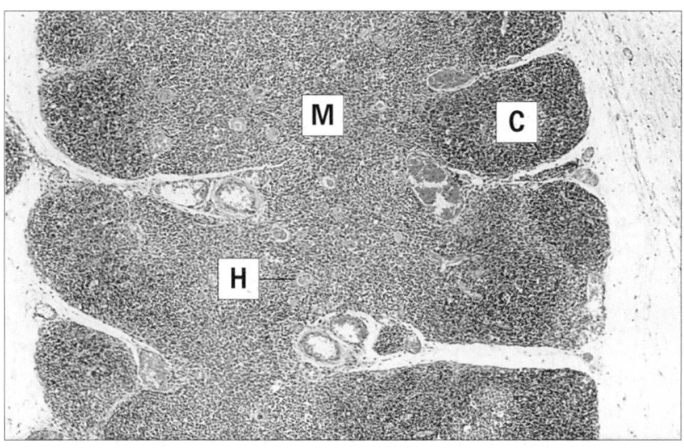

Fig. 2.37 Thymus section showing the lobular organization. This section shows the two main areas of the thymus lobule – an outer cortex of immature cells (C) and an inner medulla of more mature cells (M). Hassall's corpuscles (H) are found in the medulla. H&E stain. ×25. (Courtesy of Dr A. Stevens and Professor J. Lowe.)

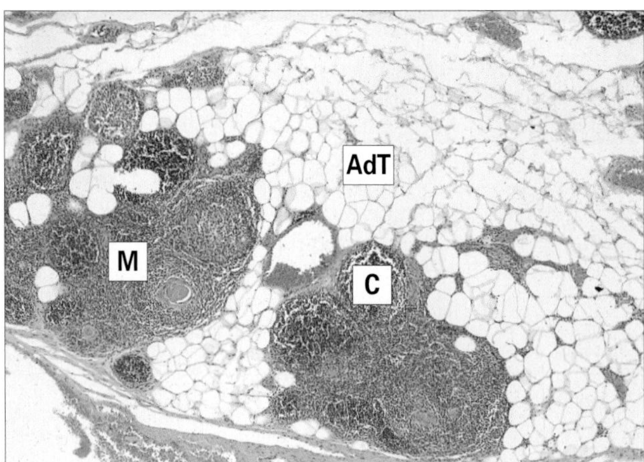

Fig. 2.38 Atrophic adult thymus. There is an involution of the thymus with replacement by adipose tissue (AdT). The cortex (C) is largely reduced and the less cellular medulla (M) is still apparent. (Courtesy of Dr A. Stevens and Professor J. Lowe.)

Three types of epithelial cells are present in the thymic lobules

At least three types of epithelial cells can be distinguished in the thymic lobules according to distribution, structure, function and phenotype. The epithelial nurse cells are in the outer cortex, the cortical epithelial cells form an epithelial network, and the medullary epithelial cells are mostly organized into clusters. In addition, interdigitating dendritic cells (IDC) and macrophages (both derived from bone marrow) are found in thymic lobules, particularly at the corticomedullary junction. Epithelial cells, IDCs and macrophages express MHC molecules which are crucial to T-cell development and selection.

Hassall's corpuscles are found in the thymic medulla. Their function is unknown, but they appear to contain degenerating epithelial cells rich in high molecular weight cytokeratins.

The mammalian thymus involutes with age (*Fig. 2.38*). In man, atrophy begins at puberty and continues throughout life. Thymic involution begins within the cortex and this region may disappear completely, whereas medullary remnants persist. Cortical atrophy is related to corticosteroid sensitivity of the cortical thymocytes. Thus, all conditions associated with acute increase in steroids, for example pregnancy and stress, promote thymic atrophy. However, it is conceivable that T-cell generation within the thymus continues into adult life, albeit at a low rate.

Stem-cell immigration initiates T-cell development

The thymus develops from the third (and in some species also from the fourth) pharyngeal pouch, as an epithelial rudiment which becomes seeded with blood-borne stem cells. Relatively few stem cells appear to be needed to give rise to the enormous repertoire of mature T cells with diverse antigen receptor specificities. At least in the mouse, two layers of embryonic tissue are involved in the formation of the thymic anlage: the ectoderm of the third branchial cleft that forms the epithelium of the thymic cortex, and the endoderm of the third pharyngeal pouch that differentiates into the epithelium of the thymic medulla.

From experimental studies, migration of stem cells into the thymus is not a random process but results from chemotactic signals periodically emitted from the thymic rudiment. β_2-microglobulin, a component of the MHC class I molecule, is one such putative chemoattractant. In birds, stem cells enter the thymus in two or possibly three waves but it is not clear that there are such waves in mammals. Once in the thymus, the stem cells begin to differentiate into thymic lymphocytes (called thymocytes), under the influence of the epithelial microenvironment. Whether or not the stem cells are 'pre-T cells', i.e. are committed to becoming T cells before they arrive in the thymus, is controversial. Although the stem cells express CD7, substantial evidence exists that they are in fact multipotent. Granulocytes, APCs, NK cells, B cells and myeloid cells have all been generated, *in vitro*, from haemopoietic precursors isolated from the thymus. This means that the prethymic bone marrow-derived cell entering the thymic rudiment is multipotent. Epithelial cells, macrophages and bone marrow-derived IDCs, rich in MHC class II antigens, are important in the differentiation of T lymphocytes from this multipotent stem cell. For example, specialized epithelial cells in the peripheral areas of the cortex (thymic 'nurse' cells) contain thymocytes within pockets in their cytoplasm. These cells support lymphocyte proliferation by producing a cytokine termed IL-7. The subcapsular region of the thymus is the first to be colonized by stem cells arriving from the bone marrow. These cells develop into large, actively proliferating, self-renewing lymphoblasts which generate the thymocyte population.

There are many more developing lymphocytes (85–90%) in the thymic cortex than in the medulla. Moreover, studies of function and cell surface markers have indicated that cortical thymocytes are less mature than medullary thymocytes. This reflects the fact that cortical cells migrate to, and mature in, the medulla. Most mature T cells leave the thymus via postcapillary venules located at the corticomedullary junction. However, other routes of exit may exist, including lymphatic vessels.

T cells change their phenotype during maturation

As with the development of granulocytes and monocytes, 'differentiation' markers of functional significance appear or are lost during the progression from stem cell to mature T cell. Analyses of genes encoding $\alpha\beta$ and $\gamma\delta$ T-cell receptors, and other studies examining changes in surface membrane antigens, suggest that there are at least two pathways of T-cell differentiation in the thymus. It is not known whether these pathways are distinct, but it seems more likely that they diverge from a common pathway. As mentioned earlier, only a small proportion, less than 1%, of mature thymic lymphocytes express the $\gamma\delta$ TCR. Most thymocytes differentiate into $\alpha\beta$ TCR cells, which account for the majority (>95%) of T lymphocytes found in the secondary lymphoid tissues and in the circulation. Phenotypic analyses have shown sequential changes in surface membrane antigens during T-cell maturation (*Fig. 2.39*). The phenotypic variations can be simplified into a three-stage model.

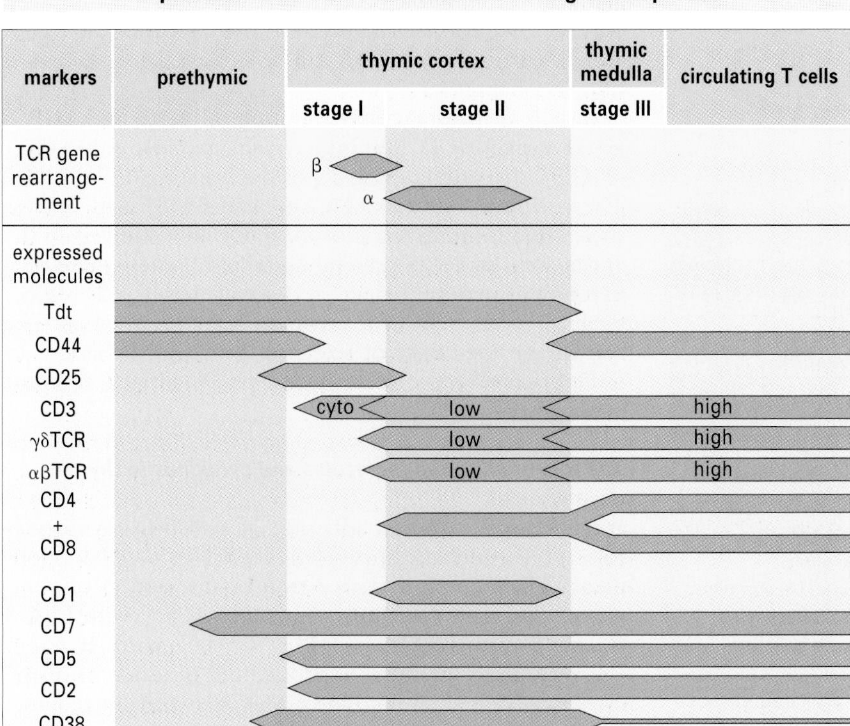

Fig. 2.39 Terminal deoxynucleotidyl transferase (Tdt) is an enzyme which is present in thymic stem cells, decreases in stage II and is lost altogether in the medulla. Several surface glycoproteins appear during differentiation. CD1 is present on stage II cortical thymocytes and is lost in the medulla. CD2 and CD7 (the pan-T marker) appear very early in differentiation and are maintained through to the mature T-cell stage. CD5 appears at an early stage and persists on mature T cells. CD3 is expressed first in the cytoplasm in stage I cells (cyto), and then on the surface simultaneously with the TCR. In most stage II cells, both surface CD3 and the αβ TCR are expressed at low density, but are present at high density on stage III cells. CD4 and CD8 are co-expressed on stage II cells (double positives). One of these molecules is lost during differentiation into mature stage III cells (single positives).

Stage I (early) thymocytes – There are two phases of stage I. In the first phase, the cells express CD44, CD25 and are $CD4^-$, $CD8^-$ (i.e. double negative cells), and the TCR genes are in the germ-line configuration. In this phase the cells are capable of giving rise to other lineages (see above). In the second phase they become $CD44^-$, are $CD25^+$ but still remain double negative for CD4 and CD8, and re-arrange the β chain of the TCR. They express cytoplasmic but not surface TCR-associated CD3 and are now committed to become T cells. They continue to express CD7 together with CD2 and CD5. Proliferation markers such as the transferrin receptor (CD71) and CD38 (a marker common to all early haemopoietic precursors) are also expressed at this stage. Note that none of the proliferation markers are T lineage-specific.

Stage II (intermediate or common) thymocytes – These account for around 80% of lymphoid cells in the fully developed thymus. They are characteristically $CD1^+$, $CD44^-$, $CD25^-$ but become $CD4^+$, $CD8^+$ (double positives). Genes encoding the TCR α chain are rearranged in these intermediate thymocytes; both chains of the αβ receptor are expressed at low density on the cell surface in association with polypeptides of the $CD3^-$ antigen receptor complex.

Stage III (mature) thymocytes – These show major phenotypic changes, namely loss of CD1, cell surface CD3 associated with the high density αβ TCR, and the distinction of two subsets of cells expressing either CD4 or CD8 (i.e single positives). The majority of thymocytes at this stage lack CD38 and the transferrin receptor, and they are virtually indistinguishable from mature, circulating T cells. All these cells express the receptor CD44, thought to be involved in migration and homing to peripheral lymphoid tissues. L-selectin (CD62L) is also expressed at this time.

T-cell receptor diversity is generated in the thymus

T cells have to recognize a wide variety of different antigens. The genes of the αβ and γδ TCR undergo somatic recombination during thymic development to produce functional genes for the different T-cell receptors (see Chapter 5). This takes place within the subcapsular and outer cortex of the thymus, where there is active cell proliferation. Through a random assortment of different gene segments, a large number of different T-cell receptors are made, but thymocytes that fail to make a functional receptor die. The T-cell receptors associate with peptides of the CD3 complex, which transduces activating signals to the cell.

'Alternative' forms of the TCR during development

From studies in transgenic mice, it has been shown that early in ontogeny, T cells can express alternative forms of the TCR complex which may be involved in generating signals that drive development. TCRβ dimers associate with CD3 in the absence of TCRα; TCRβ chains can be found on the cell surface as PI-linked proteins that do not associate with CD3; surface TCRβ chains can be associated with an incomplete CD3 complex. Finally, a 33-kD glycoprotein linked to TCRβ chains in pre-T cells acts as a 'surrogate' chain (pre-Tα chain). These receptors, like the surrogate pre-B-cell receptors (see *Fig. 8.2*), are probably

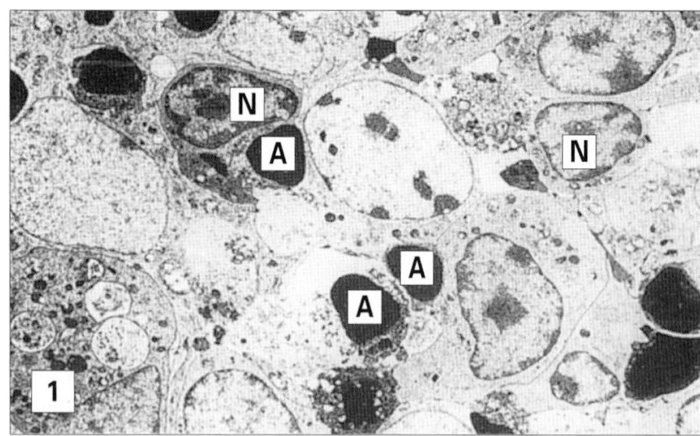

Fig. 2.40 Thymic cell apoptosis. (**1**) Fetal thymic lobes in culture were treated with anti-CD3 antibodies – this simulates activation via the TCR and therefore triggers programmed cell death (apoptosis). This electron micrograph shows the heavy condensation of nuclear chromatin in apoptotic nuclei (A) compared with the dispersed chromatin of normal cells (N). (Courtesy of Dr C. Smith.) (**2**) Analysis of the DNA from apoptotic cells by agarose gel electrophoresis shows the characteristically ordered, ladder-like pattern created by bands of digested DNA fragments.

involved in proliferation, maturation and selection during the early phases of lymphocyte development.

Positive and negative selection of developing T cells occurs in the thymus

Positive selection – T cells recognize antigenic peptides only when presented by self-MHC molecules on APCs. In fact, T cells show 'dual recognition' of both the antigenic peptides and the polymorphic part of the MHC molecules. (CD4, found on a subset of T cells, also recognizes the class II molecule, but its non-polymorphic portion.) Positive selection (also called thymic education) ensures that only those TCRs with a moderate affinity for self MHC are allowed to develop further. There is evidence that positive selection is mediated by thymic epithelial cells, acting as APCs. T cells displaying very high or very low receptor affinities for self MHC undergo apoptosis and die in the cortex. Apoptosis is a pre-programmed 'suicide', achieved by activating endogenous nucleases that cause DNA fragmentation (*Fig. 2.40*). T cells with receptors with intermediate affinities are rescued from apoptosis, survive, and continue along their pathway of maturation.

Negative selection – Some of the positively selected T cells may have receptors that recognize self components other than self MHC. These cells are deleted by a 'negative selection' process, which occurs in the deeper cortex, at the corticomedullary junction and in the medulla. Thymocytes interact with antigen, interdigitating cells and macrophages. Only thymocytes that fail to recognize self antigen are allowed to proceed in their development. The rest undergo apoptosis and are destroyed. These, and all the other apoptotic cells generated in the thymus, are phagocytosed by (tingible body) macrophages in the deep cortex. The processes involved in the education of T cells are shown in *Figure 2.41* and self tolerance is discussed fully in Chapter 12.

T cells at this stage of maturation ($CD4^+$ $CD8^+$ TCR^{lo}) go on to express TCR at high density and lose either CD4 or CD8, becoming 'single positive' mature thymocytes. These separate subsets of $CD4^+$ and $CD8^+$ cells possess specialized homing receptors (e.g. CD44), and exit to the T-cell areas of the peripheral lymphoid tissues where they function as mature 'helper' and 'cytotoxic' T cells respectively. Less than 5% of thymocytes leave the thymus. The rest die as the result of selection processes or failure to undergo productive rearrangements of antigen receptor genes.

The role of adhesion molecules and cytokines in thymic development

It has been shown that adhesion of maturing thymocytes to epithelial and accessory cells is crucial for T-cell development. This adhesion is mediated by interaction of complementary adhesion molecules, such as CD2 with LFA-3 (CD58), and LFA-1 (CD11a, CD18) with ICAM-1 (CD54). Such interactions induce the production of the cytokines IL-1, IL-3, IL-6 and GM–CSF, which are required for T-cell maturation in the thymus. Early thymocytes also express receptors for IL-2. This cytokine, together with IL-7, promotes cell proliferation which mainly occurs in the subcapsular and outer cortex.

Negative selection may also occur in the periphery

Not all self-reactive T cells are eliminated during intrathymic development. This probably occurs because not all self antigens are able to be presented in the thymic tissues. The thymic epithelial barrier that surrounds blood vessels may also limit access to some circulating antigens. Given the survival of some self-reacting T cells, a separate mechanism is required to prevent them attacking the body. Recent experiments with transgenic mice have suggested that peripheral inactivation of self-reactive T cells (peripheral tolerance) could occur via two mechanisms:

- Downregulation of TCR and CD8 (in cytotoxic cells), so that the cells are unable to interact with target autoantigens.
- Anergy, due to the lack of crucial secondary activation signals provided by the target cells, followed by induction of apoptosis after interaction with autoantigen

Peripheral tolerance is discussed in more detail in Chapter 12.

Extrathymic T-cell development

Although the vast majority of T cells require a functioning thymus for their differentiation, small numbers of cells (often oligoclonal in nature) carrying T-cell markers have been found in athymic ('nude') mice. The possibility that these mice possess thymic remnants cannot be ruled out. However, there is accumulating evidence to suggest that bone marrow precursors can home to mucosal epithelia and mature to form functional T cells with $\gamma\delta$ TCRs, and probably also T cells with $\alpha\beta$ TCRs, without the need for a thymus. The importance of extrathymic development in

T-cell differentiation within the thymus

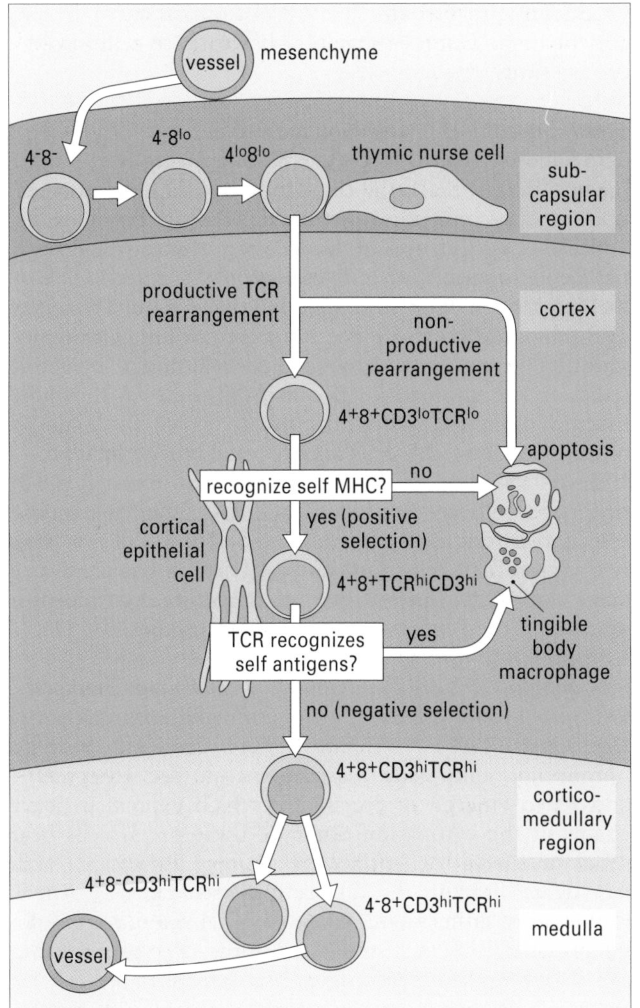

Fig. 2.41 In this model, pre-thymic T cells are attracted to and enter the thymic rudiment. They proliferate below the subcapsular region as large lymphoblasts, which replicate and give rise to a pool of cells entering the differentiation pathway. Many of these cells are associated with epithelial thymic nurse cells, although the significance of this interaction is still debated. Cells in this region first acquire CD8 and then CD4 at low density. They also rearrange their TCR genes and may express the products of these genes at low density on the cell surface. Maturing cells move deeper into the cortex and adhere to cortical epithelial cells. These epithelial cells are elongated and branched, and thus provide a large surface area for contact with thymocytes. The TCRs on the thymocytes are exposed to epithelial MHC molecules through these contacts. This leads to positive selection. Those cells which are not selected undergo apoptosis and are phagocytosed by macrophages. There is an increased expression of CD3, TCR, CD4 and CD8 during thymocyte migration from the subcapsular region to the deeper cortex. Those TCRs with self reactivity are now deleted through contact with autoantigens presented by interdigitating cells and macrophages at the corticomedullary junction – a process called negative selection. Medullary epithelial cells might also contribute to this process. Following this stage, cells expressing either CD4 or CD8 appear and exit to the periphery via specialized vessels at the corticomedullary junction. (A process of negative selection may also occur in the cortex, leading to the elimination of those cells with TCRs having high affinity for self MHC.)

animals that are euthymic (i.e. that have a normal thymus) is at present unclear.

T cells in the neonate are immature

Most T cells in neonatal blood are CD45RA$^+$, an observation that is consistent with the idea that they have not yet encountered their antigen. Furthermore, exposure of neonatal T cells to a variety of antigens results in the production of less IFNγ (and probably other cytokines) than adult T cells.

Mammalian B cells develop in the bone marrow and fetal liver

Mammals do not have a specific discrete organ for B-cell lymphopoiesis. Instead, these cells develop directly from lymphoid stem cells in the haemopoietic tissue of the fetal liver (*Fig. 2.42*), from 8 to 9 weeks of gestation in humans, and by about 14 days in the mouse. Later, the site of B-cell production moves from the liver to the bone marrow, where it continues through adult life. This is also true of the other haemopoietic lineages, giving rise to erythrocytes,

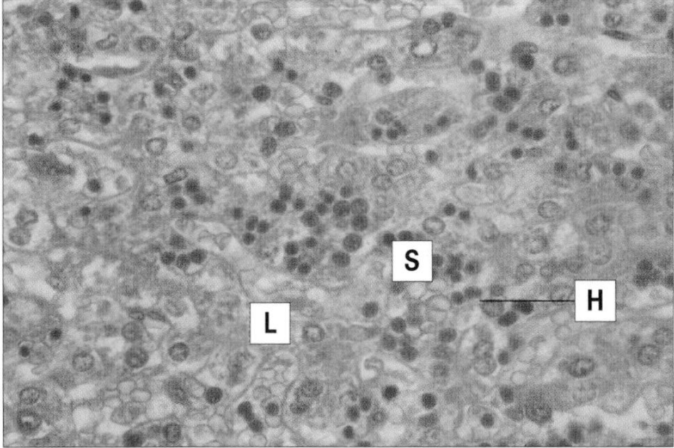

Fig. 2.42 Haemopoiesis in fetal liver. Section of human fetal liver showing islands of haemopoiesis (H). Haemopoietic stem cells are found in the sinusoidal spaces (S) between plates of liver cells (L). (Courtesy of Dr A. Stevens and Professor J. Lowe.)

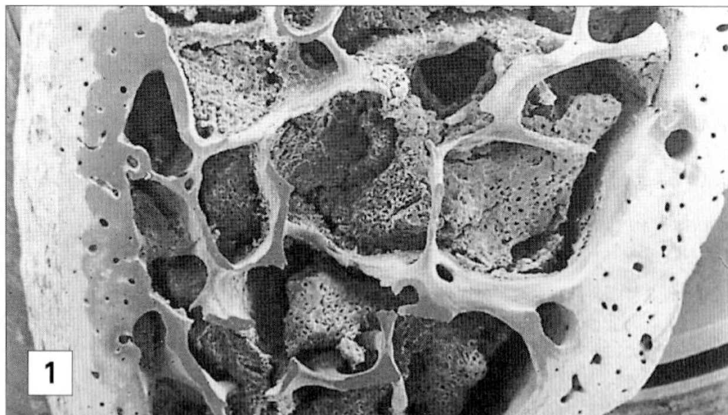

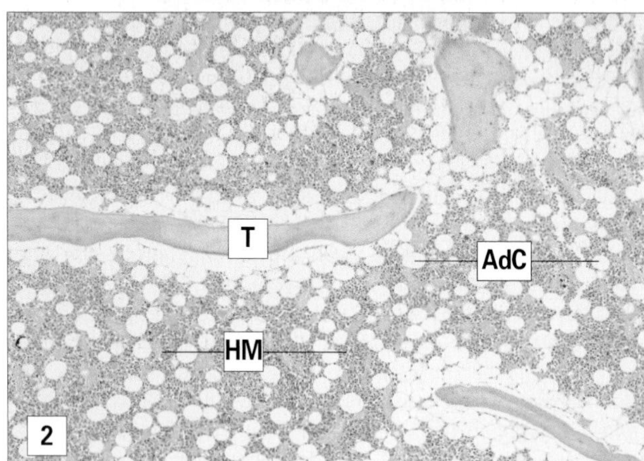

Fig. 2.43 Bone marrow. (**1**) Low-power scanning electron micrograph showing the architecture of bone and its relationship to bone marrow. Within the cavities of spongy bone between the bony trabeculae, B-cell lymphopoiesis takes place, with maturation occurring in a radial direction towards the centre (from the endosteum to the central venous sinus). (**2**) The biopsy below shows haemopoietic bone marrow (HM) in the spaces between the bony trabeculae (T). Some of the space is also occupied by adipocytes (AdC). (Courtesy of A. Stevens and J. Lowe.)

granulocytes, monocytes and platelets. Recent data have shown that B-cell progenitors are also present in the omental tissue of murine and human fetuses. Whether or not these B-cell progenitors precede those in the fetal liver remains to be established.

B-cell production in the bone marrow does not occur in distinct domains

B-cell progenitors in the bone marrow are seen adjacent to the endosteum of the bone lamellae. Each B-cell progenitor, at the stage of immunoglobulin gene rearrangement, may produce up to 64 progeny. These migrate towards the centre of each cavity of the spongy bone and reach the lumen of a venous sinusoid. In the bone marrow, B cells mature in close association with stromal reticular cells. The latter are found both adjacent to the endosteum and in close association with the central sinus, where they are termed adventitial reticular cells (*Fig. 2.43*). Reticular cells have mixed phenotypic features with some similarities to fibroblasts, endothelial cells and myofibroblasts. They produce type IV collagen, laminin and the smooth-muscle form of actin. Experiments *in vitro* have shown that reticular cells sustain B-cell differentiation, possibly by producing the cytokine IL-7. Adventitial reticular cells may be important for the release of mature B cells into the central sinus.

B cells are subject to selection processes

The majority of B cells (over 75%) maturing in the bone marrow do not reach the circulation but (like thymocytes) undergo a process of programmed cell death or apoptosis, and are phagocytosed by bone marrow macrophages. It has been suggested that B-cell–stromal interactions may mediate a form of positive selection that rescues a minority of B cells with productive rearrangements of their immunoglobulin genes from programmed cell death. Negative selection of autoreactive B cells may occur in the bone marrow or in the spleen, the site to which the majority of newly produced B cells are exported during fetal life.

From kinetic data, it is estimated that about 5×10^7 murine B cells are produced each day. Since the mouse spleen contains approximately 7.5×10^7 B cells, a large proportion of B cells must die, probably at the pre-B-cell stage due to non-productive rearrangements of receptor genes or if they express self-reactive antibodies.

Immunoglobulins are the definitive B-cell lineage markers

Lymphoid stem cells expressing terminal deoxynucleotidyl transferase (TdT) proliferate, differentiate and undergo immunoglobulin gene rearrangements (see Chapters 4 and 8) to emerge as pre-B cells which express μ heavy chains in the cytoplasm. Some of these pre-B cells bear small numbers of surface μ chains, associated with 'surrogate' light chains $V_{\text{pre B}}$ and γ5 (see *Fig. 8.2*). Allelic exclusion of either maternal or paternal immunoglobulin genes has already occurred by this time. The proliferating pre-B cells are thought to give rise to smaller pre-B cells. Once a B cell has synthesized light chains, which may be either κ- or λ-type, it becomes committed to the antigen-binding specificity of its sIgM antigen receptor. Thus, one B cell can make only one specific antibody, a central tenet of the clonal selection theory for antibody production. Surface immunoglobulin-associated molecules Igα and Igβ (CD79a and b) are present by the pre-B-cell stage of development.

Developing B cells acquire characteristic surface molecules

A sequence of immunoglobulin gene rearrangements and phenotypic changes takes place during B-cell ontogeny, similar to that described above for T cells. Heavy chain gene rearrangements occur in B-cell progenitors and represent the earliest indication of B-lineage commitment. This is followed by light chain gene rearrangements which occur at later pre-B-cell stages. The development of B cells and the expression of surface markers and cytokine receptors is discussed in Chapter 8.

B cells migrate and function in the secondary lymphoid tissues

Early B-cell immigrants into fetal lymph nodes (17 weeks in man) are $sIgM^+$ and are B-1 cells. $CD5^+$ B-cell precursors are found in the fetal omentum. $CD5^+$ B cells are also found in the mantle zone of secondary follicles in adult lymph nodes (*Fig. 2.53*).

Following antigenic stimulation, mature B cells can develop into memory cells or antibody-forming cells (AFCs). Surface immunoglobulins (sIg) are usually lost in plasma cells (the terminally differentiated form of an AFC), since their function as a receptor is no longer required. Like any other terminally differentiated haemopoietic cell, the plasma cell has a limited lifespan, and eventually undergoes apoptosis.

Secondary lymphoid organs and tissues

The generation of lymphocytes in primary lymphoid organs is followed by their migration into peripheral secondary tissues. The secondary lymphoid tissues comprise well-organized encapsulated organs, the spleen and lymph nodes (systemic organs) and non-encapsulated accumulations of lymphoid tissue. Lymphoid tissue that is found in association with mucosal surfaces is called the mucosa-associated lymphoid tissue (MALT). Systemic organs and the mucosal system have different functions in immunity. The spleen is responsive to blood-borne antigens and patients who have had their spleens removed are much more susceptible to pathogens that reach the blood stream. The lymph nodes protect the body from antigens that come from skin or from internal surfaces and are transported via the lymphatic vessels. Responses to antigens encountered via these routes result in secretion of antibodies into the circulation and in local cell-mediated responses. By contrast, the mucosal system protects mucosal surfaces. It is the site of first encounter (priming) of immune cells with antigens entering via mucosal surfaces. Thus, lymphoid tissues are associated with surfaces lining the intestinal tract (gut-associated lymphoid tissues, or GALT), the respiratory tract (bronchus-associated lymphoid tissue, or BALT) and the genitourinary tract. The major effector mechanism at mucosal surfaces is secretory IgA antibody (sIgA), actively transported via the mucosal epithelial cells to the lumen of the tracts. It is perhaps not surprising that the bulk of the body's lymphoid tissues (>50%) is found associated with the mucosal system, especially the GALT, since this is a major pathway of entry for external antigens. Likewise, IgA is the most abundant immunoglobulin in the body.

The systemic immune system: the spleen

The spleen lies at the upper left quadrant of the abdomen, behind the stomach and close to the diaphragm. The adult spleen is around 13 × 8 cm in size and weighs about 180–250 g. Its outer layer consists of a capsule of collagenous bundles of fibres which enter the parenchyma of the organ as short trabeculae. These, together with a reticular framework, support two main types of splenic tissue – the white pulp and the red pulp (*Fig. 2.44*).

The white pulp – The white pulp consists of lymphoid tissue, the bulk of which is arranged around a central arteriole to form the periarteriolar lymphoid sheaths (PALS; *Fig. 2.45*). PALS are composed of T- and B-cell areas. The T cells are found around the central arteriole; the B cells may be organized into either primary 'unstimulated' follicles (aggregates of virgin B cells), or secondary 'stimulated' follicles (which possess a germinal centre with memory cells). The germinal centres also contain follicular dendritic cells and phagocytic macrophages. Specialized macrophages and a subset of B cells, which respond to type II thymus-independent antigens, i.e. polysaccharides (see Chapter 8), are found in the marginal zone, the area overlying the mantle of secondary follicles. Macrophages and the follicular dendritic cells (FDCs) present antigen to B cells in the spleen. B cells and other lymphocytes are free to leave and enter the PALS via capillary branches of the central arterioles that enter the marginal zone.

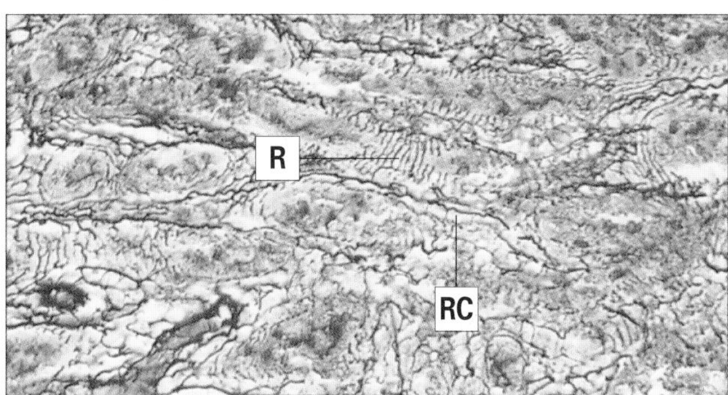

Fig. 2.44 Spleen. Spleen section showing the reticular framework of the red pulp. This section is stained for reticulin and shows the ring fibres (R) that support the endothelial cells of the venous sinuses. These blood vessels lack a continuous basement membrane and holes in the endothelial layer allow free flow of plasma into their lumen, and selective passage of cells from the red pulp cords (RC). ×125.

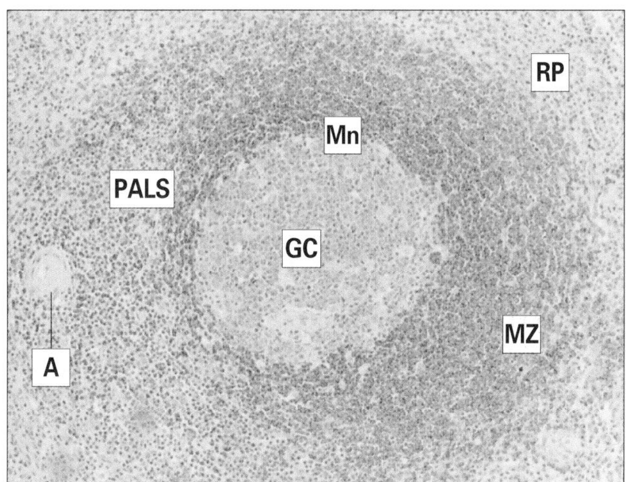

Fig. 2.45 White pulp of spleen. Spleen section showing a white pulp lymphoid aggregate. A secondary lymphoid follicle, with germinal centre (GC) and mantle (Mn), is surrounded by the marginal zone (MZ) and red pulp (RP). Adjacent to the follicle, an arteriole (A) is surrounded by the periarteriolar lymphoid sheath (PALS) consisting mainly of T cells. Note that the marginal zone is only present at one side of the secondary follicle. (Courtesy of Professor I. Maclennan.)

Schematic organization of lymphoid tissue in the spleen

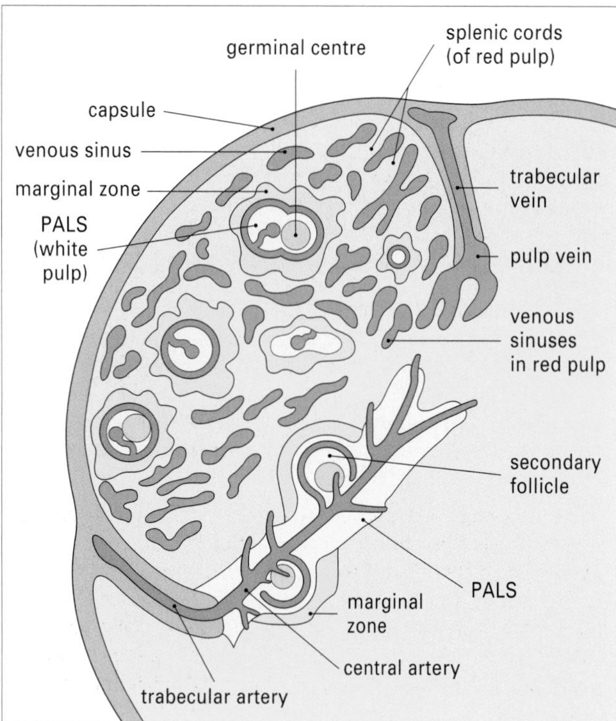

Fig. 2.46 The white pulp is composed of periarteriolar lymphoid sheaths (PALS), frequently containing lymphoid follicles. The white pulp is surrounded by the marginal zone which contains numerous macrophages, APCs, slowly recirculating B cells and NK cells. The red pulp contains venous sinuses separated by splenic cords. Blood enters the tissue via the trabecular arteries which give rise to the many-branched central arteries. Some end in the white pulp, supplying the germinal centres and mantle zones of the follicle, but most empty into or near the marginal zones. Some arterial branches run directly into the red pulp, mainly terminating in the cords. The venous sinuses drain blood into the pulp veins, trabecular veins and then the splenic vein.

Some lymphocytes, especially maturing plasmablasts, can pass across the marginal zone via bridges into the red pulp (*Fig. 2.46*).

The red pulp – This tissue consists of venous sinuses and cellular cords containing resident macrophages, erythrocytes, platelets, granulocytes, lymphocytes and numerous plasma cells. Note that, in addition to immunological functions, the spleen serves as a reservoir for platelets, erythrocytes and granulocytes. Aged platelets and erythrocytes are destroyed in the spleen. This process is carried out in the red pulp and is referred to as 'haemocatheresis'. These functions are made possible by the vascular organization of the spleen (*Fig. 2.46*). Central arteries surrounded by PALS end with arterial capillaries which open freely into the red pulp cords. Thus, circulating cells reach these cords and become trapped. Aged platelets and erythrocytes are recognized and phagocytosed by macrophages. Blood cells that are not ingested and destroyed can re-enter the blood circulation by squeezing through holes in the discontinuous endothelial wall of the venous sinuses (*Fig. 2.47*), whereas plasma flows freely through them.

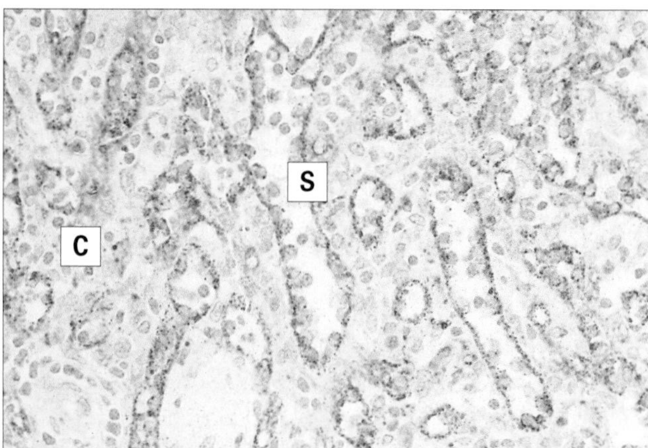

Fig. 2.47 Venous sinuses and cords of the red pulp. Macrophages, immunostained for cathepsin D, are associated with the sinus walls (S) and distributed throughout the splenic cords (C). (Courtesy of Dr A. Stevens and Professor J. Lowe.)

Lymph nodes and the lymphatic system

The lymph nodes form part of a network which filters antigens from the interstitial tissue fluid and lymph during its passage from the periphery to the thoracic duct and the other major collecting ducts (*Fig. 2.48*). Lymph nodes frequently occur at branches of the lymphatic vessels. Clusters of lymph nodes are strategically placed in areas such as the neck, axillae, groin, mediastinum and the abdominal cavity, which drain various superficial and deep regions of the body. Lymph nodes protect the skin (superficial, subcutaneous nodes) and mucosal surfaces of the respiratory, digestive and genitourinary tracts (visceral or deep nodes).

Human lymph nodes are 2–10 mm in diameter, are round or kidney shaped, and have an indentation called the hilus where blood vessels enter and leave the node. Lymph arrives at the lymph node via several afferent lymphatic vessels, and leaves the node through one efferent lymphatic vessel at the hilus. A typical lymph node is surrounded by a collagenous capsule (*Fig. 2.49*). Radial trabeculae, together with reticular fibres, support the various cellular components. The lymph node consists of a B-cell area (cortex), a T-cell area (paracortex) and a central medulla, consisting of cellular cords containing T cells, B cells, abundant plasma cells and macrophages (*Figs 2.50* and *2.51*).

The paracortex contains many APCs (interdigitating cells) which express high levels of MHC class II surface antigens. These are cells migrating from the skin (Langerhans' cells) or from mucosae (dendritic cells), which transport processed antigens into the lymph nodes from the external and internal surfaces of the body (*Fig. 2.52*). The bulk of the lymphoid tissue is found in the cortex and paracortex. The paracortex contains specialized postcapillary vessels – high endothelial venules (HEV) that allow traffic of lymphocytes out of the circulation into the lymph node (see 'Lymphocyte traffic' below and *Fig. 2.62*). The medulla is

The lymphatic system

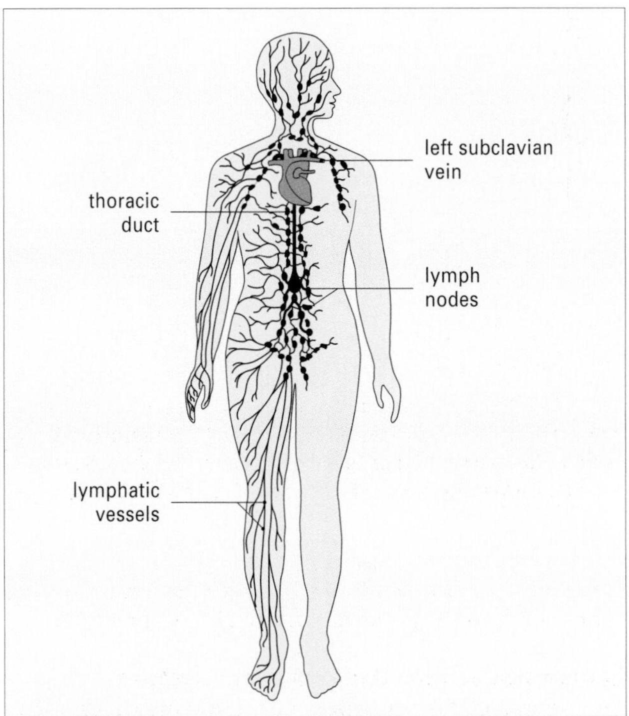

Fig. 2.48 Lymph nodes are found at junctions of lymphatic vessels and form a network, the latter draining and filtering interstitial fluid from the tissue spaces. They are either subcutaneous or visceral, the latter draining the deep tissues and internal organs of the body. The lymph eventually reaches the thoracic duct, which opens into the left subclavian vein and thus back into the circulation.

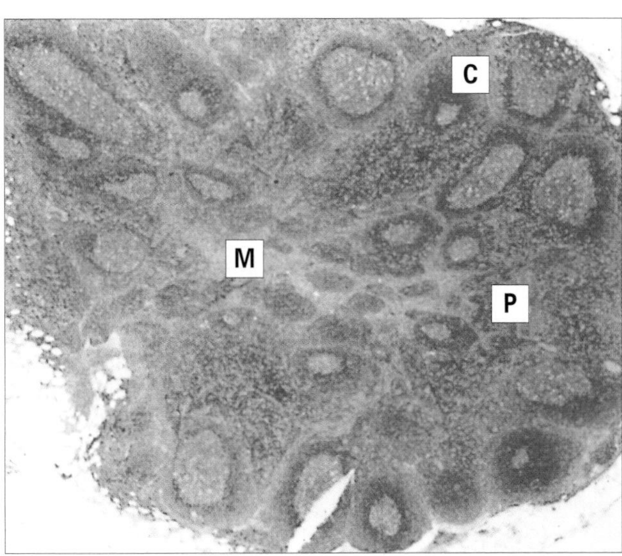

Fig. 2.49 Lymph node section. The lymph node is surrounded by a connective tissue capsule and is organized into three main areas: C, the cortex (B-cell area); P, the paracortex (T-cell area); M, the medulla, which contains cords of lymphoid tissue (T- and B-cell area rich in plasma cells and macrophages). H&E stain. ×10. (Adapted from Zucker-Franklin D *et al. Atlas of Blood Cells: Function and Pathology*. Vol II. 2nd edn. Philadelphia: Lea and Febiger, 1988.)

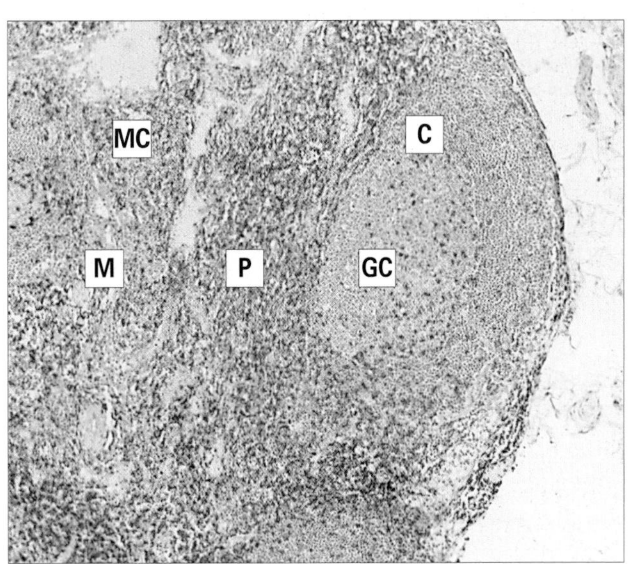

Fig. 2.50 Histological structure of the lymph node. Cortex (C), paracortex (P) and medulla (M) are shown. The section has been stained to show localization of T cells. They are most abundant in the paracortex, but a few are found in the germinal centre (GC) of the secondary lymphoid follicle, in the cortex and in the medullary cords (MC). (Courtesy of Dr A. Stevens and Professor J. Lowe.)

organized into cords separated by lymph (medullary) sinuses which drain into a terminal sinus, the origin of the efferent lymphatic vessel (*Fig. 2.51*). Scavenger phagocytic cells are arranged along the lymph sinuses, especially in the medulla. As the lymph passes across the nodes from the afferent to the efferent lymphatic vessels, particulate antigens are removed by the phagocytic cells and transported into the lymphoid tissue of the lymph node.

The cortex contains aggregates of B cells in the form of primary or secondary follicles, whilst T cells are mainly found in the paracortex. Thus, if an area of skin or mucosa is challenged by a T-dependent antigen, the lymph nodes draining that particular area show active T-cell proliferation in the paracortex. Further evidence for this localization of T cells comes from patients with congenital thymic aplasia (DiGeorge syndrome), who have fewer cells in the paracortex than normal. Similar features are found in neonatally thymectomized or congenitally athymic ('nude') mice or rats.

Germinal centres in secondary follicles are seen in antigen-stimulated lymph nodes. These are similar to the germinal centres seen in the B-cell areas of the splenic PALS and of MALT. Germinal centres are surrounded by a mantle of lymphocytes (*Fig. 2.53*). Mantle zone B cells (*Fig. 2.54*) co-express surface IgM, IgD and CD44. This is taken as evidence that they are virgin and actively recirculating B cells. In most secondary follicles, this thickened mantle or corona is oriented towards the capsule of the

Schematic structure of the lymph node

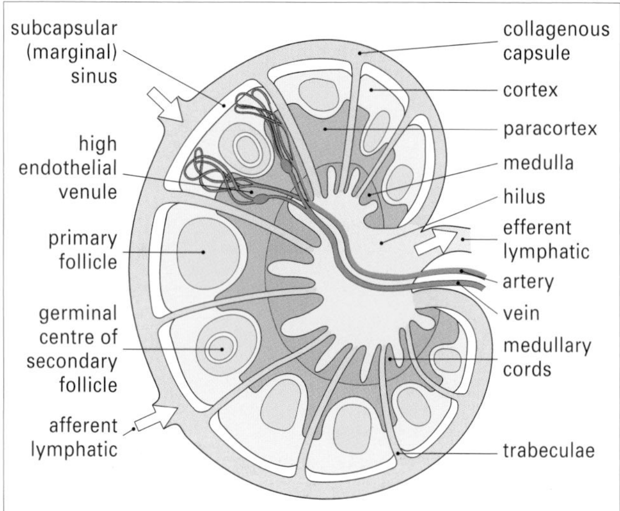

Fig. 2.51 Beneath the collagenous capsule is the subcapsular sinus, which is lined by endothelial and phagocytic cells. Lymphocytes and antigens from surrounding tissue spaces or adjacent nodes pass into the sinus via the afferent lymphatics. The cortex is mainly a B-cell area. B cells are organized into primary or, more commonly, secondary follicles – that is, with a germinal centre. The paracortex contains mainly T cells. Each lymph node has its own arterial and venous supply. Lymphocytes enter the node from the circulation through the highly specialized high endothelial venules (HEVs) in the paracortex. The medulla contains both T and B cells in addition to most of the lymph node plasma cells organized into cords of lymphoid tissue. Lymphocytes leave the node through the efferent lymphatic vessel.

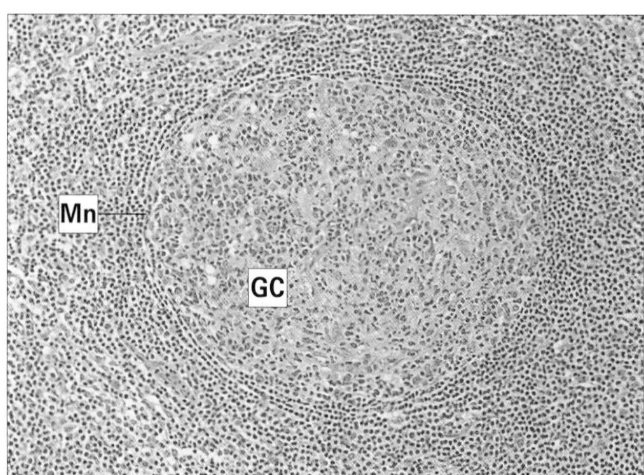

Fig. 2.53 Structure of the secondary follicle. A large germinal centre (GC) is surrounded by the mantle zone (Mn).

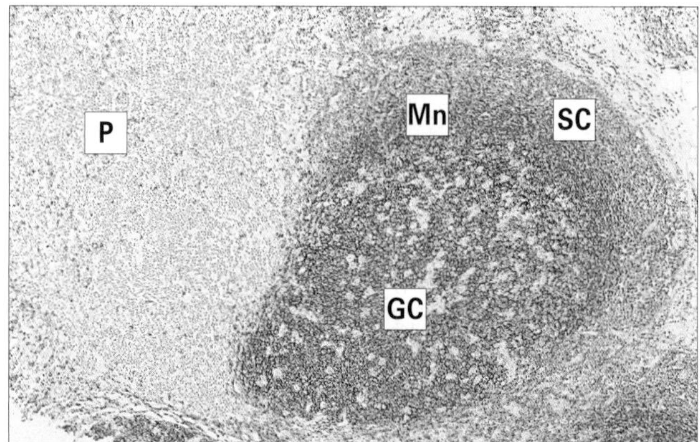

Fig. 2.54 Distribution of B cells in the lymph node cortex. Immunohistochemical staining of B cells for surface immunoglobulin shows that they are largely concentrated in the secondary follicle, germinal centre (GC), mantle zone (Mn) and between the capsule and the follicle – the subcapsular zone (SC). A few B cells are seen in the paracortex (P) which mainly contains T cells (see *Fig. 2.50*).

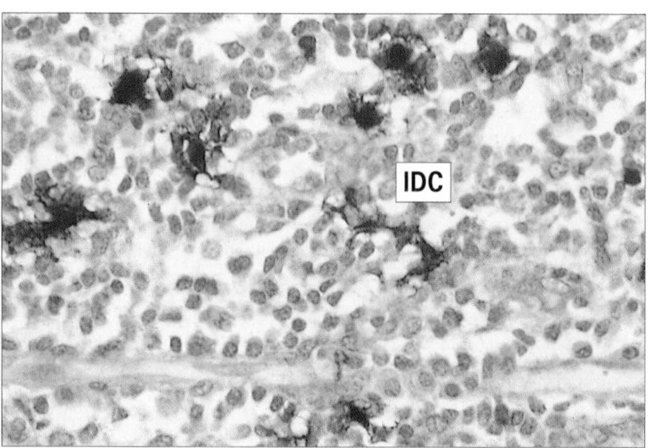

Fig. 2.52 Interdigitating cells in the lymph node paracortex. Interdigitating dendritic cells (IDC) form contacts with each other and paracortical T cells. (Courtesy of Dr A. Stevens and Professor J. Lowe.) (See also *Fig. 2.19*.)

node. Secondary follicles contain FDCs (*Fig. 2.55*), some macrophages (*Fig. 2.56*) and a few CD4$^+$ T cells which interact with the germinal centre dendritic cells. All these cells, together with specialized marginal sinus macrophages, appear to play a role in generating B-cell responses and, in particular, in the development of B-cell memory, which is the primary function of germinal centres.

Mucosa-associated lymphoid tissue (MALT)

Aggregates of non-encapsulated lymphoid tissue are found especially in the lamina propria and submucosal areas of the gastrointestinal, respiratory and genitourinary tracts (*Fig. 2.36*). The tonsils contain a considerable amount of lymphoid tissue, often with large secondary follicles and intervening T-cell zones with high endothelial venules. There are three main kinds of tonsils, palatine, pharyngeal (called adenoids when diseased) and lingual, which constitute the Waldeyer's ring. A section of a lingual tonsil is shown in *Figure 2.57*. Similar aggregates of lymphoid tissue are seen lining the bronchi and along the genitourinary tract. The digestive, respiratory and genitourinary

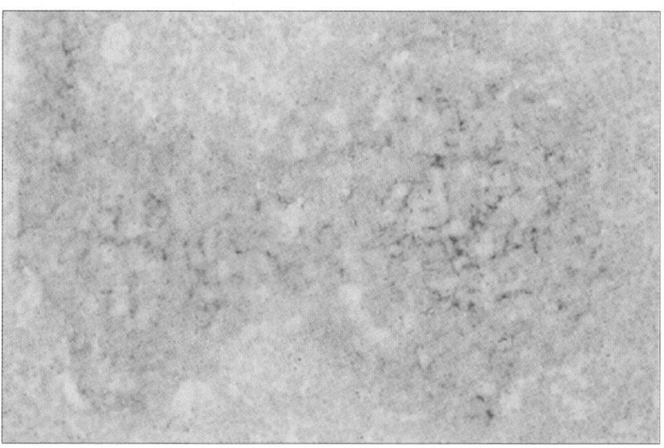

Fig. 2.55 Secondary lymphoid follicle. This lymph node follicle is stained with enzyme-labelled monoclonal antibody to demonstrate follicular dendritic cells.

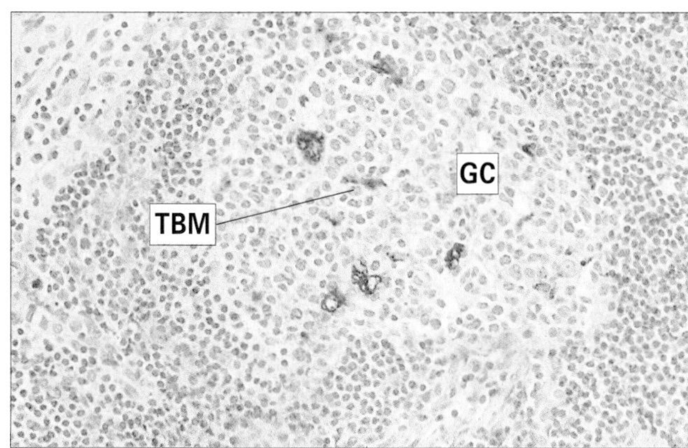

Fig. 2.56 Germinal centre macrophages. Immunostaining for cathepsin D shows several macrophages localized in the germinal centre (GC) of a secondary follicle. These cells, which phagocytose apoptotic B cells, are called tingible body macrophages (TBM). (Courtesy of Dr A. Stevens and Professor J. Lowe.)

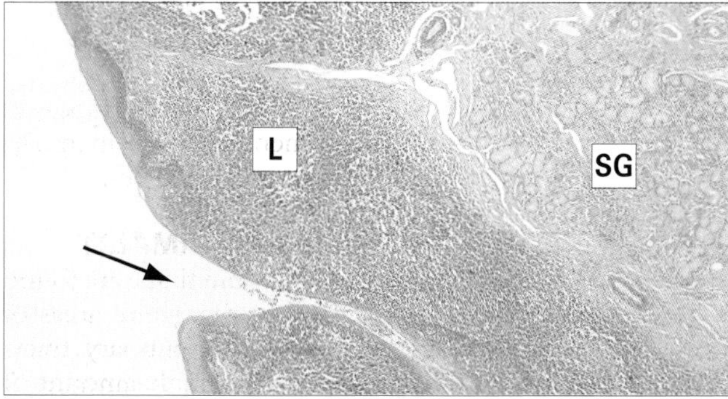

Fig. 2.57 Structure of the lingual tonsil. The lingual tonsil, situated in the posterior third of the tongue, consists of accumulations of lymphoid tissue (L) with large secondary follicles associated with a mucosa forming deep cleft-like invaginations (arrow). Mucous-containing salivary glands (SG) are seen around the tonsil. These are common features of all types of tonsil. (Courtesy of Dr A. Stevens and Professor J. Lowe.)

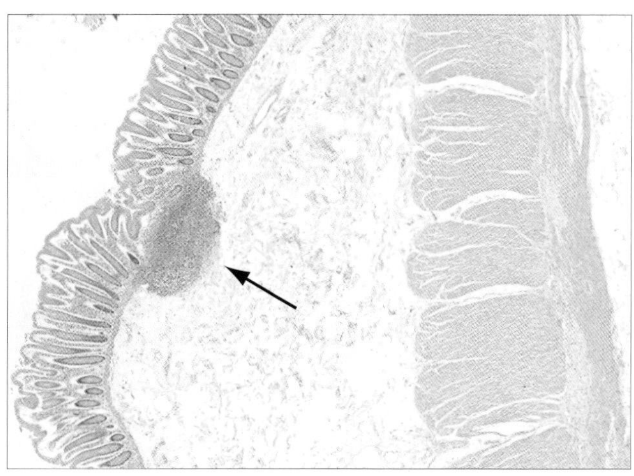

Fig. 2.58 A solitary lymphoid nodule in the large intestine. This nodule is localized in the mucosa and submucosa of the intestinal wall (arrow). (Courtesy of Dr A. Stevens and Professor J. Lowe.)

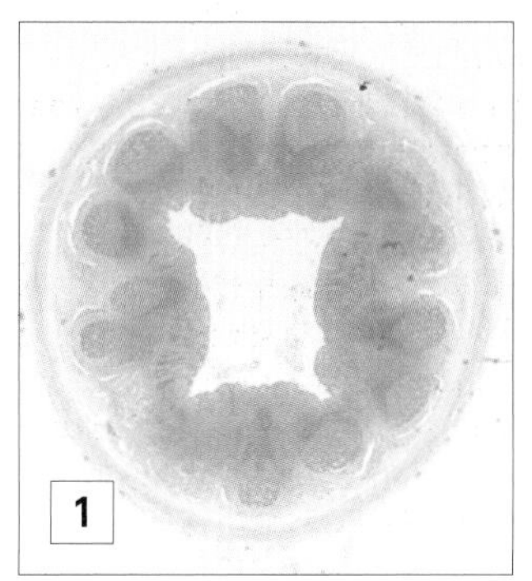

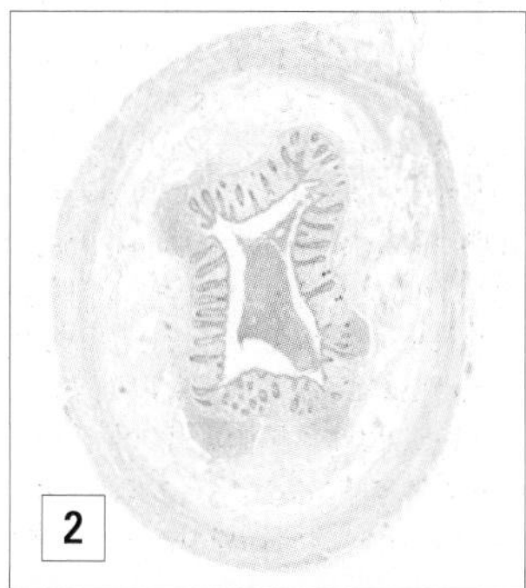

Fig. 2.59 Lymphoid nodules in the human appendix. (**1**) Appendix of a 10-year-old child, showing large lymphoid nodules extending into the submucosa. (**2**) Appendix from a 36-year-old man. Note the dramatic reduction of lymphoid tissue, with virtual disappearance of lymphoid follicles. This illustrates the atrophy of lymphoid tissues during ageing, which is not limited to the appendix. (Courtesy of Dr A. Stevens and Professor J. Lowe.)

mucosae contain dendritic cells for uptake, processing and transport of antigens to the draining lymph nodes. Lymphoid tissues seen in the lamina propria of the gastrointestinal wall often extend into the submucosa and are found either as solitary nodules (*Fig. 2.58*) or aggregated nodules such as in the appendix (*Fig. 2.59*). The Peyer's patches are found in the lower ileum. The intestinal epithelium (follicle associated epithelium – FAE) overlying the Peyer's patches is specialized to allow the transport of pathogens into the lymphoid tissue. This particular function is carried out by epithelial cells termed 'M' cells, scattered amongst enterocytes and so called because they have numerous microfolds on their luminal surface (*Fig. 2.60*). M cells contain deep invaginations of the basolateral plasma membrane which form pockets containing B and T lymphocytes, dendritic cells and macrophages (*Fig. 2.61*). Antigens and microorganisms are transcytosed

Structural organization of a Peyer's patch

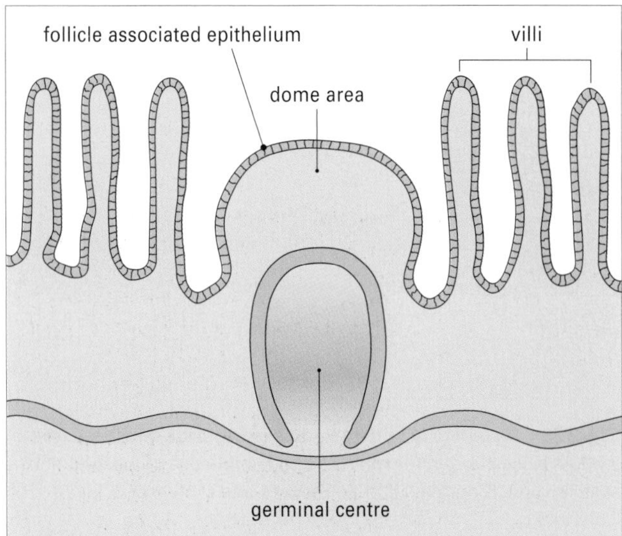

Fig. 2.60 The intestinal mucosa bulges in an area devoid of villi. The surface epithelium contains scattered M cells and is called follicle-associated epithelium (FAE). The deep region of the mucosa contains a cluster of secondary follicles with large germinal centres surrounded by T-cell-dependent interfollicular zones with interdigitating cells and high endothelial venules. The dome area is found between the FAE and the follicular area and contains mainly B cells, the majority of which are memory cells.

Location of M cells

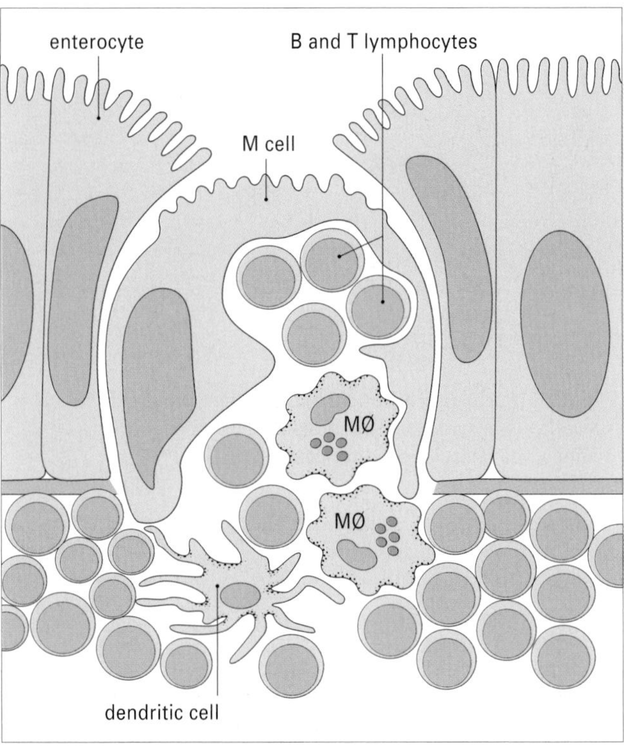

Fig. 2.61 The intestinal FAE contains M cells. Note the lymphocytes and occasional macrophages (MØ) in the intracellular pocket. Endocytosed antigens are passed via this pocket into the subepithelial tissues.

into the pocket and to the organized mucosal lymphoid tissue under the epithelium. M cells are not exclusive to Peyer's patches but are also found in epithelia associated with lymphoid cell accumulations at 'antigen sampling' areas in other mucosal sites.

Humoral immune responses at the mucosal level are mostly of the IgA isotype. Secretory IgA is an antibody that can traverse epithelial membranes and helps prevent entry of infectious microorganisms (see *Fig. 4.21*).

Mucosal lymphocytes

In addition to organized lymphoid tissue forming the MALT system, a large number of lymphocytes and plasma cells are found in the mucosa of the stomach, of the small and large intestine, of the upper and lower respiratory airways and of several other organs. Lymphocytes are found both in the connective tissue of the lamina propria and within the epithelial layer:

- Lamina propria lymphocytes (LPLs) are predominantly activated T cells, but numerous activated B cells and plasma cells are also detected. These plasma cells secrete mainly IgA, which is transported across the epithelial cells and released into the lumen.
- Intra-epithelial lymphocytes (IELs) are mostly T cells; but, the population is different from the LPLs, as it includes a high proportion of $\gamma\delta$ T cells (10–40%) and $CD8^+$ cells (70%).

Most LPL and IEL T cells belong to the CD45RO subset of memory cells. They respond poorly to stimulation with antibodies to CD3, but may be triggered via other activation pathways (e.g. via CD2 or CD28). The integrin αE chain HML-1 (CD103) is not present on resting circulating T cells but is expressed following phytohaemagglutinin (PHA) stimulation. Antibodies to this molecule are mitogenic and induce expression of the low affinity IL-2 receptor α chain (CD25) on peripheral blood T cells. αE is coupled with a β_7-chain to form an $\alpha E/\beta_7$ heterodimer, an integrin expressed by IELs and other activated leucocytes. IELs are known to release cytokines including IFNγ and IL-5. One function suggested for IELs is immune surveillance against mutated or virus-infected host cells.

LYMPHOCYTE TRAFFIC

The migration of lymphocytes from primary to secondary lymphoid tissues has already been described. Once in the secondary tissues the lymphocytes do not simply remain there; many move from one lymphoid organ to another via the blood and lymph (*Fig. 2.62*).

Lymphocytes leave the blood via high endothelial venules

Although some lymphocytes leave the blood through non-specialized venules, the main exit route in mammals is through a specialized section of the postcapillary venules known as the high endothelial venules or HEV (*Figs 2.63*

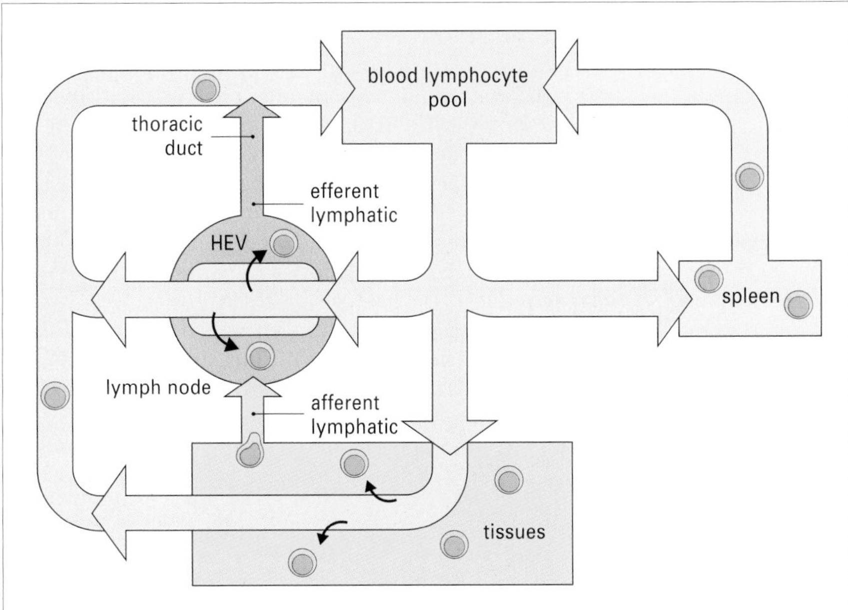

Fig. 2.62 The lymphocytes move through the circulation and enter the lymph nodes and MALT via the specialized endothelial cells of the postcapillary venules (HEVs). They leave through the efferent lymphatic vessels and pass through other nodes, finally entering the thoracic duct which empties into the circulation at the left subclavian vein (in humans). Lymphocytes enter the white pulp areas of the spleen in the marginal zones; they pass into the sinusoids of the red pulp and leave via the splenic vein.

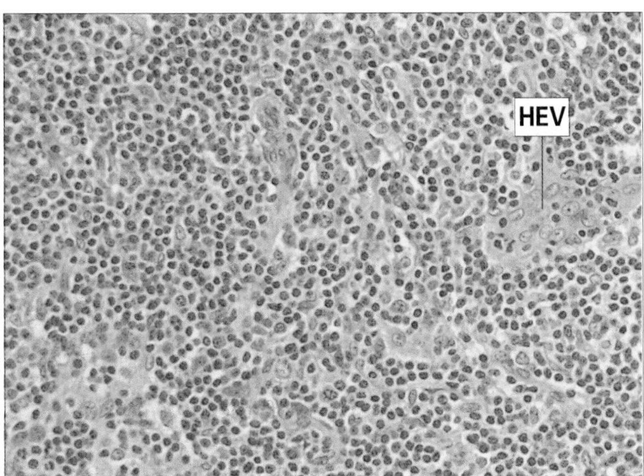

Fig. 2.63 Lymph node paracortex showing high endothelial venules (HEV). Lymphocytes leave the circulation through HEVs and enter the node. H&E. ×200. (Courtesy of Dr A. Stevens and Professor J. Lowe.)

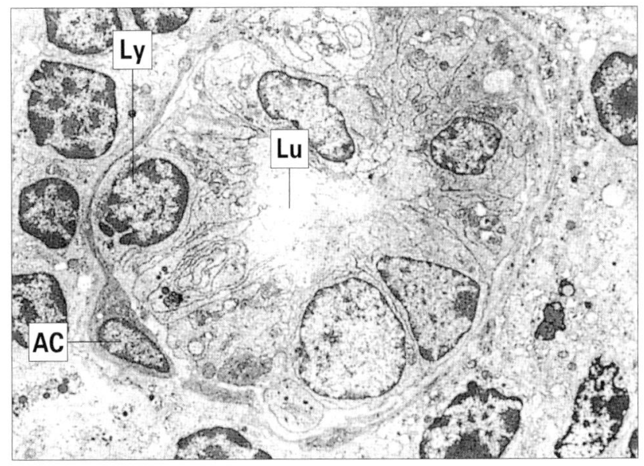

Fig. 2.64 Electron micrograph showing a high endothelial venule in the paracortex of a lymph node. A lymphocyte (Ly) in transit from the lumen (Lu) of the HEV can be seen close to the basal lamina. The HEV is partly surrounded by an adventitial cell (AC). ×1600.

and *2.64*). In the lymph nodes these are mainly in the paracortex with fewer in the cortex and none in the medulla. Some lymphocytes, primarily T cells, arrive from the drainage area of the node through the afferent lymphatics, not via HEV; this is the main route by which antigen enters the nodes. Besides the lymph nodes, HEV are found in MALT and in the thymus.

HEVs are permanent features of secondary lymphoid tissues, but they can also develop from normal endothelium at sites of chronic inflammatory reactions, for example in the skin and in the synovium. This, in turn, may direct specific T-lymphocyte subsets to the area where HEVs have formed. The movement of lymphocytes across endothelium is controlled by adhesion molecules and chemokines. For example, the adhesion molecule MadCAM-1 is expressed on endothelial cells in intestinal tissues, while VCAM-1 is present on endothelial cells in the lung and skin. Homing molecules on lymphocytes selectively direct lymphocytes to particular organs by interaction with these adhesion molecules. In the case of the intestine, a critical role is played by $\alpha_4\beta_7$-integrins that mediate adherence of lymphocytes to HEVs of Peyer's patches that express MadCAM-1. The mechanisms which control lymphocyte migration are discussed in detail in Chapter 3.

Lymphocyte trafficking exposes antigen to a large number of lymphocytes

Lymphoid cells within lymph nodes return to the circulation by way of the efferent lymphatics, which pass via the thoracic duct into the left subclavian vein. About 1–2% of the lymphocyte pool recirculates each hour. Overall, this process allows a large number of antigen-specific lymphocytes to come into contact with their appropriate antigen in the microenvironment of the peripheral lymphoid organs. This is particularly important, as lymphoid cells are monospecific and there is only a limited number of lymphocytes capable of recognizing any particular antigen.

Under normal conditions there is continuous lymphocyte traffic through the nodes, but when antigen enters the lymph nodes of an animal already sensitized to that antigen there is a temporary shut down in the traffic which lasts for approximately 24 hours. Thus, antigen-specific lymphocytes are preferentially retained in the lymph nodes draining the source of antigen. In particular, blast cells do not recirculate but appear to remain in one site.

One reason for considering the MALT as a system distinct from the systemic lymphoid organs is that mucosa-associated lymphoid cells mainly recirculate within the mucosal lymphoid system. Thus, lymphoid cells stimulated in Peyer's patches pass via regional lymph nodes to the blood stream and then 'home' back into the intestinal lamina propria (*Fig. 2.65*). Specific recirculation is made possible because the lymphoid cells expressing homing molecules attach to adhesion molecules specifically expressed on endothelial cell adhesion molecules of the mucosal postcapillary venules, but which are absent from lymph node HEVs (see above). Thus, antigen stimulation at one mucosal area elicits an antibody response largely restricted to the MALT.

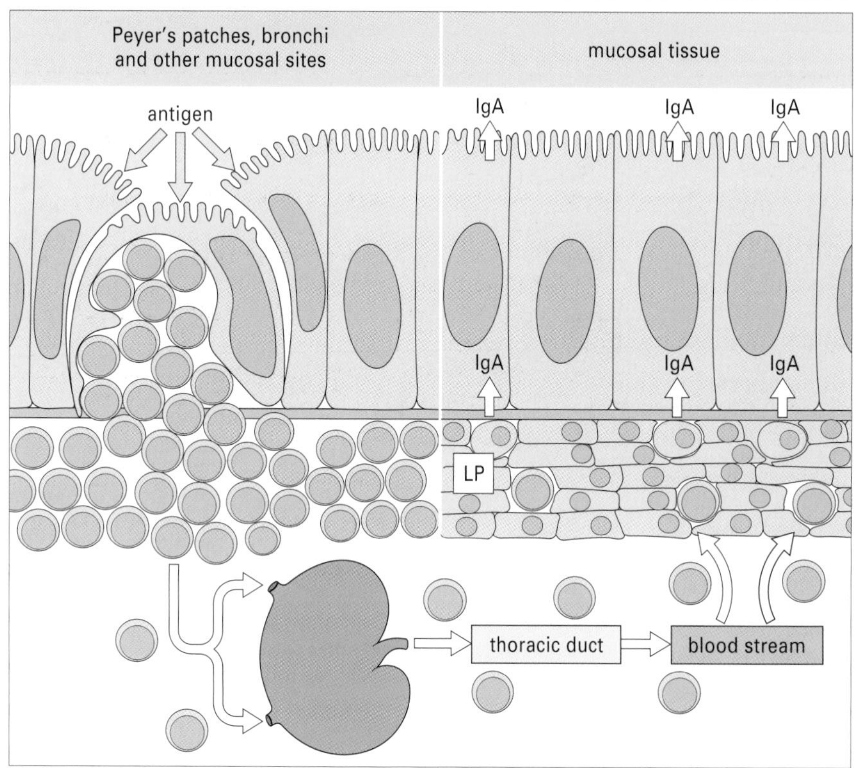

Fig. 2.65 Lymphoid cells which are stimulated by antigen in Peyer's patches (or the bronchi or another mucosal site) migrate via the regional lymph nodes and thoracic duct into the blood stream and hence to the lamina propria (LP) of the gut or other mucosal surfaces which might be close to or distant from the site of priming. Thus lymphocytes stimulated at one mucosal surface may become distributed selectively throughout the MALT system. This is mediated through specific adhesion molecules on the lymphocytes and mucosal HEV.

CRITICAL THINKING • Development of the immune system (Explanations on p. 453)

Immunodeficiencies can tell us a lot about the way the immune system functions normally. Mice which congenitally lack a thymus (and have an associated gene defect which produces hairlessness), termed 'nude mice', are often used in research.

2.1 What effect would you expect this defect to have on numbers and types of lymphocytes in the blood? How would this affect the structure of the lymph nodes? What effect would this have on the ability of the mice to fight infections?

Occasionally adult patients develop tumours in the thymus (thymoma), and it is necessary to completely remove the thymus gland.

2.2 What effect would you expect adult thymectomy to have on the ability of such patients to fight infections?

With the development of modern techniques in molecular biology, it is possible to produce animals which completely lack individual genes. Such animals are called 'gene knockouts'. Sometimes these knockouts can have quite surprising effects on development, and sometimes only minor effects. Others, like the immunodeficiencies, are very informative. Based on the information provided in this chapter, what effects would you expect the following 'knockouts' to have on the development of leucocytes and/or lymphoid organs?

2.3 *RAG1*. (The *RAG1* and *RAG2* genes are involved in the recombination processes which generate antigen receptors on B cells and T cells.)

2.4 Interleukin-7.

2.5 The β_7-integrin chain.

FURTHER READING

Abbas AK, Rao A. CD4 and CD8 T-cell subsets. *Immunologist* 1999;**7**:14–15.

Banchereau J, Steinman RM. Dendritic cells and the control of immunity. *Nature* 1998;**392**:245–52.

Butcher EC, Williams M, Youngman K, Rott L, Briskin M. Lymphocyte trafficking and regional immunity. *Adv Immunol* 1999;**72**:209–53.

Ganz T, Lehrer RI. Antimicrobial peptides of leukocytes. *Curr Opin Hematol* 1997;**4**:53–8.

Goldsby RA, Kindt TJ, Osborne BA, Kuby J. *Kuby Immunology,* 4th edn. Oxford: WH Freeman, 2000.

Lydyard PM, Whelan A, Fanger MW. *Instant Notes in Immunology.* Oxford: Bios Scientific, 2000.

Ogra P (ed). *Mucosal Immunity,* 2nd edn. London: Academic Press, 1998.

Perry M, Whyte A. Immunology of the tonsils. *Immunol Today* 1998;**19**:414–21.

Playfair JHL. *Immunology at a Glance,* 6th edn. Oxford: Blackwell Scientific Publications, 1996.

Roitt IM, Delves P. *Essential Immunology,* 10th edn. Oxford: Blackwell Scientific Publications, 2001.

Romagnani S, Kapsenberg M, Radbruch A, Adorini L. TH1 and TH2 cells. *Res Immunol* 1998;**149**:871–3.

3 Cell migration and inflammation

- **Cellular migration is a complex process,** which depends on the population of leucocytes, their state of activation and how they interact with endothelium in different vascular beds throughout the body. The process is controlled by adhesion molecules and chemokines expressed on the surface of the endothelium.
- **Adhesion molecules which control leucocyte migration** fall into families which are structurally related. They include the cell adhesion molecules (CAMs) of the immunoglobulin supergene family, the selectins and their carbohydrate ligands and the integrins.
- **Chemokines are a large group of signalling molecules,** which initiate chemotaxis and/or cellular activation. Most chemokines act on more than one receptor, and most receptors respond to more than one chemokine.
- **Resting or naïve lymphocytes** tend to migrate across high endothelial venules into lymphatic tissues, whereas activated lymphocytes tend to migrate to inflammatory sites. Which cells migrate where is determined by the chemokine receptors on different leucocyte populations and the sets of chemokines present in each tissue.
- **Phagocytes, including neutrophils and monocytes,** leave the bone marrow and migrate to peripheral tissues, particularly at sites of infection or inflammation. Neutrophils make a one-way trip, but monocytes differentiate into macrophages, and may recirculate back to the secondary lymphoid tissues to act as antigen presenting cells.
- **Inflammation is a response which brings leucocytes and plasma molecules to sites of infection or tissue damage.** The principle effects are an increase in blood supply, an increase in vascular permeability to large serum molecules and enhanced migration of leucocytes across the local endothelium and towards the inflammatory site.
- **The complement system is an important mediator of acute inflammation.** It can be activated by the classical, alternative or lectin pathways. The classical pathway is activated by immune complexes, the lectin pathway by carbohydrates and the alternative pathway by activator surfaces on microorganisms.
- **The effector mechanisms of the complement system** include: (i) opsonization of microorganisms for phagocytosis; (ii) direct killing of microorganisms by lysis; (iii) chemotactic attraction of phagocytes to sites of inflammation; (iv) processing of immune complexes; (v) activation of mast cells and basophils to release inflammatory mediators.
- **Cells of the body are protected against complement-mediated attack** by the actions of control proteins.
- **The kinin system and mediators from mast cells including histamine,** contribute to the enhanced blood supply and increased vascular permeability at sites of inflammation.

MECHANISMS OF CELL MIGRATION

The patterns of leucocyte migration through the body are determined by interactions between circulating leucocytes and endothelium of blood vessels. This process is controlled by signalling molecules which are expressed on the surface of the endothelium and it occurs principally in venules (*Fig. 3.1*). There are three reasons for this:

1. The signalling molecules and adhesion molecules which control migration are selectively expressed in venules.
2. The haemodynamic shear force in the venules is relatively low, and this allows time for leucocytes to receive signals from the endothelium and allows adhesion molecules on the two cell types to interact effectively.
3. The endothelial surface charge is lower in venules (*Fig. 3.2*).

Although the patterns of leucocyte migration are complex, the basic mechanism appears to be universal. The initial interactions are represented by a three-step model (*Fig. 3.3*):

1. Leucocytes are slowed as they pass through a venule and roll on the surface of the endothelium before being halted. This is mediated primarily by adhesion molecules called selectins interacting with carbohydrates on glycoproteins.
2. The slowed leucocytes now have the opportunity to respond to signalling molecules held at the endothelial surface. Particularly important are the large group of cytokines, termed chemokines, which activate particular populations of leucocytes that have the appropriate chemokine receptors.
3. Activation upregulates the affinity of the leucocytes' integrins which now engage the cellular adhesion molecules on the endothelium to cause firm adhesion and initiate a programme of migration.

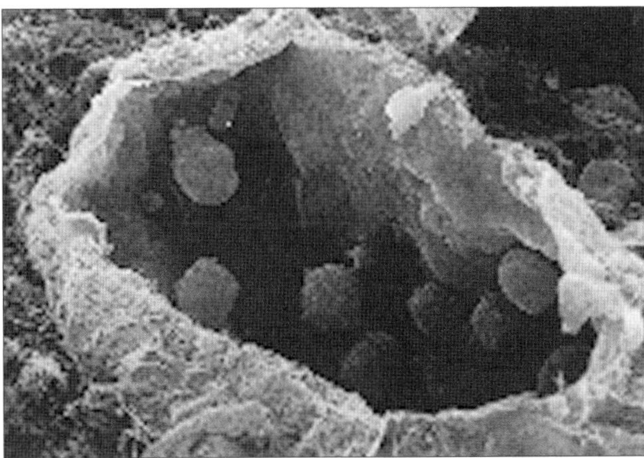

Fig. 3.1 Scanning electronmicrograph, showing leucocytes adhering to the wall of a venule in inflamed tissue. × 16 000 (Courtesy of Professor M.J. Karnovsky).

Leucocyte migration across endothelium

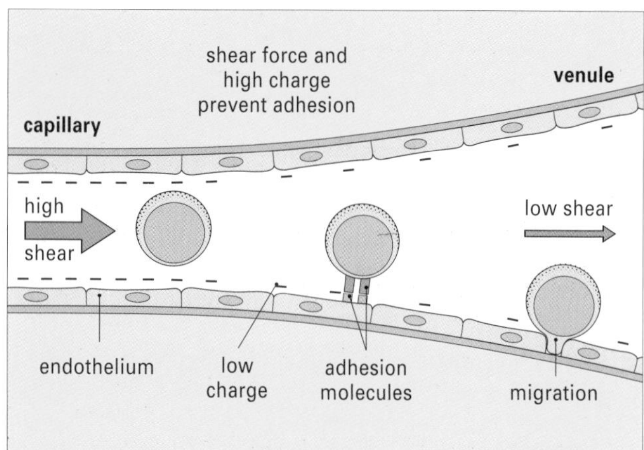

Fig. 3.2 Leucocytes circulating through a vascular bed may interact with venular endothelium via sets of surface adhesion molecules. In the venules, haemodynamic shear is low, surface charge on the endothelium is lower and adhesion molecules are selectively expressed.

Three-step model of leucocyte adhesion

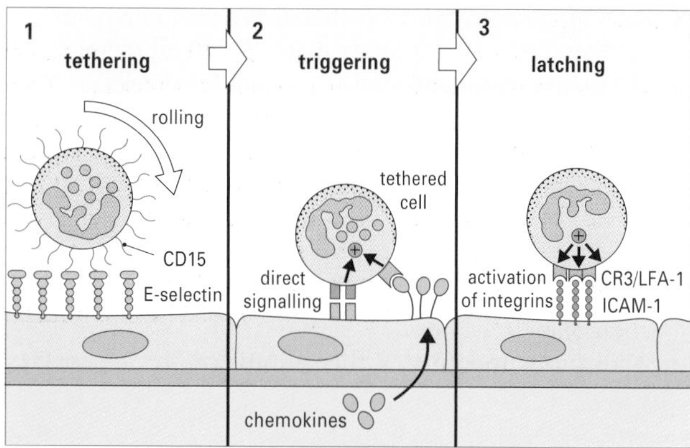

Fig. 3.3 The three-step model of leucocyte adhesion and activation is illustrated by a neutrophil, although different sets of adhesion molecules would be used by other leucocytes in different situations. (**1**) Tethering: the neutrophil is slowed in the circulation by interactions between E-selectin and carbohydrate groups on CD15, causing it to roll along the endothelial surface. (**2**) Triggering: the neutrophil can now receive signals from chemokines bound to the endothelial surface, or by direct signalling from endothelial surface molecules. The longer a cell rolls along the endothelium, the longer it has to receive sufficient signal to trigger migration. (**3**) Adhesion: The triggering upregulates integrins (CR3 and LFA-1), so that they bind to ICAM-1 induced on the endothelium by inflammatory cytokines.

Transendothelial migration is an active process involving both cell types and occurs near the junctions between endothelial cells (*Fig. 3.4*). There has been much controversy concerning whether leucocytes migrate through the junctions between endothelial cells or across the endothelium itself. In specialized tissues such as the brain and

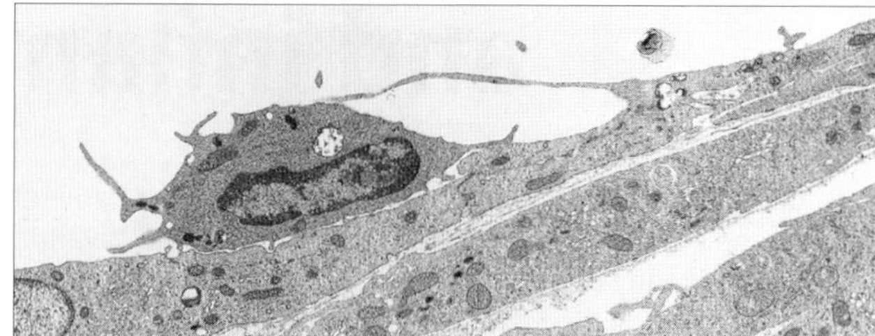

Fig. 3.4 Lymphocyte migration. Electronmicrograph showing a lymphocyte adhering to brain endothelium close to the interendothelial cell junction, in an animal with experimental allergic encephalomyelitis. Adhesion precedes transendothelial migration into inflammatory sites. (Courtesy of Dr C. Hawkins.)

thymus, where the endothelium is connected by continuous tight junctions, it is clear that lymphocytes migrate across the endothelium in vacuoles, and the junctions do not break apart. There is increasing evidence that this process also occurs in other tissues.

Migrating cells extend pseudopods down to the basement membrane and move beneath the endothelium using new sets of adhesion molecules. Enzymes are now released which digest the collagen and other components of the basement membrane, allowing cells to migrate into the tissue. Once there, the cells can respond to new sets of chemotactic stimuli, which allow them to position themselves appropriately in the tissue.

The following section describes the adhesion molecules and signalling molecules in more detail. Where and when these molecules are expressed determine the patterns of leucocyte traffic into different tissues.

Intercellular adhesion molecules

Intercellular adhesion molecules are membrane-bound proteins which allow one cell to interact with another. Often these molecules traverse the membrane and are linked to the cytoskeleton, so that the cell can use them to gain traction on other cells, or on the extracellular matrix, as they move. In many cases, a particular adhesion molecule can bind to more than one ligand, using different binding sites. Although the binding affinity of individual adhesion molecules to their ligands is usually low, clustering of the molecules in patches on the cell surface means that the avidity of the interaction can be high.

Cells can modulate their interactions with other cell types, either by increasing the numbers of adhesion molecules on the surface, or by altering their affinity/avidity. There are two ways in which cells can alter the level of expression of adhesion molecules: many cells retain large intercellular stores of these molecules in vesicles, which can be directed to the cell surface within minutes following cellular activation. Alternatively, new molecules can be synthesized and transported to the cell surface, a process which usually takes several hours.

Step 1: selectins bind to carbohydrates to slow the circulating leucocytes

The selectins include the molecules E-selectin and P-selectin, expressed on endothelium and platelets, and

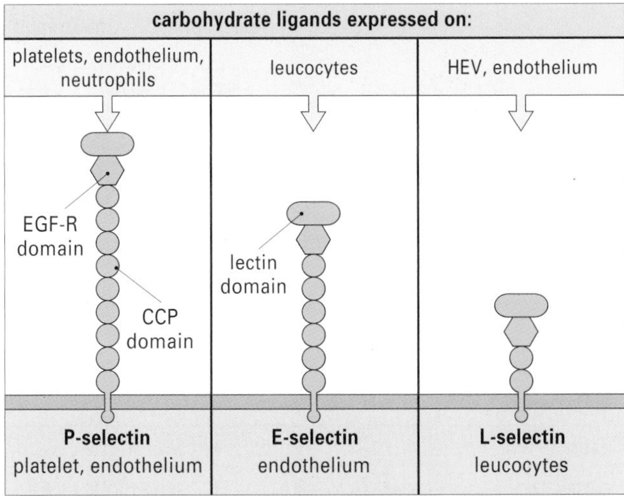

Fig. 3.5 The structures of three selectins are shown. They have terminal lectin domains which bind to carbohydrates on the cells listed. The EGF-R domain is homologous to a segment in the epidermal growth factor receptor. The CCP domains are homologous to domains found in complement control proteins, such as factor H, decay accelerating factor and membrane cofactor protein.

L-selectin, which is expressed on some leucocytes (*Fig. 3.5*). They are transmembrane molecules, with a number of extracellular domains homologous to those seen in complement control proteins (see below). The extracellular region also has a domain related to the epidermal growth factor (EGF) receptor and an N-terminal domain which has lectin-like properties (i.e. it binds to carbohydrate residues), hence the name selectins.

The carbohydrate ligands for the selectins may be associated with several different proteins. For example, Sgp-200 expressed on HEV has numerous O-linked carbohydrates which bind to L-selectin on lymphocytes and directs these cells to peripheral lymph nodes. At sites of inflammation E-selectin and P-selectin, which are induced on activated endothelium, bind to the sialyl Lewis-X carbohydrate associated with CD15, present on many leucocytes. Some of the selectin ligands are selectively expressed on particular populations of leucocytes. For example, the molecule PSGL-1 (P-selectin glycoprotein ligand) present on type-1 T helper (TH1) cells binds to E- and P-selectin, but a variant found on type-2 T helper (TH2) cells does not.

When selectins bind to their ligands the circulating cells are slowed within the venules. Video pictures of cell migration show that the cells stagger along the endothelium. During this time the leucocytes have the opportunity of receiving migration signals from the endothelium. This is a process of signal integration – the more time the cell spends in the venule, the longer it has to receive sufficient signals to activate migration. If a leucocyte is not activated, then it will detach from the endothelium and return to the venous circulation. Thus a cell may circulate hundreds of times, before it finds an appropriate place to migrate into the tissues.

Step 2: chemokines and other chemotactic molecules trigger the tethered leucocytes

Chemokines

The chemokines are a group of at least 40 small cytokines involved in cell migration, activation and chemotaxis. They determine which cells will cross the endothelium, and where they will move within the tissue. Most chemokines have two binding sites, one for their specific receptors and a second for carbohydrate groups on proteoglycans, such as heparan sulphate. This allows them to attach to the lumenal surface of endothelium (blood side), ready to trigger any tethered leucocytes (*Fig. 3.6*). The chemokines

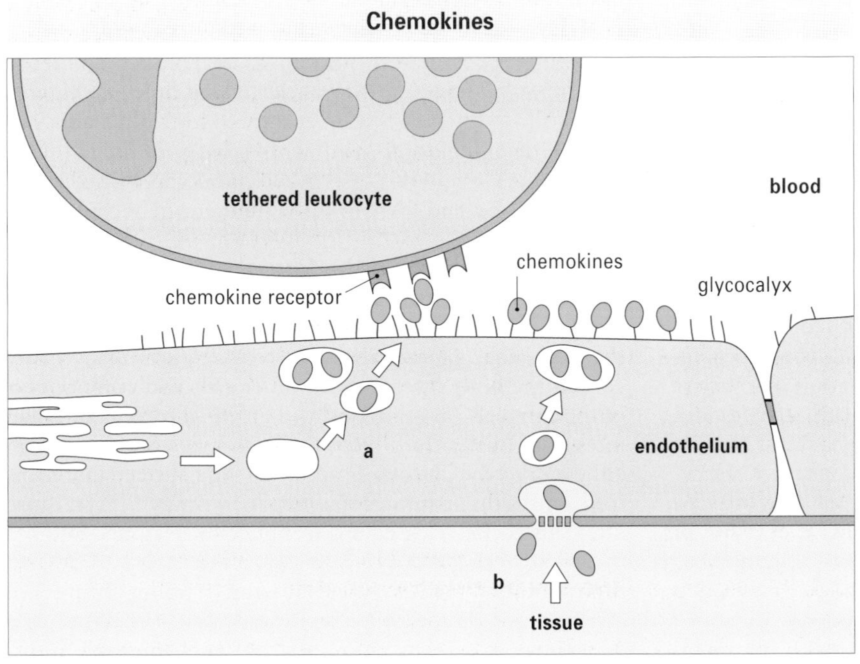

Fig. 3.6 Chemokines bind to glycosaminoglycans on endothelium via one binding site while a second site interacts with chemokine receptors expressed on the surface of the leucocyte. (a) Chemokines may be synthesized by the endothelial cell and stored in vesicles (Weibel Palade bodies) to be released to the lumenal surface (blood side) following activation. (b) Alternatively chemokines may be produced by cells in the tissues, and be transported across the endothelium. Thus, cells in the tissue can signal either directly or indirectly to circulating leucocytes.

may be produced by the endothelium itself. This depends on several factors including: (i) the tissue; (ii) the presence of inflammatory cytokines; and (iii) haemodynamic forces. In addition chemokines produced by cells in the tissues can be transported to the lumenal side of the endothelium. Thus, immune reactions or events occurring within the tissue can induce the release of chemokines, which signal the inward migration of required populations of leucocytes.

Chemokine receptors

Chemokines fall into four different families, based on the spacing of conserved cysteine (C) residues. For example, the α-chemokines have a CXC structure and β-chemokines a CC structure. All of the chemokines act via 'serpentine receptors', which have seven transmembrane segments and are linked to GTP-binding proteins (G-proteins) that cause cell activation. Most chemokines act on more than one receptor, and most receptors will respond to several chemokines. Because of this complexity, it is easiest to understand what chemokines are doing by considering their receptors. The receptors for the CXC chemokines are called CXCR1, CXCR2 and so on, while those for the CC chemokines are called CCR1, CCR2, etc. *Figure 3.7* lists the chemokine receptors and some of their principal ligands. A full list is given in Appendix 4. The receptors are selectively expressed on particular populations of leucocytes, and this determines which cells can respond to signals coming from the tissues. The profile of chemokine receptors on a cell depends on its type and state of differentiation. For example, all T cells express CCR1 while TH2 cells preferentially express CCR3 and TH1 cells CCR5 and CXCR3. Once a cell has crossed the endothelium, it is capable of responding to a new set of chemokines, which direct its migration through the tissues. Thus, cell migration resembles the sport of orienteering. Cells move from one place to another, receiving successive signals for the next destination. Which of the chemokines are involved in each type of cell migration will be considered below.

Other chemotactic molecules

Several other molecules are chemotactic for neutrophils and macrophages. Both of these cells have an fMet-Leu-Phe (fMLP) receptor. This receptor binds to peptides blocked at the N terminus by formylated methionine. As prokaryotes (e.g. bacteria) initiate all protein translation with this amino acid, whereas eukaryotes do not, this provides a simple specific signal for the presence of bacteria, towards which phagocytes should move. These cells also have receptors for C5a, a fragment of a complement component, and leukotriene-B_4 (LTB_4), both of which are generated at sites of inflammation, C5a following complement activation and LTB_4 following activation of a variety of cells, particularly macrophages and mast cells. In addition, molecules generated by the blood clotting system, notably fibrin peptide B and thrombin, attract phagocytes. However, many molecules such as these only act indirectly by inducing chemokines. The first cells to arrive at a site of inflammation, if activated, are able to release chemokines which attract others. For example, IL-8 released by activated monocytes can induce neutrophil and basophil chemotaxis. Similarly, macrophage activation leads to the metabolism of arachidonic acid with release of LTB_4. Like chemokines, many of these other chemotactic molecules, including C5a and f.MLP, act via serpentine receptors.

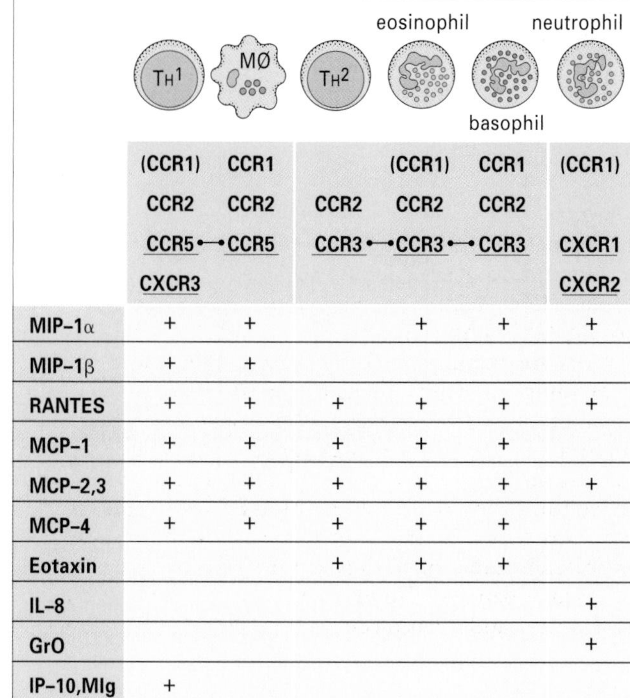

Chemokine receptors

	TH1	MØ	TH2	eosinophil	basophil	neutrophil
	(CCR1) CCR2 CCR5 CXCR3	CCR1 CCR2 CCR5	CCR2 CCR3	(CCR1) CCR2 CCR3	CCR1 CCR2 CCR3	(CCR1) CXCR1 CXCR2
MIP-1α	+	+		+	+	+
MIP-1β	+	+				
RANTES	+	+	+	+	+	+
MCP-1	+	+	+	+	+	
MCP-2,3	+	+	+	+	+	+
MCP-4	+	+	+	+	+	
Eotaxin			+	+	+	
IL-8						+
GrO						+
IP-10,Mlg	+					

Fig. 3.7 The table lists somes of the chemokine receptors found on particular leucocytes and the chemokines they respond to. The cells are grouped according to the principle types of effector response. Note that TH1 cells and mononuclear phagocytes both express CCR5 which allows them to respond to MIP-1β, while TH2 cells, eosinophils and basophils express CCR3 which allows them to respond to eotaxin. This allows selective recruitment of sets of leucocytes into areas with particular types of immune/inflammatory response. Both groups of cells express CCR1 and CCR2, which allow responses to macrophage chemotactic proteins (MCPs). Neutrophils express CXCR1 and CXCR2 which allows them to respond to IL-8 and Gro. Bracketed entries indicate that only a subset of cells express that receptor. Full details are given in Appendix 4.

Step 3: integrins on the leucocytes bind to cell adhesion molecules on the endothelium

Activation of cells via their chemokine receptors initiates the next stage of migration. Leucocytes and many other cells in the body interact with other cells and components of the extracellular matrix using a group of molecules called integrins. In the third step, the leucocytes develop a firm adhesion to the endothelium using their surface integrins. Cell activation promotes this step in two ways; it can cause integrins to be released from intracellular stores, and/or it can cause clustering of integrins on the cell surface into high avidity patches. Normally the binding affinity of integrins for the cell adhesion molecules (CAMs) on the endothelium is relatively weak, but when multiple interactions take place, the cells adhere firmly. Many of the CAMs on the endothelium have immunoglobulin-like domains, i.e. they belong to the immunoglobulin superfamily. Some of the CAMs are constitutively expressed, while other are specifically induced on particular endothelia, or at sites of inflammation. The integrins and CAMs are very important groups of molecules and their structures are considered below.

Integrins

Integrins comprise a major group of adhesion molecules, present on many cells, including leucocytes. Each member of this large family of molecules consists of two non-covalently bound polypeptides (α and β), both of which traverse the membrane. They fall into three major families depending on which β-chain they have, because any β-chain can associate with several α-chains. Broadly, the β_1-integrins are involved in binding of cells to extracellular matrix, the β_2-integrins are involved in leucocyte adhesion to endothelium or to other immune cells, and the β_3-integrins (cytoadhesins) are involved in the interactions of platelets and neutrophils at inflammatory sites or sites of vascular damage. However, there are several exceptions to this rule, and it has more recently been found that some α-chains can associate with more than one β-chain (*Fig. 3.8*). The ability of integrins to bind to their ligands depends on divalent cations. For example, LFA-1 (lymphocyte functional antigen-1 $\alpha_L\beta_2$ integrin) has a Mg^{2+} ion coordinated at the centre of a binding site which accommodates an aspartate residue from the ligand. In addition, Ca^{2+} ions binding to leucocyte functional antigen-1 (LFA-1) at another site cause it to dimerize at the cell surface, thus increasing the effective affinity for its ligand intercellular adhesion molecule-1 (ICAM-1).

Many of the integrins can bind to more than one ligand. For example, LFA-1 present on most lymphocytes binds to both ICAM-1 and ICAM-2, which are expressed on endothelium. Another example is VLA-4 ($\alpha_4\beta_1$-integrin) which binds to both vascular cell adhesion molecule-1 (VCAM-1), expressed on endothelium and fibronectin, which is an extracellular matrix component.

Cell adhesion molecules

The cell adhesion molecules on the endothelium which interact with integrins are all members of the immunoglobulin supergene family. They include ICAM-1 and ICAM-2, VCAM-1 and mucosal addressin cell adhesion molecule (MAdCAM-1) (*Fig. 3.9*). All members of this family are expressed, or inducible, on vascular endothelium. ICAM-1 and VCAM-1 are both induced by inflammatory cytokines, while ICAM-2 is constitutively expressed at low levels on some endothelia and is down-regulated by inflammatory cytokines. The two N-terminal domains of ICAM-1 are homologous to those of ICAM-2 and both molecules interact with LFA-1. (There is a third ligand for LFA-1, called ICAM-3, which is expressed on lymphocytes.) MAdCAM-1 is a composite molecule which includes two

Integrins

integrin general structure

α

β

leucocyte

integrin	ligands	expression
VLA-1 $\alpha_1\beta_1$	?	T cells, fibroblasts
VLA-2 $\alpha_2\beta_1$	collagen	activated T cells, platelets
VLA-3 $\alpha_3\beta_1$	laminin, collagen, fibronectin	kidney, thyroid
VLA-4 $\alpha_4\beta_1$	VCAM-1, fibronectin	lymphocytes, some phagocytes
VLA-5 $\alpha_5\beta_1$	fibronectin	some leucocytes, platelets
VLA-6 $\alpha_6\beta_1$	laminin	widely distributed
LPAM-1 $\alpha_4\beta_7$	MAdCAM-1 (VCAM-1)	some T cells
LFA-1 $\alpha_L\beta_2$	ICAM-1, ICAM-2 (ICAM-3)	most leucocytes
CR3 $\alpha_M\beta_2$	C3b, C4b, ICAM-1	mononuclear phagocytes, neutrophils
CR4 $\alpha_X\beta_2$	C3b, C4b, ICAM-1 ?	macrophages

Fig. 3.8 The general structure of an integrin consisting of two non-covalently linked chains is shown at the top. The table gives the properties of some of the integrins involved in leucocyte binding to endothelium or extracellular matrix. A gene for an additional integrin, $\alpha D,\beta 2$, has recently been discovered. It is closely linked to $\alpha X,\beta 2$.

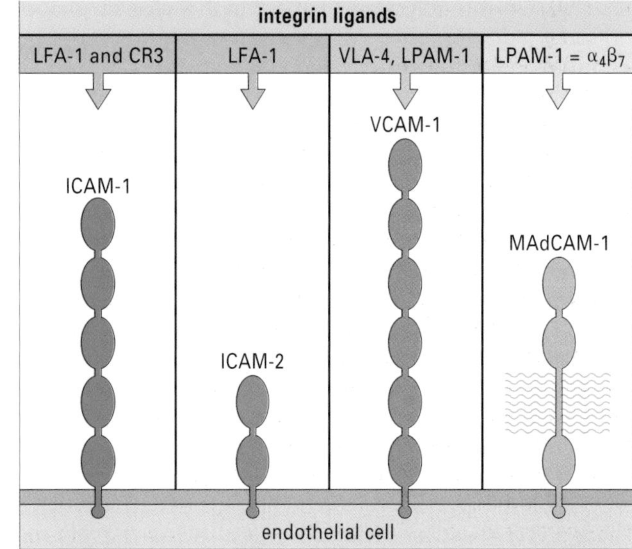

Fig. 3.9 The molecules ICAM-1, ICAM-2, VCAM-1 and MAdCAM-1, are illustrated diagrammatically with their immunoglobulin-like domains. Their integrin ligands are listed above. MAcdCAM-1 also has a heavily glycosylated segment which binds L-selectin.

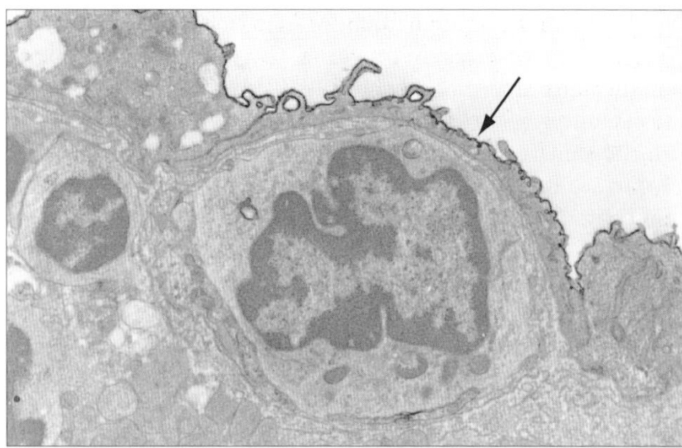

Fig. 3.10 Mucosal addressin on endothelium. The immunoelectron micrograph has been stained to show MAdCAM-1 as a dark border (arrow), on the lumenal surface of endothelium. In this instance the molecule is expressed on brain endothelium in chronic relapsing experimental allergic encephalomyelitis, induced by immunization of Biozzi AB/H mice with myelin basic protein. (Courtesy of Drs J. K. O'Neill and C. Butter, with permission from *Immunology* 1991; **72**: 520–525.)

Ig-like domains which interact with an integrin and a glycosylated segment which can interact with selectins. It was first identified on mucosal lymph node endothelium, but it can also be induced at sites of chronic inflammation (*Fig. 3.10*).

PATTERNS OF CELL MIGRATION

The patterns of migration are controlled by both leucocytes and endothelium

To explain the complex and varied patterns of cell migration, one must consider the large numbers of factors which modulate it. They include:

1. The state of activation of the lymphocytes or phagocytes – the expression of adhesion molecules and their functional affinity vary depending on the type of cell and whether it has been activated by antigen, cytokines or cellular interactions.
2. The types of adhesion molecules expressed by the vascular endothelium, which is related to its anatomical site, and to whether it has been activated by cytokines.
3. The particular chemotactic molecules and cytokines present – receptors vary between leucocyte populations, so that particular chemotactic agents act selectively on some cells only.

Different patterns of movement occur at different stages of a lymphocyte's life span. For example, resting T cells tend to migrate across high endothelial venules into secondary lymphoid tissues, while activated TH1 cells tend to migrate into sites of inflammation. Moreover, there is selective migration to particular regions. Thus, lymphocytes isolated from Peyer's patches tend to relocalize to the gut on reinfusion.

Migration of cells into lymphoid tissues

Migration into lymph nodes, Peyer's patches and mucosal lymphoid tissues occurs across high endothelial venules (see Chapter 2). Up to 25% of lymphocytes which enter a lymph node via the blood may be diverted across the high endothelial venule (HEV). By contrast, only a tiny proportion of those circulating through other tissues will cross the regular venular endothelium at each transit. High endothelial venules are therefore particularly important in controlling lymphocyte recirculation. Normally they are only present in the secondary lymphoid tissues, but they may be induced at sites of chronic inflammation. In addition to their peculiar shape, these cells express distinct sets of heavily glycosylated, sulphated adhesion molecules, which bind to circulating T cells, and direct them to the lymphoid tissue. The HEVs in different lymphoid tissues have different sets of adhesion molecules. In particular, there are separate molecules controlling migration to Peyer's patches, mucosal lymph nodes and other lymph nodes. These molecules were previously called vascular addressins, and their expression on different HEV, accounts for the way in which lymphocytes relocalize to their own lymphoid tissue.

Naïve lymphocytes express L-selectin which contributes to their attachment to carbohydrate ligands on HEV in mucosal and peripheral lymph nodes. Once they have stopped on the HEV, migrating lymphocytes may use the integrin $\alpha_4\beta_7$ (LPAM-1) to bind to MAdCAM on the HEV of mucosal lymph nodes or Peyer's patch. Since the expression of $\alpha_4\beta_7$ allows migration to mucosal lymphoid tissue, while $\alpha_4\beta_1$ allows attachment to VCAM-1 on activated endothelium, or fibronectin in tissues, expression of one or the other of these molecules can alternately be used by naïve lymphocytes migrating to lymphoid tissue or activated T cells to inflammatory sites.

Chemokines are also important in controlling cell traffic to lymphoid tissues. Naïve T cells express CCR7 and CXCR4 which allow them to respond to chemokines expressed in lymphoid tissues. They also interact with chemokines (DC-CK1 and ELC) produced by dendritic cells, which is thought to direct them to the appropriate T-cell areas of the lymph node where dendritic cells can present antigen to them. Once T cells have been activated they lose CXCR4 and CCR7, but gain new chemokine receptors which allow them to respond to different chemokines, e.g. those produced at sites of inflammation.

Naïve B cells also express CCR7 and CXCR4, and migrate to secondary lymphoid tissues. In addition they express CXCR5, a receptor for a chemokine (BCA-1) which appears to be required for localization to lymphoid follicles within the lymph nodes. Thus cells moving into lymphoid tissue respond sequentially to signals on the endothelium and signals from the different areas within the tissue (*Fig. 3.11*).

INFLAMMATION

Inflammation is the local response of a tissue to damage or infection. It has three principle components:

1. An increased blood supply to the area, bringing leucocytes and serum molecules to the affected site.
2. An increase in capillary permeability allowing exudation of the serum proteins (antibody, complement, kininogens, etc.) required to control the infection.
3. An increase in leucocyte migration into the tissue.

Chemokines and cell migration into lymphoid tissue

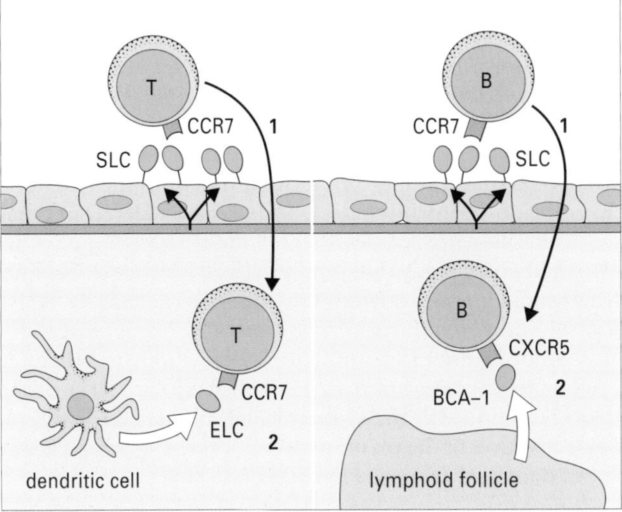

Fig. 3.11 Cell migration occurs in stages. Naïve T cells express CCR7 which allows them to respond to SLC (secondary lymphoid tissue chemokine) produced by the endothelium in lymphoid organs. Once the cells have migrated across the endothelium the same receptor can respond to signals from ELC, a chemokine produced by dendritic cells, which is thought to promote interaction with these cells in the T-cell areas of the nodes. B cells also express CCR7 and can therefore use similar mechanisms to migrate into secondary lymphoid tissues. However, they express CXCR5, which allows them to respond to BCA-1, a chemokine produced by cells within the lymphoid follicles. Thus B cells are directed to the B-cell areas of the tissue. Mice lacking CXCR5 do not develop normal lymphoid follicles.

There is a clear distinction between the cell traffic which occurs to lymphoid tissues and that which occurs into sites of inflammation. The types of cells which are seen at sites of inflammation, their preponderance and their time of arrival, depend primarily on the nature of the antigenic challenge and on the site where the reactions occur. In general, neutrophils are the first cells into sites of acute inflammation caused by infection. They represent the major cell type for several days. From the first day onwards mononuclear phagocytes and activated lymphocytes start to arrive. $CD8^+$ T cells and small numbers of B cells usually arrive later. The outcome of an acute reaction depends on whether antigen or the infectious agent is cleared; if not a chronic inflammatory reaction develops. In this case, few neutrophils are seen, but there are large numbers of $CD4^+$ T cells and mononuclear phagocytes. Reactions to parasite infections (e.g. schistosomiasis) often lead to an accumulation of eosinophils. Eosinophils, together with basophils and macrophages, are also prevalent in the wall of the bronchus following asthmatic attacks.

Leucocyte migration

Different sets of adhesion molecules and chemotactic agents are used for each type of cell movement. When damage occurs in the tissue, cells including mononuclear phagocytes release inflammatory cytokines such as TNFα or IL-1, which induce synthesis and expression of E-selectin. *In vitro*, cells transfected with the gene for E-selectin bind neutrophils strongly, and this suggests that the slowing of neutrophils by E-selectin is a critical first step in their migration. P-selectin acts similarly, but is held ready-made in the Weibel–Palade bodies of endothelium and released to the cell surface if the endothelium becomes activated or damaged. Both E-selectin and P-selectin can slow circulating platelets, or leucocytes.

In the second step of migration, neutrophils are triggered by chemokines such as IL-8, synthesized by cells in the tissue or by the endothelium itself. IL-8 acts on two different chemokine receptors CXCR1 and CXCR2 to initiate neutrophil migration. In some tissues different sets of chemokines will cause the local accumulation of different groups of leucocytes. For example, in the bronchii of individuals with asthma, the chemokine eotaxin is released, which causes the accumulation of eosinophils. Eotaxin acts on CCR3, which is also present on TH2 cells and basophils; thus by releasing one chemokine, the tissue can signal to three different kinds of cell to migrate into the tissue. This particular set of cells is characteristic of TH2-type immune responses, such as asthma (see Chapter 7). Another example of this is the selective expression of CXCR3 on TH1 cells, which allows them to respond to chemokines produced at sites of chronic inflammation (see Chapter 11).

Some of the endothelial adhesion molecules, particularly ICAM-1 and VCAM-1, are also induced at sites of inflammation by the cytokines tumour necrosis factor-α (TNFα), IL-1 and interferon-γ (IFN-γ) (*Fig. 3.12*). Their level of expression is also tissue specific. For example, ICAM-1 is expressed at higher levels on brain endothelium than VCAM-1, while VCAM-1 is equally expressed in skin endothelium. By contrast, ICAM-2 is not induced by inflammatory cytokines, and it has been suggested that ICAM-2 determines the basal level of binding of leucocytes to different types of endothelium. In addition, a clear role has

Expression and induction of endothelial adhesion molecules

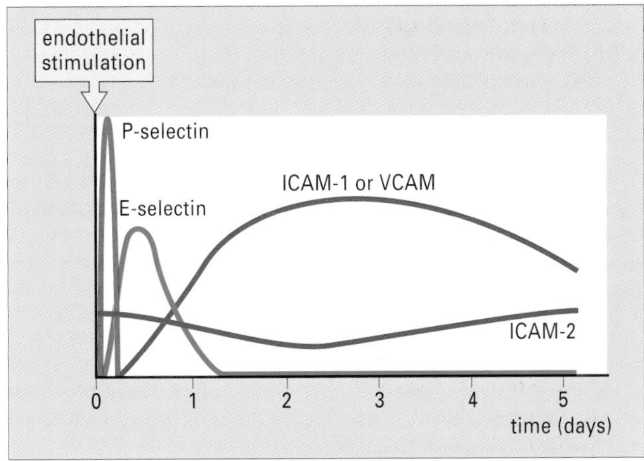

Fig. 3.12 The graph shows the time course of induction of different endothelial molecules on human umbilical vein endothelium *in vitro*, following stimulation by TNFα.

been shown for ICAM-2 in development, as it appears on blood vessels in the brain at the time when the brain is first colonized by mononuclear phagocytes.

ICAM-1 and ICAM-2 both interact with LFA-1 ($\alpha_L\beta_2$)-integrin), which is present on most leucocytes, whereas VCAM-1 interacts with VLA-4 ($\alpha_4\beta_1$-integrin). Both of these integrins are upregulated on activated lymphocytes, so the process of cell activation induces both the chemokine receptors which allow them to respond to inflammatory cytokines and the integrins which allow them to migrate. Another important integrin is CR3 ($\alpha_M\beta_2$-integrin), which is expressed on monocytes. The function of CR3 in phagocyte accumulation has been pinpointed by studies *in vivo* using antibodies to CR3, which inhibit phagocyte migration. It is notable that a group of patients who suffer from leucocyte adhesion deficiency (LAD) syndrome, and who suffer from severe infections due to poor phagocyte accumulation, are deficient in all the β_2-integrins (LFA-1, CR3, etc.). CR3 recognizes a site on ICAM-1, distinct from that recognized by LFA-1. Lymphocyte binding to endothelium can be modulated using antibodies to adhesion molecules or inactive analogues of chemokines, and this holds out prospects for therapy of diseases where immunopathological inflammation occurs.

Once they have crossed the endothelium and entered the tissues, the cells must interact with the proteins of the extracellular matrix (collagen, laminin, fibronectin, etc.), as well as the tissue cells. As lymphocytes leave the blood vessel, they lose some of their surface molecules (e.g. L-selectin) which are no longer required. The functional phenotype changes from that of a circulating cell to one adapted to move through tissues.

Many of the molecules which allow interaction with extracellular matrix belong to the β_1-integrin group, and are known as very late antigens (VLAs), so called because they were first identified on the T-cell surface at a late stage after T-cell activation. The whole group of β_1-integrins is now referred to as VLA molecules, even though most of them are not just expressed on lymphocytes. This group includes receptors for collagen (VLA-2 and VLA-3), laminin (VLA-3 and VLA-6) and fibronectin (VLA-3, VLA-4 and VLA-5). The fact that some of these molecules appear late after lymphocyte activation suggests that cells go through a programme of differentiation, and that the ability to interact with extracellular matrix is one of the last functions to develop.

Movement of molecules into tissues is controlled by the plasma enzyme systems and mediators released from mast cells and basophils

In addition to the enhanced cell migration, detailed above, serum molecules also leak into inflammatory sites. However, whereas cell migration occurs across venules, serum exudation occurs primarily across capillaries where blood pressure is higher and the vessel wall is thinnest. This event is controlled in two ways:

1. Blood supply to the area increases.
2. There is an increase in capillary permeability, caused by retraction of the endothelial cells and possibly also by increased vesicular transport across the endothelium. This permits larger molecules to traverse the endothelium than would ordinarily be capable of doing so and thus allows antibody and molecules of the plasma enzyme systems to reach the inflammatory site.

Four major plasma enzyme systems have an important role in haemostasis and control of inflammation. These are the clotting system, the fibrinolytic (plasmin) system, the kinin system and the complement system. The complement system has many important functions in immune reactions, in addition to inflammation, and it is considered in detail in the following sections. The kinin system generates the mediators bradykinin and lysyl-bradykinin, or kallidin. Bradykinin is a very powerful vasoactive nonapeptide, which causes venular dilatation, increased vascular permeability and smooth muscle contraction. Bradykinin is generated following the activation of Hageman factor (XII) of the blood clotting system, whereas kallidin is generated following activation of the plasmin system, or by enzymes released from damaged tissues (*Fig. 3.13*).

COMPLEMENT

Complement is central to the development of inflammatory reactions

The complement system consists of approximately 30 serum molecules constituting nearly 10% of the total serum proteins and forming one of the major defence systems of the body. In evolutionary terms this system is very ancient and antedates the development of the adaptive immune system. The functions of the system include control of inflammatory reactions and chemotaxis, clearance of immune complexes, cellular activation and antimicrobial defence. The system also plays a role in the development of antibody responses, and it is a major effector in immuno-

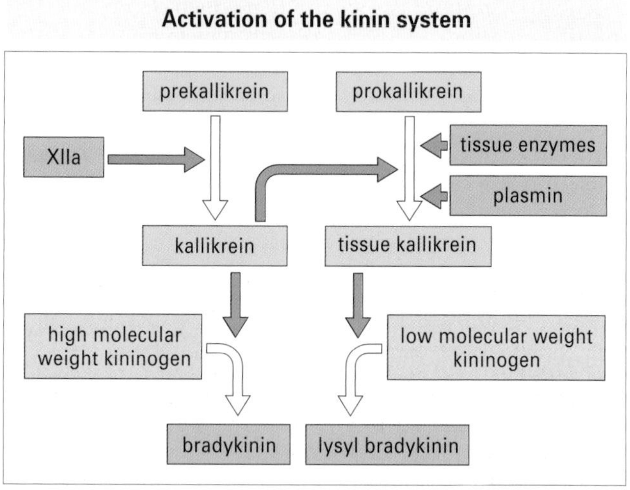

Activation of the kinin system

Fig. 3.13 Activated Hageman factor (XIIa) acts on prekallikrein to generate kallikrein, which in turn releases bradykinin from high molecular weight kininogen (HMWK). Prekallikrein and HMWK circulate together in a complex. Various enzymes activate prokallikrein to tissue kallikrein which releases lysyl-bradykinin from low molecular weight kininogen. Bradykinin and lysyl-bradykinin are both extremely powerful vasodilators.

pathological diseases. The importance of complement is illustrated by individuals who lack particular components. For example, children who lack the third component C3 are subject to overwhelming bacterial infections, while a deficiency of the eighth component C8 is associated with neisserial infections (see Chapter 19).

Three principle pathways are involved in complement activation, all of which converge on the activation of the third component C3. These are the classical pathway which is activated by antibody bound to antigen, the lectin pathway activated by carbohydrates and the alternative pathway activated in the presence of various microbial pathogens (*Fig. 3.14*). These are considered in more detail below. The proteins of the system act in enzyme cascades, where each step generates enzymes which act in the following step of the cascade. Thus a small initial stimulus can rapidly generate a large effect. All three pathways generate enzymes which cleave C3 into two fragments, C3a and C3b. This is the central step in the process of complement activation – the smaller fragment C3a activates phagocytes and mast cells, while the larger fragment can attach covalently to whatever happens to be nearby. The details of complement activation, the nomenclature and the ways in which the pathways are controlled are summarized in

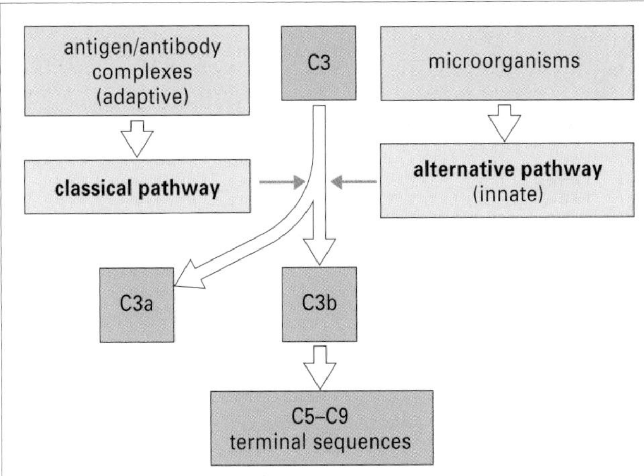

Fig. 3.14 Both classical and alternative pathways generate a C3 convertase, which converts C3 to C3b, the central event of the complement pathway. C3b in turn activates the terminal, lytic sequence, C5–C9. The first stage in the classical pathway is the binding of antigen to antibody. The alternative pathway does not require antibody and is initiated by the covalent binding of C3b to hydroxyl and amine groups on the surface of various microorganisms. The alternative pathway provides non-specific 'innate' immunity, whereas the classical pathway represents a more recently evolved link to the adaptive immune system.

Figure 3.15. This figure contains a large amount of information and you should refer back to it as you read the following sections on complement function.

The principle functions of the complement system are described below.

Opsonization and cell activation – involves complement components coating the surface of a target such as a bacteria. Phagocytic cells carrying receptors for these complement components are then able to bind to the bacteria, which triggers phagocytosis and cell activation.

Chemotaxis – Polymorphs and macrophages have specific receptors for small complement fragments that are generated during complement activation. The fragments diffuse away from the site of activation and stimulate chemotaxis, in a similar way to the chemokines.

Lysis of target cells – The final step in complement activation causes the assembly of a membrane attack complex (MAC), which can insert itself into lipid bilayers, such as the outer membrane of Gram-negative bacteria or a viral envelope. If the complement system attacks mammalian cells, e.g. erythrocytes from an incompatible blood transfusion, then osmotic disruption of the target cell ensues causing lysis.

C3b acts as an opsonin

C3 belongs to a family of proteins containing an unusual structure, an internal thioester bond formed between a glutamine and a cysteine residue. The bond is only partly stable, and is susceptible to attack by nucleophilic groups such as hydroxyl groups (–OH) and amine groups (–NH2) in proteins and carbohydrates. When C3 is cleaved into C3a and C3b, a conformational change takes place that makes the internal thioester bond very unstable, so that it can now react with nearby amine and hydroxyl groups (*Fig. 3.16*). If activated C3 fails to react with one of these groups, then the active site is neutralized by interaction with water. The activated state, C3b*, lasts for only a few milliseconds, therefore C3b deposition will be confined to the immediate vicinity of the activation site. Bound C3b can act as a focus for further complement activation by the alternative pathway, and it can act as an opsonin, i.e. it facilitates binding to phagocytes (*Fig. 3.17*). Phagocytes including monocytes, macrophages and neutrophils have several different types of receptor for C3b, which allow them to bind to immune complexes or pathogens which have C3b deposited on their surface. For example the immune adherence receptor, CR1 (complement receptor 1: CD35), is present on all mononuclear phagocytes and neutrophils as well as B cells and follicular dendritic cells. Binding of immune complexes to phagocytes via CR1 mediates both phagocytosis and cell activation, a process described fully in Chapter 9.

Summary of the complement activation pathways

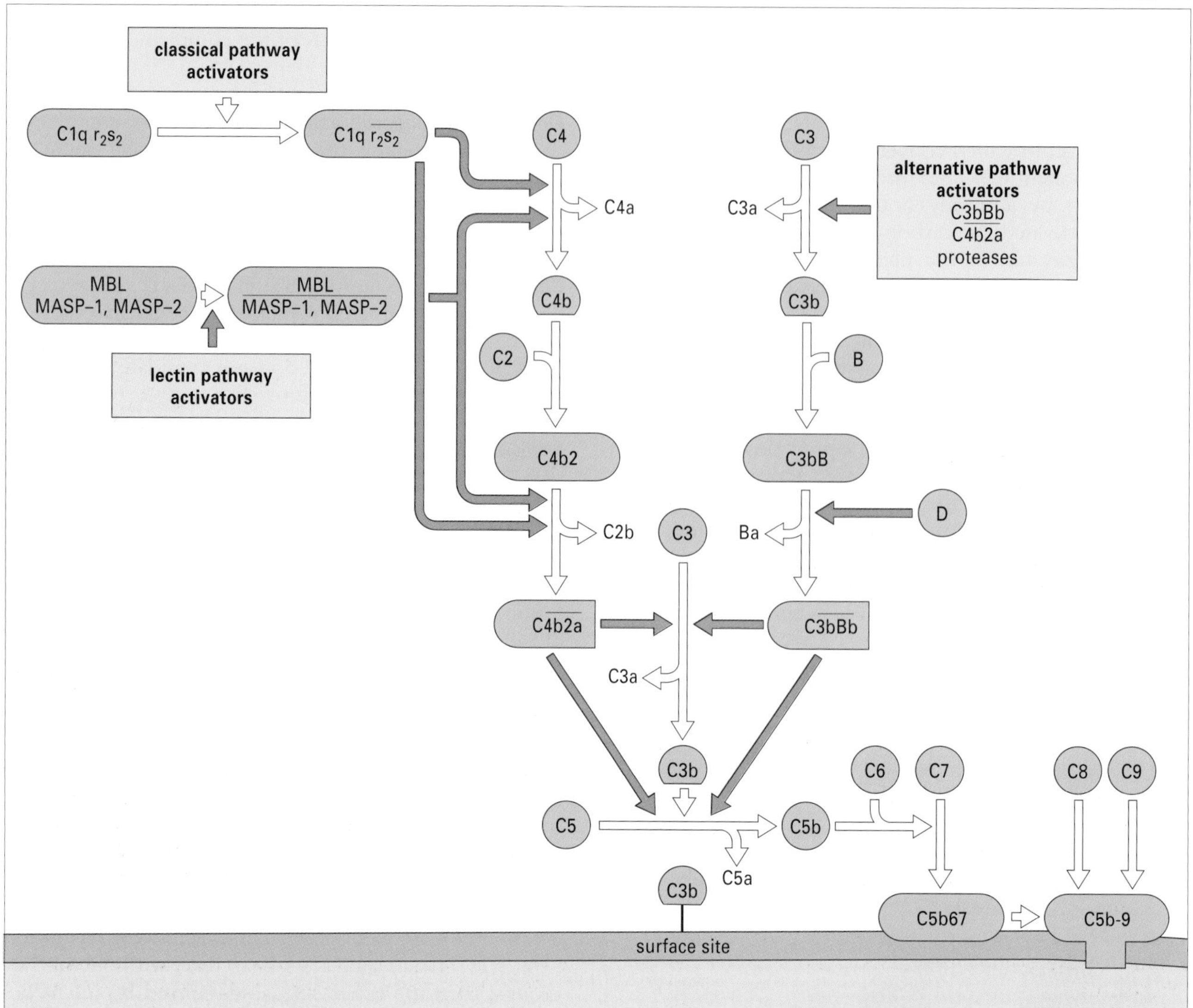

Fig. 3.15 The proteins of the classical and lytic pathways are assigned numbers, C1, C2, etc. Many of the proteins are zymogens, i.e. pro-enzymes which require proteolytic cleavage to become active. The enzymatically active form is distinguished from its precursor by a bar drawn above. The cleavage products of complement proteins are distinguished from parent molecules by suffix letters, C3a, C3b, etc. The proteins of the alternative pathway are called 'factors' and are identified by single letters, e.g. factor B, which may be abbreviated to FB or just 'B'. Components are shown in green, conversion steps as white arrows and activation/cleavage steps as red arrows.

The classical pathway is activated by the cleavage of C1r and C1s following association of C1qr2s2 with classical pathway activators including immune complexes. Activated C1s cleaves C4 and C2 to form the classical pathway C3 convertase C4b2a. Cleavage of C4 and C2 can also be effected via MASP-1 and MASP-2 of the lectin pathway, which are associated with mannan-binding lectin (MBL).

The alternative pathway is activated by the cleavage of C3 to C3b, which associates with factor B and is cleaved by factor D to generate the alternative pathway C3 convertase C3bBb. The initial activation of C3 happens to some extent spontaneously, but this step can also be effected by classical or alternative pathway C3 convertases or a number of other serum or microbial proteases. Note that the activation pathways are functionally analogous and the diagram emphasizes these similarities. For example C3 and C4 are homologous, as are C2 and factor B. MASP-1 and MASP-2 are homologous to C1r and C1s respectively.

Either the classical or alternative pathway C3 convertases may associate with C3b bound on a cell surface to form C5 convertases, C4b2a3b or C3bBb3b, which split C5. The larger fragment, C5b associates with C6 and C7, which can then bind to plasma membranes. The complex of C5b67 assembles C8 and a number of molecules of C9 to form a membrane attack complex (MAC), C5b–9.

Activation of the C3 thioester bond

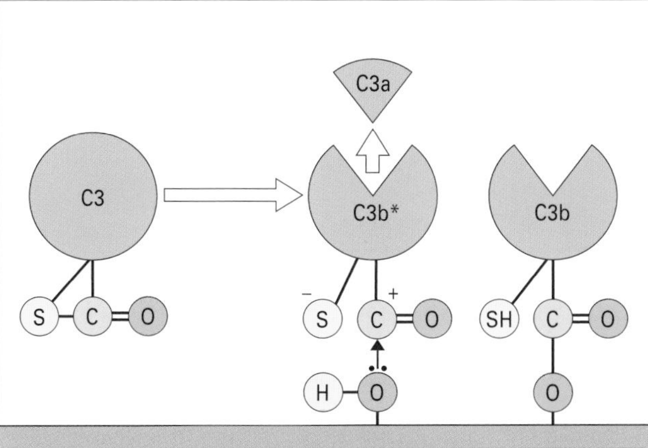

Fig. 3.16 The α-chain of C3 contains a thioester bond formed between a cysteine and a glutamine residue, with the elimination of ammonia. Following cleavage of C3 into C3a and C3b*, the bond becomes unstable and susceptible to nucleophilic attack by electrons on –OH and $-NH_2$ groups, allowing the C3b to form covalent bonds with proteins and carbohydrates – the active group decays rapidly by hydrolysis, if such a bond does not form. C4 also contains a thioester bond which becomes activated similarly when C4 is split into C4a and C4b.

Opsonization, binding and phagocytosis

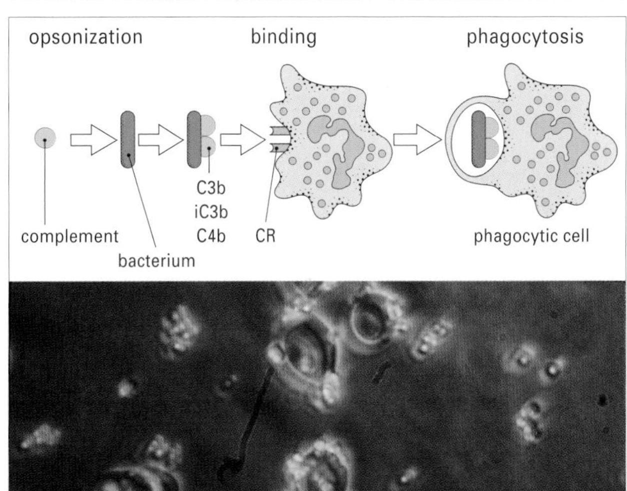

Fig. 3.17 Upper panel: A bacterium is sensitized by the covalent binding of C3b, iC3b and C4b, which allow it to be recognized by complement receptors (CR) on neutrophils and mononuclear phagocytes. This promotes phagocytosis and activation of the phagocyte. In primates, erythrocytes also express CR1, which allows them to bind opsonized bacteria and immune complexes. In the lower panel fluoresceinated bacteria which have been opsonized with antibody and complement are seen adhering to human erythrocytes. (Courtesy of Professor G.D. Ross.)

CR1 is also present on erythrocytes in man, and this allows immune complexes in the circulation to attach to erythrocytes for transport to phagocytes in the liver and spleen, leading to their subsequent clearance. Rodent platelets express CR1, which performs a similar transport function in these species. C3b is broken down by enzymatic cleavage successively by factor I and serum proteases (see *Fig. 3.24*), generating the fragments C3bi, C3d and C3g. Some of the complement receptors also bind to these fragments.

The function of complement receptors on follicular dendritic cells (FDCs) is rather different. They allow the FDCs to take up immune complexes for storage and subsequent presentation to B cells. This process is very important in the development and maturation of the antibody response – the secondary antibody response does not develop normally in animals which have been artificially depleted of C3. B cells also have receptors for C3 (CR1 and CR2) which allow them to take up immune complexes, and this facilitates B-cell activation. These roles of complement in the development of the antibody responses are described in Chapters 8 and 11.

C5a and C3a cause chemotaxis and mast cell activation

C5a and C3a are protein fragments released following enzymatic cleavage of C5 and C3 respectively. Both are involved in recruiting leucocytes to sites of inflammation and activating their effector systems. Both of these mediators are relatively small and can therefore diffuse away from the site of production. They both act on specific receptors, C5aR and C3aR, which belong to the same superfamily of G-protein-coupled receptors as the chemokine receptors. When they were first investigated, it was noted that production of these mediators in the circulation, or direct injection could produce the symptoms of anaphylaxis – bronchoconstriction and cardiovascular collapse, leading sometimes to death. For this reason, C5a and C3a are often referred to as 'anaphylatoxins'. Despite their structural and functional similarities, the actions of the two fragments are slightly different.

Actions of C5a – C5a is a potent activator of all cells of the myeloid lineage – granulocytes and mononuclear phagocytes (*Fig. 3.18*). Neutrophils respond to C5a by increased movement (chemokinesis) and directional movement (chemotaxis). They induce degranulation, and activate the respiratory burst leading to the production of free oxygen radicals. Because neutrophil granules contain stores of adhesion molecules, degranulation leads to increased expression of adhesion molecules at the cell surface, which promotes adhesion to the endothelium and migration of neutrophils into the tissue. Monocytes and macrophages show similar chemotactic responses to neutrophils.

C5a plays another important role in inflammation by causing degranulation of mast cells and basophils, with

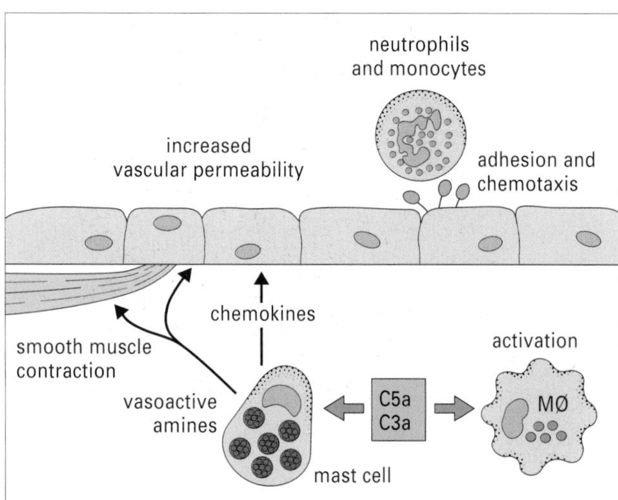

Fig. 3.18 C5a and C3a both act on mast cells to cause degranulation and release of vasoactive amines, including histamine and 5-hydroxytryptamine, which enhance vascular permeability and local blood flow. The secondary release of chemokines from mast cells causes cellular accumulation and C5a itself acts directly on receptors on monocytes and neutrophils to induce their migration to sites of acute inflammation and subsequent activation.

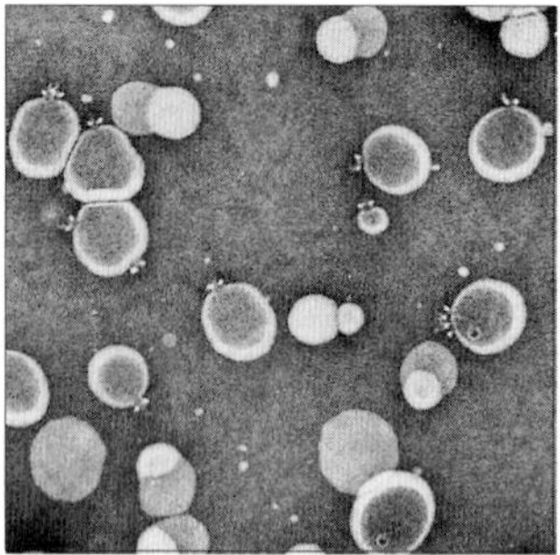

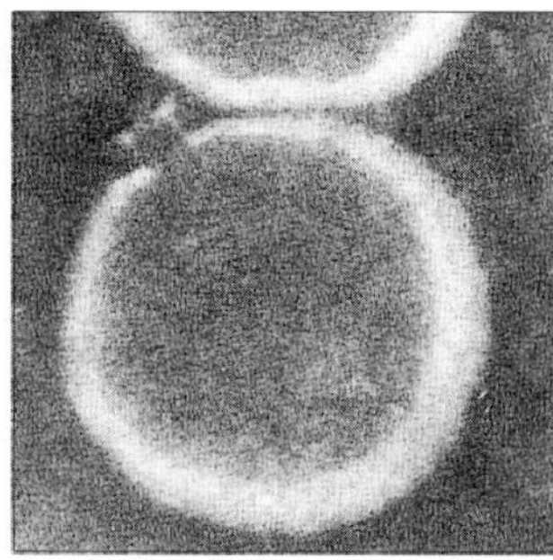

Fig. 3.19 Electronmicrographs of the membrane attack complex (MAC). The complex consists of a cylindrical pore, in which the walls of the cylinder, formed by C9, traverse the cell membrane. In these micrographs the human C5b–9 complex has been reincorporated into a lecithin liposomal membrane. ×234 000. (Courtesy of Professor J. Tranum-Jensen and Dr S. Bhakdi.)

release of histamine and other vasoactive mediators (see below). As a consequence, there are indirect effects on blood vessels, vasodilation of arterioles and increased permeability of capillaries. C5a is very short lived in serum. It is rapidly inactivated by carboxypeptidase N which removes the N-terminal arginine residue leaving C5a desArg, which is much less potent as a mediator than C5a itself. C5a which has bound to receptors on cells is internalized and rapidly proteolysed to inactive fragments.

Actions of C3a – C3a is much less active than C5a. It induces weak neutrophil aggregation and activation of the respiratory burst, and also causes mast cell degranulation. In contrast to C5a, it is not significantly chemotactic.

Note that in addition to the complement pathways, several other enzymes can activate complement C3, C5 and C4. These include the serum enzymes plasmin and kallikrein, enzymes from leucocytes such as neutrophil elastase and bacterial proteases (e.g. gingipain-1 from *P. gingivalis*, which causes periodontal disease).

The membrane attack complex causes lysis of cells

The membrane attack complex (MAC) consists of the components C5b,6,7,8, and a variable number of C9 molecules. Once C5 has been cleaved, the rest of the complex is assembled non-enzymatically. C5b binds C6 and C7, and this complex is amphiphilic, allowing it to insert into cell membranes. C8 now joins the complex and unwinds into the cell membrane. This complex of C5b–8 can itself cause disruption and lysis of membranes, an effect which is greatly enhanced by the incorporation of C9. If more than six molecules of C9 enter the complex, typical doughnut-shaped pores are seen, first observed in electronmicrographs by Humphrey and Dourmashkin (*Fig. 3.19*). These pores allow the flow of solutes and electrolytes across the cell membrane. The degree of damage caused depends on the cell type. A small number of pores can cause lysis of an erythrocyte, but nucleated cells tolerate more MACs before they are killed, although the presence of the MACs can compromise cell function.

Membrane attack complexes are regulated by proteins in serum and on host cell membranes

The assembly of MACs is moderated by vitronectin, a protein present in serum. If C5b–7 does not attach to a membrane, then it binds vitronectin and is subsequently inactive. A lipoprotein found in serum can also inhibit the binding of C5b–7 to membranes.

It has been known for some time that erythrocytes are poorly lysed by homologous complement, but readily lysed by complement derived from other species. This observation is explained by the finding that host cells express membrane proteins that protect against MACs. Protectin (CD59) is a protein anchored by a glycophospholipid anchor. It is widely distributed on cell membranes, binds to C8 in C5b–8 complexes and inhibits insertion of C9 into cell membranes (*Fig. 3.20*). Another protein, homologous restriction factor (HRF), has similar but weaker activity to CD59. It too is GPI anchored on the cell membrane and is expressed on erythrocytes and platelets. It limits formation of the MAC on these cells by interaction with C8 and C9.

Let us look now in more detail at how the system becomes activated.

The complement system can be activated by the classical, alternative or lectin pathways

The classical pathway is activated by immune complexes

Classical pathway activation is initiated by the binding of C1 to domains in IgG or IgM which are complexed with

CD59 inhibits C9 binding to C5b–8

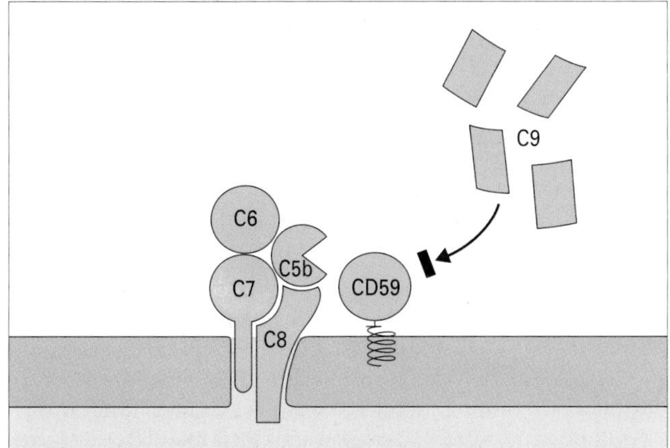

Fig. 3.20 CD59 binds to C8 in the C5b–8 complex and blocks attachment of C9, and thus formation of the MAC.

Structure of C1

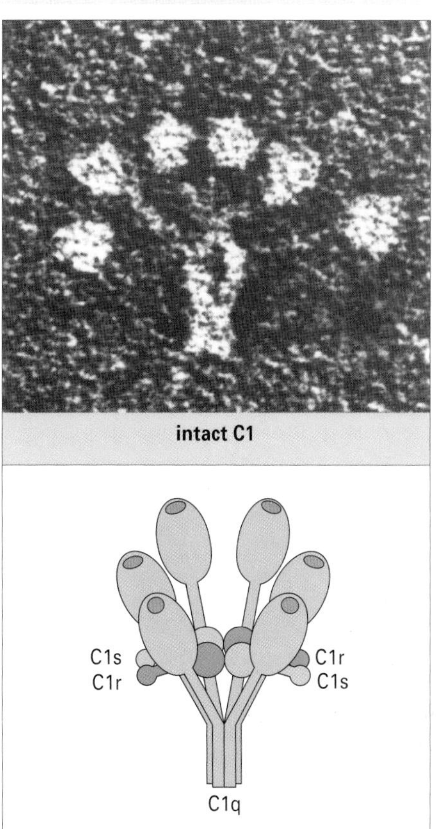

Fig. 3.21 Electronmicrograph of a human C1q molecule demonstrates six subunits. Each subunit contains three polypeptide chains, giving 18 in the whole molecule. The receptors for the Fc regions of IgG and IgM are in the globular heads. The connecting stalks contain regions of triple helix and the central core region contains collagen-like triple helix. The lower panel shows a model of intact C1 with two C1r and two C1s proenzymes positioned within the ring. The catalytic heads of C1r and C1s are closely apposed and conformational change induced in C1q following binding to complexed immunoglobulin causes mutual activation/cleavage of each C1r unit followed by cleavage of the two C1s units. The cohesion of the entire complex is dependent on Ca^{2+}. (Electronmicrograph, reproduced by courtesy of Dr N. Hughes-Jones.)

antigen. C1 is a molecular complex consisting of C1q and two molecules each of C1r and C1s (*Fig. 3.21*). The six heads of C1q each contain a binding site for a domain in IgG (CH2 domain). C1r and C1s are proenzymes. An immune complex presents a cluster of IgG molecules to which the C1q binds. This leads to a conformational change in C1 which causes the two C1r molecules to activate each other (autocatalysis) and then to cleave the two C1s molecules. This activates the C1s molecules, so that they can carry out the steps in the activation sequence shown in *Fig. 3.15*, resulting in the production of a C3 cleaving enzyme $\overline{C4b2a}$, which is the classical pathway C3 convertase.

Different classes of antibodies are more or less efficient at activating the classical pathway (see Chapter 4, for a full explanation of antibody classes). Only some of the IgG classes are able to activate complement. However IgM is very efficient at complement activation as it contains potentially 10 C1q binding sites in its CH3 domains. When IgM forms part of an immune complex the planar molecule is flexed into a 'staple' configuration, which exposes the C1q binding sites. Thus a single molecule of complexed IgM can activate complement, whereas it needs at least two molecules of complexed IgG. In effect, the bigger an immune complex is, the more efficiently it activates the classical pathway.

The lectin pathway is activated by bacterial carbohydrates

The lectin pathway is similar to the classical pathway. The molecule which initiates the pathway mannan-binding lectin (MBL) belongs to the same family as C1q – a family called the collectins. MBL is associated with two proenzymes MASP-1 and MASP-2 (MBL-associated serine proteases) which are homologous to C1r and C1s, although the stoichiometry of the complex is not yet known. When MBL binds to terminal mannose groups on bacterial carbohydrates it activates MASP-1 and MASP-2, which go on to activate the classical pathway in an antibody-independent fashion (*Figure 3.15*). The functions of MASP-1 and MASP-2 are roughly analagous to C1r and C1s, but it has been shown that activated MASP-2 cleaves C4 and C2 while activated MASP-1 cleaves C3 and C2.

Interestingly, C1q itself is also able to bind directly to some microorganisms, including mycoplasmas and retroviruses, in an antibody-independent fashion.

The alternative pathway is activated near 'protected' surfaces

The activation of the alternative pathway is rather different from the lectin and classical pathway. In fact, the alternative pathway is continuously being activated, at a very low rate, but this increases dramatically in the presence of suitable activator surfaces, such as bacterial and fungal cell walls. The internal thioester bond of native C3 is susceptible

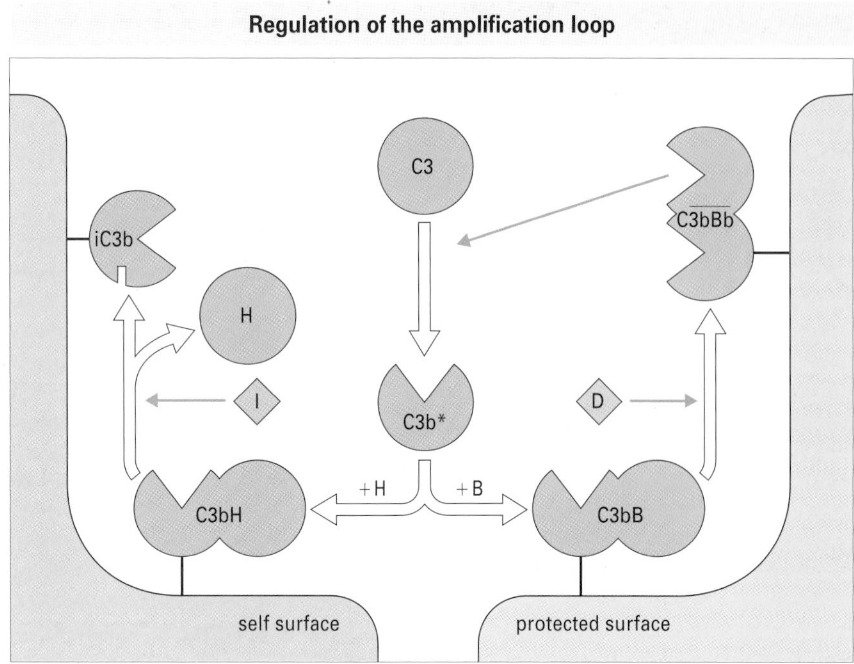

Fig. 3.22 Alternative pathway activation depends on the presence of protected surfaces. 'Protected' means that bound C3b is protected from proteolytic degradation. C3b which is bound to an activator surface binds factor B, which is cleaved by factor D to produce the alternative pathway C3 convertase $\overline{C3bBb}$, which drives the amplification loop, by cleaving more C3. However on self surfaces the binding of factor H is favoured and C3b is inactivated by factor I. Thus the binding of factor B or factor H controls the development of the alternative pathway reactions. In addition, proteins such as CR1 and DAF also limit complement activation on self cell membranes (see *Fig. 3.25*).

to spontaneous hydrolysis by water, which produces an activated form of C3 called C3i. This is termed 'tickover' activation. Potentially, the activated C3 can bind to factor B, which is then cleaved to form a C3 convertase. Whether this will happen depends on local environment. In serum and at the surface of the body's own cells, the C3 convertase is hydrolysed by water and inactivated, but near activator surfaces the C3 convertase remains to convert more C3 (*Fig. 3.22*).

Another feature which should be clear in *Figure 3.21* is that a small amount of activated C3b forms part of the C3 convertase $\overline{C3bBb}$, which can then activate more C3. This is a positive amplification step. Because of this the alternative pathway is often called the amplification loop. It does not matter whether the initial C3b is generated by the classical, lectin or alternative pathway, the amplification loop can ratchet up the reactions, if they take place near an activator surface.

Surfaces that are good activators of complement are often called 'protected' surfaces, meaning that they protect C3b from proteolytic degradation. Cells of the body express a number of proteins which favour the breakdown and dissociation of $\overline{C3bBb}$, the alternative pathway C3 convertase. These proteins include decay accelerating factor (DAF, CD55), and complement receptor 1 (CR1, CD35). In serum and body fluids C3b tends to bind to factor H and become inactivated, rather than binding factor B to initiate the amplification loop. Although the structural requirements of a protected surface are not fully understood, the carbohydrate components and the lack of protective molecules are critical. In particular, the presence of acidic sugars, such as sialic acid, seem to help in protecting self membranes from deposition of C3b.

Figure 3.23 compares the molecules which activate the classical, lectin and alternative pathways.

The activation pathways and amplification loop are tightly controlled

Regulation of the amplification loop is important for the host – this is a positive feedback system and it will cycle until all the C3 is exhausted, unless it is regulated. Regulation occurs in two principle ways:

1. Dissociation of the C3 convertase $\overline{C3bBb}$.
2. Enzymatic breakdown of C3b.

As noted above, on autologous cell membranes both DAF and CR1 promote dissociation of $\overline{C3bBb}$. Although CR1 is only expressed on populations of leucocytes, all cells of the body express DAF, although the amount varies between different cells. Enzymatic breakdown of C3b is mediated by factor I, which breaks down C3b into smaller fragments (*Fig. 3.24*). In the fluid phase breakdown is controlled by factor H and a related protein (FHLP-1), which act as cofactors for an enzyme, factor I, which cleaves C3b; at cell surfaces CR1 or MCP (membrane cofactor protein), act as cofactors. Thus the alternative pathway amplification loop is normally regulated by CR1, factor H, DAF and MCP.

In contrast to these proteins, factor P or properdin upregulates the amplification loop. Factor P is an acute phase protein whose synthesis is enhanced during inflammatory diseases. It acts by stabilizing $\overline{C3bBb}$ – the complex $\overline{C3bBbP}$ lasts longer before it decomposes. In fact the alternative pathway was originally called the properdin pathway, because it was thought that properdin initiated the reactions. Now we know that it just promotes the reactions which are initiated by C3b.

The classical pathway is also closely regulated, in three principle ways. In the fluid phase a serine protease inhibitor (serpin) called C1 inhibitor binds to and inactivates $\overline{C1r}$ and $\overline{C1s}$. C1 inhibitor (C1inh) can also inactivate $\overline{MASP\text{-}1}$ and $\overline{MASP\text{-}2}$ of the lectin pathway. A second mechanism blocks the formation of the classical pathway C3 convertase

Activators of complement

	immunoglobulins	microorganisms: viruses	microorganisms: bacteria	microorganisms: other	other
classical pathway	complexes containing IgM, IgG1, IgG2 or IgG3	murine retroviruses, vesicular stomatitis virus	–	*Mycoplasma*	polyanions, esp. when bound to cations, PO_4^{3-} (DNA, lipid A, cardiolipin), SO_4^{2-} (dextran sulphate, heparin, chondroitin sulphate)
lectin pathway			many Gram-positive and Gram-negative organisms		arrays of terminal mannose groups
alternative pathway	complexes containing IgG, IgA or IgE (less efficient than the classical pathway)	some virus-infected cells (e.g. EBV)	many strains of Gram-positive and Gram-negative organisms	trypanosomes, *Leishmania*, many fungi	dextran sulphate, heterologous erythrocytes, carbohydrates (e.g. agarose)

Fig. 3.23 The table summarizes the activators of the classical, lectin and alternative pathways.

Breakdown of C3b

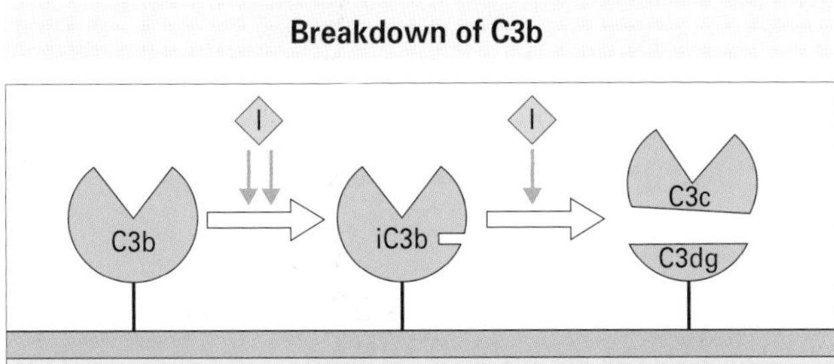

Fig. 3.24 Factor I cleaves C3b in three places to release C3c, leaving C3dg, a fragment of the α-chain, still bound to the substrate. The first two cleavages are promoted by factor H, MCP or CR1 and produce an intermediate iC3b. The third cleavage is promoted by CR1.

$\overline{C4b2a}$. In fluid phase the formation of this enzyme is inefficient, because of the action of factor I which breaks down C4b. This function is promoted by C4 binding protein (C4bp) which acts as a cofactor for factor I, in much the same way as factor H acts as a cofactor for factor I in the alternative pathway.

Classical pathway activation is also regulated by inhibiting complement binding to host surfaces. This is achieved through the actions of DAF, CR1 and MCP. The actions of these molecules in controlling the classical and alternative pathways are summarised in *Figure 3.25.*

AUXILIARY CELLS IN ACUTE INFLAMMATION

Auxiliary cells, including mast cells, basophils and platelets, are also very important in the initiation and development of acute inflammation. They act as sources of the vasoactive

Control proteins

	number of CCP domains	dissociation of C3 and C5 convertases: classical pathway	dissociation of C3 and C5 convertases: alternative pathway	cofactor for factor I on: C4b	cofactor for factor I on: C3b	localization
C4bp	52 or 56	+	–	+	–	serum
H	20	–	+	–	+	serum
DAF (CD55)	4	+	+	–	–	erythrocytes leucocytes platelets
MCP (CD46)	4	–	–	+	+	B cells neutrophils T cells macrophages
CR1 (CD35)	28 or 35	+	+	+	+	erythrocytes B cells follicular dendritic cells macrophages

Fig. 3.25 The five proteins listed are widely distributed and control aspects of C3b and C4b dissociation or breakdown. Each of these proteins contains a number of 'complement control protein' (CCP) domains. They act by either enhancing the dissociation of C3 and C5 convertases, or by acting as cofactors for the action of factor I on C3b or C4b.

mediators histamine and 5-hydroxytrypytamine (serotonin), which produce vasodilatation and increased vascular permeability. Many of the proinflammatory effects of C3a and C5a result from their ability to trigger mast-cell granule release, because they can be blocked by antihistamines. Mast cells and basophils are also a route by which the adaptive immune system can trigger inflammation – IgE sensitizes these cells by binding to their surface and the cells can then be activated by antigen. Mast cells are also an important source of slow-reacting inflammatory mediators, including the leukotrienes and prostaglandins which contribute to a delayed component of acute inflammation. They are synthesized and act some hours after mediators like histamine which are pre-formed and released immediately following mast cell activation (see Chapter 19). *Figure 3.26* lists the principle mediators of acute inflammation and the interaction of the systems is shown in *Figure 3.27.*

Platelets may also be activated by the immune system by immune complexes or by platelet-activating factor (PAF) from neutrophils, basophils and macrophages. This is thought to be important in type II and type III hypersensitivity reactions.

Once lymphocytes and monocytes have arrived at a site of infection or inflammation, they can also release mediators which control the later accumulation and activation of other cells. For example, activated macrophages release the chemokine macrophage inflammatory protein-1α (MIP-1α) and the leukotriene LTB_4, both of which are

Inflammatory mediators

mediator	origin	actions
histamine	mast cells, basophils	increased vascular permeability, smooth muscle contraction, chemokinesis
5-hydroxy-tryptamine (5HT – serotonin)	platelets, mast cells (rodent)	increased vascular permeability, smooth muscle contraction
platelet activating factor (PAF)	basophils, neutrophils, macrophages	mediator release from platelets, increased vascular permeability, smooth muscle contraction, neutrophil activation
neutrophil chemotactic factor (NCF)	mast cells	neutrophil chemotaxis
IL-8	monocytes and lymphocytes	polymorph and monocyte localization
C3a	complement C3	mast-cell degranulation, smooth muscle contraction
C5a	complement C5	mast-cell degranulation, neutrophil and macrophage chemotaxis, neutrophil activation, smooth muscle contraction, increased capillary permeability
bradykinin	kinin system (kininogen)	vasodilation, smooth muscle contraction, increased capillary permeability, pain
fibrinopeptides and fibrin breakdown products	clotting system	increased vascular permeability, neutrophil and macrophage chemotaxis
prostaglandin E_2 (PGE_2)	cyclo-oxygenase pathway mast cells	vasodilation, potentiates increased vascular permeability produced by histamine and bradykinin
leukotriene B_4 (LTB_4)	lipoxygenase pathway mast cells	neutrophil chemotaxis, synergizes with PGE_2 in increasing vascular permeability
leukotriene D_4 (LTD_4)	lipoxygenase pathway	smooth muscle contraction, increasing vascular permeability

Fig. 3.26 The table lists major inflammatory mediators, which control blood supply and vascular permeability or modulate cell movement. The main sources are given (centre block).

The immune system in acute inflammation

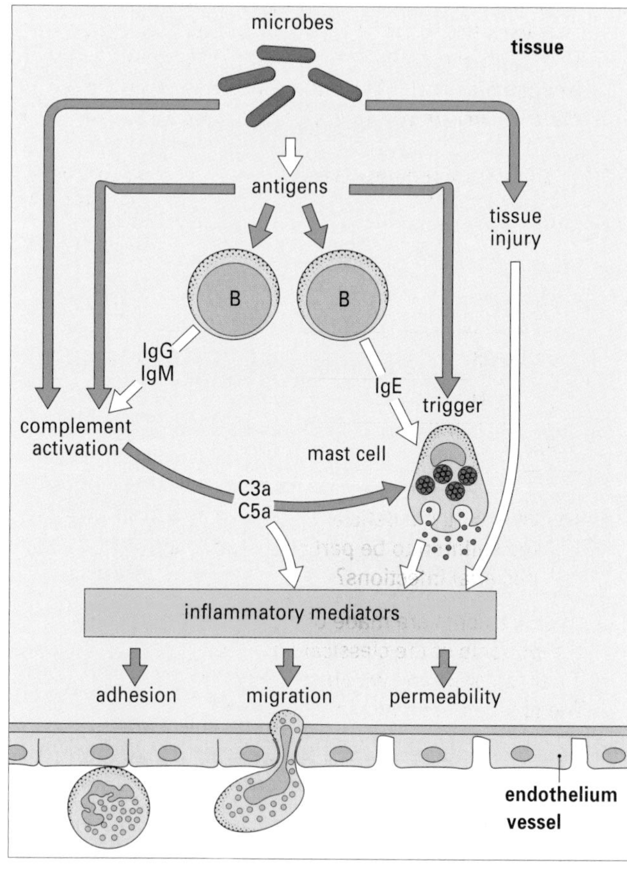

Fig. 3.27 The adaptive immune system modulates inflammatory processes via the complement system. Antigens (e.g. from microorganisms) stimulate B cells to produce antibodies including IgE, which binds to mast cells, while IgG and IgM activate complement. Complement can also be activated directly via the alternative pathway. When triggered by antigen, the sensitized mast cells release their granule-associated mediators and eicosanoids (products of arachidonic acid metabolism, including prostaglandins and leukotrienes). In association with complement (which can also trigger mast cells via C3a and C5a) the mediators induce local inflammation, facilitating the arrival of leucocytes and more plasma enzyme system molecules.

chemotactic and encourage further monocyte migration. Likewise lymphocytes can modulate later lymphocyte traffic by the release of chemokines and inflammatory cytokines, particularly IFN-γ.

Ultimately the outcome of an acute inflammatory response is related to the fate of antigen. If the initiating antigen or pathogen persists, then leucocyte accumulation continues and a chronic inflammatory reaction develops: if the antigen is cleared then no further leucocyte activation occurs and the inflammation resolves. In recurrent inflammatory reactions and in chronic inflammation the patterns of cell migration are different from those seen in an acute response. In particular macrophages and lymphocytes are usually more prevalent in chronic reactions, and neutrophils more so in acute reactions, although this also depends on the tissue involved. It is now known that the pattern of inflammatory cytokines and chemokines varies over the time-course of an inflammatory reaction and this can be related to the successive waves of migration of different types of leucocyte into the inflamed tissue. Chronic inflammation is particularly seen at sites of persistent infection, or in autoimmune reactions (where the antigen cannot ultimately be eradicated). This is considered more fully in Chapter 9.

CRITICAL THINKING • Complement deficiency (Explanations on p. 453)

A family has been identified in which three of the seven children have had repeated upper respiratory tract infections since early childhood. Of these, one has developed bacterial meningitis, and another a fatal septicaemia. In all of the children, the levels of antibodies in the serum are within the normal range. However when an assay for haemolytic complement is carried out, the three affected children are all found to be deficient in this functional assay. (This assay detects the ability of the patient's serum to lyse red cells which have been sensitized with antibody; this could be due to a deficiency in any of the components of the classical or lytic pathways.)

Complement component	Normal concentration (μg/ml)	Levels in affected children
C4	600	480–520
C2	20	15–22
C3	1300	10–80
Factor B	210	Not detectable
Factor H	480	20–35
Factor I	35	Not detectable

3.1 Why would a deficiency in complement cause the children to be particularly susceptible to bacterial infections?

Measurements are made of individual complement components of the classical and alternative pathways, in order to determine which of the components is defective. The results are shown in the table below.

3.2 Using knowledge of the complement reaction pathways, how can you explain the apparent deficiencies in C3 and several of the components of the alternative pathway?

3.3 What is the fundamental deficiency in this family and how would you treat the affected children?

FURTHER READING

Cell migration

Binnerts M E, van Kooyk Y. How LFA-1 binds to different ligands. *Immunol Today* 1999;**20**:234–9.

Davies P, Bailey P J, Goldenberg M M, Ford-Hutchinson A W. The role of arachidonic acid oxygenation products in pain and inflammation. *Annu Rev Immunol* 1984;**2**:335–58

Hemler M E. VLA proteins in the integrin family: structures, functions and their role on leukocytes. *Annu Rev Immunol* 1990;**8**:365–400.

Hynes R O. Integrins: versatility, modulation and signalling in cell adhesion. *Cell* 1992;**69**:11–25.

Lindhout E, Vissers J L M, Figdor C G, Adema G J. Chemokines and lymphocyte migration. *Immunologist* 1999;**7**:147–52.

Male D K. Cell traffic and inflammation. In: Male D K, Champion B, Cooke A, Owen M., Trowsdale J (eds). *Advanced Immunology*, 3rd London: Mosby, 1995; chap 14.

Proud D, Kaplan A P. Kinin formation: mechanism and role in inflammatory disorders. *Annu Rev Immunol* 1988;**6**:49–83.

Shimizu Y, Newman W, Gopal T V, et al. Four molecular pathways of T cell adhesion to endothelial cells. Roles of LFA-1, VCAM-1 and ELAM-1 and changes of pathway hierarchy under different activation conditions. *J Cell Biol* 1991;**113**:1203–12.

Springer T A. Adhesion receptors in the immune system. *Nature* 1990;**346**:425–34.

Springer T A. Traffic signals for lymphocyte recirculation and leukocyte emigration: the multistep paradigm. *Cell* 1994;**76**:301–14.

Complement

Aulak K S, Donaldson V H, Coutinho M, *et al.* Cl-inhibitor: structure/ function and biologic role. *Behring Inst Mitt* 1993;**93**:204–13.
Bhakdi S, Tranum-Jensen J. Complement lysis: a hole is a hole. *Immunol Today* 1991;**12**:318–20.
Campbell R D, Law S K A, Reid K B M, et al. Structure, organization, and regulation of the complement genes. *Annu Rev Immunol* 1988;**6**:161–95.
Colten H R, Rosen F S. Complement deficiencies. *Annu Rev Immunol* 1992;**10**:809–34.
Cooper N R. The classical complement pathway: activation and regulation of the first complement component. *Adv Immunol* 1985;**37**:151–216.
Dodds A W, Ren X D, Willis A C, et al. The reaction mechanism of the internal thioester in the human complement component C4. *Nature* 1996; **379**:177–9.
Farries T C, Atkinson J P. Evolution of the complement system. *Immunol Today* 1991;**12**:295–300.
Frank M M, Fries L F. The role of complement in inflammation and phagocytosis. *Immunol Today* 1991;**12**:322–6.
Gerard C, Gerard N P. C5a anaphylatoxin and its seven transmembrane-segment receptor. *Annu Rev Immunol* 1994;**12**:775–808.
Holmskov U, Maltotra R, Sim R B, et al. Collectins: collagenous C-type lectins of the innate immune defense system. *Immunol Today* 1994;**14**:67–74.
Hourcade D, Holers V M, Atkinson J P. The regulators of complement activation (RCA) gene cluster. *Adv Immunol* 1989;**45**:381–416.
Lambris J D, Reid K B M, Volanakis J E. The evolution, structure, biology and pathophysiology of complement. *Immunol Today* 1999; **20**:207–11.
Liszewski M K, Farries T C, Lublin D M, et al. Control of the complement system. *Adv Immunol* 1996;**61**:201–83.
Moffitt M C, Frank M M. Complement resistance in microbes. *Springer Semin Immunopathol* 1994;**15**:327–44.
Morgan B P. Complement regulatory molecules: application to therapy and transplantation. *Immunol Today* 1995;**16**:257–9.
Morgan B P, Meri S. Membrane proteins that protect against complement lysis. *Springer Semin Immunopathol* 1994;**15**:369–96.
Morgan B P, Walport M J. Complement deficiency and disease. *Immunol Today* 1991;**12**:301–6.
Muller-eberhard H J. The membrane attack complex of complement. *Annu Rev Immunol* 1986;**4**:503–28.
Muller-eberhard H J, Schreiber R D. Molecular biology and chemistry of the alternative pathway of complement. *Adv Immunol* 1980;**29**:1–53.
Reid K B M, Day A J. Structure–function relationships of the complement components. *Immunol Today* 1989;**10**:177–80.
Reid K B, Turner M W. Mammalian lectins in activation and clearance mechanisms involving the complement system. *Springer Semin Immunopathol* 1994;**15**:307–26.
Walport M J. Inherited complement deficiency – clues to the physiological activity of complement *in vivo*. *Q J Med* 1993;**86**:355–8.

4 Antibodies

- **Circulating antibodies** recognize antigen in serum and tissue fluids.
- **There are five classes of antibody – IgG, IgA, IgM, IgD and IgE.**
- **Immunoglobulins have a basic unit of two light chains and two heavy chains in a light-heavy-heavy-light arrangement.** The heavy chains differ between classes. IgA and IgM occur as oligomers of the four-chain unit.
- **The chains are folded into discrete regions called domains.** There are two domains in the light chain and four or five in the heavy chain, depending on their class.
- **Hypervariable regions form the antigen-binding sites.** There are three such regions in the V domains of each light and heavy chain. The folding of the domains causes them to be clustered at the distal tips of the molecule, producing two antigen-binding sites for each four-chain unit.
- **All antibodies are bifunctional.** They exhibit one or more **effector functions** in addition to antigen binding. These biological activities (e.g. complement activation and cell binding) are localized to sites that are distant from the antigen-binding sites (mostly in the Fc region).
- **Receptors for immunoglobulins** are expressed by mononuclear cells, neutrophils, natural killer (NK) cells, eosinophils and mast cells. They interact with the Fc regions of different classes of immunoglobulins and promote activities such as phagocytosis, tumour cell killing and mast cell degranulation. Most of the Fcγ receptors are members of the **immunoglobulin superfamily** and have two or three extracellular immunoglobulin domains.
- **Antibodies are highly specific for the three-dimensional conformation of the epitope.**
- **Antibody affinity** is a measure of the strength of the bond between an antibody's combining site and a single epitope. The functional affinity or avidity of the interaction additionally depends on the number of binding sites on the antibody and their ability to react with multiple epitopes on the antigen.
- **The immune system is able to recognize and respond to many antigens** by generating great diversity in the antibodies produced by the B cells.
- **Immunoglobulin light chains are encoded by V and J gene segments**; heavy chains are also encoded by V and J gene segments with additional diversity provided by the D gene segment.
- **Diversity is achieved by the recombination of a limited number of V, D and J gene segments** to produce a vast number of variable domains.
- **Immunoglobulin heavy and light chains** undergo structural modifications called somatic mutation following antigen stimulation which fine tunes their affinity.
- **Recombination of V, D and J gene segments** of immunoglobulins is controlled, at least in part, by two recombination activating genes (RAG-1 and RAG-2).
- **In addition to simple combinations of V, D and J regions**, diversity in immunoglobulins depends upon N-region diversification, joining-site variation and multiple D regions.
- **Immunoglobulin class-switching involves recombination of VDJ genes** with various C region genes and differential RNA splicing.

The recognition of foreign antigen is the hallmark of the specific adaptive immune response. Two distinct types of molecules are involved in this process – the immunoglobulins and the T-cell antigen receptors (TCRs). Diversity and heterogeneity are characteristic features of these molecules. In both cases there is evidence of extensive gene rearrangements which generate immunoglobulins or TCRs capable of recognizing many different antigens. T-cell receptors are discussed in detail in Chapter 5.

The immunoglobulins are a group of glycoproteins present in the serum and tissue fluids of all mammals. Some are carried on the surface of B cells, where they act as receptors for specific antigens. Others (antibodies) are free in the blood or lymph. Contact between B cells and antigen is needed to cause the B cells to develop into antibody forming cells (AFCs), also called plasma cells, which secrete large amounts of antibody. ('Plasma cell' is the original histological term used to describe AFCs seen in blood and tissues.) The membrane-bound immunoglobulin on a precursor B cell has the same binding specificity as the antibody produced by the mature AFC (*Fig. 4.1*).

IMMUNOGLOBULINS – A FAMILY OF PROTEINS

Five distinct classes of immunoglobulin molecule are recognized in most higher mammals, namely IgG, IgA, IgM, IgD and IgE. They differ in size, charge, amino acid composition and carbohydrate content. In addition to the difference between classes, the immunoglobulins within each class are also very heterogeneous. Electrophoretically the immunoglobulins show a unique range of heterogeneity which extends from the γ to the α fractions of normal serum (*Fig. 4.2*).

Immunoglobulins are bifunctional molecules

Each immunoglobulin molecule is bifunctional. One region of the molecule is concerned with binding to antigen while a different region mediates so-called effector functions. Effector functions include binding of the immunoglobulin to host tissues, to various cells of the immune system, to some phagocytic cells, and to the first component (C1q) of the classical complement system.

Surface and secreted antibodies

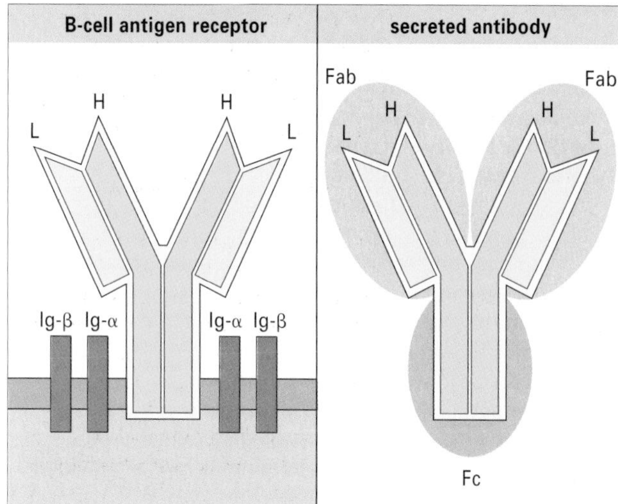

Fig. 4.1 The B-cell antigen receptor (left) consists of two identical heavy (H) chains and two identical light (L) chains. In addition, secondary components (Ig-α and Ig-β) are closely associated with the primary receptor and are thought to couple it to intracellular signalling pathways. Circulating antibodies (right) are structurally identical to the primary B-cell antigen receptors, except that they lack the transmembrane and intracytoplasmic sections. Many proteolytic enzymes cleave antibody molecules into three fragments – two identical Fab (antigen binding) fragments and one Fc (crystallizable) fragment.

Distribution of the major human immunoglobulins

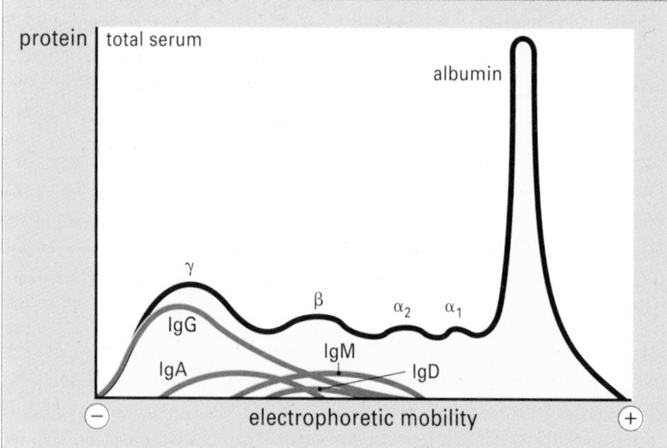

Fig. 4.2 Electrophoresis of human serum showing the distribution of the four major immunoglobulin classes. Serum proteins are separated according to their charges in an electric field, and classified as α_1, α_2, β and γ, depending on their mobility. (The IgE class has a similar mobility to IgD but cannot be represented quantitatively because of its low level in serum.) IgG exhibits the most charge heterogeneity, the other classes having a more restricted mobility in the β and fast γ regions.

Immunoglobulin class and subclass depends on the structure of the heavy chain

The basic structure of all immunoglobulin molecules is a unit consisting of two identical light polypeptide chains and two identical heavy polypeptide chains. These are linked together by disulphide bonds. The class and subclass of an immunoglobulin molecule are determined by its heavy chain type. Thus the four human IgG subclasses (IgG1, IgG2, IgG3 and IgG4) have heavy chains called γ1, γ2, γ3 and γ4 that differ slightly, although all are recognizably γ heavy chains.

The four subclasses of human IgG (IgG1–IgG4) occur in the approximate proportions of 66%, 23%, 7% and 4%, respectively. There are also known to be subclasses of human IgA (IgA1 and IgA2), but none have been described for IgM, IgD or IgE. This range of immunoglobulin class and subclass reflects isotypic variations in the immunoglobulin genes (see below). Immunoglobulin subclasses appear to have arisen late in evolution. Thus, the human IgG subclasses are very different from the four known subclasses of IgG that have been identified in the mouse. All immunoglobulins are glycoproteins, but the carbohydrate content ranges from 2–3% for IgG, to 12–14% for IgM, IgD and IgE. The physicochemical properties of the immunoglobulins are summarized in *Figure. 4.3.*

IgG – The major immunoglobulin in normal human serum, accounting for 70–75% of the total immunoglobulin pool, IgG consists of a single four-chain molecule with a sedimentation coefficient of 7S and a molecular weight of 146 000. However, IgG3 proteins are slightly larger than the other subclasses; due to the slightly heavier γ3 chain.

IgM – Accounts for approximately 10% of the immunoglobulin pool. The molecule is a pentamer of the basic four-chain structure. The individual heavy chains have a molecular weight of approximately 65 000 and the whole molecule has a molecular weight of 970 000.

IgA – Represents 15–20% of the human serum immunoglobulin pool. In humans more than 80% of IgA occurs as a monomer of the four-chain unit, but in most mammals the IgA in serum is mainly polymeric, occurring mostly as a dimer. IgA is the predominant immunoglobulin in seromucous secretions such as saliva, colostrum, milk, and tracheobronchial and genitourinary secretions. Secretory IgA (s-IgA), may be of either subclass (IgA1 or IgA2), exists mainly in the 11S, dimeric form and has a molecular weight of 385 000 due to its association with another protein, known as the secretory component.

IgD – Accounts for less than 1% of the total plasma immunoglobulin but is a major component of the surface membrane of many B cells.

IgE – Though scarce in serum, is found on the surface membrane of basophils and mast cells in all individuals.

Physicochemical properties of human immunoglobulin classes

property	immunoglobulin type									
	IgG1	IgG2	IgG3	IgG4	IgM	IgA1	IgA2	sIgA	IgD	IgE
heavy chain	γ_1	γ_2	γ_3	γ_4	μ	α_1	α_2	α_1/α_2	δ	ϵ
mean serum conc. (mg/ml)	9	3	1	0.5	1.5	3.0	0.5	0.05	0.03	0.00005
sedimentation constant	7s	7s	7s	7s	19s	7s	7s	11s	7s	8s
mol. wt (× 10^3)	146	146	170	146	970	160	160	385	184	188
half-life (days)	21	20	7	21	10	6	6	?	3	2
% intravascular distribution	45	45	45	45	80	42	42	trace	75	50
carbohydrate (%)	2–3	2–3	2–3	2–3	12	7–11	7–11	7–11	9–14	12

Fig. 4.3 Each immunoglobulin class has a characteristic type of heavy chain. Thus IgG posesses γ chains; IgM, μ chains; IgA, α chains; IgD, δ chains; and IgE, ε chains. Variation in heavy chain structure within a class gives rise to immunoglobulin subclasses. For example, the human IgG pool consists of four subclasses reflecting four distinct types of heavy chain. The properties of the immunoglobulins vary between the different classes. Note that in secretions, IgA occurs in a dimeric form (s-IgA) in association with a protein chain termed the secretory component. The serum concentration of s-IgA is very low, whereas the level in intestinal secretions can be very high.

The basic structure of IgG1

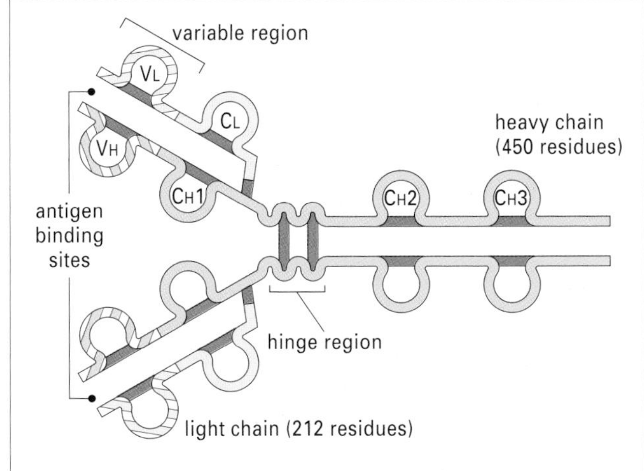

Fig. 4.4 The N-terminal end of IgG1 is characterized by sequence variability (V) in both the heavy and light chains, referred to as the VH and VL regions respectively. The rest of the molecule has a relatively constant (C) structure. The constant portion of the light chain is termed the CL region. The constant portion of the heavy chain is further divided into three structurally discrete regions: CH1, CH2 and CH3. These globular regions, which are stabilized by intrachain disulphide bonds, are referred to as 'domains'. The sites at which the antibody binds antigen are located in the variable domains. The hinge region is a segment of heavy chain between the CH1 and CH2 domains. Flexibility in this area permits the two antigen-binding sites to operate independently. There is close pairing of the domains except in the CH2 region (see *Fig. 4.6*). Carbohydrate moieties are attached to the CH2 domains.

The basic four-chain model for immunoglobulin molecules (*Fig. 4.4*) is based on two distinct types of polypeptide chain. The smaller (light) chain has a molecular weight of 25 000 and is common to all classes, whereas the larger (heavy) chain has a molecular weight of 50 000–77 000 and is structurally distinct for each class or subclass. The polypeptide chains are linked together by covalent and non-covalent forces.

All light chains have one variable and one constant region

The light chains of most vertebrates have been shown to exist in two distinct forms called kappa (κ) and lambda (λ). These are isotypes, being present in all individuals. Either of the light chain types may combine with any of the heavy chain types, but in any one immunoglobulin molecule both light chains and both heavy chains are of the same type.

Hilschmann, Craig and others in 1965 established that light chains consist of two distinct regions. The C-terminal half of the chain (approximately 107 amino acid residues) is constant except for certain allotypic and isotypic variations (see *Fig. 4.27*) and is called the CL (Constant : Light chain) region, whereas the N-terminal half of the chain shows much sequence variability and is known as the VL (Variable : Light chain) region.

IgG has a 'typical' antibody structure

The IgG molecule may be thought of as a 'typical' antibody (Fig. 4.4). It has two intrachain disulphide bonds in the light chain – one in the variable region and one in the constant region (*Fig. 4.5*). There are four such bonds in the heavy (γ) chain, which is twice the length of the light chain. Each disulphide bond encloses a peptide loop of 60–70 amino acid residues; if the amino acid sequences of these loops are compared a striking degree of homology is revealed. Essentially this means that each immunoglobulin peptide chain is composed of a series of globular regions with very similar secondary and tertiary structure (folding). This is shown for the light chain in *Figure 4.5*.

The peptide loops enclosed by the disulphide bonds represent the central portion of a 'domain' of about 110 amino acid residues. In both the heavy and the light chains

Basic folding in the light chain

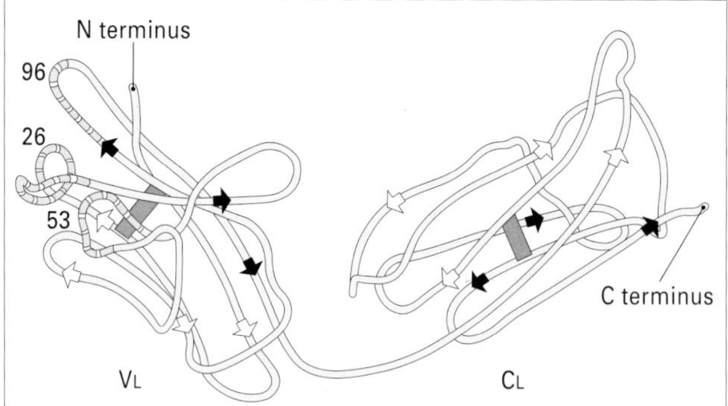

Fig. 4.5 The immunoglobulin domains in the light chain share a basic folding pattern with several straight segments of polypeptide chain lying parallel to the long axis of the domain. Light chains have two domains – one constant and one variable. Within each domain, the polypeptide chain is arranged in two layers, running in opposite directions, with many hydrophobic amino acid side-chains between the layers. One of the layers has four segments (arrowed white), the other has three (arrowed black); both are linked by a single disulphide bond (red). Folding of the VL domains causes the hypervariable regions to become exposed in three separate but closely disposed loops. One numbered residue from each hypervariable region is identified.

the first of these domains corresponds to the variable region, VH and VL respectively. In the heavy chain of IgG, IgA and IgD there are three further domains, which make up the constant part of the chain, CH1, CH2 and CH3. In both μ and ε chains there is an additional domain immediately after CH1 (*Fig. 4.6*). Thus, the C-terminal domains of IgM and IgE heavy chains (referred to as Cμ4 and Cε4) are homologous to the CH3 domain of IgG (Cγ3).

X-ray crystallography has provided structural data on complete IgG molecules, making it possible to construct both α-carbon backbone and computer-generated atomic models for this class of immunoglobulin (*Fig. 4.7*). These show the Y-shaped and T-shaped structures that have also been visualized by electron microscopy.

Homologous domains of the light and heavy chains are paired in the Fab region (indicated in *Fig. 4.6*). The Cγ3 domains of the γ heavy chains are also paired, but the Cγ2 domains are separated by carbohydrate moieties. Despite the structural similarities between domains there are striking differences at the level of domain interaction. For example, the variable domains associate with each other through their three-segment layers, whereas the constant domains associate through their four-segment layers. (See *Fig. 4.5* for an explanation of the layers in light chain domains.)

IgG – With human IgG, the four subclasses differ only slightly in their amino acid sequences. Most of the differences are clustered in the hinge region and give rise to differing patterns of interchain disulphide bonds between the four proteins. The most striking structural difference is the elongated hinge region of IgG3, which accounts for its higher molecular weight and possibly for some of its enhanced biological activity (*Fig. 4.6(2)*).

IgM – Human IgM is usually found as a pentamer of the basic four-chain unit (*Fig. 4.6(3)*). The μ chains of IgM differ from γ chains in amino acid sequence and have an extra constant region domain. The subunits of the pentamer are linked by disulphide bonds between the Cμ3 domains, and possibly by disulphide bonds between the C-terminal 18-residue peptide tailpieces. The complete molecule consists of a densely packed central region with radiating arms, as seen in electron micrographs.

Photographs of IgM antibodies binding to bacterial flagella show molecules adopting a 'crab-like' configuration (*Fig. 4.8*). This suggests that flexion readily occurs between the Cμ2 and Cμ3 domains, although note that this region is not structurally homologous to the IgG hinge. The dislocation resulting in the 'crab-like' configuration appears to be related to the activation of complement by IgM.

Two other features characterize the IgM molecule: an abundance of oligosaccharide units associated with the μ chain, and an additional peptide chain, the J (joining) chain, thought to assist the process of polymerization prior to secretion by the AFC. The J chain is an Ig-like domain of 137 amino acid residues. One J chain is incorporated into the IgM structure by disulphide bonding to the 18-residue peptide tailpiece of the separate monomers. Binding is to the penultimate cysteine residues of the tailpieces. If J chains are not freely available, there is evidence that hexameric IgM becomes the preferred form.

Fig. 4.6 In each of the structures shown the carbohydrate side-chains are shown in blue. Inter heavy chain disulphide bonds are shown in red but interchain bonds between H and L chains are omitted.
(1) A model of IgG1 indicating the globular domains of heavy (H) and light (L) chains. Note the apposition of the CH3 domains and the separation of the CH2 domains. The carbohydrate units lie between the CH2 domains.
(2) Polypeptide chain structure of human IgG3. Note the elongated hinge region.
(3) IgM heavy chains have five domains with disulphide bonds cross-linking adjacent Cμ3 and Cμ4 domains. The possible location of the J chain is shown. IgM does not have extended hinge regions, but flexion can occur about the Cμ2 domains.
(4) The secretory component of s-IgA is probably wound around the dimer and attached by two disulphide bonds to the Cα2 domain of one IgA monomer. The J chain is required to join the two subunits.
(5) This diagram of IgD shows the domain structure and a characteristically large number of oligosaccharide units. Note also the presence of a hinge region and short octapeptide tailpieces.
(6) IgE can be cleaved by enzymes to give the fragments $F(ab')_2$, Fc and Fc'. Note the absence of a hinge region.

Structural characteristics of various human immunoglobulins

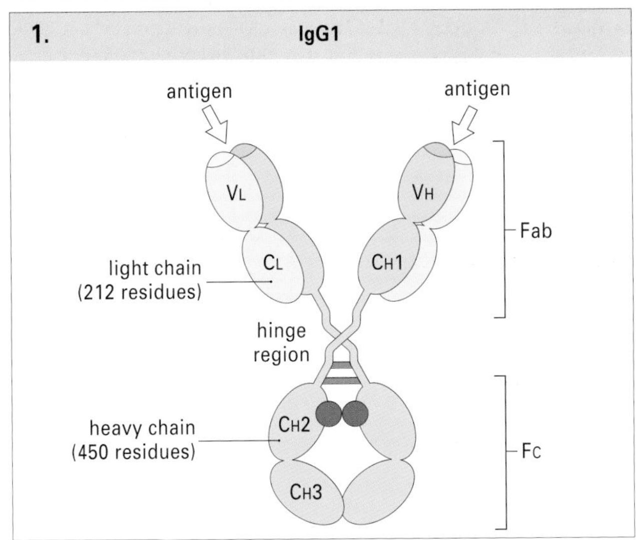

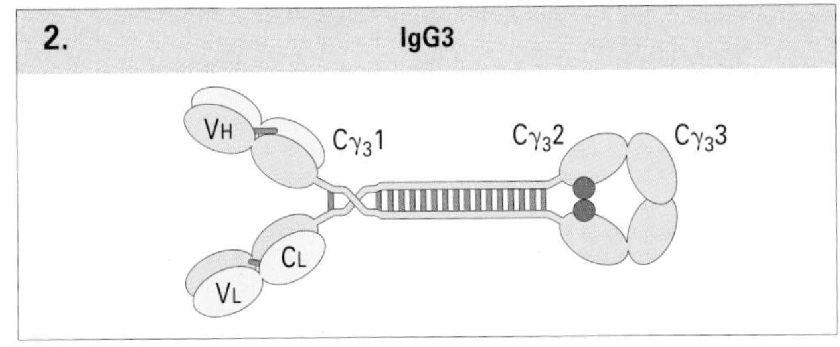

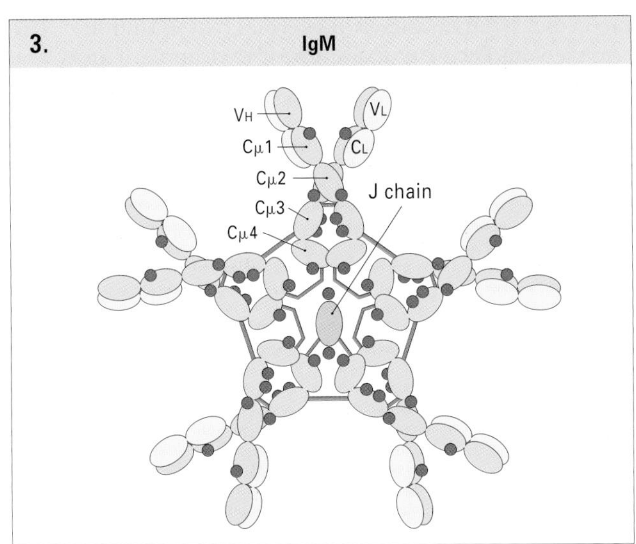

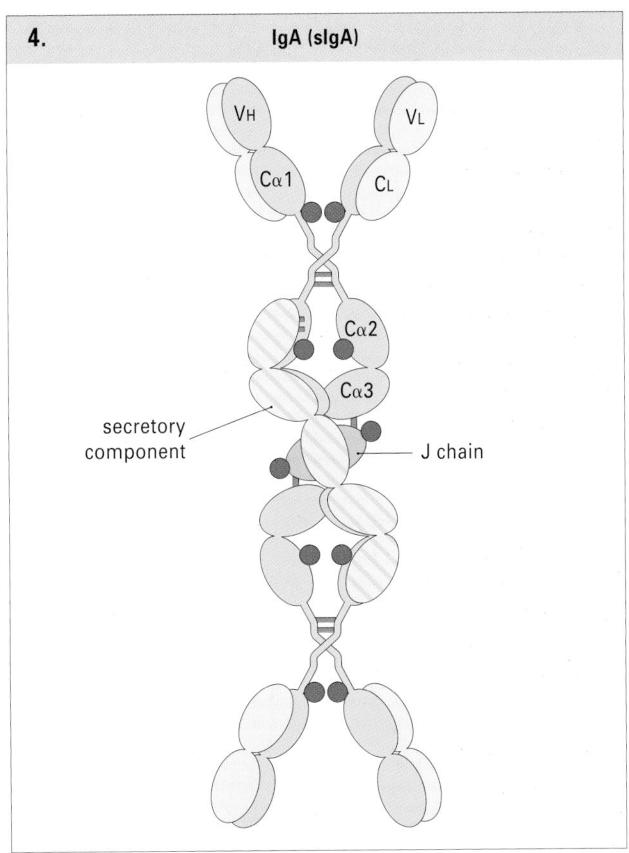

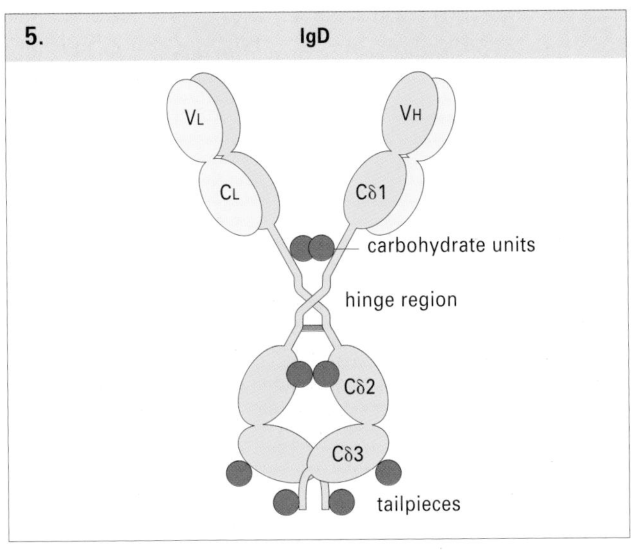

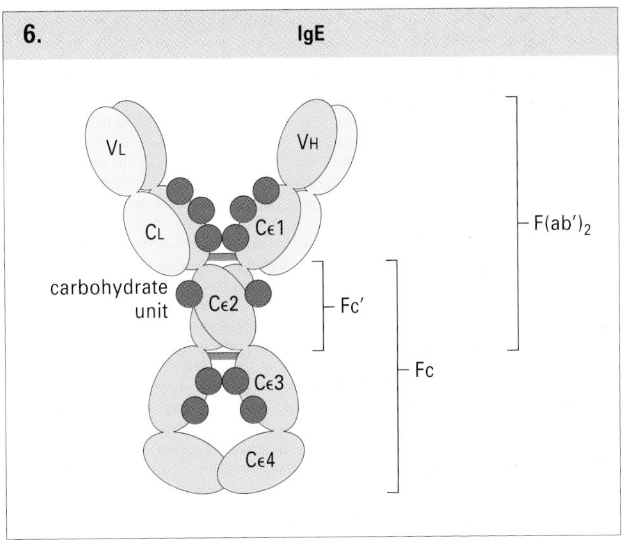

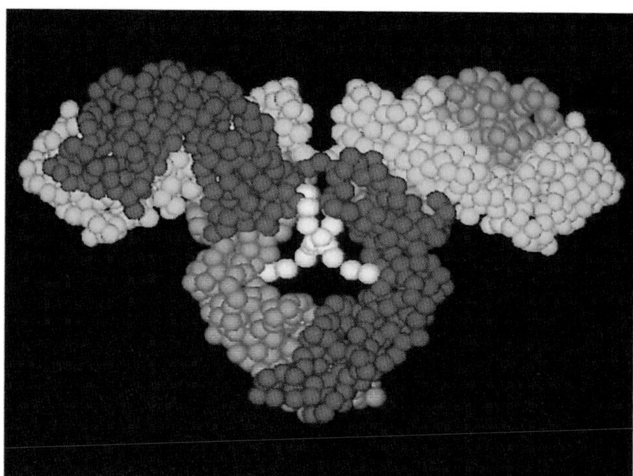

Fig. 4.7 Computer-generated model of the hinge-deleted human IgG1 protein Dob. Such proteins lack the flexibility characteristic of normal IgG molecules. Their rigidity permits structural determinations at a higher resolution. One heavy chain is shown in blue and one in red, with two light chains being depicted in green. Carbohydrate bound to the Fc portion of the molecule is shown in turquoise. The model suggests that interactions between the Cγ2 domains are weak whereas those between Cγ3 domains are strong. (The structure of this immunoglobulin was determined by David R. Davies *et al. Proc Natl Acad Sci USA* 1977; **74**; the computer graphics were generated using the system developed by Richard J. Feldmann at the National Institutes of Health.)

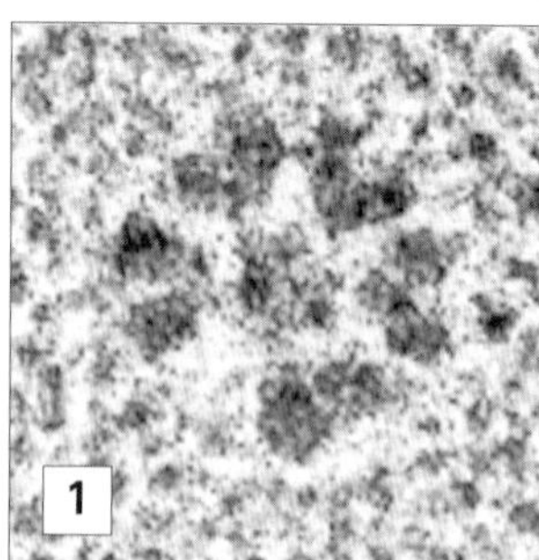

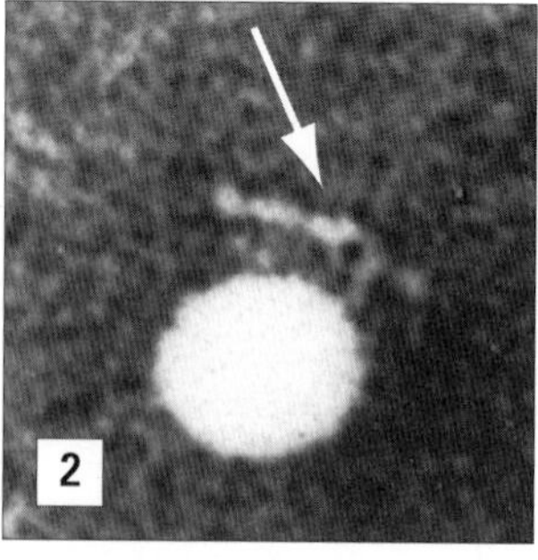

Fig. 4.8 Electron micrographs of IgM molecules. (1) In free solution, deer IgM adopts the characteristic star-shaped configuration. ×195 000. (Courtesy of Drs E. Holm Nielson P. Storgaard and Prof S-E. Svehag.) **(2)** Rabbit IgM antibody (arrowed) in 'crab-like' configuration with partly visible central ring structure bound to a poliovirus virion ×190 000. (Courtesy of Dr B. Chesebro and Professor S-E Svehag.)

IgA – The 472 amino acid residues of the α chain are arranged in four domains: VH, Cα1, Cα2 and Cα3. A feature shared with IgM is an additional C-terminal 18-residue peptide with a penultimate cysteine residue, which is able to bind covalently to a J chain to form dimers. Electron micrographs of IgA dimers show double Y-shaped structures, suggesting that the monomeric subunits are linked end-to-end through the C-terminal Cα3 regions (*Fig. 4.9*).

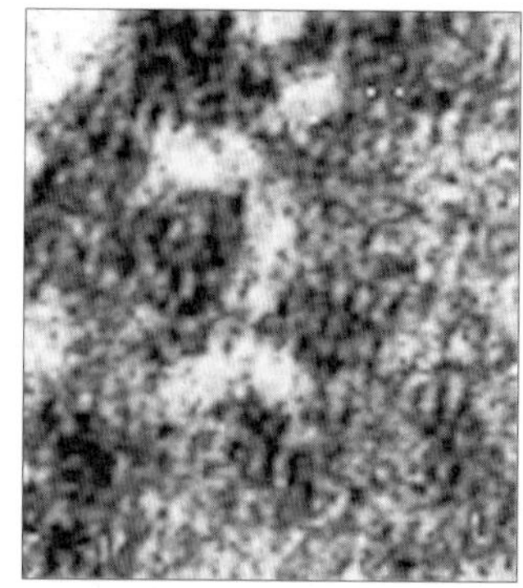

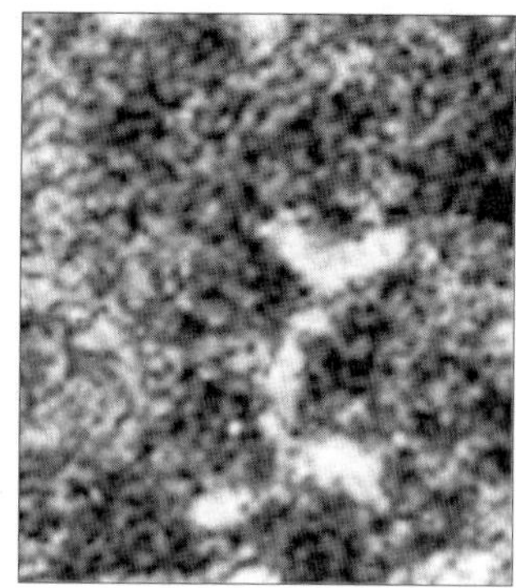

Fig. 4.9 Electron micrographs of human dimeric IgA molecules. The double Y-shaped appearance suggests that the monomeric subunits are linked end to end through the C-terminal Cα3 domain ×250 000. (Courtesy of Professor S-E. Svehag.)

Secretory IgA (s-IgA) exists mainly in the form of a molecule sedimenting at 11s (mol. wt 380 000). The complete molecule is made up of two units of IgA, one secretory component (mol. wt 70 000) and one J chain (mol. wt 15 000) (*Fig. 4.6(4)*). It is not clear how the various peptide chains are linked together. In contrast to the J chain, secretory component is not synthesized by plasma cells but by epithelial cells. IgA held in dimer configuration by a J chain, and secreted by submucosal plasma cells, actively binds secretory component as it traverses epithelial cell layers. Bound secretory component facilitates the transport of s-IgA into secretions, as well as protecting it from proteolytic attack.

IgD – Less than 1% of the total immunoglobulin in serum is IgD. This protein is more susceptible to proteolysis than IgG1, IgG2, IgA or IgM, and also has a tendency to undergo spontaneous proteolysis. There appears to be a single disulphide bond between the δ chains and a large amount of carbohydrate distributed in multiple oligosaccharide units (*Fig. 4.6(5)*).

IgE – The structure of IgE is shown in *Figure 4.6(6)*. The higher molecular weight of the ε chain (72 500) is explained by the larger number of amino acid residues (approximately 550) distributed over five domains (VH, Cε1, Cε2, Cε3 and Cε4).

Immunoglobulins are the prototypes of the immunoglobulin superfamily of molecules

The basic domain structure first identified in antibodies also occurs in a number of other molecules, including many cell surface molecules involved in immune reactions. Examples of such molecules are the adhesion molecules ICAM-1 and VCAM-1 (see Chapter 3), the T-cell antigen receptor and MHC molecules (see Chapter 5), as well as several receptors for antibodies, encountered later in this chapter. Such molecules are said to belong to the immunoglobulin supergene family (IgSF). The principle elements of the domain are two β-pleated sheets arranged opposite each other and usually stabilized by one or more disulphide bonds. This is sometimes referred to as a β-barrel. The domain structure must have developed early in evolution and has been used since as the basis for different molecules as vertebrates have radiated and developed.

INTERACTION OF ANTIBODIES WITH ANTIGENS

Antibodies form multiple non-covalent bonds with antigen

X-ray crystallography studies of antibody V domains show that the hypervariable regions are clustered at the end of the Fab arms; particular residues in these regions interact specifically with antigen. The framework residues do not usually form bonds with the antigen. However, they are essential for producing the folding of the V domains and maintaining the integrity of the binding site. The binding of antigen to antibody involves the formation of multiple non-covalent bonds between the antigen and amino acids of the binding site. Considered individually, the attractive forces (hydrogen and electrostatic bonds, Van der Waals and hydrophobic forces) are weak by comparison with co-valent bonds. However, the large number of interactions results in a large total binding energy.

The conformations of target antigen and binding site are complementary

The strength of a non-covalent bond is critically dependent on the distance (d) between the interacting groups. The force is proportional to $1/d^2$ for electrostatic forces, and to $1/d^7$ for Van der Waals forces. Thus the interacting groups must be close (in molecular terms) before these forces become significant (*Fig. 4.10*). In order for an antigenic determinant (epitope) and an antibody-combining site (paratope) to combine (*Fig. 4.11*), there must be suitable atomic groupings on opposing parts of the antigen and antibody, and the shape of the combining site must fit the epitope, so that several non-covalent bonds can form simultaneously. If the antigen and the combining site are complementary in this way, there will be sufficient binding energy to resist thermodynamic disruption of the bond. However, if electron clouds of the antigen and antibody overlap, steric repulsive forces come into play which are inversely proportional to the 12th power of the distance between the clouds: $F \propto 1/d^{12}$. These forces have a vital role in determining the specificity of the antibody molecule for a particular antigen, and its ability to discriminate between antigens, as any variation from the ideal complementary shape will cause a decrease in the total binding energy through increased repulsive forces and decreased attractive forces (*Fig. 4.11*). This is not to say that the antigen-binding site is completely inflexible; when antigen binds to antibody individual amino acid residues may become slightly displaced from their position in the free state. This is referred to as 'induced fit', but it will only occur when the energy gain in the overall antigen–antibody bond offsets that needed to induce the fit.

An examination of the interaction between lysozyme and the Fab of an antibody to lysozyme has shown that the antigen epitope and the binding site have complementary surfaces. These surfaces extend beyond the hypervariable regions. In total, 17 amino acid residues on the antibody contact 16 residues on the lysozyme molecule (*Fig. 4.12*). All the hypervariable regions contribute to the antibody-

Intermolecular attractive forces

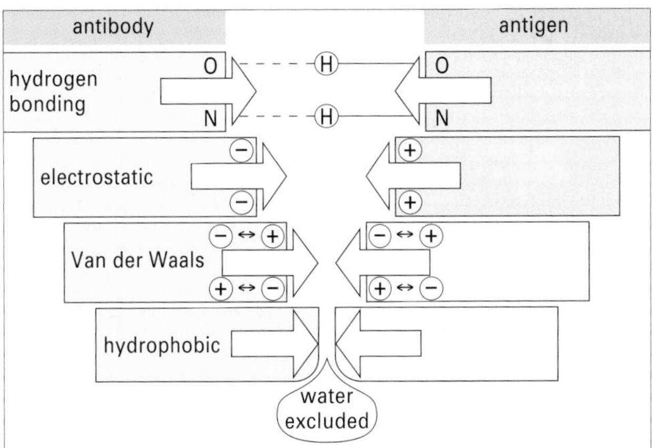

Fig. 4.10 The forces binding antigen to antibody require the close approach of the interacting groups. Hydrogen bonding results from the formation of hydrogen bridges between appropriate atoms. Electrostatic forces derive from the attraction of oppositely charged groups located on two protein side-chains. Van der Waals bonds are generated by the interaction between electron clouds (here represented as induced oscillating dipoles). Hydrophobic bonds (which may contribute up to half the total strength of the antigen–antibody bond) rely on the association of non-polar, hydrophobic groups so that contact with water molecules is minimized. The distance between the interacting groups that gives optimum binding depends on the type of bond.

Good fit and poor fit

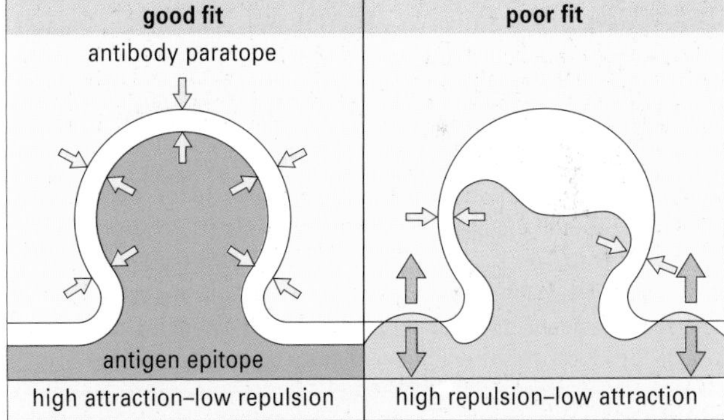

Fig. 4.11 A good fit between the antigenic determinant and the binding site of the antibody will create ample opportunities for intermolecular attractive forces to be created and few opportunities for repulsive forces to operate. Conversely, when there is a poor fit, the reverse is true. When electron clouds overlap, high repulsive forces are generated which override any small forces of attraction.

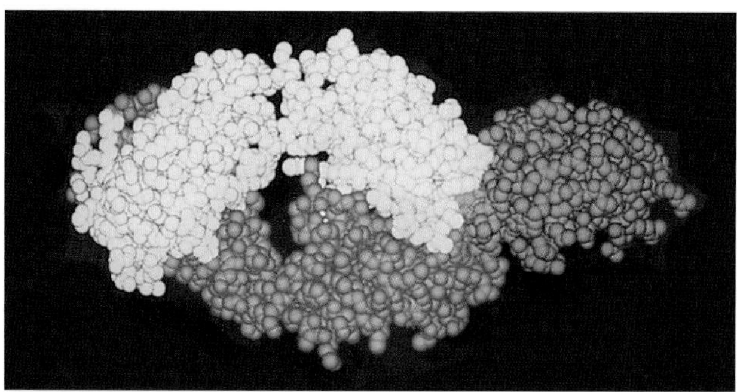

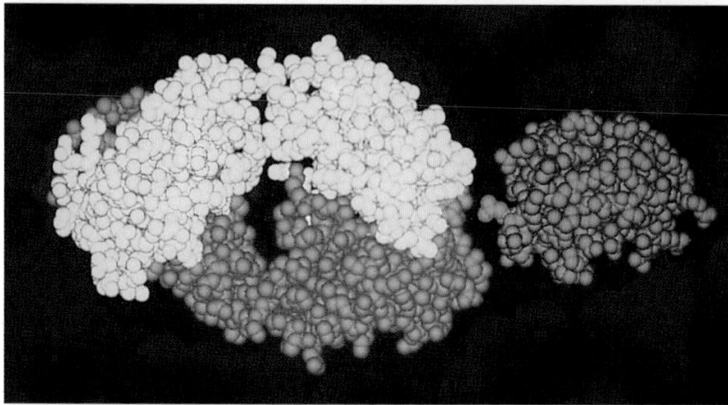

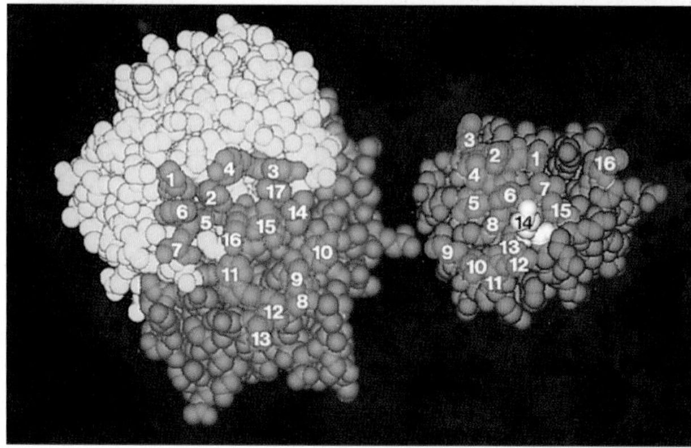

Fig. 4.12 The Fab–lysozyme complex. Upper: Lysozyme (green) binds to the hypervariable regions of the heavy (blue) and light (yellow) chains of the Fab fragment of antibody D1.3. Centre: The separated complex with Glu 121 visible (red). This residue fits into the centre of the cleft between the heavy and light chains. Lower: The same molecules rotated 90° to show the contact residues which contribute to the antigen–antibody bond. (Courtesy of Dr R. J. Poljak, from Science 1986;**233**:747–53, with permission.)

binding site, although the third hypervariable region, formed by the V–D–J junction in the heavy chain gene, lying at the centre of the combining site, appears to be most important. This may also be related to the greater variability generated by recombination of the V, D and J segments.

Antibody affinity indicates the strength of a single antigen–antibody bond

The strength of the bond between an antigen and an antibody is known as the antibody affinity. It is the sum of the attractive and repulsive forces described above (*Fig. 4.13*). Interaction of the antibody-combining site with antigen

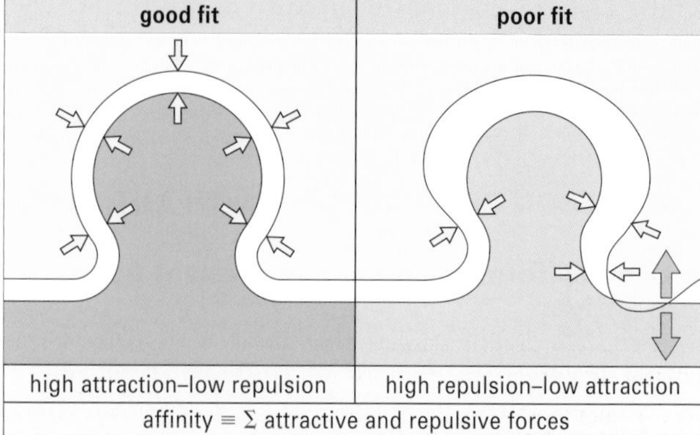

Fig. 4.13 The affinity with which antibody binds antigen is the sum of the attractive and repulsive forces between them. A high-affinity antibody implies a good fit and, conversely, a low-affinity antibody implies a poor fit.

can be investigated thermodynamically. To measure the affinity of a single combining site, it is necessary to use a monovalent antigen, or even a single isolated antigenic determinant (a hapten). Because the non-covalent bonds between antibody and epitope are dissociable, the overall combination of an antibody and antigen must be reversible; thus the Law of Mass Action can be applied to the reaction and the equilibrium constant, K, can be determined. This is the affinity constant (*Fig. 4.14*).

Antibody avidity indicates the overall strength of interaction between antibody and antigen

Because each antibody unit of four polypeptide chains has two antigen-binding sites, antibodies are potentially multivalent in their reaction with antigen. In addition, antigen can also be monovalent (e.g. haptens) or multivalent (e.g. microorganisms). The strength with which a multivalent antibody binds a multivalent antigen is termed avidity, to differentiate it from the affinity of a single antigenic determinant for an individual combining site. The avidity of

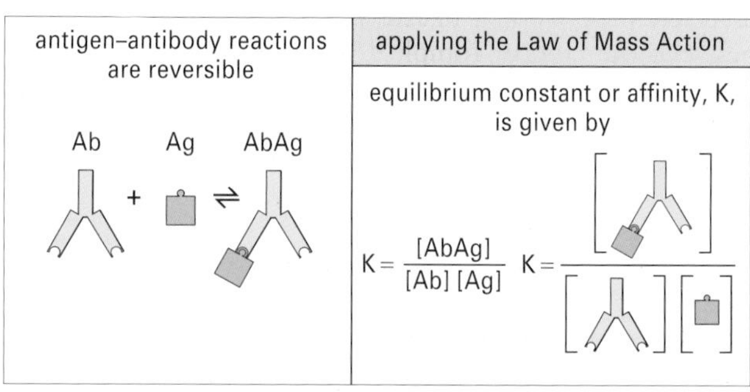

Fig. 4.14 All antigen–antibody reactions are reversible. The Law of Mass Action can therefore be applied, and the antibody affinity (given by the equilibrium constant, K) can be calculated. (Square brackets refer to the concentrations of the reactants.)

Affinity and avidity

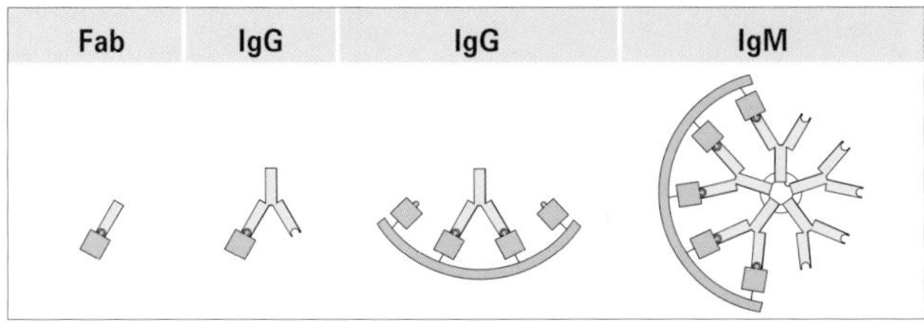

antibody	Fab	IgG	IgG	IgM
effective antibody valence	1	1	2	up to 10
antigen valence	1	1	n	n
equilibrium constant (L/M)	10^4	10^4	10^7	10^{11}
advantage of multivalence	–	–	10^3-fold	10^7-fold
definition of binding	affinity	affinity	avidity	avidity
	intrinsic affinity		functional affinity	

Fig. 4.15 Multivalent binding between antibody and antigen (avidity or functional affinity) results in a considerable increase in stability as measured by the equilibrium constant, compared with simple monovalent binding (affinity or intrinsic affinity, here arbitrarily assigned a value of 10^4 L/M^{-1}). This is sometimes referred to as the 'bonus effect' of multivalency. Thus there may be a 10^3-fold increase in the binding energy of IgG when both valencies (combining sites) are utilized and a 10^7-fold increase when IgM binds antigen in a multivalent manner.

an antibody for its antigen is dependent on the affinities of the individual combining sites for the determinants on the antigen. It is greater than the sum of these affinities if both antibody-binding sites can combine with the antigen. This is because all the antigen–antibody bonds must be broken simultaneously before the antigen and antibody dissociate (*Fig. 4.15*). In normal physiological situations, avidity is likely to be more relevant than affinity, as naturally occurring antigens are multivalent. However, the precise measurement of hapten–antibody affinity is more likely to give an insight into the immunochemical nature of the antigen–antibody reaction.

Kinetics of antibody–antigen reactions

Measurements of antibody affinity relate to equilibrium conditions. Affinity indicates the tendency of the antibodies to form stable complexes with the antigen. However, for many biological activities of antibodies, it is possible that the kinetics of the reaction may also be significant. Kinetics measures the forward rate (on-rate) constant $K_{1,2}$ ($mol^{-1}s^{-1}$) and the reverse rate (off-rate) constant $K_{2,1}$ (s^{-1}). At equilibrium, the ratio of the two constants gives the equilibrium constant, or affinity, of the antibody. It has been claimed that differences in affinity are primarily the result of differences in off-rates, but more recently it has been shown that affinity can also be influenced by differences in on-rates.

It has been suggested that B-cell selection and stimulation during a maturing antibody response depend upon both selection for the ability of antibodies to bind to antigens rapidly (kinetic selection) and selection for the ability to bind antigens tightly (thermodynamic selection).

Antibody specificity and affinity

Antigen–antibody reactions can show a high level of specificity. For example, antibodies to measles virus will bind to the measles virus and confer immunity to this disease, but will not combine with, or protect against, an unrelated virus such as polio. The specificity of an antiserum is equal to the sum of the actions of every antibody in that antiserum. The antibody population may contain many antigen-binding sites, each reacting with a different epitope, or even with different parts of the same epitope (*Fig. 4.16*). However, when some of the epitopes of an antigen, A, are shared by another antigen, B, then a proportion of the antibodies directed to A will also react with B. This phenomenon is termed cross-reactivity.

Antibodies recognize the overall conformation of antigens

Clearly, antibodies recognize the overall shape of an epitope rather than particular chemical residues (*Fig. 4.17*). Antibodies are capable of expressing remarkable specificity, and are able to distinguish between small differences in the primary amino acid sequence of protein antigens, in addition to differences in charge, optical configuration and steric conformation. One consequence of this specificity is that many antibodies will bind only to native antigens, or to fragments of antigens that retain sufficient tertiary structure to permit the multiple interactions required for bond formation (*Fig. 4.18*).

When considering antibodies which bind to protein antigens, we can distinguish some which interact with epitopes consisting of a single contiguous stretch of amino acids (a continuous epitope) from others which bind to epitopes formed from separated segments of the polypeptide chain (discontinuous epitopes). Antibodies which bind to discontinuous epitopes often do not bind to denatured antigens e.g. in Western blots.

Specificity can also create a problem when one wishes to produce antibodies for immunological assays. It is often

Specificity, cross-reactivity and non-reactivity

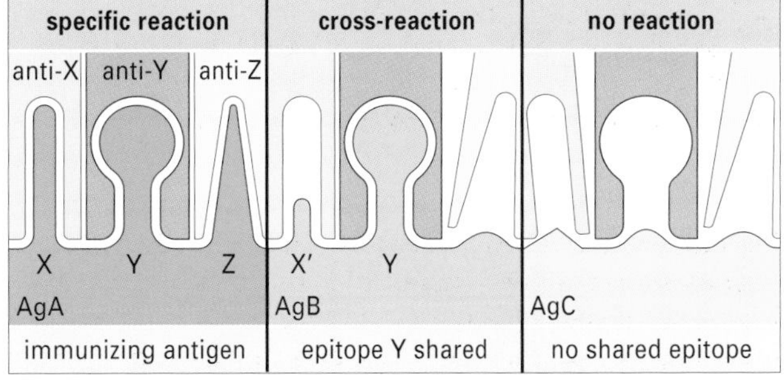

Fig. 4.16 Antiserum specificity results from the action of a population of individual antibody molecules (anti-X, anti-Y, anti-Z) directed against different epitopes (X, Y, Z) on the same or different antigen molecules. Antigen A (AgA) and antigen B (AgB) have epitope Y in common. Antiserum raised against AgA (anti-XYZ) not only reacts specifically with AgA, but cross-reacts with AgB (through recognition of epitopes Y and X'). The antiserum gives no reaction with AgC because there are no shared epitopes.

Specificity and cross-reactivity

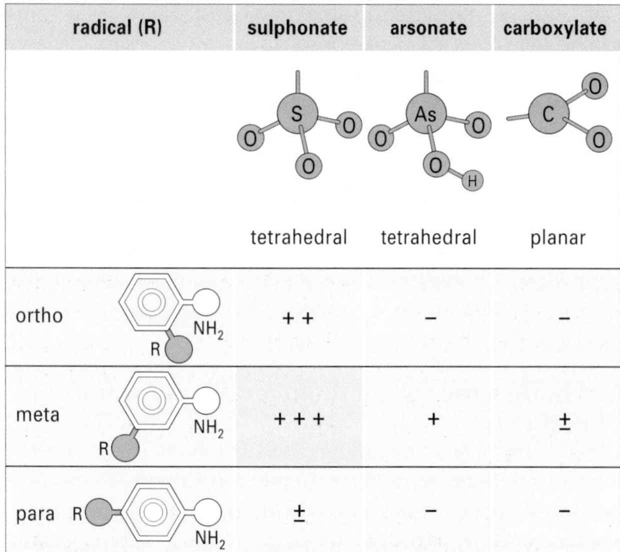

radical (R)	sulphonate	arsonate	carboxylate
	tetrahedral	tetrahedral	planar
ortho	+ +	–	–
meta	+ + +	+	±
para	±	–	–

Fig. 4.17 Antiserum raised to the meta isomer of aminobenzene sulphonate (the immunizing hapten), is mixed with ortho and para isomers of aminobenzene sulphonate, and also with the three isomers (ortho, meta, para) of two different but related antigens: aminobenzene arsonate and aminobenzene carboxylate. The antiserum reacts specifically with the sulphonate group in the meta position, but will cross-react (although more weakly) with sulphonate in the ortho position. Further, weaker cross-reactions are possible when the antiserum is reacted with either the arsonate group or the carboxylate group in the meta, but not in the ortho or para position. Arsonate is larger than sulphonate and has an extra hydrogen atom, while carboxylate is the smallest. These data suggest that an antigen's configuration is as important as the individual chemical groupings that it contains.

Configurational specificity

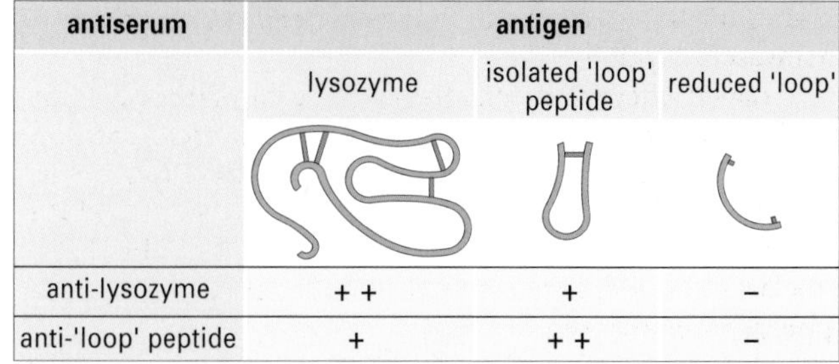

antiserum	antigen		
	lysozyme	isolated 'loop' peptide	reduced 'loop'
anti-lysozyme	+ +	+	–
anti-'loop' peptide	+	+ +	–

Fig. 4.18 The lysozyme molecule possesses an intrachain bond (red) which produces a loop in the peptide chain. Antisera raised against whole lysozyme (anti-lysozyme) and the isolated loop (anti-'loop' peptide), are able to distinguish between the two. Neither antiserum reacts with the isolated loop in its linear, reduced form. This demonstrates the importance of tertiary structure in determining antibody specificity.

easier to synthesize short polypeptide antigens of known primary structure than it is to purify sufficient amounts of the native antigen for immunization. However, antibodies to the synthetic polypeptides often do not bind well or predictably to the antigen in its native form.

FUNCTIONS OF ANTIBODIES

The primary function of an antibody is to bind antigen. In a few cases this has a direct effect, for example by neutralizing bacterial toxin, or by preventing viral attachment to host cells. In general, however, the interaction of antibody and antigen is without significance unless secondary 'effector' functions come into play (*Fig. 4.19*).

Selected effector functions of human immunoglobulins

Function		immunoglobulin									
		IgG1	IgG2	IgG3	IgG4	IgM	IgA1	IgA2	sIgA	IgD	IgE
complement fixation (classical pathway)		++	+	+++	–	+++	–	–	–	–	–
placental transfer		+	+	+	+	–	–	–	–	–	–
Binding to cell surface receptors on:											
mononuclear cells	FcγRI	++	–	+++	++	–	–	–	–	–	–
	FcγRIIa	+	(+)	++	–	–	–	–	–	–	–
	FcγRIIIa	+	–	+	–	–	–	–	–	–	–
	FcμR	–	–	–	–	+	–	–	–	–	–
	FcεRII	–	–	–	–	–	–	–	–	–	++
	FcαR	–	–	–	–	–	++	++	++	–	–
neutrophils	FcγRIIa	+	–	+	–	–	–	–	–	–	–
	FcγRIIIb	+	–	+	–	–	–	–	–	–	–
	FcαR	–	–	–	–	–	++	++	++	–	–
mast cells/ basophils	FcεRI	–	–	–	–	–	–	–	–	–	+++

Fig. 4.19 These effector functions are associated with different parts of the Fc region. Placental transfer of IgG in man and intestinal transport in rodents are mediated by an MHC class-I-like receptor molecule (see *Fig. 4.24*). A complex family of receptor molecules able to bind immunoglobulin continues to be discovered (selected examples are listed here). FcμR is expressed by activated B cells but not by T cells or monocytes. FcεRII is also expressed on eosinophils, platelets, T cells and B cells.

IgG class – IgG is the most important class of immunoglobulin in secondary immune responses and, unlike IgM, is distributed evenly between the intravascular and extravascular pools.

A major effector mechanism of the human IgG1 and IgG3 subclasses is the activation of the classical pathway of complement. The latter is a complex group of serum proteins involved in the elimination of pathogens and the mediation of inflammation (see Chapter 3). The IgG2 subclass is less effective at complement activation and IgG4 appears to be inactive.

In humans IgG molecules of all subclasses cross the placenta and confer a high degree of passive immunity to the newborn (*Fig. 4.20*). In some species, e.g. the pig, maternal immunoglobulin is only transferred to the offspring postnatally. In such cases there is a selective transport of such IgG across the gastrointestinal tract via a specific receptor. The IgG subclasses also interact with a complex array of Fc receptors expressed on various cells, as summarized in *Figure 4.19* and discussed further in the section below.

IgM class – IgM is the predominant antibody in primary immune responses. The protein is largely confined to the intravascular pool and is frequently associated with the immune response to antigenically complex, blood-borne infectious organisms.

Once bound to its target, IgM is a potent activator of the classical pathway complement. Unlike IgG-mediated activation where two antibody molecules in close apposition are required, a single molecule of bound IgM is able to initiate the cascade because adjacent Fc regions are intrinsic to the structure.

IgA class – Although there are significant levels of IgA in human serum it is generally accepted that the secretory form of the protein is, in a functional sense, the most important. Secretory IgA is assembled during an active transport process as locally produced dimeric IgA passes across mucosal epithelium (*Fig. 4.21*).

In human serum IgA1 is the predominant subclass (approximately 90% of total IgA) and in many secretions such as nasal secretions, tears, saliva and milk IgA1 will account for 70–95% of total IgA. However, in the colon IgA2 predominates (approximately 60% of the total IgA). It is of interest that many microorganisms in the upper respiratory tract have adapted to their environment by releasing proteases that cleave IgA1.

IgD class – The precise biological function of this class of immunoglobulin remains unclear although it may play a role in antigen-triggered lymphocyte differentiation.

IgE class – Despite its low serum concentration, the IgE class is characterized by its ability to bind avidly to

Immunoglobulins in the serum of the fetus and newborn child

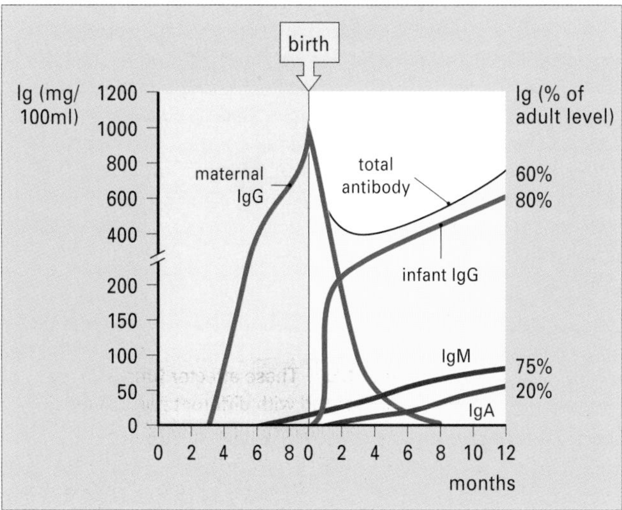

Fig. 4.20 IgG in the fetus and newborn infant is derived solely from the mother. This maternal IgG has disappeared by the age of 9 months, by which time the infant is synthesizing its own IgG. The neonate produces its own IgM and IgA; these classes cannot cross the placenta. By the age of 12 months, the infant produces 80% of its adult level of IgG, 75% of its adult IgM level and 20% of its adult IgA level.

Transport of IgA across the mucosal epithelium

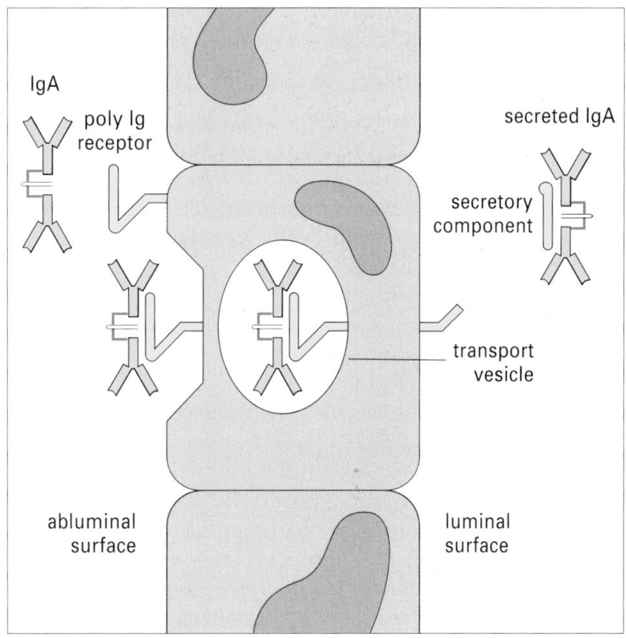

Fig. 4.21 IgA dimers secreted into the intestinal lamina propria by plasma cells bind to poly-Ig receptors on the internal (abluminal) surface of the epithelial cells. The s-IgA–receptor complex is then endocytosed and transported across the cell while still bound to the membrane of transport vesicles. These vesicles fuse with the plasma membrane at the luminal surface, releasing IgA dimers with bound secretory component derived from cleavage of the receptor. The dimeric IgA is protected from proteolytic enzymes in the lumen by the presence of this secretory component.

circulating basophils and tissue mast cells through the high affinity FcεRI receptor (see next section). It also sensitizes cells on mucosal surfaces such as the conjunctival, nasal and bronchial mucosae. This class of immunoglobulin may have evolved to provide immunity against helminthic parasites but in developed countries it is now more commonly associated with allergic diseases such as asthma and hay fever.

Fc RECEPTORS

There are three types of cell surface receptor for IgG

IgG receptors mediate several effector functions and have overlapping biological activities, which are triggered by cross-linking with the appropriate immunoglobulin. The major activities are phagocytosis, antibody-dependent cell-mediated cytotoxicity (ADCC), mediator release and enhancement of antigen presentation.

Three groups of human IgG receptor are now recognized on cell surfaces: FcγRI (CD64), FcγRII (CD32) and FcγRIII (CD16). They are all characterized by extracellular domains showing significant homology with immunoglobulin V regions (*Fig. 4.22*), i.e. they belong to the immunoglobulin superfamily, as does FcαR, a receptor specific for IgA molecules.

FcγRI (CD64) in man binds monomeric IgG with high affinity (10^8–10^9 M^{-1}) and has a more restricted distribution than the other receptors. Primarily, it is expressed on all cells of the mononuclear phagocyte lineage, and is involved in the phagocytosis of immune complexes (see Chapter 9).

FcγRII (CD32) is broadly distributed on cells and is frequently the only receptor to be expressed. It binds only complexed or polymeric IgG with a low intrinsic affinity ($<10^7$ M^{-1}). On B cells, it has a particular function of moderating cell activation when the levels of specific antibody are high (see *Fig. 11.5*).

FcγRIII (CD16) is extensively glycosylated and is expressed as a molecule with a range of molecular weights (50 000–80 000). FcγRIIIa is expressed on macrophages, NK cells and some T cells and interacts with complexed as well as monomeric IgG (intrinsic affinity 3×10^7 M^{-1}). The GPI-linked FcγRIIIb is selectively expressed on granulocytes and has a low affinity for IgG ($<10^7$ M^{-1}).

The three Fcγ receptors generate 12 different isoforms and genetic polymorphism has been described for both FcγRII and FcγRIII. In addition to this intrinsic heterogeneity there is evidence that the receptors are expressed on cell surfaces as complexes in association with other chains. Two such chains have been identified to date in unrelated receptor complexes:

- FcγRI is associated with disulphide-linked dimers of the γ chain also seen in FcεRI.
- FcγRIIIa can associate with the same dimers of γ chains, or with dimers of ζ chains from the TCR complex, or with γ–ζ heterodimers.

In addition to preventing degradation of the FcγRIIIa complex in the endoplasmic reticulum, these associated chains appear to be essential for signal transduction. In the case of the GPI-anchored FcγRIIIb there appears to be no requirement for either γ or ζ chains (*Fig. 4.22*).

Selected phagocyte receptors interacting with IgG

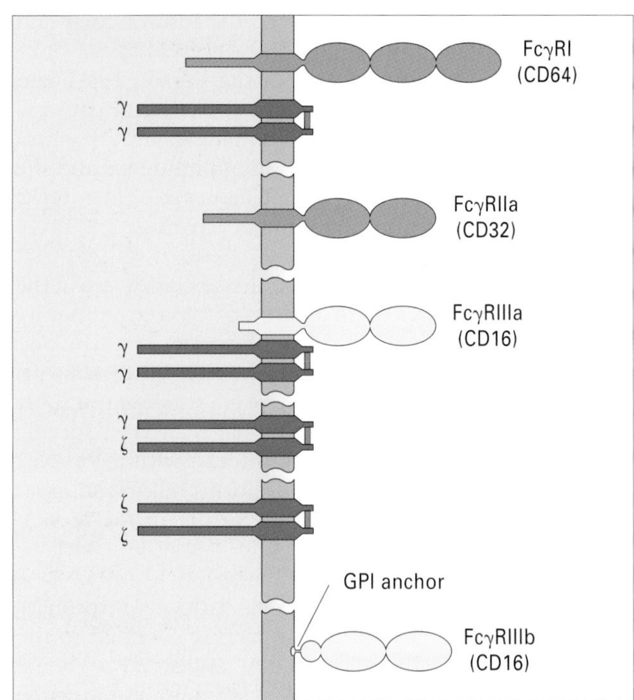

Fig. 4.22 The human Fcγ receptor structures shown are those for FcγRI (expressed by monocytes), FcγRIIa (expressed by monocytes and neutrophils), FcγRIIIa (expressed by monocytes and attached as a normal transmembrane protein) and FcγRIIIb (expressed by neutrophils and attached by a phosphatidyl inositol glycan [GPI] membrane anchor). Each receptor belongs to the immunoglobulin superfamily and expresses two or three extracellular immunoglobulin-like domains. Several of the receptors are now known to exist as complexes with various disulphide-linked subunits. FcγRI and FcγRIIIa both associate with dimers of the γ chain originally described as part of the high-affinity FcεRI complex (see *Fig 4.23*). FcγRIIIa has also been shown to associate with dimers of the ζ chain found in the TCR–CD3 complex. In the case of FcγRIIIa these subunits can associate as either homodimers (γ–γ or ζ–ζ) or as heterodimers (γ–ζ). They appear to be essential for surface expression and signal transduction. In FcγRI interactions, the receptor appears to bind a structural motif centred around Leu 235 in the CH2 domain, present in IgG1, IgG3 and IgG4.

Two distinct Fcε receptors bind to IgE

Two different receptors for IgE on cells are now known (*Fig. 4.23*). The high affinity receptor (FcεRI) is found on mast cells and basophils and is the 'classical' IgE receptor. This receptor is part of the immunoglobulin supergene family and quite distinct from the low affinity Fc receptor for IgE (FcεRII) found on leucocytes and lymphocytes. The low-affinity receptor has not evolved from the immunoglobulin superfamily, but has substantial homology with several animal lectins such as mannose-binding lectin (MBL).

IgE Fc receptors

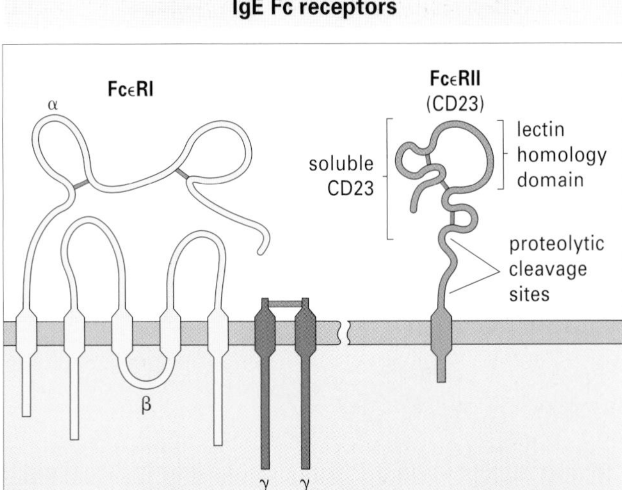

Fig. 4.23 The model for FcεRI proposes a tetramer consisting of one α chain with two disulphide-linked immunoglobulin-like loops. The β chain has two extracellular portions near two γ chains which are linked by disulphide bonds (red). The α chain is crucial for IgE binding. The model for FcεRII is hypothetical, and is based on sequence data and the homology with animal lectins. Proteolytic cleavage can release several types of IgE-binding factors, including the 25-kDa soluble CD23 molecule, which contains the lectin domain. This cleavage is inhibited by IgE, accounting for the apparent increase of FcεRII expression on lymphocytes cultured in the presence of IgE.

FcεRI is the high-affinity IgE receptor

FcεRI has a tetrameric structure (*Fig. 4.23*). The α chain (45 kDa) is glycosylated and exposed on the cell surface. Antibodies against the α chain can block IgE binding to the receptor and trigger histamine release from rat basophil leukaemia cells. The carbohydrate probably protects the α chain from serum protease activity, as it does with many other cell-surface proteins. It is unlikely that the carbohydrate on the α chain plays a role in IgE binding and IgE-mediated histamine release. The single β chain (33 kDa) and the two disulphide-linked γ chains (9 kDa) are essential components of the $\alpha\beta\gamma_2$ receptor unit. They are required for receptor expression on the cell surface, and may have a role in signal transduction.

The receptor interacts with the distal portion of the IgE heavy chain, that is, regions of the Cε2 and/or Cε3 domains. The interaction is highly specific and the binding constant for IgE is very high (approximately 10^{10} M^{-1}). Neither the interaction of monovalent IgE with the receptor complex, nor the binding of substrate to a single IgE, appear to activate mast cells or basophils, since no histamine release occurs. It is the cross-linking of several surface-bound IgEs, by antigen or by other molecules, that stimulates degranulation.

The carbohydrate associated with IgE itself does not seem to be of importance in its interaction with FcεRI. Its role seems to be in the secretion of IgE from B cells. The high-affinity receptor was thought to be limited to mast cells and basophils, but some data suggest that receptors may also be found on Langerhan's cells and stem cells.

FcεRII is the low-affinity IgE receptor

The human lymphocyte FcεRII or CD23 antigen (45 kDa) shows the characteristics of a membrane-bound molecule, i.e. a transmembrane domain, but it is unusual in that it lies 'upside-down' in the cell membrane, the C-terminus being extracellular (*Fig. 4.23*).

Two forms of the human FcεRII have now been identified, cloned and sequenced. They differ only in the N-terminal cytoplasmic region, the extracellular domains being identical. The FcεRIIa is normally expressed on B cells, whereas expression of FcεRIIb is inducible on T cells, B cells, monocytes and eosinophils by the cytokine IL-4. Expression of FcεRIIb is often increased on B cells and monocytes of individuals with eczema, and on lymphocytes of hayfever sufferers.

Many of the sites of effector functions in antibodies have been identified

In contrast to the rapid progress made in localizing the antigen-binding sites of antibodies, the precise structural locations of most effector functions have proved to be elusive. Enzymic subfragments and peptide inhibition studies provided provisional data, but further progress was slow until the technique of site-directed mutagenesis was introduced. This allowed researchers to selectively alter amino acids at different positions in the known peptide sequence, and thus to assess the importance of specific residues for particular functions. An investigation of complement activation by IgG was one of the first uses of this technique. Earlier studies had already suggested that the C1q subcomponent of C1 interacted with the Cγ2 domain of IgG. Site-directed mutagenesis was used to localize the binding site for C1q to three side chains in the Cγ2 domain, Glu 318, Lys 320 and Lys 322. This IgG sequence motif appears to be the common feature in interactions between C1q and IgG molecules.

In the case of IgM, complement activation seems to involve a different mechanism. Free circulating IgM in the star-shaped configuration is clearly incapable of activating complement, whereas IgM bound to antigen is a potent activator. Feinstein and colleagues suggested that the process of IgM binding to a polymeric or latticed antigen dislocates the $F(ab')_2$ units out of their original plane and leads to the so-called crab-like configuration visualized by electron microscopy (*Fig. 4.8*). These conformational changes would unveil a ring of C1q binding sites that are hidden in the star-shaped configuration of IgM by the close juxtaposition of the subunits. Candidate residues are His 430, Asp/Gly 432 and Pro 436, which occupy a structural location in the Cμ3 domain that is analogous to the proposed C1q binding site in the Cγ2 domain of IgG.

IgG molecules interact with a wide range of cellular Fc receptors. Site-directed mutagenesis studies suggest that the high-affinity FcγRI receptor of monocytes interacts with a motif centred around a leucine residue at position 235 of the IgG heavy chain, between the Cγ2 domain and the hinge region.

The interactions between maternal IgG and the MHC class-I-like FcRn expressed on the intestinal epithelium of the neonatal rat have now been studied at high resolution (*Fig. 4.24*) and are believed to mimic closely the binding

The intestinal Fc receptor FcRn

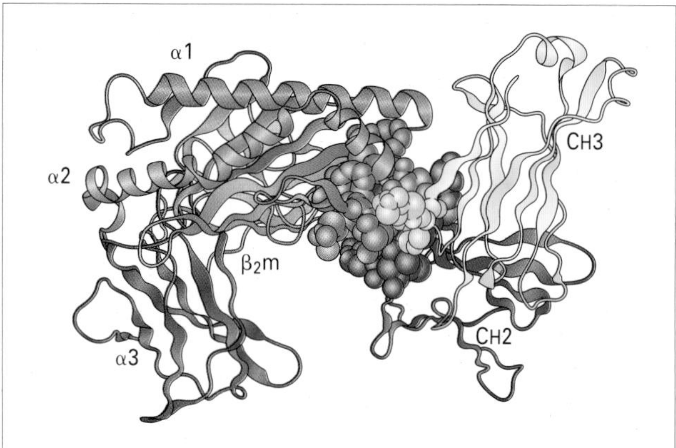

Fig. 4.24 Principal interactions between neonatal rat intestinal FcRn and the Fc of maternal IgG (derived from milk) are illustrated by ribbon diagrams of FcRn (domains α1, α2, α3 and β_2m are shown in red, light green, purple and grey respectively) and of Fc (CH2 and CH3 domains are shown in blue and yellow). The main contact residues of the FcRn (α1 domain, 90; α2 , 113–119 and 131–135; β_2m 1–4 and 86) are depicted as space-filling structures. (Reproduced with permission from Ravetch and Margulies. New tricks for old molecules. *Nature* 1994;**372**:323–4.)

Interaction of IgE with IgE receptors

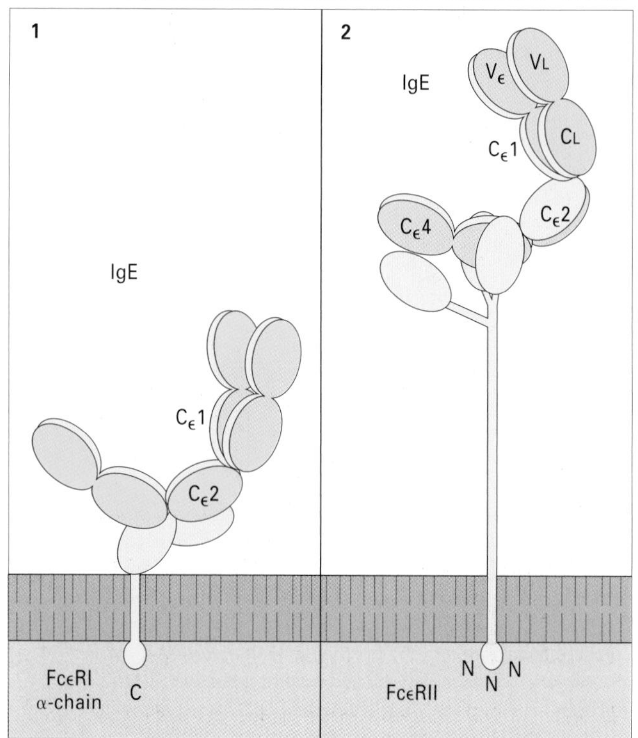

Fig. 4.25 Possible models for IgE interactions with (**1**) the FcεRI receptor and (**2**) the FcεRII receptor. The model shown in (**1**) envisages the α chain of the FcεRI receptor oriented at an angle to the membrane and interacting through the membrane-proximal Ig-like domain with the convex surface of an IgE molecule at the Cε2 and Cε3 interface. Such a model explains why IgE can, apparently, bind only a single FcεRI α-chain. The model shown in (**2**) illustrates the interaction of the Cε3 domains of the IgE molecule with two of the three lectin domains of the membrane-bound FcεRII receptor.

of the human placental counterpart hFcRn with maternal IgG. Fc contacts FcRn mainly in the junction between the CH2 and CH3 domains, overlapping the Fc binding site for Protein A. It is probable that three or four histidine residues on the Fc interface are critical. Titration of histidines could account for the binding of IgG to FcRn at pH 6.5 (the pH of ingested milk) and its release at pH 7.5 (the pH of blood).

The interaction between Protein A of *Staphylococcus aureus* and the Fc region of IgG has also been mapped in some detail. The data suggest a binding site spanning the Cγ2–Cγ3 junction in the Fc region.

A genetic engineering approach has been used to study the sites on the IgE molecule that interact with mast cells through the FcεRI receptor, or with B cells through the FcεRII receptor. Recombinant peptides containing ε-chain sequences were synthesized and then used to inhibit IgE–receptor interactions. In the case of FcεRI interactions, a 76-residue peptide spanning the Cε2–Cε3 junction appears to be critical. By contrast, the FcεRII site appears to recognize a motif involving residues in the Cε3 domains of both ε chains. Possible models for the interaction of IgE with the FcεRI and FcεRII receptors are illustrated in *Figure 4.25*.

GENERATION OF ANTIBODY DIVERSITY

Antibodies are remarkably diverse and provide enough different combining sites to recognize the millions of antigenic shapes in the environment. Each class of antibody also has a characteristic effector region so that, for instance, IgE can bind to Fc receptors on mast cells, whereas IgG can bind to phagocytes. It has been estimated that an individual produces more different forms of antibody than all the other proteins of the body put together. In fact, we produce more types of antibody than there are genes in our genome. How can all this diversity be generated? Ideas about the formation of antibodies have changed considerably over the years, but it is perhaps surprising how close Ehrlich came with his side-chain hypothesis at the beginning of the twentieth century (*Fig. 4.26*). His idea of antigen-induced selection is close to our present view of clonal selection, except that he placed several different receptors on the same cell.

Theories of antibody formation

After Ehrlich the situation became more complicated. The problem was that many new organic compounds were being synthesized and Landsteiner was showing that the immune system could react with the production of specific antibody for each new compound. It was not thought possible that the immune system could, by natural selection, have maintained genes for all these antibodies directed at

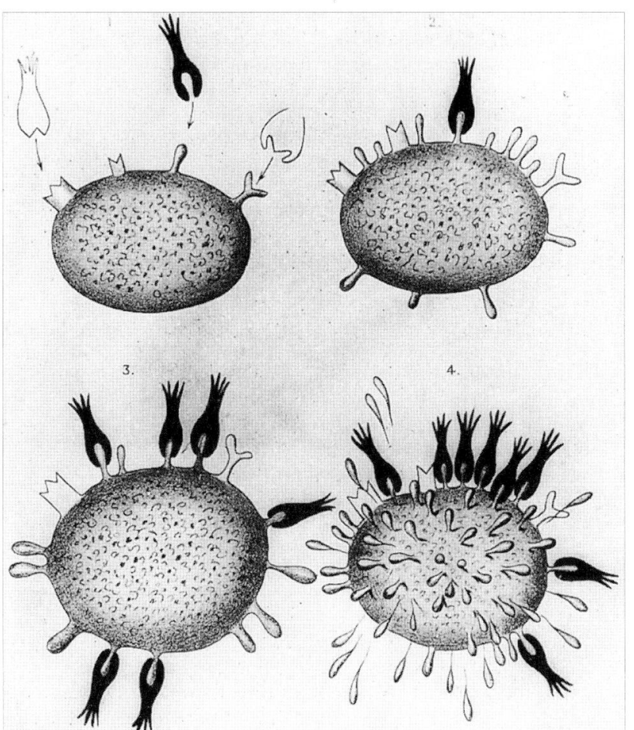

Fig. 4.26 Ehrlich's side-chain theory. Ehrlich proposed that the combination of antigen with a preformed B-cell receptor (now known to be antibody) triggered the cell to produce and secrete more of those receptors. Although the diagram indicates that he thought a single cell could produce antibodies to bind more than one type of antigen, it is evident that he anticipated both the clonal selection theory and the idea that the immune system could generate receptors before contact with antigen.

novel, artificial compounds. This led to the development of the instructive hypothesis, which proposed a flexible antibody molecule that is acted on by antigen to form a complementary binding site. With the spectacular progress in molecular biology in the 1950s and 1960s the instructive hypothesis became untenable, as it became clear that the mechanism for the proposed 'instruction' simply did not exist. The circle turned and selective theories came back into favour, with both Jerne and Burnet putting forward the idea of clonal selection. Each lymphocyte produces one type of immunoglobulin only, and the antigen selects and stimulates cells carrying that immunoglobulin type.

This still left the problem of antibody diversity. One solution was to postulate the existence of a separate gene for each antibody specificity. This immediately presented a problem. Looking at the structure of a light chain, half the chain is variable in amino acid sequence but the other half is constant; similarly with heavy chains, a quarter of the chain is variable while the rest is constant. How, if there are so many genes, is it possible to maintain this constancy of sequence in the constant regions? Dreyer and Bennett proposed a solution to this problem by suggesting that the constant and variable portions of the chains are coded for by separate genes, with one or only a few genes coding for the constant (C) region and many genes coding for the variable (V) region. At this point, the theory still needed to account for the multiple variable regions. A solution to this aspect of the diversity problem was suggested by the idea of somatic mutation, which proposes that relatively few germ line genes give rise to many mutated genes during the lifetime of the individual. It was also suggested that a number of gene segments could recombine to give a complete V gene. During cutting and joining of the DNA, extra nucleotides may be inserted at the cut ends to give further variability. This is called N-region diversity because the sequence is non-germ-line encoded. Rather than mutation, a panel of pseudogenes can also be used to alter the sequences within the variable region by a process of gene conversion. This gave five possible solutions to the problem of generating diversity:

- Multiple V-region genes in the germ line.
- Somatic recombination between elements forming a V-region gene.
- Gene conversion.
- Nucleotide addition.
- Somatic mutation.

It is now known that mammals may use all five mechanisms to generate diversity. Interestingly, sharks rely on having a large number of antibody genes, and do not use somatic recombination, while chickens have small numbers of antibody genes that undergo a very high level of gene conversion (see *Figs 13.20, 13.21*)

Immunoglobulins show isotypic, allotypic and idiotypic variation

Immunoglobulins are composed of heavy and light chains, the light chains being either kappa (κ) or lambda (λ) type. Because virtually any light chain can combine with any heavy chain, the number of possible antigen-binding sites is the product of the number of heavy and light chains. Part of the variability in immunoglobulin structure is derived from the interaction of these separate polypeptide chains. For example, if there are 10^4 different light chains each capable of binding with any of 10^4 different heavy chains, then 10^8 different antibody specificities are theoretically possible. Separate diversification mechanisms exist for each of the chains, as they are encoded on separate chromosomes. For example, in humans the genes encoding kappa and lambda light chains are found on chromosomes 2 and 22 respectively whereas the heavy chain gene locus is found on chromosome 14.

Polymorphic forms of immunoglobulins derive from variation in many parts of the molecule (*Fig. 4.27*).

Isotypic variation

The genes for isotypic variants are present in all healthy members of a species. For example, the genes for γ1, γ2, γ3, γ4, μ, α1, α2, δ, ε, κ and λ chains are all present in the human genome, and are therefore isotypes.

Allotypic variation

This refers to genetic variation between individuals within a species, involving different alleles at a given locus. For example, the variant of IgG3 called G3m(b^0) is characterized by a phenylalanine at position 436 of the γ3 heavy chain. It is not found in all people and is therefore an

Variability of immunoglobulin structure

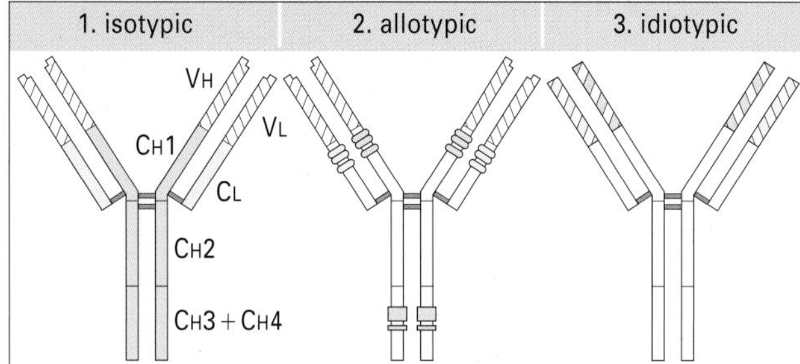

Fig. 4.27 All immunoglobulins have the basic four-chain structure. There are three types of immunoglobulin variability:
(**1**) Isotypic variation is present in the germ line of all members of a species, producing the heavy (μ, δ, γ, ε, α) and light chains (Igκ, λ) and the V-region frameworks (subgroups).
(**2**) Allotypic variation is intraspecies allelic variability.
(**3**) Idiotypic variation refers to the diversity at the antigen-binding site (paratope) and in particular relates to the hypervariable segments.

allotype. Allotypes occur mostly as variants of heavy chain constant regions.

Idiotypic variation

Variation in the variable domain, particularly in the highly variable segments known as hypervariable regions, produces idiotypes. These determine the binding specificity of the antigen-binding site. Idiotypes are usually specific for individual B-cell clones (private idiotypes), but are sometimes shared between different B-cell clones (public, cross-reacting or recurrent idiotypes).

Hypervariable sequences in the antigen-binding site allow antibodies to bind a range of antigens

Within the variable regions of both heavy and light chains, some short polypeptide segments show exceptional variability. Termed hypervariable regions, these segments are located near amino acid positions 30, 50 and 95 (*Fig. 4.28*). Because they create the antigen-binding site, hypervariable regions are sometimes referred to as complementarity determining regions (CDRs). The intervening peptide segments are called framework regions (FRs). In both light and heavy chain V regions there are three CDRs (CDR1–CDR3) and four FRs (FR1–FR4).

The variable regions of the light and heavy chains are folded in such a way that the regions of hypervariability are brought together to create the surface structure that binds antigen. These regions are, in the main, associated with bends in the peptide chain (see *Fig. 4.5*).

IMMUNOGLOBULIN GENE RECOMBINATION

Light chain genes recombine V and J segments to make a gene for the VL domain

With the advent of recombinant DNA techniques, it became possible to attempt analysis of the genes encoding antibodies. In accord with the Dreyer and Bennett hypothesis, it was found that two separate segments of DNA code for the constant and variable regions of light chains. In cells not producing antibody, these gene segments are far apart on the chromosomes, but in antibody-forming cells they are brought closer together. However, even in a fully differentiated B cell, the two gene segments do not join directly, but remain about 1500 base pairs apart. Between the V and C segments, and joined onto the V segment in rearranged chromosomes, is a short section of DNA known as the J (joining) segment. (Not to be confused with the J chain present in IgM and dimeric IgA.)

Amino acid variability in the variable regions of immunoglobulins

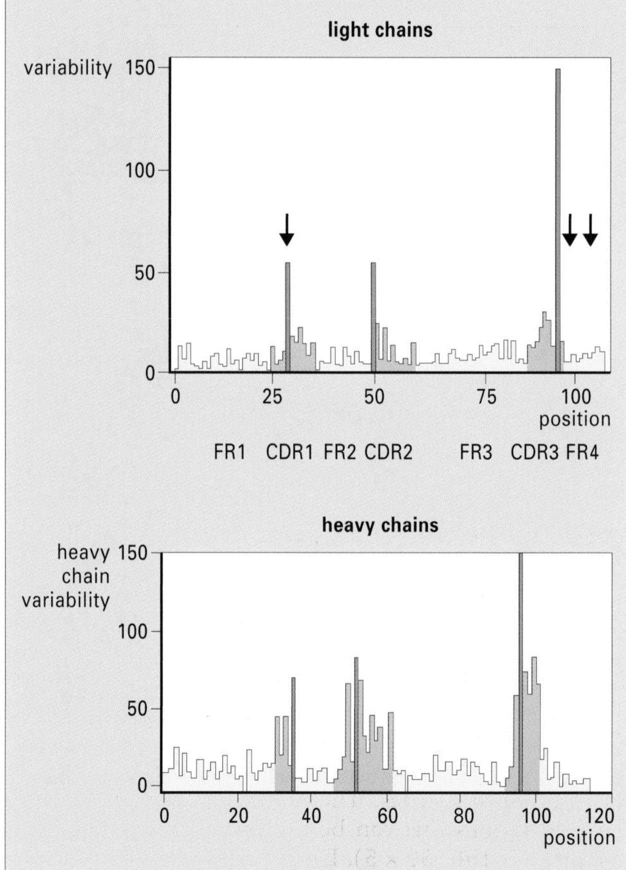

Fig. 4.28 Variability is calculated by comparing the sequences of many individual chains and, for any position, is equal to the ratio of the number of different amino acids found at that position, to the frequency of the most common amino acid. The areas of greatest variability, of which there are three in the VL domain, are termed the hypervariable regions. In some sequences studied, extra amino acids have been found, but these are excluded here to enhance comparison; their positions are indicated by arrows. The areas shaded pink denote regions of hypervariability (CDR), and the most hypervariable positions are shaded red. The four framework regions (FR) are shown in yellow. (Courtesy of Professor E. A. Kabat.)

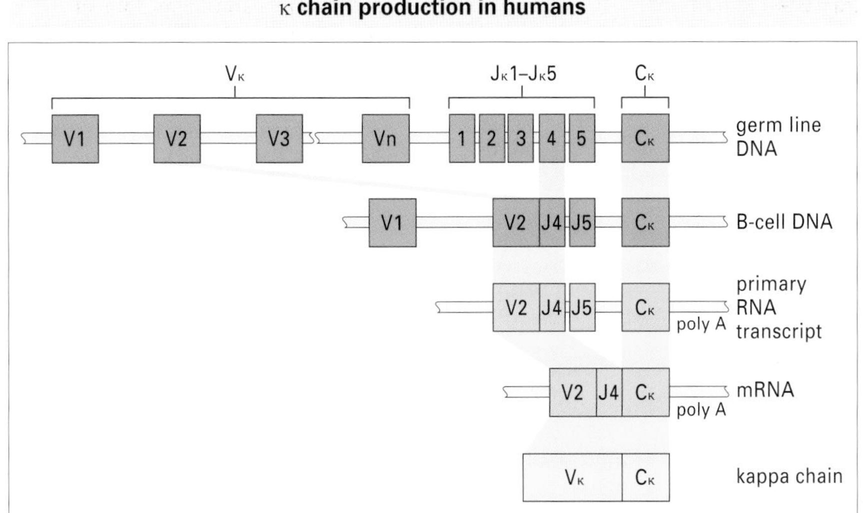

Fig. 4.29 During differentiation of the pre-B cell one of several Vκ genes on the germ line DNA (V1–Vn) is recombined and apposed to a Jκ segment (Jκ1–Jκ5). The B cell transcribes a segment of DNA into a primary RNA transcript that contains a long intervening sequence of additional J segments and introns. This transcript is processed into mRNA by splicing the exons together, and is translated by ribosomes into kappa (κ) chains; B-cell DNA is coloured light brown; RNA is coloured green; and immunoglobulin peptides are coloured yellow. The rearrangement illustrated is only one of the many possible recombinations.

Structure of the light chain systems

The Vκ-gene segment codes for the V region of the antibody light chain, up to and including amino acid 95; the Jκ-gene segment codes for the rest of the V region (*Fig. 4.29*). There is only one constant-region gene but in humans, of 76 Vκ genes, 16 have minor defects and 25 are pseudogenes leaving 35 potentially functional genes. During differentiation of lymphoid cells, there is rearrangement of the DNA such that one of the V genes is joined to one of five J genes. The number of possible κ-chain variable regions that can be produced in this way is approximately 150 (30 × 5). Each V segment is preceded by a leader or signal sequence, a short hydrophobic segment responsible for targeting the chain to the endoplasmic reticulum. The leader sequence is cleaved in the endoplasmic reticulum and the antibody molecule is then processed through the intracellular secretory pathway.

The λ-gene locus in humans contains a set of V genes, but each of seven C genes is accompanied by just one J gene. Despite the difference, the overall process of V–J recombination is similar to that of the κ genes (*Fig. 4.30*).

Following rearrangement of the V and J genes, there is still an intron (a non-coding intervening sequence) between the recombined VJ gene and the gene for the C region. This whole stretch of DNA (from the leader to the end of the C gene, including introns) is then transcribed into heterogeneous nuclear RNA (hnRNA), that is, unprocessed mRNA. A process of RNA splicing then removes the introns, leaving mRNA that can be translated into protein.

Heavy chain genes recombine V, D and J gene segments to make a gene for the VH domain

The heavy chain variable region is also encoded by V- and J-segment genes. Additional diversity is provided by a third gene segment, the D (diversity)-segment gene (*Fig. 4.31*). The D segment is highly variable both in the number of codons and in the sequence of base pairs. In antibodies

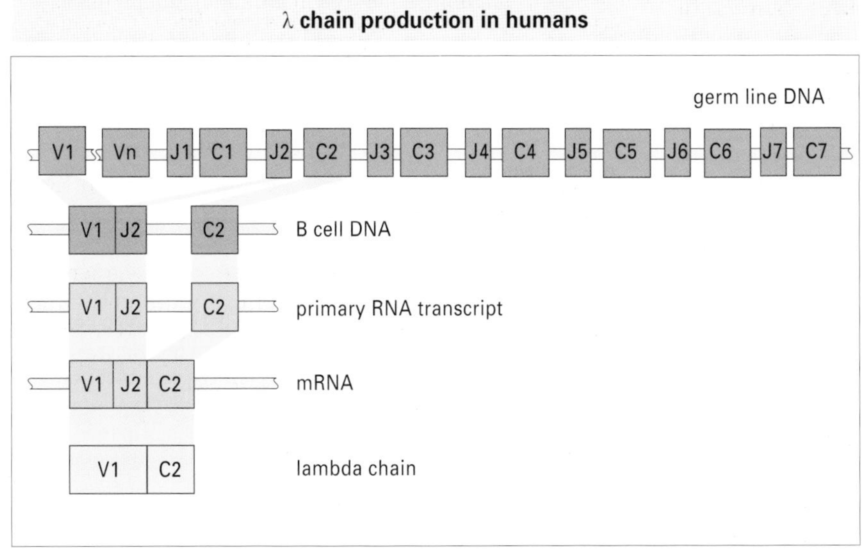

Fig. 4.30 During B-cell differentiation, one of the germ line Vλ genes recombines with a J-segment to form a V–J combination. The rearranged gene is transcribed into a primary RNA transcript complete with introns (non-coding segments occurring between the genes), exons (which code for protein) and a poly-A tail. This is spliced to form messenger RNA (mRNA) with loss of the introns, and then translated into protein.

Heavy chain VDJ recombination in humans

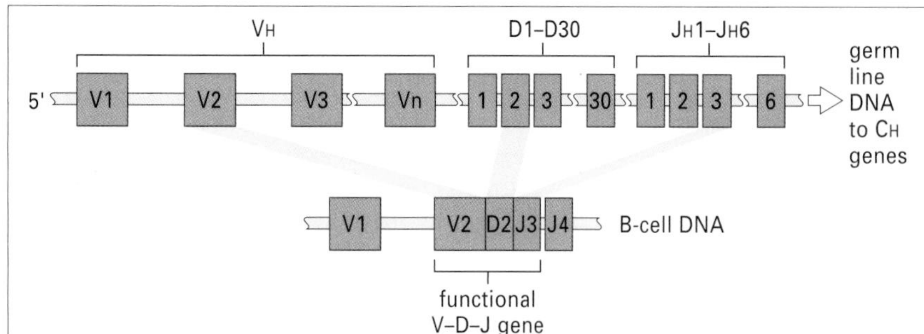

Fig. 4.31 The heavy chain gene loci combine three segments to produce the exon (V–D–J gene) which codes for the VH domain. Of some 80 V genes, about 50 are functional, and the others are pseudogenes. The V gene recombines with one of 30 D segments and one of six J segments, to produce a functional V–D–J gene in the B cell.

binding dextran this section comprises two amino acids; in those binding phosphorylcholine up to eight amino acids are inserted; in anti-levan antibodies this section is completely missing. More than one D segment may join to form an enlarged D region. The D region may be read in three possible reading frames without generating stop codons, so adding to diversity. So far, 30 germ line D segments have been identified. Eighty-seven VH segments are found on chromosome 14, of which at least 32 are pseudogenes. The recombination junction of V, D and J segments in the heavy chain is largely responsible for variability in the complementarity-determining region, CDR-3, which forms an essential part of the antigen-binding site. In some systems, such as the family of anti-dextran antibodies, the differences between antibodies are nearly all situated in this region.

V regions are rearranged and expressed in a programmed manner during early fetal life

When animals are immunized with selected antigens during fetal life or soon after birth, the ability to respond to each antigen develops in a precise order, suggesting a programmed pattern of development. In humans the V region nearest to the J regions is utilized first, and it is interesting that V6-1, the nearest V gene, is a single conserved sequence. In all primate species examined, only a single copy is present, and no sequence variation occurs within a species. Between humans and other primates, only 2% of the nucleotides vary.

This fetal repertoire is overrepresented in autoantibodies, indicating that autoimmunity might, in part, be the result of dysregulation of these early sequences. There is similar overrepresentation of particular V segments in tumours of early B cells, 20 V segments being present in 85% of chronic lymphocytic leukaemias.

Recombination sequences flanking the V, D and J genes direct joining of the gene segments

The recombination of gene segments is a key feature of the generation of a functional gene for both light and heavy chain variable regions. The precise mechanism by which this recombination occurs is now becoming clear, and specific base sequences that act as recombination signal sequences (RSS) have been identified. A signal sequence is found downstream (3′) of V- and D-segment genes. It consists of a heptamer CACAGTG or its analogue, followed by a spacer of unconserved sequence (12 or 23 bases), and then a nonamer ACAAAAACC or its analogue. Immediately upstream (5′) of all germ line D and J segments is a corresponding signal sequence of a nonamer and then a heptamer, again separated by an unconserved sequence (12 or 23 bases). The heptameric and nonameric sequences following a VL, VH or D segment are complementary to those preceding the JL, D or JH segments with which they recombine. The 12 and 23 base spacers correspond to either one or two turns of the DNA helix (*Fig. 4.32*).

The recombination process is controlled at least in part by two recombination-activating genes (RAG-1 and RAG-2). Mice whose RAG-1 and RAG-2 genes have been 'knocked out' lack mature T and B cells, because of a failure to produce the T-cell receptors and immunoglobulins respectively. Interleukin-7 (IL-7), a cytokine produced by bone-marrow stromal cells, has been shown to influence levels of RAG-1 and RAG-2 expression. Studies with synthetic DNA substrates containing heptamer and nonamer sequences, together with 12b and 23b spacers and purified RAG-1 and RAG-2, have established that these proteins are able to mediate the formation of a synaptic complex between two RSS. Initially, RAG-1 binds to the nonamer sequence, then RAG-2, which cannot bind

Recombination sequences in immunoglobulin genes

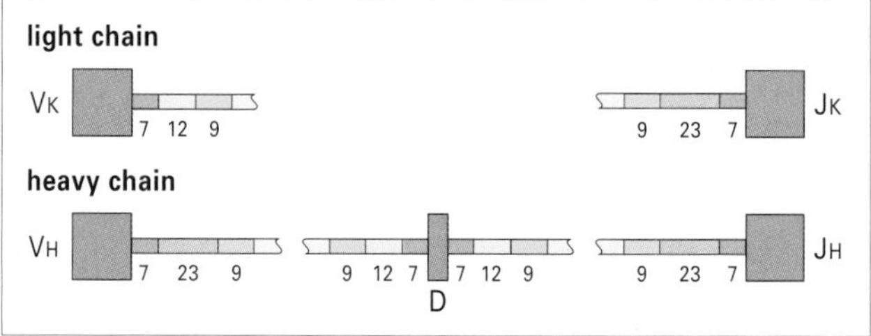

Fig 4.32 The recombination sequences in the light chain genes (top) and heavy chain genes (bottom) consist of heptamers (7), 12 or 23 unconserved bases and nonamers (9). The sequences of heptamers and nonamers are complementary and the nonamers act as signals for the recombination activating genes to form a synapsis between the adjoining exons. Similar recombination sequences are present in the T-cell receptor V, D and J gene segments (see Chapter 5).

to DNA on its own, binds to the RAG-1–DNA complex, particularly next to a 12b spacer. Synapsis then occurs between 12b and 23b spacers. It is possible that this is mediated between the RAG-1–RAG-2 complex on the nonamer–12b spacer sequence and a RAG-1 complex on the nonamer–23b sequence. After binding, cleavage is directed by the heptamer sequences at the borders between the V–(D–)J coding regions and the heptamers.

Cleavage is initiated by introducing a nick in the area bordering the 5′ end of the signal heptamer and the coding region. This is then converted, by the RAG proteins, into a double-strand break, generating a hairpin coding end. *In vitro*, hairpin formation is clearly seen at the cut coding ends. This also occurs *in vivo*, but is less obvious, as the hairpins are often further modified before joining.

The place at which V and J segment genes join may vary slightly

Slight variations in the positions at which recombination takes place generate additional diversity. For example, the 95th residue of the κ light chain is usually encoded by the last codon of the V-segment gene; the 96th is frequently encoded by the first Jκ triplet. Sometimes, however, the 96th amino acid is encoded by a composite triplet formed by the second and third bases, or third base alone, of the first Jκ triplet, with the other bases of the triplet coming from the intron 3′ to the V-segment gene (*Fig. 4.33*). This will lead to variations in amino acid sequence. Obviously, to produce a functional light chain the correct reading frame must be preserved; if the gene segments join out of phase, non-functional antibodies are produced.

In the case of the heavy chain, similar imprecision in joining occurs between the D and JH segment genes and can extend over as many as 10 nucleotides (*Fig. 4.34*). Furthermore, a few nucleotides may be inserted between D and JH and between VH and D by means of the enzyme, terminal deoxynucleotidyl transferase, without the need for a template. The addition of these N-nucleotides is called N-region diversity. In mice, terminal deoxynucleotidyl transferase activity increases with age, giving rise to long N segments in adult animals. Thus the recombinational variability of the D region can be so great that no recognizable D-gene segment remains.

Light chain diversity created by variable recombination

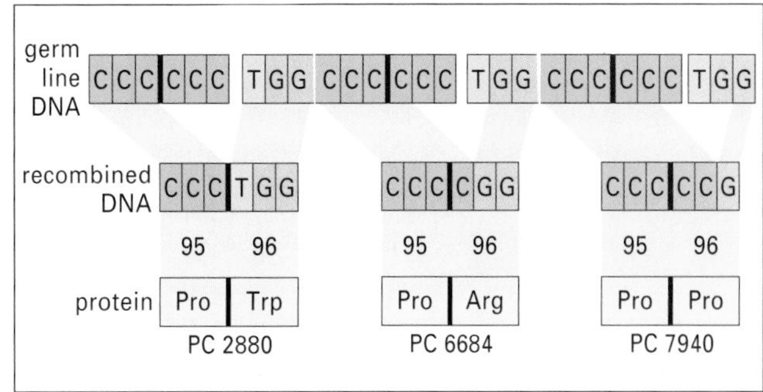

Fig. 4.33 The same Vκ21 and J1 sequences of the germ line create three different amino acid sequences in the proteins PC2880, PC6684 and PC7940 by variable recombination. PC2880 has proline and tryptophan at positions 95 and 96, caused by recombination at the end of the CCC codon. Recombination one base down produces proline and arginine in PC6684. Recombination two bases down from the end of Vκ21 produces proline and proline in PC7940.

Severe combined immune deficiency (SCID) mice do not generate functional T or B cells because of a defect in V–(D)–J recombination.

SOMATIC MUTATION

Immunoglobulin heavy and light chain genes undergo structural modifications after antigen stimulation

The idea that somatic mutations could occur during the lifetime of an individual and thus increase the diversity of antibodies has been strongly argued for many years. Most sequences in the murine λ1 light chain system are identical, with a few variations in the complementarity-determining regions giving eight sequences in all. However, only one Vλ1 gene segment has been found per haploid genome, and this corresponds to the main shared prototype sequence; thus, all variant sequences must be generated by

Heavy chain diversity created by variable recombination and N region diversity

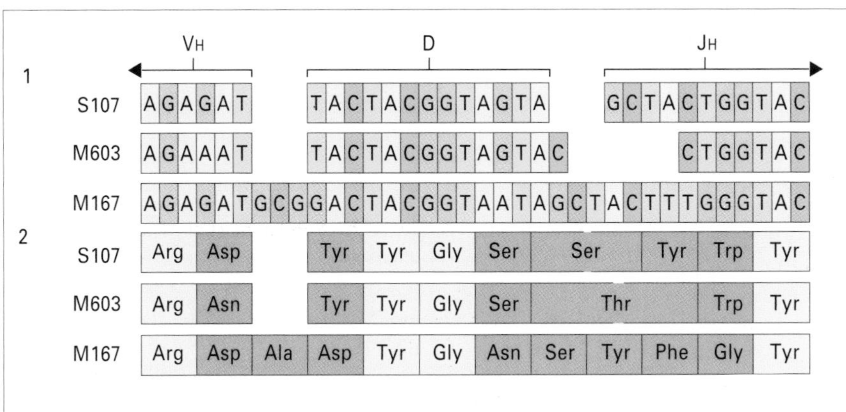

Fig. 4.34 The DNA sequence (**1**) and amino acid sequence (**2**) of three heavy chains of anti-phosphorylcholine are shown. Variable recombination between the germ line, V, D and J regions and N region insertion causes variation (orange) in amino acid sequences. In some cases (e.g. M167) there appear to be additional inserted codons. However, these are in multiples of three, and do not alter the overall reading frame.

somatic mutations produced by single base changes. Somatic mutants have also been identified in κ light chains and in heavy chains.

There is some evidence that the region of DNA encoding the variable region may be particularly susceptible to mutation. For example, examination of the nucleotide sequences of two anti-phosphorylcholine antibodies shows them to have numerous mutations from the germ line sequence. These mutations are found in both introns and exons of the V region, but not in adjoining sequences, implying that the whole V region is particularly mutable (*Fig. 4.35*). Somatic mutation occurs in germinal centres, and cells which have produced a higher-affinity antibody are selected for survival (see Chapter 8). This process is dependent on both T cells and germinal centres. Athymic mice lack T cells and germinal centres and there is no affinity maturation.

Antibody diversity thus arises at several levels. First there are the multiple V genes recombining with J and D segments. The imprecision with which recombination occurs achieves further variation. Note that the structures of the first and second hypervariable regions are coded for entirely by germ line genes. CDR-2 (HV2) already has wide diversity encoded in the genome, CDR-1 is diversified by somatic mutation, and variability in CDR-3 is largely the result of recombination. As virtually any light chain may pair with any heavy chain the combinatorial binding of heavy and light chains amplifies the diversity enormously (*Fig. 4.36*). Somatic hypermutation probably contributes less than 5% of total sequence variability, but up to 90% of B cells express VH genes which have undergone somatic mutation.

Mutations in the DNA of two heavy chain genes

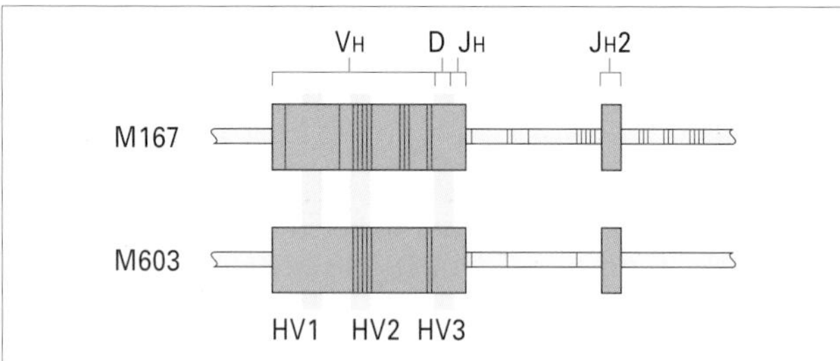

Fig. 4.35 DNA of two IgG antibodies to phosphorylcholine are illustrated. Both antibodies share the T15 idiotype. Black lines indicate positions where the sequence has mutated from the germ line sequence. There are large numbers of mutations in both the introns and exons of both genes, but particularly in the second hypervariable region (HV2). By comparison, there are no mutations in the regions encoding the constant genes, which implies that the mutational mechanism is highly localized.

Seven mechanisms for the generation of antibody diversity

1. multiple germ line V genes
2. V–J and V–D–J recombinations
3. N–nucleotide addition
4. gene conversion
5. recombinational inaccuracies
6. somatic point mutation
7. assorted heavy and light chains

Fig. 4.36 Since each mechanism can occur with any of the others, the potential for increased diversity multiplies at each step of immunoglobulin production.

CRITICAL THINKING • The specificity of antibodies (Explanations on pp. 453–454)

The human rhinovirus HRV14 is formed from four different polypeptides: one of them (VP4) is associated with viral RNA in the core of the virus, while the other three polypeptides (VP1–VP3) make up the shell of the virus – the capsid.

4.1 When virus is propagated in the presence of neutralizing anti-viral antiserum it is found that mutated forms of the virus develop. Mutations are detected in VP1, VP2 or VP3, but never in VP4. Why should this be so?

The most effective neutralizing antibodies are directed against the protein VP1 – this is termed an immunodominant antigen. Two different monoclonal antibodies against VP1 were developed and used to induce mutated forms of the virus. When the sequences of the mutated variants were compared with the original virus, it was found that only certain amino acid residues became mutated (see table below).

Antibody	Amino acid number	Residue in wild type	Observed mutations
VP1-a	91	Glu	Ala, Asp, Gly, His, Asn, Val, Tyr
	95	Asp	Gly, Lys
VP1-b	83	Gln	His
	85	Lys	Asn
	138	Glu	Asp, Gly
	139	Ser	Pro

4.2 What can you tell about the epitopes which are recognized by the two different monoclonal antibodies?

4.3 When the binding of the antibody VP1-a is measured against the different mutant viruses, it is found that it binds with high affinity to the variant with Glycine (Gly) at position 138, with low affinity to the variant with Gly at position 95 and it does not bind to the variant with Lysine (Lys) at position 95.

How can you explain these observations?

DISCUSSION POINT How could you use this information to design a vaccine against a common cold virus?

FURTHER READING

Blackwell TK, Alt FW. Mechanism and developmental program of immunoglobulin gene rearrangement in mammals. *Annu Rev Genet* 1989;**23**:605–36.

Burton DR. Antibody: the flexible adaptor molecule. *Trends Biochem Sci* 1990;**15**:64–9.

Conrad DH. The low affinity receptor for IgE. *Annu Rev Immunol* 1990;**8**:623–45.

Davies AC, Schulman MJ. IgM – molecular requirements for its assembly and function. *Immunol Today* 1989;**10**:118–22, 127–8.

Davies DR, Metzger H. Structural basis of antibody function. *Annu Rev Immunol* 1984;**1**:87–117.

Feinstein A, Richardson N, Taussig MJ. Immunoglobulin flexibility in complement activation. *Immunol Today* 1986;**7**:169–73.

Harriman W, Volk H, Defanoux N, *et al.* Immunoglobulin class switch recombinations. *Annu Rev Immunol* 1993;**11**:361–84.

Honjo T, Alt FW. *Immunoglobulin Genes.* London: Academic,1995.

Hunkapiller T, Hood L. Diversity of the immunoglobulin gene superfamily. *Adv Immunol* 1990;**44**:1–63.

Kerr MA. The structure and function of human IgA. *Biochem J* 1990;**271**:285–96.

Kilian M, Russell MW. Function of mucosal immunoglobulins. In: Ogra P, Mestecky J, Lamm ME, *et al.* (eds). *Handbook of Mucosal Immunology.* San Diego: Academic, 1994:127–37.

Lewis SM. The mechanism of V(D)J joining: lessons from molecular, immunological and comparative analyses. *Adv Immunol* 1994;**56**:27–150.

Möller G. (ed). Immunoglobulin D: structure, synthesis, membrane representation and function. *Immunol Rev* 1977;**37**.

Möller G. (ed). Immunoglobulin E. *Immunol Rev* 1978;**41**.

Möller G. (ed). Fc receptors. *Immunol Rev* 1992;**125**.

Möller G. (ed). The B-cell antigen receptor complex. *Immunol Rev* 1993;**132**.

Nisonoff A. *Introduction to Molecular Immunology.* 2nd edn. Baltimore: Sinauer Associates, 1984:326.

Pascual V, Capra JD. Human immunoglobulin heavy-chain variable region genes: organization, polymorphism and expression. *Adv Immunol* 1991;**49**:1–74.

Ravetch JV, Kinet J-P. Fc receptors. *Annu Rev Immunol* 1991;**9**:457–92.

Ravetch JV, Margulies DH. New tricks for old molecules. *Nature* 1994;**372**:323–4.

Shakib F. (ed). *The Human IgG Subclasses. Molecular analysis of structure, function, and regulation.* Oxford: Pergamon, 1990.

Van de Winkel JGJ, Capel PJA. Human IgG Fc receptor heterogeneity: molecular aspects and clinical implications. *Immunol Today* 1993;**14**:215–21.

INTERNET REFERENCES

The ImMunoGeneTics database IMGT was originally established in 1989 and the IMGT/LIGM-DB is a comprehensive database of Ig and TcR sequences from human and other vertebrates
http://www.ebi.ac.uk/imgt

V base contains the germline variable region sequences of more than 1000 published sequences
http://www.mrc-cpe.cam.ac.uk/imt-doc/public

The Kabat database contains sequences of proteins of immunological interest
http://immuno.bme.nwu.edu

5 T-cell receptors and major histocompatibility complex molecules

- **The T-cell antigen receptor (TCR)** is a disulphide-linked heterodimer having either $\alpha\beta$ or $\gamma\delta$ chains that enables T cells to recognize a diverse array of antigens. It is associated at the cell surface with a complex of polypeptides known collectively as CD3.
- **The TCR is generated by four different sets of genes:** α and β genes are expressed in the majority of peripheral T cells; γ and δ genes are expressed in a subpopulation of thymic T cells and in a minor population of peripheral T cells.
- **Diversification of the TCR** occurs by recombination between V, D and J gene segments, with minor variations in detail for each locus.
- **The major histocompatibility complex (MHC)** encodes two sets of highly polymorphic cell-surface molecules, termed MHC class I and MHC class II. The $\alpha\beta$ TCR recognizes processed antigen as peptide fragments bound to MHC class I or class II molecules. Both MHC and peptide residues associate with the TCR.
- **A peptide binding cleft** is formed by the folding of an MHC molecule. This accommodates peptides that have been processed by the cell, to be presented to T cells. Peptides of eight or nine residues can bind to class I molecules, whereas longer peptides can bind to class II molecules.
- **Binding pockets** within the clefts are able to accommodate different peptides depending on the haplotype. Because MHC molecules are highly polymorphic, and because a cell can express several different MHC molecules, this explains how the cell can present many different antigenic peptides to a T cell.
- **The binding affinity of an antigenic peptide** within the TCR–MHC–peptide complex determines whether the T cell will be activated. High-affinity interactions promote activation, while low-affinity interactions may antagonize activation.
- **CD4 and CD8 molecules** bind to the TCR–MHC–peptide complex and recruit tyrosine kinases that phosphorylate CD3, thereby initiating T-cell activation.
- **CD1 is an MHC class-I-like molecule which presents glycolipid antigens.** CD1 molecules are not polymorphic and are encoded outside the MHC.

Antigen recognition by T lymphocytes is central to the generation and regulation of an effective immune response. Many important questions in immunology have centred on the nature of the receptor on T cells that mediates specific antigen recognition. As T cells recognize antigens which are presented by other cells of the body, the way in which the T-cell receptor (TCR) recognizes antigen is quite different from antigen recognition by antibody. The most important distinction, is that T cells recognize antigen fragments which are bound and presented by specialized antigen-presenting molecules. They do not recognize free antigen. The most important group of antigen-presenting molecules are the class I and class II molecules of the major histocompatibility complex (MHC) which present polypeptides to T cells. More recently other antigen-presenting molecules have been identified, such as CD1 which presents lipid and glycolipid antigens.

Despite the differences, antibody and the TCR have many similarities. They are structurally related as they are both folded into Ig superfamily domains. They are both clonally distributed, i.e. each lymphocyte has a receptor with its individual specificity. Moreover the way in which the receptors are generated by somatic recombination from a limited number of germline genes is similar.

THE T-CELL RECEPTOR

A T-cell receptor (TCR) was first purified using specific antibodies directed against a clone-specific molecule on T cells. It was called the $\alpha\beta$ TCR because it was a heterodimeric molecule comprising an α chain and a β chain linked by a disulphide bond. Independently, genes which might encode TCR chains were isolated from cDNA libraries, on the basis of their being expressed in some clones but not others. The amino acid sequence deduced from the nucleotide sequence of the genes matched the partial sequence obtained from α and β TCR proteins purified using monoclonal antibodies. Thus, the two different approaches had identified the same entity. In further experiments, a second TCR, called $\gamma\delta$, was isolated. Any one T cell has either an $\alpha\beta$ or a $\gamma\delta$ receptor, and the great majority of cells generate an $\alpha\beta$ receptor,

The $\alpha\beta$ TCR heterodimer forms the recognition unit of the receptor

The $\alpha\beta$ TCR comprises a disulphide-linked heterodimer of α (40–50 kDa) and β (35–47 kDa) subunits. The structural features of the $\alpha\beta$ heterodimer have been determined by X-ray crystallography and are shown in *Figure 5.1.* Each polypeptide chain comprises two extracellular immunoglobulin-like domains of approximately 110 amino acids, anchored into the plasma membrane by a transmembrane peptide which has a short cytoplasmic tail. The difference in molecular weights of the human α and β chains is accounted for by the presence of extra N-linked carbohydrate on the α chain. The overall features of the structure clearly show that the α and β chains fold into a structure that resembles the Fab region of antibodies.

The amino acid sequence variability of the TCR resides

The T-cell antigen receptor

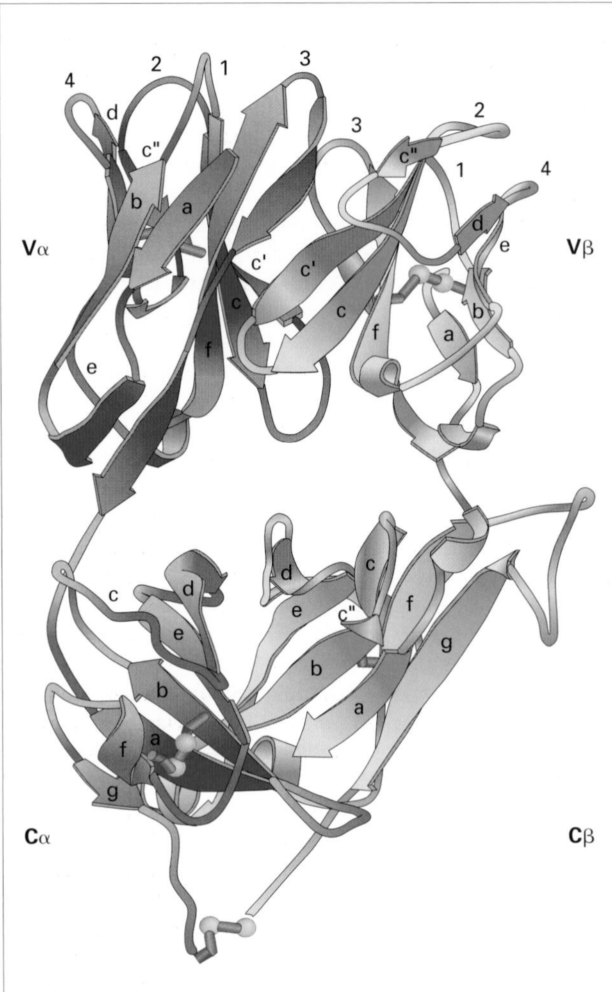

Fig. 5.1 Three-dimensional structure of an αβ TCR. The α chain is coloured blue (residues 1–213), and the β chain is coloured green (residues 3–247). The β strands are represented as arrows and labelled according to the standard convention used for the Ig fold. The disulphide bonds (yellow balls for sulphur atoms) are shown within each domain and for the COOH-terminal interchain disulphide. The CDRs lying at the top of the diagram are numerically labelled (1–4) for each chain. These form the binding site for antigen/MHC. (Adapted from Garcia KC, Degano M, Stanfield RL, *et al. Science* 1996;**274**:209–19.)

in the N-terminal domains of the α and β polypeptides and the regions of greatest variability correspond to immunoglobulin hypervariable regions, also known as complementarity-determining regions (CDRs). These are clustered together to form an MHC–antigen-binding site which is analogous to the antigen-binding site on antibodies. Notice however that there are two additional hypervariable loops in the TCR, by comparison with the three in antibodies, and that CDR3 from both the α chain and the β chain lie at the centre of the antigen-binding site.

The disulphide bond that links the α and β chains is in a peptide sequence between the constant domain and the transmembrane peptide. An unusual feature of both α- and β-chain transmembrane regions is the inclusion of positively charged residues. These charged residues are essential for the assembly and intracellular transport of the TCR complex.

The CD3 complex associates with the αβ and γδ forms of the T-cell receptor

The αβ and γδ forms of the TCR are both associated physically with a series of polypeptides, collectively called CD3. This association is required for surface expression of the TCR complex at the cell surface. The CD3 components show no amino acid variability on different T cells and thus cannot generate the diversity associated with TCRs. Rather, the CD3 component of the TCR is required for signal transduction following antigen recognition by the TCR heterodimer. CD3 comprises four invariant polypeptides, called γ, δ, ε and ζ. (Do not confuse the γ and δ chains of CD3 with the γδ form of the antigen/MHC-binding chains described above) The stoichiometry of the CD3–TCR complex is (αβ)2,γ,δ,ε2,ζ2, with the CD3 chains organized as heterodimers of γε and δε and a homodimer of ζζ. Using immunoprecipitation, it was found that both the γε unit and the δε unit associate with the αβ TCR, and that separate subunits are linked by the ζζ dimer. This suggests that the TCR complex exists as a dimeric structure, and a model which conforms to these data is shown in *Figure 5.2*.

The CD3 γ, δ and ε chains are the products of three closely linked genes and are clearly related in their primary sequences. The polypeptides are members of the immunoglobulin superfamily, each containing an external domain followed by a transmembrane region and a highly conserved cytoplasmic tail of 40 or more amino acids. An unusual feature of the transmembrane regions is that they each contain a negatively charged amino acid, rather than being completely apolar. We know that the negatively charged residues are essential for the assembly of the TCR complex, because *in vitro* mutation of the residues prevents the assembly of the complex. It is thought that the negatively charged residues in the transmembrane region of CD3 chains interact with the positively charged residues on the αβ units, via the generation of hydrogen bonds, or ion pairs within the membrane (*Fig. 5.2*).

The CD3 ζ gene is on a different chromosome from the CD3 γδε gene complex and the ζ and γδε polypeptides are structurally unrelated. The ζ chains comprise a small extracellular domain of only nine amino acids which includes the disulphide bond, a transmembrane segment including a negatively charged residue, and a large cytoplasmic tail. An alternatively spliced form of CD3ζ called CD3η is also produced having an intracytoplasmic domain which is 42 amino acids longer at the C terminus. The chains may associate in all three possible combinations (ζζ, ζη or ηη). The intracytoplasmic sections of the CD3 ζ and η chains contain particular amino acid sequences called 'immunoreceptor tyrosine activation motifs' or ITAMs. The tyrosine residue in these motifs is a target for phosphorylation by specific protein kinases. There are three such ITAMs in each of the chains. It is clear that ITAMs are essential for T-cell activation, as mutation of the tyrosines in

The T-cell receptor complex

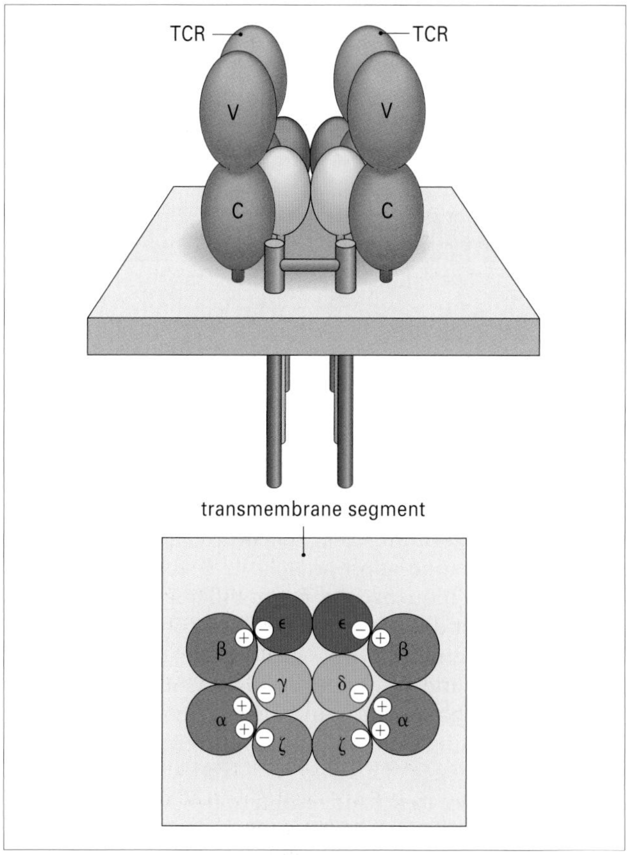

TCR TCR V V C C transmembrane segment β ε ε β γ δ α α ζ ζ

Fig. 5.2 The TCR α and β (or γ and δ) chains each comprise an external V and C domain, a transmembrane segment containing positively charged amino acids and a short cytoplasmic tail. The two chains are disulphide linked on the membrane side of their C domains. The CD3 γ, δ and ε chains comprise an external immunoglobulin-like C domain, a transmembrane segment containing a negatively charged amino acid and a longer cytoplasmic tail. A dimer of ζζ, ηη or ζη is also associated with the complex. Several lines of evidence support the notion that the TCR–CD3 complex exists at the cell surface as a dimer. The transmembrane charges are important for the assembly of the complex. A plausible arrangement which neutralizes opposite charges is shown.

the motif prevents activation. When the TCR is bound to antigen–MHC, these motifs become phosphorylated within minutes, and this is the first step in the process of T-cell activation described fully in Chapter 6. ITAMs are not confined to CD3ζ and η; they are also present in Igα and Igβ (CD79) which are involved in B-cell activation, and CD3ζ itself can form a complex with the Fc receptor (CD16) which is involved in the activation of macrophages and natural killer (NK) cells (see *Fig. 4. 22*).

The polypeptide chains of CD3 γ, δ or ε may also become phosphorylated following ligation of the TCR. Notably phosphorylation of the CD3γ chain causes down-regulation of receptor expression at the cell surface. This can be equated with association of the phosphorylated γ chain with adaptor proteins which increase the rate of receptor internalization.

The γδ TCR structurally resembles the αβ TCR

The overall structure of the γδ TCR is similar to that of its αβ counterpart, each chain being organized into external V and C domains, a transmembrane segment containing positively charged residues and a short cytoplasmic tail. The structure of γδ TCRs is more variable in humans than in the mouse. Human γ and δ chains can be disulphide linked, or can exist as monomers, the disulphide link correlating with the presence of a cysteine in the Cγ2 constant region exon. TCR γ chains containing a Cγ2 constant region vary in molecular weight due to duplication or triplication of this second exon. However, the biological significance of these structural differences remains unclear.

The two forms of TCR show quite distinct anatomical locations. The αβ TCR is present on more than 95% of peripheral T cells and on the majority of TCR-expressing thymocytes. By contrast, T cells expressing the γδ receptor often have defined anatomical locations. Although γδ T cells form only a small proportion of T cells in the thymus and secondary lymphoid organs, they are abundant in various epithelia, such as the epidermis (in mice but not humans), intestinal epithelium, uterus and tongue.

There has been considerable research into the question of whether γδ T cells recognize different classes of antigen to αβ T cells. Animals which are genetically deficient in γδ cells generally have impaired resistance to infection, and animals which lack αβ T cells still have some level of protection, showing that γδ cells make a contribution to host defence against pathogens. As information has accumulated, it has become clear that γδ T cells recognize both exogenous antigens such as viral and protozoal peptides, and autoantigens such as heat shock proteins. Moreover, the peptides can be presented by either class I or class II MHC molecules (see below), and there are several studies which suggest that γδ cells do not require antigen to be presented by classical MHC molecules at all. There is also evidence that γδ T cells produce lower levels of some cytokines than αβ T cells, but whether this is a fundamental difference, or related to their preferential location in particular tissues, is not yet known. Taken together, the data show that γδ T cells have a clear role in host defence against some pathogens, and may also be involved in the control and modulation of responses mediated by αβ T cells.

GENES OF THE T-CELL ANTIGEN RECEPTOR

The general arrangement of genes for the α, β, γ and δ chains of the TCR is remarkably similar to immunoglobulin heavy chains. *Figure 5.3.* illustrates the murine TCR genes which are similar to those in man. The nomenclature is simple enough – the TCRA locus encodes the α chain, TCRB the β chain and so on. The gene loci are quite distinct from the immunoglobulin gene loci, but interestingly the TCRD locus is nested inside the TCRA genes. The α and γ loci have sets of V genes and J genes (which is analagous to Ig light chains) while the β and δ loci have sets of V, D and J genes, which is similar to the Ig heavy chain locus.

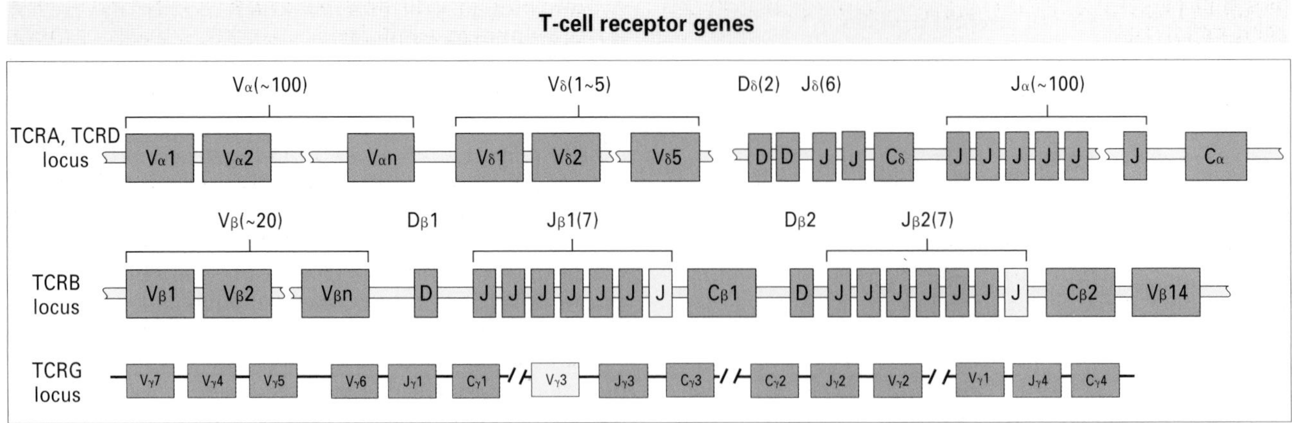

Fig. 5.3 The genes of the murine TCR chains are shown. The δ chain loci are embedded within the α loci and tandem duplication has occurred in the β chain loci. The last of each set of Jβ genes and the Vγ3 gene are pseudogenes.

Diverse TCRs are generated by recombination of V, D and J gene segments

Diversification of the TCR gene occurs by recombination between V, D and J segments, with minor variations in detail for each locus. TCRA is superficially simple, except for the complication of the TCRD locus embedded between V and J loci. As in the IGK locus (κ chain), a complete variable region is produced by rearrangement of a Vα segment to a Jα segment. Diversity is markedly increased by the unusually large number of Jα segments.

The TCRB locus includes two sets of D, J and C genes. Most of the Vβ genes are grouped together, but one (Vβ14) is present at the extreme 3′ end of the locus. The tandem duplication of Dβ, Jβ and Cβ must have occurred early in the evolution of mammals, as it is present in both mice and humans. Extensive diversity is generated in the joining process, as not only are V–D–J arrangements possible, but also V–J and V–D–D–J joins. The D segments are used in all three reading frames, adding even further to β-chain diversity.

The arrangement of the γ-chain loci in mice and in humans is rather different. The murine locus bears a striking similarity to the antibody light chain locus, with four Cγ genes (including a pseudogene), each associated with one J gene, and one to four Vγ genes. There are no D genes. In man there are eight Vγ genes, followed upstream (5′) by three Jγ and the first Cγ; then there are two additional Jγ genes before Cγ2. Imprecise joining of V with J, together with insertions in the joins, is important in generating diversity.

The TCRD locus was discovered during studies on the TCRA locus. Although relatively simple, with only five Vδ, two Dδ and six Jδ genes, it has been calculated that 1014 different δ chains could be generated by imprecision in joining, insertion of additional residues and use of the D genes in all three reading frames.

The mechanisms for TCR gene recombination appear to be similar to those of B cells, because the genes have similar patterns of heptamer- (12 or 23 base/spacer)–nonamer sequences flanking them (see Chapter 4). Similar or identical rearrangement enzymes operate in B and T cells; experiments have shown that transfected TCR Dβ and Jγ genes can rearrange appropriately in B cells. Analysis of the amino acid sequences of many different TCRs shows that the greatest diversity is in the third complementarity-determining region (CDR3) which is created by somatic recombination and N-region development is particularly marked. Although somatic mutation is an important mechanism in generating immunoglobulin diversity, it does not occur in TCR genes. This may be linked with the need to maintain tolerance to self and recognition of MHC by T cells.

Hunkapiller and Hood have estimated that it is possible to make about 4.4×10^{13} different forms of Vβ and 8.5×10^{12} forms of Vα, and estimate that if only 1% of the sequences coded for viable proteins, this would still give 2.9×10^{22} receptors. Making the assumption that 99% of these are rejected owing to coding for autoantigens or other defects, this would still give 2.9×10^{20} possible murine TCRs. As fewer than 10^9 thymocytes leave the thymus in the lifetime of a mouse, this raises the question: how random is the generation of receptors?

Once the TCRs have been generated the cells are subjected to selection within the thymus, and then may be selected further by interactions with antigen-presenting cells. For these reasons even if TCRs are generated by random recombinations of gene segments, the expressed repertoire will be skewed towards usage of particular genes. A major area of research in recent years has been to determine which sets of TCR V genes are used in the responses against different antigens, and this depends not just on the antigen, but also on the MHC molecules within the individual, since T cells recognize antigenic peptides on a particular MHC molecule.

Furthermore, the expression of different V-gene segments by distinct T-cell subsets may reflect their ontogeny. For example, γδ T cells residing in mouse skin (dendritic epidermal cells or DECs) express exclusively the Vγ3 and Vδ1 regions, whereas intraepithelial lymphocytes (IELs) from the gut epithelium express Vγ5 almost exclusively (in combination with predominantly Vδ4, Vδ5, Vδ6 or Vδ7). It is thought that these populations may arise at distinct stages during intrathymic T-cell development.

MAJOR HISTOCOMPATIBILITY COMPLEX (MHC) MOLECULES

The molecules which present antigen to T cells are mostly encoded within the MHC. This gene complex was first identified, when it was observed that histocompatibility, i.e. the ability to accept grafts from another strain, depended on the donor and recipient sharing the same MHC haplotype. It transpired that the gene complex is very large, containing more than 100 separate gene loci, but the molecules which determine graft rejection are a limited group termed class I and class II MHC molecules and these are the molecules that present antigen. This gene complex has been identified in all mammalian species, although it varies in detail between species.

MHC class I and II molecules are highly polymorphic cell-surface structures. They were initially identified using alloantibodies produced by one inbred strain of mouse in response to immunization with cells of other strains differing genetically only at the MHC. Subsequently, specific antibodies to molecules encoded in subregions of the MHC, defined from crossovers in inbred strains, were used to map the MHC in detail. The gene complex in mouse is called H-2. Similar techniques were used to define the human MHC, which is known as the human leucocyte antigen (HLA) system. The nomenclature reflects the way in which these molecules were characterized, i.e. as antigens that could be recognized by antibodies or lymphocytes from another strain.

The overall organization of the human and murine MHCs is presented in *Figure 5.4*. Class I and class II molecules represent distinct structural entities; that is, although multiple class I and class II genes exist within the MHC, all class I and class II gene products have similar overall structures. The remaining genes in the complex are very diverse. They include some that encode complement system molecules (C4, C2, Factor B), some cytokines (TNF), enzymes, heat-shock proteins and some molecules involved in antigen processing. There are no functional or structural similarities between these other genes; they have collectively been called class III gene products, although this term is gradually falling into disuse. Only those loci involved in antigen presentation are described in this chapter.

MHC class I molecules consist of an MHC-encoded heavy chain bound to β_2-microglobulin

The overall structure of the extracellular portion of an MHC class I molecule is presented in *Figure 5.5*. It comprises a glycosylated heavy chain (45 kDa) non-covalently associated with β_2-microglobulin (12 kDa), a polypeptide that is also found free in serum. The class I heavy chain consists of three extracellular domains, designated α_1 (N-terminal), α_2 and α_3, a transmembrane region and a cytoplasmic tail. The three extracellular domains each comprise about 90 amino acids and can be cleaved from the surface with the proteolytic enzyme papain. The α_2 and α_3 domains both have intrachain disulphide bonds enclosing loops of 63 and 86 amino acids respectively. The α_3 domain is structurally homologous to immunoglobulin C domains, and contains a site which interacts with CD8 on cytotoxic T cells. The extracellular portion of the class I heavy chain is glycosylated, the degree of glycosylation depending on the species and haplotype. The predominantly hydrophobic transmembrane region comprises 25 amino acid residues and traverses the lipid bilayer most probably in an α-helical conformation. The hydrophilic cytoplasmic domain, 30–40 residues long, may be phosphorylated *in vivo*.

β_2-microglobulin is essential for expression of MHC class I molecules

β_2-microglobulin is non-polymorphic in humans, but is dimorphic in mice (a single amino acid change at position 85). It has the structure of an immunoglobulin constant region domain. This molecule also associates with a number of other class I-like molecules, for example the products of the CD1 genes on chromosome 1 in man, and the Fc receptor that mediates the uptake of IgG from milk in

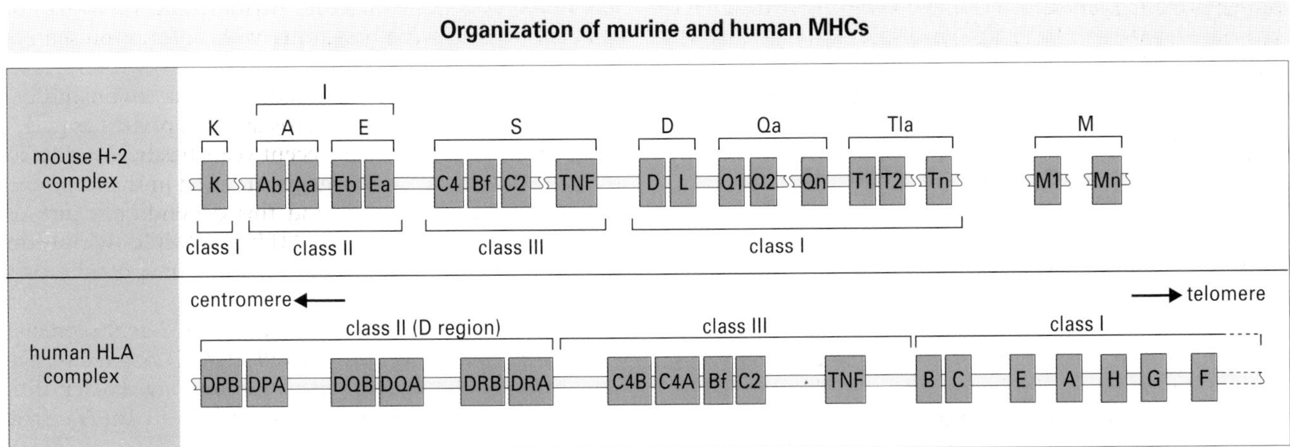

Fig. 5.4 Diagram showing the locations of subregions of the murine and human MHCs and the positions of the major genes within these subregions. The human organization pattern, in which the class II loci are positioned between the centromere and the class I loci, occurs in every other mammalian species so far examined. The regions span 3–4 Mbp of DNA.

A model of an MHC class I molecule

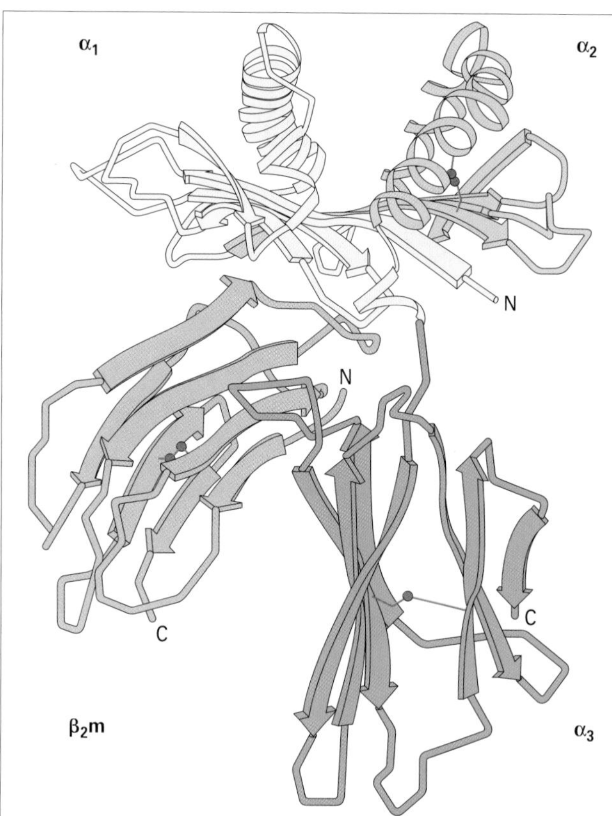

Fig. 5.5 The peptide backbone of the extracellular portion of HLA-A2 is shown. The three globular domains (α_1, α_2 and α_3) of the heavy chain are shown in green or turquoise and are closely associated with the non-MHC encoded peptide, β_2-microglobulin (grey). β_2-microglobulin is stabilized by an intrachain disulphide bond (red) and has a similar tertiary structure to an immunoglobulin domain. The groove formed by the α_1 and α_2 domains is clearly visible.

The antigen-binding site of HLA-A2

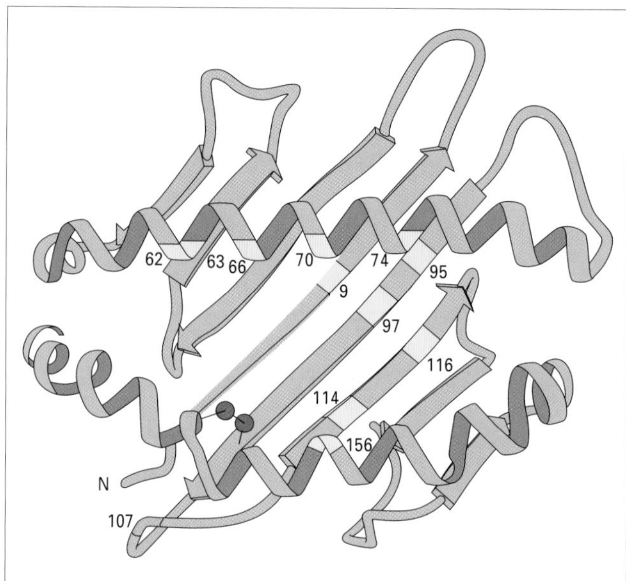

Fig. 5.6 The view of the peptide antigen-binding groove in HLA-A2 as 'seen' by the TCR. The α_1 and α_2 domains each consist of four antiparallel β strands followed by a long helical region. The domains pair to form a single eight-stranded β sheet topped by α helices. The locations of the most polymorphic residues are highlighted. Residues around the binding site are highly polymorphic. For example, HLA-2 and HLA-Aw68 differ from each other by 13 amino acid residues. Ten of these differences occur around the antigen binding site (yellow). (Modified from Bjorkman *et al. Nature* 1987;**329**:512–16, with additional data from Parham. *Nature* 1989;**342**:617–18.)

intestinal cells of neonatal rats. Such molecules which have a structural similarity to the MHC class I genes are referred to as 'class-1b molecules'. β_2-microglobulin is essential for expression of all class I molecules at the cell surface – mutant mice lacking β_2m do not express class I.

Heavy chain α_1 and α_2 domains form the antigen-binding groove

X-ray crystallography has shown that the α_1 and α_2 domains constitute a platform of eight anti-parallel β strands supporting two anti-parallel α helices (*Fig. 5.6*). The disulphide bond in the α_2 domain connects the N-terminal β strand to the α helix of the α_2 domain. A long groove separates the α helices of the α_1 and α_2 domains. The original crystal structure of the HLA-A2 molecule revealed the presence of diffuse 'extra electron density' in the groove, suggesting that it was the binding site for processed antigen. This contention is strengthened by the observation that the majority of polymorphic residues and T-cell epitopes on class I molecules are located in or near the groove.

Variations in amino acid sequence change the shape of the binding groove

Comparisons of the structures of HLA-A2 and HLA-Aw68 have further refined our understanding of the structural basis for the binding of peptide to class I antigens. The differences between HLA-A2 and HLA-Aw68 result from amino acid side-chain differences at 13 positions: six in α_1, six in α_2, and one (residue 245, which contributes to interactions with CD8) in α_3. Ten of the α_1 and α_2 differences are at positions lining the floor and side of the peptide-binding groove (*Fig. 5.6*). These differences give rise to dramatic differences in the shape of the groove and on the antigen peptides that it will bind. Seen in detail, the groove forms a number of ridges and pockets with which amino acid side-chains can interact. Typically the groove on an MHC class I molecule will accommodate peptides of eight or nine residues. Amino acid variations within the groove can vary the positions of the pockets, providing the structural basis for differences in peptide-binding affinity that in turn govern exactly what is presented to a T cell (*Fig. 5.7*).

Class II molecules resemble class I molecules in their overall structure

The products of the class II genes (A and E in the mouse, DP, DQ and DR in humans) are heterodimers of heavy (α)

Peptide-binding grooves of HLA-Aw68 and HLA-A2

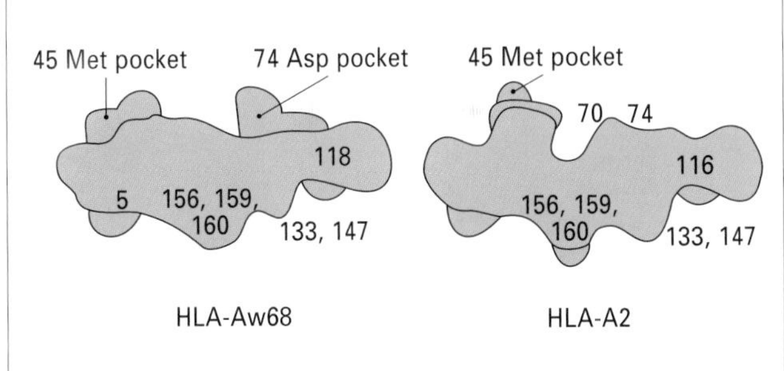

Fig. 5.7 The diagram illustrates the shape of the antigen-binding groove on each molecule. Differences in amino acids around the groove create different antigen-binding sites. For example, residues around position 45 produce a methionine-binding pocket in both molecules, but the aspartate-binding pocket around residue 74 is only present in HLA-Aw68.

Comparison of the extracellular domains of class I and class II molecules

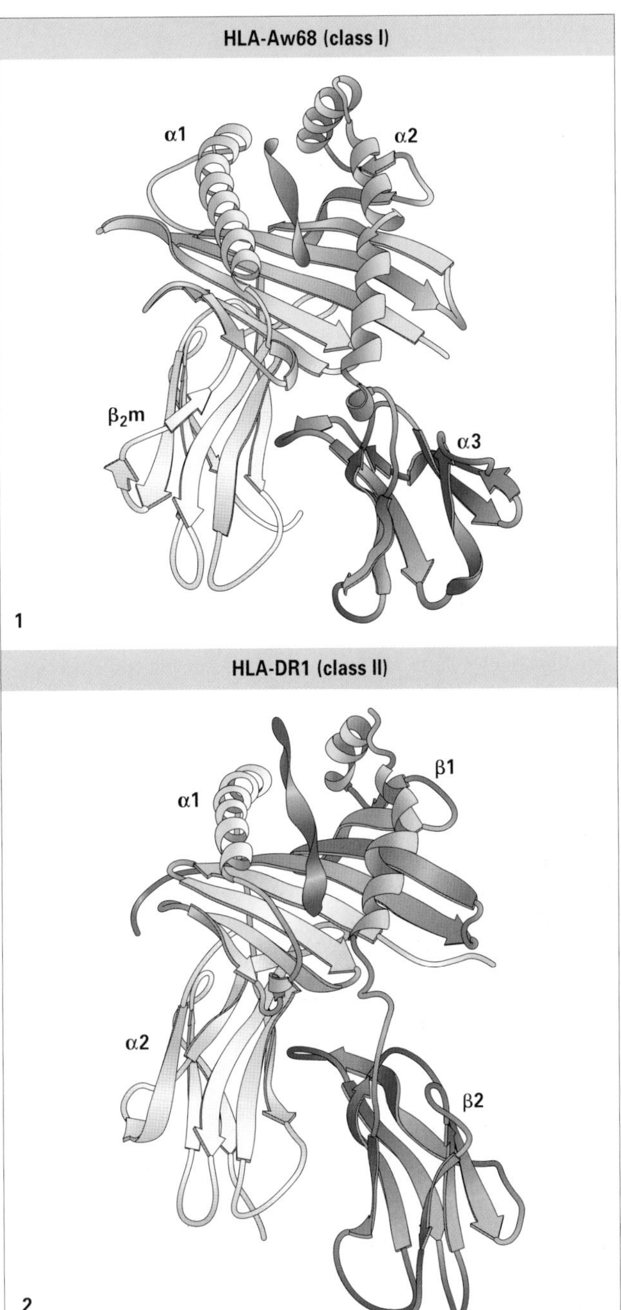

Fig. 5.8 Ribbon diagrams of the extracellular domains of class I HLA-Aw68 (**1**) and class II HLA-DR1 (**2**) histocompatibility antigens. The binding cleft is shown with a resident peptide. These diagrams emphasize the similarity in the three-dimensional structures of class I and class II antigens. (Redrawn with permission from Stern LJ. *Structure* 1994;**2**:245–51.)

and light (β) glycoprotein chains. Both of the chains are encoded in the MHC. The α chains have molecular weights of 30–34 kDa. The β chains range from 26 to 29 kDa, depending on the locus involved. A number of lines of evidence indicate that the α and β chains have the same overall structures. An extracellular portion comprising two domains (α_1 and α_2, or β_1 and β_2) is connected by a short sequence to a transmembrane region of about 30 residues and a cytoplasmic domain of about 10–15 residues.

The α_2 and β_2 domains are similar to the class I α_3 domain and β_2m, possessing the structural characteristics of immunoglobulin constant domains. The β_1 domain contains a disulphide bond generating a 64 amino acid loop. The difference in molecular weights of the class II α and β chains is primarily due to differential glycosylation. The α_1, α_2 and β_1 domains are N-glycosylated, and the β_2 domain is not. The β_2 domain does however contain a binding site for CD4, and class II molecules on antigen-presenting cells interact with CD4 on T cells in an analagous way to the interaction of class I molecules with CD8. As will be explained below, CD4 and CD8 are important elements in antigen presentation, because they are involved in the recruitment of kinases, which signal T-cell activation.

Despite the differences in length and organization of the polypeptide chains, the overall three-dimensional structure of class II molecules is very similar to that of class I (*Fig. 5.8*).

INTERACTIONS OF MHC MOLECULES WITH ANTIGENIC PEPTIDES

The MHC class II binding groove accommodates longer peptides than class I

Notwithstanding their similarities, differences are seen in the class I and II molecules. Notably, the class II groove is more open than that of class I, so that longer peptides can be accommodated (*Fig. 5.9*). The structural features of the class II antigen-binding site have been illuminated by the determination of the crystal structure of HLA-DR1 complexed with an influenza virus peptide (*Fig. 5.10*). Pockets were clearly visible within the peptide-binding site

The peptide binding sites of class I (H–2K^b) and class II (HLA-DR1) molecules

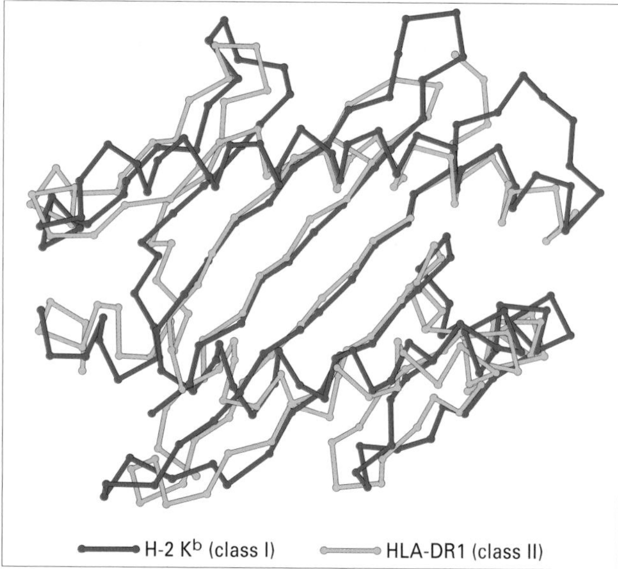

Fig. 5.9 The peptide binding sites of class I (H–2K^b) and class II (HLA–DR1) are shown as α-carbon atom traces in a top view of the peptide-binding clefts. The similarities between the two sites can clearly be seen, although there are also some differences, some of which account for the difference in peptide length preference between class I (8–10 amino acid residues) and class II (>12 amino acid residues). (Redrawn with permission from Stern LJ. *Structure* 1994;2:245–51.)

Peptides bind non-covalently within the antigen-binding groove

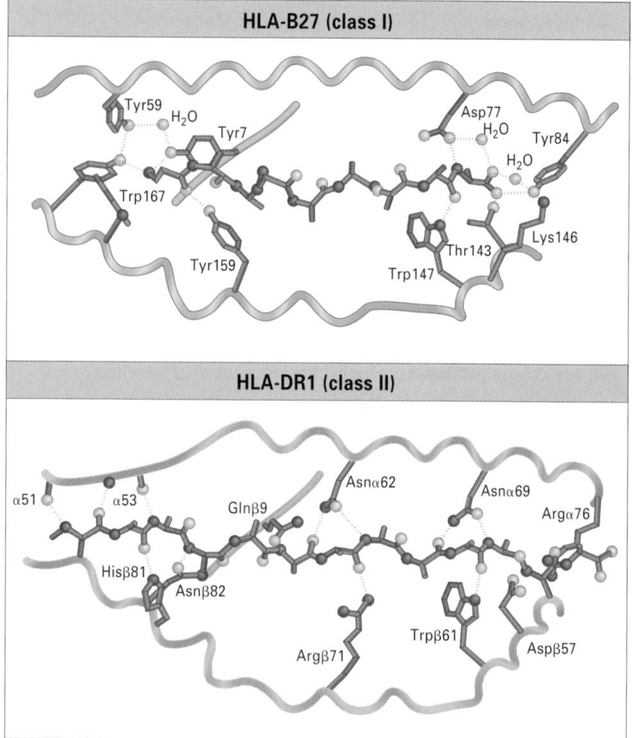

Fig. 5.10 The hydrogen bonds made by the main chain of a bound peptide with class I (HLA-B27) or class II (HLA-DR1) are shown. The major difference between the two hydrogen-bonding patterns is the clustering of conserved class I hydrogen bonds at the ends of the peptide. By contrast, conserved class II hydrogen bonds are distributed throughout the length of the peptide. (Redrawn with permission from Stern LJ. *Structure* 1994;2:245–51.

that accommodate five side-chains of the bound peptide and explain the peptide specificity of HLA-DR1.

As was noted above, the precise topology of the MHC peptide-binding groove depends partly on the nature of the amino acids within the groove, and thus varies from one haplotype to the next. Which peptide can bind to a particular MHC molecule depends on the nature of the side-chains of the peptide and their complementarity with the MHC molecule's binding groove. Some amino acid side-chains of the peptide stick out of the groove and are available to contact the TCR.

Peptides are held in the MHC molecules' binding cleft by characteristic anchor residues

It is possible to purify and sequence peptides that have been generated by a cell and then bound by MHC molecules at the cell surface. These peptides include not just foreign peptides from internalized antigens or viral particles, but also self molecules produced within the cell or endocytosed from extracellular fluids. Self peptides eluted from MHC class I molecules have been purified and sequenced. They were shown to be nine amino acids in length. Remarkably, these peptides were precisely defined. A number of peptides bound by particular MHC molecules were sequenced, and characteristic residues were identified – one at the C terminus and another close to the N terminus of the peptide. These characteristic motifs distinguish sets of binding peptides for different class I molecules (*Fig. 5.11*).

The significance of these conserved residues has become clear by analysis of the three-dimensional structures of several class I molecules. These studies have generated a particularly clear picture of the peptide residing in the binding groove. The ends of the peptide binding groove are closed. The peptide is an extended (not α-helical) chain of nine amino acids and the N and C termini are buried at the ends of the groove. Some of the side-chains also extend into the pockets formed within the variable region of the class I heavy chain and numerous hydrogen bonds are formed between residues on the class I molecule and those of the peptide along its length. In particular, tyrosine residues commonly found at the N terminus of the peptide and a conserved lysine in the class I binding groove stabilize peptide binding (*Fig. 5.10*). The centres of the peptide bulge out of the groove, thus presenting different structures to TCRs. This picture is consistent with the characteristic motifs found at the ends of peptides eluted from class I molecules.

The groove on the MHC class II molecule also incorporates a number of binding pockets, although the location is somewhat different from that on class I molecules. As the class II groove is not closed at the ends, peptides bound

Allele-specific motifs in peptides eluted from MHC class I molecules

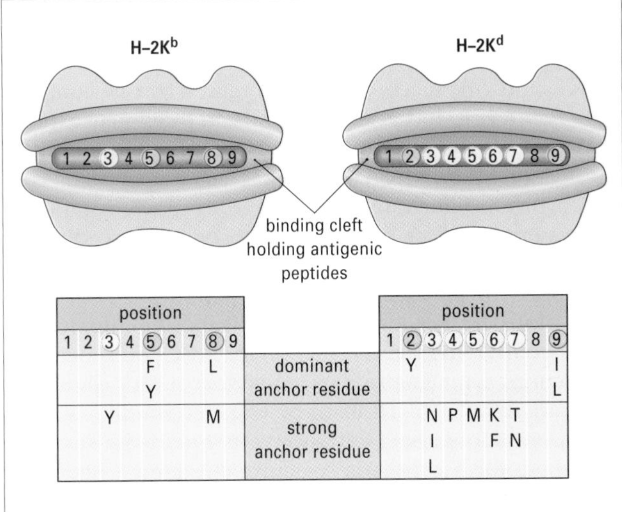

H-2K^b position 1	2	3	4	5	6	7	8	9		H-2K^d position 1	2	3	4	5	6	7	8	9
				F Y			L		dominant anchor residue		Y							I L
		Y					M		strong anchor residue			N I L	P	M	K F	T N		

Fig. 5.11 Class I molecules from either H-2K^b or H-2K^d haplotypes were immunoprecipitated. Peptides bound to these molecules were purified and sequenced. Amino acid residues that were commonly found at a particular position are classified as 'dominant' anchor residues. Residues that are fairly common at a site are shown as 'strong'. Positions for which no amino acid is shown could be occupied by several different amino acids with equal frequency. The one-letter amino acid code is used. The diagram represents the MHC class I binding cleft, viewed from above with anchor positions of each haplotype highlighted.

Allele-specific motifs in peptides eluted from MHC class II molecules

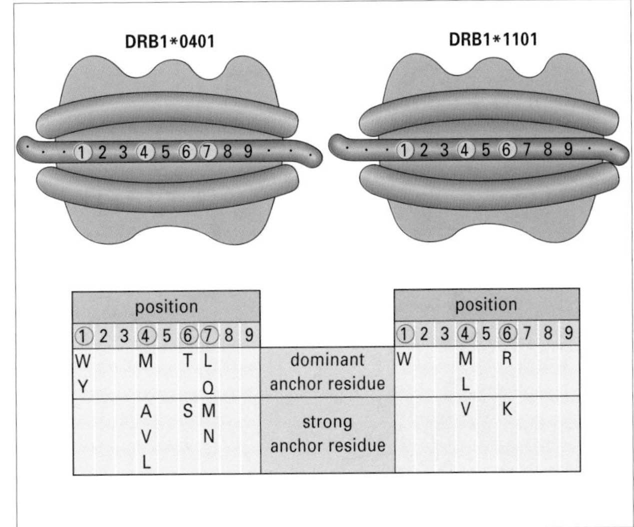

DRB1*0401 position 1	2	3	4	5	6	7	8	9		DRB1*1101 position 1	2	3	4	5	6	7	8	9
W Y			M		T	L Q			dominant anchor residue	W			M L		R			
			A V L		S	M N			strong anchor residue				V		K			

Fig. 5.12 HLA-DR molecules of two haplotypes (DRB1*0401 and DRB1*1101) were purified and incubated with a library of peptides (generated in phage M13). After multiple rounds of selection, peptides that bound effectively to the class II molecules were identified and sequenced. Residues having a frequency greater than 20% are shown as 'dominant' anchor residues. Other fairly common residues are shown as 'strong'. (Data abstracted from Hammer, Valsasnini, Tolba, *et al. Cell* 1993;**74**:197–203.) Note that the binding site on class II molecules accommodates longer peptides than that on class I.

to class II molecules extend out of the ends of the groove. Consistent with this observation, peptides eluted from class II molecules tend to be longer – more than 15 residues. Conserved anchor residues in class II peptides have been identified, although these are more difficult to detect than those of class I peptides because of the ragged ends and the more even distribution of bonds tethering the peptide to the class II binding groove (*Fig. 5.12*). A major difference occurs at the ends of the peptide binding groove: in class I antigens, interactions at the N and C termini confine the peptide to the cleft; for class II molecules, peptides may extend beyond the ends of the cleft.

The peptides which bind to MHC class I molecules come from proteins synthesized within the cell, which are broken down and transported to the endoplasmic reticulum. The mechanism of antigen processing will be explained fully in Chapter 6, but it should be noted here that the internal antigen-processing pathways generally produce peptides of an appropriate size to occupy the class I antigen binding groove. By contrast, peptides which bind to MHC class II come from proteins which have been internalized by the cell and then degraded. These peptides are less uniform in size and may be trimmed once they have bound to the MHC class II molecule. The class II antigen processing pathway is quite distinct from the class I pathway (see Chapter 6).

INTERACTION OF THE T-CELL RECEPTOR WITH MHC AND ANTIGEN

Once the structures of the T-cell receptor and the MHC–peptide complex had been established, the next question was to determine how they interact. The first crystallographic data was derived using a co-crystal of a mouse class I molecule bound to an endogenous cellular peptide and an $\alpha\beta$ T-cell receptor (*Fig. 5.13*). This structure showed that the axis of the T-cell receptor was roughly aligned with the peptide-binding groove on the MHC molecule, but set at 20–30° askew. This means that the first and second complementarity-determining regions (CDR) of the TCR α and β chains are positioned over residues near the N and C termini of the presented polypeptide, and the third CDRs of each chain, lying at the centre of the TCR-binding site, are positioned over the central residues of the peptide which protrude from the groove. This is very logical, since the first two CDRs are encoded in the germ line, while CDR3α and CDR3β are generated by recombination, are therefore more variable and thus are best suited for interactions with diverse antigenic peptides. Residues from each of the CDRs are positioned to interact with residues from the MHC molecule. Hence the molecular structure underpins the experimental findings that T cells recognize antigenic peptides bound to particular

Interaction of a T-cell receptor and MHC–peptide complex

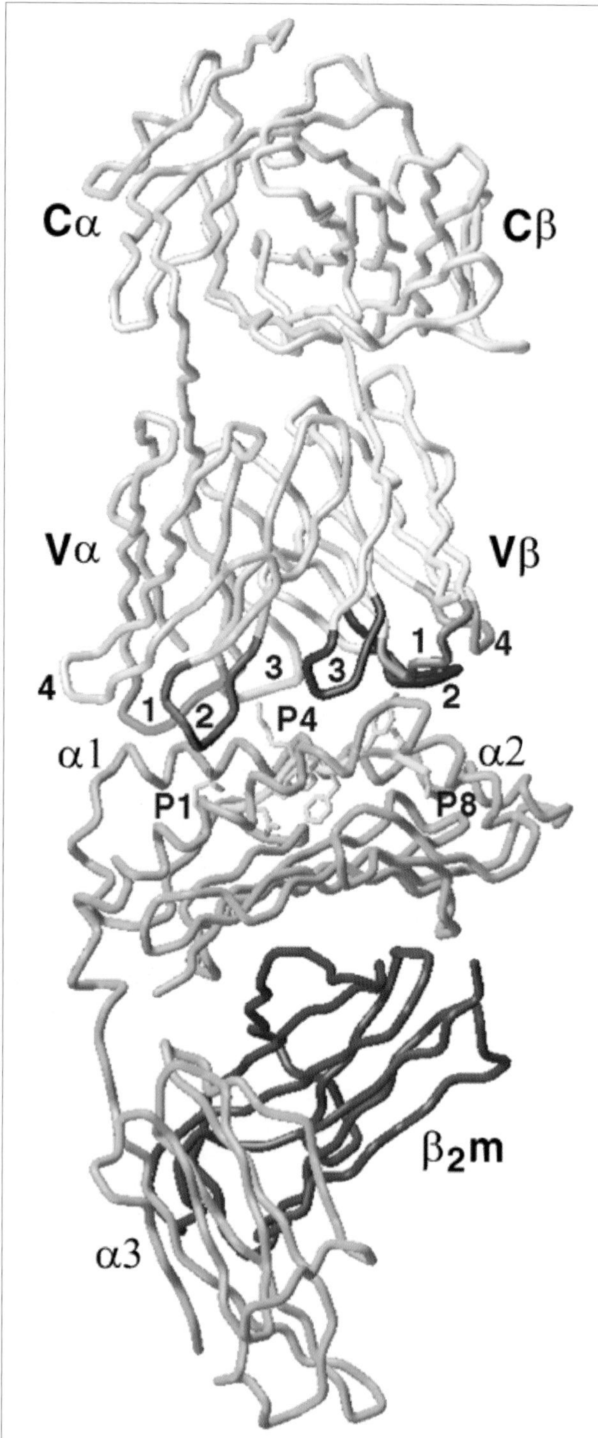

Fig. 5.13 The structure of an MHC class I molecule (H-2K[b]), complexed to an octapeptide (yellow tube) is shown bound to an αβ TCR. The six CDRs which contact the peptide (1, 2, 3, 1, 2) are highlighted in deeper colours. Residues from αHV4 (pink) and βHV4 (orange) are not positioned to take part in the intermolecular interactions. (Illustration was kindly provided by Dr Christopher Garcia, and is reproduced with permission: *Science* 1996;**274**:209–19.)

MHC molecules. This arrangement of TCR and MHC–antigen is broadly similar, for the small number of of receptors which have been analysed by X-ray crystallography.

Aggregation of TCRs initiates T cell activation

Although basic models of T cell activation by antigen/MHC show one receptor being triggered by one complex (e.g. *Fig. 1.12*)., this is simplistic. Each T cell may express 10^5 receptors and each antigen presenting cell has a similar number of MHC molecules. If a T cell engages an APC only a tiny proportion of the MHC/antigen complexes on its surface will be of the correct type to be recognised by the T cell. What then, is the minimum signal for T cell activation? In practice, only a few peptide/MHC/TCR interactions are needed, perhaps 100 specific interactions or 0.1% of the MHC molecules on the APC. Moreover the interactions can take place over a period of time – it is not necessary for all 100 TCRs to be engaged simultaneously.

The model of the TCR shown in *Figure 5.2* suggests that it can form a dimeric structure clustered around the signalling molecules of the CD3 complex. Interestingly there is some evidence that MHC molecules can also dimerize, and that TCRs which are bound to MHC–peptide complexes tend to form dimers or aggregates. These observations have lead to the view that T-cell activation requires the cooperative aggregation of specific TCRs with MHC–peptide complexes. The auxiliary molecules CD4 and CD8 are also important in T-cell activation. The presence of CD4 or CD8 can help stabilize the interaction of the TCR and MHC–peptide. In addition, kinases which are associated with these molecules are brought into proximity with CD3, so that they can phosphorylate the ζζ dimer which initiates activation (*Fig. 5.14*). The ensuing steps are described in Chapter 6 (see *Fig. 6.21*).

Antigenic peptides can induce or antagonize T-cell activation

The affinity of TCRs for antigen peptides expressed on MHC molecules is typically 10^{-5}–10^{-6}M, which is much lower than the affinity of antibody for an epitope on an antigen. The affinity of antigen–MHC for the TCR is very important because it determines the degree to which the T cell becomes activated. Peptides which activate a T cell are called agonist peptides. By changing one or two amino acids in an agonist peptide it is possible to generate peptides which antagonize the normal activation by the original peptide. The antagonist peptides typically have a lower affinity for the TCR than the original agonist peptide. They are thought to act either by interfering with the binding of the agonist peptide for the MHC molecule, and/or by binding less effectively to the TCR. Occasionally, a modified peptide will be more effective in activating the T cell than the agonist. These strong agonist (or superagonist) peptides produce higher affinity binding in the TCR–MHC–peptide complex. The distinctions between these three different types of peptide is not purely academic. For example, researchers are attempting to use antagonist peptides to block adverse immune responses. Also an understanding of T-cell receptor affinity is important in understanding how T cells may become tolerant to self antigens during development, a process described in Chapter 12.

The role of CD4 and CD8 in T-cell activation

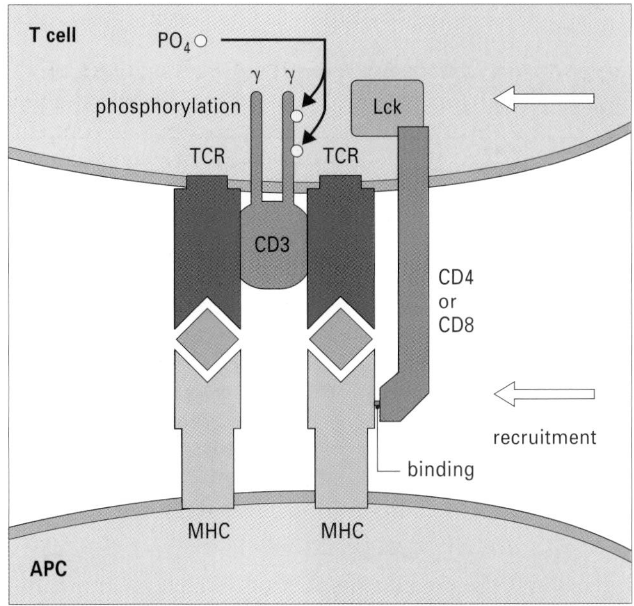

Fig. 5.14 After aggregation of MHC–peptide on the antigen-presenting cell with the T-cell's receptor, either CD4 or CD8 can join the complex. CD4 binds to MHC class II molecules and CD8 to class I. The kinase lck is attached to the intracytoplasmic portion of CD4 or CD8. Binding of these molecules to specific sites in the MHC brings the kinase into proximity with the ITAMs on the CD3 ζζ dimer. The kinase phosphorylates the motifs, as the first step in T-cell activation.

Finally we should consider the question of what constitutes T-cell specificity. When the specificity of lymphocytes was first explained in Chapter 1, it was stated that each lymphocyte binds to just one antigen using its receptor. Although this is a good starting point for understanding immune reactions it is not strictly true. In Chapter 4 it was seen that immunoglobulins could bind to different antigens if they had epitopes which were sufficiently similar. This chapter has shown that antigenic peptides can be mutated and still bind and trigger T-cell activation. One question, then, is how far a peptide can be mutated and still bind to its own TCR? In some cases it has been possible to change every single amino acid in a peptide without destroying its ability to bind to the MHC molecule or the TCR. Provided the peptide can form part of the TCR–MHC–peptide complex and provide sufficient binding energy, its precise amino acid sequence does not matter. This is a very important observation. Later, when we consider how antigenic peptides from microorganisms could trigger autoimmune diseases (see Chapter 26), one proposed mechanism is that a self peptide and a foreign peptide are similar and bind to the same T cell, thus causing a breakdown in self tolerance. One conclusion from the work cited above is that such peptides do not have to be identical to be cross-reactive.

MHC GENOMIC ORGANIZATION AND EXPRESSION

The numbers of gene loci for class I and class II molecules varies between species and between different haplotypes within each species. Many polymorphic variants have been described at each of the loci. Much of the original work on the MHC was done using mice and this has been broadly applicable to man.

There are three human class I loci

The human class I region contains three principle class I loci, called HLA-A, HLA-B and HLA-C. Each locus encodes the heavy chain of a classical MHC class I antigen and the whole region extends over 1.8 million bases of DNA and includes 118 genes (*Fig. 5.15*). Closer analysis of this region has revealed multiple additional class I genes. The HLA-E, -F, -G and -H genes also encode MHC class I proteins, and these are called class 1b genes. They are much less polymorphic than the A, B and C locus gene products and recent work has ascribed various functions to them. For example, HLA-E and HLA-G gene products can bind to antigenic peptides but are involved in recognition by NK cells (see Chapter 10).

Mice have two or three class I loci

The mouse MHC (H–2) has three class I loci, but the number of class I genes varies between haplotypes (*Fig. 5.16*). Class I genes involved in antigen presentation to T cells are located in H–2K, H–2D and H–2L loci. The organization of the H–2K region is similar in all strains that have been studied. It contains two class I genes, termed K and K2.

Genes within the human class I region

principal class I genes
B C E A H G F
other class I genes
17 X 30 92 J 80 P5-3 21 70 16 90 75

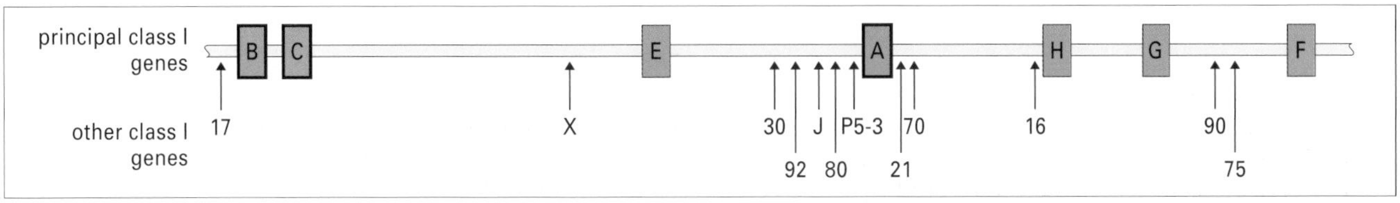

Fig. 5.15 The human class I region lies telomeric to the class II–class III region. In addition to the genes encoding the classic transplantation antigens (HLA-A, HLA-B and HLA-C), several other principle class I-like genes have been identified (HLA-E, HLA-F and HLA-G). Mutations in the HLA-H gene are associated with haemochromatosis. A number of other non-classical class I genes and pseudogenes are present, mostly with unknown functions.

Genes within the murine class I region

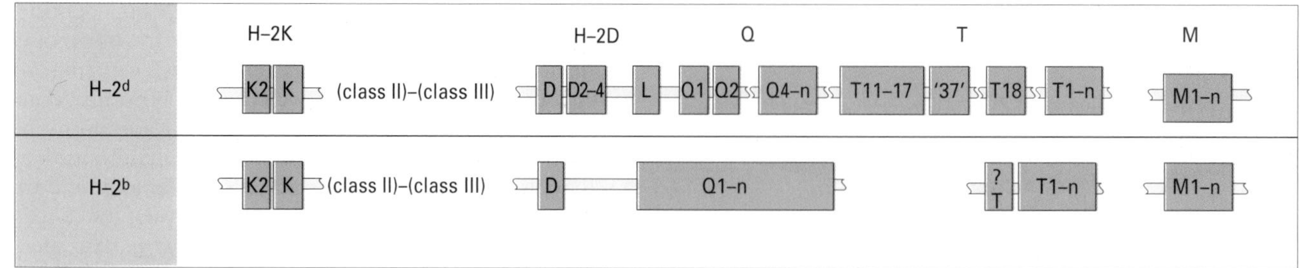

Fig. 5.16 The organization of the MHC class I region of two haplotypes, BALB/c (H–2^{d}) and B10 (H–2^{b}), is shown. The class II–class III region lies between the H–2K and H–2D regions. The brackets denote gaps added to align alleles between the two haplotypes. H–2^{d} and H–2^{b} haplotypes have different numbers of class I genes in the H–2D/H–2L region. Five class I genes map to the D/L region of BALB/c (H–2^{d}) mice. Two of these genes encode the serologically detectable H–2D^{d} and H–2L^{d} antigens. Three additional class I genes are found in the region between the proximal H–2D^{d} and distal H–2L^{d} genes. These genes, called D2^{d}, D3^{d} and D4^{d}, are of unknown function. Only one class I gene has been identified in the H–2D region of B10 mice. The Q, T and M regions contain a large number of class Ib genes, the functions of which are mostly unknown.

The H–2K gene encodes the H–2K antigen expressed on most cell types and recognized serologically, whereas the H–2K2 gene exhibits varied patterns of expression, depending on the strain. The numbers of genes in the H–2D and H–2L loci are variable (*Fig. 5.16*).

The Qa, Tla and M regions encode class 1b molecules, of which the functions are mostly unknown. The Qa locus comprises about 200 kb of DNA distal to H–2D/L (*Fig. 5.16*). This region encodes the serologically detectable molecules Qa-1, 2, 3, 4 and 5 and encompasses a cluster of eight (BALB/c) to ten (B10) class I genes. Qa-1b coresponds to HLA-E which is involved in NK cell recognition. The murine Tla region, although defined initially as encoding the TL (thymus leukaemia) antigen, has subsequently been shown to contain the largest number of class I genes and the greatest number of differences in organization between the B10 and BALB/c haplotypes. The M region is located between the K and A regions and contains a number of new class I genes, termed M1–M7. The class 1b genes exhibit a low degree of polymorphism.

Human class II genes are located in the HLA–D region

The HLA-D region encodes at least six α and ten β chain genes for MHC class II molecules (*Fig. 5.17*). Three loci, DR, DQ and DP, encode the major expressed products of the human class II region, but additional genes have also been identified. The DR family comprises a single α gene (DRA) and up to nine β genes (DRB1–9) including pseudogenes. Several different gene arrangements occur

Genes within the human and murine class II regions

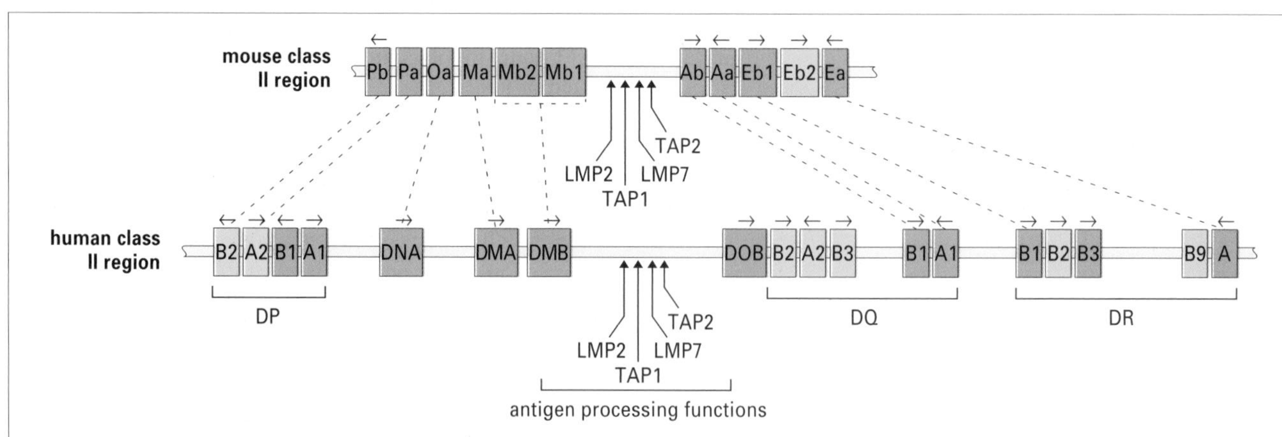

Fig. 5.17 The arrangement of the genes within the human and murine MHCs is shown. Homologous genes between the two species are indicated. Expressed genes are coloured orange and pseudogenes are shown yellow. Mice of the b, s, f and q haplotypes fail to express I-E molecules. The b and s haplotypes fail to transcribe the Ea gene but make normal cytoplasmic levels of Eb chain. Mice of f and q haplotypes fail to make both Ea and Eb chains.

The number of DRB loci varies with different haplotypes

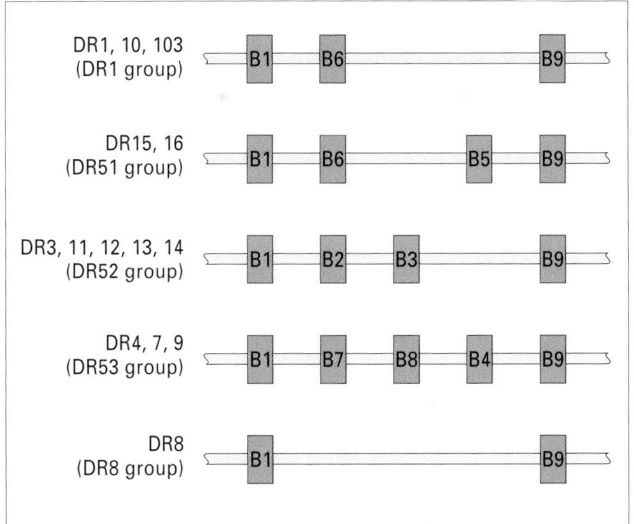

Fig. 5.18 The numbers of DRB loci varies between individuals. For example a person who has a haplotype producing molecules of the type DR1 (see Appendix I) has three loci for DRB (top line).Not all these loci produce mRNA for DRβ chains.

within this locus. The DQ and DP families each have one expressed gene for α and β chains, and an additional pair of pseudogenes. DR, DQ and DP α chains associate in the cell primarily with β chains of their own loci. For example the DPA1 and DPB1 gene products associate to generate the HLA-DP class II molecules detected using specific antibodies. Similarly, DQA1 and DQB1 encode the HLA-DQ antigens. The organization and length of the DRB region varies in different haplotypes (*Fig. 5.18*), with different numbers of β chains expressed.

The class II region also contains genes that encode proteins involved in antigen presentation that are not expressed at the cell surface. These genes including their gene products are discussed in Chapter 6. The class II region spans about 1000 kb of DNA and the order and orientation of the various loci is similar to that of the homologous loci in the murine class II region.

Murine class II genes are located in the H–2I region

The α and β chains of murine class II molecules are encoded by separate genes located in the I region of the H–2 complex (*Fig. 5.17*). The Ab and Aa genes encode the β and α chains of the A molecule. Eb and Ea genes likewise encode the two chains of the E molecule. (The gene nomenclature indicates first of all the locus and then the type of chain it encodes.) Several other class IIa and b genes have been cloned, for which no protein product is known. One of these, Pb, is a pseudogene whereas two others, called Ob and Eb2, are potentially functional. These latter genes display a low level of polymorphism and are transcribed, but it is not known whether they are translated. Different strains of mice vary in their expression of some of the class II genes (*Fig. 5.17*).

MHC polymorphism is concentrated in and around the peptide-binding cleft

A hallmark of the MHC is the extreme degree of polymorphism (structural variability) of the molecules encoded within it. Polymorphism is not evenly spread throughout the MHC. The class 1b molecules are much less polymorphic than the classical class I and class II antigens. A list of allelic variants of HLA class I and class II molecules is given in Appendix I.

Within a particular class I or class II molecule, the structural polymorphisms are clustered in particular regions of the molecule. The amino acid sequence variability in class I antigens is clustered in three main regions of the α_1 and α_2 domains. The α_3 domain appears to be much more conserved.

In class II molecules, the extent of variability depends on the subregion and on the polypeptide chain. For example, most polymorphism occurs in DRβ and DQβ chains while DPβ chains are slightly less polymorphic. DQα is polymorphic whereas DRα chains are virtually invariant, being represented by just two alleles. In outbred populations where individuals have two MHC haplotypes, hybrid class II molecules, with one chain from each haplotype, can be produced. This generates additional structural diversity in the expressed molecules.

Most of the polymorphic amino acids in class I and class II antigens are clustered on top of the molecule around the peptide binding site. Thus, variation is almost exclusively centred in the base of the antigen-binding groove or pointing in from the sides of the α helices. Thus as noted above (*Fig. 5.6*), the polymorphism affects the ability of the different MHC molecules to bind antigenic peptides.

An individual's MHC haplotype affects their susceptibility to disease

Genetic variations in MHC molecules would be of specialist interest only, were it not for the following facts. Different MHC molecules affect:

- The ability to make immune responses, including the level of antibody production.
- Resistance or susceptibility to infectious diseases.
- Resistance or susceptibility to autoimmune diseases and allergies.

Knowing this, we can start to answer the question why the MHC is so polymorphic. The immune system must handle many different pathogens. By having several different MHC molecules an individual can present a diverse range of antigens and therefore is likely to be able to mount an effective immune response. Thus, there is a selective advantage in having different MHC molecules. Going beyond this, we know that different pathogens are prevalent in different areas of the world. Consequently evolutionary pressures from pathogens will tend to select for different MHC molecules in each area. This is indeed what is found. Different ethnic groups in various geographical areas have differing profiles of MHC haplotypes. These ideas will be further developed in Chapter 11.

Expression of MHC molecules

All nucleated cells of the body express MHC class I molecules. The function of MHC class I molecules is to present antigens which have originated inside the cell, such as viral peptides (see *Fig. 1.12*). Because any cell of the body may become infected with a virus or intracellular pathogen, all cells need to sample their internal molecules and present them at the cell surface to cytotoxic T cells. By contrast, MHC class II molecules are used by antigen-presenting cells to present antigens to helper T cells. Consequently the distribution of class II molecules is much more limited (see *Fig. 6.3*).

MHC molecules are co-dominantly expressed. This means that in one individual, all of the principle gene loci are expressed from both the maternal and paternal chromosomes. As there are three class I loci in man (HLA-A, -B and -C), and as each of the loci are highly polymorphic, most individuals will have genes for six different class I molecules, all of which will be present at the cell surface. Each MHC molecule will have a slightly different shape and present a different set of antigenic peptides. A similar argument applies to class II molecules. There are three principle loci in man (HLA-DP, -DQ and -DR), all of which are polymorphic. At first sight, it would appear that an antigen-presenting cell could express six different class II molecules as well as its class I molecules. However, this is probably an underestimate. As mentioned above, hybrid class II molecules (using one polypeptide encoded by the maternal chromosome and one by the paternal chromosome) also occur.

MHC restriction of cytotoxic T cells

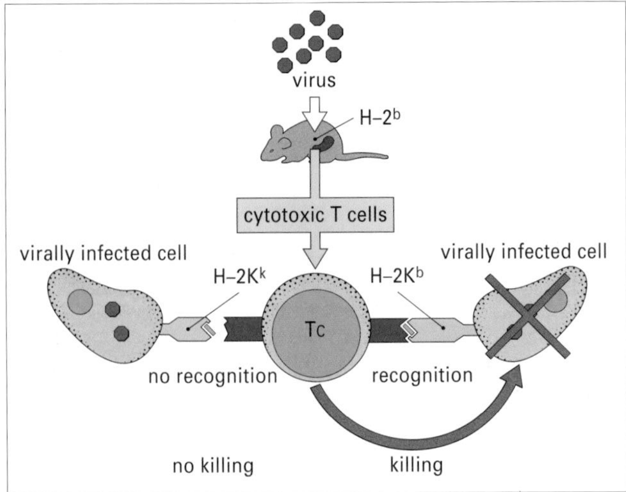

Fig. 5.19 A mouse of the H-2^b haplotype is primed with virus and the Tc cells thus generated are isolated and tested for their ability to kill H-2^b and H-2^k cells infected with the same virus. The Tc cells kill H-2^b, but not H-2^k cells. In this instance, it is the H-2K class I gene product which is presenting the antigen to the T cells. The T cell is recognizing a specific structure produced by the association of a specific MHC molecule with a specific viral antigen.

The specificity of the TCR and MHC explains genetic restriction in antigen presentation

Much of the original work on antigen presentation was carried out using inbred strains of mice. These have been inbred to the point where both maternal and paternal chromosomes are identical; consequently any offspring always inherit the same set of autosomes from each parent and offspring are genetically identical to their parents. Clearly the level of diversity in the MHC molecules is much less than in an outbred human population. However, the relative simplicity of the system allowed immunologists to dissect out exactly how antigens were presented to T cells, in a whole animal. This was at a time when the molecular structures of the MHC molecules and the TCR were completely unknown.

The key experiment which demonstrated the importance of the MHC in antigen presentation revealed a phenomenon called genetic restriction. In essence, it was noted that cytotoxic T cells from an animal infected with a virus are primed to kill cells of the same H-2 haplotype infected with that virus; they will not kill cells of a different haplotype infected with the same virus (*Fig. 5.19*). This data, and similar experiments using antigen-presenting cells and T-helper cells, showed that T cells that have been primed to recognize antigen presented on MHC molecules of one haplotype, will normally only respond again when they see the same antigen on the same MHC molecule. We can now understand these results in terms of the molecular interactions – a T-cell receptor recognizes a particular antigenic peptide presented by a specific MHC molecule, because it interacts with both the antigenic peptide and residues on the MHC molecule.

ANTIGEN PRESENTATION BY CD1

CD1 molecules are structurally related to MHC class I, consisting of a transmembrane chain which is non-covalently bound to β_2-microglobulin. However, the CD1 genes are located outside the MHC and are not polymorphic. In man, they consist of five closely linked genes, of which four are expressed (*Fig. 5.20*), encoding proteins which fall into two separate groups. Group 1 molecules in man include CD1a, CD1b and CD1c, while CD1d forms the second group. Originally CD1 was identified on cortical thymocytes, and was noted as a T-cell differentiation marker. However, CD1 molecules were subsequently found on B cells and dendritic cells.

Human CD1 genes

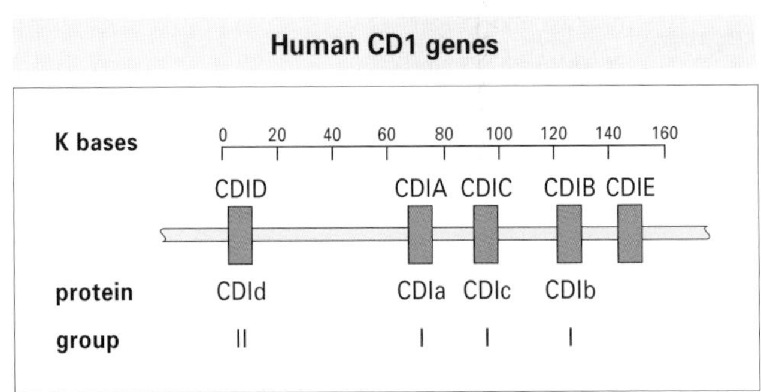

Fig. 5.20 The genes of the human CD1 cluster extend over 160 kilobases on chromosome 1. A gene product for CD1E has not yet been identified.

CD1 is an MHC class I-like molecule which presents lipid antigens

CD1d from mouse has been crystallized and analysed by X-ray crystallography. This shows that the molecule has a deep electrostatically neutral antigen-binding groove, which is highly hydrophobic and can accommodate lipid or glycolipid antigens (*Fig. 5.21*). One model for the binding places hydrophobic acyl groups of the lipids into the large hydrophobic pockets, leaving the more polar groups of the antigens, such as the phosphate and carbohydrate, on the top, where they can interact with the TCR. The binding requirements of the hydrophobic pockets on CD1 are fairly tolerant, as they will accommodate acyl groups of different lengths, but the interactions with the TCR are much more specific – small changes in the structure of the carbohydrate moiety will destroy the ability to stimulate a T cell.

The antigens presented by the group 1 CD1 molecules and CD1d are different; e.g. group 1 molecules present lipo-arabinomannan, a component of the cell wall of mycobacteria (see *Fig. 15.1*), whereas CD1d cannot do this. Another difference between CD1 and conventional MHC molecules is the way in which antigen is loaded into the antigen-binding groove. As will be explained in the next chapter, class I molecules are loaded with antigenic peptides in the endoplasmic reticulum, and this requires transport of the peptides from the cytoplasm. By contrast, group 1CD1 molecules appear to be loaded in an acidic endosomal compartment, as they do not bind to lipid antigens unless they are partially unfolded at low pH.

There is some debate as to the physiological functions of the CD1 molecules in host defence. Group 1CD1 molecules present lipids from mycobacteria and *Haemophilus influenzae* and can stimulate both $CD4^+$ and $CD8^+$ cytotoxic T cells. Hence they appear to have a role in antimicrobial defence. By contrast, most CD1d molecules appear to bind self antigens, although they also present lipids from parasites such as *Plasmodium falciparum* and *Trypanosoma brucei* (see Chapter 16) to T cells which use a restricted group of T-cell receptors. This indicates a role in defence against single-celled protozoal parasites.

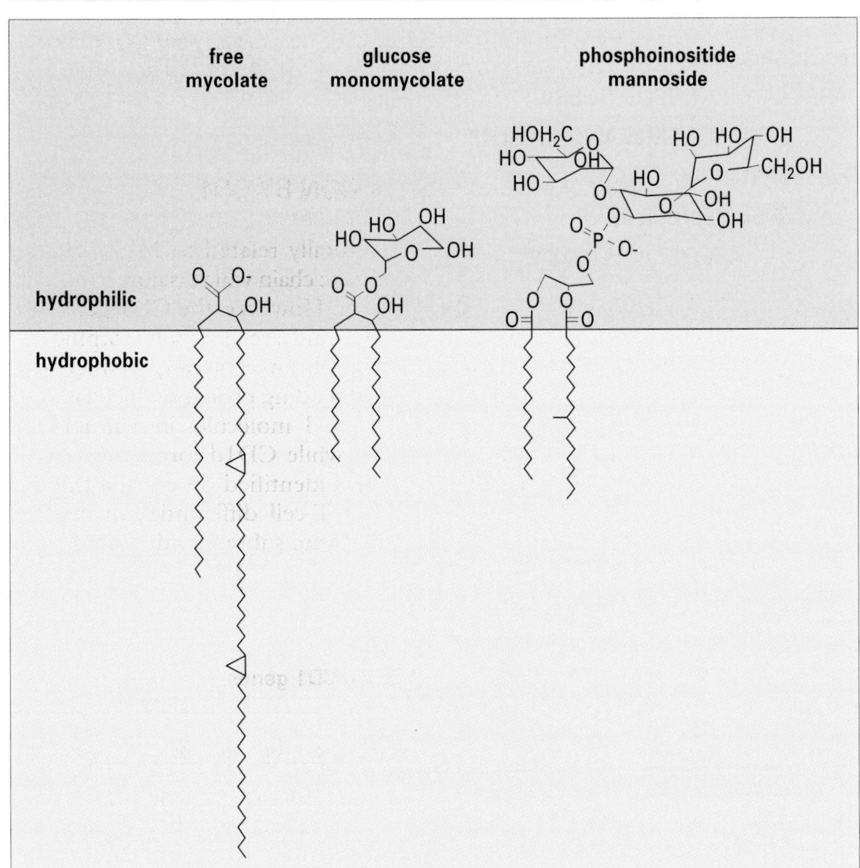

Fig. 5.21 Some of the antigens presented by CD1b are shown, each of which is a component of mycobacterial cell walls. Each of the antigens has two aliphatic tails which are thought to be buried in the two hydrophobic binding pockets on CD1b. This leaves the hydrophilic segments exposed in the centre of the binding groove, where they can contact the TCR. (Information based on Porcelli *et al. Immunol Today* 1998;**19**:362–8.)

CRITICAL THINKING • The specificity of T cells (Explanations on p. 454)

SM/J mice of the haplotype H–2^{v} were immunized with the λ repressor protein, a molecule having 102 amino acid residues. After 1 week, T cells were isolated from the animals and set up in culture with antigen-presenting cells (APCs) and antigen. The ability of APCs to activate the T cells was determined in a lymphocyte proliferation assay (see Fig. 27.25, for the basic methodology). It was found that when APCs from SM/J mice were used in the culture, the T cells were activated, but that when APCs from Balb/c mice were used (H–2^{d}) they were not activated. APCs from F1 (SM/J × Balb/c) mice were able to activate the T cells just as well as the APCs from the parental SM/J strain.

5.1 Explain why the SM/J cells and the F1 cells can present antigen to the T cells, but why the Balb/c cells cannot.

Using the primed T cells from the SM/J mouse and APCs from the same strain, the investigation continues, but peptides of the λ repressor protein are used instead of intact antigen. It is found that a peptide corresponding to residues 80–94 of the intact protein is able to stimulate the T cells, but that other peptides are much less effective or ineffective. The table below shows the sequences of some of these peptides and their ability to activate the T cells, when included in the culture at a concentration of 10 μM.

5.2 Explain why peptides 80–102 and 80–94 activate the T cells while the others do not.

In a final experiment the T cells are stimulated with a mutated variant of peptide 80–94 with aspartate (D) substituted for isoleucine (I) at position 87 (bold). It is found that the mutated peptide is able to stimulate the T cells as well as the original peptide, even when present at lower concentrations (1 μM).

5.3 What term is used to describe this kind of mutated peptide? What would you predict about the binding affinity of this peptide within the TCR–MHC–peptide complex?

Peptide	Amino acid sequence	T-cell activation
12–36	QLEDARRLKAIYEKKKNELGLSQESV	–
80–102	SPSIAREIYEMYEAVSMQPSLRS	+++
73–88	ILKVSVEEFSPSIAREIY	–
80–94	SPSIARE**I**YEMYEAVS	++
84–98	AREIYEMYEAVSMQP	–

FURTHER READING

Bentley GA, Mariuzza RA. The structure of the T cell antigen receptor. *Annu Rev Immunol* 1996;**14**:563–90.

Bjorkman PJ, Parham P. Structure, function and diversity of Class I major histocompatibility complex molecules. *Annu Rev Biochem* 1990;**59**:253–88.

Bjorkman PJ, Saper MA, Samraoui B, *et al.* The structure of the human Class I histocompatibility antigen HLA-A2. *Nature* 1987;**329**:506–12.

Bjorkman PJ, Samraoui B, Bennett WS, *et al.* The foreign antigen binding site and T-cell recognition regions of Class I histocompatibility antigens. *Nature* 1987;**329**:512–16.

Bodmer JG, Marsh, SE, Albert ED, *et al.* Nomenclature for factors of the HLA system, 1994. *Tissue Antigens* 1994;**44**:1–18.

Brenner MB, MacLean J, Dialynas DP, *et al.* Identification of a putative second T-cell receptor. *Nature* 1986;**322**:145–9.

Brown JH, Jardetzky TS, Gorga JC, *et al.* Three-dimensional structure of the human class II histocompatibility antigen HLA-DR1. *Nature* 1993;**364**:33–9.

Burdin N, Kronenberg M. CD1-mediated immune responses to glycolipids. *Curr Opin Immunol* 1999;**111**:326–31.

Carosella ED, Dausett J, Kirzenbaum H. HLA–G revisited. *Immunol Today* 1996;**17**:407–9.

Chien Y-H, Jores R, Crowley MP. Recognition by γδ T cells. *Annu Rev Immunol* 1996;**14**:511–32.

Davis MM, Bjorkman PJ. T-cell antigen receptor genes and T-cell recognition. *Nature* 1988;**334**:395–402.

Davis MM, Boniface JJ, Reich Z, *et al.* Ligand recognition by αβ T cells. *Annu Rev Immunol* 1998;**16**:523–44.

Garcia KC, Degano M, Stanfield RL, *et al.* An αβ T cell receptor structure at 2.5Å and its orientation in the TCR–MHC. *Complex Sci* 1996;**274**:209–19.

Garcia KC, Teyton GL, Wilson IA. Structural basis of T cell recognition. *Annu Rev Immunol* 1999;**17**:369–398.

Garratt TPJ, Saper MA, Bjorkman PJ, *et al.* Specificity pockets for the side chains of peptide antigens in HLA-w68. *Nature* 1989;**342**:692–6.

Hass W, Pereira P, Tonegawa S. Gamma/delta cells. *Annu Rev Immunol* 1993;**11**:637–85.

Lefranc M-P, Rabbitts TH. The human T-cell receptor γ (TRG) genes. *Trends Biochem Sci* 1989;**14**:214–18.

Leiden JM. Transcriptional regulation of T cell receptor genes. *Annu Rev Immunol* 1993;**11**:539–70.

Madden DR, Gorga JC, Strominger L, *et al.* The structure of HLA-B27 reveals nonamer self-peptides bound in an extended conformation. *Nature* 1991;**353**:321–5.

Manning TC, Kranz DM. Binding energetics of T-cell receptors: correlation with immunological consequences. *Immunol Today* 1999;**20**:417–22.

Porcelli SA, Segelke BW, Sugita M, Wilson IA, Brenner MB. The CD1 family of lipid antigen-presenting molecules. *Immunol Today* 1998;**19**:362–8.

Powis SH, Trowsdale J. Human major histocompatibility complex genes. *Behring Inst Mitt* 1994;**94**:17–25.

Raulet DH. How $\gamma\delta$ T cells make a living. *Curr Biol* 1994;**4**:246–51.

Salter RD, Benjamin RJ, Wesley PK, *et al.* A binding site for the T-cell co-receptor CD8 on the α_3 domain of HLA-A2. *Nature* 1990;**345**:41–6.

San José E, Sahuquillo AG, Bragado R, Alarcón B. Assembly of the TCR/CD3 complex: CD3 epsilon/delta and CD3 epsilon/gamma dimers associate indistinctly with both TCR alpha and TCR beta chains. Evidence for a double TCR heterodimer model. *Eur J Immunol* 1998;**28**:12–21.

Sloan-Lancaster J, Allen PM. Altered peptide–ligand induced partial T cell activation: molecular mechanisms and role in T cell biology. *Annu Rev Immunol* 1996;**14**:1–27.

Stern LJ, Brown JH, Jardetzky TS, *et al.* Crystal structure of the human class II MHC protein HLA-DR1 complexed with an influenza virus peptide. *Nature* 1994;**368**:215–21.

Stern LJ, Wiley DC. Antigenic peptide binding by class I and class II histocompatibility proteins. *Structure* 1994;**2**:245–51.

Weiss A, Littman DR. Signal transduction by lymphocyte antigen receptor. *Cell* 1994;**76**:263–74.

Zeng ZH, Castaño LH, Segelke B, Stura EA, Peterson PA, Wilson IA. The crystal structure of mouse CD1: an MHC-like fold with a large hydrophobic binding groove. *Science* 1997;**277**:339–45.

6 Antigen presentation

- **T cells recognize peptide fragments which have been processed and become bound to major histocompatibility complex (MHC) class I or II molecules.** These MHC–antigen complexes are presented at the cell surface.
- **MHC class I molecules bind to peptides produced by degradation of the cells' internal molecules.** This type of antigen processing is carried out by proteasomes which cleave the proteins and transporters which take the fragments to the endoplasmic reticulum.
- **MHC class II molecules bind to peptides produced following breakdown of proteins which the cell has endocytosed.** The peptides produced by degradation of these external antigens are loaded onto class II molecules in a specialized endosomal compartment called MIIC.
- **CD4 binds to MHC class II and CD8 to MHC class I.** These interactions increase the affinity of T-cell binding to the appropriate MHC–antigen complex.
- **Intercellular adhesion molecules also contribute to the interaction between a T cell and an antigen-presenting cell (APC).** Interactions between intercellular adhesion molecule-1 (ICAM-1) or ICAM-3 and leucocyte functional antigen-1 (LFA-1) and between CD2 and its ligands extend the interaction between T cell and APC.
- **Co-stimulatory molecules are essential for T-cell activation.** Molecules such as B7 on the APC bind to CD28 on the T cell to cause activation. Antigens presented without co-stimulation usually induce T-cell anergy.
- **T-cell activation induces enzyme cascades, leading to the production of interleukin-2 (IL-2) and the high affinity IL-2 receptor on the T cell.** IL-2 is required to drive T-cell division.

Antigens recognised by T cells are degraded or processed in some way, so that the determinant recognized by the TCR is only a small fragment of the original antigen. Antigen processing refers to the degradation of antigen into peptide fragments which become bound to MHC class I or class II molecules (see Chapter 5). These are the critical fragments involved in triggering T cells. T-cell receptors (TCRs) are sensitive to the sequences of amino acids in the MHC groove, rather than the conformational determinants recognized by antibodies.

Antigen presentation plays a central role in initiating and maintaining an appropriate immune response to antigen. The process is tightly controlled at several levels. Different types of APCs are brought into play depending on the situation, dendritic cells being crucial for initiating responses. A complex series of molecular interactions takes place to ensure that small fragments of antigens are recognized in a highly specific manner by T cells. Another level of control is exerted by co-stimulatory molecules on APCs resulting in T-cell activation only when appropriate, such as in an infection. Signals from the cell surface are transmitted by invoking a series of signal transduction pathways which are interpreted by regulation of gene expression in the nucleus.

ANTIGEN-PRESENTING CELLS

Interaction with antigen-presenting cells is essential for T-cell activation

The interaction between T cells and the heterogeneous group of cells collectively termed 'antigen presenting cells', or APCs, is the most extensively studied example of cell interaction in the immune system. It is the first such interaction to occur after antigen challenge and its outcome largely dictates the subsequent course of events: if a sufficient number of $CD4^+$ T -helper (TH) cells are triggered, then the activation of B cells or the development of cell-mediated immunity follows. If TH cells are not triggered, a form of immunological tolerance can develop (see Chapter 12), so that no other immunological events follow.

Several cell types can act as antigen-presenting cells

A wide spectrum of cells can present antigen, depending on how and where the antigen is first dealt with by cells of the immune system. In a lymphoid organ, the three main types of APC are dendritic cells, macrophages and B cells (*Fig. 6.1*). Activation of naïve T-cells on first encounter with antigen on the surface of an APC is called *priming*, to distinguish it from the responses of effector T cells to antigen on the surface of their target cells and the responses of primed memory T cells. Dendritic cells (DCs), which are found in abundance in the T-cell areas of lymph nodes and spleen, are the most effective cells for the initial activation of naïve T cells. DCs pick up antigens in peripheral tissues then migrate to lymph nodes, where they express high levels of adhesion and co-stimulatory molecules, as well as MHC class II antigens, which interact with the T-cell receptor (TCR) and CD4 on helper T cells. Once they have migrated, DCs stop synthesis of class II but maintain high levels of stable expression of class II molecules containing peptides from antigens derived from the tissue where the DCs originated.

Interdigitating DCs are believed to be the major APCs involved in primary immune responses because they induce T-cell proliferation more effectively than any other APC. Remarkably, DCs are able to present *internalized* antigens to T cells via class I as well as class II molecules, in a phenomenon called *cross-priming*. This results in activation of cytotoxic T cells which are then available for killing of infected cells. Macrophages and B cells can also express MHC class II, so this alone cannot explain the greater effectiveness of DCs in antigen presentation.

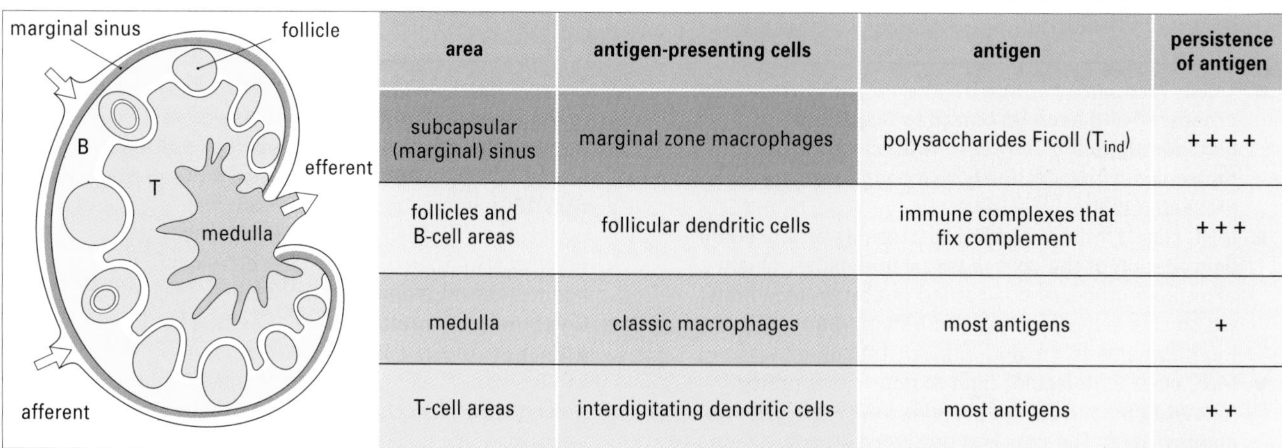

Localization of APCs in lymph nodes

area	antigen-presenting cells	antigen	persistence of antigen
subcapsular (marginal) sinus	marginal zone macrophages	polysaccharides Ficoll (T_{ind})	+ + + +
follicles and B-cell areas	follicular dendritic cells	immune complexes that fix complement	+ + +
medulla	classic macrophages	most antigens	+
T-cell areas	interdigitating dendritic cells	most antigens	+ +

Fig. 6.1 A lymph node represented schematically shows afferent and efferent lymphatics, follicles, the outer cortical B-cell area and the paracortical T-cell area. Different antigen-presenting cells predominate in these areas and selectively take up different types of antigen, which then persist on the surface of the cells for variable periods. Polysaccharides are preferentially taken up by marginal zone macrophages and may persist for months or years, whereas antigens on recirculating macrophages in the medulla may last for only a few days or weeks. Note that recirculating 'veiled' cells (Langerhans' cells), which originally come from the skin, change their morphology to become interdigitating dendritic cells within the lymph node. Both these cells, and the follicular dendritic cells, have long processes which are in intimate contact with lymphocytes.

Macrophages and B cells express appropriate co-stimulatory molecules for activation of naïve T cells only upon infection. Macrophages ingest microbes and particulate antigens for presentation. They destroy microorganisms as part of the innate immune system and this process of removal of invading microbes does not require T-cell help. Like DCs, phagocytic cells (mononuclear phagocytes or macrophages) also present antigens very effectively on class II molecules. High levels of MHC as well as co-stimulatory molecules such as B7 (see later) are induced on macrophages by uptake of bacteria which is enhanced by receptors specific to certain surface components of bacteria. Once engulfed, the microorganisms are digested in phagolysosomes to generate peptides for presentation.

B cells can bind to a specific antigen, internalize it and then degrade it into peptides which associate with class II molecules. If antigen concentrations are very low B cells with high-affinity antigen receptors (IgM or IgD) are the most effective APC, because other APCs simply cannot capture enough antigen. Thus, for secondary responses, when the number of antigen-specific B cells is high, B cells may be a major type of APC. B cells do not normally express co-stimulatory molecules such as B7, but these can be induced by bacterial constituents.

The properties and functions of some APCs are summarized in *Figures 6.2* and *6.3*.

ANTIGEN PROCESSING AND PRESENTATION

Antigens are processed before they are presented to T cells

Antibody responses and cell-mediated immune reactions are generally directed against different determinants on the antigen. For example, mouse B cells recognize an epitope at the N terminus of glucagon, whereas T cells recognize determinants near the C terminus (*Fig. 6.4*). This is because, as explained above, antigens are not presented by MHC molecules as intact proteins, but rather as processed peptides. The cells that process antigen in this way may be either specialized antigen-presenting cells (APCs), which are capable of stimulating T-cell division, or may be virally infected cells within the body which then become targets for effector T cells.

Antigen processing involves degrading the antigen into peptide fragments. The vast majority of epitopes recognized by T cells are fragments from a peptide chain. Only a minority of peptide fragments from a protein antigen are able to bind to a particular MHC molecule. Furthermore, different MHC molecules bind different sets of peptides. For example, studies using a viral antigen that is recognized by mouse strains of several different haplotypes (that is, having different MHC molecules) showed that TH cells from each haplotype recognized a distinct peptide from that antigen (*Fig. 6.5*). This depended largely on the ability of a peptide to bind to a particular MHC class II molecule.

Antigens are partially degraded into peptide before binding to MHC molecules

The processing of antigens to generate peptide that can bind to MHC molecules occurs in intracellular organelles (*Fig. 6.6*). For the purposes of laboratory studies, the internal degradation by APCs can be circumvented by the use of synthetic peptides. This ability to use laboratory-synthesized peptides of known sequences has enabled researchers to identify epitopes recognized by T cells with different specificities (*Fig. 6.7*). The relative importance of different amino acids within a defined epitope can also be

Antigen presentation

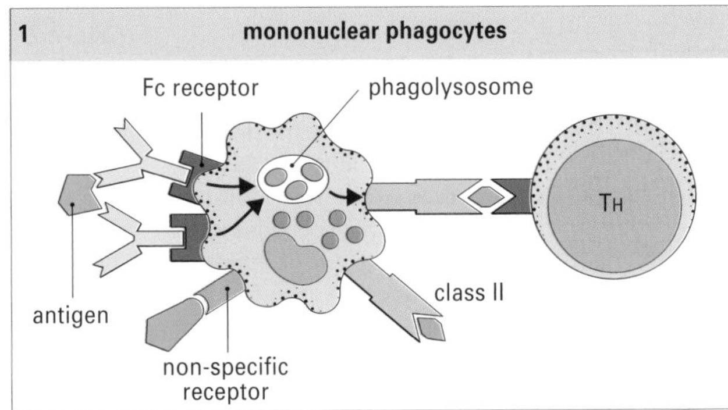

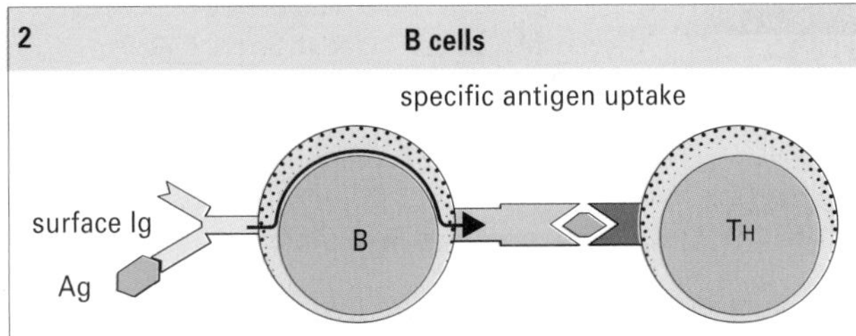

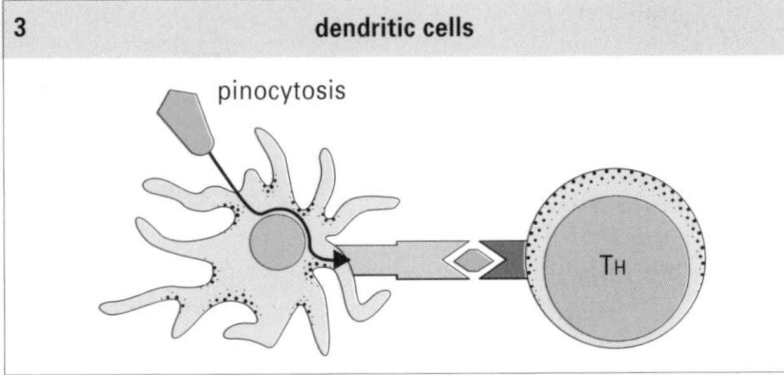

Fig. 6.2 Mononuclear phagocytes (**1**), B cells (**2**) and dendritic cells (**3**) can all present antigen to MHC class II-restricted T-helper (TH) cells. Macrophages take up bacteria or particulate antigen via non-specific receptors or as immune complexes, process it and return fragments to the cell surface in association with class II molecules. Activated B cells can take up antigen via their surface immunoglobulin and present it to T cells associated with their class II molecules. Dendritic cells constitutively express class II MHC molecules and take up antigen by macropinocytosis.

Antigen-presenting cells

	phago-cytosis	type	location	class II expression
phagocytes (monocyte/macrophage lineage)	+	monocytes	blood	(+)→+++ inducible
		macrophages	tissue	
		marginal zone macrophages	spleen and lymph node	
		Kupffer cells	liver	
		microglia	brain	
non-phagocytic constitutive antigen-presenting cells	–	Langerhans' cells	skin	++ constitutive
		interdigitating dendritic cells (IDCs)	lymphoid tissue	
		follicular dendritic cells	lymphoid tissue	–
lymphocytes	–	B cells and T cells	lymphoid tissues and at sites of immune reactions	–→++ inducible
facultative antigen-presenting cells	+	astrocytes	brain	inducible
		follicular cells	thyroid	inducible
	–	endothelium	vascular and lymphoid tissue	–→++ inducible
		fibroblasts	connective tissue	
		other types in appropriate tissue		

Fig. 6.3 Many APCs are unable to phagocytose antigen, but can take it up in other ways, such as by pinocytosis. Endothelial cells (not normally considered APCs), which have been induced to express class II molecules by interferon-γ (IFNγ), are also capable of acting as APCs, as are some epithelial cells. Another example is the thyroid follicular cell, which acts as an APC in the pathogenesis of Graves' autoimmune thyroiditis.

investigated by amino acid replacements at different sites. Using defined peptides, direct binding to both MHC class I as well as class II molecules has been demonstrated. In the case of class I, mutant cells lacking TAP, the molecule that transports peptides into the ER (see below), are useful for studying peptide binding because they only express class I molecules receptive to peptides. A comparison of the effects of an amino acid substitution on MHC binding and T-cell reactivity has enabled conclusions to be drawn as to which amino acids contact the MHC molecule and which contact the TCR. For example, a peptide representing residues 52–61 of egg-white lysozyme is recognized by A^k-restricted T cells. This peptide binds to A^k molecules and functional data have implicated three amino acid residues within this peptide as interacting with MHC class II and yet another three residues as contacting the TCR. Crystal

T-cell and B-cell epitopes are distinct

glucagon	N 1 – 17	18 – 29
antibody response	+++	+
lymphocyte stimulation	–	+++
DTH response	+	+++

Fig. 6.4 The immune responses to two peptides of the antigen glucagon are shown. Antibody (a B-cell response) is primarily directed to epitopes at the N terminus, while the C-terminal peptide 18–29 stimulates T-cell responses, including lymphocyte stimulation *in vitro* and the delayed type hypersensitivity (DTH) response *in vivo*.

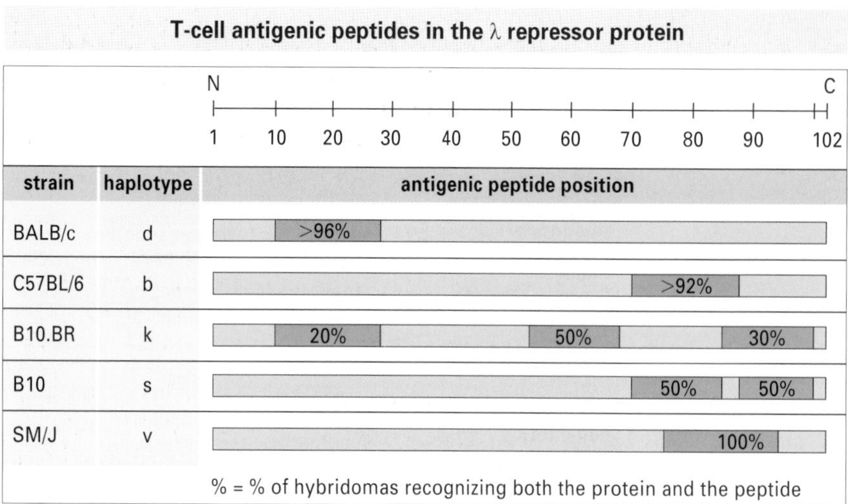

Fig. 6.5 Diversity of antigenic peptides in relation to MHC class II. Mice were immunized with λ repressor protein. T-cell hybridomas generated from mouse cells were tested against a panel of overlapping peptides which spanned the entire protein. Positions of antigenic peptides are shown in dark blue. One peptide was always immunodominant, although more than one peptide was antigenic in some mouse strains. (Adapted from data of Roy S, Scherer MT, Briner TJ, *et al. Science* 1989; **244**: 572–5.)

structures of MHC and TCR, in some cases as co-crystals, now reveal in great detail the interaction between the distal ends of the two proteins, with the peptide enclosed within the groove of the MHC molecule.

Class I molecules associate with endogenously synthesized peptides

Class I-restricted T cells (Tc) recognize endogenous antigens synthesized within the target cell, whereas class II-restricted T cells (TH) recognize exogenous antigen. Manipulation of the location of a protein can determine whether it elicits a class I- or class II-restricted response. For example, influenza virus haemagglutinin (HA), a glycoprotein associated with the membranes of the host cell, normally elicits only a weak Tc response. However, influenza HA can be generated in the cytoplasm by deleting that

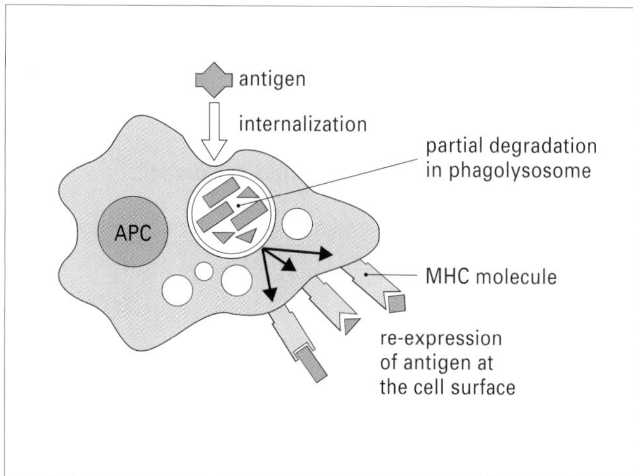

Fig. 6.6 Exogenous antigens are internalized by APCs and are then degraded by proteolytic enzymes in specialized intracellular compartments. Antigenic peptides associate with class II MHC molecules in vesicles that intersect the endocytic pathway on their way to the cell surface.

T-cell peptides in proteins

peptide	amino acid sequence
myoglobin	69–78 102–118 132–145
flu haemagglutinin	109–119 130–140 302–313
hepatitis B surface Ag	38–52 95–109 140–154
hepatitis B pre-S	120–132
FMDV VPI	141–160
rabies spike precursor	32–44

Fig. 6.7 The table shows peptides that are known to stimulate T cells. The peptides come from a number of proteins. Synthetic peptides corresponding to the entire amino acid sequence of a protein antigen can be used to stimulate specific T cells. Usually, only one or a few peptides from a protein are stimulators.

part of the transfected cDNA sequence coding for the N-terminal signal peptide. When this is done, there is a strong Tc-cell response to HA. Similarly, the introduction of ovalbumin into the cytoplasm of a target cell (using an osmotic shock technique) generates Tc cells recognizing ovalbumin, whereas the addition of exogenous ovalbumin generates exclusively a TH-cell response.

Proteasomes are cytoplasmic organelles that degrade cytoplasmic proteins

Although the assembly of class I antigens occurs in the endoplasmic reticulum of the cell, peptides destined to be presented by class I molecules are generated from cytosolic proteins. The initial step in this process involves an organelle called the proteasome. This is a complex of 14–17 different subunits that form a barrel-like structure (*Fig. 6.8*).

Generation of immunoproteasomes by replacement of active subunits

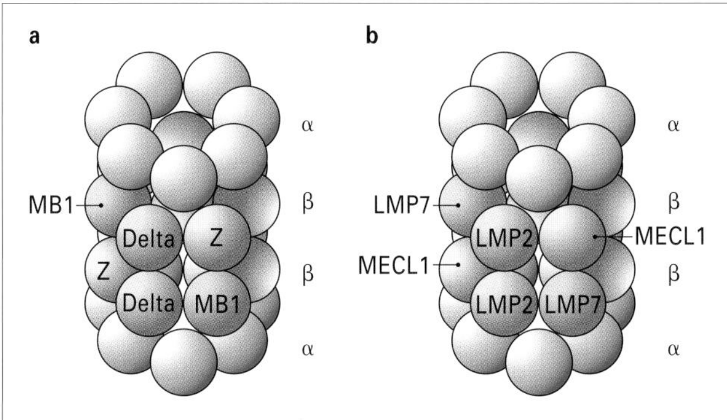

Fig. 6.8 The 20S proteasome, shown in cartoon form, is composed of four stacked disks, two identical outer discs, of α-subunits and two similar inner discs, comprising of β-subunits. Each disc has seven different subunits. Peptides enter into the body of the proteasome for cleavage into peptides. Only three of the β-subunits are active. In normal proteasomes, these are called MB1, delta and z. IFNγ treatment of cells results in replacement of these three subunits by the two MHC-encoded proteins, LMP2 and LMP7, as well as a third inducible protein, MECL1. These subunits are shown adjacent to each other here, whereas they are actually in separate parts of the β-ring and some would be hidden at the back of the structure shown.

Proteasomes provide the major proteolytic activity of the cytosol. They have a range of different endopeptidase activities and they degrade denatured or ubiquitinated proteins to peptides of about 5–15 amino acids. Ubiquitin is a protein that tags other proteins for degradation. Two genes, *LMP2* and *LMP7*, located in the class II region of the MHC (*Fig. 6.9*), encode proteasome components that subtly modify the range of peptides produced by proteasomes. The expression of these genes is induced by interferon-γ (IFNγ) and the protein products displace constitutive subunits of the proteasome. *LMP2* and *LMP7*, along with a third inducible proteasome component encoded on a different chromosome, influence processing of peptides by creating peptide fragments suitable for binding class I molecules and possibly preventing cleavage of such peptides derived from pathogens such as viruses. Additional interferon-inducible proteins, called PA28 molecules, associate with the ends of proteasomes. These also influence antigen processing.

How do the peptides that are produced by proteasomes traverse the endoplasmic reticulum (ER)? The products of two genes, *TAP1* and *TAP2*, that map adjacent to *LMP2* and *LMP7* (*Fig. 6.9*), function as a heterodimeric transporter that translocates peptides into the lumen of the ER. TAP is a member of the large ATP-binding cassette (ABC) family of transporters localized in the ER membrane. Microsomes from cells lacking TAP1 or TAP2 could not take up peptide in experiments *in vitro*. Using a similar system it was shown that the most efficient transport occurred with peptide substrates of 8–15 amino acids. Although this size is close to the length preference of class I binding sites, it suggests that some additional trimming may be required in the lumen of the ER.

Recent evidence has suggested that some of the various components of the processing pathway are physically associated in the ER (*Fig. 6.10*). For example, newly synthesized class I-β_2-microglobulin complexes are associated with TAP in the endoplasmic reticulum. Another MHC-encoded protein, called TAPASIN, appears to form a bridge between class I and TAP, until peptide is associated with the class I molecule. Dissociation occurs upon transport to the cis-Golgi. Peptide loading involves other proteins such as calnexin, calreticulin and ERP57. These chaperones promote and guide the assembly of stable class I/β_2-microglobulin–peptide complexes. Class I complexes lacking peptide are unstable, ensuring that only functionally useful complexes are available for interaction with TCRs.

The location of antigen-processing genes in the MHC may not be fortuitous

The finding of a cassette of antigen-processing genes such as the *LMPs* and *TAPs* in the class II region of the MHC is striking. There is some evidence, particularly from studies in rats, that particular alleles of *TAP* are genetically

MHC genes involved in antigen processing and presentation

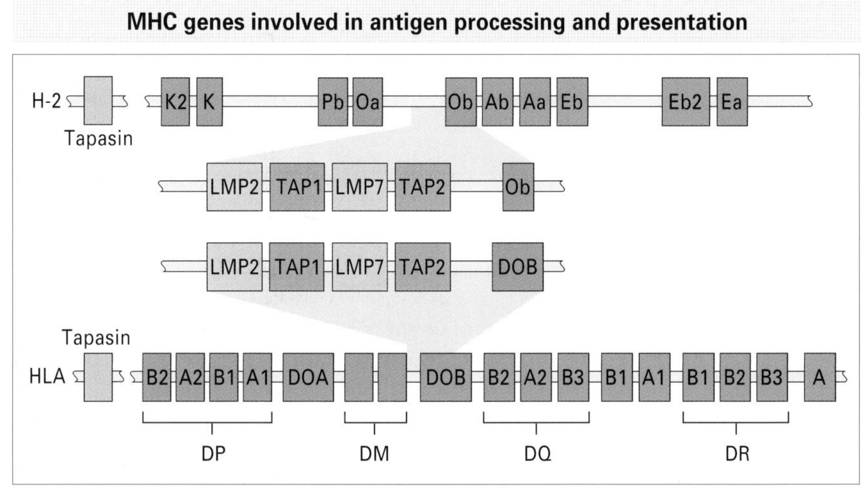

Fig. 6.9 Genes encoding a peptide transporter (TAP) and components of a multisubunit organelle called a proteasome (LMP) are located in the murine and human class II regions. The *TAPASIN* gene is located just centromeric (left) of the MHC.

Assembly of endogenous peptides with MHC class I antigens

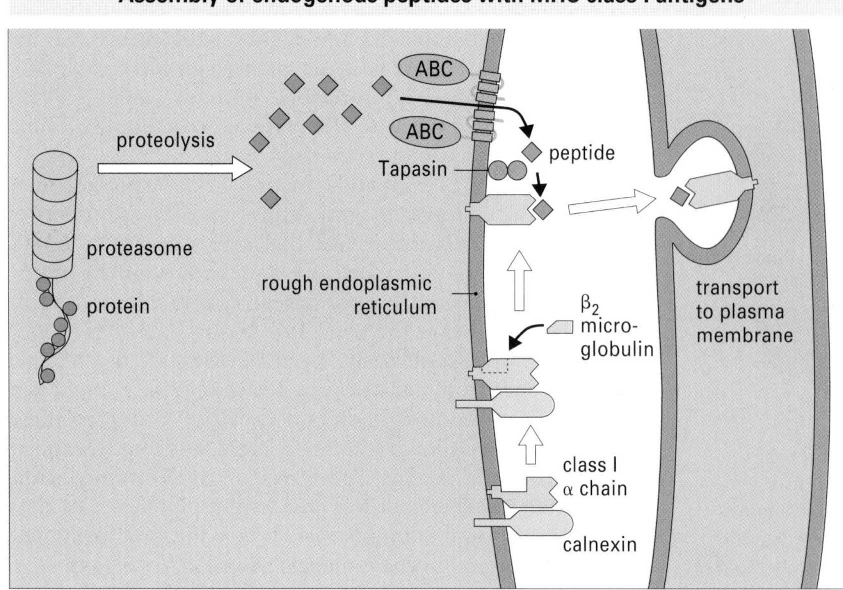

Fig. 6.10 Proposed assembly pathway of antigen–MHC complex. Cytoplasmic antigens are processed by proteasomes. Peptides are transported by two members of the 'ABC' superfamily of transporters, also encoded within the MHC (TAP1 and TAP2). Antigenic peptides associate with class I heavy chains and β_2-microglobulin (β_2m) in the ER. Molecular chaperones, such as calnexin, associate with partially assembled class I complexes. The Ig-superfamily molecule Tapasin forms a bridge between TAP and the class I molecule waiting to be loaded with peptide. Fully assembled class I molecules are then transported to the cell surface.

linked with alleles of class I genes that are most suited to receive the kind of peptides preferentially transported (*Fig. 6.11*). The rat data suggest that recruitment of antigen-processing genes into the MHC provided a selective advantage. However, other data suggest that the arrangement of MHC genes found within the MHC may have developed before the emergence of the adaptive immune system, revealing that the positioning of antigen-processing genes in the MHC could be fortuitous. Human and mouse *TAP* and *LMP* genes exhibit a low degree of polymorphism and there is little evidence to suggest that this is functionally significant.

In rats, TAP genes are polymorphic and different alleles are linked in *cis* to the appropriate class I allele

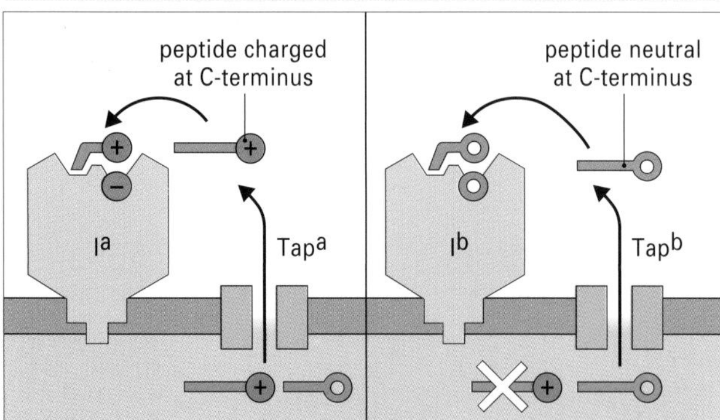

Fig. 6.11 Different class I molecules in rats can accommodate peptides (blue bars) with either a positive charge at the –COOH terminus (+), or a neutral amino acid (o). Similarly, TAP molecules (orange) come in two forms, which differ in the types of peptide they preferentially transport into the ER. Most rat strains have the appropriate *TAP* allele on the same haplotype as the class I gene that it serves best.

Class II molecules are loaded with exogenous peptides in an endosomal compartment

Class II α- and β-chains are found in the ER complexed to a polypeptide called the invariant chain (Ii), as shown in *Figure 6.12*. This protein is encoded outside the MHC. The αβ–Ii complex is transported through the Golgi complex to an acidic endosomal or lysosomal compartment called MIIC (*Fig. 6.13*). These MIIC vesicles appear to be specialized for the transport and loading of class II molecules. They have characteristics of both endosomes and lysosomes and have an onion-skin appearance under the electronmicroscope, comprising multiple membrane structures. The αβ complex spends 1–3 hours in this compartment before reaching the cell surface. The Ii chain is cleaved to small fragments, one of which, termed CLIP (*cl*ass II associated *i*nvariant *p*eptide), is located in the groove of the class II molecule until being replaced by peptides destined for presentation.

How do antigenic peptides derived from exogenous proteins meet MHC molecules in the appropriate compartment? The answer to this question lies in the intracellular traffic routes of MHC molecules. After synthesis in the ER both types of MHC molecule are transported through the Golgi compartment, class I in association with antigenic peptide and class II bound to invariant chain. Class II molecules segregate from class I in the trans-Golgi network. They then join the endosomal/lysosomal MIIC compartment en route to the plasma membrane. Exogenous antigen can also enter APCs via an endocytic route (either receptor mediated or fluid phase) where in some cells, such as DCs, it can load onto class II in MIIC vesicles and class I molecules in the ER, in a TAP-dependent manner. These findings reveal variation in antigen-processing pathways in APCs.

The exchange of CLIP for other peptides is orchestrated by a class II-related molecule called HLA-DM. This glycoprotein consists of an α-chain and a β-chain, both

Proposed routes of intracellular trafficking of MHC molecules involved in antigen presentation

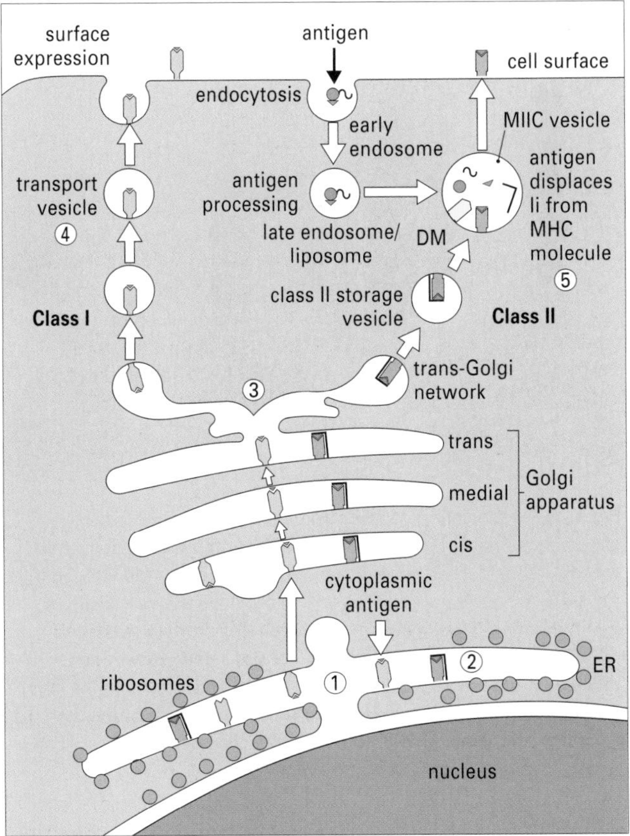

Fig. 6.12 Newly synthesized class I molecules are loaded with peptide (**1**). Class II molecules associate with Ii in the ER (**2**). Ii prevents loading with peptide and contains sequences that enable the class II molecule to exit from the rough endoplasmic reticulum (RER). Class I and class II molecules segregate after transit through the Golgi (**3**). Class I molecules go directly to the cell surface (**4**). Class II molecules enter an acidic compartment called MIIC, where they are loaded with peptide derived from exogenous antigen, and the CLIP peptide that occupies the binding groove dissociates (**5**).

Class II processing compartment

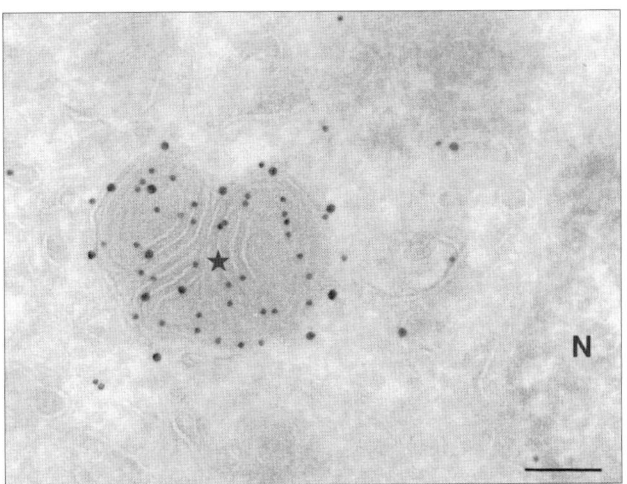

Fig. 6.13 Electronmicrograph of ultrathin cryosections from B cells showing multilaminar MIIC vesicle. The bar represents 100 nm. Class II molecules are revealed by antibodies coupled to 10 nm gold particles and HLA-DM by large gold particles (15 nm). (Courtesy of Dr Monique Kleijmeer.)

of which are encoded in the class II region of the MHC (*Fig. 6.9*). In cell lines lacking *DMA* and *DMB* genes, class II molecules are unstable and the cells no longer process and present proteins. When class II is purified from these mutant cells and bound peptides are extracted, they are found mostly to consist of the CLIP peptide from the invariant chain itself. Conceptually, -DM acts by stabilizing empty class II molecules so that as CLIP is released other peptides get a chance to associate (*Fig. 6.14*). In mutant cells lacking DM, class II molecules end up at the cell surface occupied by CLIP fragments of the invariant chain (*Fig. 6.15*). In *in vitro* assays, HLA-DM can catalyse the replacement of CLIP from class II molecules, with other peptides, at acidic pH, recapitulating conditions in MIICs. Enzymatic degradation of the endocytosed proteins occurs in the endosomal/lysosomal compartments and peptides are transferred to class II molecules in an HLA-DM

HLA-DM acts like a catalyst to influence binding of peptides in exchange for CLIP

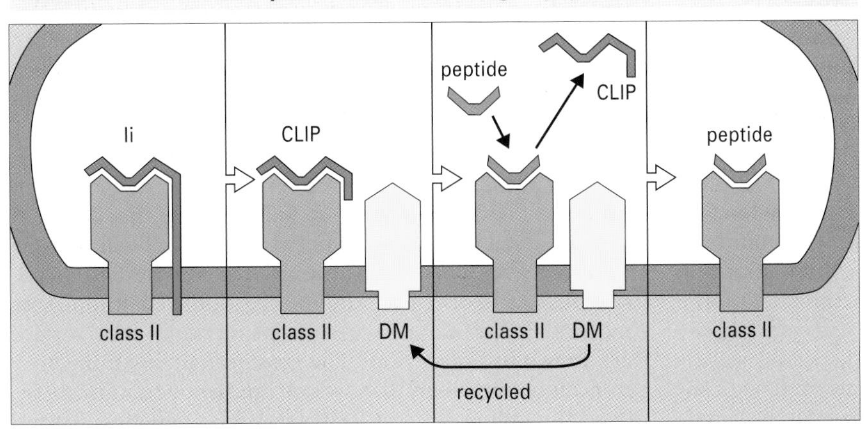

Fig. 6.14 A class II molecule is shown loaded with the Ii chain. The Ii chain is cleaved to the CLIP fragment. Association of the complex with HLA-DM then allows CLIP to be exchanged for other peptides, derived from endocytosed proteins, which are present in MIIC vesicles.

Absence of HLA-DM leads to failure of class II molecules to bind appropriate peptides

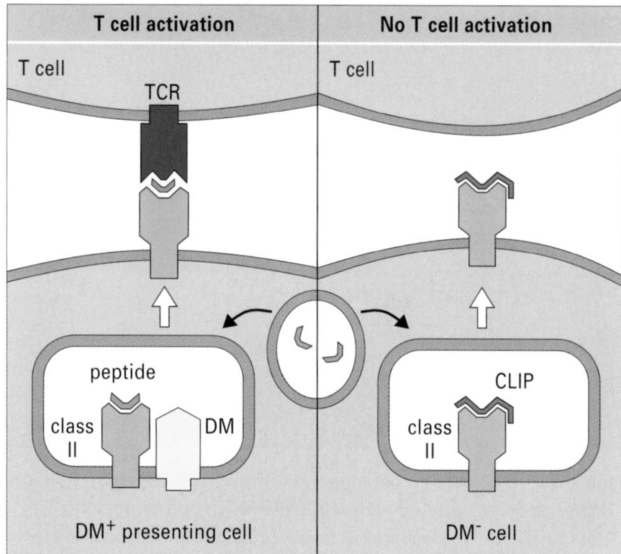

Fig. 6.15 In normal APCs (left) peptides are loaded onto class II molecules, as shown in *Figure 6.14*. In the absence of HLA-DM (right), the CLIP fragment is not removed, and the blocked MHC molecule is unable to activate T cells.

Summary of the key intercellular signals in T-cell activation

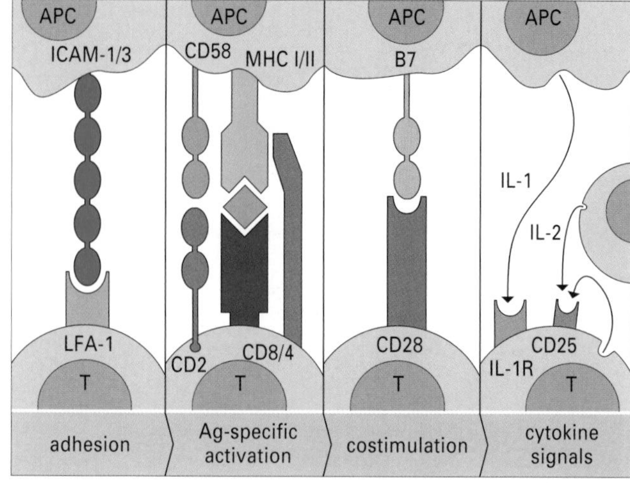

Fig. 6.16 Association of APCs and T cells first involves non-specific, reversible binding through adhesion molecules, such as the LFA-1/ICAM interaction. Recognition of the peptide antigen in the MHC molecule by the TCR, which provides the specificity of the interaction, results in prolonged cell–cell contact. A second signal (co-stimulation) is necessary for the T cell to respond efficiently, otherwise tolerance may result. Activation results in upregulation of cytokines and their receptors, which boost the activatory signals and help to decide the cell fate.

catalysed process resulting in the dissociation of invariant chain at a stage at which the biosynthetic and endocytic pathways intersect. A further MHC-encoded molecule, HLA-DO (*Fig. 6.9*), which associates with -DM, is also involved. Like conventional class II molecules, HLA-DO is a heterodimer, consisting of the DOA (formerly DNA) and DOB chains. DM and DO are class II-related heterodimeric structures that do not bind or present antigens. Similar genes and molecules are found in other species, in mouse encoded by the *Ma, Mb* and *Oa, Ob* genes respectively.

CO-STIMULATORY MOLECULES

The process of activating T cells generally takes place in the nearest lymph node to the infection. The TCRα- and β-chain dimer complex recognizes a specific peptide lodged in the peptide binding groove of the MHC molecule. This interaction dictates immunological specificity, as a peptide associated with an MHC molecule of one particular haplotype forms a unique structure to be recognized by the TCR. Other molecules are involved in this interaction. The initial encounter of T cells with APCs is by non-specific binding through adhesion molecules. This transient binding by adhesion molecules permits the T cell to encounter a large number of different MHC/peptide combinations on different APCs. In the absence of a specific interaction the APC and T cell rapidly dissociate. Crucially, co-stimulatory molecules act together with the antigen-specific signals before the T cell is sanctioned for proliferation. Co-stimulatory and antigen-specific signals must be present simultaneously on the same cell. Overall, antigen presentation through class I or class II molecules can be split into four stages: adhesion, antigen-specific activation, co-stimulation and cytokine signalling (*Fig. 6.16*).

Multiple cell-surface molecules interact during antigen presentation to T cells

Intercellular adhesion molecules, particularly ICAM-1 (CD54) and ICAM-3 (CD50), which are members of the Ig superfamily, interact with the integrin, lymphocyte functional antigen-1 (LFA-1 or CD11a/CD18), present on all immune cells. If mouse cells are transfected with both human MHC and human ICAM-1, their capacity to act as human APCs is augmented. When the T cell happens to encounter the appropriate MHC/peptide, which happens rarely except during an ongoing infection, a conformational change in LFA-1 on the T cell, signalled via the TCR, results in tighter binding to ICAM-1, which results in prolonged cell–cell contact. The joined cells can exist as a pair for long periods, allowing time for the T cell to proliferate and differentiate.

The specific MHC/peptide–TCR interaction, although necessary, is not sufficient to fully activate the T cell. A second signal is required, otherwise the T cell will become unresponsive. This second signal, also referred to as co-stimulation, is of crucial importance. Some co-stimulatory molecules that interact with ligands on the T-cells' surface are shown in *Figure 6.17*. The most potent co-stimulatory molecules known are B7s, which are Ig superfamily molecules, including B7-1 (CD80) and B7-2 (CD86). Several

Critical molecules involved in antigen presentation

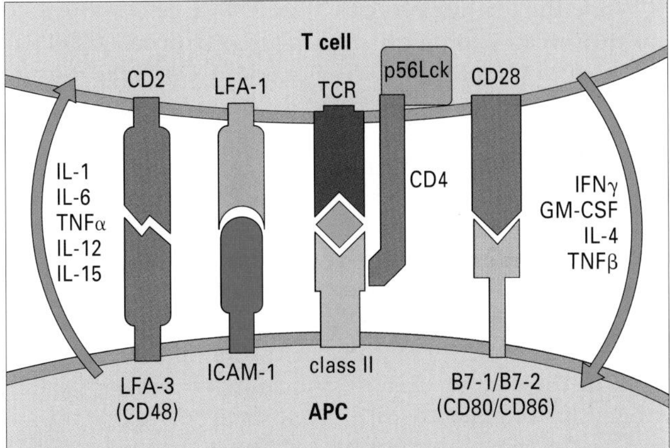

Fig. 6.17 The molecules involved in the interaction between T cells and APCs. The various cytokines and their direction of action are also shown. In man LFA-3 (CD58) acts as a ligand for CD2, but in rodents CD48 performs this function.

Role of CTLA-4 in controlling T-cell activation

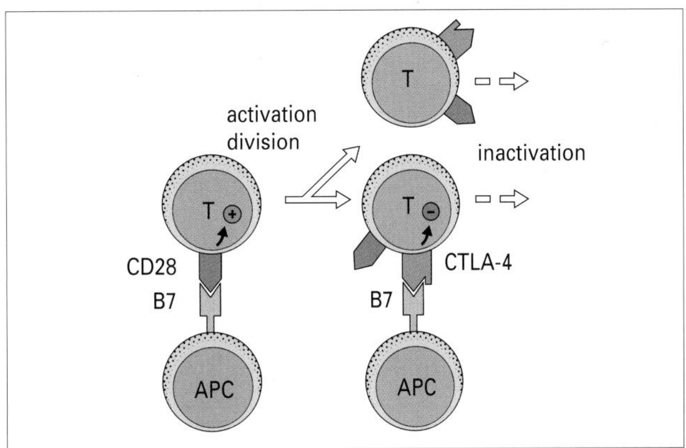

Fig. 6.18 Before activation, T cells express CD28 which ligates B7-1 and B7-2 on APCs (e.g. B cells). After activation, CTLA-4 is expressed, which is an alternative high-affinity ligand for B7. CTLA-4 ligates B7, so the T cells no longer receive an activation signal.

other B7-related molecules are beginning to emerge. B7s exist as homodimers on the cell surface. These proteins are constitutively expressed on DCs, but can be upregulated on monocytes, B cells and probably other APCs. They are the ligands for other Ig superfamily molecules, CD28 and its homologue CTLA-4 (CD152) – which is expressed after T-cell activation. CD28 is the main co-stimulatory ligand expressed on naïve T cells. CD28 stimulation has been shown to prolong and augment the production of IL-2 and other cytokines, and is probably important in preventing the induction of tolerance. Although the CD28/B7 interaction is extremely important, CD28 knockout mice do respond to antigen, although they require higher doses, so CD28 triggering is not obligatory, even for naïve T cells. Probably, in CD28 knockout mice other co-stimulatory signals replace that delivered by CD28/B7.

CTLA-4, the alternative ligand for B7, is an inhibitory receptor limiting T-cell activation, resulting in less IL-2 production. Thus CD28, constitutively expressed, initially interacts with B7, leading to T-cell activation, but once this has peaked, the upregulation of CTLA-4 with its higher affinity limits the degree of activation, as available B7 will interact with CTLA-4 (*Fig. 6.18*). The importance of CTLA-4 is seen in CTLA-4 knockout mice, which suffer from an aggressive lymphoproliferative disorder, because they do not inactivate dividing T cells efficiently.

The CD2 molecule on T cells is also involved in T-cell activation, in conjunction with the TCR. CD2 is a receptor for LFA-3 (LFA-3, CD58), which is widely distributed on cells and is present on all APCs. In rodents CD48 binds to CD2 and appears to be functionally equivalent to LFA-3 in man. Incidentally, the presence of LFA-3 on sheep red cells is responsible for the sheep red-cell rosetting reaction (the E rosette), widely used to purify T cells before the advent of monoclonal antibodies. Both CD2 and LFA-3 are members of the Ig superfamily.

Molecules such as B7, which reinforce the signal from the TCR and induce positive activation of T cells, have been identified as the second signal mentioned above. Resting T cells cannot respond optimally without this signal, and if they recognize their antigen in a non-stimulating manner they become inactivated, producing a state of immunological tolerance (*Fig. 6.19*). This tolerance is specific, only affecting TH cells that respond to a particular antigen. Persistent tolerance without cell death is known as clonal anergy. As discussed in Chapter 12, tolerance may be induced centrally as well as peripherally. Because central tolerance to self antigens is not absolute, many autoreactive T cells are present in circulation. These cells are tolerized peripherally, as although they are specific for self MHC–peptide this is first encountered on cells which lack the appropriate co-stimulatory signals.

CD4 and CD8 are co-receptors for MHC molecules

The two major subsets of T cells, TH and Tc, express either CD4 or CD8, respectively. These two molecules are only distantly related but they serve similar functions as co-receptors for MHC–peptide–TCR interactions. CD8 interacts with class I and CD4 with class II, in association with the TCR–MHC peptide. CD4 consists of four Ig domains external to the cell and the cytoplasmic tail has a docking site for the tyrosine kinase, Lck (see below). CD8 consists of two chains with Ig-like domains on long stalks, coupled by a disulphide bridge. CD8 co-receptor binds to conserved portions of the α_3 domains of class I molecules, leaving the portion enclosing peptide free to interact with TCR. Like CD4, CD8 associates with Lck. Both CD4 and CD8 co-receptors increase the sensitivity of T cells to antigen-presenting molecules by about 100-fold.

Interleukin-2 drives T-cell division

Apart from the cell-surface interactions, cytokines, acting locally, are also involved in T-cell activation. IL-2 is responsible for promoting cell division in a resting T cell (*Fig. 6.19*). Triggering of the TCR along with co-receptors results in IL-2 synthesis by the T cell itself. This binds to low-affinity

Dual signalling is necessary for full T-cell activation

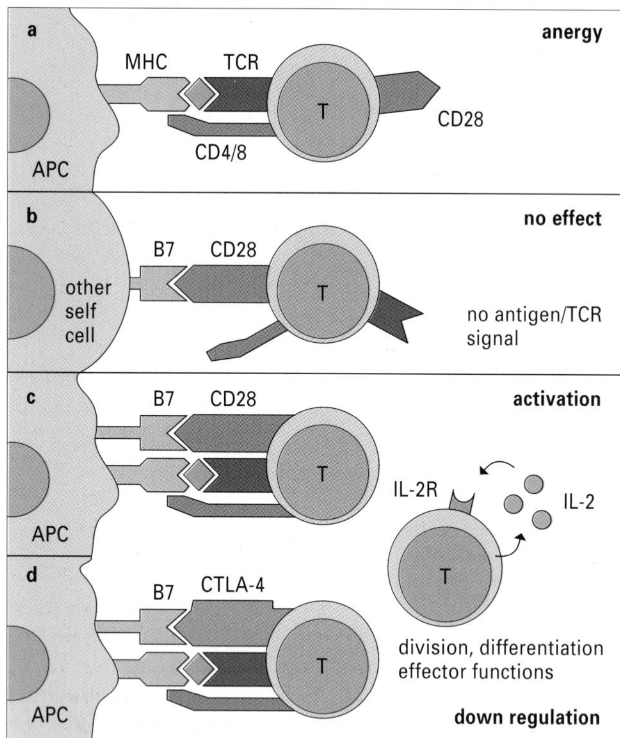

Fig. 6.19 A T cell requires signals from both the T-cell receptor and CD28 for activation.
(a) In the absence of co-stimulatory molecules inactivation or anergy results. This situation would prevail in order to tolerize T cells not removed by central tolerance to self antigens expressed on peripheral tissues.
(b) In the absence of an antigen-specific signal (wrong peptide for example) there is no effect on the T cell.
(c) Co-reception of both signals, from the surface of a professional APC, activates the T cell to produce IL-2 and its receptor. The cell divides and differentiates into an effector T cell, which no longer requires signal 2 for its effector function.
(d) At the termination of the immune response, CTLA-4 replaces CD28 and downregulates T-cell function.

IL-2 receptors on the T-cell surface that consist of two chains, β and γ. TCR triggering also results in expression of the α-chain of the IL-2 receptor, which, in conjunction with the other two chains, results in a high-affinity receptor. T cells activated by this self-propagating loop divide actively in the space of a few days. The interaction of the co-receptor pair CD28/B7 is vital for IL-2 induction. In the absence of co-stimulation there is little IL-2 produced and T cells do not proliferate and may become tolerized.

Interest has focused on other cytokines such as IL-1 and IL-6, molecules produced by certain APCs, including macrophages. T cells do not always require stimulation by these molecules, especially if they are already dividing. In resting T cells, IL-1 and IL-6 induce the expression of IL-2R. IL-12 is also of major importance in T-cell activation, helping to enhance IFNγ production, and it directs naïve T cells to develop into TH1 cells. IL-15 made by antigen-presenting cells can also induce T-cell proliferation and may be very important before IL-2 is produced.

While the interaction between $CD4^+$ T cells and APCs has been reasonably well studied, that between $CD8^+$ T cells and APCs is less well understood. $CD4^+$ cells help in the activation of most $CD8^+$ T cells. Because a single interdigitating dendritic cell (IDC) can bind many T cells, it has been proposed that activation takes place in a cluster of $CD4^+$ and $CD8^+$ T cells gathered on the surface of IDCs.

Antigen presentation affects the subsequent course of an immune response

Antigen-presenting cells may be activated rapidly in an immune response, for example by the immunogenic entity itself, in the case of bacteria and some viruses, or by the antigen in conjunction with the adjuvant component of a vaccine. Antigen presentation is not a unidirectional process. T cells, as they become activated, release cytokines such as IFNγ and granulocyte-macrophage–colony-stimulating factor (GM–CSF), in addition to expressing surface molecules such as CD40 ligand, which enhance antigen presentation. When APCs are activated, they express more MHC class I and II, more Fc receptors and more co-stimulatory adhesion molecules, including B7-1 and -2, CD11a/b/c, ICAM-1 and -3. They also produce numerous cytokines (e.g. IL-1, IL-6, TNFα), enzymes and other mediators.

Activation of lymphocytes leads to two partially competing processes: cell proliferation and differentiation into effector cells. Cells at the end stage of differentiation, such as plasma cells, may become so specialized that they lose surface molecules such as class II, and are unable to respond to regulatory signals or to proliferate.

The fate of lymphocytes responding to antigen is varied. Some can persist for a long time as memory cells. The lifespan of memory cells can be more than 40 years in humans, as judged by the chromosome abnormalities (e.g. cross-linking of DNA which would prevent mitosis) found in the blood cells of Hiroshima survivors. Other lymphocytes have a short lifespan, which explains why moderate antigenic stimulation does not lead to lymphoid enlargement. This is nevertheless sufficient for generating effective cell-mediated and antibody responses. Apoptosis is critically important for disposing of unwanted cells after an immune response.

Self/non-self and danger

In recent years it has become appreciated that APCs must respond appropriately, to an infection for example, but would not necessarily respond to high levels of harmless substances that may fluctuate in the environment. APC activation is generally a response to infection, or at least the presence of substances, such as constituents of bacterial cell walls, characteristic of infection. This requirement neatly explains the need for adjuvants, which are typically derived from bacterial components. Adjuvants are generally necessary in vaccines in order to stimulate a robust immune response. The concept of immune activation only in response to infection, (or adjuvant as a surrogate for infection) and not to other antigens, has been popularized as the 'danger' hypothesis. This idea proposes that the immune system does not merely distinguish self from non-self, as mentioned

Diagram of an immunological synapse, or raft

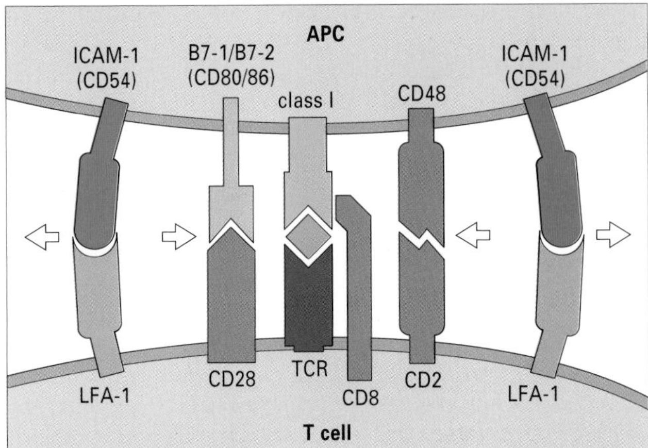

Fig. 6.20 Sets of receptors and their ligands: TCR/peptide MHC;CD2/CD48;CD28/CD80 all contribute to the formation of a synapse or raft. The TCR assembles with MHC/antigen peptide molecules and this moves to form a cluster. LFA-1/ICAM-1 interactions are relegated to the perimeter of the raft.

in some textbooks. It responds to clues that an infection has taken place before responding strongly to antigens. In other words, foreign substances may be innocuous or invisible to the immune system unless accompanied by danger signals, such as infection. These signals may be transduced by co-stimulatory molecules, upregulated by microbial products.

The highly ordered area of contact between the T cell and APC is an 'immunological synapse'

The junction between a T cell and an APC apparently does not just consist of ligand–receptor interactions of molecules arranged randomly on the cell surface. There is a clustering of T-cell receptors in a patch on the cell surface, in an area of membrane with distinct properties, surrounded by a ring of adhesion molecules. Immunological synapse formation is thought to be an active, dynamic process that helps T cells to distinguish potential antigenic ligands. Experiments show that initially TCR ligands are relegated to the outer ring of the nascent synapse. Subsequently, there is transport of the complexes to a central cluster, which is dependent, in an unknown way, on TCR–ligand interaction kinetics. Productive T-cell proliferation appears to depend on the formation of a stable central cluster of TCR interacting with MHC molecules (*Fig. 6.20*). The final configuration of the synapse or raft has MHC/peptide–TCR interactions at the hub of the synapse, ringed by ICAM-1/LFA-1. Large CD45 molecules, also known as the leukcocyte common antigen, are excluded to an outer ring.

T-CELL ACTIVATION

Receptors on the surface of T cells signal to the interior of the cell using signal transduction pathways that are common to many other cell types, including B cells. A key principle is the clustering of receptors upon ligand binding. This leads to activation of associated tyrosine kinases which phosphorylate tyrosine residues in the cytoplasmic tails of the clustered receptors, followed by recruitment of additional kinases and signalling molecules, in cascades. The end result of these complex pathways is the induction of gene synthesis by the activation of transcription factors (*Fig. 6.21*).

Activation is initiated by the actions of tyrosine kinases

TCR α- and β-chains are associated with the CD3γ, δ, and ε molecules, the ζ- and η-chains, and the enzyme Lck ($p56^{lck}$) that is attached to the intracellular portions of CD4 or CD8. The label $p56^{lck}$ signifies a lymphocyte-specific tyrosine kinase of 56 kDa. Recognition of an antigen–MHC complex by the TCR and ligation of co-stimulatory molecules initiates the signalling events. The earliest events comprise tyrosine phosphorylation, involving tyrosine kinases of the Src family, particularly Lck associated with CD4 and CD8, and Fyn which phosphorylate target sequences found in the ζ-chain (also present on Igα, Igβ and FcγR), termed immunoreceptor tyrosine-based activation motifs (ITAMs). Phosphorylation of the ITAMs initiates a series of steps detailed in *Figure 6.21*, which lead to the activation of transcription factors and their translocation to the nucleus. The transcription factors act on genes required for T-cell activation, including the *IL-2* and *IL-2R* genes. Cell division occurs after IL-2 production and is secondary to ligation of the IL-2 receptor. In summary, TCR stimulation results in activation of a variety of tyrosine kinases and downstream effectors that regulate cellular responses, resulting in the regulation of IL-2 gene expression, which is largely responsible for activating the T cell.

B-cell activation and T-cell activation follow similar patterns

In B cells, the function of CD3 is replaced by Igα and Igβ, which also carry ITAM motifs in their cytoplasmic tails. Cross-linking of surface Ig leads to activation of the Src family kinases, which in B cells are Fyn, but also Lyn and Blk. A series of analagous activation steps occurs in B cells, which are explained in Chapter 8.

An activating signal is integrated from both the antigen receptor and co-stimulatory molecules

It is still not clear exactly what is an effective antigenic signal. For a T cell, interaction at a single TCR is not sufficient, but exactly how many interactions are necessary may depend on other lymphocyte stimulatory signals and the type and activation state of the T cell being stimulated. Murine T-cell hybrids (derived from the fusion of a normal T cell with a T-cell tumour cell) are known to be easily triggered. To stimulate a T-cell hybrid, an effective APC, such as a macrophage, need carry no more than 60 MHC class II–antigen fragment complexes. A weak APC, such as a class II-transfected fibroblast, needs 5000 such complexes. Recent work has suggested that about 8000 TCR molecules need to interact with MHC–peptide complexes and become activated, as judged by their loss from the T-cell surface, in order for T-cell clones to be triggered.

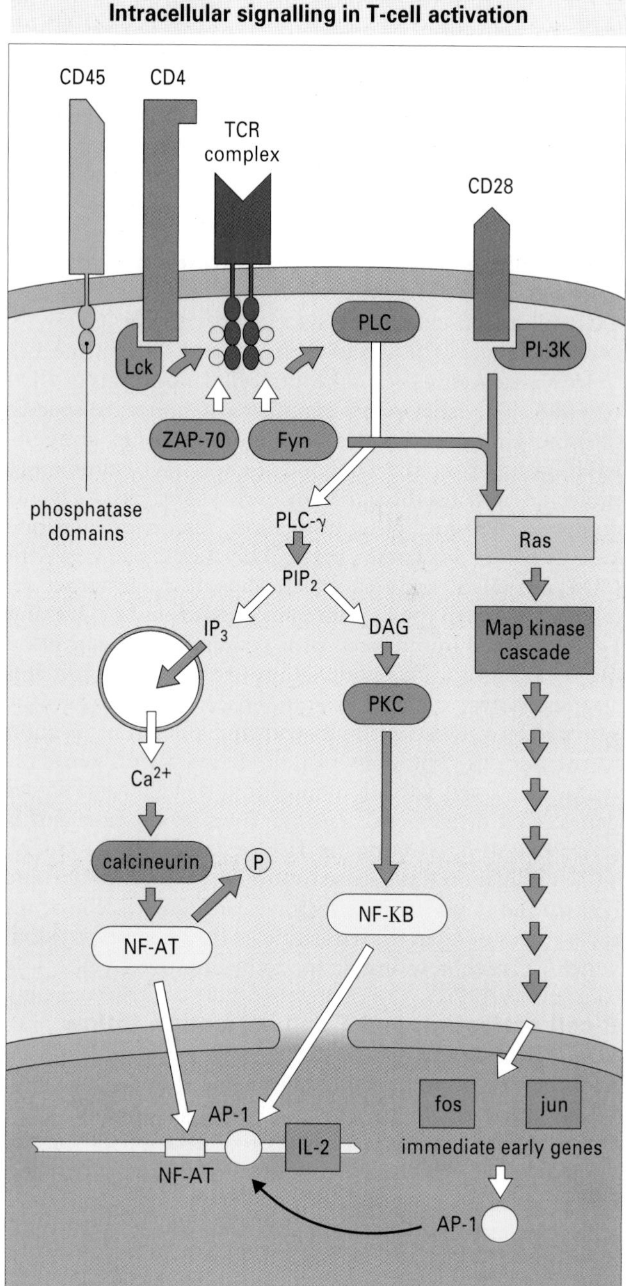

Fig. 6.21 T-cell activation involves the transduction of signals from both the T-cell receptor and CD28. Clustering of surface receptors such as TCR/CD4/CD28 and CD45 results in activation of tyrosine kinases Fyn and Lck. CD4, which is associated with the TCR complex, binds to the kinase, Lck. Such kinases become activated by dephosphorylation, possibly by phosphatase domains on CD45 (leucocyte common antigen). Lck can now phosphorylate the ITAM domains on the γ chains of CD3, which allows them to associate with other kinases including Fyn and ZAP-70. Fyn activates phospholipase C (PLC-γ), which leads to two pathways by the cleavage of phosphatidylinositol bisphosphate (PIP2) into diacylglycerol (DAG) and inositol trisphosphate (IP3). IP3 releases Ca^{2+} from intracellular (ER) stores to activate calcium-dependent enzymes such as calcineurin. Calcineurin dephosphorylates phosphate from the transcription factor NF-AT which causes its translocation to the nucleus. DAG activates protein kinase C, which then activates the transcription factor NF-κB. Meanwhile, ZAP-70, Fyn and PI-3 kinase (PI-3K) (associated with CD28) integrate signals via kinase cascades in the cytoplasm, which activate specific transcription factors. Adaptor proteins are used to link the various receptors to the common intracellular signalling components. GTP-binding proteins (G proteins) are involved in activating a set of protein kinases in the MAP kinase cascade. The transcription factors translocate to the nucleus to activate genes, including 'immediate early genes' *fos* and *jun* for cell division and the promotor AP-1 which acts with NF-AT on the *IL-2* gene.

As TCR–MHC interactions are of low affinity, one MHC–peptide complex could activate multiple TCRs. In the presence of a co-stimulatory signal such as CD28/B7 ligation, 1500 activated and internalized TCRs are sufficient for the activation of T-cell clones.

As discussed above, interaction at the TCR or membrane immunoglobulin alone cannot mediate a positive activation signal for T or B cells, on the contrary it may induce a negative or tolerogenic signal. Co-stimulatory molecules such as CD2, CD11a/CD18 are not only responsible for binding, their cytoplasmic domains are also involved in signalling. For example, experimental deletion of the intracytoplasmic domain of CD2 interfered with activation, but left its adhesion function unaltered. CD28 ligation appears to result in induction of IL-2 synthesis by a pathway distinct from that regulated by calcineurin.

As shown in *Figure 6.21*, the induction of IL-2 gene expression requires integrated signals from the activation of PLC, Ras and the calcium-dependent serine phosphatase calcineurin. The IL-2 enhancer contains a binding site for a nuclear factor, NF-AT (nuclear factor of activation of T cells), that is induced upon T-cell activation. NF-AT is activated by calcineurin. It then translocates to the nucleus where it interacts with Fos/Jun to induce IL-2 gene expression. IL-2 expression is dependent on the additional signals initiated upon ligation of CD28 by B7 (*Figs 6.19, 6.21*). How the signal from CD28 complements the TCR signal is not established but it may act by stabilizing IL-2 mRNA as well as increasing transcription. Cyclosporin, an immunosuppressive drug, causes inhibition of the phosphatase activity of calcineurin. Rapamycin, on the other hand, blocks signalling downstream of IL-2 activation.

Mitogens and superantigens can also activate T cells

T cells can also be activated by some mitogens. Most T cells are stimulated by phytohaemagglutinin (PHA) a lectin isolated from red kidney beans, or by concanavalin-A, extracted from castor beans. These molecules are able to bind to T cell surface molecules including the TCR complex and CD2, causing them to cluster on the cell surface, thereby mimicking the clustering caused by antigen presentation. Such mitogens however will activate the T cells regardless of their antigen specificity.

Another group of molecules which can activate T cell non-specifically are the 'superantigens' which are mostly of bacterial origin. They include the staphylococcal enterotoxins (responsible for some types of acute food poisoning) toxic shock syndrome toxin (responsible for tampon-sepsis induced shock) and exfoliative dermatitis toxin. Superantigens bind to class II molecules on APCs and are recognized by TCRs, but not in the same way as an MHC/ peptide complex. Binding is to the Vβ chain of the TCR alone: depending on experimental conditions, the effects are the same as with antigen in that either activation or clonal anergy may occur (*Fig. 6.22*). A key point about superantigens is that they stimulate families of clones using common Vβ gene segments.

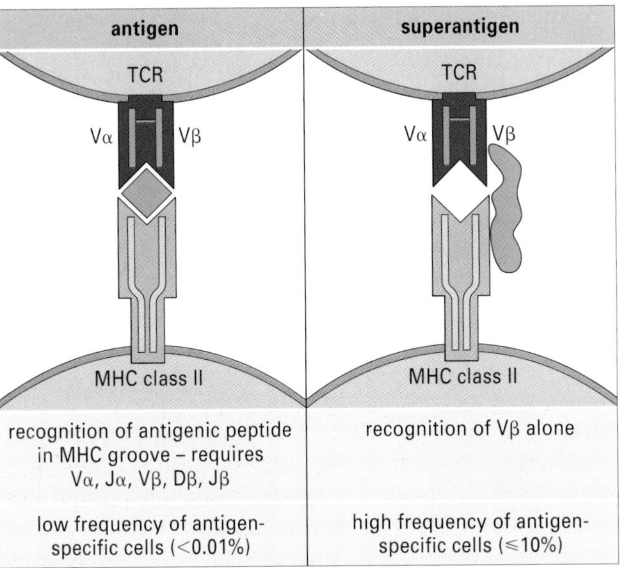

Fig. 6.22 Antigenic peptides must normally be processed and presented on MHC molecules in order to trigger the TCR. However, superantigens, such as staphylococcal enterotoxins are not processed, but bind directly to class II and Vb. Each superantigen activates a distinct set of Vβ-expressing T cells, depending on which Vb gene segment the T cell is expressing.

CTLA-4 expression downregulates T cells

The role of the B7 counter-receptor CTLA-4 (CD152) in downregulating T cell activation has been referred to above (*Fig. 6.19*). The negative signal generated by CTLA-4 may be propagated through the cytoplasmic tail of the molecule, which bears a motif known as an ITIM (immunoreceptor tyrosine-based inhibitory motif), which has the characteristic sequence IxYxxL. ITIM motifs are thought to work by recruiting inhibitory phosphatases such as SHIP, which remove phosphate groups added by tyrosine kinases. Other inhibitory receptors with similar motifs include the Killer Inhibitory Receptors (KIRs), which are expressed on NK cells as well as T cells.

IL-2 is central to T cell activation

Expression of the IL-2 receptor is a critical step in T cell activation. The IL-2 receptor may be a low affinity form consisting of 2 polypeptide chains or a high affinity form with 3 chains. The low affinity form has the β chain (p75) which binds IL-2 and is associated with a γ chain, which signals to the cell. When the T cell is activated, it produces an α chain (p55 = CD25) which contributes to IL-2 binding and, together with the β and γ chains, forms the high affinity receptor (*Fig. 6.23*). The structures and functions of the cytokine receptors are described more fully in Chapter 7.

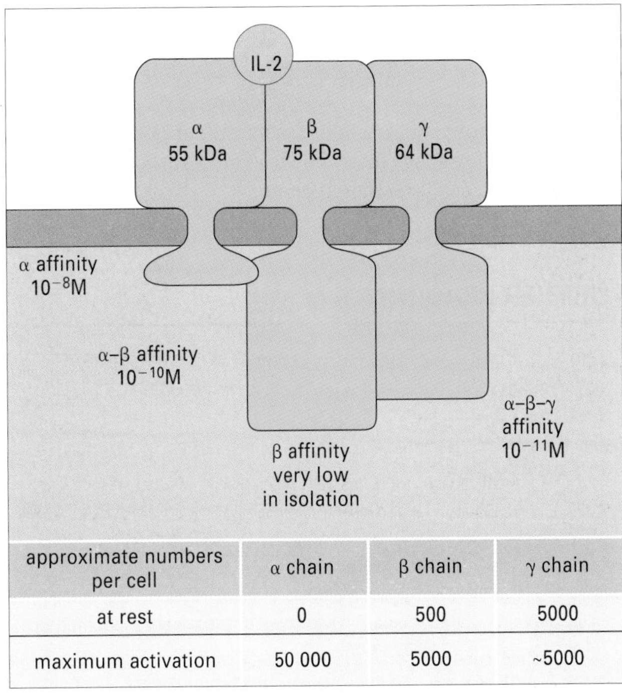

approximate numbers per cell	α chain	β chain	γ chain
at rest	0	500	5000
maximum activation	50 000	5000	~5000

Fig. 6.23 The high affinity IL-2 receptor consists of 3 polypeptide chains, shown schematically. Resting T cells do not express the α chain, but after activation they may express up to 50,000 α chains per cell. Some of these associate with the β chain to form the high affinity IL-2 receptor.

In all T cells, TCR activation induces the production of cytokines. In most CD4+ cells and some CD8+ T cells, there is a transient production of IL-2 for 1-2 days. During this time the interaction of IL-2 with the high affinity IL-2 receptor results in T cell division. Other cytokines may also contribute to T cell proliferation. For example IL-1 enhances the expression of the IL-2 receptor, while IL-4 and IL-15 may also provide stimulatory signals through their own receptors.

The transient expression of the high affinity IL-2 receptor for about 1 week after stimulation of the T cell, together with the induction of CTLA-4 helps limit T cell division. In the absence of positive signals, the T cells will start to die by apoptosis.

CRITICAL THINKING • Antigen processing and presentation (Explanations on p. 454)

Two T-cell clones have been produced from a mouse infected with influenza virus. One of the clones reacts to a virus peptide when it is presented on APCs which have the same MHC class I (H-2K) locus as the original mouse, i.e. the clone is MHC class I restricted. The other clone is MHC class II restricted. The two clones are stimulated in tissue culture using syngeneic macrophages as APCs. The macrophages have either been infected with live flu virus or have been treated with inactivated virus. The patterns of reactivity of the two clones are shown in the table below.

In the last two lines of the table the macrophages are pretreated with either emetine or chloroquine before they are infected with flu virus. Emetine is a protein synthesis inhibitor. Chloroquine inhibits the fusion of lysosomes with phagosomes.

Antigen	APCs treated with	Reactivity of clone: Clone 1	Clone 2
None	–	–	–
Live flu virus	–	+	+
Inactivated flu	–	–	+
Live flu virus	Emetine	–	+
Live flu virus	Chloroquine	+	–

6.1 Why are macrophages used as APCs in this experiment? Would you get the same results if you used infected fibroblasts?

6.2 Why does the live flu virus stimulate both clones, while the inactivated flu virus only stimulates the MHC class II-restricted clone.

6.3 Why does emetine prevent the macrophages presenting antigen to the class I-restricted T cells, while chloroquine prevents them from presenting to class II-restricted cells.

6.4 One of these clones expresses CD4 and the other CD8. Which way around is it?

FURTHER READING

Alberola I J, Takaki S, Kerner J D, Perlmutter R M. Differential signalling by lymphocyte antigen receptors. *Ann Rev Immunol* 1997;**15**:125–54.

Bell D, Young J W, Banchereau J. Dendritic cells. *Ann Rev Immunol* 1999;**17**:255–305.

Clements J L, Boerth N J, Ran Lee J, Koretzky G A. Integration of T cell receptor-dependent signalling pathways by adapter proteins. *Ann Rev Immunol* 1999;**17**:89–108

Germain R N, Stefanova I. The dynamics of T cell receptor signalling: complex orchestration and the key roles of tempo and cooperation. *Ann Rev Immunol* 1999;**17**:467–522.

Grakoui A, Bromley S K, Sumen C, *et al.* The immunological synapse: a molecular machine controlling T cell activation. *Science* 1999;**285**:221–7.

Healy J I, Goodnow C C. Positive versus negative signalling by lymphocyte antigen receptors. *Ann Rev Immunol* 1998;**16**:645–70.

Lehner P J, Trowsdale J. Antigen processing: coming out gracefully. *Curr Biol* 1998;**8**:R605–8.

Mellman I, Turley S J, Steinman R M. Antigen processing for amateurs and professionals. *Trends Cell Biol* 1998;**8**:231–7.

Nelson C A, Fremont D H. Structural principles of MHC class II antigen presentation. *Rev Immunogenet* 1999;**1**:47–59.

Pamer E, Cresswell P. Mechanisms of MHC Class I-restricted antigen processing. *Annu Rev Immunol* 1998;**16**:323–58.

Parham P. Accessory molecules in the immune response. *Imm Revs* 1996;**153**.

Parham P. Mechanisms of antigen-processing. *Imm Revs* 1996;151 (see other more recent *Imm Revs*).

Rodriguez A, Regnault A, Kleijmeer M, Ricciardi-Castagnoli P, Amigorena S. Selective transport of internalized antigens to the cytosol for MHC class I presentation in dendritic cells. *Nature Cell Biol* 1999;**1**:362–8.

Terhorst C, Spits H, Staal F, Exley M. T lymphocyte signal transduction. In: Hames B D, Glover D M (eds). *Molecular Immunology.* Oxford: IRL Press, 1996.

Watts C, Powis S. Pathways of antigen processing and presentation. *Rev Immunogenet* 1999;**1**:60–74.

7 Cytokines and cytokine receptors

- **Cytokines are small protein, signalling molecules.** They principally act in an autocrine or paracrine way.
- **Cytokine receptors fall into four principal families.** Chemokine receptors are a separate group, belonging to the seven-transmembrane domain family.
- **Many cytokines act by causing aggregation of receptors at the cell surface.** This leads to the activation of second messenger systems.
- **The type I cytokine receptors activate the Janus kinases, leading to the production of STATs.** STATs are transcription factors which induce synthesis of new proteins. Activation pathways are not mututally exclusive or specific for an individual cytokine – pathways can intersect, or be used by more than one cytokine. Many of the type I receptors also induce the MAP kinase pathways.
- **T helper cells can be divided into TH1 and TH2 subsets according to the cytokines they produce.** TH1 cells secrete interferon-γ (IFNγ), tumour necrosis factor-β (TNF-β) and interleukin-2 (IL-2). TH2 cells typically produce IL-4, IL-5, IL-10 and IL-13. TH1 cells help macrophages and cell-mediated immunity. TH2 cells tend to promote antibody responses.
- **TH1 cells can downregulate TH2 cells and vice versa.** Thus an immune response tends to settle into one type of effector response or the other.
- **Cytokines act in a network.** The response of an individual cell will depend on the pattern of cytokines it is subjected to and on the set of cytokine receptors which it expresses.

Direct cell–cell interaction and local production of soluble mediators control communication between cells of the immune system. The cell–cell interactions involve a number of different classes of molecules: major histocompatibility complex (MHC), accessory molecules, integrins, co-stimulatory molecules and membrane forms of cytokines. Cytokines are also released from cells, forming important soluble 'messenger' proteins. They generally act over very short distances, being 'autocrine' (acting on cells that produced them) or 'paracrine' (acting on cells close by) rather than 'endocrine' (acting on cells at a distance).

Thus cytokines are part of an extracellular signalling network that controls every function of the innate and specific immune response including: inflammation, defence against virus infection, proliferation of specific T- and B-cell clones and regulation of their differentiated function.

CYTOKINES AND CYTOKINE RECEPTOR FAMILIES

Cytokines can be defined as small proteins (approx. 8–80 kDa) that usually act in an autocrine or paracrine manner. They are extremely potent, acting at picomolar and sometimes even femtomolar levels. *Figure 7.1* shows an example of the virus protective action of an interferon. In this case 1picogram (10^{-12} g), was able to protect one million cells from ten million virus particles in a tissue culture experiment. The production of these potent regulatory molecules is usually transient and tightly regulated. Well over 200 different human cytokines have now been identified. The human genome mapping project is revealing new members of existing cytokine gene families, and identifying completely new families. Analysis of a data set

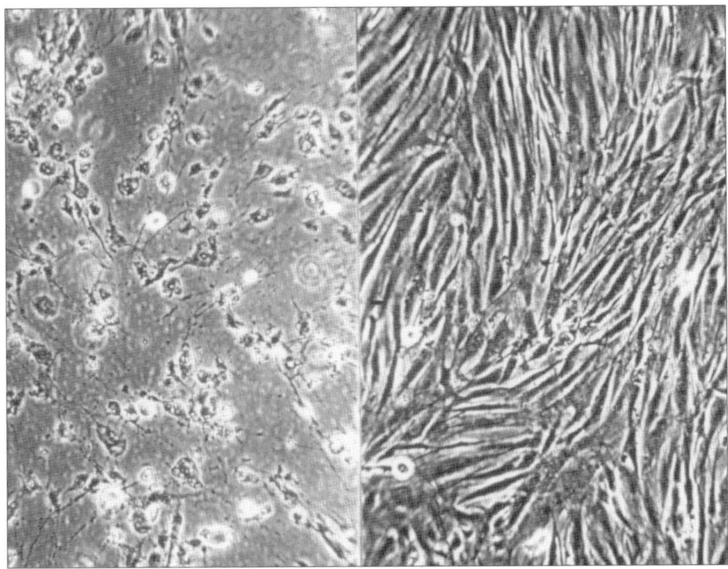

Fig. 7.1 Antiviral action of interferon. Fibroblasts in tissue culture were infected with a cytopathic virus. Cells on the right pre-treated with interferon survive while untreated cells are killed by the replicating virus.

Nomenclature of cytokines

name	abbreviation	examples
interleukins	IL	IL-1, IL-2 etc
interferons	IFN	IFNα, IFNβ, IFNγ
tumour necrosis factors	TNF	TNFα, TNFβ
growth factors	GF	NGF, EGF
colony stimulating factors	CSF	M-CSF, G-CSF, GM-CSF
chemokines	–	RANTES, MCP-1, MIP-1α

Fig. 7.2 The nomenclature of cytokines partly reflects their first-described function and also the order of their discovery. There is no single unified nomenclature, and individual cytokines may belong to two groups, e.g. the chemokine interleukin-8 (IL-8).

corresponding to about 10% of the human genome shows that there are many more cytokines to be discovered.

Cytokines have a wide variety of names. This is not surprising, as they have been discovered in disciplines ranging from immunology, virology and haematology to cell biology and oncology. Interleukins (currently numbered 1–22), interferons, colony-stimulating factors, tumour necrosis factors, growth factors and chemokines (see Chapter 3) can all be considered cytokines (*Fig. 7.2*). Much of the confusion in the nomenclature stems from the fact that, at least *in vitro*, cytokines can have multiple functions – for example TNFα has diverse actions on a wide variety of cells (*Fig. 7.3*). It is not unusual for a cytokine to be isolated independently by scientists working with entirely different experimental systems. Not only that, but several cytokines share similar functions, the cytokine IL-1, for instance, has many actions in common with TNFα. Another complication in studying these molecules is they are rarely produced alone, and rarely act alone. Put simply, cytokines function in a complex network where production of one cytokine will influence the production of, or response to, several others. Individual cytokines can be considered as letters of an alphabet where the ultimate behaviour of a cell depends on the cytokine 'words' spelt out on its surface receptors.

The preceding chapter explained how the production of IL-2 and expression of IL-2 receptors on T cells was an essential step in cell activation leading to division. This chapter introduces the basic aspects of cytokine biology and explains their role in the events that occur after antigen

TNF α a cytokine with many functions

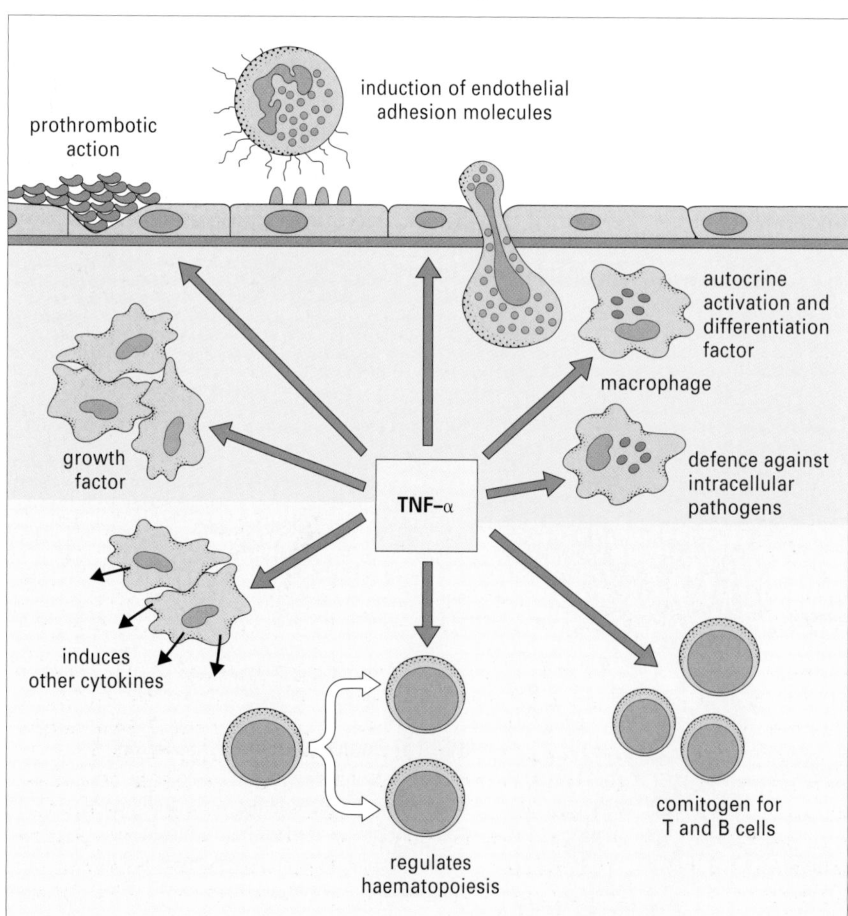

Fig. 7.3 TNFα has several functions in inflammation. It is prothrombotic and promotes leucocyte adhesion and migration (top). It has an important role in the regulation of macrophage activation and immune responses in tissues (centre) and also modulates haematopoiesis and lymphocyte development (bottom).

presentation. The complexity of the cytokine network may seem rather daunting to both student and experienced researcher, but over the past few years the field has been unified and simplified by three aspects of cytokine biology: crystallographic determination of the three-dimensional structure of ligands and receptors; elucidation of intracellular signalling pathways; and identification of new cytokines using molecular genetics.

Cytokine receptors fall into four families

Although there is little similarity between most of the individual cytokines or cytokine groups in terms of DNA or amino acid sequence, there are a number of families of closely related cytokines: most notably the alpha interferons, (IFNα), with at least 15 functional members; chemokines with more than 50 different mediators being predicted from genomic analysis; and a family of about 30 cytokines related to tumour necrosis factor, (TNFα) (*Fig. 7.4*).

However, in terms of three-dimensional structure, it is easier to divide the cytokines into distinct groups according to the structure and sequence similarities of their cell-surface receptors (*Fig. 7.5*). The largest family of cytokine receptors is called the cytokine or Type I receptor superfamily and is characterized by an extracellular region of structural homology approximately 200 amino acids long. Receptors for cytokines such as IL-2, IL-3 IL-4, IL-5, IL-6, IL-7, IL-9, IL-12, granulocyte and granulocyte and macrophage colony-stimulating factors (G–CSF and GM–CSF) belong to this family. Despite their sequence differences, some cytokines belonging to this family have overall structural similarities (*Fig. 7.6*). Other members are receptors for factors known to act outside the immune system such as growth hormone and prolactin.

The Type II family of related cytokine receptors can be considered part of the immunoglobulin superfamily and contains receptors for all IFN types as well as IL-10 and macrophage colony-stimulating factor (M–CSF) (*Fig. 7.5*).

TNF family cytokines bind to Type III cytokine receptors which all have multiple cysteine-rich repeats of about 40 amino acids in the extracellular domain. Apart from receptors for TNFα and TNFβ (also called lymphotoxin) this family includes important molecules such as CD40, CD27 and the death signalling receptors Fas/CD95, DR4 and DR5. (The fact that CD40 is classified as a Type III cytokine receptor is an example of a co-stimulatory molecule that is also a cytokine receptor.)

Molecular structures of IL-8 and TNFα

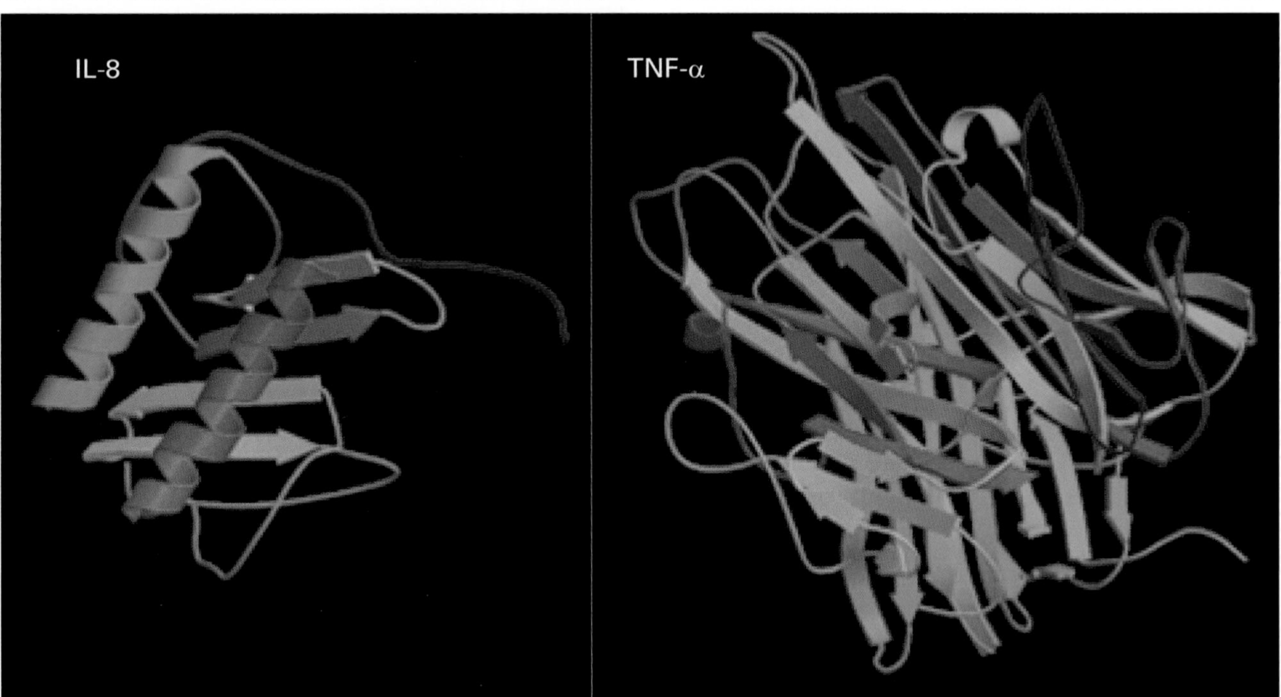

Fig. 7.4 IL-8 has a common structure, shared with many chemokines. The cytokine is shown in its normal dimeric form with two sections of α-helix lying above a region of β-pleated sheet. This bears a remarkable resemblance to the binding groove of the MHC molecules. Many chemokines attach to extracellular matrix via sites in the α-helix and to their specific receptors via sites in the β-sheet. TNFα is shown in its normal trimeric form. Note that many cytokines have their effects by polymerizing their receptors at the cell surface, thus TNF and related molecules trimerize their receptors. (The molecules were rendered using data provided by the Research Collaboratory for Structural Bioinformatics (RCSB). Berman HM, Westbrook J, Feng Z, Gilliland G, Bhat TN, Weissig H, Shindyalov IN, Bourne PE. The Protein Data Bank. *Nucl Acids Res*, **28** pp 235–242 (2000). IL-8: Clore GM, Appella E, Yamada M, Matsushima K, Gronenborn AM. Three-dimensional structure of interleukin 8 in solution. *Biochemistry* **29** pp 1689 (1990). TNFα: Eck MJ, Sprang SR. The structure of tumor necrosis factor-alpha at 2.6 Å resolution. Implications for receptor binding. *J Biol Chem* **264** pp 17595 (1989).)

Families of cytokine receptors

class	example	typical members
I	IL-3R	IL-2R IL-3R IL-5R IL-6R IL-7R GM-CSFR IL-9R IL-12R G-CSFR erythropoietin receptor growth hormone receptor
II	IFNα R	type 1 IFN receptor type 2 IFN receptor IL-I0R M-CSFR
III	TNFR-1	TNFR-1 TNFR-2 CD40L NGFR TRAIL FASL
IV	IL-IR1	IL-IR1 IL-IR2

Fig. 7.5 Four families of cytokine receptors are identified. Examples are given of each type. Type I is the cytokine-receptor family, typically consisting of separate binding and signalling subunits. The binding subunits have domains containing conserved motifs (WSXWS). The type III family consists of molecules which have cysteine-rich domains of the NGF-receptor type. Type IV receptors have immunoglobulin superfamily domains.

Receptors for IL-1α and β are representative of the Type IV cytokine receptor family (*Fig. 7.5*).

Regardless of these subtypes, cytokine receptors have several common characteristics. They usually consist of two or more subunits, and receptors for different cytokines may even share common subunits. A common pattern is for an individual cytokine to bind to a 'private' and highly specific subunit and a 'public' subunit that is shared by other related cytokines (*Fig. 7.7*). For instance, the functional complexes that make receptors for IL-2, IL-4, IL-7, IL-9 and IL-15 all possess a gamma common chain γc. Similarly, the β-chain of the IL-6 receptor (also known as gp 130) is used by cytokines such as LIF (leukaemia inhibitory factor), oncostatin M and IL-11.

The functional redundancy of certain cytokines may be partially explained by their common receptor subunits. For instance, IL-6, IL-11 and oncostatin M all act in a similar way on hepatocytes, megakaryocytes and osteoclasts and sharing of the IL-2 Rγ chain may explain the redundant actions of IL-2 and IL-4 as cell growth factors. However, each cytokine still has a unique function on some cell types. This may be due to differential expression of private ligand-specific receptors. For example, LIF can maintain embryonic stem cells in an undifferentiated state, but IL-6 is unable to do this as embryonic stem cells do not express IL-6 receptors.

Structures of IL-2 and IL-4

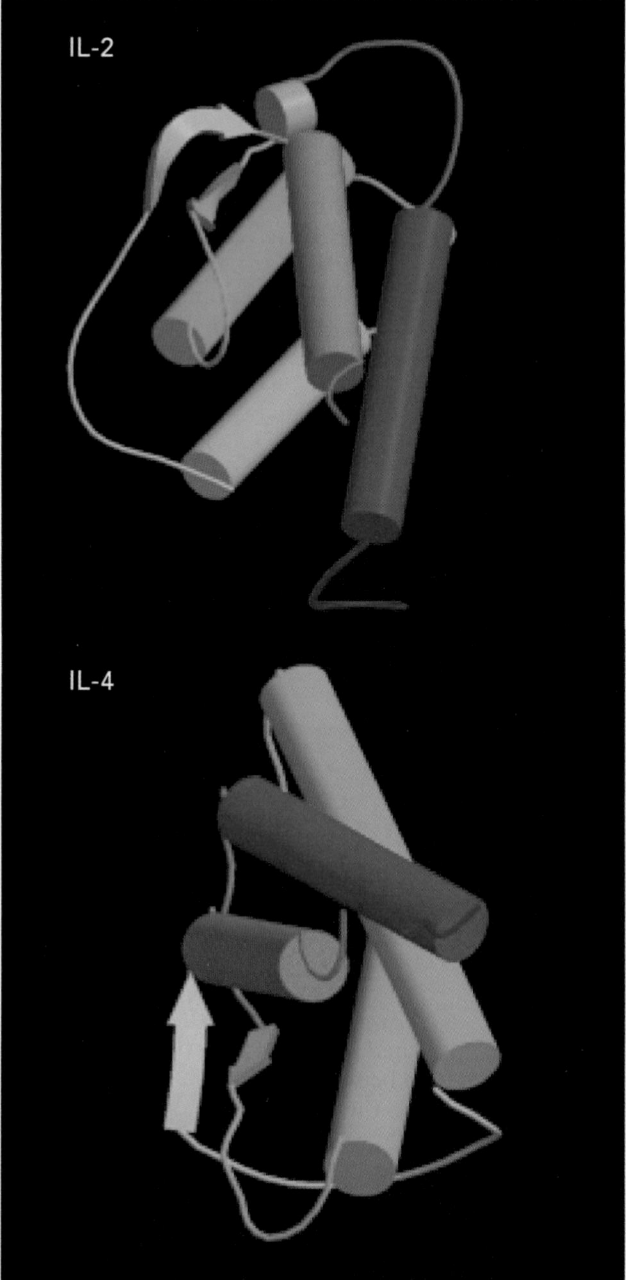

Fig. 7.6 IL-2 and IL-4 both bind to type I cytokine receptors. Despite their sequence differences, they are clearly structurally related. (The molecules were rendered using data provided by the Research Collaboratory for Structural Bioinformatics (RCSB). Berman HM, Westbrook J, Feng Z, Gilliland G, Bhat TN, Weissig H, Shindyalov IN, Bourne PE. The Protein Data Bank. *Nucl Acids Res* **28** pp 235–242 (2000). IL-2: Mott HR, Baines BS, Hall RM, Cooke RM, Driscoll PC, Weir MP, Campbell ID. The solution struture of the F42A mutant of human interleukin 2. *J Mol Biol* **247** pp 979 (1995). IL-4: Redfield C, Smith LJ, Boyd J, Lawrence GM, Edwards RG, Gershater CJ, Smith RA, Dobson CM. Analysis of the solution structure of human interleukin-4 determined by heteronuclear three-dimensional nuclear magnetic resonance techniques. *J Mol Biol* 238 pp 23 (1994).)

Structures of the IL-2 and IL-4 receptors

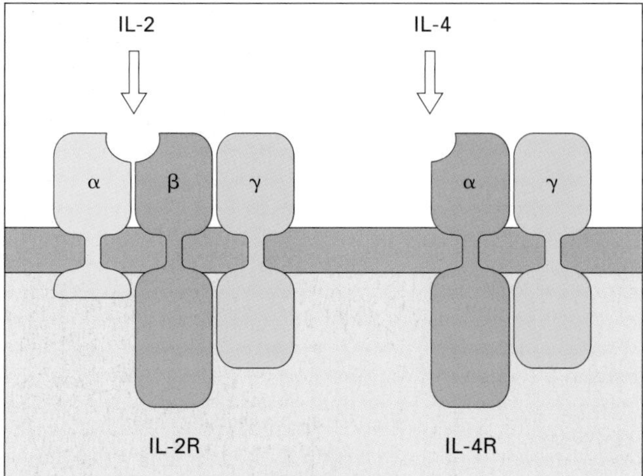

Fig. 7.7 The high-affinity IL-2 receptor is formed by three polypeptide chains, of which the α and β chains bind to the cytokine, while the γ chain is involved in signalling to the cell. The IL-4 receptor shares the γ signalling chain, but has a unique α chain which specifically recognizes IL-4.

Chemokine receptors belong to the seven-transmembrane domain family

Chemokines bind to a distinct class of receptors called seven transmembrane domain proteins because of their unique structure. A few of these receptors are specific with only one chemokine known to bind; others are shared with several ligands (see Chapter 3 and Appendix 4). There is also one 'promiscuous' receptor, known as the Duffy antigen, on red blood cells, which binds many different chemokines. The Duffy antigen may be involved in 'mopping-up' excess chemokine at sites of inflammation, containing and localizing these mediators. The chemokine receptor group also includes the related β-adrenergic receptor, once again showing the overlap between cytokines and other soluble signalling networks in the body.

MECHANISMS OF CELL ACTIVATION

Engagement of cytokine receptors activates intracellular signalling pathways

The binding of a cytokine to its appropriate receptor sets off a cascade that leads to induction or inhibition of transcription of a number of cytokine regulated genes. This occurs via a chain of protein–protein recognition events leading to binding of diverse transcription factors to DNA. Cytokines initiate intracellular signals through ligand-induced aggregation of receptor components (*Fig. 7.8*). Cytokine binding can cause hetero- or homo-dimerization of receptors, or receptor trimerization, depending on the particular family member. However the aggregation occurs, the common outcome is activation of kinases associated with the cytoplasmic domains of the receptors. This is followed by phosphorylation of cellular substrates.

Two families of receptor-associated tyrosine kinases are particularly involved in cytokine signalling from Type I and II cytokine receptors, the JAK and Src kinases. The JAK kinases (named after the Roman god with two faces, Janus) have two catalytic domains and are involved in signalling from both Type I and II cytokine receptors. JAK kinases associate with the cytoplasmic tails of cytokine receptors, close to the membrane, and are activated by cross-phosphorylation after receptor aggregation. JAK kinases then couple ligand binding to tyrosine phosphorylation of various cytoplasmic signalling proteins especially STATs (signal transducers and activators of transcription). The overlapping and yet unique functions of individual cytokines reflect the different intracellular signalling pathways involved. For instance, in T cells, IL-2, IL-4 and IL-9 use the IL-2Rγ (γc) chain and all activate Jak1 and Jak3; IL-10 activates Jak1 and Tyk2 and IL-12 activates Jak2 and Tyk2. Several Src kinases, including Src, Lck, Lyn and Fyn, have also been implicated in cytokine signalling and are important in phosphorylation of specific receptor subunits.

Type III cytokine receptors bind adapter proteins which do not have catalytic activity. These adapter proteins are involved in recruitment and activation of kinase cascades (see *Fig. 10.9*).

A basic model for cytokine action

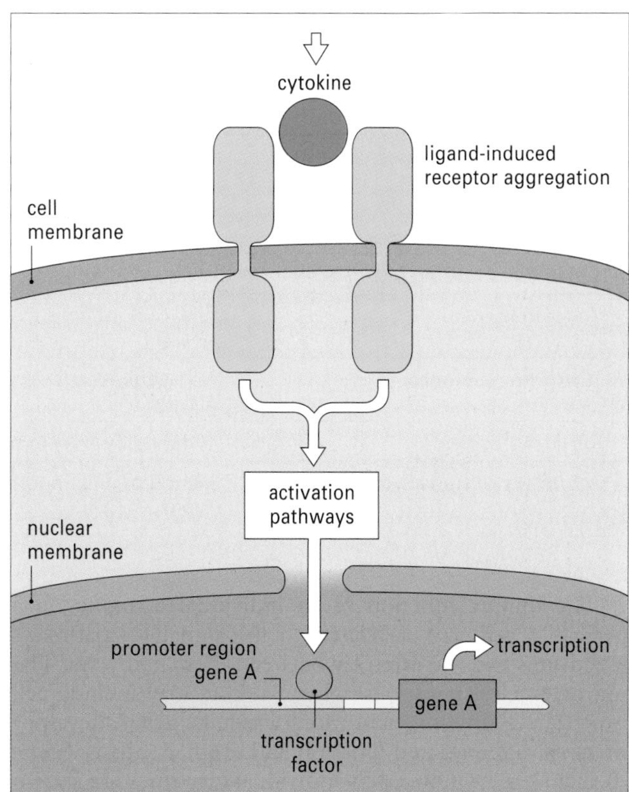

Fig. 7.8 A simple model for cytokine activation of a cell is shown. Cytokine binds to its receptor on the cells and induces dimerization or polymerization of receptor polypeptides at the cell surface. This causes activation of intracellular signalling pathways (e.g. kinase cascades), resulting in the production of active transcription factors which migrate to the nucleus and bind to the promotor or enhancer regions of genes induced by that cytokine.

Typical proteins induced by cytokines

Induced molecules	Example
• Cell to cell adhesion molecules	Actions of TNFα, and IL-1 on endothelium.
• Cell to matrix adhesion molecules	Induction of integrins on T cells by IL-2.
• Inducible nitric oxide synthase	Induced in macrophages by IFNβ and IFNα
• Extracellular proteases	Activation of osteoclasts by IL-1.
• Acute phase proteins	Induced in hepatocytes by IL-6.
• Lipid-metabolizing enzymes	Induced in adipocytes by TNFα.
• Cytokines	GM-CSF induces macrophage M-CSF and G-CSF
• Cytokine receptors	IL-1 enhances IL-2R synthesis in activated T cells
• MHC molecules	Induced by IFNγ in many cell types
• Inhibitors of transcription	Action of IFNα and IFNβ on many cell types

Fig. 7.9 Most cytokines have many effects and act on several different cell types. A single example of each is selected in this table.

The unique function of an individual cytokine on a particular cell type is related to the signalling pathways it activates and the interplay between these pathways. The ultimate cellular response of a cytokine may include cell growth, cell division, activation of specific genes, development of differentiated function and even apoptosis. Some of the proteins induced by individual cytokines are shown in *Figure 7.9* and their effects on cell phenotype are listed below:

- Proliferation and differentiation.
- Growth inhibition.
- Apoptosis.
- Chemotaxis and chemokinesis.
- Resistance to viral infection.
- Induction of cytotoxic effector phenotype.
- Induction of phagocytic phenotype.
- Promotion of intercellular adhesion.
- Regulation of adhesion to extracellular matrix.

The signalling pathways that elicit these responses are complex and are not mutually exclusive, intersecting at a number of control points. There are, however, four major signalling pathways activated in response to Type I–IV cytokine receptor engagement: the Ras/mitogen-activated protein kinase pathway (Ras/MAPK); the phosphoinositide-3-kinase (PI-3-kinase) pathway; STAT pathways, and those that lead to cell death.

The MAP kinase and PI-3 kinase pathways are involved in cell proliferation

The Ras/MAPK pathway is commonly associated with cell proliferation and the prevention of apoptosis. Many cytokine receptors, including all Type I receptors, activate this pathway upon ligand binding, but certain cytokines may only activate the pathway in certain cell types. The PI-3-kinase pathway is also important in stimulating cell proliferation by cytokines such as IL-2, IL-3, IL-4, IL-5 and GM–CSF (see *Fig. 6.21*). Phosphorylated lipids resulting from PI-3-kinase activation can act as second messengers interacting directly with cellular kinases.

Type I cytokine receptors induce STATs by activating Janus kinases (JAKs)

Although the mitogenic properties of cytokines are important, stimulation of gene transcription is vital to many other cytokine actions. Induction of gene transcription is mediated by latent cytoplasmic transcription factors that are activated by receptor-associated kinases. Once activated, the transcription factors translocate to the nucleus where they bind unique DNA sequences in the promoter regions of cytokine responsive genes. Of particular importance are the STATs. One or more STAT molecules are induced by all members of the Type I cytokine receptor family. JAK kinases are crucial to STAT activation, although these kinases may have other roles. The exact mechanism by which STATs activate transcription is not clear; they probably activate the machinery directly but may also make complexes with other known transcription factors such as c-Jun and C/EBPα. There are seven known STATs: STATs 1, 3 and 5 can be stimulated by multiple cytokines, but STATs 2, 4 and 6 are involved with a restricted set of cytokines. *Figure 7.10* shows JAK–STAT involvement in IFNα receptor signalling. Ligand binding aggregates the three subunits of the receptor. This leads to activation and phosphorylation of two JAK kinases, Jak1 and Tyk2, which then phosphorylate STATs 1 and 2. The two transcription factors form a complex with a DNA-binding protein called p48. The complex moves to the nucleus and activates transcription of genes bearing the interferon response element (ISRE).

The immune and inflammatory response leads to increased expression of many genes and involves a number of transcription pathways as well as STATs, and factors such as c-Jun and Elk-1. Two other transcription factors that are particularly important in the inflammatory and acute phase response are NF-IL6 and NFκB. NF-IL6 (C/EBPβ) is involved in induction of genes such as IL-1, IL-4, IL-8, TNFα and GM–CSF. It is expressed widely and also induced by IL-1, TNFα, lipopolysaccharide (LPS) and other mediators of inflammation. NFκB subunits are

Intracellular signalling pathways

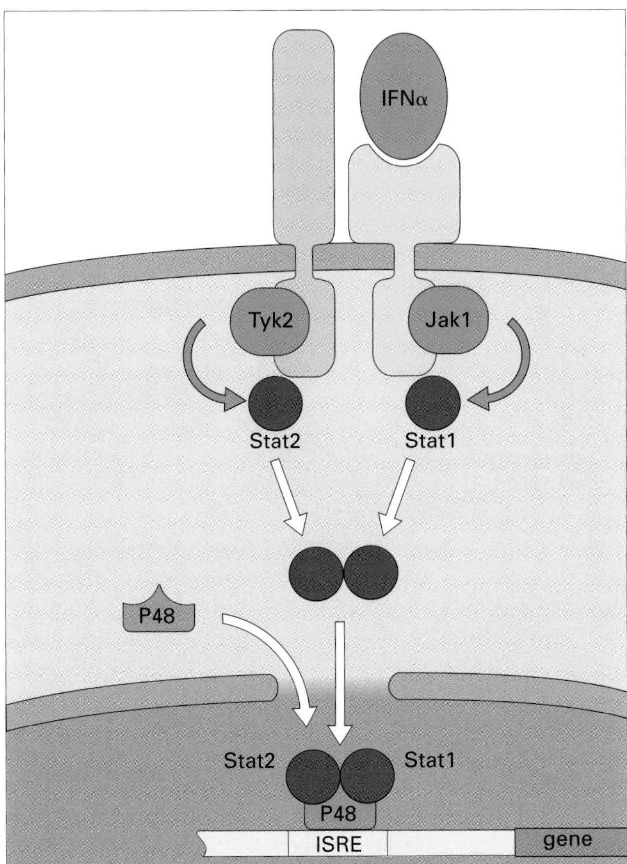

Fig. 7.10 The intracellular signalling pathways activated by IFNα are illustrated diagramatically. IFNα binding aggregates the two subunits of the receptor. This leads to activation and phosphorylation of two Jak kinases, Jak1 and Tyk2, which then phosphorylate Stat1 and Stat2. These two transcription factors form a complex with a DNA-binding protein called p48. The complex moves to the nucleus and induces transcription of genes bearing an interferon response element (ISRE).

Intracellular signalling pathways induced by TNF

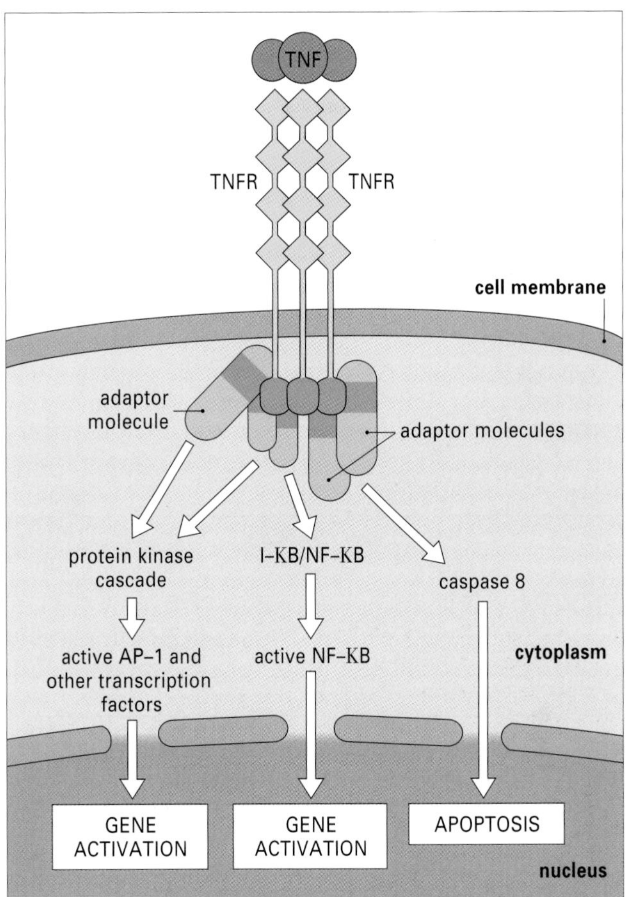

Fig. 7.11 TNF induces the trimerization of the TNF receptor on the cell surface, which causes adaptor molecules to be recruited to the receptor complex. One pathway leads to the activation of caspase-8 and apoptosis. Other pathways lead to the activation of the transcription factors AP-1 and NFκB, which cause gene activation and may offset the effects of the caspase pathway.

normally inactive, being bound to a protein called IκB-α. Signalling through cytokines such as TNFα and IL-1 causes dissociation of NFκB from IκB-α so that the transcription factor is able to translocate to the nucleus.

Other cytokines, especially members of the TNF family, TNFβ, Fas Ligand, CD40 Ligand, TRAIL and TNFα itself, are able to activate cell pathways that lead to cell death. As described above, TNFα also induces NFκB activation, which generally counterbalances the apoptotic signals unless a cell is metabolically compromised, infected with virus or simultaneously treated with other cytokines such as IFNγ. The cytoplasmic domains of some receptors of the TNF family, including TNF receptors and Fas, contain a specific interaction sequence, termed a death domain, which can bind other cytoplasmic proteins that also have death domains. These interactions lead to activation of caspase-8, which initiates a cascade of proteases that attack cell structures and degrade DNA resulting in apoptotic cell death (see *Fig. 10.9*). Other death domain containing adaptor proteins link receptor aggregation with protein kinase cascades and the dissociation of IκB from NFκB. *Figure 7.11* shows some of the signalling pathways induced by TNFα.

Thus distinct signalling pathways are activated when an individual cytokine binds to its receptor. It is important to remember that these pathways influence each other and intersect at different points forming an intracellular network that can initiate multiple events leading to a particular cellular response.

CYTOKINE PRODUCTION BY T-CELL SUBSETS

Differentiation into T helper cell subsets is an important step in selecting effector functions

It is now clear that local patterns of cytokine and hormone expression help to select the lymphocyte effector mechanism and that the polarized responses of CD4$^+$ TH cells

Differentiation of CD4⁺ TH cells

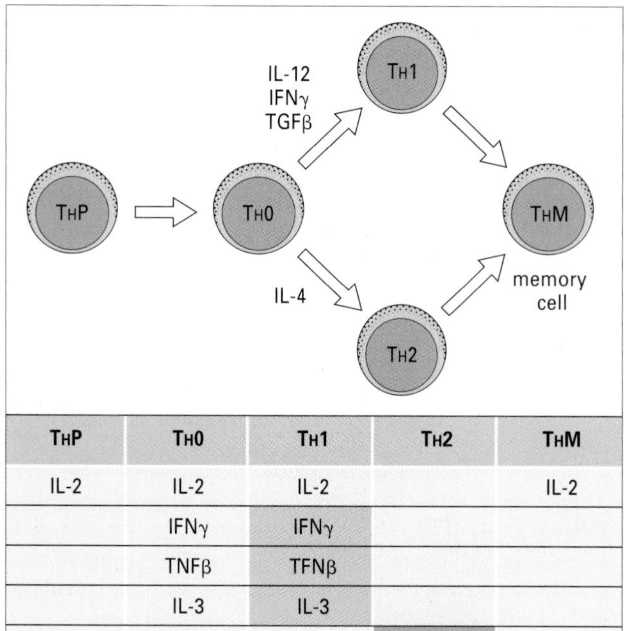

THP	TH0	TH1	TH2	THM
IL-2	IL-2	IL-2		IL-2
	IFNγ	IFNγ		
	TNFβ	TFNβ		
	IL-3	IL-3		
	IL-4		IL-4	
	IL-5		IL-5	
	IL-6		IL-6	
	IL-9		IL-9	
	IL-10		IL-10	
	IL-13		IL-13	
	GM–CSF	GM–CSF	GM–CSF	
	TNFα	TNFα	TNFα	

Fig. 7.12 The diagram illustrates the differentiation of murine TH cells into subsets with distinctive patterns of cytokine release. IL-12, IFNγ and TGFβ favour differentiation of TH1 cells and IL-4 favours TH2 cells. The cytokine patterns influence the effector functions that are activated.

seem to be based on their profile of cytokine secretion (*Fig. 7.12*). Typical human TH1 cytokines include IFNγ, TNFβ and IL-2 and these TH1 cells promote the production of IgG2a opsonizing and complement-fixing antibodies, macrophage activation, antibody-dependent cell-mediated cytotoxicity and delayed-type hypersensitivity. TH2 clones are typified by the production of IL-4 and IL-5 with IL-6, IL-9, IL-10 and IL-13 also commonly produced. These cells provide optimal help for humoral immune responses, including IgG1 and IgE isotype switching and mucosal immunity, stimulation of mast cell and eosinophil growth and differentiation and IgA synthesis. Thus TH1 cells are associated with cell-mediated inflammatory reactions and TH2 cells are associated with strong antibody and allergic responses. If polarizing signals are not present, CD4⁺ TH0 cells have a less differentiated cytokine profile and represent a heterogeneous population with individual clones that can differentiate along the TH1 or TH2 pathway.

Selection of effector mechanisms by TH1 and TH2 cells

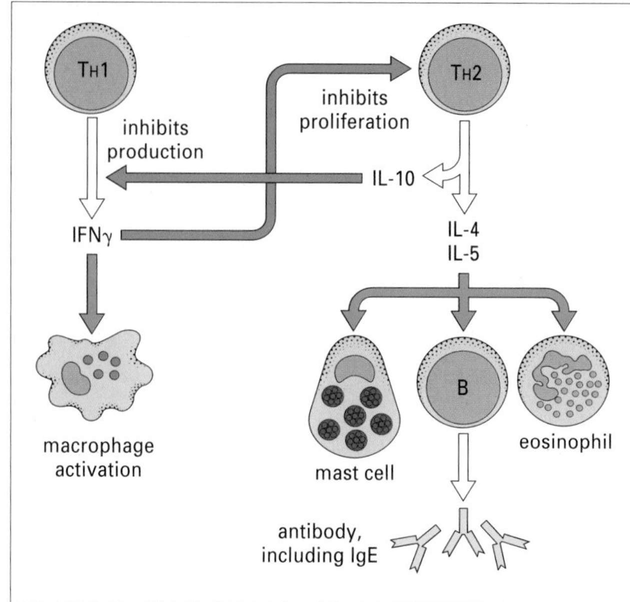

Fig. 7.13 Not only does their cytokine output drive different effector pathways, but TH1 cells tend to switch off TH2 cells, and vice versa.

Cytokines from TH1 cells inhibit the actions of TH2 cells and vice versa. Thus an immune response tends to settle into a TH1 or a TH2 type of response (*Fig. 7.13*).

Surface differences between TH1 and TH2 cells have recently been identified. For instance, CD26/LAG-3, a member of the immunoglobulin superfamily, and the chemokine receptor CCR5 are preferentially expressed by TH1 cells. Chemokine receptors CCR3 and CCR4 are associated with TH2 cells.

A single TH cell precursor is able to differentiate into either a TH1 or TH2 phenotype. The TH1-Th2 decision is crucial to effective immunity and it is likely that many inter-locking factors will contribute to that decision. Factors that may influence the differentiation of TH cells include:

- The site of antigen presentation.
- Co-stimulatory molecules.
- Properties of the immunogen.
- Peptide density and binding affinity – high MHC class II peptide density favours TH1, low densities favour TH2.
- Antigen dose.
- Antigen-presenting cells and the cytokines they produce.
- Activity of co-stimulatory molecules and hormones present in the local environment.
- Host genetic background.
- The cytokine profile and balance of cytokines evoked by antigen. This is thought to be the major stimulus. IL-12 is a potent initial stimulus for IFNγ production by T cells and natural killer (NK) cells and hence regulates TH1 cell differentiation. IFNα, a cytokine produced early during viral infection, is not only a potent IL-12 inducer but can switch TH cells from a TH2 to

TH1 profile. By contrast, early production of IL-4 will favour the generation of TH2 cells.

Immune responses are not always strongly polarized in this way. TH1 and TH2 cells are best considered as extremes on a scale. However, TH1 and TH2 responses do play different protective roles and may contribute to immunopathology. TH1 responses and isolation of TH1 T-cell clones typify organ-specific immune disorders, acute allograft rejection, unexplained recurrent abortions and multiple sclerosis. All T-cell clones from patients with atopic asthma caused by grass pollen have a TH2 profile, as do cells from Crohn's disease and systemic lupus erythematosis (SLE).

CD8$^+$ T cells can also be divided into subsets on the basis of cytokine expression

Many CD8$^+$ cytotoxic T cells make a spectrum of cytokines similar to TH1 cells and are termed Tc1 cells. CD8$^+$ cells that make TH2-associated cytokines are associated with regulatory and suppressor functions. The differentiation of these cells may be affected by the CD4$^+$ cell cytokine profile, with cytotoxic T cells commonly associated with TH1 responses and less commonly found when TH2 cells are present. Thus IFNγ and IL-12 may encourage Tc1 generation and IL-4 Tc2 cells. However, both Tc1 and Tc2 cells can be cytotoxic and kill mainly by a Ca^{++}/perforin-dependent mechanism.

THE CYTOKINE NETWORK

It has been shown above that there are many cytokines with multiple functions and apparent redundancy of action forming a complex communication network. How can this complex network be unravelled and the *in vivo* role of individual cytokines understood? Molecular genetics has proved a most powerful tool with the ability to genetically 'knock-out' a cytokine or its receptor in mice and has been another unifying force in cytokine research. By deleting one member of the network we are able to define its vital role in the whole organism in both health and disease. *Figure 7.14* shows some of the most important observations made with this technique, particularly those relating to immunity and inflammation. Some cytokines, e.g. IL-7, TNFα and TNFβ, are important in the development of the immune system before birth. The absence of others e.g. IL-2, IL-4, IL-12 and IFNγ is more obvious when animals are stressed by infection. The importance of IL-12 in IFNγ production and normal delayed type hypersensitivity (DTH) responses has been demonstrated in deficient mice. Disruption of several cytokine genes leads to intestinal lesions similar to those of human inflammatory bowel diseases, highlighting the fact that tissue under the most constant antigenic pressure in the body is the bowel mucosa. The anti-inflammatory role of TGFβ is demonstrated by multifocal inflammation in deficient animals. The importance of the IL-2Rγ (γc) as a public signalling molecule used by a number of cytokines is demonstrated by the profound immune deficiency of mice lacking this receptor subunit.

All these results must be interpreted with some caution. The role of an individual cytokine in the mature animal, for instance, cannot be properly defined if its absence during development leads to a deficient immune system. Moreover, absence of one cytokine may influence the production and action of another. For instance, mice with deletions of either TNF receptor 1 or TNF receptor 2 produce fivefold more TNF in response to LPS. If they lack both receptors they produce 10–15-fold more cytokine. This is presumably because the soluble forms of these receptors normally bind excess TNF and eliminate it from the body. However, it seems likely that among its redundant functions, an individual cytokine has one or more specific activities that have resulted in their conservation during evolution.

Cytokine and cytokine receptor knockout mice

Cytokine/receptor deleted	Mouse phenotype
TNFα	Major defects in primary B-cell function. Impaired antibody follicles and marginal zones. Abnormally susceptible to intracellular pathogens.
TNFα receptor (p55)	Readily succumb to infection Resistant to endotoxic shock
TNFβ (lymphotoxin)	No lymph nodes or Peyer's patches Abnormal segregation of B and T cells in spleen
IL-2	Increased serum IgG Raised activated B and T cells 50% die by 4–9 weeks 100% inflammatory bowel disease
IL-2Rγ	Severe combined immunodeficiency
IL-4	Low IgE, IgG1 Deficient in TH2 cytokine production
IL-7/IL-7 receptor	Profound reduction in thymic and peripheral lymphoid cells, no γδ T cells
IL-10	Growth retardation, anaemic colitis resembling Crohn's disease
IFNγ/IFNγ receptor	Abnormally susceptible to intracellular pathogens Defective macrophage function Decreased splenic NK activity and decreased MHC expression
TGFβ	Multifocal inflammatory disease Massive mononuclear cell infiltrates into organs such as heart, lungs, pancreas and liver
IL-12	Impaired production of IFNγ and impaired ability to mount a TH1 response. Enhanced IL-4 response. Reduced DTH responses but normal generation of CTL and IL-2 production

Fig. 7.14 Knockout mice shed light on the normal functions of particular cytokines. CTL = cytotoxic T lymphocyte; DTH = delayed type hypersensitivity (a largely TH1-mediated inflammatory response to antigen injected into the skin).

The functional importance of the JAKs and STATs (see above) can also be demonstrated in mice in whom these genes have been deleted. For example, Stat-1 deficient mice have quite specific defects in their responses to IFNα and β, are exquisitely sensitive to virus infection, have defective macrophage nitric oxide production and show a TH2 type response in infection. By contrast, homozygous deletion of Jak-1 is lethal at the time of birth. Mice fail to nurse and are deficient in IL-7 signalling with a global inability to generate lymphocytes. Their phenotype resembles that of SCID mice and humans.

The cytokine network is controlled *in vivo* in a number of ways (*Fig. 7.15*):

- Individual cytokine production is transient and tightly regulated.
- Cytokines act synergistically or antagonistically.
- Cytokines induce or inhibit production of other cytokines.
- Cytokines regulate expression of their own and other cytokine receptors.
- Receptor antagonists bind to a specific receptor but do not transmit a signal.
- 'Deceptors' – specifically bind ligand but do not transmit a signal.
- Extracellular domains of cytokine receptors are shed and bind soluble cytokine molecules.
- Stimulation of cell-surface shedding of membrane-associated cytokines.

Regulation of the cytokine network

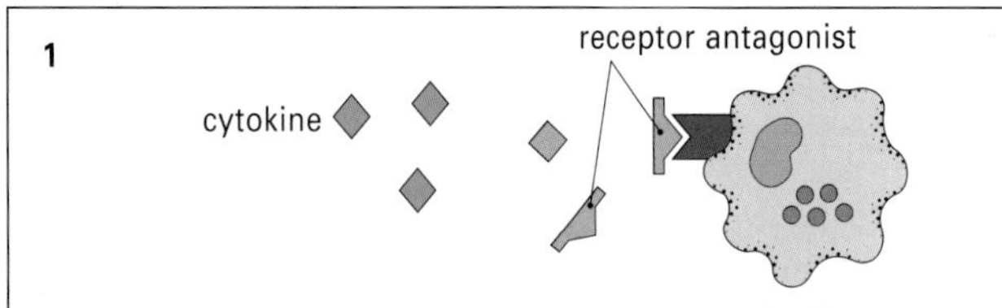

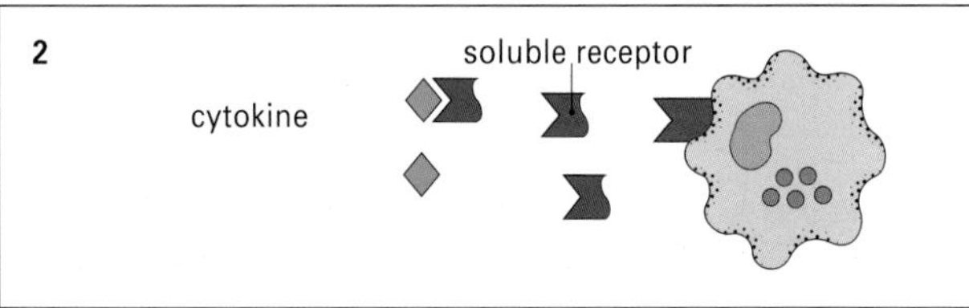

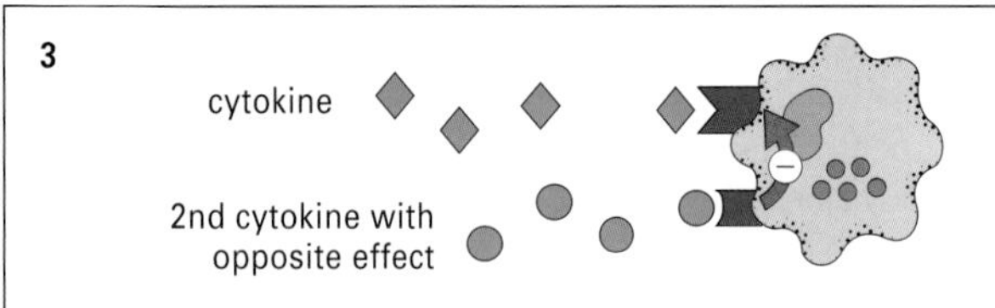

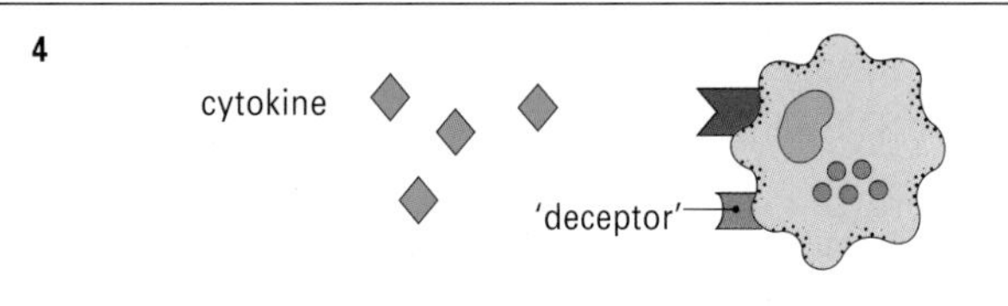

Fig. 7.15 (**1**) Molecules homologous with the cytokine and able to bind to its receptor without leading to signal transduction act as competitive inhibitors. The gene for an IL-1 inhibitor of this type has been cloned. There may also be inhibitory glycosylation variants of some mediators. (**2**) The extracellular domains of TNF and IL-1 receptors can be shed. They bind their cytokine in the fluid phase, and so stop the cytokine from reaching receptors on cell membranes. (**3**) Other mediators, acting through quite separate receptors, can exert opposite effects on the cell (**4**) Some cells express cytokine-binding molecules (deceptors) which do not activate the cell.

If we consider the inflammatory cytokine network, it is clear that there are some cytokines that are pivotal to the response and that a combination of agonist and antagonist cytokines regulates the outcome. Animal experiments and studies in human inflammatory disease have demonstrated the importance of TNFα in inflammation. Mice over-expressing TNFα develop rheumatoid arthritis, and TNFα antagonists are now being used successfully in patients with Crohn's disease and rheumatoid arthritis. Blocking the action of IL-1β and IL-6 has a similar anti-inflammatory action, at least in animal models. The cytokines IL-4, IL-10, IL-11 and TGFβ are known to be important in down-regulating the cytokine network.

The level of cytokine production and magnitude of response may also be controlled at a genetic level. Cytokine genes show a high number of polymorphisms, which are frequently in the regions that regulate transcription or post-transcriptional events. The inflammatory response, therefore, is genetically programmed both quantitatively and qualitatively, with some individuals having a more vigorous response than others. It is likely that these genetic factors contribute to disease susceptibility and clinical severity, although environmental factors are also important or essential. In particular, polymorphisms in the TNF and IL-1 locus are associated with susceptibility and/or severity in a number of inflammatory and autoimmune diseases.

The cytokine network has multiple physiological roles

The evolution and function of the immune system parallels that of the nervous system in many ways. For instance, both systems have learning and memory functions based on cell-to-cell communication, and share many mediators, receptors and antigens. Both systems need an internal communication network, and also a network that can control and interact with other organs. The nervous system is directly 'wired' to most other organs via nerves, but also uses the hypothalamus–pituitary–adrenal axis to send signals to the periphery. By contrast, the immune system is composed mostly of free, mobile cells: cell-to-cell interactions are intermittent and mostly concerned with internal communication. Thus communication with the organs is largely cytokine mediated, although it must be stressed that this control is generally localized and not systemic. In addition to these direct effects, the immune system is integrated with the nervous and endocrine systems. For example, cytokines such as IL-1, TNFα and IL-6 have direct effects on the hypothalamus or pituitary – IL-1 and IL-6 regulate body temperature, while IL-1 induces slow wave sleep and suppresses appetite. Many cells of the immune system also express receptors for neurotransmitters, opioids and neuropeptides.

The known functions of the characterized cytokines are summarised elsewhere (see Appendix III), but it is important to remember that not all of the listed functions will turn out to be physiologically relevant if they have only been defined by *in vitro* experiments.

CRITICAL THINKING • Cytokine production (Explanations on p. 454)

Peripheral blood was taken from 10 individuals. The leucocytes were isolated and cultured for 24 hours in tissue culture medium containing the mitogen/cytokine stimulator phytohaemagglutinin. An ELISA assay was then used to measure blood cell production of the cytokines TNF and IL-6. The results are shown in the table below:

Sample	TNF (pg/ml)	IL-6 (pg/ml)
1	2250	1000
2	1200	625
3	950	350
4	50	200
5	200	50
6	750	300
7	2000	650
8	600	500
9	1750	500
10	650	400

7.1 Given that culture conditions were well controlled, why do you think there is so much variability in cytokine production between individuals?

7.2 Is there a correlation between the amount of TNF and IL-6 in individual samples? If so, why is this?

7.3 A sample was also taken from the cultures at 2 hours. Only TNF was found at this time point. What could that suggest?

FURTHER READING

Balkwill FR (ed) *Frontiers in Molecular Biology. The Cytokine Network.* Oxford: Oxford University Press; 2000.

Benveniste EN. Cytokine actions in the central nervous system. *Cytokine Growth Factor Rev* 1998;**9**:259–75.

Cox A, Camp NJ, Nicklin MJ, DiGiovine FS, Duff GW. (1998) An analysis of linkage disequilibrium in the interleukin-1 gene cluster, using a novel grouping method for multiallelic markers. *Am J Hum Genet 1998;***62**:1180–8.

Cox A, Duff GW. Cytokines as genetic modifying factors in immune and inflammatory diseases. *J Pediatr Endocrinol Metabol* 1996;**9**:129–32.

Demoulin JB, Renauld JC. Signalling by cytokines interacting with the interleukin-2 receptor gamma chain. *Cytokine Cell Mol Ther* 1999;**4**:243–56

Heim MH. The Jak–Stat pathway: cytokine signalling from the receptor to the nucleus. *J Recept Signal Transduct Res* 1999;**19**:75-120

Kollias G, Douni E, Kassiotis G, Kontoyiannis D. On the role of tumor necrosis factor and receptors in models of multiorgan failure, rheumatoid arthritis multiple sclerosis and inflammatory bowel disease. *Immunol Rev* 1999;**169**:175–94.

Pfeffer LM, Dinarello CA, Herberman RB, *et al.* Biological properties of recombinant α-interferons: 40th anniversary of the discovery of interferons. *Cancer Res* 1998;**58**:2489–99.

Remick DG, Friedland JS (eds) Cytokines in Health and Disease. New York: Marcel Dekker; 1997.

Romagnani S. TH1/TH2 cells. *Inflamm Bowel Dis* 1999;**5**:285–94.

Schwarz MK, Wells TNC. Interfering with chemokine networks – the hope for new therapeutics. *Curr Opin Chem Biol* 1999;**3**:407–11.

Vaday GG, Lider O. Extracellular matrix moieties, cytokines, and enzymes: dynamic effects on immune cell behaviour and inflammation. *J Leukocyte Biol* 2000;**67**:149–59.

Vitkovic L, Bockaert J, Jacque C. Inflammatory cytokines: neuromodulators in normal brain? *J Neurochem* 2000;**74**:457–71.

Wallach D, Varolomeeve EE, Malinin NL,Kovalenko AV, Boldin MP. Tumour necrosis factor receptor and Fas signalling mechanisms. *Annu Rev Immunol* 1999;**17**:331–67.

8 Cell cooperation in the antibody response

- **The primary development of B cells is antigen independent.** Pre-B cells recombine genes for immunoglobulin heavy and light chains to generate their surface receptor for antigen.
- **T-independent antigens activate B cells without requiring T-cell help.** They can be divided into two groups. TI-1 antigens can act as polyclonal stimulators, while TI-2 antigens are polymers which activate by cross-linking the B-cell receptor.
- **T-dependent antigens are taken up by B cells, processed and presented to helper T cells.** T cells and B cells usually recognize different parts of an antigen.
- **B-cell activation requires signals from the B-cell receptor and co-stimulation.** CD40 is the most important co-stimulatory molecule on B cells. Ligation of the B-cell–coreceptor complex can lower the threshold of antigen needed to trigger the B cell. Intracellular signalling pathways are analogous in B cells and T cells.
- **Activated B cells proliferate and differentiate into antibody-forming cells.** Cytokines from T helper (TH) cells control the process of division, differentiation and class switching.
- **Mutation of immunoglobulin genes, followed by selection of high-affinity clones is the basis of affinity maturation.** These processes occur in germinal centres.
- **Class switching is effected by somatic recombination occurring within the heavy chain genes.** Differential splicing of long RNA transcripts is a second mechanism by which B cells can produce more than one type of antibody.

The antibody response is the culmination of a series of cellular and molecular interactions occurring in an orderly sequence between a B cell and a variety of other cells of the immune system. In this chapter, the principles of B-cell development, activation, proliferation and differentiation leading to the generation of plasma cells and memory cells are discussed in the context of immune cell cooperation. In addition, some of the critical molecules involved are described and the consequences of the interactions, including affinity maturation and class switching, are examined.

DEVELOPMENT OF B CELLS

Primary B-cell development is antigen independent

Within the bone marrow, a sequence of immunoglobulin rearrangements and phenotypic changes takes place during B-cell ontogeny, analogous to that described for T cells in the thymus which leads to the production of the B cell's antigen receptor (*Fig. 8.1*). The molecular processes involved in immunoglobulin gene rearrangement have been

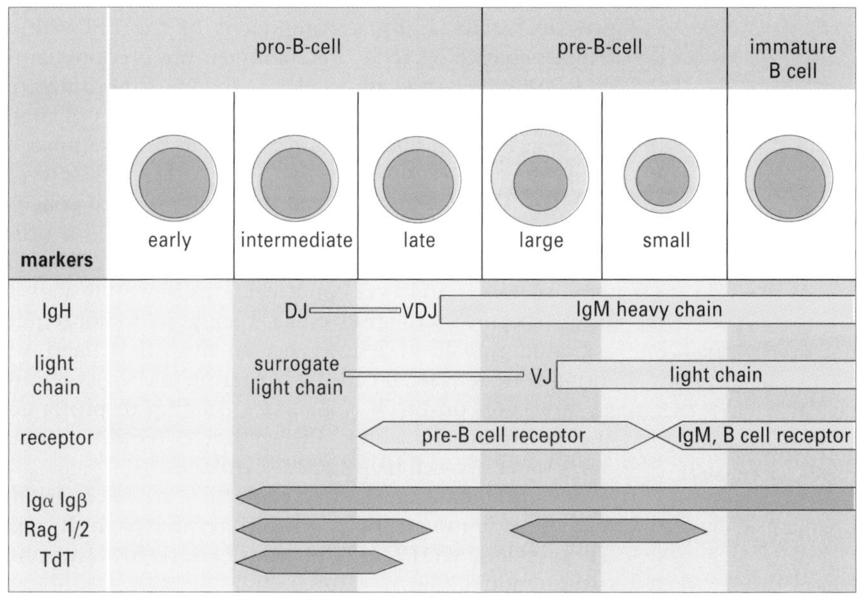

Fig. 8.1 During early B-cell development, the heavy chain gene (IgH) undergoes a DJ recombination, followed by a VDJ recombination. The recombined heavy chain is initially expressed with a surrogate light chain and the Igα and Igβ chains (CD79) to produce the pre-B-cell receptor. Later, light chain genes undergo a VJ recombination and surface IgM is produced as the B-cell receptor. Recombination events are associated with expression of the recombination activating genes (RAG-1 and RAG-2), but TdT expression only occurs during heavy chain recombination.

described in Chapter 4, and this section relates these events to B-cell development.

The earliest stage of antigen-independent B-cell development identified is the progenitor B (pro-B) cell stage. Pro-B cells can be divided into three groups based on the expression of terminal deoxynucleotidyltransferase (TdT), an intranuclear enzyme uniquely expressed during VH-gene rearrangement, and a marker called B220. This identifies a particular splice-variant of leucocyte common antigen (CD45R in humans), a tyrosine phosphatase that appears to be important in regulating B-cell receptor signalling. Early pro-B cells express TdT alone, intermediate pro-B cells express both TdT and B220, and late pro-B cells express B220 and have downregulated TdT. B220 remains expressed on the surface throughout the remainder of B-cell ontogeny. As the cells progress through the pro-B cell stage, they rearrange their Ig heavy chain genes and begin to express CD43 (leukosialin), CD19, RAG (recombination-activating gene)-1 and RAG-2. As late pro-B cells pass into the pre-B-cell stage, they downregulate TdT, RAG-1, RAG-2 and CD43.

Pre-B cells can be divided into large mitotically active pre-B cells and small non-dividing pre-B cells. Both large and small pre-B cells express Ig μ heavy chains in the cytoplasm (cμ) and the pre-B cell–receptor complex on their surface (*Fig. 8.2*). Large pre-B cells have successfully rearranged their Ig heavy chain genes. As these cells pass from the large pre-B cell group into the small pre-B cell group, they begin to rearrange their Ig light chain genes and upregulate RAG-1 and RAG-2. The final stage of B-cell development is the immature B-cell stage. Immature B cells have successfully rearranged their light chain genes and express IgM. Once again, RAG-1 and RAG-2 expression has been downregulated. As immature B cells develop further into mature B cells, they begin to express both IgM and IgD on their surface. These mature B cells are then free to exit the bone marrow and migrate into the periphery.

Other phenotypic markers such as CD25 (IL-2Rα chain), CD79a (Igα), CD79b (Igβ) and c-Kit can help to identify particular populations of pro-B, pre-B or immature B cells (*Fig. 8.3*). Transcription factors such as E2A, EBF and Pax5 have been shown to be specifically regulated within the B-cell lineage.

In addition, a number of growth and differentiation factors are required to drive the B cells through early stages of development. Receptors for these factors are expressed at various stages of B-cell differentiation. IL-4, IL-3 and low-molecular-weight B cell growth factor (L-BCGF) are important in initiating the process of B-cell differentiation, whereas other factors are active in the later stages.

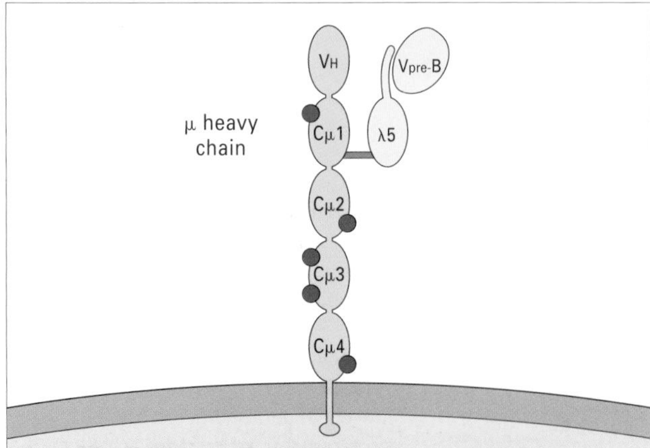

Fig. 8.2 The surrogate B-cell receptor complex is composed of a μ heavy chain and a $V_{pre\text{-}B}$ and λ5 proteins (surrogate light chains). The receptor has a role in early differentiation and development of B cells. The unit shown here associates with the signalling molecules Igα and Igβ.

ACTIVATION OF B CELLS BY T-INDEPENDENT ANTIGENS

Naïve mature B cells are free to exit the bone marrow and migrate into the periphery. If these cells do not encounter antigen, they soon die within a few weeks by apoptosis. If, however, these mature B cells encounter specific antigen, they undergo activation, proliferation and differentiation leading to the generation of plasma cells and memory B cells.

T-independent antigens do not require T-cell help to stimulate B cells

The immune response to most antigens depends on both T cells and B cells recognizing the antigen in a linked fashion. This type of antigen is called T-dependent (TD). There are, however, a small number of antigens capable of activating B cells without MHC class II-restricted T-cell help, referred to as T-independent (TI) antigens (*Fig. 8.4*). Importantly, many TI antigens are particularly resistant to degradation. TI antigens can be divided into two groups (TI-1 and TI-2) based on the manner in which they activate B cells. TI-1 antigens are predominantly bacterial cell wall components. The prototypical TI-1 antigen is lipopolysaccharide (LPS), a component of the cell wall of Gram-negative bacteria. TI-2 antigens are predominantly large polysaccharide molecules with repeating antigenic determinants. Bacterial cell wall polysaccharides, polymeric bacterial flagellin and poliomyelitis virus are examples of such.

Many TI-1 antigens possess the ability in high concentrations to activate B-cell clones that are specific for other antigens, a phenomenon known as polyclonal B-cell activation. However, in lower concentrations they only activate B cells specific for themselves. TI-1 antigens do not require a second signal. TI-2 antigens, on the other hand, are thought to activate B cells by clustering and cross-linking Ig molecules on the B cell surface, leading to prolonged and persistent signalling. TI-2 antigens require residual non-cognate T-cell help such as cytokines.

Several signal transduction molecules are necessary for mediating T-independent antigen responses in B cells. These include CD19, HS1 protein, Lyn, IL-5Rα, lymphotoxin α, and TNFα.

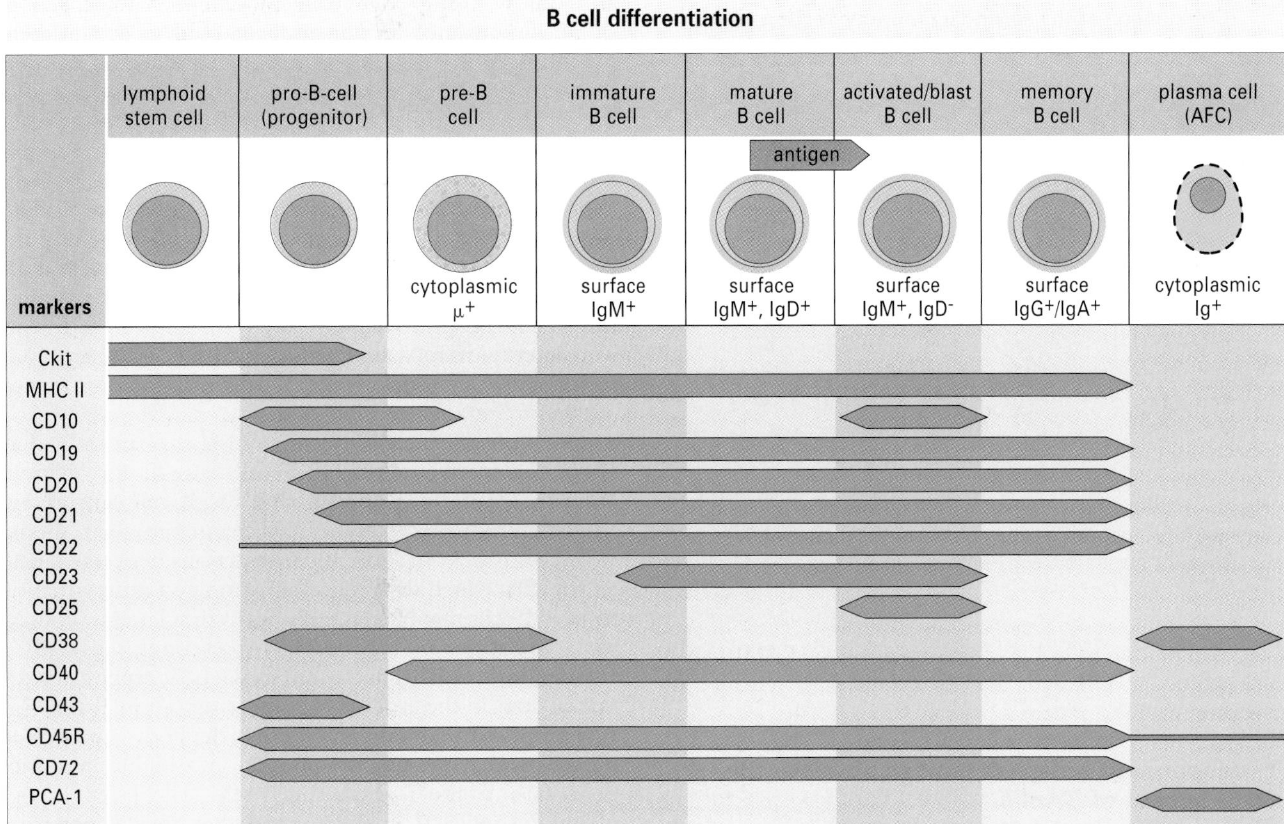

Fig. 8.3 B cells differentiate from lymphoid stem cells into virgin B cells and may then be driven by antigen to become memory cells or plasma cells. The cellular location of immunoglobulin is shown in yellow. Pre-B cells express cytoplasmic μ chains only. The immature B cell has surface IgM, and the mature B cell other immunoglobulin isotypes. Upon antigen stimulation, the B cell proliferates and develops into a plasma cell or a memory cell after a phase of proliferation, activation and blast transformation. Memory cells and plasma cells are found at different sites in lymphoid tissue. TdT is expressed very early in ontogeny.

T-independent antigens

antigen	polymeric	polyclonal activation	resistance to degradation
lipopolysaccharide (LPS)	+	+++	+
Ficoll	+++	–	+++
dextran	++	+	++
levan	++	+	++
poly-D amino acids	+++	–	+++
polymeric bacterial flagellin	++	++	+

Fig. 8.4 The major common properties of some of the main T-independent antigens are listed. T-independent antigens induce the production of cytokines IL-1, TNFα and IL-6 by macrophages. (Note: both poly-L amino acids and monomeric bacterial flagellin are T-dependent antigens, demonstrating the role of antigen structure in determining T-independent properties.)

T-independent antigens induce poor memory

Primary antibody responses to TI antigens *in vitro* are generally slightly weaker than those to TD antigens. They peak fractionally earlier and both generate mainly IgM. However, the secondary responses to TD and TI antigens differ greatly. The secondary response to TI antigens resembles the primary response, whereas the secondary response to TD antigens is far stronger and has a large IgG component (*Fig. 8.5*). It seems, therefore, that TI antigens do not usually induce the maturation of a response leading to class switching or to an increase in antibody affinity, as seen with TD antigens. This is most likely due to the lack of CD40 activation (see below). Memory induction to TI antigens is also relatively poor.

There are potential survival advantages if the immune response to bacteria does not depend on complex cell interactions, as it could be more rapid. Many bacterial antigens bypass T-cell help because they are very effective inducers of cytokine production by macrophages – they induce IL-1, IL-6 and tumour necrosis factor-α (TNFα) from macrophages. The short-lived response and lack of IgG

Comparison of the secondary immune response to T-dependent and T-independent antigens *in vitro*

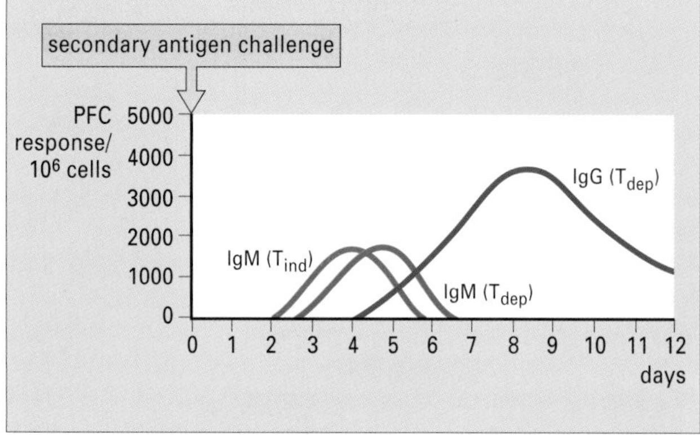

Fig. 8.5 The secondary response to T-dependent antigens is stronger and induces a greater number of IgG-producing cells, as measured by plaque-forming cells (see Chapter 26).

may also be due to lack of co-stimulation via CD40L and lack of IL-2, IL-4 and IL-5, which T cells produce in response to TD antigens.

T-independent antigens tend to activate the CD5⁺ subset of B cells

TI antigens predominantly activate the B-1 subset of B cells found mainly in the peritoneum. These B-1 cells can be identified by their expression of CD5, which is induced upon binding of TI antigens. In contrast to conventional B cells, B-1 cells have the ability to replenish themselves.

ACTIVATION OF B CELLS BY T-DEPENDENT ANTIGENS

T cells and B cells recognize different parts of antigens

In the late 1960s and early 1970s, studies by Mitchison and others, using chemically modified proteins, led to significant advances in our understanding of the different functions of T cells and B cells. To induce an optimal secondary antibody response to a small chemical group or hapten (which is only immunogenic if bound to a protein carrier), it was found that the experimental animal must be immunized and then challenged using the same hapten–carrier conjugate – not just the same hapten. This was referred to as the 'carrier effect'. By manipulating the cell populations in these experiments, it was shown that TH cells are responsible for recognizing the carrier, whereas the B cells recognize hapten (*Fig. 8.6*). These experiments were later reinforced by details of how B cells use antibody to recognize epitopes, while T cells recognize processed antigen fragments (see *Fig. 6.4*).

One consequence of this system is that an individual B cell can receive help from T cells specific for different antigenic peptides, provided that the B cell can present those determinants to each T cell. In an immune response *in vivo*, it is believed that the interactions between T cells and B cells which drive B-cell division and differentiation involve T cells that have already been stimulated by contact with the antigen on other antigen-presenting cells (APCs; e.g. dendritic cells). This has led to the basic scheme for cell interactions in the antibody response set out in *Figure 8.7*. It is proposed that antigen entering the body is processed by cells which present the antigen in a highly immunogenic form to the TH cells and B cells. The T cells recognize determinants on the antigen that are distinct from those recognized by the B cells, which differentiate and divide into antibody-forming cells. Thus two processes are required to activate a B cell:

- Antigen interacting with B-cell Ig receptors. This involves 'native' antigen.
- Stimulating signal(s) from TH cells that respond to processed antigen bound to MHC class II molecules.

B-cell activation and T-cell activation follow similar patterns

In B cells, the signalling function of CD3 is carried out by a heterodimer of Igα and Igβ. Two molecules of the

Carrier priming

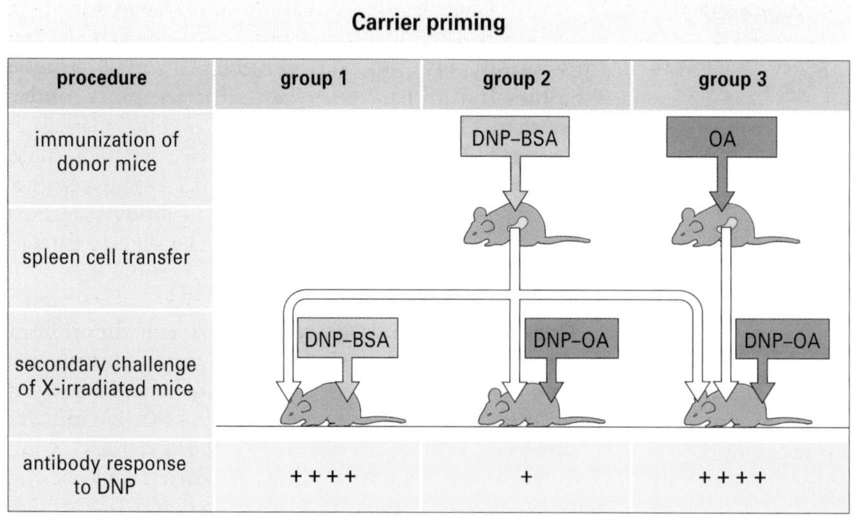

Fig. 8.6 Three groups of X-irradiated mice were given antigen-primed spleen cells and challenged with antigen: (**1**) Mice that received DNP-BSA-primed cells and were then challenged with DNP-BSA gave a strong antibody response to DNP. (**2**) Mice that received DNP-BSA-primed cells and were then challenged with DNP-OA, gave a weak antibody response (no carrier effect). (**3**) Mice that received DNP-BSA-primed cells and OA-primed cells and were then challenged with DNP-OA gave a strong response to DNP. This shows that the need for carrier priming can be circumvented by supplying carrier-primed spleen cells.

Cell cooperation in the antibody response

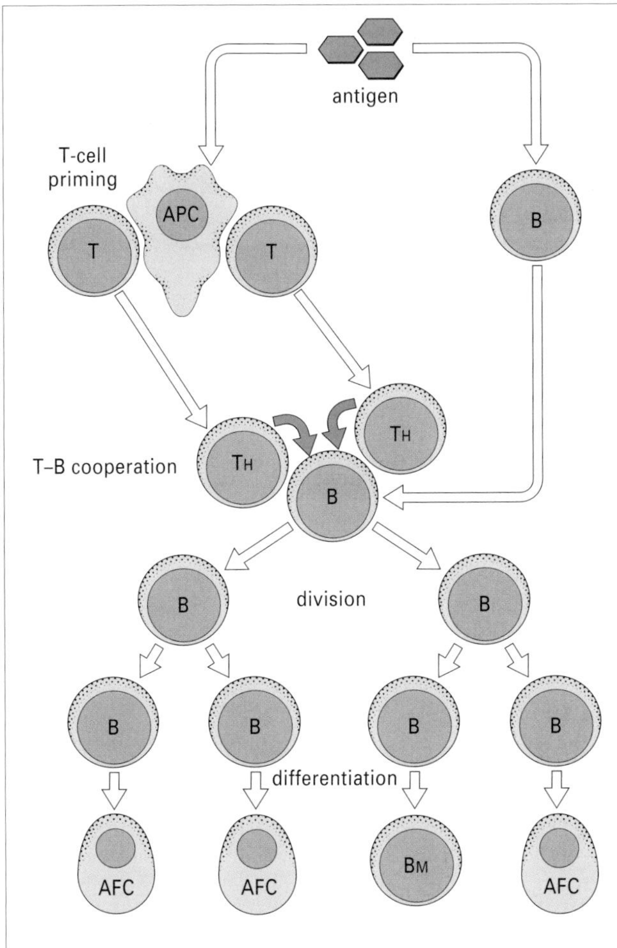

Fig. 8.7 Antigen is presented to virgin T cells by antigen-presenting cells (APCs) such as dendritic cells. B cells also take up antigen and present it to the T cells, receiving signals from the T cells to divide and differentiate into antibody-forming cells (AFCs) and memory B (BM) cells.

Intracellular signalling in B-cell activation

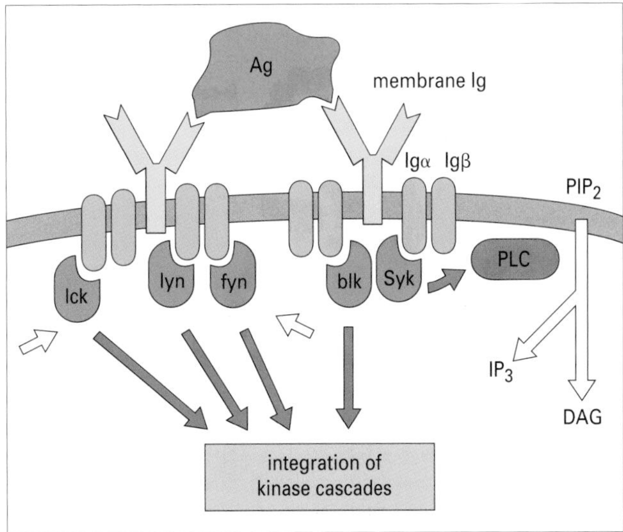

Fig. 8.8 B-cell activation is similar to T-cell activation. If membrane Ig becomes cross-linked (e.g. by a T-independent antigen), tyrosine kinases, including Lck, Lyn, Fyn and Blk, become activated. They phosphorylate the ITAM domains in the Igα and Igβ chains of the receptor complex. These can then bind another kinase, Syk, which activates phospholipase C. This acts on membrane PIP_2 to generate IP_3 and diacyl glycerol (DAG) which activates protein kinase C. Signals from the other kinases are transduced to activate nuclear transcription factors.

Igα/Igβ heterodimer associate with surface Ig to form the B-cell receptor (BCR). The cytoplasmic tails of Igα and Igβ carry immunoreceptor tyrosine activation motifs (ITAM). Cross-linking of surface Ig leads to activation of the src family kinases, which in B cells are Fyn, but also Lyn and Blk. Syk is analogous to ZAP-70 in T cells, and binds to the phosphorylated ITAMs of Igα and Igβ (*Fig. 8.8*). This leads to activation of a kinase cascade and translocation of nuclear transcription factors analogous to the process that occurs in T cells (see *Figure 6.21*).

B-cell activation is also markedly augmented by the 'co-receptor complex' comprising three proteins – CD21 (complement receptor-2, CR2), CD19 and CD81 (target of anti-proliferative antibody, TAPA-1) (*Fig. 8.9*). Follicular dendritic cells are known to retain antigen on their surface for prolonged periods of time as immune complexes (iccosomes). The antigen in such complexes can bind to CD21 (via the complement molecule C3d), and surface Ig on the B cells. Phosphorylation of the cytoplasmic tail of CD19 can then occur, leading to binding and activation of Lyn. It is likely that these kinases enhance the activation signal through the phospholipase C and phosphatidylinositol 3-kinase pathways, particularly when antigen concentration is low.

Direct interaction of B cells and T cells involves co-stimulatory molecules

Antigen-specific T-cell populations can be obtained by growing and cloning T cells with antigens, APCs and IL-2. It is thus possible to visualize directly B-cell and T-cell clusters interacting *in vitro*. The T cells become polarized, with the T-cell receptors concentrated on the B-cell side. The B cells also become polarized and express most of their MHC class II molecules and ICAM-1 in proximity to the T cells. The interactions in these clusters strongly suggest an intense exchange of information, which leads to two important events in the B-cell life cycle: induction of proliferation and differentiation into antibody forming cells (AFCs).

The initial interaction between a naïve B cell and a cognate antigen via the BCR in the presence of cytokines or other growth stimuli induces activation and proliferation of the B cell. This then leads to processing of the T-dependent antigen and presentation to T cells (see Chapter 6). The interaction between B cells and T cells is a two-way process in which B cells present antigen to T cells and receive signals from the T cells for division and

B cell–coreceptor complex

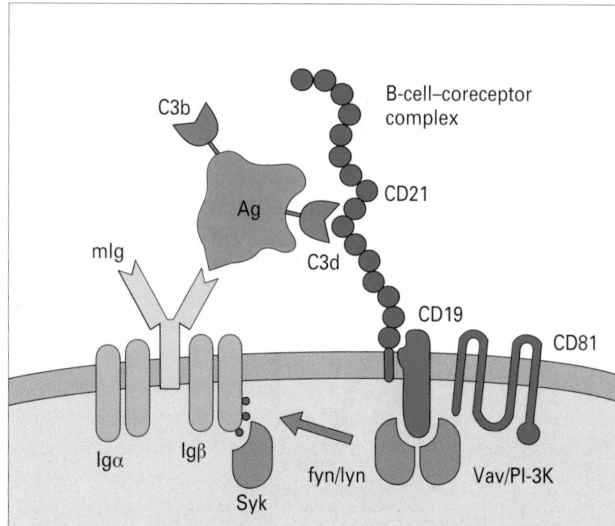

Fig. 8.9 The B cell–co-receptor complex consists of CD21 (the complement receptor type-2), CD19 and CD81 (a molecule with four transmembrane segments). Antigen with covalently bound C3b or C3d can cross-link the membrane Ig to CD21 of the co-receptor complex. This greatly reduces the cell's requirement for antigen to activate it. CD19 can associate with tyrosine kinases including Lyn, Fyn, Vav and PI-3 kinase (PI-3K). Compare this with CD28 on the T cell. Receptor cross-linking causes phosphorylation of the Igα and Igβ chains of the antigen–receptor complex and recruitment and activation of Syk.

Cell-surface molecules involved in the interaction between B cells and TH cells

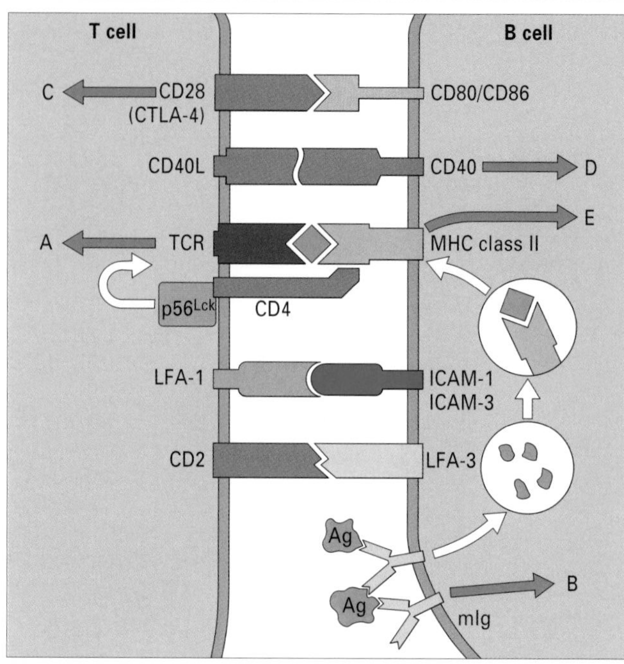

Fig. 8.10 Membrane immunoglobulin (mIg) takes up antigen (Ag) into an intracellular compartment where it is degraded and peptides can combine with MHC class II molecules. Other arrows show the discrete signal transduction events that have been established. A and B are the antigen–receptor signal transduction events involving tyrosine phosphorylation and phosphoinositide breakdown. The antigen receptors also regulate LFA-1 affinity for ICAM-1 and ICAM-3, possibly through the signal transduction events. In the T cell, CD28 also sends a unique signal to the T cell (C). In the later phases of the response CTLA-4 can supplant CD28 to cause downregulation. In the B cell, stimulation via CD40 is the most potent activating signal (D). In addition, class II MHC molecules appear to induce distinct signalling events (E). Not shown is the exchange of soluble interleukins and binding to the corresponding receptors on the other cell. (Adapted with permission from DeFranco A, *Nature* 1991; **351**: 603–5.)

differentiation (*Fig. 8.10*). The central, antigen-specific interaction is that between the MHC class II–antigen complex and the TCR. This interaction is augmented by interactions between LFA-3 and CD2 and between ICAM-1 or ICAM-3 and LFA-1. Other cell-surface molecules are also involved. The CD80 (B7-1) and CD86 (B7-2) molecules on B cells interact with CD28 and CTLA-4 on the T cell, which causes stabilization of mRNA for IL-2 and other cytokines in the T cells, thereby augmenting and prolonging the delivery of the activation signals through the TCR.

It is now recognized that CD40, a member of the TNF receptor family, delivers the most potent activating signal to B cells, more potent even than signals transmitted via surface Ig. Upon activation, T cells transiently express a ligand, termed CD40L, which interacts with CD40. CD40L is a member of the TNF family. CD40/CD40L interaction helps to drive B cells into cell cycle. Transduction of signals through CD40 also induces upregulation of CD80/CD86 and thus helps to provide co-stimulatory signals to the responding T cells. Signalling through CD40 is also essential for germinal centre development and antibody responses to T-cell-dependent antigens. This is confirmed by hyper-IgM syndrome, an immunodeficiency disease caused by a genetic mutation of CD40L. This disorder is characterized by a failure to form germinal centres and absence of isotype switch to IgG, IgE or IgA production.

Cytokine secretion from CD4 T cells is important in B-cell proliferation and differentiation

Recent work has shown that $CD4^+$ T cells in both mouse and man can be divided into different subsets, depending on their cytokine profile (see *Figure 7.12*).

- TH1 cells: $CD4^+$ T cells that produce IL-2 and interferon-γ (IFNγ), but not IL-4, are designated TH1 and are chiefly responsible for delayed-type hypersensitivity responses, but can also help B cells to produce IgG2a, but not much IgG1 or IgE.
- TH2 cells: $CD4^+$ T cells that produce IL-4, IL-5, IL-6, IL-10 and IL-13, but not IL-2 or IFNγ, are designated TH2 and are very efficient helper cells for production of antibody, especially of IgG1 and IgE.
- TH0 cells: Many $CD4^+$ T cells, especially in humans, have cytokine profiles intermediate between the above,

Stages in B-cell activation and development

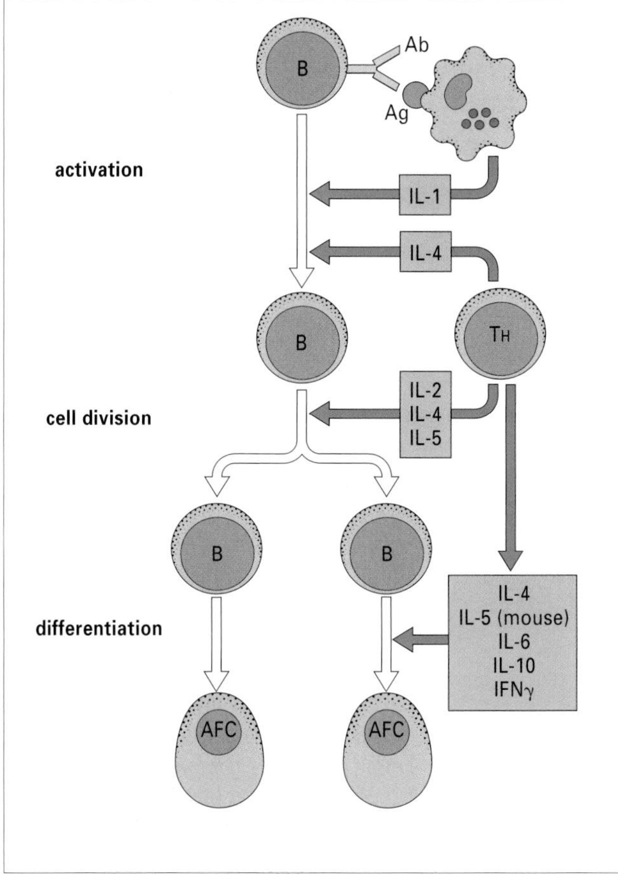

Fig. 8.11 B cells are activated by antigen on antigen-presenting cells (APCs) such as macrophages in the presence of IL-4 and IL-1. This causes expression of receptors for IL-2 and other cytokines. IL-2, IL-4 and IL-5 drive cell division. Only one cycle of cell division is illustrated, although many cycles will usually occur. Differentiation into antibody-forming cells (AFCs) is effected by IL-4, IL-5, IL-6, IL-10 and IFNγ.

and are known as 'TH0' cells. These cells are capable of producing both the TH1 cytokine IFNγ and the TH2 cytokine IL-4. However, classic TH1 and TH2 cells have been well documented in humans, especially in diseased tissues.

During B-cell–T-cell interaction, T cells can secrete a number of cytokines that have a powerful effect on B cells (*Fig. 8.11*). IL-2, for example, is an inducer of proliferation for B cells. The specific cytokines produced by TH2 cells also affect B cells. These cytokines include IL-4, IL-5, IL-6, IL-10 and IL-13. IL-4 (previously known as B-cell activating or differentiation factor-1) acts on B cells to induce activation and differentiation. It also acts on T cells as a growth factor and promotes differentiation of TH2 cells, thus reinforcing the antibody response. At the same time, it inhibits the production of pro-inflammatory cytokines such as IL-1 and TNFα by macrophages.

Excess IL-4 plays a part in allergic disease, causing production of IgE. IL-5 in humans is chiefly a growth and activation factor for eosinophils and it is responsible for the eosinophilia of parasitic disease. In the mouse it also acts on B cells to induce growth and differentiation. IL-6, previously know as B-cell-differentiating factor or hepatocyte-stimulating factor, is produced by many cells including T cells, macrophages, B cells, fibroblasts and endothelial cells. It acts on most cells, but is particularly important in inducing B cells to differentiate into antibody-forming cells. In the liver, it stimulates the production of acute phase proteins. IL-6 is considered to be an important growth factor for multiple myeloma, a malignancy of plasma cells. IL-10 acts as a growth and differentiation factor for B cells. IL-13, which shares a receptor component and signalling pathways with IL-4, acts on B cells to produce IgE. Other cytokines such as IL-7, originally isolated from a stromal cell line as a factor supporting pre-B-cell growth, has been shown to be indispensable for B-cell development.

Cytokines can also influence antibody affinity. Antibody affinity to most T-dependent antigens increases during an immune response, and a similar effect can be produced by certain immunization protocols. For example, high-affinity antibody subpopulations are potentiated after immunization with antigen and IFNγ (*Fig. 8.12*). A number of adjuvants are capable of enhancing levels of antibody,

Cytokine influence on antibody affinity

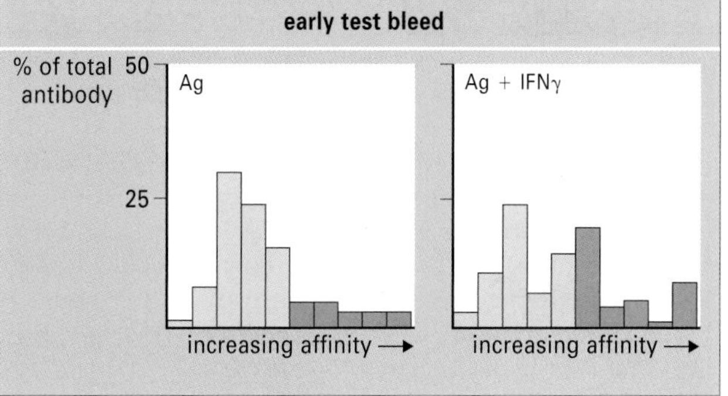

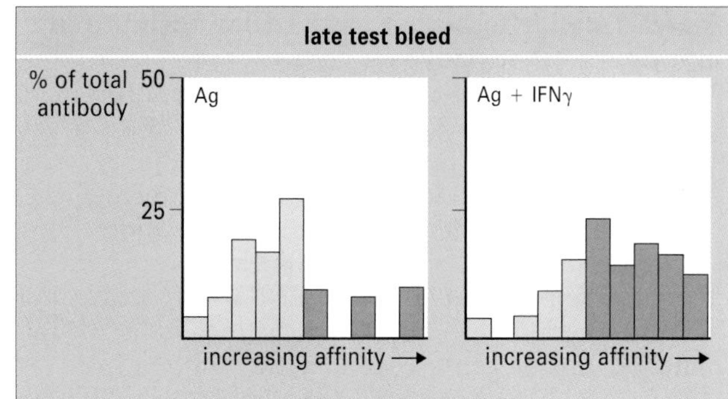

Fig. 8.12 Mice were immunized either with antigen alone (Ag) or with antigen plus 30 000 units of IFNγ (Ag + IFNγ). The affinity of the antibodies was measured either early or late after immunization. Mice receiving IFNγ show more high-affinity antibody (darker bars) in both the early and late bleeds than those mice that received antigen alone. (Adapted from Holland, Holland & Steward. *Clin Exp Immunol* 1990;**82**:221–26.)

Cytokine receptor expression during B-cell development

markers	lymphoid stem cell	pro-B cell (progenitor)	pre-B cell	immature B cell	mature B cell	activated/blast B cell	memory B cell	plasma cell
L-BCGFR								
H-BCGFR								
IL-1R								
IL-2R								
IL-3R								
IL-4R								
IL-5R								
IL-6R								
IL-7R								

Fig. 8.13 The whole life history of B cells from stem cell to mature plasma cell is regulated by cytokines present in their environment. Receptors for these cytokines are selectively expressed by B cells at different stages of development. IL-7 plays an important part in initiating events in B-cell differentiation. Some of these receptors now have CD markers (see Appendix 2). BCGFR = B-cell growth factor receptor.

but few have this characteristic of also potentiating affinity. As affinity markedly influences the biological effectiveness of antibodies, IFNγ may be an important adjuvant for use in vaccines.

In addition to the effects of cytokines on B-cell proliferation and differentiation, cytokines are capable of influencing the class switch from IgM to other immunoglobulin classes (see below).

Cytokine receptors aid in B-cell growth and differentiation

Receptors for the many growth and differentiation factors required to drive the B cells through early stages of development are expressed at various stages of B-cell differentiation. Receptors for IL-7, IL-3 and low-molecular-weight B-cell growth factor are important in the initial stages of B-cell differentiation, whereas other receptors are more important in the later stages (*Fig. 8.13*)

B-cell–T-cell interaction may either activate or inactivate (anergize)

The above description of B-cell–T-cell interaction suggests that the only possible outcome is activation of the B cell. However, this is not the case. It has already been seen that APC–T-cell interaction may yield two diametrically opposing results, namely activation or inactivation (clonal anergy). In the same way, B cells frequently become anergic. This is an important process because affinity maturation of B cells during the immune response, as a result of rapid mutation in the genes encoding the antibody variable regions, could easily result in high-affinity autoantibodies. Clonal anergy and other forms of tolerance in the periphery are important for silencing these potentially damaging clones. However, the molecular details of this process are still unclear. Moreover, the respective roles of IgM and IgD, the two cell-surface receptors for antigen on B cells, are also not understood in terms of activation or inactivation. Both IgM and IgD appear to be capable of transmitting signals for both functions.

ACTIVATION AND DIFFERENTIATION OF B CELLS IN THE GERMINAL CENTRE

Following activation, antigen-specific B cells can follow either of two separate developmental pathways. The first pathway involves proliferation and differentiation into antibody forming cells (AFCs) in the lymph nodes or in the periarteriolar lymphoid sheath of the spleen. These AFCs function to rapidly clear antigen. However, the great majority of these cells die via apoptosis within 2 weeks. Therefore, it is unlikely that these AFCs are responsible for long-term antibody production. Consequently, a second pathway exists whereby some members of the expanded B-cell population migrate into adjacent follicles to form germinal centres before differentiating into memory B cells. The mechanism that determines which path a B cell takes is unknown. However, it is likely that the decision can be influenced by the nature of the naïve B cells initially recruited into the response, the affinity and specificity of the BCR, the type of antigen driving the response, and the levels of T-cell help.

Memory B cells, producing high-affinity antibody, develop in germinal centres

The germinal centre is important in that it provides a microenvironment whereby B cells can undergo developmental events that ultimately result in an affinity-matured, long-lived memory B-cell compartment of the immune system (*Fig. 8.14*). These developmental events come about due to complex interactions between B cells, CD4 helper T cells, and follicular dendritic cells. These events include clonal proliferation, antibody variable region somatic hypermutation, receptor editing, isotype switch recombination, affinity maturation and positive selection.

The germinal centre (GC) initially contains only dividing centroblasts. Shortly thereafter, the GC polarizes itself into a dark zone containing centroblasts and a light zone containing non-dividing (resting) centrocytes (*Fig. 8.15*). Centroblasts proliferate rapidly in the dark zone and

B-cell development in germinal centres

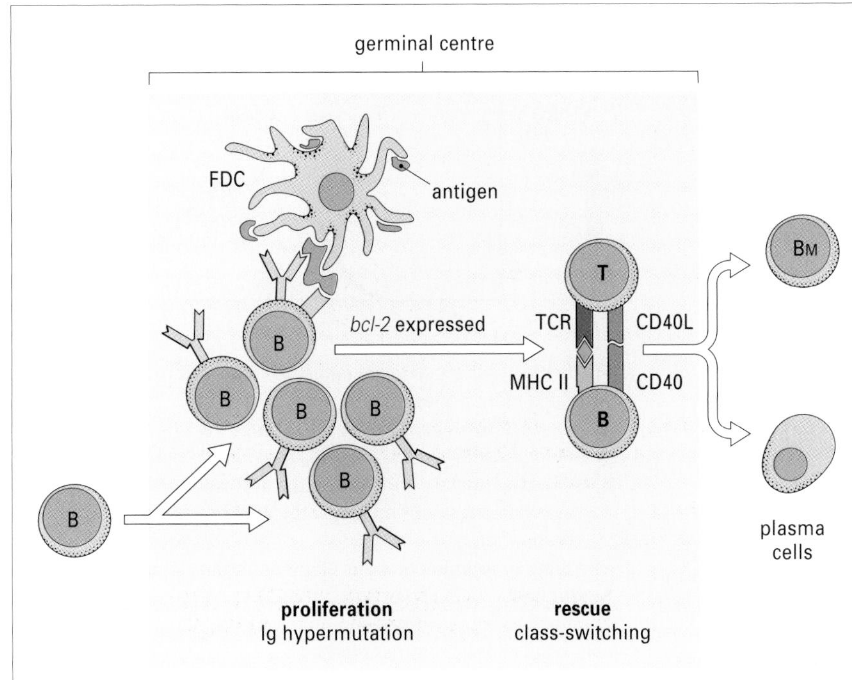

Fig. 8.14 A B cell enters a germinal centre and undergoes rapid proliferation and hypermutation of its immunoglobulin genes. Antigen is presented by the follicular dendritic cell (FDC), but only B cells with high-affinity receptors will compete effectively for this antigen. B cells, which do have a higher-affinity immunoglobulin, express Bcl-*2* and are rescued from apoptosis by interaction with T cells (i.e. the B-cell-presenting antigen to the T cell). Interaction with T cells promotes class switching. The class switch that takes place depends on the T cells present, which partly relates to the particular secondary lymphoid tissue and the type of immune response current (TH1 versus TH2). B cells leave the germinal centre to become either plasma cells or B memory cells (BM).

downregulate the expression of their surface immunoglobulin. Somatic hypermutation then occurs in order to diversify the rearranged variable region genes. Somatic hypermutation allows a single B cell to give rise to a clone that contains variants with different affinities for the antigen. Isotype switch recombination occurs following somatic hypermutation and requires cell cycling. Receptor editing of immunoglobulin light chain genes also occurs in centroblasts.

Somatic mutation of Ig genes and B-cell selection occur in the germinal centre

Following these developmental changes, the centroblasts migrate to the follicular dendritic cell- (FDC-) light zone of the GC and give rise to centrocytes which then re-express surface immunoglobulin BCR. In the light zone, centrocytes encounter antigen bound to the FDCs and antigen-specific TH2 cells. FDCs and T cells interact with centrocytes through surface molecules such as the BCR, CD40, CD80 (B7-1), CD86 (B7-2), LFA-1, VLA-4, CD54 (ICAM-1) and CD106 (VCAM-1), and through cytokines such as IL-2, IL-4, IL-5, IL-6, IL-10, IL-13 and lymphotoxin-α. After the centrocytes have stopped dividing, they are selected according to their ability to bind antigen. Those with high-affinity receptors for foreign antigen are positively selected, while those without adequate affinity undergo Fas-dependent apoptosis (see *Figs 10.8* and *10.9* for an explanation of how Fas (CD95) is involved in apoptosis).

Self-reactive B cells generated by somatic mutation are deleted

Those centrocytes that respond to soluble antigen or that do not receive T-cell help are negatively selected and undergo Fas-independent apoptosis. In this way, selection provides a mechanism for elimination of self-reactive antibodies that may be generated during somatic hypermutation. Positively selected centrocytes can re-enter the dark zone for successive rounds of expansion, diversification and selection. Somatic hypermutation and selection improve the average affinity of the GC B-cell population for presented antigen. Following these B-cell developmental stages, the GC centrocytes exit the GC and lose their apoptotic phenotype by downregulating Fas and increasing the expression of Bcl-2. Three possible outcomes are associated with exit from the GC – antibody-secreting bone marrow homing effector B cells, marginal zone memory B cells or recirculating memory B cells. The factors that regulate the decision to exit the GC are poorly understood.

ANTIBODY RESPONSES *IN VIVO*

The earliest studies on antibody responses followed the development of specific antibodies in animals immunized with T-dependent or T-independent antigens. With our improved knowledge of B-cell development and maturation, it is now possible to understand the features of immune responses *in vivo* in terms of the underlying cellular events. Features of antibody responses *in vivo* include:

- The enhanced secondary response.
- Isotype switching.
- Affinity maturation.
- The development of memory.

However, some of these events can be understood only by viewing the B-cell population as a whole, rather than as a

Schematic organization of the germinal centre

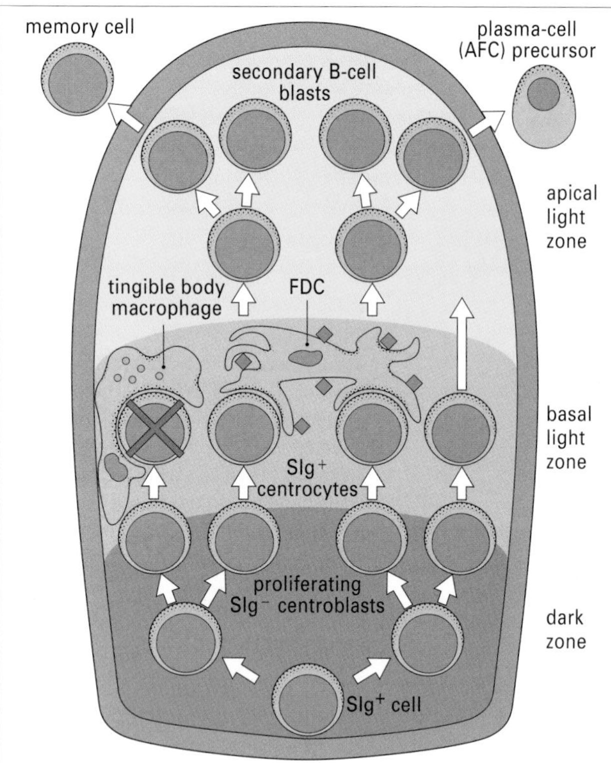

Fig. 8.15 The functions of the germinal centre are clonal proliferation, somatic hypermutation of Ig receptors, receptor editing, isotype class switching, affinity maturation and selection by antigen. In this model, the germinal centre is composed of three major zones: a dark zone, a basal light zone and an apical light zone. These zones are predominantly occupied by centroblasts, centrocytes and secondary blasts, respectively. Primary B-cell blasts carrying surface immunoglobulin receptors (SIg^+) enter the follicle and leave as memory B cells or AFCs. Antigen-presenting follicular dendritic cells (FDCs) are mainly found in the two deeper zones, and cell death by apoptosis occurs primarily in the basal light zone where tingible body macrophages are also located. Blue squares are iccosomes on FDC. (Adapted from Roitt IM. *Essential Immunology*, 7th edn. Oxford: Blackwell Scientific Press, 1991.)

The four phases of a primary antibody response

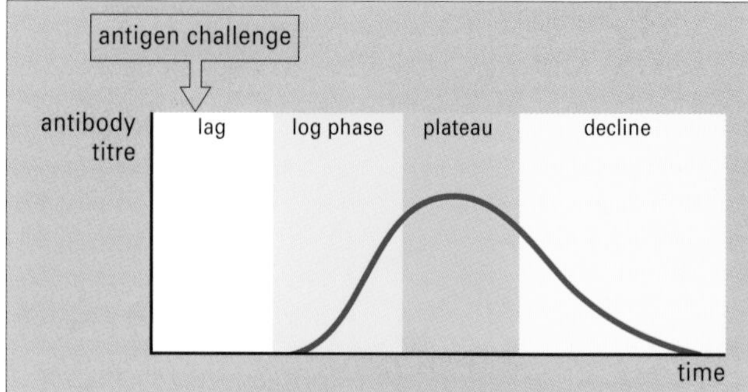

Fig. 8.16 After antigen challenge, the antibody response proceeds in four phases:

1. A lag phase when no antibody is detected.
2. A log phase when the antibody titre increases logarithmically.
3. A plateau phase during which the antibody titre stabilizes.
4. A decline phase during which the antibody is cleared or catabolized.

In a primary immune response, IgM antibodies initially predominate, followed by IgG antibodies. The actual time course and titres reached will depend on the nature of the antigenic challenge and the nature of the host.

collection of individual cells. The elements of the antibody response *in vivo* are detailed below.

Following primary antigenic challenge, there is an initial lag phase when no antibody can be detected. This is followed by phases in which the antibody titer increases logarithmically to a plateau and then declines. The decline occurs because the antibodies are either naturally catabolized or bind to the antigen and are cleared from the circulation (*Fig. 8.16*).

An examination of the responses following primary and secondary antigenic challenge shows that the responses differ in four major respects:

Time course – The secondary response has a shorter lag phase and an extended plateau and decline.

Antibody titre – The plateau levels of antibody are much greater in the secondary response, typically 10-fold or more than plateau levels in the primary response.

Antibody class – IgM antibodies form a major proportion of the primary response, whereas the secondary response consists almost entirely of IgG, with very little IgM.

Antibody affinity – The affinity of the antibodies in the secondary response is usually much higher. This is referred to as 'affinity maturation'.

The characteristics of primary and secondary antibody responses are compared in *Figure 8.17*.

Different immunoglobulin classes have different functions

Each of the different immunoglobulin classes perform different functions, as detailed in Chapter 4 and summarized below.

IgG – This is the major immunoglobulin in serum, acting as an anti-toxin and as an opsonin, by its ability to bind to Fc receptors on macrophages and neutrophils. It is also important in conferring immunity to neonates and in the first months of life.

IgM – Accounts for approximately 10% of the serum immunoglobulin. It is largely confined to the intravascular pool and is the predominant 'early' antibody, frequently seen in the immune response to antigenically complex infectious organisms.

IgA – The predominant immunoglobulin in seromucous

Primary and secondary antibody responses

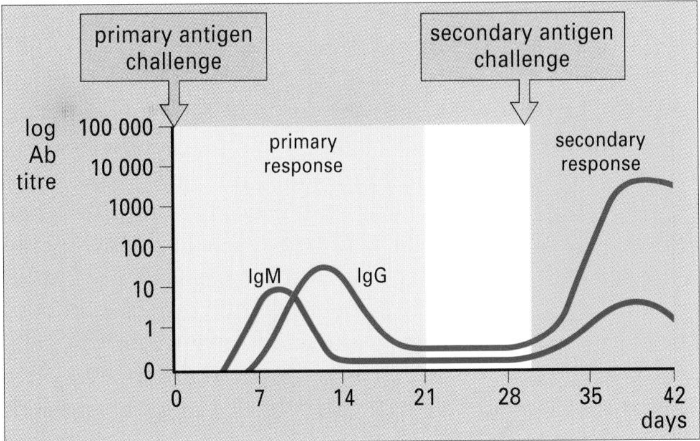

Fig. 8.17 In comparison with the antibody response after primary antigenic challenge, the antibody level after secondary antigenic challenge in a typical immune response:

- Appears more quickly.
- Persists for a longer period of time.
- Attains a higher titre.
- Consists predominantly of IgG antibodies.

Affinity maturation

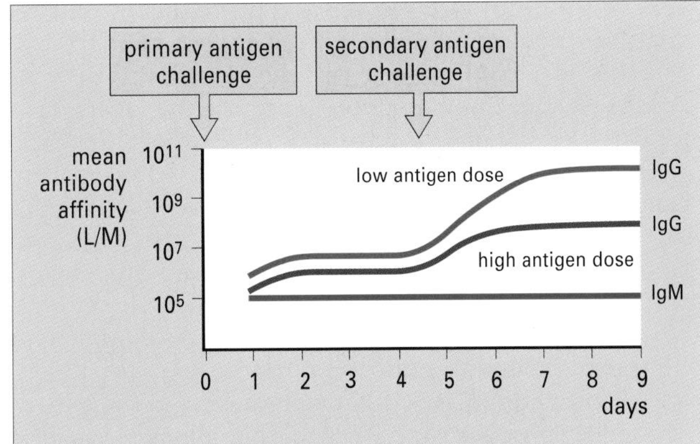

Fig. 8.18 The average affinity of the IgM and IgG antibody responses after primary and secondary challenge with a T-dependent antigen is shown. The affinity of the IgM response is constant throughout. The affinity maturation of the IgG response depends on the dose of the secondary antigen. Low antigen doses produce higher-affinity immunoglobulin than do high antigen doses, because the high-affinity clones compete effectively for the limiting amount of antigen.

secretions such as saliva, colostrum, breast milk, and tracheobronchial and genitourinary secretions.

IgD – Thought to play a role in B-cell differentiaiton.

IgE – Found predominantly on the surface of basophils and mast cells. It sensitizes these cells for triggering by antigen. It plays a role in mediating immediate hypersensitivity reactions, but is also important in defences against helminthic parasites.

The production of different immunoglobulin classes during an immune response can be related to isotype class switching by individual B cells, which is explained in the following section. Within the body, these processes can also be related to different tissues. For example, B cells which produce IgA predominate in mucosa-associated lymphoid tissues, which is related to the tissue environment and the presence of T cells which promote switching to IgA production. This is thought to be directed by distinct signals and cytokines within each tissue.

DIFFERENTIATION OF B CELLS

Affinity maturation depends on cell selection

The antibodies produced in a primary response to a TD antigen generally have a low average affinity. However, during the course of the response, the average affinity of the antibodies increases or 'matures.' As antigen becomes limiting, the clones with the higher affinity will have a selective advantage. This process is called affinity maturation.

The degree of affinity maturation is inversely related to the dose of antigen administered. High antigen doses produce poor maturation compared with low antigen doses (*Fig. 8.18*). It has been suggested that, in the presence of low antigen concentrations, only B cells with high-affinity receptors bind sufficient antigen and are triggered to divide and differentiate. However, in the presence of high antigen concentrations, there is sufficient antigen to bind and trigger both high- and low-affinity B cells.

Although individual B cells do not usually change their overall specificity, the affinity of the antibody produced by a clone may be altered. Affinity maturation is achieved through two processes:

- Somatic mutation of the variable (V), diversity (D) and joining (J) gene segments encoding the variable regions of antibodies (see Chapter 4).
- Antigen-driven selection and expansion of mutant clones expressing higher affinity antibodies.

The mechanism by which affinity maturation occurs is thought to involve B-cell progeny binding to antigen on FDCs in order to proliferate and differentiate further. It is thought that unprocessed antigen in immune complexes is captured by the FDCs via their Fc and complement receptors and held there. As B cells encounter the antigen, there is competition for space on the surface of the FDC, leading to selection. When a cell with higher affinity arises, it will stay there longer and presumably be given a stronger signal. B cells with higher affinity will thus have a selective advantage. An alternative theory is that B cells with higher affinity receptors will compete more effectively to bind and internalize antigen and therefore they have a greater potential of presenting antigen to T cells, and receiving T-cell help.

Somatic mutation and receptor editing lead to changes in the B-cell receptor

Somatic hypermutation is a common event in antibody-forming cells during T-dependent responses and is important in the generation of high-affinity antibodies. Somatic hypermutation introduces point mutations at a very high rate into the variable regions of the rearranged heavy and light chain genes (see *Fig. 4.35*). This results in mutated immunoglobulin molecules on the surface of the B cell. Mutants that bind antigen with higher affinity than the original surface immunoglobulin provide the raw material for the selection processes mentioned above.

In this context, somatic hypermutation is a normal and beneficial event. However, the same process could occasionally yield high-affinity IgG autoantibodies (e.g. anti-DNA), which would be highly deleterious. This type of mutation has been demonstrated experimentally in long-term tissue culture, but its role in the development of common autoimmune diseases is not known.

Receptor editing is another mechanism by which diversity can be introduced into B cells during affinity maturation. Secondary V(D)J recombination can occur in immature B cells whose antigen receptors bind self antigen. The resulting immunoglobulin rearrangement converts these cells into non self-reactive cells. In this way, specificity for foreign antigens can be improved and self reactivity avoided.

B cells switch to another immunoglobulin class by recombining heavy chain genes

B cells produce antibodies of five major classes: IgM, IgD, IgG, IgA and IgE. In man, there are also four subclasses of IgG and two of IgA (see Chapter 4). Each terminally differentiated plasma cell is derived from a specific B cell and produces antibodies of just one class or subclass.

All classes of immunoglobulin use the same set of variable region genes. The first B cells to appear during development carry surface IgM as their antigen receptor (see above). Upon activation, other classes of immunoglobulin are seen, each associated with different effector functions. When a mature antibody-forming cell switches antibody class, all that changes is the constant region of the heavy chain. The expressed V(D)J region and light chain do not change. Thus, antigen specificity is retained. This has been shown by the analysis of double myelomas, in which two monoclonal antibodies are present in the serum at the same time. IgM and IgG antibodies from a patient with multiple myeloma have been found to have identical light chains and VH regions; only the constant regions are switched, from μ to γ. Similarly, IgM and IgD

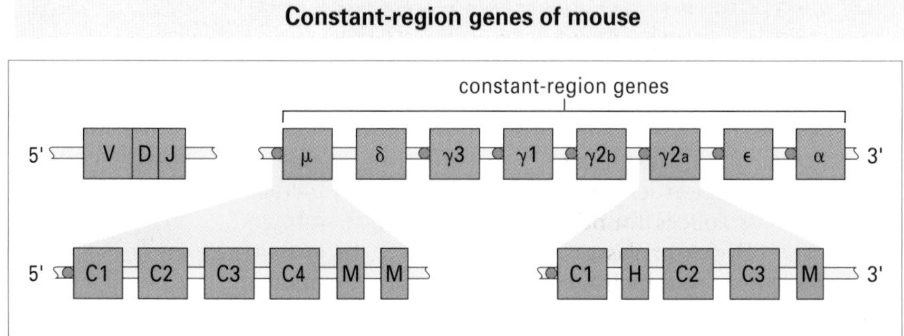

Fig. 8.19 The constant-region genes of the mouse are arranged 8.5 kb downstream from the recombined VDJ segment. Each C gene (except Cδ) has one or more switching sequences at its start (red circles), which correspond to a sequence at the 5′ end of the μ gene. This allows any of the C genes to be expressed together with the VDJ segment. δ genes appear to use the same switching sequences as μ, but the μ gene transcript is lost in RNA processing to produce IgD. The C genes (expanded below for μ and γ2a) contain introns separating the exons for each domain (C1, C2, etc.). The γ genes also have a separate exon coding for the hinge (H), and all the genes have one or more exons coding for membrane-bound immunoglobulin (M).

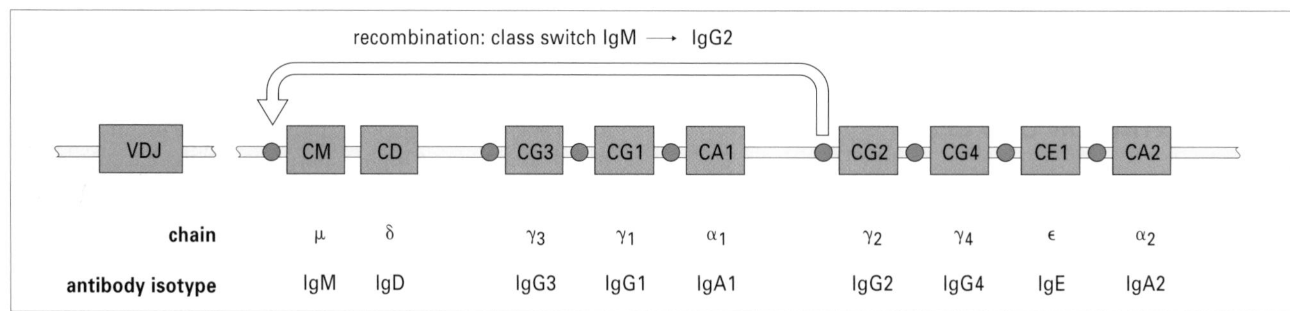

Fig. 8.20 The human immunoglobulin heavy chain gene locus (IGH) is shown. Initially, B cells transcribe a VDJ gene and a μ heavy chain that is spliced to produce mRNA for IgM. Under the influence of T cells and cytokines, class switching may occur, illustrated here as a switch from IgM to IgG2. Each heavy chain gene except CD (which encodes IgD) is preceded by a switch region. When class switching occurs, recombination between these regions takes place, with the loss of the intervening C genes – in this case CM, CD, CG3, CG1 and CA1. (Note that pseudogenes have been omitted from this diagram.)

are often found on the surface of a lymphocyte at the same time. Again, although the classes are different, the antigen-binding specificities are identical.

The constant region genes encoding the different heavy chains (CH) are responsible for the generation of antibody classes and subclasses. These genes are clustered at the 3′ end of the immunoglobulin heavy chain (IGH) locus, downstream of the J-segment genes. In man, they appear in a determined sequence along chromosome 14. In the mouse there is one gene for each of the IgM, IgE and IgA (μ, ε, α) isotypes and one γ gene for each of the four different IgG isotypes (γ1, γ2,a γ2b, γ3) (*Fig. 8.19*). In the human, there is one gene for each of the IgM and IgE isotypes, one gene for each of the two IgA isotypes and one gene for each of the four different IgG isotypes (*Fig. 8.20*).

Upstream of the μ genes is a switch sequence (S) which is repeated upstream to each of the other constant-region genes except δ. These sequences are important in the recombination events which occur during class switching, as will be explained below.

Class switching occurs during maturation and proliferation

Most class switching occurs during proliferation. However, it can also take place before encounter with exogenous antigen during early clonal expansion and maturation of the B cells (*Fig. 8.21*). This is known because some of the progeny of immature B cells synthesize antibodies of other immunoglobulin classes, including IgG and IgA. Further B-cell differentiation results in synthesis of surface IgD, an antibody class that is found almost exclusively on B-cell membranes. Different classes of sIg on the same B cell have the same antigen specificity, that is to say, they express the same V-region genes, although later additional diversity within a single clone may be generated by somatic mutation after class switching. Evidence that some class switching occurs independently of antigen comes from experiments with vertebrates raised in gnotobiotic (virtually sterile) environments, where exposure to exogenous antigens is severely restricted.

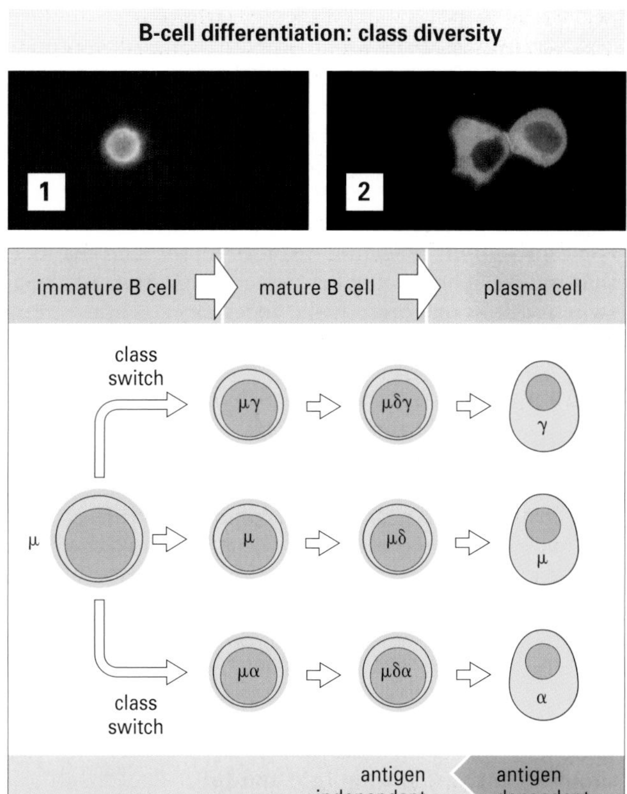

Fig. 8.21 Immature B cells produce IgM only, but mature B cells can express more than one cell surface antibody, because mRNA and cell surface immunoglobulin remain after a class switch. IgD is also expressed during clonal maturation. Maturation can occur in the absence of antigen, but the development into plasma cells (which have little surface immunoglobulin but much cytoplasmic immunoglobulin) requires antigen and (usually) T-cell help. The photographs show B cells stained for surface IgM (green, 1) and plasma cells stained for cytoplasmic IgM and IgG (green and red, 2). IgM is stained with fluorescent anti-μ chain and IgG with rhodaminated anti-γ chain.

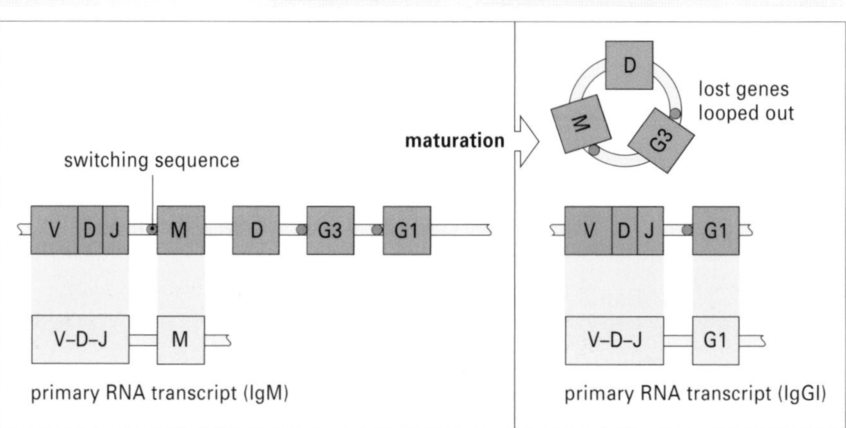

Fig 8.22 Initially the VDJ region is transcribed together with the M gene for the IgM heavy chain (left). After removal of introns during processing, mRNA for secreted IgM is produced. During B-cell maturation, class-switch recombination occurs between the Sμ recombination region and a downstream switch region (G1 in this example). The intervening region (containing genes for IgM, IgD and IgG3 in this instance) is looped out and then cut, with deletion of the intervening regions and joining of the two switch regions.

Class switching is achieved by gene recombination

B cells switch from IgM to the other classes or subclasses by an intrachromosomal deletion process in which the intervening genetic material between highly repetitive switch regions 5′ to each CH gene is excised as a circle (*Fig. 8.22*, see also *Fig. 8.20*). Switching involves cytokine-dependent transcription of DNA in the region of the new constant region, reflecting changes in the chromatin in that region. This occurs before recombination of the 5′ switch regions that precede the genes for each of the heavy chain isotype constant region domains.

Class switching may also be achieved by differential splicing of mRNA

Class switching is important in the maturation of the immune response and may be accompanied or preceded by somatic mutation. Initially, a complete section of DNA that includes the recombined VDJ region and the δ and μ constant regions is transcribed. Two mRNA molecules may then be produced by differential splicing, each with the same VDJ segment, but having either μ or δ constant regions. It is suggested that much larger stretches of DNA are sometimes also transcribed together, with differential splicing giving other immunoglobulin classes sharing VH regions (*Fig. 8.23*). This has been observed in cells simultaneously producing IgM and IgE.

Membrane and secreted immunoglobulins are produced by differential splicing of RNA transcripts of heavy chain genes

Membrane-bound immunoglobulin (B-cell antigen receptor) is identical to secreted immunoglobulin (antibody), except for an extra stretch of amino acids at the C terminus of each heavy chain. Membrane immunoglobulins are therefore slightly larger than their secreted counterparts. Their additional amino acids traverse the cell membrane and anchor the molecule in the lipid bilayer. In membrane IgM, for example, a section of hydrophobic (lipophilic) amino acids are sandwiched between hydrophilic amino acids, which lie on either side of the membrane (*Fig. 8.24*). The hydrophobic residues are thought to form a stretch of α helix within the membrane. Membrane immunoglobulins only exist as the basic four-chain unit, do not polymerize further and are associated with molecules involved in signal transduction (e.g. Igα and Igβ).

Production of the two forms of immunoglobulin occurs by differential transcription of the germ line C region (*Fig. 8.25*) It is thought that the poly-A sequence is important in determining which RNA transcript is produced, but exactly how this is controlled is uncertain.

Immunoglobulin class expression is influenced by cytokines and type of antigenic stimulus

During a T-dependent immune response, there is a progressive change in the predominant immunoglobulin class of the specific antibody produced, usually to IgG. This

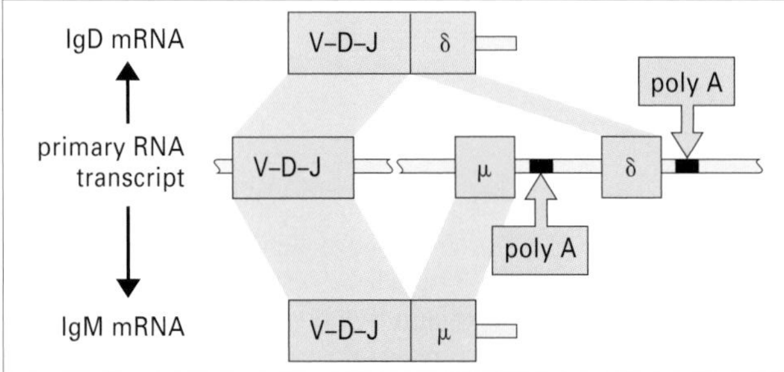

Fig. 8.23 Single B cells produce more than one antibody isotype from a single long primary RNA transcript. A transcript containing μ and δ is shown here. Polyadenylation can occur at different sites, leading to different forms of splicing, producing mRNA for IgD (top) or IgM (bottom). Even within this region, there are additional polyadenylation sites that determine whether the translated immunoglobulin is the secreted or membrane-bound form.

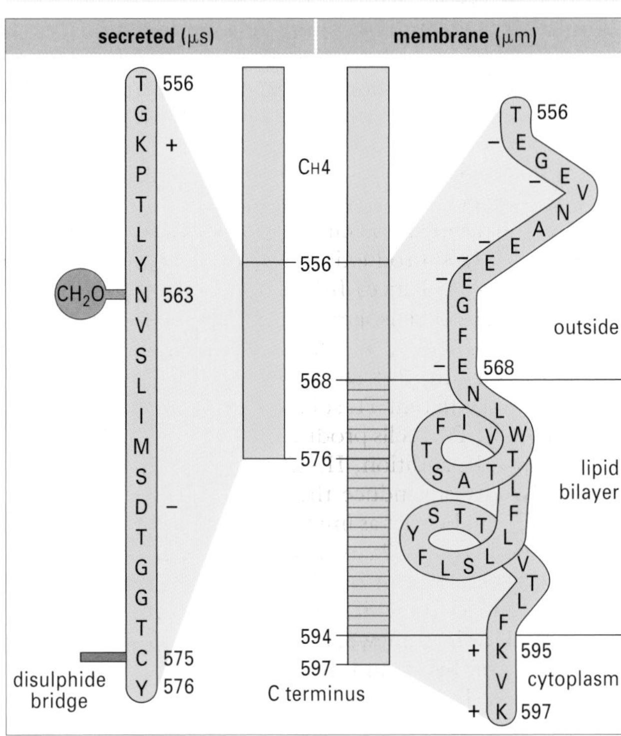

Fig. 8.24 C-terminal amino acid sequences for both secreted and membrane-bound IgM are identical up to residue 556. Secreted IgM has 20 further residues. Residue 563 (asparagine) has a carbohydrate unit attached to it, while residue 575 is a cysteine involved in the formation of interchain disulphide bonds. Membrane IgM has 41 residues beyond 556. A stretch of 26 residues between 568 and 595 contains hydrophobic amino acids sandwiched between sequences containing charged residues. This hydrophobic portion may traverse the cell membrane as two turns of α helix. A short, positively charged section lies inside the cytoplasm. Mouse IgM is shown in this example.

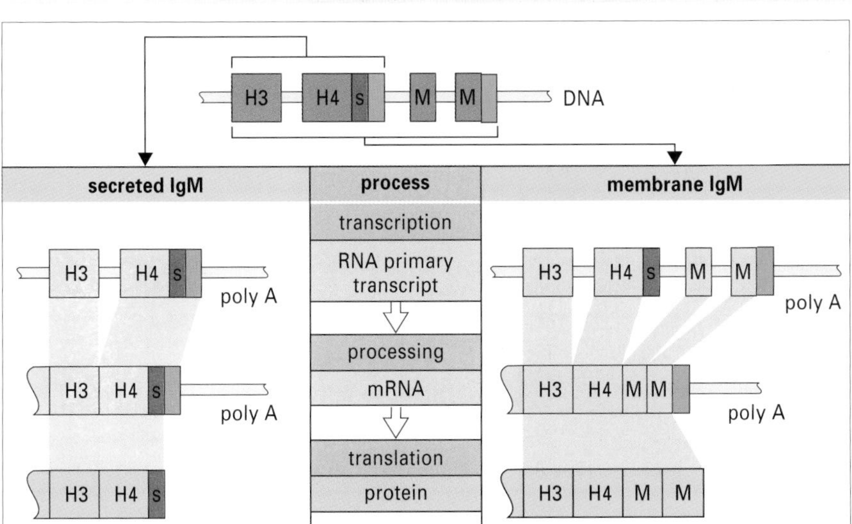

Fig. 8.25 Part of the DNA coding for IgM is shown diagrammatically. The exons for the μ3 and μ4 domains (H3 and H4) and the transmembrane and cytoplasmic segment of membrane IgM (M) are indicated. The 3′ untranslated sequence is present at the end of the H4 and second membrane segments (S = stop codons). The DNA can be transcribed in two ways. If transcription stops after S, the transcript with a poly-A tail is processed to produce mRNA for secreted IgM. If transcription runs through to include the membrane segments, processing removes the codons for the terminal amino acids and the stop signal of H4, so that translation yields a protein with a different C terminus.

class switch is not seen in T-independent responses, in which the predominant immunoglobulin usually remains IgM. There is now considerable evidence for the involvement of T cells and their cytokines in the *de novo* isotype switching. In mice, T cells in mucosal sites have been shown to stimulate IgA production. IL-4 preferentially switches B cells that have been either polyclonally activated (by LPS) or specifically activated by antigen, to the IgG1 or IgE isotype, with concomitant suppression of other isotypes. In a similar system, IL-5 induces a 5- to 10-fold increase in IgA production with no change in other isotypes. IFNγ enhances IgG2a and IgG3 responses, but suppresses all other isotypes (*Fig. 8.26*). It is interesting that IL-4 and IFNγ, which act as reciprocal regulatory cytokines for the expression of antibody isotypes, are derived from different TH subsets. TH1 cells produce IFNγ in the mouse; TH2 cells produce IL-4, IL-5 and IL-10 (see Chapter 7). In addition, IL-12 and IL-18 stimulation of mouse B cells can induce the production of IFNγ. Thus these cells can then act as immunoregulatory cells by differentially inducing IgG2a expression, while inhibiting IgG1, IgE and IgG2b expression. Transforming growth factor-β (TGFβ) induces the switch to IgA or IgG2b. In humans, the situation is somewhat different. IL-4 induces the expression of IgG4 and IgE, while TGFβ induces the expression of IgA alone.

Isotype regulation by mouse T-cell cytokines

TH	cytokines	immunoglobulin isotypes					
		IgG1	IgE	IgA	IgG3	IgG2b	IgG2a
TH2	IL-4	↑	↑	↓	↓	↓	↓
	IL-5	=	=	↑	=	=	=
TH1	IFNγ	↓	↓	↓	↓	↓	↑

Fig. 8.26 The effects of IFNγ (product of TH1 cells) and IL-4 and IL-5 (products of TH2 cells) which result in an increase (↑), a decrease (↓) or no change (=) in the frequency of isotype-specific B cells after stimulation with the polyclonal activator LPS, *in vitro*.

CRITICAL THINKING • Development of the antibody response (Explanations on pp 454–455)

A project is underway to develop a vaccine against mouse hepatitis virus, a pathogen of mice, which may become a serious problem in colonies of mice. The vaccine consists of capsid protein of the virus, which is injected subcutaneously as a depot in alum on day 0. At days 5 and 14, the group of six mice is bled and the serum is tested for the presence of antibodies against the viral capsid protein. Separate assays are done for each of the immunoglobulin classes, IgM, IgG and IgA. The amounts, expressed in μg/ml of antibody, are shown in *Figure 8.27* opposite.

When the data is analyzed it appears that two of the animals (diamonds) have high titres of antibody particularly of IgG and IgA, at both days 5 and 14.

8.1 Why do the titres of IgG antibodies increase more rapidly between days 5 and 14 than do IgM antibodies, in all animals?

8.2 Propose an explanation for the high titres of IgG antibodies in the two animals indicated at day 5. Can this explanation also account for the relatively high levels of IgA antibodies also seen in these mice?

The spleens from mice taken at day 14 are used to produce B cells making monoclonal antibodies against the viral protein (see Chapter 26 for the methodology). Of the clones produced, 15 produce IgG, three produce IgM and none produce IgA.

8.3 Why do you suppose there are no IgA-producing clones, despite the good IgA response?

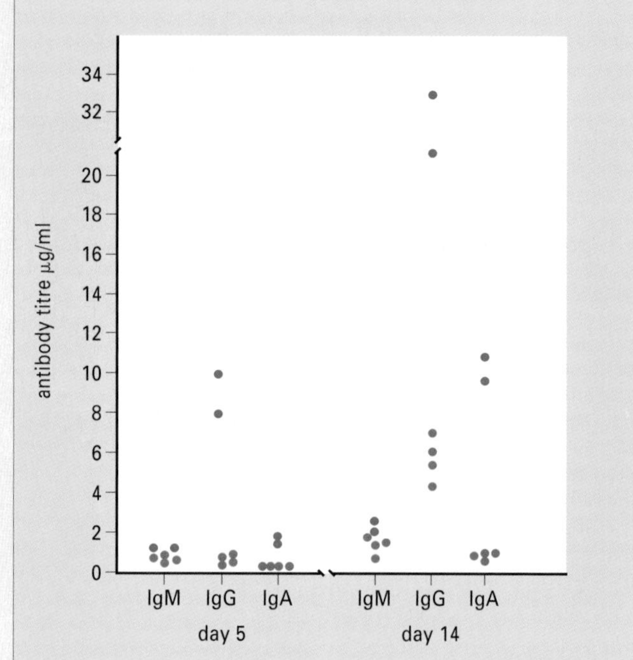

Fig. 8.27

8.4 You want a high-affinity antibody for use in an assay. Which of the clones you have produced are likely to be of higher affinity?

FURTHER READING

Henderson A, Calamé K. Transcriptional regulation during B cell development. *Annu Rev Immunol* 1998;**16**:163–200.

Lane P. Development of B cell memory and effector function. *Curr Opin Immunol* 1996;**8**:331–36.

Lipsky PE, Attrep JF, Grammer AC, McIlraith MJ, Nishioka Y. Analysis of CD40–CD40 ligand interactions in the regulation of human B cell function. *Ann N Y Acad Sci* 1997;**815**:372–83.

Liu Y-J, de Bouteiller O, Fugier-Vivier I. Mechanisms of selection and differentiation in germinal centers. *Curr Opin Immunol* 1997;**9**:256–62.

McHeyzer-Williams MG, Ahmed R. B cell memory and the long-lived plasma cell. *Curr Opin Immunol* 1999;**11**:172–9.

Osmond DG, Rolink A, Melchers F. Murine B lymphopoiesis: towards a unified model. *Immunol Today* 1998;**19**:65–8.

Przylepa J, Himes C, Kelsoe G. Lymphocyte development and selection in germinal centers. *Curr Top Microbiol Immunol* 1998;**229**:85–104.

Smith KG, Fearon DT. Receptor modulators of B-cell receptor signalling – CD19/CD22. *Curr Top Microbiol Immunol* 2000;**245**:195–212.

Snapper CM, Mond JJ. A model for induction of T cell-independent humoral immunity in response to polysaccharide antigens. *J Immunol* 1996;**157**:2229–33.

Stavnezer J. Antibody class switching. *Adv Immunol* 1996;**61**:79–146.

Tarlington D. Germinal centers: form and function. *Curr Opin Immunol* 1998;**10**:245–51.

9 Mononuclear phagocytes in immune defence

- **Macrophages, myeloid dendritic cells and osteoclasts** all differentiate from circulating blood monocytes.
- **Resident macrophages are widely distributed throughout the body.** Phenotypically distinct populations are present in each organ and within the different zones of spleen and lymph nodes.
- **Resident and recruited macrophages respond according to locally produced cytokines.** Cytokines from TH1 cells such as interferon-γ (IFNγ) enhance inflammation and anti-microbial activity. TH2 cytokines induce an alternative activation with efficient antigen presentation to B cells. Transforming growth factor-β (TGFβ), corticosteroids and interleukin-10 (IL-10) can induce an anti-inflammatory phenotype.
- **Resident macrophages clear apoptotic cells using scavenger receptors and the vitronectin receptor.** Endocytosis by this pathway does not activate the macrophage killing mechanisms.
- **Macrophages internalize pathogens using a variety of specific and opsonic receptors.** These include the lipopolysaccharide (LPS) receptor and Toll-like receptors, the mannose receptor, the Fc receptors and complement receptors CR1, CR3 and CR4.
- **Activated macrophages secrete cytokines, enzymes, complement system molecules and procoagulants.**
- **Activated macrophages produce reactive oxygen and nitrogen intermediates which are highly toxic for endocytosed bacteria and fungi.** Recently recruited cells are most effective at anti-microbial killing, whereas resting macrophages have only a limited killing activity.

Mononuclear phagocytes comprise a family of cells that share common haematopoietic precursors and are distributed via the blood stream as monocytes to all tissues of the body, including secondary lymphoid organs, even in the absence of an overt inflammatory stimulus. Within tissues they undergo maturation, adapt to their local microenvironment and differentiate into various cell types (macrophages, myeloid-derived dendritic cells, osteoclasts) which perform specific housekeeping, trophic and immunological functions (*Fig. 9.1*). The macrophages for the most part become and remain highly efficient phagocytes and play an important role in pathogen recognition and clearance, as well as removal of senescent and dying cells (*Fig. 9.2*). In response to particulate and other potential antigenic stimuli, the dendritic cells are uniquely efficient inducers of primary immune responses by naïve T lymphocytes, whereas macrophages produce a range of secretory products which affect the migration and activation of other immune cells. Macrophages are actively endocytic and degrade antigens, but can present peptides to already primed T lymphocytes in secondary responses, after MHC and other accessory molecules have been induced by cytokines such as IFNγ derived from TH1 cells and NK cells. Once recruited and activated by such interactions, the macrophage plays a major role in the effector limb of cell-mediated immunity to intracellular pathogens such as mycobacteria, often within focal accumulations of cells known as granulomas.

Macrophages are extremely heterogeneous in their gene expression and cellular activities, with beneficial as well as destructive roles in tissue homeostasis and host defence. Through their varied plasma membrane receptor repertoire and secretory responses they interact with other leucocytes as well as non-haematopoietic cells in all tissues, thus regulating both innate and acquired immunity. Whilst the concept of the mononuclear phagocyte system is central to

Differentiation of monocytes

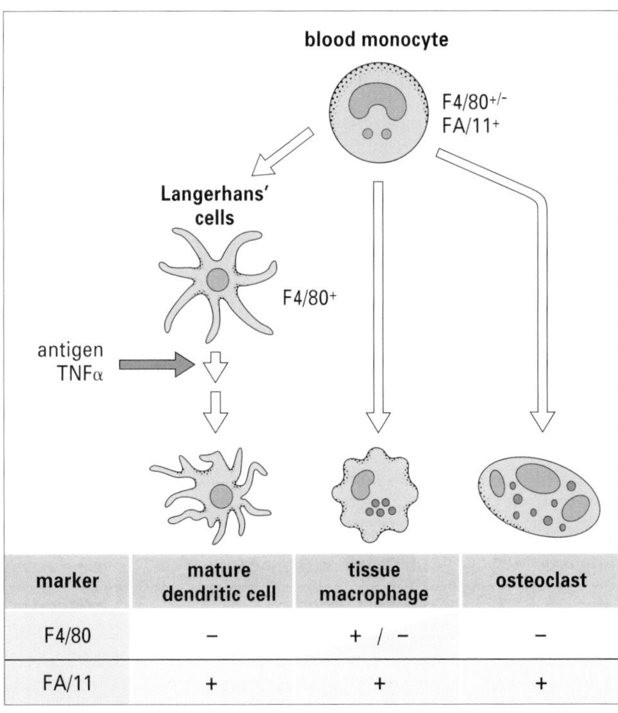

marker	mature dendritic cell	tissue macrophage	osteoclast
F4/80	–	+ / –	–
FA/11	+	+	+

Fig. 9.1 Circulating monocytes give rise to myeloid dendritic cells (distinct from lymphoid dendritic cells), tissue macrophages and osteoclasts. F4/80 and FA/11 (macrosialin, the murine homologue of CD68) are differentiation antigens of mouse macrophages and closely related cells.

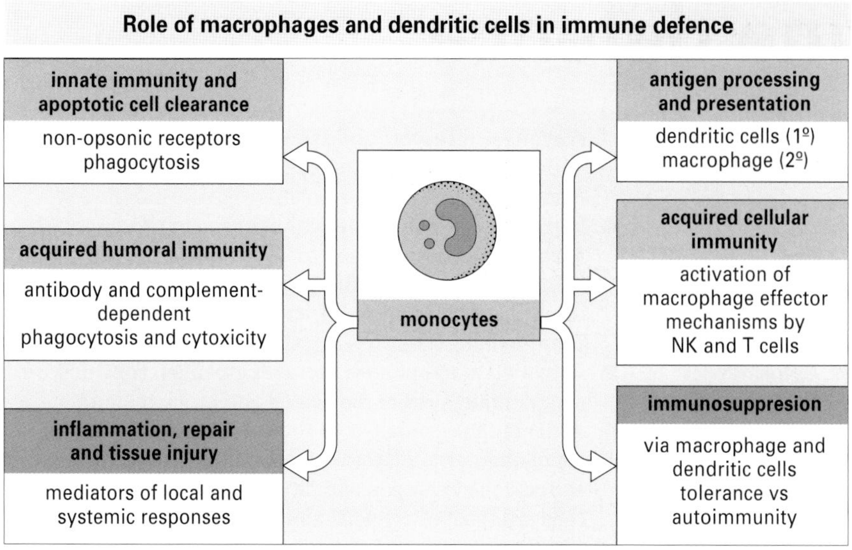

Fig. 9.2 Both macrophages and dendritic cells play important roles in innate immune responses, inflammation and tissue remodelling as well as specific immune responses.

our understanding of immunity, this is but one role in a wider context of physiological and pathological contributions to tissue maintenance, response to injury and repair.

RESIDENT AND MOBILE POPULATIONS OF MACROPHAGES

Resident macrophages are widely distributed throughout the body

Some of the key features of resident macrophage populations in tissues are shown in *Figure 9.3*. The cells vary in their lifespan, morphology and phenotype. They have usually ceased to proliferate, but retain the ability to express a range of mRNA and protein species, often as relatively long-lived cells, with low turnover, unlike neutrophils. Plasma membrane differentiation markers such as the F4/80 antigen have proved useful in defining the distribution of mature macrophages in many (but not all) murine tissues (*Fig. 9.4*); in man, the CD68 antigen, an intracellular vacuolar marker, is widely expressed; the murine homologue (macrosialin) is a pan-macrophage marker, also present in many myeloid dendritic cells and osteoclasts, unlike F4/80. It is possible to reconstruct a

Resident tissue macrophage populations

organ	name/site	functions/properties
bone marrow	stromal macrophage	interacts with haematopoietic cells removes erythroid nuclei
liver	Kupffer cells	clearance of cells and complexes from blood
spleen	red pulp macrophages white pulp tingible body macrophages marginal zone macrophages	clearance of senescent blood cells phagocytosis of apoptotic B cells interface between circulation and immune system
lymph node	subcapsular sinus macrophages medullary macrophages	interface with afferent lymph interface with efferent lymph
thymus	thymic macrophage	clearance of apoptotic cells
gut	lamina propria	endocytosis
lung	alveolar macrophage	clearance of particulates
brain	microglia in neutrophil choroid plexus	interacts with neurons interface with cerebrospinal fluid
skin	Langerhans' cells	antigen capture
reproductive tract	ovary, testis	clearance of dying cells
endocrine organs	adrenal, thyroid, pancreas, etc.	metabolic homeostasis
bone	osteoclasts	bone remodelling

Fig. 9.3

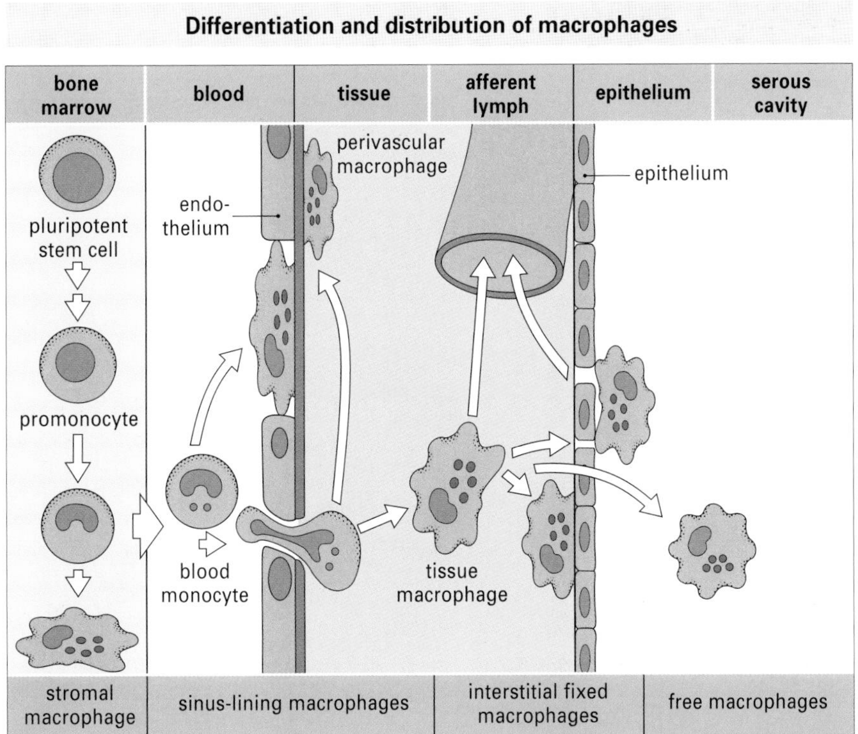

Fig. 9.4 Blood monocytes are derived from bone marrow in the adult host and enter tissues initially as sinus-lining or extravascular mature cells. Interstitial or intraepithelial adherent macrophages and serosal macrophages can enter afferent lymphatics. Stromal macrophages in bone marrow may also derive from the circulating monocyte population.

constitutive migration pathway in which monocytes become endothelial like and line vascular sinusoids, as in the liver (Kupffer cells), or penetrate between endothelial cells. They underlie endothelia or epithelia, which can also be penetrated for example by Langerhans' cells (F4/80$^+$ precursors of dendritic cells), or enter the interstitial space, or serosal cavities. Whilst macrophages are often regarded as sessile cells, compared with freely migratory dendritic cells, they readily migrate to draining lymph nodes after an inflammatory stimulus and become arrested there. They are therefore absent from efferent lymph and do not, as a rule, re-enter the circulation.

Mature macrophages are themselves part of the stromal microenvironment in bone marrow. They associate with developing haematopoietic cells to perform poorly defined non-phagocytic trophic functions, as well as removing effete cells and erythroid nuclei.

Secondary lymphoid organs contain several distinct types of macrophage and related cells, which are still poorly understood. *Figure 9.5* illustrates the complexity of macrophage-like cells in rodent spleen (red and white pulp, marginal zone) and normal lymph nodes (subcapsular sinus, medulla). Differentiation antigens such as sialoadhesin, a lectin-like receptor for sialylated glycoconjugates, are particularly strongly present on marginal metallophils (inner marginal zone) and on subcapsular sinus macrophages. These cells are present at the interface between blood (spleen), afferent lymph (lymph nodes) and organized lymphoid structures. They play a role in capture of organisms, particulates, polysaccharides and soluble antigens, as well as of circulating host cells or migrating dendritic cells, which have their own characteristic distribution in T- and B-cell-dependent areas. The relationship between migrating and resident antigen capture cells is ill defined, but may include a newly described antigen transport system defined by the mannose receptor (see below).

The molecular mechanisms of constitutive macrophage distribution and induced migration are beginning to be defined, involving cellular adhesion molecules, cytokines and growth factors, as well as chemokines and chemokine receptors, as summarized in *Figure 9.6*. Macrophage colony stimulating factor (M-CSF or CSF-1) is a major growth, differentiation and survival factor selective for macrophages, whereas granulocyte macrophage colony stimulating factor (GM–CSF) regulates myeloid cell production and function. Chemokines are produced by a range of haematopoietic and tissue cells, including macrophages themselves, and act on various leucocyte subpopulations depending principally on their chemokine receptor profile.

Resident and recruited macrophages respond to injury and immune stimuli

Inflammatory stimuli, for example local infection, enhance the recruitment of monocytes (and often other myeloid cells) from blood, and ultimately from bone marrow stores. Monocytes adhere to activated endothelium through a

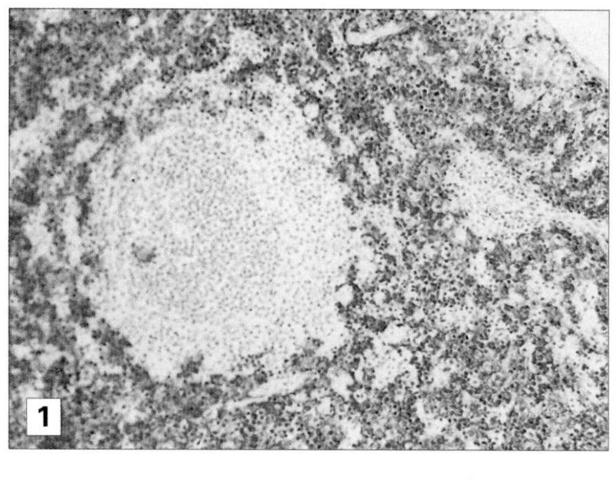

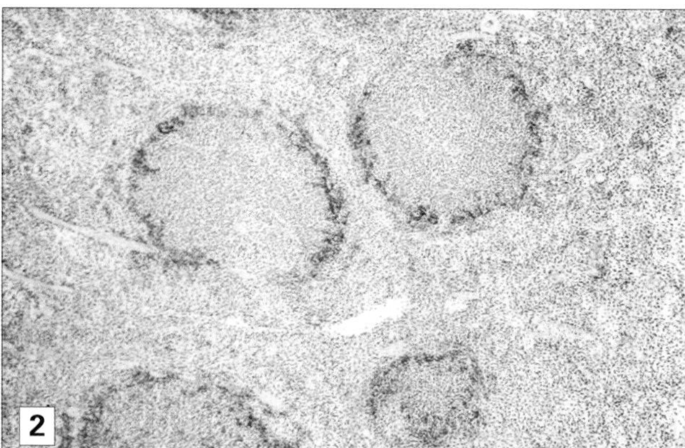

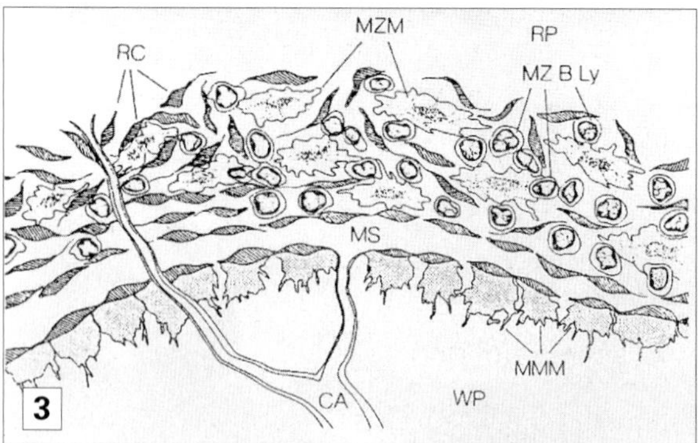

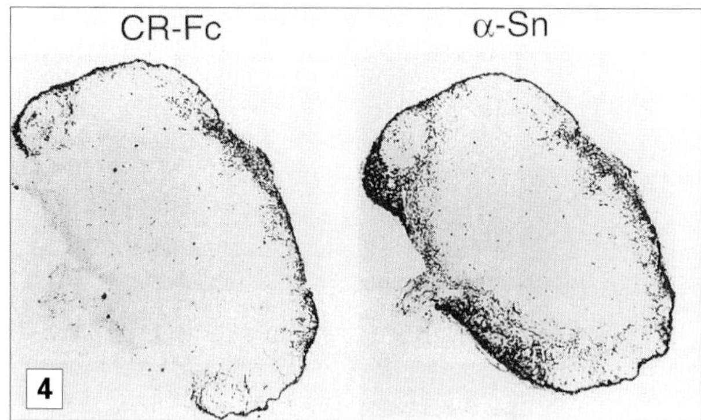

Fig. 9.5 Macrophages in secondary lymphoid tissues. Heterogeneity of macrophages in secondary lymphoid organs of mouse: (**1**) Red pulp of spleen stained with the 4/80 antibody. Macrophages stain strongly positive. (Courtesy of Dr D.A. Hume.) (**2**) Mouse spleen stained with antibody to sialoadhesin. The marginal metallophils of spleen are strongly sialoadhesin positive. (Courtesy of Dr P.R. Crocker.) (**3**) The marginal zone contains inner metallophilic and outer zones. In the diagram of the marginal zone of the spleen, the central arteriole (CA) branches into small capillaries that either pass through the marginal zone and end in the red pulp (RP) or open into the marginal sinus (MS). The marginal zone is composed of reticular cells (RC). Within this reticular framework, the large marginal zone macrophages (MZM) and marginal zone B cells (MZB) are localized. At the inner border of the marginal sinus and the white pulp (WP), the marginal metallophilic macrophages (MMM) are situated. (Courtesy of G. Kraal.) (**4**) Lymph node contains subcapsular sinus macrophages, which are sialoadhesin positive and strongly express sulphated glycoconjugates which bind CR-Fc, a chimeric probe of the mannose receptor cysteine-rich domain and human Fc (left); only medullary macrophages also express sialoadhesin (right). (Courtesy of Dr L. Martinez-Pomares.)

series of well-described interactions involving β_2 integrins and CD31, as well as chemokines acting on their receptors (see Chapter 3). Diapedesis results in local tissue interactions and accumulation of macrophages with enhanced turnover and an altered phenotype, for example the up-regulation of endocytic receptors and production of pro-inflammatory mediators. Phagocytosis by recently recruited monocytes profoundly alters their differentiation into migratory dendritic cells or more sessile macrophages. Recent studies have confirmed the potential of monocytes to differentiate into either of these cell types *in vivo*, as they do in cell culture.

It is convenient to distinguish the macrophages 'elicited' by a non-specific inflammatory stimulus from 'immunologically activated' macrophages. The latter cells respond to IFNγ by acquiring enhanced anti-microbial properties and express enhanced MHC class II antigens, whereas other genes, for example the mannose receptor, are down-regulated. Cytokines produced by natural killer (NK) cells, lymphocytes and various antigen-presenting cells influence the pattern of gene expression by macrophages. Work *in vitro*, and some studies *in vivo*, especially with cytokine/receptor knockout mouse strains, have made it possible to classify macrophages differing in their functional state (*Fig. 9.7*). The initial and further interactions with endocytic and phagocytic stimuli give rise to further heterogeneity in phenotype. It should be emphasized that whilst the evidence for individual molecules as mediators of activation is good, we have little insight into the complex interactions which pertain *in vivo*. *Figure 9.8* illustrates a mycobacteria-induced granuloma, rich in macrophages. Cytokines, for example tumour necrosis factor-α (TNFα) and receptors such as the type 3 complement receptor (CR3), play an important role in granuloma formation. Immunologically activated macrophages express the capacity to produce anti-microbial products including lysozyme and reactive oxygen and nitrogen species. However, characteristic morphological features such as epithelioid cell and giant cell formation, hallmarks of mycobacterial granulomas, remain mysterious in origin.

Environmental influences on macrophages

stimulus	example/receptors	response
growth factors	M–CSF, GM–CSF	growth, differentiation, survival
cytokines	IFNγ TNFα IL-4, IL-13 IL-10	activation activation alternate activation deactivation
chemokines	macrophage chemotactic protein-1 (MCP-1)	migration
extracellular matrix	fibronectin (β_1 integrin)	adhesion, phagocytosis
peptides	vasoactive peptide (VIP)	modulation of various functions
eicosanoids	prostaglandin E_2 (PGE_2), leukotriene B_4 (LTB_4)	modulation of various functions
cellular interactions endothelium T lymphocytes	 CR3 (β2 integrin) accessory molecules (CD80, CD86)	 recruitment antigen presentation
microbial interactions	LPS (CD14)	secretion, activation
proteases	neutral proteinases, e.g. plasmin	adhesion, secretion

Fig. 9.6 The table lists some of the mediators which act on macrophages.

Activation of macrophages

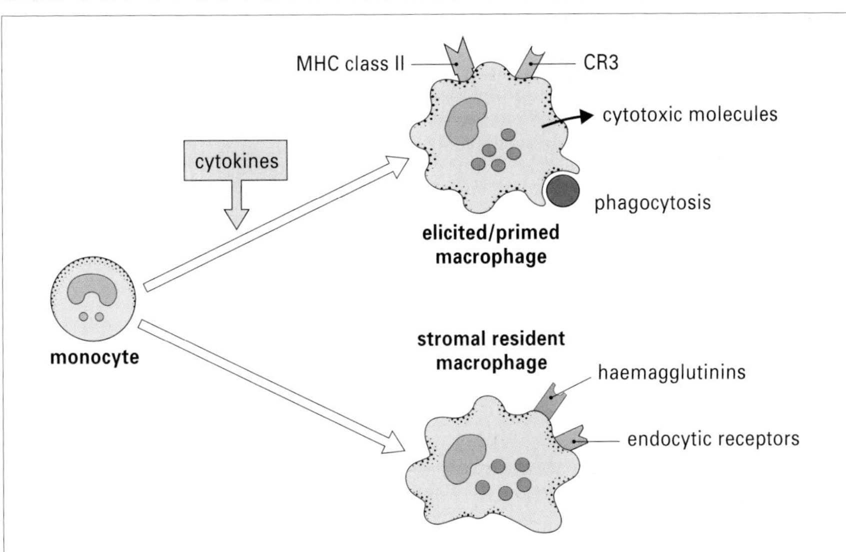

Fig. 9.7 Elicited and immunologically primed macrophages differ from resident macrophages. Monocyte recruitment is enhanced and yields macrophages with pro-inflammatory and cytotoxic properties. Activation by cytokines enhances expression of MHC class II and the complement receptor CR3. Phagocytosis and the production of pro-inflammatory mediators and cytotoxic products are increased. By contrast, resident macrophages (e.g. in bone marrow) lack inflammatory functions but participate in trophic reactions, for example, with developing haemopoietic cells, as well as performing endocytosis.

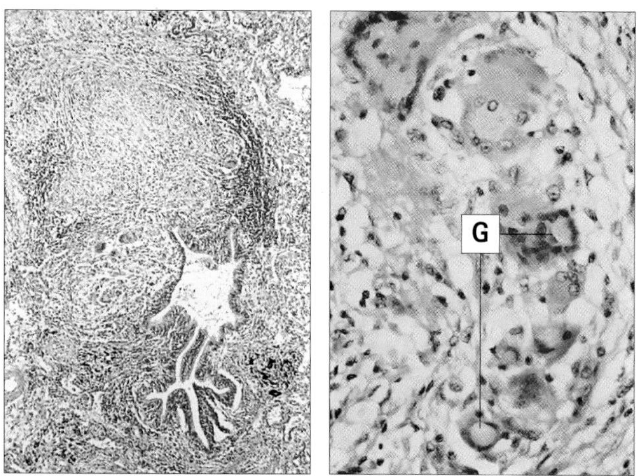

Fig. 9.8 A granulomatous reaction in pulmonary tuberculosis. The central area of caseous necrosis, in which much of the cellular structure is destroyed, is characteristic of tuberculosis in the lung. Apart from this necrosis, the histology is typical of chronic T-cell-dependent 'tuberculoid' granulomas. The lesion is surrounded by a ring of epithelioid cells and mononuclear cells. Multinucleate giant cells, believed to be derived from the fusion of epithelioid cells, are also present (left ×170). Giant cells (G) are illustrated at a higher magnification (right). Haematoxylin and eosin stain. (Courtesy of Dr G. Boyd.)

Cytokines modulate the phenotype of macrophages

A further level of heterogeneity derives from the distinct effects of TH1- and TH2-type cytokines on monocyte/macrophage differentiation (*Fig. 9.9*). *In vitro* studies with macrophages treated with different cytokines have indicated that there is a spectrum of gene expression induced by different cytokines (*Fig. 9.10*). Whilst IFNγ characteristically enhances pro-inflammatory and anti-microbial activities ('immune activation') and IL-10 efficiently counteracts these properties ('deactivation'), IL-4 and IL-13 exert distinctive effects on MHC class II and mannose receptor expression, which we have termed 'alternate activation', rather than focusing on the modest inhibition of pro-inflammatory products. Broadly speaking, while 'activated' macrophages mediate cellular immunity, 'alternatively activated' macrophages may promote humoral immunity, including repair processes.

It is well established that macrophages and myeloid dendritic cells produce IL-12 and IL-18, which enhance the production of IFNγ by NK cells and T cells. There is, as yet, no comparable IL-4/13 inducing activity which can be ascribed to the antigen presenting cells, although subsets of dendritic cells have been implicated in TH2 differentiation, which has also been postulated to constitute a 'default' pathway. The links between innate and acquired immune responses are therefore only understood in part; nor is the role of plasma membrane receptors and

Modulation of macrophage activation

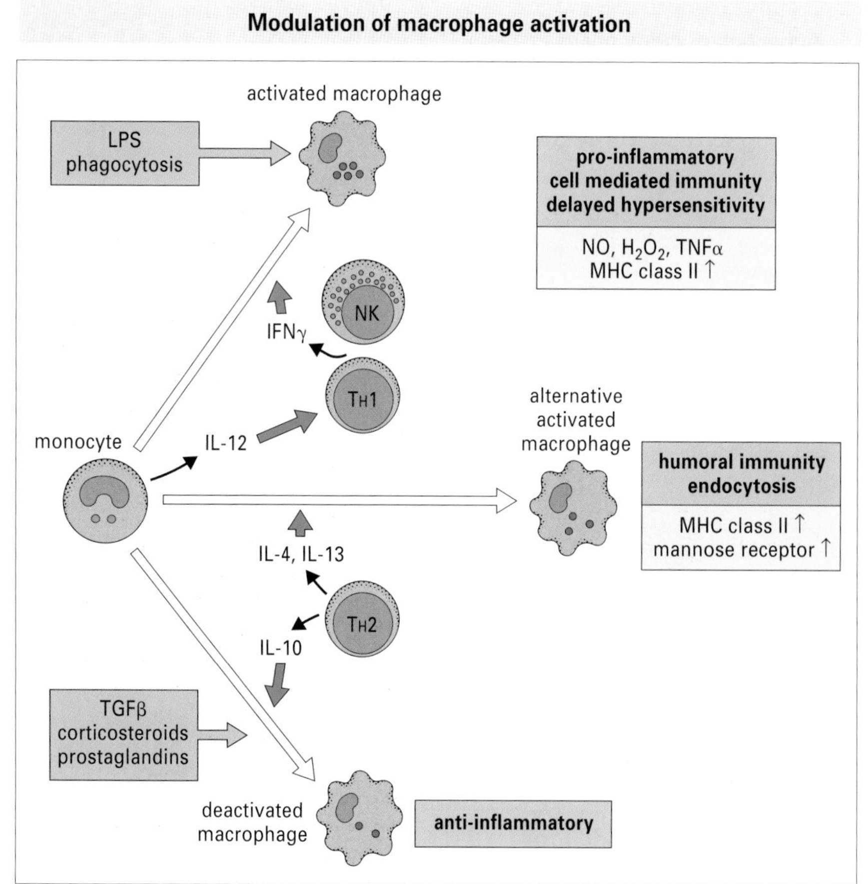

Fig. 9.9 Signals from microbial products, phagocytosis and cytokines result in changes to the surface and secretory properties of macrophages, which can be classified as activated, deactivated or alternatively activated.

Regulation of macrophage phenotype

TH1 type		TH2 types		
	IFNγ	IL-4/13	IL-10	significance
MHC class II (IA)	++	+	–	immune cell interactions
respiratory burst	++	(–)	–	cell-mediated immunity
NO	++	(–)	–	tissue injury, e.g. tuberculosis
TNFα IL-1 IL-6	++	(–)	–	pro-inflammatory
mannosyl receptor	–	++	0	phagocytosis/ endocytosis, e.g. antigens
growth	–	+	0	local growth of MØ in immune lesions
fusion	0	++	0	giant cell formation – granulomata, e.g. tuberculosis
growth factor secretion	–	++	+	healing of lesions

Fig. 9.10 TH1 and TH2 cytokines act on macrophages to induce distinctive functions which can be described as 'activation' (TH1 type) or 'alternate activation' (TH2 type). + = increase, – = decrease, 0 = no effect.

signals in the differential activation of T-lymphocyte subsets evident.

RECEPTORS ON MACROPHAGES

Macrophages are involved in the clearance of apoptotic cells as well as inflammation

Macrophages express a very wide range of plasma membrane receptors, which underlie their interactions with other cells, extracellular ligands derived from plasma, extracellular matrix and microorganisms. It is useful to distinguish opsonic receptors (e.g. for antibody and complement) from 'non-opsonic' receptors. The processes of phagocytosis mediated by opsonic receptors are shown in *Figure 9.11.*

Whereas neutrophils express similar opsonic receptors, they lack most of the opsonin-independent receptors for phagocytosis. Unlike the clonally expressed receptors of T and B lymphocytes which undergo somatic rearrangement, the receptors of macrophages (and, where known, myeloid dendritic cells) are germ-line encoded and recognize classes of common host or microbial structures, such as antibody, complement, glycoconjugates and lipids. The term 'pattern recognition' has entered wide use, and emphasizes the exogenous 'non-self' ligands found on a range of microorganisms. However, pattern recognition clearly extends to endogenous, host-derived molecules (self, which may be modified), although there may be intriguing differences in the outcome of these receptor–ligand

Phagocytosis mediated by opsonic receptors

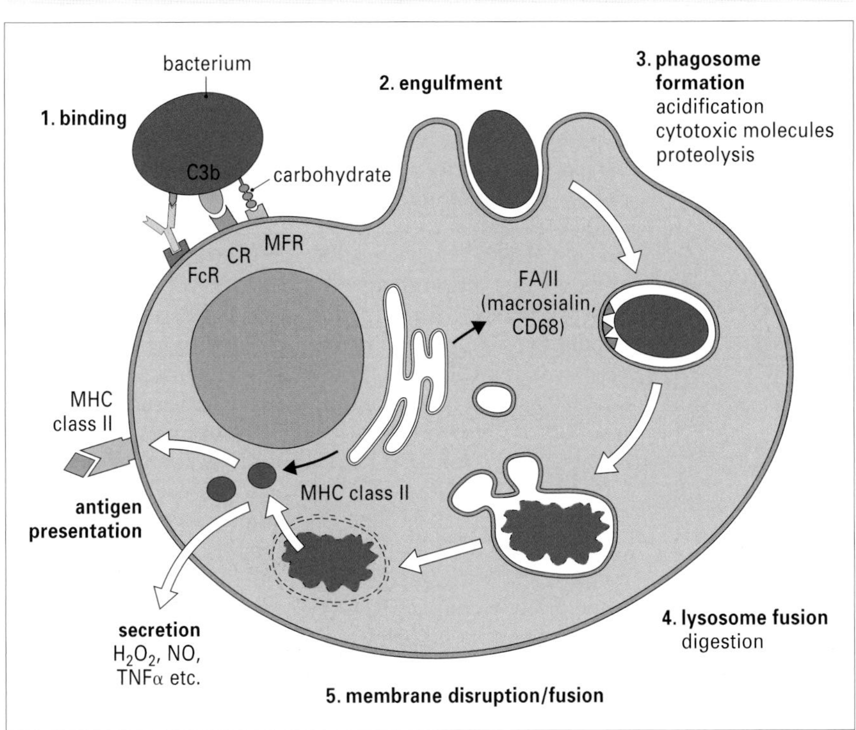

Fig. 9.11 (**1**) Pathogens such as bacteria are taken up by binding to opsonic receptors including the Fc receptor, complement receptors and receptors for carbohydrate (MR). (**2**) The particle is engulfed and the phagosome forms (**3**). Acidification of the phagosome follows as toxic molecules (reactive oxygen and nitrogen intermediates) are pumped into the phagosome. The marker FA/11 is located in the phagosome membrane. (**4**) Lysosomes fuse with the phagosome releasing proteolytic enzymes into the phagolysosome which digest the bacteria. (**5**) On occasion the membrane of the phagolysosome is disrupted. Antigenic fragments may – then bind MHC class T molecules or become diverted to the acidic endosome compartment for interaction with MHC class II molecules and antigen presentation. The process induces secretion of toxic molecules and cytokines.

interactions regarding cytokine responses and the inflammatory consequences. In particular, macrophage receptors play a dual role in clearance of both macromolecules and apoptotic cells, which differs from their role in uptake of microbial invaders, or foreign antigens. In the first case there is no or even a suppressed inflammatory response, whereas in the second, the immune system may need to be alerted. The roles of cell type, receptor profile, signal pathway and mediator release in these dual responses are all under investigation.

Receptors involved in the clearance of apoptotic cells

In order to maintain appropriate numbers of all cell types in development and normal tissue homeostasis, as well as during immune, inflammatory and other pathological responses, cells die naturally by programmed death (apoptosis), or by necrosis, the latter releasing potentially injurious products. Cellular and biochemical pathways resulting in apoptosis are conserved in evolution; apoptotic cells are rapidly and efficiently cleared by macrophages, for example in thymus (*Fig. 9.12*), although they can also be engulfed by non-professional phagocytes. The receptors implicated in apoptotic cell recognition show considerable redundancy, and include a range of so-called 'scavenger receptors' (e.g. SR-A-I) (*Fig. 9.13*), vitronectin receptor, an ATP-transporter and CD14, to be discussed further below. Thrombospondin and C1q can act as opsonins. The ligands expressed by apoptotic cells are not well defined; but recently a conserved, widely distributed receptor has been identified for phosphatidyl serine, displayed on the outer leaflet of apoptotic cells. Ligation of the vitronectin receptor results in the production of anti-inflammatory products (e.g. prostaglandin (PGE_2) and TGFβ) which can overcome proinflammatory responses induced by potent stimuli such as lipopolysaccharide (LPS). Indeed, intracellular pathogens can induce and exploit this downregulation, presumably a host-protective reaction, to promote their own survival. Inefficient clearance of apoptotic cells may also contribute to autoimmune disorders such as systemic lupus erythematosus, and may explain their association with genetic deficiencies of complement components. Macrophages are more efficient than dendritic cells in capture and digestion of apoptotic cells; during their maturation dendritic cells become able to present antigens acquired by less mature stages to T cells. Macrophages and dendritic cells may express different receptor profiles, but other differ-ences could also contribute to a different fate for ingested dying cells. The recognition mechanisms of normally senescent haematopoietic cells (e.g. erythrocytes, platelets) and of necrotic cells are still obscure.

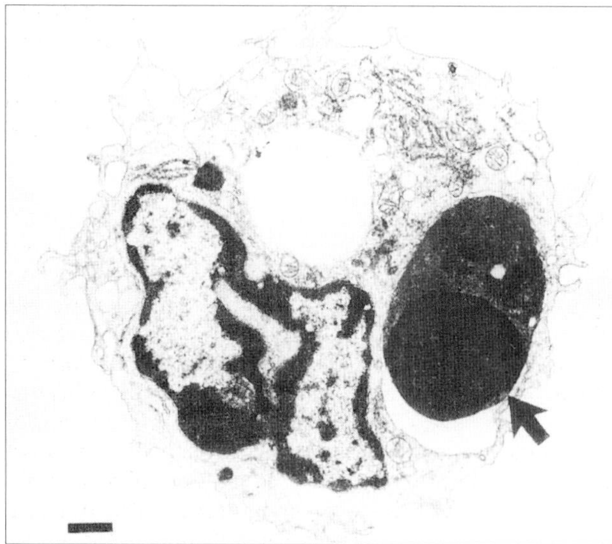

Fig. 9.12 Phagocytosis of apoptotic thymocyte by thymic macrophage. Thymic macrophages phagocytose the large numbers of thymocytes which die during T-cell development. The arrow indicates the nucleus of a phagocytosed thymocyte.

Mannose receptor

Whilst macrophages can express a range of lectins, specific for various sugar ligands, the mannose receptor (MR) is the best studied and may play a unique role in tissue homeostasis, as well as host defence. The receptor contains eight C-type lectin domains responsible for endocytosis and phagocytosis of mannosylated, or related, glycoconjugates.

Endogenous ligands include lysosomal hydrolases and myeloperoxidase, whereas a range of pro- and eukaryotic organisms express mannose-rich structures which serve as ligands. In addition, an N-terminal cysteine-rich domain of the mannose receptor is a distinct lectin for sulphated glycoconjugates highly expressed in secondary lymphoid organs (marginal metallophils, subcapsular sinus macrophages and follicular dendritic cells). The structure of the mannose receptor is illustrated diagrammatically in *Figure 9.14*. A novel antigen transport pathway has been postulated, by which cell-associated or soluble MR could deliver antigen to B and/or T lymphocytes, modulating their immune response. The cysteine-rich domain may also contribute to clearance of hormones such as lutropin, which contains similar sulphated structures.

CD14 and Toll-like receptors

Monocytes and to a lesser extent tissue macrophages express a GPI-anchored molecule, CD14, implicated in the cellular response to bacterial LPS. A plasma LPS binding protein (LBP) enhances LPS responses markedly; genetic ablation of CD14 in mice renders them highly resistant to septic shock, mainly mediated by TNFα release into the circulation. Toll-like receptors (TLR), discovered recently, play a major role in LPS signalling in macrophages, by analogy with a microbial and fungal recognition mechanism first described in *Drosophila* development. The signalling pathways for IL-1 and TLR show many similarities (*Fig. 9.15*), resulting in NFκB activation. The apparent ability of different TLR to discriminate between different classes of organism is poorly understood; the TLR can be recruited to early phagosomes, but has not been shown to be directly coupled to CD14, or pathogen recognition. Other receptors involved in LPS clearance, such as SR-A, may serve to downregulate responses induced via the CD14 pathway, and thus limit systemic release of TNFα and resultant septic shock.

Scavenger receptors

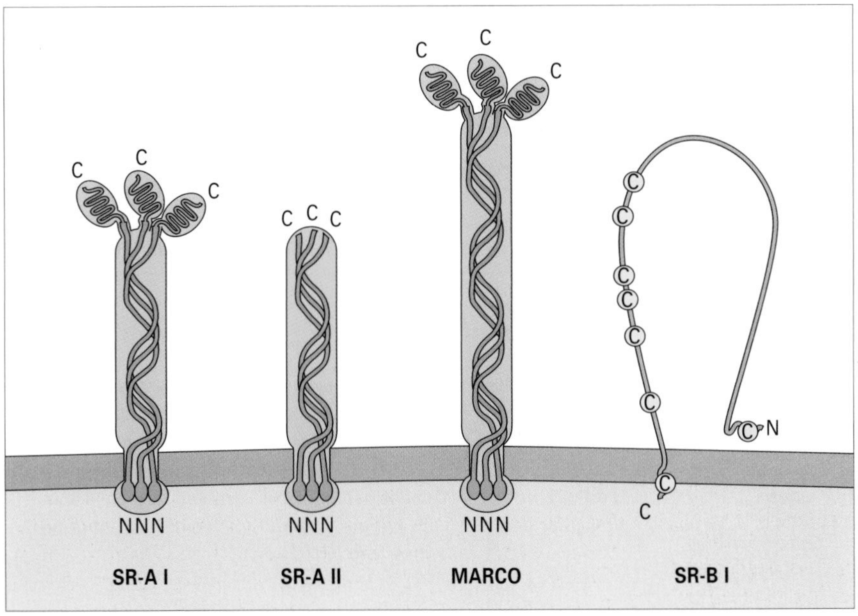

C C C C C C
C C C
NNN NNN NNN
C N
SR-A I SR-A II MARCO SR-B I

Fig. 9.13 Two classes of scavenger receptor are shown. Type A scavenger receptors (SR-A) of macrophages are responsible for the uptake of apoptotic cells and of modified lipoproteins and other polyanionic ligands, including lipopolysaccharide (LPS) and lipoteichoic acids (LTA).

Mannose receptor

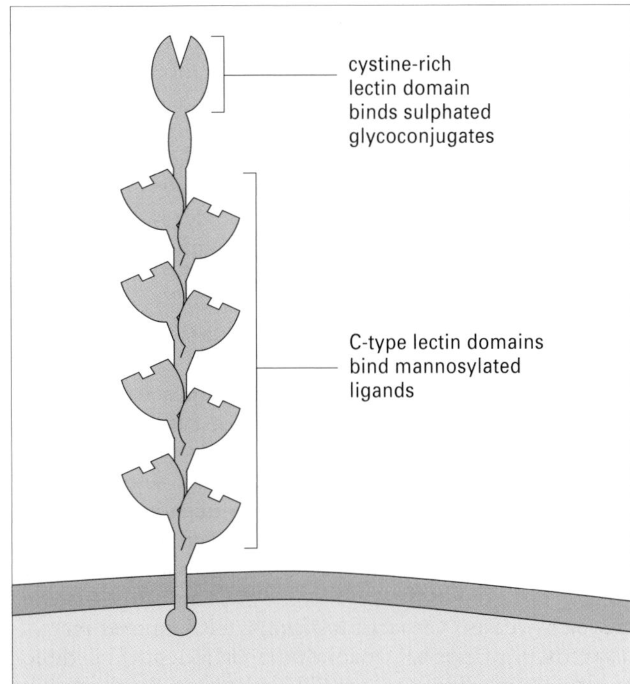

Fig. 9.14 The mannose receptor contains eight C-type lectin domains, involved in binding to mannosylated carbohydrates and related glycoconjugates. A distinct lectin domain is located in the distal (C-terminal) segment, which binds sulphated glycoconjugates.

Complement receptors

Monocytes and macrophages express a range of heterodimeric receptors for C3 cleavage products (CR1, CR3, CR4) and interact with other components of the classical, alternate or lectin-induced pathways of complement activation (*Fig. 9.16*). CR3 contributes to myelomonocytic cell recruitment by adhesion to induced endothelial ligands, including intercellular adhesion molecule-1 (ICAM-1), as shown in human and murine genetic deficiency syndromes. CR3 is a promiscuous receptor with other ligands than iC3b, including fibrinogen. Its role in regulated phagocytosis has been well studied, and the mechanism of CR3-mediated ingestion differs strikingly from that mediated by Fc receptors (see below). Inflammatory and secretory responses also differ after complement and antibody-dependent uptake. Complement receptors contribute to apoptotic cell clearance as well as to host defence to infection, but also serve as a 'safe' entry receptor for organisms such as mycobacteria by direct interaction with microbial ligands, or after opsonization.

Fc receptors

These are various opsonic receptors for immunoglobulin subclasses, especially IgG. The receptors are themselves Ig superfamily members, with two or three domains (see *Fig. 4.22*). They contain immune receptor tyrosine-based activation motifs (ITAM) or inhibitory (ITIM) motifs, which, by interaction with other membrane molecules (e.g. γ chain) and cytoplasmic kinases (e.g. Syk) and/or phosphatases, regulate complex signalling pathways. Apart from the activation of effector responses (phagocytosis, endocytosis, antibody-dependent cytotoxicity), different Fc receptors can also downregulate inflammatory cascades and may provide a link between innate and adaptive immunity.

The mechanism for the ingestion of antibody-coated particles is distinct from that mediated by CR3 (*Fig. 9.17*). FcR-mediated uptake proceeds by a zipper-like process,

Activation of macrophages by LPS and IL-1

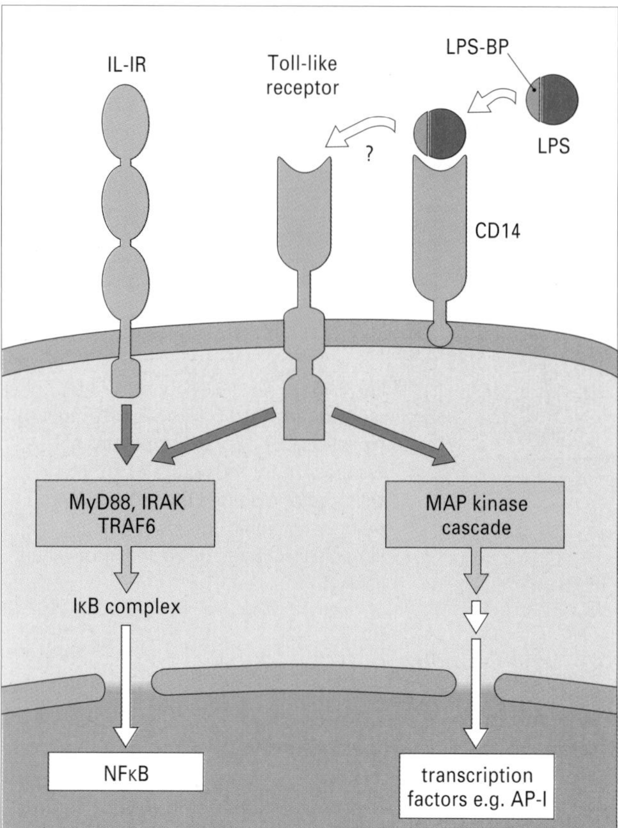

Fig. 9.15 LPS binds leucocyte CD14 (which is GPI-anchored to the membrane) through LPS binding protein and interacts with Toll-like transmembrane receptors by an unknown mechanism to initiate signal transduction. Signalling pathways of the receptor share signalling elements with the IL-1 receptor pathway, e.g. IRAK (IL-1 receptor-associated kinase). Cell activation proceeds via both the MAP-kinase pathways and the induction of NFκB (see *Fig. 7.11*). Different Toll-like receptors are involved in signalling induced by different microorganisms.

where sequential attachment between receptors and ligands guides pseudopod flow around the circumference of the particle; CR3 contact sites are discontinuous for complement-coated particles which 'sink' into the macrophage cytoplasm. Small GTPases play distinct roles in actin cytoskeleton engagement by each receptor-mediated process.

Inhibitory receptors

Recent studies have discovered several new receptors with ITIM motifs expressed on macrophages, which deactivate their effector functions (e.g. SIRPs) or resemble NK inhibitory receptors in their ability to ligate MHC class I molecules. Transmembrane glycoproteins such as DAP-12 promote the surface expression of C-type lectins, analogous to NK cell receptors. These may play an important regulatory function in monocytes and macrophages, for example in deactivation of cellular cytotoxicity.

Complement receptors

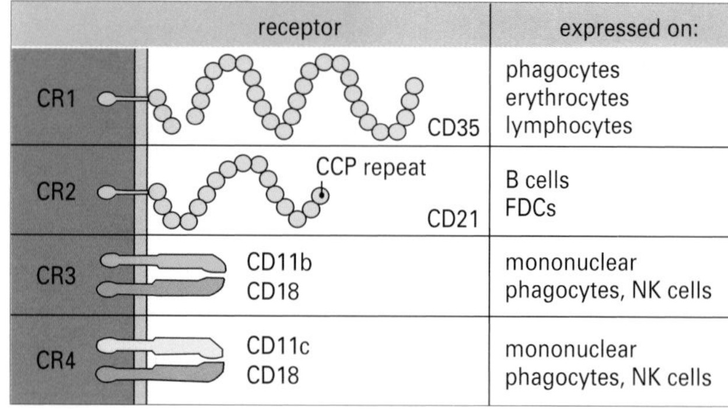

Fig. 9.16 The complement receptors CR1 and CR2 are formed from numerous repeated complement control protein (CCP) domains. CR3 and CR4 are integrins which share a common β chain (CD18). CR1, CR3 and CR4 are expressed on macrophages and other phagocytic cells, while CR2 is confined to B cells and follicular dendritic cells, where it has a function in the maturation of the antibody response (see *Fig. 8.9*).

G-protein-coupled receptors

Macrophages express a range of G-protein-coupled receptors including multispan receptors for f-met-leu-phe chemokines such as MCP-1 (see Appendix III), and C5a. Particular chemokine receptors, especially CCR5, have been implicated in HIV infection of macrophages. The F4/80 antigen contains a seven-transmembrane spanning portion, homologous to a family of peptide receptors (e.g. vasoactive intestinal peptide, VIP) and a large extracellular domain consisting of multiple epidermal growth factor (EGF) domains. Related molecules expressed by myeloid cells include CD97; its ligand CD55 (decay accelerating factor, DAF) protects cells from complement-induced lysis.

Non-opsonic phagocytosis can lead to intracellular infection

In the absence of opsonins, macrophages use multiple receptors to recognize and engulf a range of microorganisms, parasites and viruses directly. These include CR3, SR-As, MR and CD14. SR-As use selected polyanionic ligands including LPS (Gram-negative) and lipoteichoic acid (Gram-positive) for bacterial recognition. MR ligands are found on mycobacteria (intracellular pathogen), HIV gp120, *Pneumocystis carinii*, *Klebsiella*, as well as yeasts (*Candida albicans*). CR3 ligands include phosphatidyl inositol mannoside (PIM) and a direct saccharide binding site on CR3 has been implicated in opsonin-independent recognition. Different receptors often collaborate, for example CR3 and MR in the uptake of *Leishmania* promastigotes. Non-opsonic uptake, or invasion, result in a range of survival strategies by intracellular pathogens, enabling them to avoid phagosome maturation, inhibit fusion with lysosomes and acidification (*Mycobacteria*), or conversely to promote invasion by rapid recruitment of lysosomes (*Candida albicans*, *Trypanosoma cruzi*).

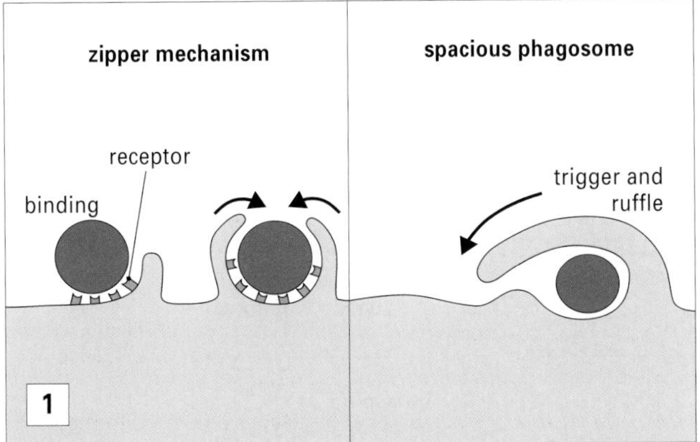

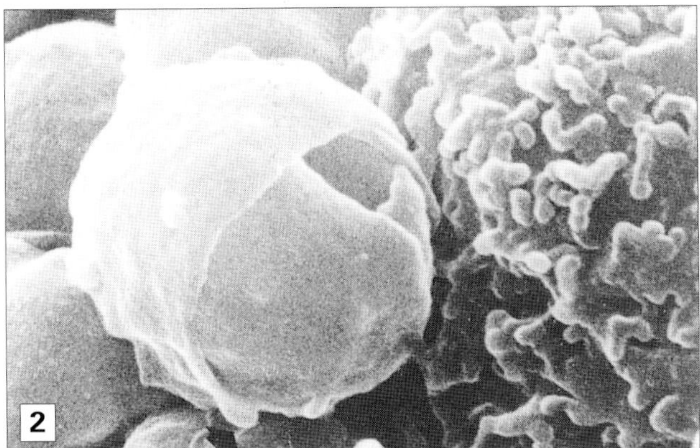

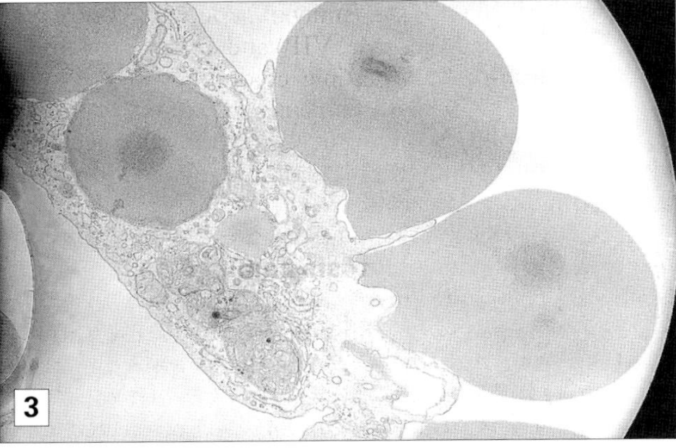

Fig. 9.17 During phagocytosis, receptor–ligand interactions guide the extension of tightly apposed pseudopods around the particle's total circumference until a fusion of the plasma membrane occurs at the tip (**1**). This is known as the zipper mechanism. Alternate 'trigger' mechanisms, in which spacious phagosomes result from flipping over of ruffles back onto the plasma membrane, have also been described. The cytoskeleton of phagocytes plays a key role in engulfment, during which there is extensive remodelling of actin filaments. Some microorganisms and intracellular parasites induce novel mechanisms, to recruit cell membranes during entry into phagocytes. Electron micrograph of ingestion of antibody (IgG) coated sheep erythrocytes by peritoneal macrophage by the zipper mechanism. (Scanning electron micrograph (**2**), courtesy of Dr G.G. MacPherson. Transmission electron micrograph (**3**), courtesy of Dr S.C. Silverstein.)

Legionella pneumophila induces a coiling phagocytosis, and recruits various intracellular organelles (ER, mitochondria), whereas *Salmonella* induces the formation of spacious phagosomes. Once within vacuoles the organism can replicate in secondary lysosomes (*Leishmania*) or escape into the cytosol by membrane dissolution (*Listeria monocytogenes*). Interferon-γ can overcome many of these evasion strategies, resulting in killing or stasis of the organisms, by the mechanisms described below. Opsonization by antibody and/or complement can alter the fate of the organism by extracellular lysis, or by targeting it to a different compartment, viz. lysosomes. Some organisms (e.g. *Salmonella*) induce apoptosis in macrophages, and/or spread between cells by fusion (e.g. *HIV*) or by intercellular infection (e.g. *Listeria*).

The ability of macrophages to present processed peptide antigens derived from intracellular pathogens to T cells is poorly defined; it is possible that they collaborate with dendritic cells by releasing breakdown products, thus activating naïve T lymphocytes. Once MHC class II molecules are induced by IFNγ, exogenous antigens are presented by the MHC class II pathway; endogenous antigens are presented by the MHC class I pathway so that infected macrophages can become targets for $CD8^+$ cytotoxic T cells. Lipid antigens derived from mycolic acids of mycobacteria are presented by dendritic cells via CD1 molecules (see *Fig. 5.20*), which are also inducible on selected macrophage populations.

RESPONSES OF MACROPHAGES

Activated macrophages produce both pro-inflammatory and suppressive cytokines

Following encounters with microorganisms and antigens, resident macrophages are able to enhance their transcription and translation of a wide range of gene products, including secreted molecules which often act locally, close to the cell surface. Secretory products include a range of low molecular weight metabolites, eicosanoids, cytokines, complement proteins and enzymes, especially lysozyme (*Fig. 9.18*). After priming by IFNγ, macrophages triggered by surface-acting stimuli such as LPS release increased levels of various products, which promote an inflammatory reaction, recruit other cells, regulate their activities and induce adhesion. Macrophages also release inhibitory molecules (e.g. TGFβ, PGE_2, IL-10) which suppress inflammatory and immune responses, including T-cell proliferation. IFNγ, IL-1 and TNFα are potent regulators of leucocyte and other cellular activities. These cytokines are all capable of inducing endothelial cell adhesion molecules and selectins, and in association with macrophage-derived chemokines such as macrophage inflammatory protein-1α (MIP-1α) and macrophage chemotactic protein-1 (MCP-1), they induce the accumulation of further inflammatory cells. IL-6 and IL-1 act as circulating mediators of the acute phase response. Distant targets of these macrophage-derived cytokines include thermoregulatory centres in the CNS, muscle and fat stores, and the neuroendocrine system. Cytotoxic products and powerful neutral proteinases such as elastase, collagenase and urokinase (generating

Secretory products of macrophages

category	example	function
low molecular weight metabolites	reactive oxygen intermediates reactive nitrogen intermediates eicosanoids – prostaglandins, leukotrienes platelet activating factor (PAF)	killing, inflammation killing, inflammation regulation of inflammation clotting
cytokines	IL-1β, TNFα, IL-6 IFNα/IFNβ IL-10 IL-12, IL-18 TGFβ MIP1α/β, MCP-1, RANTES, IL-8	local and systemic inflammation antiviral, innate immunity, immunomodulation deactivation of MØ, B-cell activation IFNγ production by NK and T cells repair, modulation, inflammation chemokines
adhesion molecules	fibronectin thrombospondin	opsonization, matrix adhesion, phagocytosis apoptotic cells
complement	C3, all others	local opsonization
procoagulant	tissue factor	clotting cascade
enzymes	lysozyme urokinase (plasminogen activator) collagenase elastase	Gram-positive bacterial lysis fibrinolysis matrix catabolism matrix catabolism

Fig. 9.18 Macrophages produce a wide range of secreted molecules.

Actions of macrophage neutral proteinases

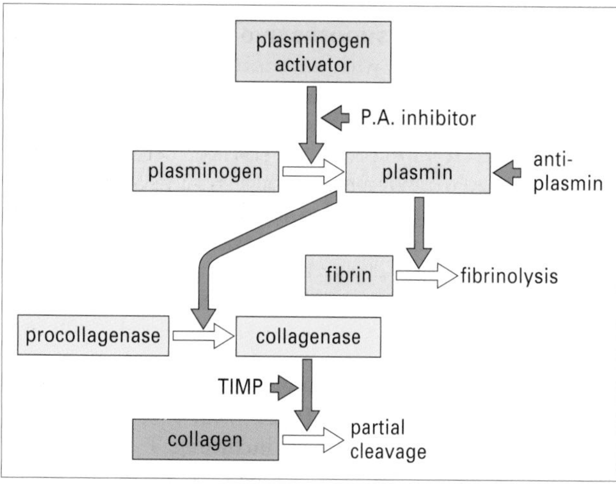

Fig. 9.19 Macrophage-derived neutral proteinases interact with plasma and tissue enzymes and their inhibitors (which can also be generated by macrophages) to regulate fibrinolysis and matrix catabolism. TIMP = Tissue inhibitor of metalloproteinases.

plasmin) (*Fig. 9.19*) are able to induce tissue injury and contribute to destructive chronic inflammation in joints and lung. Monocyte-derived procoagulant/tissue factor can also induce vascular occlusion and tissue damage. Macrophages themselves express receptors for cytokines, as well as producing molecules which are cleaved by metalloproteinases and shed into the circulation. By contrast, soluble receptors and receptor antagonists (e.g. IL-1Ra, soluble TNF-R) are potential inhibitors of receptor–ligand interactions.

New DNA chip methods to analyse gene expression generate complex profiles of selective induction and inhibition of large numbers of genes, some highly restricted to macrophages, others shared with different cell types. Patterns of macrophage mRNA and protein expression will provide insights into intrinsic and extrinsic regulation of macrophage differentiation and activation.

Resting macrophages have limited anti-microbial killing activity

Following phagocytosis, pathogens are subjected to a variety of killing mechanisms, which are generally more diverse and more effective in activated macrophages. Following lysosome fusion, there is a transient rise in the pH of the phagolysosome, followed by a fall in pH, which occurs within 10–15 minutes. The acidification of the phagolysosome by itself may contribute to the killing of some organisms, but the additional killing mechanisms, described below, may be more effective at specific pH values. For example the production of reactive oxygen intermediates (ROIs) in activated macrophages occurs immediately after internalization, whereas cationic proteins are most active during the early alkaline phase and many lysosomal enzymes are more active in the later acidic phase (*Fig. 9.20*).

The resident macrophage has a relatively limited killing capacity which may be sufficient to restrict the growth of many, if not most organisms, including viruses. Lysozyme

Mechanism involved in bacterial killing

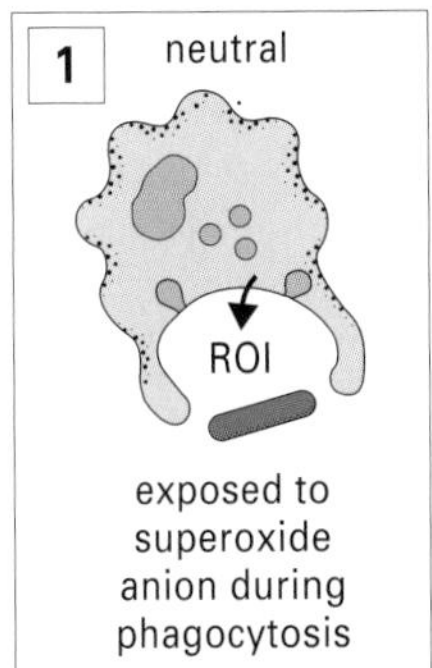

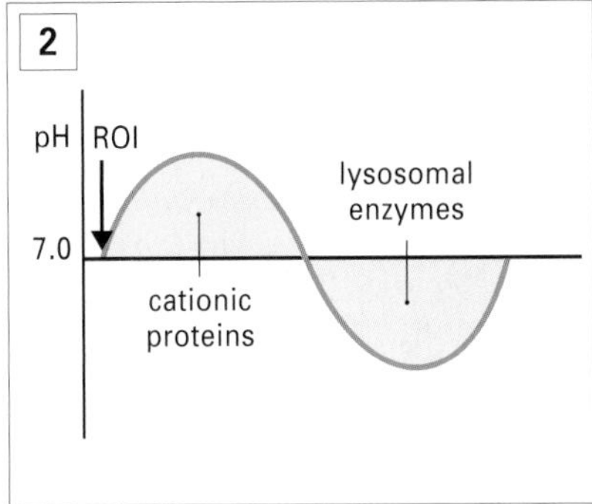

Fig. 9.20 During phagocytosis there is immediate exposure to reactive oxygen intermediates (ROIs) (**1**). This leads to a transient increase in pH, when cationic proteins may be most effective (**2**). Subsequently the pH falls as H^+ ions are pumped into the phagolysosome and lysosomal enzymes with low pH optima become effective. Lactoferrin acts by chelating free iron and can do so at alkaline or acidic pH.

Action of lysozyme on the cell wall of *Staph. aureus*

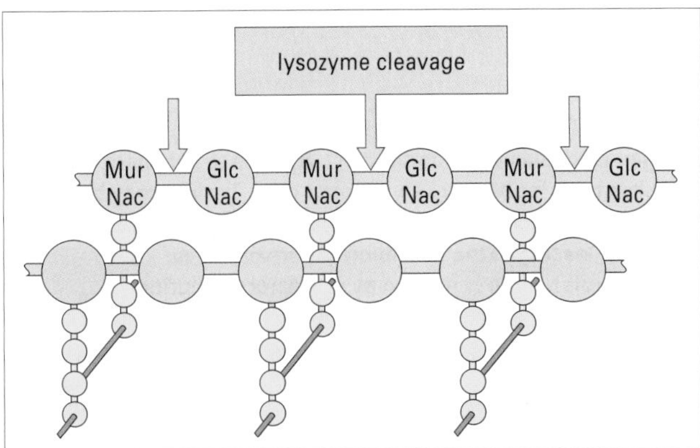

Fig. 9.21 The structure of the cell wall of Gram-positive bacteria such as *Staph. aureus* include a backbone of *N*-acetylglucosamine (GlcNac) alternated with *N*-acetylmuramic acid (MurNac) cross-linked by amino acid side-chains (yellow) and bridges of five glycine residues (orange). Lysozyme splits the molecules at the places indicated.

acts directly on the bacterial cell wall proteoglycans, present in the exposed cell wall of Gram-positive bacteria (*Fig. 9.21*). The cell walls of Gram-negative bacteria may also become exposed to lysozyme if they have been damaged by complement membrane attack complexes. Lysozyme is constitutively produced by macrophages.

A group of highly cationic proteins and polypeptides called defensins also contribute to macrophage anti-bacterial activities. The defensins are small peptides (30–33 amino acids) found in some macrophages of many species and also in human neutrophils, where they comprise up to 50% of the granule proteins. They form ion-permeable channels in lipid bilayers (cf. C9 and perforin), and probably act before acidification of the phagolysosome. They are able to kill a range of pathogens, including bacteria (*Staph. aureus, Pseudomonas aeruginosa, E. coli*), fungi (*Cryptococcus neoformans*) and enveloped viruses (herpes simplex).

In resident macrophages, endocytosis, lysosome delivery and fusion, and acidification favour the destruction of phagocytosed pathogens, but may facilitate the escape of an organism from vacuole to cytosol. The N-ramp multispanning glycoprotein found in macrophage phagosomes contributes to cellular, and ultimately host resistance or susceptibility to a range of intracellular pathogens (mycobacteria, *Leishmania, Salmonella* sp.) by influencing iron transport into or possibly out of the vacuole. Other ion transporters and channels are unlikely to be cell specific.

Activated macrophages deploy oxygen-dependent killing mechanisms and synthesize nitric oxide

Elicited and immunologically activated macrophages produce higher levels of lysozyme, as well as pro-inflammatory cytokines, chemokines, growth factors and proteases. One major difference between resting and activated macrophages is the ability to generate H_2O_2, and other metabolites generated by the respiratory burst. The phagocyte oxidase (Phox) membrane and cytosolic proteins found in neutrophils and activated macrophages assemble to form an NADPH oxidase complex, which contains a novel B cytochrome (*Fig. 9.22*). In the presence of myeloperoxidase, released by myelomonocytic cells, the Klebanoff reaction generates even higher levels of reactive oxygen metabolites. Patients with chronic granulomatous disease lack essential oxidase components and suffer from repeated infections.

Macrophages in mouse as well as man can be activated by IFNγ to express high levels of inducible nitric oxide synthase (i-NOS) which catalyses the production of nitric oxide from arginine (*Fig. 9.23*). Release of NO by macrophages affects neighbouring vessels and leucocytes, and contributes to the killing of intracellular pathogens such as *Leishmania* either directly or by the production of peroxynitrites. Failure of macrophage activation in AIDS contributes to opportunistic pathogen infections and persistence of HIV, as well as reactivation of latent tuberculosis. Rare inborn errors in man for IL-12 and IFN receptors have confirmed experimental gene ablation studies in mouse, which render the host susceptible to infection by intracellular bacteria (see *Fig. 7.14*).

Recently recruited cells are particularly effective in microbial killing

Macrophages vary considerably in their anti-microbial activity. Monocytes produce more reactive oxygen metabolites and myeloperoxidase than differentiated tissue macrophages. It is the recently recruited and further activated cell which is primarily responsible for host defence. *In situ* analysis shows that granuloma macrophages are the major source of newly produced proteins such as lysozyme, TNFα and IL-1. The latter is more tightly regulated and further exposure to microbial components such as LPS is needed to induce the majority of macrophages to express these mediators. Once effector mechanisms are activated,

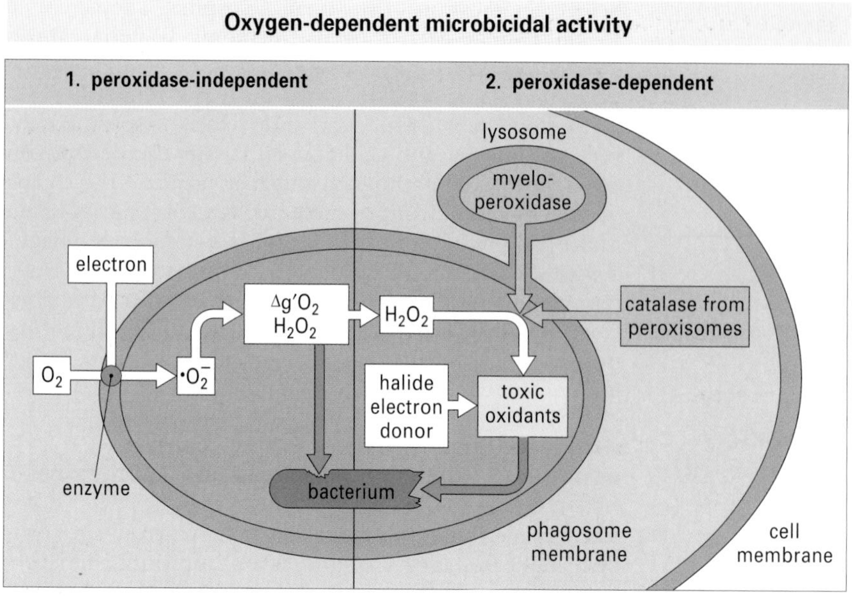

Oxygen-dependent microbicidal activity

1. peroxidase-independent
2. peroxidase-dependent

lysosome
myelo-peroxidase
electron
$\Delta g'O_2$ H_2O_2
H_2O_2
catalase from peroxisomes
O_2
$\bullet O_2^-$
halide electron donor
toxic oxidants
enzyme
bacterium
phagosome membrane
cell membrane

Fig. 9.22 (**1**) An enzyme in the phagosome membrane reduces oxygen to the superoxide anion ($\bullet O_2^-$). This can give rise to hydroxyl radicals ($\bullet OH$), singlet oxygen ($\Delta g'O_2$) and hydrogen peroxide (H_2O_2), all of which are potentially toxic. Lysosome fusion is not required for these parts of the pathway, and the reaction takes place spontaneously following formation of the phagosome. (**2**) If lysosome fusion occurs, myeloperoxidase (or under some circumstances, catalase from peroxisomes) acts on peroxides in the presence of halides. Then additional toxic oxidants, such as hypohalite (HIO, HClO), are generated.

The nitric oxide pathway

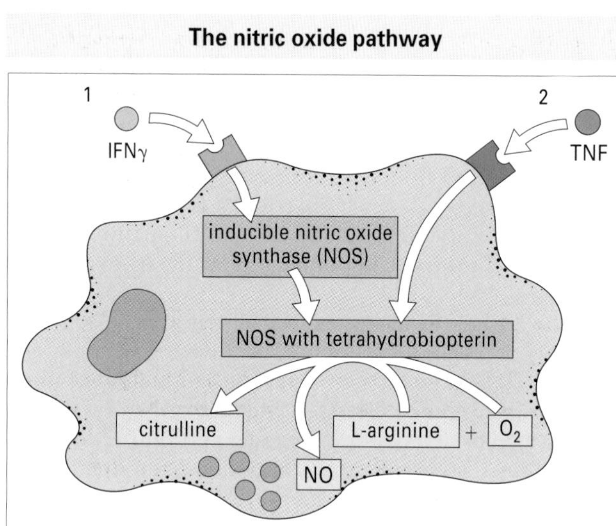

Fig. 9.23 The inducible nitric oxide synthase (i-NOS) combines oxygen with guanidino nitrogen of L-arginine to give nitric oxide, which is toxic for bacteria and tumour cells. Toxicity may be increased by interactions with products of the oxygen reduction pathway, leading to the formation of peroxynitrites. Tetrahydrobiopterin is needed as a cofactor. In murine macrophages IFNγ activates the pathway (**1**), which is then optimally triggered by TNF (**2**). Triggering release of NO from human macrophages is more complex and usually involves cross-linking of membrane CD23. Human macrophages can sometimes express i-NOS but they contain little tetrahydrobiopterin, and maximal NO release may require interaction with other cell types.

local surface reactions also influence the release of potentially injurious macrophage molecules. If ligands are presented on a non-internalizable surface ('frustrated phagocytosis') secretory products can be released into the extracellular environment. Activated macrophages contribute considerably to tissue damage in autoimmune and chronic inflammatory diseases in joints, lung and the nervous system (*Fig. 9.24*).

CONCLUSION

The macrophage is able to initiate, promote, prevent, suppress or terminate an immune response. Its actions may seem antigen non-specific, although antigen dependent. Apart from a major role in host defence, macrophages are neglected participants in autoimmunity (failure to prevent immunity) and peripheral tolerance. They may contribute to T-cell downregulation in placenta, a macrophage-rich organ, and at immunologically privileged sites such as the anterior chamber of the eye. Macrophages can nurse or kill neighbouring cells and partners, and we need to learn more about how they discriminate friend from foe, danger from safety. The host is not viable without macrophages, which perform vital functions within and beyond the immune system.

Role of activated macrophages in immunopathology

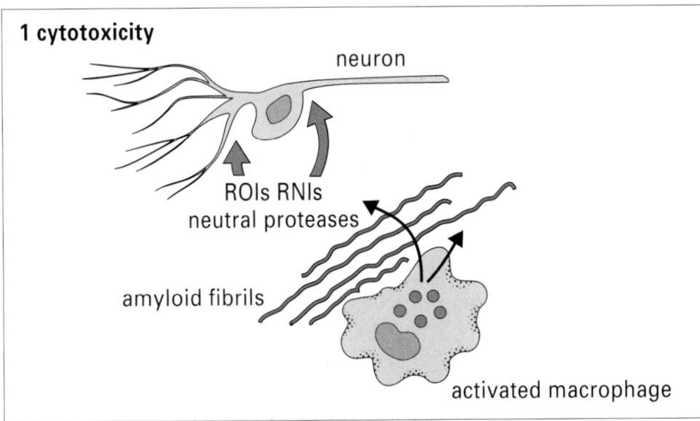

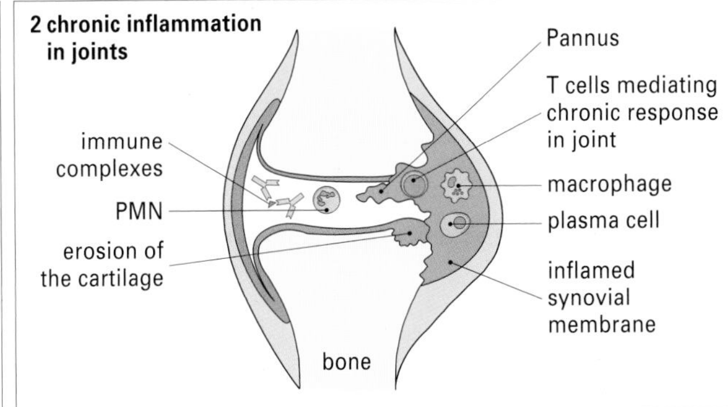

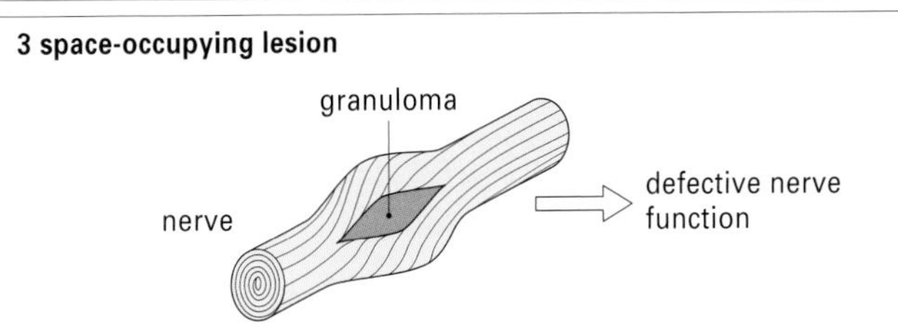

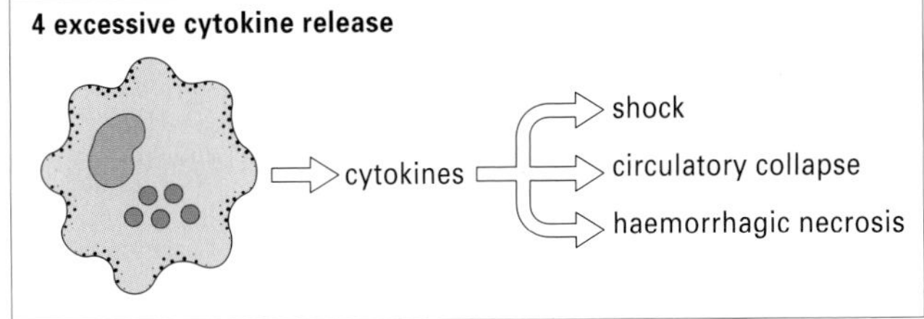

Fig. 9.24 (**1**) Activated microglia may recognize, but be unable to degrade, extracellular β amyloid fibrils and release cytotoxic products that affect neuronal function and survival. (**2**) The response may be directed towards autoantigens (or perhaps to unidentified cryptic infections or commensal organisms), leading to chronic inflammation, as is seen in rheumatoid arthritis. Non-internalizable immune complexes may perpetuate inflammation and antibody/complement-dependent cytotoxicity. (**3**) A granuloma may cause a bulky space-occupying lesion, impairing the function of sensitive tissues such as brain, retina and nerve. (**4**) Excessive release of cytokines can lead to several tissue-damaging syndromes, especially toxic shock syndromes with TNFα.

CRITICAL THINKING • Mononuclear phagocytes in immune defence (Explanations on p. 455)

Problem 1: the role of macrophages in toxic shock syndrome

In an experimental model of septic shock, mice are infected systemically with Bacille Calmette Guerin (BCG), a non-lethal vaccine strain of mycobacteria. After 12 days, the mice are challenged intraperitoneally with graded doses of lipopolysaccharide (LPS). Blood samples are taken at 2 hours and the clinical condition of the mice monitored for up to 24 hours. Experiments are terminated earlier if mice show severe signs of distress.

9.1 What cytokines would you measure in the 2-hour serum sample?

9.2 What clinical signs would be indicative of incipient septic shock?

9.3 What mechanisms contribute to septic shock?

9.4 What outcome would you expect if the following knockout mouse strains were used instead of wild type controls: CD14, scavenger receptor Class A (SR-A), IFNγ?

9.5 Interpret your results.

9.6 Suggest further experiments.

9.7 What is the clinical significance of this experiment?

Problem 2: the distinction between inflammatory responses and house-keeping of apoptotic cells

Mouse peritoneal macrophages are fed a meal of apoptotic cells in culture, and then challenged with an intracellular pathogen, *Trypanosoma cruzi.* Subsequent single cell analysis of parasite survival shows that *T. cruzi* growth is enhanced by prior uptake of apoptotic cells, but not of necrotic cells or control particles.

9.8 How would you investigate the macrophage surface receptors responsible for apoptotic cell uptake?

9.9 Suggest a possible mechanism by which apoptotic cell uptake promotes *T.cruzi* survival.

9.10 How would you investigate this experimental model?

9.11 What is the possible *in vivo* and clinical significance of this observation?

Problem 3: the role of macrophages in TH1 and TH2 responses

Isolated mouse peritoneal macrophages are treated for 2 days with selected cytokines (IFNγ, IL-4, IL-13, IL-10) in culture and a range of assays for cell activation employed. It is found that IFNγ enhances the respiratory burst (after LPS challenge), MHC class II expression and pro-inflammatory cytokine production, but downregulates mannose receptor (MR) mediated endocytosis. IL-10 is an efficient antagonist of the above effects. IL-4 and IL-13, however, are weak antagonists of respiratory burst and pro-inflammatory cytokine production and induce MHC class II molecules and MR activity markedly.

9.12 Interpret the significance and possible functional relevance of these results in relation to concepts of TH1/TH2 differentiation.

9.13 What further work could be done to investigate the possibility that macrophage activation could by analogy be classified as M1/M2?

9.14 How would you investigate the role of macrophages and dendritic cells as possible inducers of $CD4^+$ T lymphocyte subset differentiation?

FURTHER READING

Reviews

Aderem A, Underhill DM. Phagocytosis. *Ann Rev Immunol* 1999;**17**:593–623.

Gordon S. Macrophages and the immune response. In: Paul W (ed.) *Fundamental Immunology,* 4th edn. Philadelphia: Lippincott-Raven; 1999: chap 15, pp 533–45.

Gordon S. Development and distribution of mononuclear phagocytes: relevance to inflammation. In: Gallin R, Snyderman D, Fearon D, Haynes B, Nathan C (eds) *Inflammation: Basic Principles and Clinical Correlates,* 3rd edn. Philadelphia: Lippincott-Raven; 1999:35–48.

Gordon S (ed.). *Advances in Cell and Molecular Biology of Membranes and Organelles. Phagocytosis,* Vol. 5. Stanford, CT: JAI Press.

Gordon S (ed.). *Advances in Cell and Molecular Biology of Membranes and Organelles. Microbial Invasion.* Vol. 6. Stanford, CT: JAI Press.

Gordon S, McKnight AJ. Innate recognition systems. *Forum Immunol Microbes Infection* 2000;**3**:239–336.

Linehan SA, Martinez-Pomares L, Gordon S. Macrophage lectins in host defence. *Microbes Infection* 2000;**2**:279–88.

Luster AD. Chemokines – chemotactic cytokines that mediate inflammation. *New Engl J Med* 1988;**338**:436–45.

Martinez-Pomares L, Gordon S. The mannose receptor and its role in antigen presentation. *Immunologist* 1999;**7**:119–23.

McKnight AJ, Gordon S. Membrane molecules as differentiation antigens of murine macrophages. *Adv Immunol* 1998;**68**:271–314.

Medzhitov R, Janeway CA. Innate immunity impacts on the adaptive immune response. *Curr Opin Immunol* 1997;**9**:4–9.

Mosser DM, Karp CL. Receptor mediated subversion of macrophage cytokine production by intracellular pathogens. *Curr Opin Immunol* 1999;**11**:406–11.

O'Neil LAJ, Dinarello CA. The IL-1R receptor toll-like receptor superfamily: crucial receptor for inflammation & host defense. *Immunol Today* 2000;**21**:206–9.

Pearson AM. Scavenger receptors in innate immunity. *Curr Opin Immunol* 1996;**8**:20–8.

Platt N, da Silva R, Gordon S. Recognising death: the phagocytosis of apoptotic cells. *Trends Cell Biol* 1998;**8**:365–372.

Wright SD. Toll, a new piece in the puzzle of innate immunity. *J Exp Med* 1999;**189**:605–9.

Selected papers

Dalton DK, Pitts-Meek S, Keshav S, Figari IS, Bradley A, Stewart TA. Multiple defects of immune cell function in mice with disrupted interferon-γ genes. *Science* 1993;**259**:1739–42.

Gruenheid S, Pinner E, Desjardins M, Gros P. Natural resistance to infection with intracellular pathogens: the Nramp1 protein is recruited to the membrane of the phagosome. *J Exp Med* 1997;**185**:717–30.

Kindler Y, Sappino AP, Grau GE, Piquet PF, Vassali P. The inducing role of TNF in the development of bactericidal granulomas during BCG infection. *Cell* 1981;**56**:731–40.

10 Cell-mediated cytotoxicity

- **Cytotoxic T cells recognize antigen presented on MHC molecules.** Most cytotoxic T cells are CD8$^+$ and recognize antigenic peptides presented on MHC class I.
- **Natural killer (NK) cells react against cells which do not express MHC class I.** They can interact with these cells using a variety of receptors.
- **NK cells express two major classes of inhibitory receptors for MHC molecules.** These are lectin-like receptors of the CD94 family and immunoglobulin superfamily molecules (KIRs).
- **Cytotoxicity is mediated by combinations of direct cell–cell interactions, cytokines and the release of granule proteins.** Fas ligand and tumour necrosis factors can signal apoptosis to the target cell. Granules containing perforin and granzymes contribute to target cell damage.
- **Ligation of Fas or the type-1 tumour necrosis factor (TNF) receptor on the target cell leads to the activation of caspases.** The caspases are the ultimate mediators of apoptosis in the target.
- **Myeloid cells induce damage in targets principally by the release of toxic molecules.** This is a reflection of their normal function of killing pathogens.

The last two chapters dealt with the types of immune reaction which are controlled by T helper (TH) cells, namely antibody responses directed by TH2 cells and cell-mediated immunity mediated by macrophages and TH1 cells. This chapter is concerned with cytotoxicity, the ways in which leucocytes recognize and destroy other cells. Cell-mediated cytotoxicity is an essential defence against intracellular pathogens, including viruses, some bacteria and parasites. Tumour cells, eukaryotic pathogens and even cells of the body, may also become the target of cytotoxic cells. Addtionally, the process is important in the destruction of allogeneic tissue grafts. Several types of cell can execute this activity including T-cytotoxic (Tc) cells, NK cells and sometimes myeloid cells. The mechanisms of recognition and killing used by the lymphoid cells are quite distinct from those of the myeloid cells, and will be considered first.

Cytotoxic T cells and NK cells are complementary elements in the immune defence against virally infected cells

Cytotoxic T cells and NK cells recognize their targets in different ways (*Fig. 10.1*).

Cytotoxic T cells recognize specific antigens (e.g. viral peptides on infected cells) presented by MHC molecules. Most Tc cells are CD8$^+$ and recognize antigen presented on MHC class I, but about 10% of MHC-restricted cytotoxic T cells are CD4$^+$ and recognize antigen presented on class II molecules.

NK cells recognize cells which fail to express MHC class I molecules. These cells also use a variety of receptors to recognize their targets positively. For example, they can bind to antibody already attached to antigen on a target cell, using their Fc receptors (CD16): this is known as antibody-dependent cell-mediated cytotoxicity (ADCC), or killer cell (K cell) activity.

The most important role of Tc cells is the elimination of cells infected with virus (see Chapter 14). Nearly all nucleated cells express MHC class I molecules and if they become infected they can therefore present antigen to CD8$^+$ Tc cells. The detailed mechanisms of antigen presentation to Tc cells are discussed in Chapters 5 and 6 and

Recognition of target cells by Tc cells and NK cells

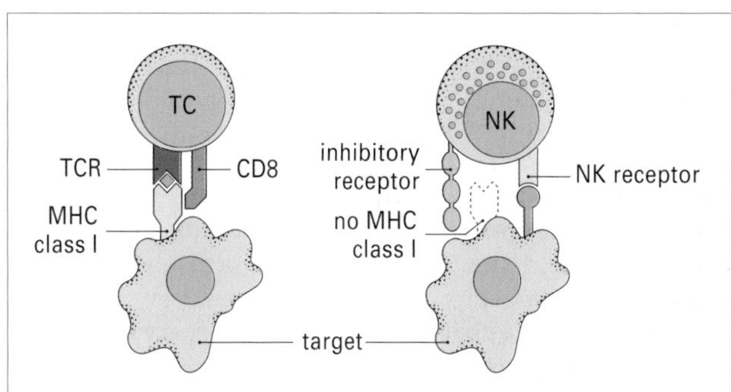

Fig. 10.1 Cytotoxic T cells recognize processed antigen presented on the target cell by MHC molecules using their T-cell receptor (TCR). Most Tc cells are CD8$^+$ and recognize antigen presented by MHc class I, but a minority are CD4$^+$ and recognize antigen presented by MHC class II. By contrast, NK cells have receptors that recognize MHC class I on the target and signal inhibition of cytotoxicity. They use a number of different receptors (NK receptors) to identify their targets positively for killing, including CD2, CD69, or antibody bound to their Fc receptor (CD16).

are summarized briefly here. Cellular molecules that have been partly degraded by proteasomes are transported to the endoplasmic reticulum to become associated with MHC class I molecules and are then transported to the cell surface. Thus each cell samples its own molecules and presents them for review by CD8$^+$ Tc cells. Both the cell's own molecules and those of intracellular pathogens will be presented in this way.

Additional interactions may be required to stabilize the bond between the Tc cell and the target (*Fig. 10.2*), and can even help to trigger the killing event. For example, by adding antibodies against CD3 or CD2 on the Tc cell *in vitro*, it is possible to trigger the killing of target cells that are bound to the Tc cell. It is probable that binding of physiological ligands to these molecules can also trigger Tc cells in this way.

Interactions between Tc cells and target cells

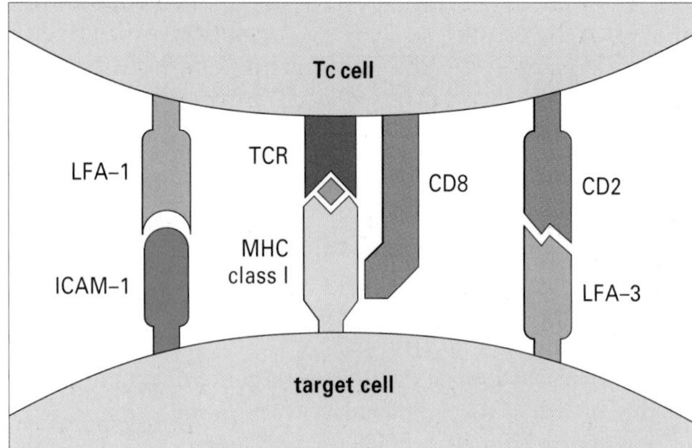

Fig. 10.2 Some of the ligands involved in the interaction between cytotoxic T cells and their targets.

Several viruses (particularly herpes viruses) have evolved mechanisms to avoid recognition by Tc cells. They reduce the expression of MHC molecules or even produce proteins which divert MHC molecules out of the endoplasmic reticulum. This reduces the likelihood that processed viral peptides will be presented at the cell surface. Because NK cells specifically recognize cells which have lost their MHC class I molecules, we can see that Tc cells and NK cells act in a complementary way to protect the body. In effect, the NK cells check that cells of the body are carrying their identity card (MHC class I) while the Tc cell checks the specific identity (antigen specificity) on that card.

Experiments involving the micromanipulation of individual cells have shown that a single cytotoxic T cell can kill several target cells sequentially. To function in this manner, Tc must be resistant to their own killing mechanisms and able to detach effectively from dying target cells.

Cytokine activated killer (LAK) cells are related to NK cells

Immunologists have experimented with several potential treatments for cancer. One approach has been to activate the patient's own lymphocytes *in vitro* with IL-2, and then to reinfuse them. These cells, which are initially derived from blood or spleen, are called cytokine activated killer cells or LAKs. Such cells show enhanced MHC non-restricted cytotoxicity, and they appear to be largely derived from precursors that are indistinguishable from NK cells. Thus LAK cells probably do not represent a separate lineage, but rather a consequence of activation. This type of cell is undergoing trials for the treatment of cancer in humans.

NATURAL KILLER CELL RECEPTORS

NK cells are mostly derived from 'large granular lymphocytes' (LGLs), which comprise about 5% of human peripheral blood lymphocytes. The majority of NK cells are $CD3^-CD16^+CD56^+CD94^+$ (see Appendix 2), and do not contain productive rearrangements of the T-cell receptor genes. Initial experiments on the specificity of NK cells showed that MHC class I expression protected cells from NK-cell mediated cytotoxicity and that particular allotypes of HLA-C were dominant genes for producing resistance. This lead to a search for receptors on NK cells which could inhibit cytotoxicity and which might be expressed in a variety of different forms, capable of reacting with MHC class I and signalling its presence to the NK cell. Two major types of molecules were identified and termed 'killer inhibitory receptors' or KIRs. One group of molecules was identified as type-2 membrane glycoproteins (C-terminus outside) with a C-type lectin domain (Ca^{2+}-dependent). The other group of molecules were members of the Ig superfamily. Subsequently, it was realized that while some members of each group did indeed act as killer inhibitory receptors, others could actually activate the killer cell. So, it was not correct to call all members of both groups 'inhibitory receptors'. Therefore it was proposed that the term 'KIR' now meaning 'killer immunoglobulin-like receptor', should be used for just the second group of molecules.

The lectin-like receptor CD94 interacts with HLA-E

The lectin-like receptor CD94 is a characteristic marker of human NK cells, but is also found on a subset of Tc cells. It covalently assembles with different members of another group of type-2 membrane molecules called NKG2, and the dimers are expressed on the cell membrane (*Fig. 10.3*). There are at least six members of the NKG2 family (NKG2A–NKG2F). The dimer of CD94-NKG2A is an inhibitory receptor, which blocks NK cell-mediated cytotoxicity. By contrast, CD94-NKG2C is an activating receptor. Although these two molecules are very similar, they differ in their intracellular segments, and this determines whether the receptor is inhibitory or activating (*Fig. 10.3*). *In vivo*, the role of the inhibitory version is clear, but that of the activating variant is not. Possibly, it may act as one of the receptors by which NK cells carrying CD94-NKG2C actively engage their targets.

CD94 is distantly related to the mouse molecule Ly-49, which is present in the NK cell gene complex (NKC). Indeed, it was partly this homology of CD94 to mouse NK cell receptors, that alerted researchers to the possibility that CD94 was an NK cell receptor in man.

HLA-E presents peptides from other MHC class I molecules

It is now known that the ligand for both CD94-NKG2A and CD94-NKG2C is the HLA-E molecule. The HLA-E gene locus encodes an MHC class I-like molecule. These are sometimes called class 1b molecules, to distinguish them from the classical MHC molecules which present antigen to Tc cells. The extraordinary function of HLA-E is to present peptides from other MHC class I molecules. The leader peptides from other MHC molecules are released in the endoplasmic reticulum, and these are required to stabilize functional HLA-E molecules (*Fig. 10.4*). Cells lacking classical MHC class I molecules do not express HLA-E at the cell surface. Hence an inhibitory signal is not passed to the NK cell. In effect HLA-E is a sensitive

Lectin-like receptors of NK cells

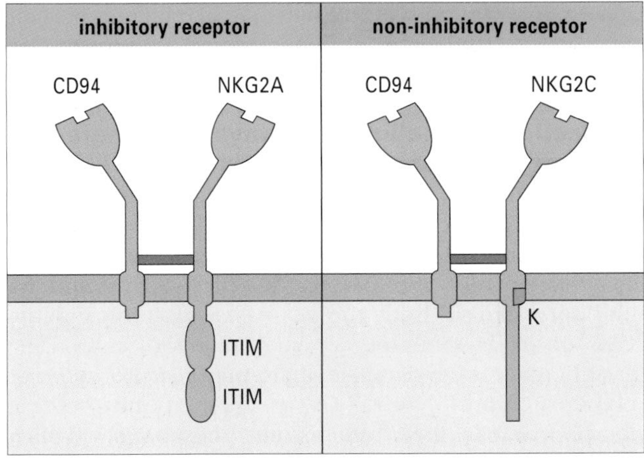

Fig. 10.3 The inhibitory receptors consist of the lectin-like CD94 disulphide bonded (red) to peptides from the NKG2 locus, such as NKG2A which have intracellular domains carrying ITIM motifs (immunoreceptor tyrosine inhibitory motif). The non-inhibitory receptors, such as CD94/NKG2C, lack ITIMs, but have a charged lysine (K) in the transmembrane segment which allows them to interact with signal transducing molecules.

HLA-E presents peptides of other MHC class I molecules

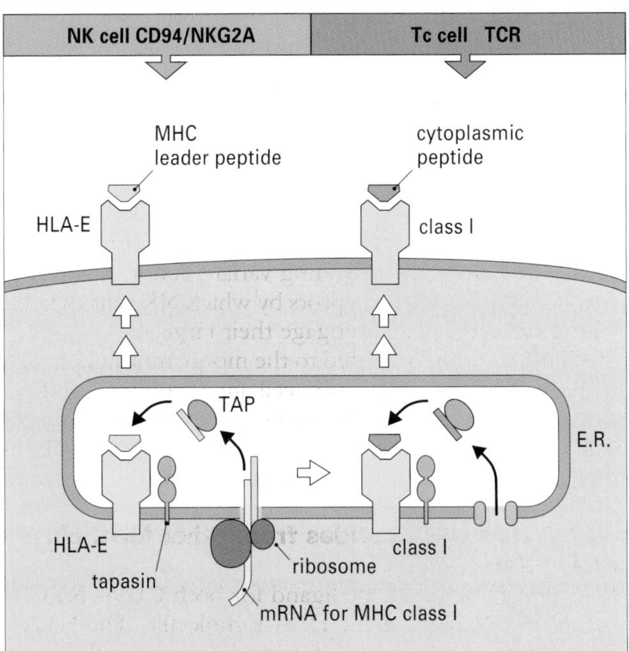

Fig. 10.4 Leader peptides from MHC class I molecules are loaded onto HLA-E molecules in the endoplasmic reticulum, a process which requires TAP transporters and tapasin to assemble functional HLA-E molecules. These are presented at the cell surface for review by the CD94 series of receptors on NK cells (left). The MHC class I molecules meanwhile present antigenic peptides from cytoplasmic proteins which have been transported into the endoplasmic reticulum. These complexes are presented to the TCR on CD8^{+} cytotoxic T cells.

mechanism for monitoring whether viruses or tumours have downregulated MHC class I expression in a cell.

Although CD94 has a lectin domain, the recognition of the HLA-E/peptide occurs via interaction with residues from the peptide and the α_1 and α_2 domains of the MHC molecule. The lectin domain could however reinforce this interaction by binding to carbohydrate associated with the MHC molecule.

KIRs are members of the immunoglobulin superfamily

The second group of NK cell receptors are members of the immunoglobulin superfamily. They fall into two subsets, having either two or three Ig domains (*Fig. 10.5*). A set of approximately 12 such genes has been identified as a cluster on chromosome 19q13.4. The two-domain members (KIR2D) are defined as CD158, while the three-domain members (KIR3D) were originally described as p70, based on their molecular weights. Two of the two-domain members have been shown to bind to allelic variants of HLA-C, and these isoforms have inibitory cytoplasmic domains (see below). The specificity of these receptors can partly explain why particular HLA-C allotypes inhibited some NK cells, as described above. It also explains why these allotypes produce dominant resistance – if a cell expresses a particular HLA-C allotype, then that is sufficient to inhibit a K cell which has engaged it.

Other isoforms of the KIRs have activating domains. These generally engage HLA molecules with a lower affinity than the inhibitory forms, and like the activating forms of CD40-NKG2, their physiological functions are uncertain.

There is also a third group of receptors clustered in the same region as the KIRs, which have either two or four

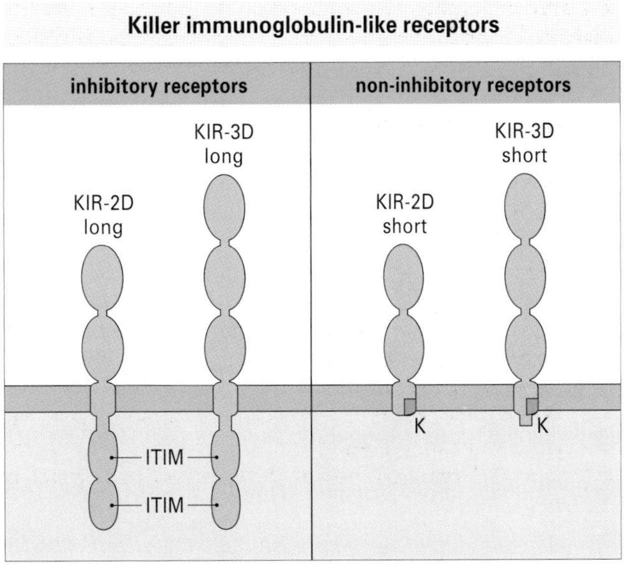

Killer immunoglobulin-like receptors

inhibitory receptors
non-inhibitory receptors
KIR-2D long
KIR-3D long
KIR-2D short
KIR-3D short
ITIM
ITIM
K
K

Fig. 10.5 These receptors consist of either two or three extracellular Ig superfamily domains. The inhibitory forms are longer and have intracellular ITIMs, while the non-inhibitory forms have the charged residue in the membrane comparable to the non-inhibitory forms of CD94/NKG2.

Ig-like domains. They are called immunoglobulin-like transcripts or ILTs and they have a wider cellular distribution than the other NK cell receptors, Some of these interact with a broad spectrum of MHC molecules, and others with none at all, hence their functions are still uncertain.

HLA-G inhibits NK cell action against the placenta

An intriguing recent discovery is that the HLA-G molecule, which is expressed only on placental trophoblasts, is a dominant NK-cell inhibitor that confers resistance to all types of NK cells (HLA-G is another MHC class 1b molecule). Trophoblast cells are derived from the fetus and invade the maternal circulation as the placenta is established. They are therefore allogeneic in the mother, because they contain paternal MHC genes. However, all conventional MHC genes are downregulated in these cells, and the HLA-G expression is therefore required to protect the placenta from attack by NK cells. There is some debate as to which of the inhibitory receptors recognize HLA-G. Both CD94 and several of the better-defined KIRs have been excluded, but a likely candidate is ILT2.

NK cells and K cells use several different receptors to positively identify their targets

NK cells may engage their targets using a variety of receptors, including CD2, CD16, CD69 and receptors related to those which inhibit cytotoxicity. The Fc receptor, CD16, binds antibody bound to target cells and mediates ADCC (*Fig. 10.6*). It is customary to refer to this as killer (K) cell activity, but this function may also be performed by several other cell types with Fc receptors, including T cells. Myeloid cells expressing Fc receptors can also show K-cell activity, but probably use killing mechanisms different from those of T cells and NK cells (discussed later).

Potential targets for K-cell action include viral antigens on cell surfaces, MHC molecules and some epitopes present on tumours. Thus monocytes and (according to some controversial reports) polymorphs may also be active against antibody-coated tumour targets. Some myeloid cells (monocytes and eosinophils) are certainly important effectors of damage to antibody-coated schistosomulae (see Chapter 18).

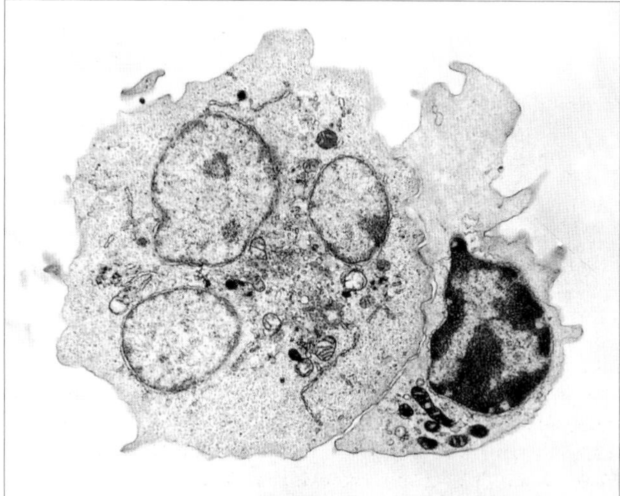

Fig. 10.6 K-cell activity. Electron micrograph of a lymphocyte (right) engaging a target cell sensitized with antibody (left). × 2500. (Courtesy of Dr P. Penfold.)

Intracellular signalling pathways coordinate inhibitory and activating signals

The next question is how a NK cell decides between cytotoxic action or inaction. This decision is thought to depend on the coordination of intracellular signalling pathways, and may involve the balance between activating and inhibitory signals. Both the lectin-like receptor and the KIRs occur as inhibitory or activating molecules. The key difference is the presence of 'immunoreceptor tyrosine inhibitory motifs' or ITIMs. If these motifs become phosphorylated, they can recruit phosphatases which downregulate the activity of the NK cell (*Fig. 10.7*).

By contrast, other KIRs which lack the ITIMs can associate with a molecule (DAP12) which is related to the ζ chain of the T-cell receptor complex. This molecule has 'immunoreceptor tyrosine activation motifs' (ITAMs), which allow it to phosphorylate and recruit tyrosine kinases including ZAP-70 (*Fig. 10.7*, and compare with figure 6.21), which lead to cell activation. At present, it is not known how the balance of activation and inhibition is resolved. In particular it is uncertain how a ligand such as HLA-C will act when it can bind to both inhibitory and activating receptors on the same cell.

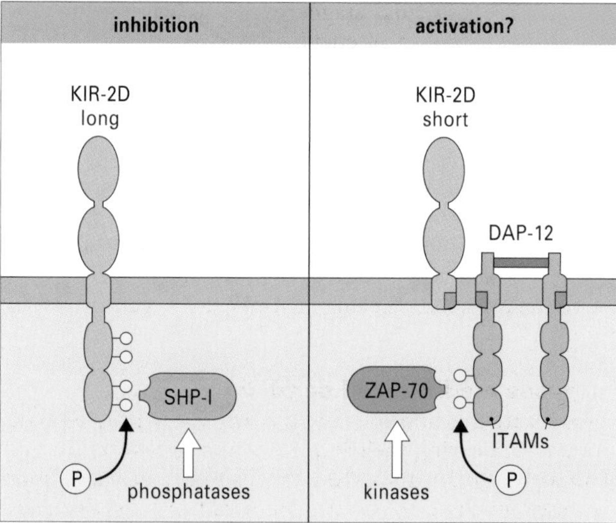

Fig. 10.7 Following phosphorylation of its ITIMs, the inhibitory receptors of NK cells can bind to phosphatases, including SHP-1 and SHP-2, which inhibit killing. The non-inhibitory forms of the receptor associate with a dimeric molecule DAP12, via the complementary charged residues in their membanes. DAP12 has activation motifs (ITAMs). When phosphorylated this recruits kinases of the syk family or ZAP-70 (cf. T-cell activation, Chapter 6). Whether this leads to NK cell activation, or whether it modulates the inhibitory signals is not known.

MECHANISMS OF CYTOTOXICITY

Cytotoxicity is effected by direct cellular interactions, cytokines and granule exocytosis

Cytotoxic T cells, NK cells and K cells use a variety of different mechanisms to kill their targets. These include direct cell–cell signalling via surface molecules and indirect signalling via cytokines. In addition, many $CD8^+$ cytotoxic T cells and large granular lymphocytes (NK cells and K cells) have granules which contain proteins that damage target cells if they are released directly against the target cell plasma membrane. Exactly which combination of these three mechanisms is used depends on the Tc cell involved.

Cytotoxic T cells and NK cells induce apoptosis in their targets

Cells can die in two principle ways – by necrosis or apoptosis. Apoptosis is a highly ordered process in which cells are systematically disassembled. The cells detach from their neighbours and the cytoplasm and nucleus condense. Mitochondria lose their membrane potential and leak cytochrome c into the cytoplasm. As the chromatin condenses, it is cleaved into regular-sized fragments by endonucleases. Finally the cell membrane starts to form blebs and the cell may fragment into condensed apoptotic bodies. Dead cells attract mononuclear phagocytes and are rapidly taken up by phagocytosis to be broken down in phagolysomes. Apoptosis is a feature of normal physiology. For example, T cells which fail thymic selection die by apoptosis (see Chapters 2, 12), as do B cells which are not selected during affinity maturation in germinal centres (see Chapter 8). This type of cell death also occurs extensively during organ development, particularly in the central nervous system. In each case the final stages of cell death involve the activation of a group of enzymes called caspases, but the events which trigger apoptosis are different for each process.

By comparison necrosis is a less orderly event, in which dying cells fall apart releasing their contents. This tends to provoke macrophage activation and inflammation. Another difference is that apoptosis requires energy (ATP) while necrosis does not. The damage caused by pathogens and the colateral damage caused by granulocytes and macrophages acting against them induce cell death by necrosis.

Caspases mediate cell death by apoptosis

Caspases are a group of proteases which have the unusual property of cleaving their substrates on the C-terminal side of an aspartate residue. More than 10 caspases have been identified in man. They are produced in a pro-enzyme form and become activated by cleavage into two or three subunits. The caspases have very wide-ranging effects within a cell. They can affect cell structure, intracellular signalling, cell cycle control, DNA integrity and repair, and intercellular adhesion. Studies with caspase gene knockout mice have shown that different caspases are associated with particular forms of apoptosis. For example, caspase-3-deficient mice die shortly after birth due to a failure of normal CNS development, but the mechanisms of cell death induced by cytotoxic cells are unaffected. Notably, however, caspase-8-deficient mice are not susceptible to cell killing by the mechanisms outlined below.

Cytotoxicity may be signalled via Fas or a TNF receptor on a target cell

Cytotoxic T cells signal to their targets using members of the TNF receptor group of molecules. These include Fas (CD95) and the type 1 TNF receptor, TNFR-1, which are widely distributed in the body (*Fig. 10.8*). Other members of the group are CD30 and CD40 which are involved in lymphocyte differentiation The ligand for Fas (FasL) is expressed on mature $CD4^+$ and $CD8^+$ T cells after activation. Ligation of Fas induces trimerization of the Fas molecules on the cell surface, which causes them to associate with a transducing molecule which recruits and activates caspases 8 or 10 (*Fig. 10.9*). Note that cell killing mediated by Fas also occurs as part of the normal processes of lymphocyte selection, during development. For cytotoxic lymphocytes which lack granules the Fas pathway is thought to be the principle means of signalling to the target.

Most $CD8^+$ Tc cells, NK cells (and macrophages) have vesicles containing TNF and lymphotoxin which can be released onto a target cell. TNF acts in a very similar way to the Fas ligand. It causes trimerization of the TNFR-1 so that the receptor associates with adaptor proteins which recruit caspases. Both TNFR-1 and Fas contain intracytoplasmic domains (death domains) which are found on a number of proteins involved in cell survival. (Note however that a different form of TNF receptor, TNFR-2, lacks these intracytoplasmic segments and therefore does not transduce signals for apoptosis.)

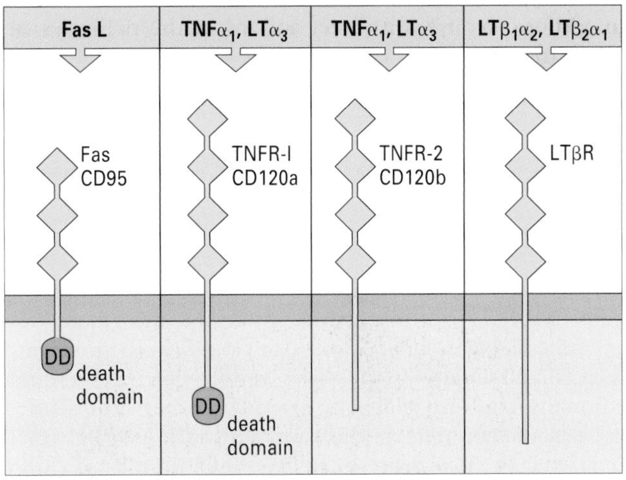

Fig. 10.8 The molecule Fas (CD95), the two TNF receptors and the lymphotoxin receptor are illustrated diagramatically. The extracellular domains are similar to those found in the NGF receptor. Both Fas and TNFR-1 have death domains which are involved in the recruitment of caspases. The ligands for these receptors are indicated at the top. Lymphotoxin-α can form homotrimers or heterotrimers with lymphotoxin-β. Up to 25 other members of these families have been identified by data-base searching.

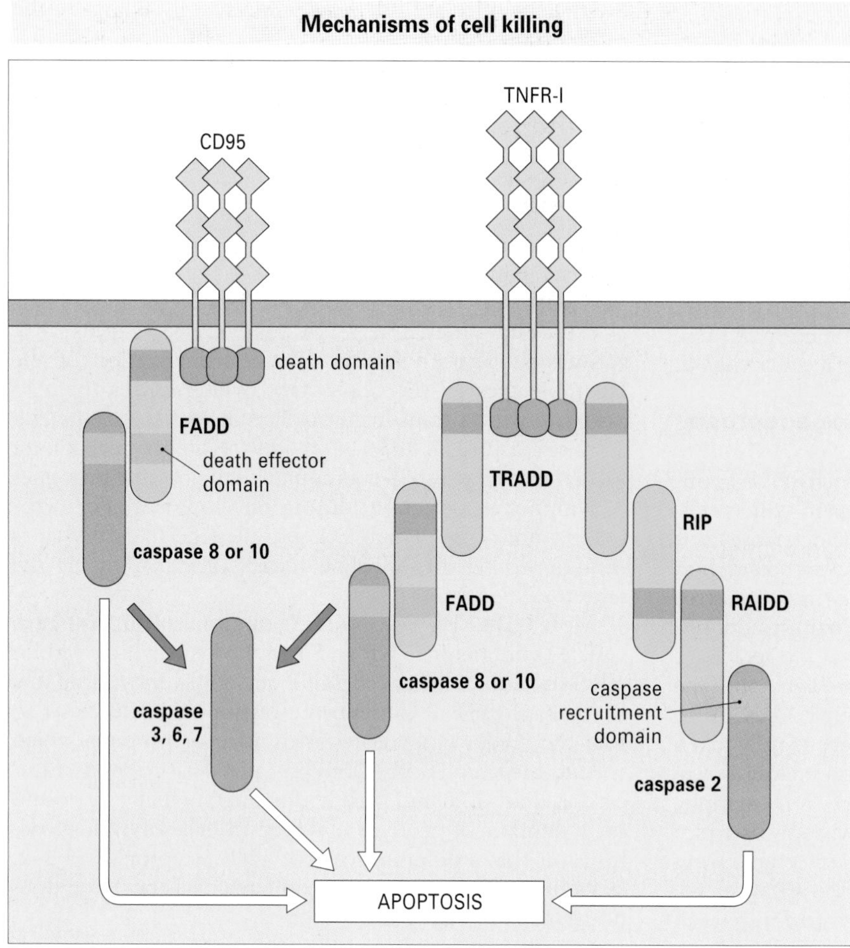

Fig. 10.9 Ligation of CD95 or TNFR-1 causes trimerization of the receptors. Death domains in the cytoplasmic portion of CD95 bind to the adaptor protein FADD (=MORT-1), which recruits caspase 8 or 10. TNFR-1 can activate either caspase 8 or 10, via TRADD and FADD, or caspase 2 via RIP and RAIDD. Caspase 8 can further activate other caspases, and these in concert lead to apoptosis of the target cell.

Activated caspase 8 can cleave and activate other caspases, in addition to its own direct actions in the pathways of apoptosis (*Fig. 10.9*).

Granules of cytotoxic T cells contain perforin and granzymes

It was originally thought that all cytotoxicity was caused by the release of granule proteins onto the target cell. Indeed the processes described above were only identified when it was realized that cells which lack granules could still kill targets. The specific granules of NK cells and Tc cells contain several proteins, including perforin and granzymes (granule-associated enzymes). After binding to its target, the Tc cell directs its granules towards the membrane adjoining the target. Then, in a Ca^{2+}-dependent phase, the granule contents are discharged into the cleft between the two cells. This process can be seen in time-lapse video microscopy (*Fig. 10.10*).

Perforin is a monomeric pore-forming protein that is related both structurally and functionally to the complement component, C9. The vesicles also contain a serine esterase that may be involved in the assembly of the lytic complex. In the presence of Ca^{2+}, the perforin monomers bind to the target cell membrane and polymerize to form transmembrane channels. Although in close contact with the perforin, the Tc cell survives and can continue to kill further targets. It is thought to be protected from autodestruction by a proteoglycan (chondroitin sulphate A) which is also present in the vesicles, and which may bind to and inactivate the perforin. Perforin-knockout mice have Tc cells which display reduced but still functional cytotoxicity, implying that perforin cannot be the only mechanism used by these cells.

Granzymes are a collection of serine esterases (enzymes) which are also released upon granule exocytosis and become active after release. They are not essential for cytotoxicity, as cells lacking granzymes may still be cytotoxic. Some of the granzymes may interact with intracellular pathways in the target cell to activate mechanisms which trigger apoptosis and DNA degradation. In fact, it is notable that granzyme B has the same unusual specificity as the caspases (see above). In order to activate apoptosis pathways in the target cell, the granzymes need to gain access to the cytoplasm. It has been proposed that perforin and granzymes act synergistically; the granzymes enter the target cell via pores created by perforin. The ways in which granule proteins can contribute to cytotoxicity are shown in *Figure 10.11*.

To summarize, $CD8^+$ Tc cells use both FasL and granule release to kill their targets, $CD4^+$ Tc cells use principally FasL, and NK cells use primarily their granules. TNF may contribute to the cytotoxic damage produced by any of these cells.

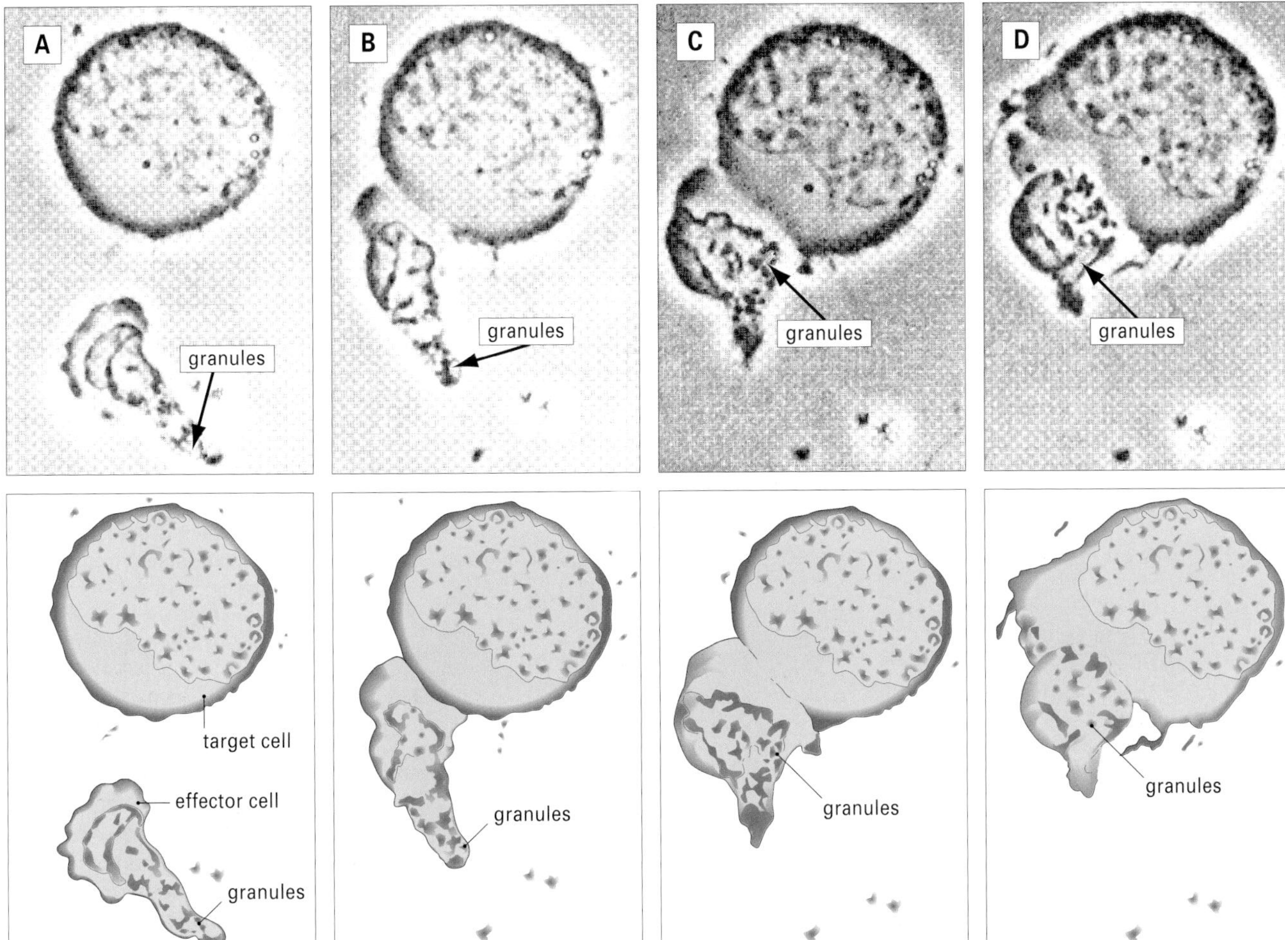

Fig. 10.10 Intracellular reorganizations during effector–target cell interaction. Early events in the interaction of Tc with specific targets were studied with high-resolution cinematographic techniques. Four frames (together with interpretative drawings) are shown, taken at different times, of a Tc interacting with its target. The location of the granules within the effector cell is indicated in each case. Before contact with the target (a), the effector had granules located in a uropod at the rear, and was seen to move randomly by extending pseudopods from the organelle-free, broad leading edge of the cell. Within 2 minutes of contacting the target (b), the Tc had begun to round up and initiate granule reorientation (c). After 10 minutes (d), the granules occupied a position in the zone of contact with the target, where they appear to be in the process of emptying their contents into the i ntercellular space between the two cells. (Courtesy of Dr V.H. Engelhard.)

Granule-associated killing mechanisms

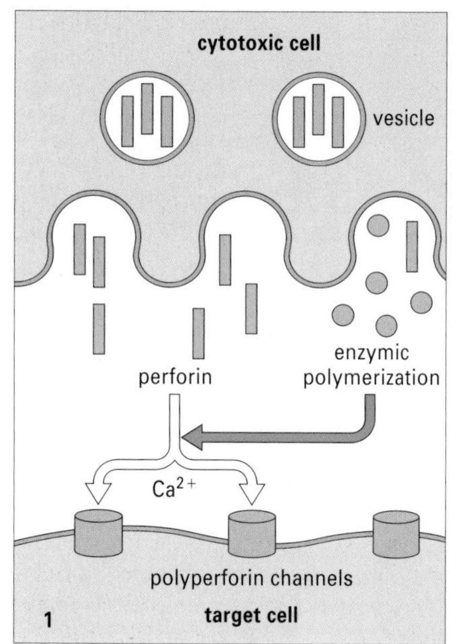

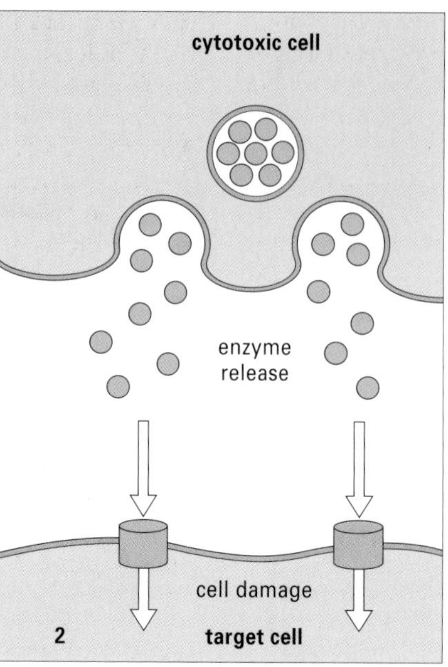

Fig. 10.11 The cytotoxic lymphoid cell degranulates, releasing perforin and various enzymes (granzymes) into the immediate vicinity of the target cell membrane. In the presence of Ca^{2+} there is enzymic polymerization of the perforin to form polyperforin channels on the target cell (**1**). Enzymes which activate the apoptosis pathways, degradative enzymes or other toxic substances released from the cytotoxic cell may pass through the channels on the target and cause cell damage or killing (**2**).

NON-LYMPHOID CYTOTOXIC EFFECTORS

Macrophages can damage targets using their non-specific toxic effector systems or via cytokines

A number of non-lymphoid cells may be cytotoxic to other cells or invading microorganisms, such as bacteria or parasites. Cytotoxicity may be triggered specifically to a target by antibody-dependent cell mediated cytotoxicity (ADCC) or may involve a range of non-specific toxic mediators. For example macrophages and neutrophils both express FcγRI and FcγRII which allows them to engage tumours by ADCC.

In general, macrophages and neutrophils aim to destroy pathogens by internalizing them and subjecting them to toxic molecules and enzymes within the phagolysosome. These include the production of reactive oxygen intermediates, toxic oxidants and NO detailed in Chapter 9, as well as the secreted molecules such as neutrophil defensins, lysosomal enzymes and cytostatic proteins. If the phagocyte fails to internalize its target, then these mediators may be released into the extracellular environment and contribute to localized cell damage. This action is referred to as 'frustrated phagocytosis', and occurs when the target is engaged by surface receptors, but is too large to phagocytose. The actions of the mediators produced by the phagocyte damage the target, rather than induce apoptosis. For this reason, the cytotoxic action of these cells tends to produce necrosis and inflammation.

Nevertheless, in the case of macrophages, activated cells secrete TNF which can induce apoptosis in a similar way to NK cells and Tc cells. For this reason, macrophages can induce necrosis, apoptosis or a combination of both, depending on the state of activation of the macrophages and the target involved. The mechanisms by which myeloid cells produce cytotoxic damage are shown in *Figure 10.12.*

Mechanisms which may contribute to the cytotoxicity of myeloid cells

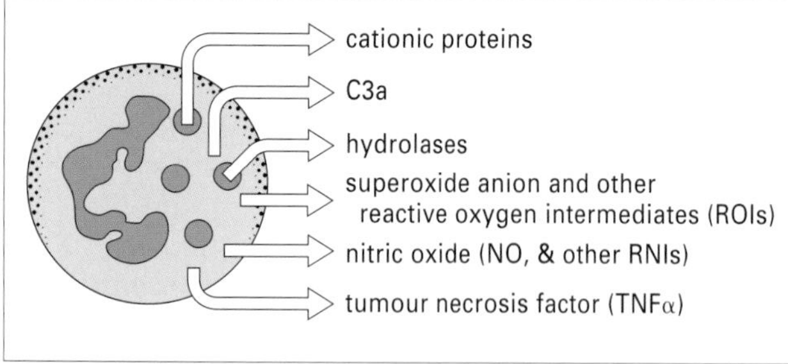

Fig. 10.12 Reactive oxygen intermediates (ROIs) and reactive nitrogen intermediates (RNIs), cationic proteins, hydrolytic enzymes and complement proteins released from myeloid cells may damage the target cell in addition to cytokine-mediated attack.

Eosinophils mediate cytotoxicity by exocytosis of their granules

Mature eosinophils are characterized by their granules, which have a crystalloid core which binds the dye eosin. Generally, eosinophils are only weakly phagocytic; they ingest some bacteria following activation, but are less efficient than neutrophils at intracellular killing. Their major function appears to be the secretion of various toxic granule constituents, following activation. They are therefore effective for the extracellular killing of microorganisms, particularly large parasites such as schistosomes (see Chapter 16).

The components of the eosinophil granule include major basic protein (MBP), eosinophil peroxidase (EPO) and eosinophil cationic protein (ECP). Major basic protein (not to be confused with myelin basic protein of oligodendrocytes) is the major component of eosinophil granules, forming the crystalloid core. It has been shown to damage, and sometimes kill, parasites, but also damages host tissue cells. Eosinophil peroxidase is a highly cationic heterodimeric 71–77-kDa haemoprotein, which is distinct from the myeloperoxidase of neutrophils and macrophages. In the presence of H_2O_2, also produced by eosinophils, EPO will oxidize a variety of substrates, including halide ions to produce hypohalite. Indeed, this may represent the eosinophils' most potent killing mechanism for some parasites. ECP is an eosinophil-specific toxin which is very potent at killing many parasites, particularly the schistosomulae of *Schistosoma mansoni*. The molecule is a ribonuclease, which because of its high charge, binds avidly to negatively charged surfaces. It is possible that it forms membrane channels, which allow other mediators access to the target organism. Other molecules produced by eosinophils are lysophospholipase and eosinophil-derived neurotoxin (EDN), which is also a ribonuclease but with strong neurotoxic activity.

Degranulation of eosinophils can be triggered in a number of ways. Binding to IgG-coated parasites via surface FcγRII triggers release of some mediators including ECP, but not EPO. By contrast, triggering via FcεRII leads to the release of EPO, but not ECP. Parasite killing may involve contact-dependent degranulation or may simply require deposition of toxins within the local tissue. Degranulation may also be triggered directly *in vitro* by several cytokines, including IL-3, IL-5, granulocyte-macrophage–colony-stimulating factor (GM-CSF), TNF, interferon-β (IFNβ) and platelet activating factor (PAF). These mediators also enhance ADCC-mediated degranulation. Eosinophils are prominent in the inflammatory lesion of a number of diseases, particularly atopic disorders of the gut, skin and respiratory tract, where they are often closely associated with fibrotic reactions. Examples are atopic exzema, asthma and inflammatory bowel disease. Although eosinophils may play some regulatory role in these conditions, such as inactivating histamine, their toxic products and cytotoxic mechanisms are a major cause of the tissue damage. For example, in asthma, eosinophil granule proteins are detectable in the blood and lungs following asthmatic attacks. MBP can kill some pneumocytes and tracheal epithelial cells while EPO kills type II pneumocytes. MBP can also induce mast cells to secrete histamine, thus exacerbating allergic inflammation.

CRITICAL THINKING • Mechanisms of cytotoxicity (Explanations on pp 455–456)

Lymphocytes from a normal individual were stimulated *in vitro* by coculture with irradiated T lymphoma cells. (Irradiation of these stimulator cells prevents them from dividing in the coculture.) After 7 days the lymphocytes were harvested and fractionated to obtain a population of cytotoxic cells (CD8$^+$), and a population of NK cells (CD94$^+$, CD16$^+$). These effector cells were set up in a cytotoxicity assay with the tumour cells as targets. The tumour cells were labelled, in order to detect both DNA fragmentation and cell lysis. The following results were obtained in these assays.

10.1 Why do the Tc cells lyse the targets and induce DNA fragmentation? What are these cells recognizing on the tumour cell surface?

10.2 Why might the NK cells cause some damage to the tumour? Why does the presence of antibody to the tumour enhance the cytotoxic capacity of the NK cells?

10.3 Explain the result with purified perforin.

Treatment	Lysis	DNA fragmentation
No effector cells	4%	1%
CD8$^+$ Tc cells	82%	80%
NK cells	12%	11%
Anti-tumour cell antibody	5%	1%
NK cells + anti-tumour cell antibody	28%	28%
Purified perforin	95%	2%

FURTHER READING

Berke G. The binding and lysis of target cells by cytotoxic lymphocytes. *Annu Rev Immunol* 1994;**12**:735.

Bleackle RC, Lobe CG, Duggan B, *et al.* The isolation of a family of serine protease genes expressed in activated cytotoxic T lymphocytes. *Immunol Rev* 1988;**103**:5.

Boyington JC, Motyka SA, Schuck P, Brooks AG, Sun PD. Crystal structure of an NK cell immunoglobulin-like receptor in complex with it class I MHC ligand. *Nature* 2000;**405**:537–43.

Kagi D, Ledermann B, Burki K, *et al.* Cytotoxicity mediated by T cells and natural killer cells is greatly impaired in perforin-deficient mice. *Nature* 1994;**369**:31–7.

Lanier LL, Phillips JH. Inhibitory MHC class I receptors on NK cells and T cells. *Immunol Today* 1996;**17**:86–91.

Lee N, Llano M, Carreto M, *et al.* HLA-E is a major ligand for the natural killer inhitory receptor CD94/NKG2A. *Proc Natl Acad Sci* 1998;**95**:5199–204.

López-Botet M, Bellón T. Natural killer cell activation and inhibition by receptors for MHC class I. *Curr Opin Immunol* 1999;**11**:301–7.

Navarro F, Llano M, Bellón T, Colona M, Geraghty DE, López-Botet M. The ILT2 (LIR-1) and CD94NKG2A cell receptors respectively recognise HLA-G1 and HLA-E molecules on coexpressed targets. *Eur J Immunol* 1999;**29**:277–83.

Rathmell JC, Thompson CB. The central effectors of cell death in the immune system. *Annu Rev Immunol* 1999;**17**:781–828.

Tormo J, Natarajan K, Margulies DH, Manuzza RA. Crystal structure of a lectin-like natural killer cell receptor bound to its MHC class I ligand. *Nature* 2000;**402**:623–31.

Trapani JA, Kwon BS, Kozak CA, Chintamaneni C, Young J D-E, Dupont B. Genomic organization of the mouse pore-forming protein (perforin) gene and localisation to chromosome 10. Similarities to and differences from C9. *J Exp Med* 1990;**171**:545.

Vassalli P. The pathophysiology of tumour necrosis factor. *Annu Rev Immunol* 1992;**10**:411–52.

Wallach D, Varfolomeev EE, Malanin NL, Goltsev YV, Kavalenko AV, Boldin MP. Tumor necrosis factor receptors and Fas signalling mechanisms. *Annu Rev Immunol* 1999;**17**:331–68.

Watanabe-Fukunga R, Brannan CI, Copeland NG, Jenkins NA, Nagata S. Lymphoproliferation disorder in mice explained by defects in Fas antigen that mediates apoptosis. *Nature* 1992;**356**:314.

Yanelli JR, Sullivan JA, Mandell GL, Engelhard VH. Reorientation and fusion of cytotoxic T cell granules after interaction with target cells as determined by high resolution cinematography. *J Immunol* 1986;**136**:377.

Yokoyama WM. Natural killer cell receptors. *Curr Opin Immunol* 1998;**10**:298–305.

11 Regulation of the immune response

- **The immune response is subject to a variety of control mechanisms** which serve to restore the immune system to a resting state when the response to a given antigen is no longer required.
- **Many factors govern the outcome of any immune response.** These include the antigen itself, its dose and route of administration, and the genetic background of the individual responding to antigenic challenge.
- **Immunoglobulins can influence the immune response positively** as anti-idiotype or through immune complex formation. They may also negatively influence immune responses by reducing antigenic challenge or by feedback inhibition of B cells.
- **The antigen-presenting cell may affect the immune response through its ability to provide co-stimulation to T cells.** Different types of antigen-presenting cell promote different modes of immune response.
- **T cells regulate the immune response.** Cytokine production by T cells influences the type of immune response elicited by antigen. $CD4^+$ T cells can deviate immune responses to TH1 (T-1 helper) or TH2 type responses. Regulatory T cells may belong to the CD4 or CD8 subpopulations. They can inhibit responses by production of suppressive cytokines such as interleukin 10 (IL-10) and transforming growth factor-β (TGFβ).
- **Selective migration of lymphocyte subsets to different sites can modulate the local type of immune response,** since TH1 cells and TH2 cells respond to different sets of chemokines.
- **Genetic factors which influence the immune system include both MHC-linked and non-MHC-linked genes.** They affect the level of immune response, susceptibility to infection and autoimmune disease. Defects in many of these genes lead to immunodeficiency or abnormal immune responses.
- **The neuroendocrine system influences immune responses.** Corticosteroids in particular downregulate TH1 responses and macrophage activation.

The immune response, like all biological systems, is subject to a variety of control mechanisms. These mechanisms restore the immune system to a resting state when responsiveness to a given antigen is no longer required. An effective immune response is an outcome of the interplay between antigen and a network of immunologically competent cells. The nature of the immune response, both qualitatively and quantitatively, is determined by many factors, including the form and route of administration of the antigen, the antigen-presenting cell (APC), the genetic background of the individual and any history of previous exposure to the antigen in question or to a cross-reacting antigen. Specific antibodies may also modulate the immune response to an antigen. Some of these factors are discussed in detail elsewhere (see Chapters 6–9) and are dealt with only briefly here.

REGULATION BY ANTIGEN

T cells and B cells are triggered by antigen after effective engagement of their antigen-specific receptors together with appropriate co-stimulation. In the case of the T cell, this engagement is not with antigen itself, but with processed antigenic peptide bound to MHC class I or class II molecules on APCs (see Chapter 5). The nature of an antigen, its dose and the route of administration have all been shown to have a profound influence on the outcome of an immune response. An effective immune response removes antigen from the system. Repeated antigen exposure is required to maintain T- and B-cell proliferation and during an effective immune response there is often a dramatic expansion of specifically reactive effector cells. At the end of an immune response reduced antigen exposure results in a reduced expression of IL-2 and its receptor leading to apoptosis of the antigen-specific T cells. The majority of antigen-specific cells therefore die at the end of an immune response and a minor population of long-lived antigen-specific T and B cells survive to give rise to the memory population of antigen-specific cells.

The nature of the antigen influences the type of immune response that occurs

Different antigens elicit different kinds of immune response. Polysaccharide capsule antigens of bacteria generally induce IgM responses, whereas proteins can induce both cell-mediated and humoral immune responses. Intracellular organisms such as some bacteria, parasites or viruses induce a cell-mediated immune response, whereas soluble protein antigens induce a humoral response. A cell-mediated immune response is also induced by agents such as silica.

However, some antigens (e.g. those of intracellular microorganisms) may not be cleared so effectively, leading to a sustained immune response that has pathological consequences (see Chapters 14 and 24).

Large doses of antigen can induce tolerance

Very large doses of antigen often result in specific T- and sometimes B-cell tolerance. It has been shown that administration of antigen to neonatal mice often results in tolerance to this antigen. It has been speculated that this may be the result of the immaturity of the immune system. However, recent studies have shown that neonatal mice can develop efficient immune responses (*Fig. 11.1*) and that non-responsiveness may in some cases be attributable, not to the immaturity of T cells, but to immune deviation whereby a non-protective type II cytokine response dominated a protective type I response. T-independent polysaccharide antigens have been shown to generate tolerance in B cells after administration in high doses.

Effect of antigen dose on the outcome of the immune response to murine leukaemia virus

virus pfu	antiviral cytotoxicity	TH1 response (IFNγ)	TH2 response (IL-4)
0.3	+ + +		
1000	+		
		80 60 40 20 0	20 40 60 80

Fig. 11.1 Newborn mice were infected with either 0.3 or 1000 plaque-forming units (pfu) of virus and the CTL response against virally infected targets was assessed together with the production of IFNγ (TH1 cytokine) or IL-4 (TH2 cytokine) in response to viral challenge. Mice infected with a low dose of virus make a TH1-type response and are protected. The results are presented as arbitrary units.

Tolerance and its underlying mechanisms are discussed in Chapter 12.

The route of administration of an antigen can determine whether or not an immune response occurs

The route of administration of antigen has been shown to influence the immune response. Antigens administered subcutaneously or intradermally evoke an immune response, whereas those given intravenously, orally or as an aerosol may cause tolerance or an immune deviation from one type of CD4$^+$ T-cell response to another. For example, rodents that have been fed ovalbumin or myelin basic protein (MBP) do not respond effectively to a subsequent challenge with the corresponding antigen. Moreover, in the case of MBP, the animals are protected from the development of the autoimmune disease, experimental allergic encephalomyelitis (EAE). This phenomenon may have some therapeutic value in allergy; recent studies have shown that oral administration of a T-cell epitope of the Der p1 allergen of house dust mite (*Dermatophagoides pteronyssimus*) could tolerize to the whole antigen. The potential mechanisms of such tolerance induction include anergy, immune deviation and the generation of regulatory T cells that act through the production of cytokines such as TGFβ.

Similar observations have been made when antigen is given as an aerosol. Studies in mice have shown that aerosol administration of an encephalitogenic peptide inhibits the development of EAE that would normally be induced by a conventional (subcutaneous) administration of the peptide (*Fig. 11.2*). This also may have therapeutic implications, as the inhibition of the response is not limited to the antigen administered as an aerosol, but also includes other antigens capable of inducing EAE such as protedipid protein.

A clear example of how different routes of administration affect the outcome of the immune response is provided by studies of infection with lymphocytic choriomeningitis virus (LCMV). Mice primed subcutaneously with peptide in incomplete Freund's adjuvant develop immunity to LCMV. However, if the same peptide is repeatedly injected intraperitoneally, the animal becomes tolerized and cannot clear the virus (*Fig. 11.3*).

Aerosol administration of antigen modifies the immune response

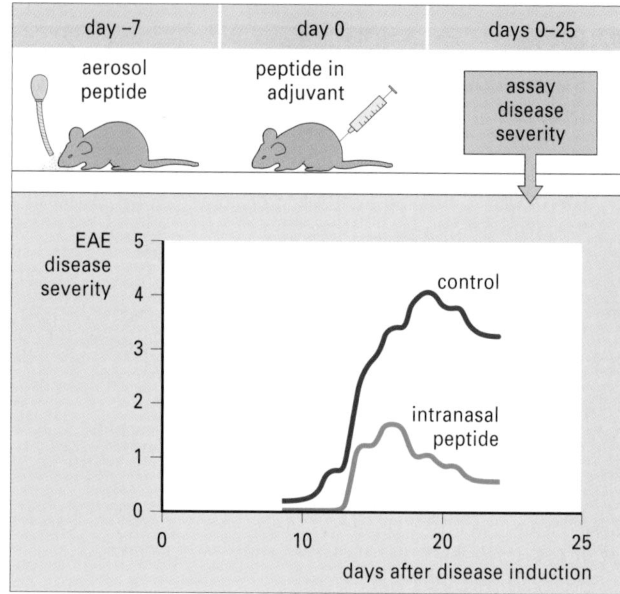

Fig. 11.2 Mice were treated with a single aerosol dose of either 100 μg peptide (residues 1–11 of myelin basic protein), or just the carrier. Seven days later the same peptide, this time in adjuvant, was administered subcutaneously. The subsequent development of EAE was significantly modified in pretreated animals.

THE ANTIGEN-PRESENTING CELL

The nature of the APC initially presenting the antigen may determine whether responsiveness or tolerance ensues. Effective activation of T cells requires the expression of co-stimulatory molecules on the surface of the APC. Thus presentation by dendritic cells or activated macrophages, which express high levels of MHC class II in addition to co-stimulatory molecules, results in highly effective T-cell activation (see *Fig. 6.19*). Furthermore, the interaction of CD40L on activated T cells with CD40 on dendritic cells is important for the high level production of IL-12 that is necessary for the generation of an effective TH1 response. However, if antigen is presented to T cells by a 'non-professional' APC that is unable to provide co-stimulation, then unresponsiveness or immune deviation results. For example, when naïve T cells are exposed to antigen by resting B cells, they fail to respond, and become tolerized. Recent experimental observations illustrate this point. It has been shown that neonatal animals are more susceptible to tolerance induction. Thus mice are resistant to the induction of EAE after administration of MBP in incomplete Freund's adjuvant during the neonatal period. This has been shown to be due to the development of a dominant TH2 response. As EAE is mediated by a TH1 response, the prior TH2 response to MBP prevents the development of the pathological response.

Peptide-induced inactivation of LCMV-specific T cells

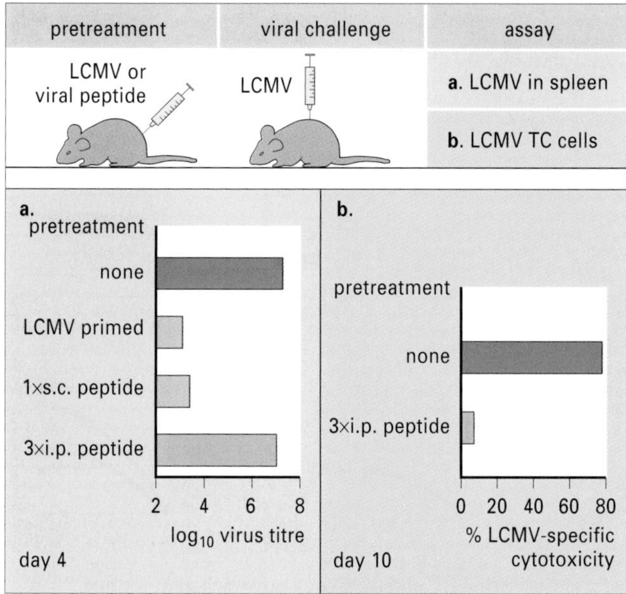

Fig. 11.3 Mice were either primed with LCMV or injected with 100 μg LCMV peptide. The peptide was given either subcutaneously (s.c.) or three times intraperitoneally (i.p.) with incomplete Freund's adjuvant. The animals were later infected with LCMV (day 0). The titre of virus in the spleen was measured on day 4. Animals that had been pretreated with subcutaneous peptide or with LCMV developed neutralizing antibody and protective immunity against the virus; animals pretreated with peptide i.p. did not develop immunity. Cytotoxic T-cell activity was assessed in the mice on day 10. Mice that had received no pretreatment demonstrated Tc cells specific for the LCMV peptide. Mice pretreated with peptide i.p. failed to show such activity.

Adjuvants may facilitate immune responses by inducing expression of high levels of MHC and co-stimulatory molecules on APCs. Their ability to activate Langerhans' cells furthermore leads to migration of these skin dendritic cells to the local draining lymph nodes where effective T-cell activation can occur. The importance of the dendritic cell in initiating a cytotoxic T lymphocyte (CTL) response is illustrated by experiments showing that newborn female mice injected with male spleen cells fail to develop a CTL response to the male antigen, H-Y. However if male dendritic cells are injected into female newborn mice, a good H-Y-specific CTL response develops.

REGULATION BY ANTIBODY

Antibody has been shown to exert feedback control on the immune response. Passive administration of IgM antibody together with an antigen specifically enhances the immune response to that antigen, whereas IgG antibody suppresses the response. This was originally shown with polyclonal antibodies, but has since been confirmed using monoclonal antibodies (*Fig. 11.4*).

The ability of passively administered antibody to enhance or suppress the immune response has certain clinical consequences and applications:

- Certain vaccines (e.g. mumps and measles) are not generally given to infants before 1 year of age. This is because levels of maternally derived IgG remain high for at least 6 months after birth; the presence of such passively acquired IgG at the time of vaccination would result in the development of an inadequate immune response in the baby.
- In cases of Rhesus (Rh) incompatibility, the administration of anti-RhD antibody to Rh^- mothers prevents primary sensitization by fetally derived Rh^+ blood cells, presumably by removing the foreign antigen (fetal erythrocytes) from the maternal circulation (see Chapter 22).

The mechanisms by which antibody modulates the immune response are not completely defined. In the case of IgM enhancing plaque-forming cells, there are thought to be two possible interpretations:

- IgM-containing immune complexes are taken up by Fc receptors or C3 receptors on APCs and are processed more efficiently than antigen alone.
- IgM-containing immune complexes stimulate an anti-idiotypic response to the IgM, which amplifies the immune response. (Idiotypic regulation is discussed below.)

Feedback control by antibody

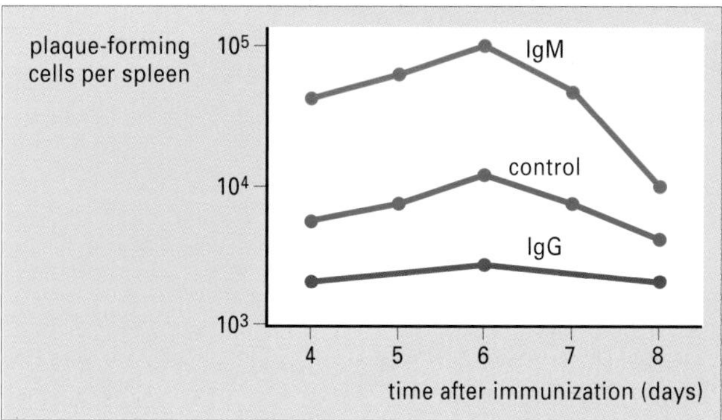

Fig. 11.4 Mice received either a monoclonal IgM anti-SRBC (sheep red blood cells), IgG anti-SRBC or medium alone (control). Two hours later, all groups were immunized with SRBC. The antibody response, measured over the following 8 days, was enhanced by IgM and suppressed by IgG.

IgG antibody can suppress specific IgG synthesis

For IgG-mediated suppression there are also various ways in which the antibody is known to act:

Antibody blocking – passively administered antibody binds antigen in competition with B cells (*Fig. 11.5*). The impact of the IgG in this case is highly dependent on the concentration of the antibody, and on its affinity for the antigen compared with the affinity of the B-cell receptors. Only high-affinity B cells compete successfully for the antigen. This mechanism is independent of the Fc portion of the antibody.

Antibody-dependent B-cell suppression

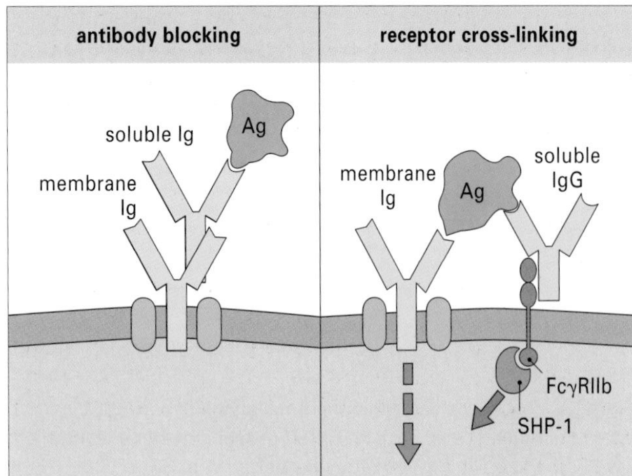

Fig. 11.5 Antibody blocking: High doses of soluble Ig block the interaction between an antigenic determinant (epitope) and membrane immunoglobulin on B cells. The B cell is then effectively unable to recognize the antigen. This receptor-blocking mechanism also prevents B-cell priming, but only antibodies which bind to the same epitope to which the B-cell's receptors bind can do this. Receptor cross-linking: Low doses of antibody allow cross-linking by antigen of a B cell's Fc receptors and its antigen receptors. The FcγRIIb receptor associates with a tyrosine phosphatase (SHP-1) which interferes with cell activation by tyrosine kinases associated with the antigen receptor. This allows B-cell priming, but inhibits antibody synthesis. Antibodies against different epitopes on the antigen can all act by this mechanism.

Antibody feedback on affinity maturation

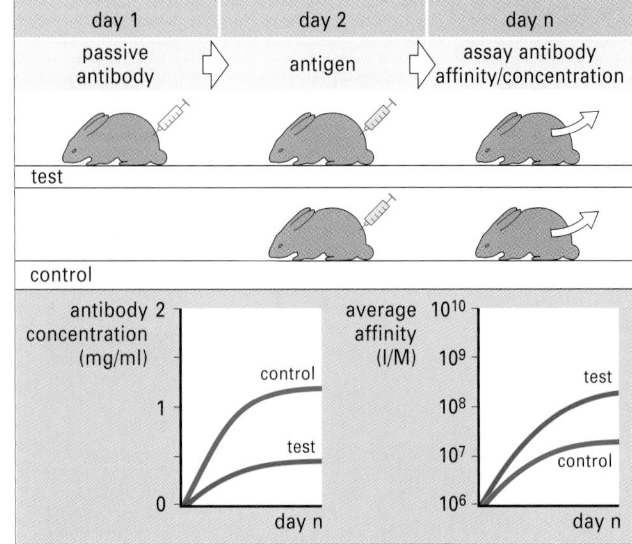

Fig. 11.6 The effect of passive antibody on the affinity and concentration of secreted antibody. One of two rabbits was injected with antibody (passive antibody) on day 1. Both rabbits were immunized with antigen on day 2 and the affinity and concentration of antibody raised to this antigen were assayed at a later time (day n). The antibody assay results show that passive antibody reduces the concentration, but increases the affinity of antibody produced.

Receptor cross-linking – IgG antibody is also known to have an effect that is Fc dependent. Experiments have demonstrated that immunoglobulin can inhibit B-cell differentiation by cross-linking the antigen receptor with the Fc receptor (FcγRIIb) on the same cell (*Fig. 11.5*). In this case, the antibodies may recognize different epitopes.

Doses of IgG that are insufficient to inhibit the production of antibodies completely have the effect of increasing the average antibody affinity; this is because only those B cells with high-affinity receptors can successfully compete with the passively acquired antibody for antigen. For this reason, antibody feedback is believed to be an important factor driving the process of affinity maturation (*Fig. 11.6*).

Immune complexes may enhance or suppress immune responses

One of the ways in which antibody (either IgM or IgG) might act to modulate the immune response involves an Fc-dependent mechanism and immune-complex formation with antigen. Immune complexes can inhibit or augment the immune response (*Fig. 11.7*). By activating complement, immune complexes may become localized via interaction with CR2 on follicular dendritic cells. This could facilitate the immune response by maintaining a source of antigen. CR2 is also expressed on B cells and, as co-ligation of CR2 with membrane IgM has been shown to activate B cells, immune complex interaction with CR2 of the B-cell–co-receptor complex and membrane Ig might lead to an enhanced specific immune response.

The immune response of patients with malignant tumours is often depressed, and it has been postulated that this is the result of the presence of circulating immune complexes composed of antibody and tumour cell antigens.

REGULATION BY LYMPHOCYTES

T cells clearly modulate the immune response in a positive sense by providing T-cell help. Furthermore, the kind of help which is generated (TH1 or TH2) affects the nature of the immune response, favouring either humoral or cell-mediated immunity. In addition, there is clear evidence that T cells are capable of downregulating immune responses (*Fig. 11.8*). Apart from the potential for TH1 and TH2 cells to regulate the immune response through an immune deviation, there is now good evidence for two further CD4$^+$ T-cell subsets, Tr1 and TH3, which are able to regulate immune responses. These differ in cytokine production; Treg or Tr1 cells make IL-10, while TH3 cells secrete high levels of TGFβ but lower levels of IL-4 and IL-10.

CD4$^+$ T cells can prevent the induction of autoimmunity

It has been shown in many experimental models of autoimmune disease that CD4$^+$ T cells can prevent the onset of disease. As mentioned previously, the route of antigen

Regulatory effects of immune complexes

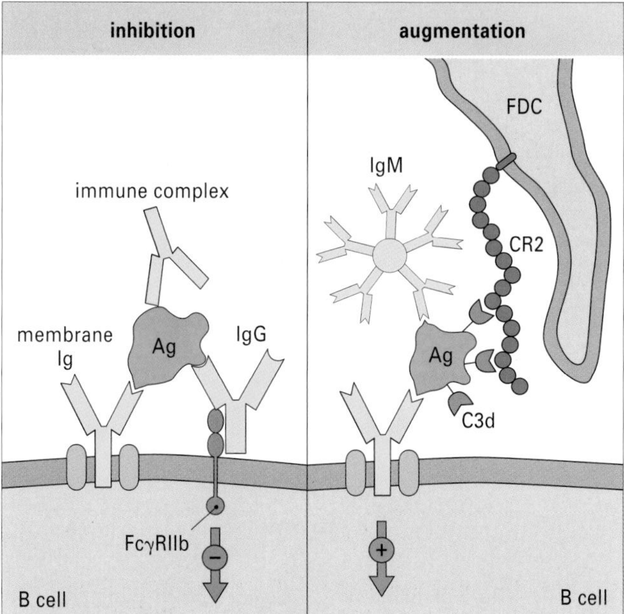

Fig. 11.7 Immune complexes can act either to inhibit or to augment an immune response. Inhibition: When the Fc receptor of the B cell is cross-linked to its antigen receptor by an antigen–antibody complex, a signal is delivered to the B cell, inhibiting it from entering the antibody production phase. Passive IgG may have this effect. Augmentation: Antibody encourages presentation of antigen to B cells when it is present on an antigen-presenting cell (APC), bound via Fc receptors or, in this case, complement receptors (CR2) on a follicular dendritic cell (FDC). Passive IgM may have this effect.

Suppressor cells in immunological tolerance

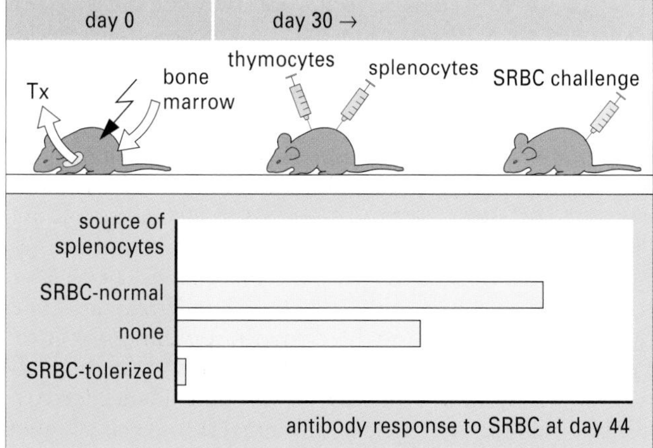

Fig. 11.8 Thymectomized and irradiated mice were reconstituted with bone marrow cells. After 30 days they were recolonized with thymocytes and splenocytes, and challenged with sheep red blood cells (SRBC). At day 44, recipients given splenocytes primed with an immunogenic dose of SRBC had made a strong response. Animals receiving no spleen cells had a moderate response. Animals receiving cells from mice tolerized to SRBC (with a high dose of antigen) did not respond, indicating that cells from tolerized animals had actively suppressed the response in the recipient.

administration and therefore the initial APC together with the nature of the antigen influence the outcome of an immune response. For example, the administration of high doses of autoantigen (often given in a soluble or deaggregated form) prevents induction of autoimmunity. Comparable observations have been made in other experimental autoimmune conditions if the antigen is given orally or as an aerosol.

This inhibition has been shown to be due to CD4$^+$ T cells which, in the case of experimentally induced autoimmune thyroid disease, have been shown to prevent both the development of autoimmune thyroiditis and autoantibodies to thyroglobulin (*Fig. 11.9*). This ability of the CD4$^+$ T cells to inhibit both autoimmune thyroiditis and autoantibody production irrespective of isotype shows that the suppression of induced autoimmunity is not attributable to an immune deviation; that is a switch from a TH1 response to a TH2 response.

Administration of a non-depleting anti-CD4 antibody at the same time as an immunogenic dose of thyroglobulin not only prevents the development of autoimmunity, but also results in the development of a population of CD4$^+$ T cells that can transfer specific tolerance to naïve recipients (*Fig. 11.10*). The exact mechanism by which these T

Transfer of tolerance by CD4$^+$ T cells

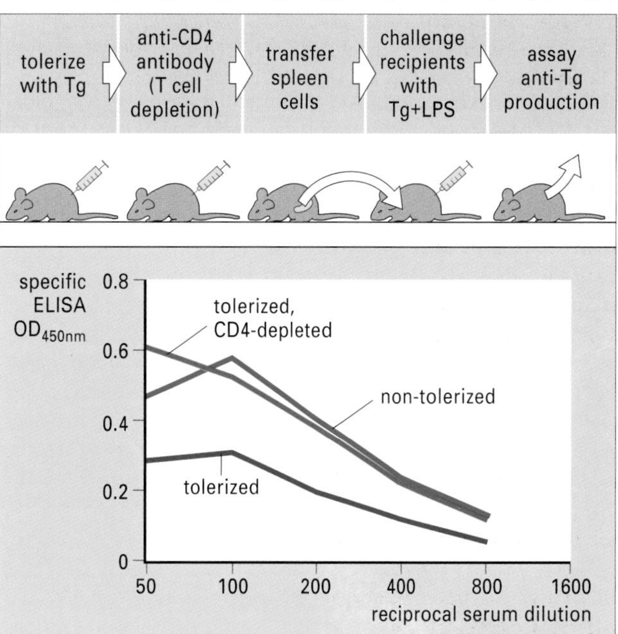

Fig. 11.9 Mice were injected intravenously with 200 μg of mouse thyroglobulin (Tg) to induce tolerance. (A control group was not tolerized.) Part of the tolerized group was further treated *in vivo* with depleting anti-CD4 antibodies, to remove CD4$^+$ T cells. For each mouse in each of these three groups (non-tolerized; tolerized; tolerized and CD4-depleted), spleen cells were transferred into an irradiated syngeneic recipient. The recipients were then challenged with mouse thyroglobulin and LPS, and their anti-Tg antibody response was assayed using ELISA (see Chapter 27). Anti-CD4 treatment removed the ability to transfer tolerance.

Anti-CD4-induced suppression of experimental allergic thyroiditis (EAT)

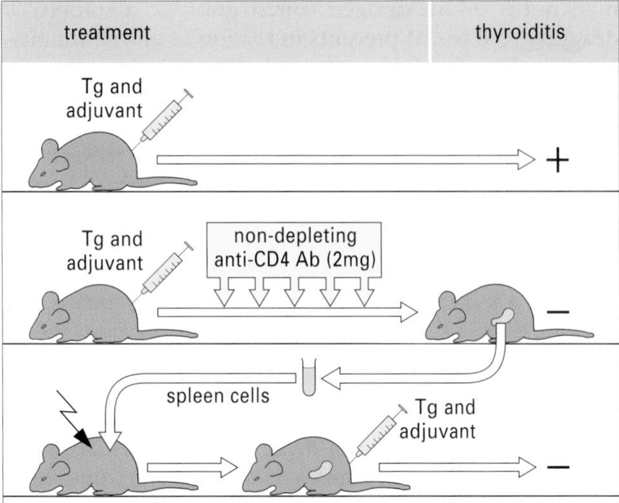

Fig. 11.10 Mice immunized with 50 μg of mouse thyroglobulin (Tg) develop thyroiditis and anti-Tg antibodies. If they are injected over a period of 11 days with a non-depleting monoclonal anti-CD4 antibody to block CD4–class II interaction, thyroiditis does not occur. Splenocytes transferred from these treated animals prevent irradiated recipients from developing thyroiditis after immunization with Tg. (Immunized mice that have received control T cells develop thyroiditis.)

Regulation of TH1 response by IL-12

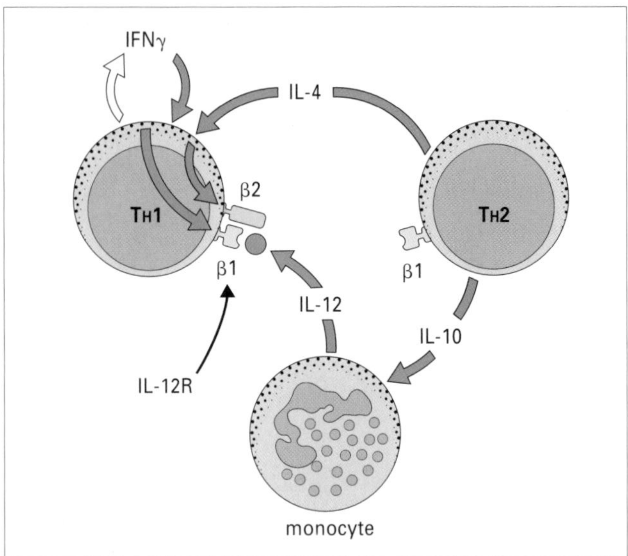

Fig. 11.11 The high-affinity IL-12 receptor consisting of the β1 and β2 chains is only expressed on TH1 cells. IL-12 released by mononuclear phagocytes promotes the development and activation of TH1 cells, but IL-12 production is inhibited by IL-10, released by TH2 cells. IFNγ from TH1 cells promotes production of the β1 chain and thus production of the high-affinity IL-12 receptor. However, this is inhibited by IL-4.

cells exert such a negative influence is not entirely clear but recent experimental results suggest an involvement of TGFβ and IL-10 in this suppression.

TH cell subsets are involved in the regulation of immunoglobulin production

The production of different cytokines by different TH ($CD4^+$) lymphocyte subpopulations probably provides an explanation for certain observations regarding the regulation of IgE synthesis. Cross-regulation of TH subsets has been demonstrated whereby cytokines such as interferon-γ (IFNγ), secreted by TH1 cells, can inhibit the responsiveness of TH2 cells (see *Fig. 7.13*). In addition, IL-10 produced by TH2 cells downregulates B7 and IL-12 expression by APCs, which in turn inhibits TH1 activation. IL-12 is important in the development of TH1 responses and the TH1/TH2 balance is modulated both by the level of expression of IL-12 and by expression of the IL-12 receptor. The high-affinity IL-12R is composed of two chains, β1 and β2, with both chains being expressed only in TH1 cells. Both TH1 and TH2 cells express the β1 chain and expression of the β2 chain is induced by IFNγ and inhibited by IL-4 (*Fig. 11.11*). T-cell subset development has also been shown to be influenced by IFNα, which favours TH1 development, even in the presence of IL-4 and neutralization of IL-12. Thus the preferential activation of TH1 or TH2 cells may result in an immune deviation – the selection of a particular type of effector response. The selective biasing of responses may prove useful in the treatment of autoimmune diseases and of allergy.

$CD8^+$ T cells can transfer resistance and tolerance

$CD8^+$ T cells have also been shown to regulate immune responses. $CD8^+$ T cells have been found in the spleens of animals tolerized to MBP by oral dosing of the antigen (see above). These cells can adoptively transfer resistance to EAE *in vivo*. The T cells not only suppress T-cell responses to MBP *in vitro*, but also perform bystander suppression of other unrelated autoantigens in the brain. This effect is thought to be mediated by TGFβ.

Regulation of the immune response by $CD4^+$ T cells is a normal physiological process

The role of such $CD4^+$ or $CD8^+$ T-cell-mediated regulatory effects in normal physiology has been questioned. However, the observation that $CD4^+$ T cells which are able to prevent autoimmunity are present in unmanipulated normal animals supports their importance in homeostasis. Peripheral T-cell lymphopenia can lead to the development of autoimmune disease. Experiments suggest that a subpopulation of T-helper cells expressing high levels of CD25 and low levels of CD45RB play a role in regulating the immune responses and maintaining peripheral tolerance to self antigens. For example it has been shown that $CD25^+CD4^+CD45RB^{Lo}$ expressing cells are able to regulate colitis. Transfer of $CD4^+CD45RB^{Hi}$ cells alone into severe combined immune deficient (SCID) mice causes colitis whereas co-transfer of $CD4^+CD45RB^{Lo}$ cells prevents the development of colitis in recipient SCID mice. Prevention of colitis by these cells is in part due to IL-10 production (*Fig. 11.12*). This role for IL-10 in the

Prevention of colitis induced in SCID mice by cytokines

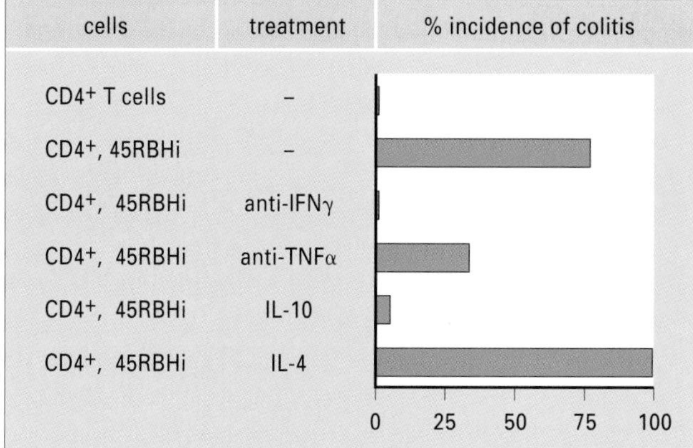

Fig. 11.12 The table shows the incidence of colitis in mice treated by transfer of different cell populations. Mice receiving unfractionated $CD4^+$ T cells are prevented from developing colitis. If they receive fractionated CD4 cells expressing high levels of CD45RB ($CD45RB^{hi}$), colitis develops. However, if the animals were also given either anti-IFNγ or anti-TNFα, then the incidence of disease was reduced. IL-10 (but not IL-4) also modulates disease in these animals. These data suggest that IFNγ and TNFα are involved in the development of colitis, and that IL-10 can switch off the effector cells.

regulation of inflammatory bowel disease (IBD) is supported by the observation that treatment of recipient mice with anti-IL-10R antibody abrogates the ability of $CD4^+CD45RB^{Lo}$ cells to prevent the development of colitis. These observations were subsequently confirmed using IL-10 knockout mice, which failed to control disease (see *Fig. 12.17*). This T-cell population which regulates the development of IBD by production of IL-10 has been termed a Treg cell or Tr1 cell. TGFβ is required for the development of these regulatory T cells. Recent experiments indicate that Treg cells constitutively express CTLA-4, a molecule associated with negative regulation of T-cell activation.

The spontaneous development of IBD in IL-10 knockout and TGFβ knockout mice is consistent with a role for these cytokines in the function of the regulatory T cells. Furthermore, the spontaneous development of multi-organ infiltrates and uncontrolled lymphocyte activation in CTLA-4 knockout mice supports a key role for this molecule in immunoregulation.

REGULATION BY NK AND NK T CELLS

Natural killer (NK) cells make cytokines and chemokines and thus play an important role in the innate immune response to infections and tumours. Their production of immunoregulatory cytokines and chemokines at early stages in the immune response influences the characteristics of the subsequent adaptive immune response and thus can influence the outcome of the immune response. These cells play a key role in the early immune response to intracellular pathogens, largely through their production of IFNγ which activates macrophages and facilitates differentiation of TH1 cells. NK cell activity itself is induced by a variety of cytokines including IFNα/β, IL-15, IL-18 and IL-12. NK cells in turn are negatively regulated by cytokines such as IL-10 and TGFβ.

In the mouse, NK T cells produce cytokines when their TCR engages glycolipids in association with CD1d. It has been suggested that these cells play an immunoregulatory role in the control of autoimmunity, parasite infection and tumour cell growth. Recent experiments suggest that NK T cells secreting IFNγ are able to induce NK cell activation, increasing both NK proliferation and cytotoxicity. They are known to to be capable of making IL-4 and IFNγ. Whether they make IL-4 or IFNγ is dependent on the cytokines present in the microenvironment when they are activated. The presence of IL-7, for example, has been shown to elicit IL-4 production in NK T cells and thus promote a TH2 response. This ability to make IL-4, particularly in the thymus, has been associated with the prevention of autoimmunity. For example, non-obese diabetic (NOD) mice have a deficit in NK T cells, and injection of NK T cells into this mouse strain has been shown to prevent the spontaneous development of autoimmune diabetes.

REGULATION BY LOCALIZATION OF CELLS

The spatial and temporal production of chemokines by different cell types is an important mechanism of immune regulation. There is good evidence to suggest that recruitment of TH1 and TH2 cells is differentially controlled thus ensuring the maintenance of locally polarized immune responses. The expression of different chemokine receptors on TH1 cells (CXCR3 and CCR5) and TH2 cells (CCR3,CCR4, CCR8) allows chemotactic signals to produce the differential localization of T-cell subsets to sites of inflammation (see *Fig. 3.7*). Since chemokines can be induced by cytokines released at sites of inflammation, this provides a mechanism for local reinforcement of particular types of response (*Fig. 11.13*). Once a response is established the T cells can induce the further migration of appropriate effector cells. This is clearly illustrated in TH1 responses where the secondary production of MCP-1, MIP-1α, IP-10 and RANTES serves to focus mononuclear phagocytes to the area of inflammation. The ability of cytokines such as TGFβ, IL-12 and IL-4 to influence chemokine or chemokine receptor expression provides a further level of control on cell migration or recruitment.

Several viruses have been shown to evade the host immune reponse by interfering with the chemokine/ chemokine receptor interactions which are pivotal for an effective inflammatory response. They do this by making chemokine receptor antagonists or chemokine receptor homologues which serve to either blockade chemokine receptors or neutralize chemokine activity .

Immune responses do not normally occur at certain sites in the body such as the anterior chamber of the eye and the testes. These sites are called immune privileged. The failure to evoke immune responses in these sites is partly due to the presence of inhibitory cytokines such

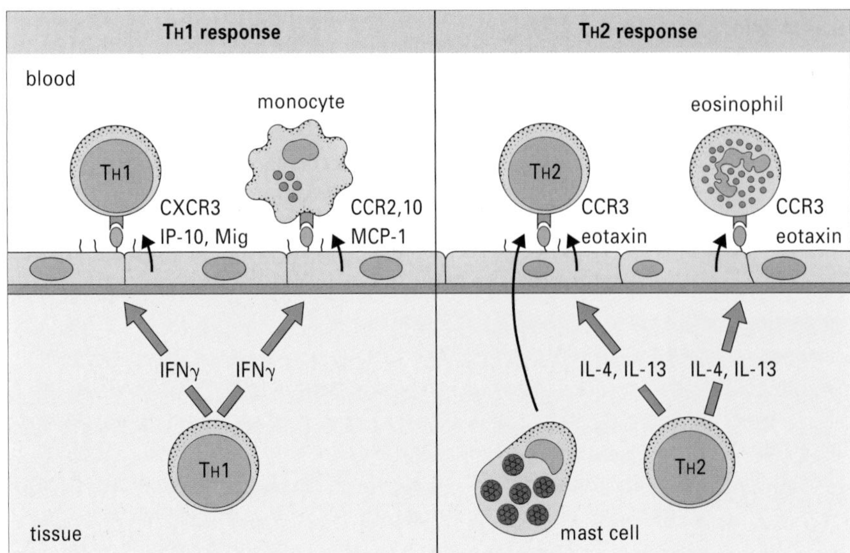

Fig. 11.13 Activated TH1 cells release IFNγ, which induces the chemokines IP-10 and Mig. These act on the chemokine receptors CXCR3 which are selectively expressed on TH1 cells, thereby reinforcing this type of response. MCP-1 which attracts macrophages and monocytes is also induced by IFNγ. Mast cells release eotaxin when activated, and endothelial cells and bronchial epithelium can also synthesize this chemokine in response to IL-4 and IL-13 from TH2 cells. Eotaxin acts on CCR3 which is selectively expressed on TH2 cells, thereby reinforcing the TH2 response. Eosinophils and basophils, which mediate allergic responses in airways, also express CCR3. Thus chemokines can potentiate both the initiation and effector phases of a specific type of immune response.

as TGFβ and IL-10 which will inhibit inflammatory responses. The presence of migration inhibition factor (MIF) in the anterior chamber of the eye would furthermore inhibit NK activity. The constitutive expression of FasL in cells of the testes and the eye has additionally been proposed as a means of eliminating Fas-expressing lymphocytes that reach these sites, through apoptosis.

IDIOTYPIC MODULATION OF RESPONSES

Tolerance to self antigens is established during ontogeny (see Chapter 12). However, during the neonatal period the unique binding regions of antigen-specific receptors on B and T cells are present at levels that are too low to generate tolerance. Similarly, although antibodies are present in the serum, tolerance only develops to their Fc portions because only these are present in sufficient concentration; tolerance does not develop to the unique determinants in the heavy and light chains that determine antigen-binding specificity. Individual T-cell receptors and immunoglobulins are therefore immunogenic by virtue of these unique sequences, known as idiotypes. Antibodies formed against these antigen-binding sites are called anti-idiotypic antibodies, and are capable of influencing the outcome of an immune response.

Idiotypic determinants may be encoded in the germ line V region genes, or they may be generated by the process of recombination and mutation involved in producing functional V-region elements (see Chapter 4). Immunogenic epitopes in or around the binding site are termed idiotopes (*Fig. 11.14*). Jerne proposed that an immune network existed within the body which interacted by means of idiotype recognition. According to this proposition, when an antibody response is induced by antigen, this antibody will in turn evoke an anti-idiotypic response to itself. This hypothesis is conceptually interesting, but

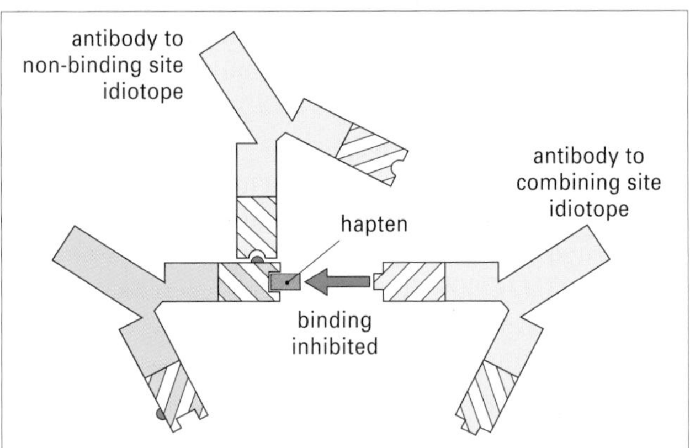

Fig. 11.14 An anti-idiotype serum may contain antibodies directed to various sites on the immunoglobulin molecule. Those associated with the combining site are site-associated idiotopes. Binding to these can be inhibited by hapten. Antibodies to non-binding-site idiotopes (non-site-associated) are not inhibited by hapten.

the role of such an idiotype network in controlling a normal immune response remains unclear.

Idiotypic interactions may enhance or suppress antibody responses

There is good evidence that anti-idiotypes can affect the representation of recognized idiotypes in an immune response. For example, when C57Bl/6 strain mice are challenged with the hapten, nitrophenyl (NP), they produce antibodies that are largely restricted to a few defined idiotypes, for example the idiotype 146. Anti-idiotype to this antibody (idiotype 146) can enhance or suppress

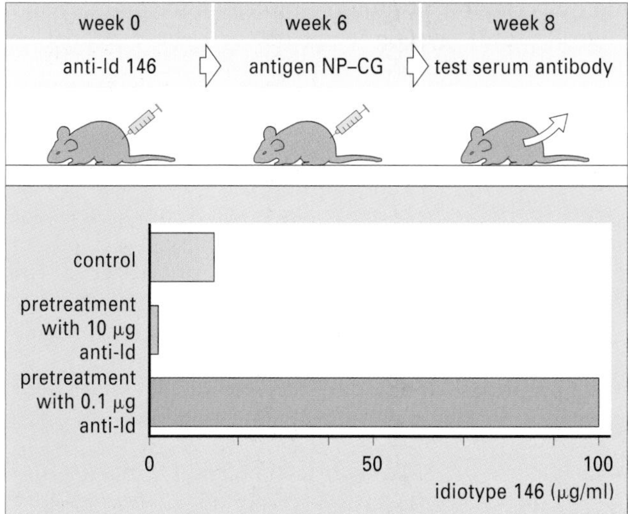

Fig. 11.15 Mice were injected at time 0 with either 10 μg or 0.1 μg of anti-idiotype (anti-Id) to the nitrophenyl (NP)-binding antibody, 146. The animals were then challenged 6 weeks later with NP on the carrier, chicken globulin (CG). Two weeks later, the serum titres of idiotype 146 (bar diagram), and total anti-NP (not shown) were assayed. Mice pretreated with 10 μg anti-Id showed suppression of idiotype 146, while mice treated with 0.1 μg showed enhanced production of idiotype 146, although the overall levels of anti-NP were similar in both groups.

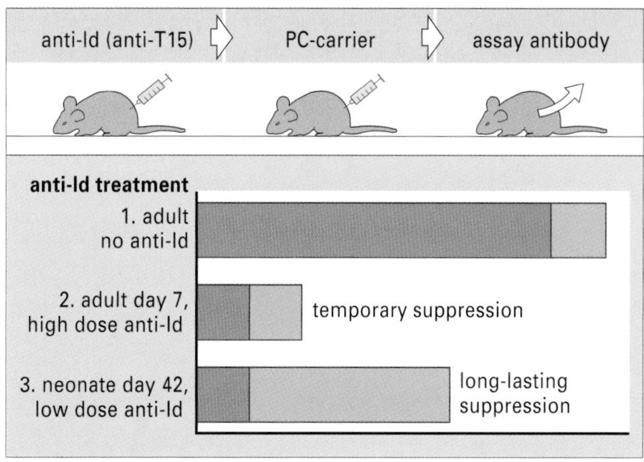

Fig. 11.16 Mice were pretreated with anti-idiotype to T15, either during the neonatal period or as adults. They were subsequently immunized with the hapten phosphoryl choline (PC) coupled to a carrier. The total antibody to PC was measured, together with the T15 component of the response (darker area). Normal adult mice make a good response to PC that is dominated by T15 (**1**). Adult mice pretreated with anti-idiotype are temporarily suppressed with the loss of the T15 component, accounting for the reduction in the total anti-PC response (**2**). Mice treated with anti-idiotype in the neonatal period undergo long-term suppression of their $T15^+$ B cells, but generate $T15^-$ PC-specific cells to compensate (**3**).

the production of idiotype 146 when the mice are subsequently challenged with NP on a carrier protein. The observed effect depends on the amount of anti-idiotype given (*Fig. 11.15*) and is idiotype specific, as the overall level of anti-NP antibody is hardly affected. Most importantly, the amounts of anti-idiotype used are within the normal physiological range for particular idiotype-bearing antibodies, which suggests that idiotypic regulation may occur *in vivo*. This kind of observation has been made in other idiotypic systems.

Dramatic effects are observed when anti-idiotype is administered neonatally, when the effect may be lifelong. For example, the ability of neonatal mice to mount an anti-phosphoryl choline response is greatly reduced after being injected with anti-idiotype to T15 (T15 is a major idiotype in the response to phosphoryl choline). The reduction lasts many months. The response which these mice subsequently make is dominated by non-T15 immunoglobulins (*Fig. 11.16*).

NEUROENDOCRINE MODULATION OF IMMUNE RESPONSES

It has long been known that stressful conditions may lead to a suppression of immune functions, for example reducing the ability to recover from infection. There is considerable evidence demonstrating that the nervous, endocrine and immune systems are interconnected (*Fig. 11.17*). Broadly, there are two main routes by which events occurring in the CNS could modulate immune function:

- Most lymphoid tissues receive direct sympathetic innervation, both to the blood vessels passing through the tissues, and directly to the lymphocytes themselves.
- The nervous system directly or indirectly controls the output of various hormones, in particular corticosteroids, growth hormone, prolactin, α-MSH, thyroxine and adrenaline.

Lymphocytes express receptors for many hormones, neurotransmitters and neuropeptides, including ones for steroids, catecholamines (adrenaline and noradrenaline), enkephalins, endorphins, substance P and vasoactive intestinal peptide (VIP). Expression and responsiveness vary between different lymphocyte and monocyte populations, such that the effect of different transmitters may vary in different circumstances. However, one particularly important control is mediated by corticosteroids, endorphins and enkephalins, all of which may be released during stress, and all of which are immunosuppressive *in vivo*. The precise *in vitro* effects of endorphins vary greatly, depending on the system and on the doses used; some levels are suppressive, and others enhance immune functions. It is certain, however, that the corticosteroids act as a major feedback control on immune responses. It has been found that lymphocytes themselves can respond to corticotrophin releasing factor to generate their own ACTH, which in turn induces corticosteroid release.

Corticosteroids have been shown to inhibit TH1 cytokine production while sparing TH2 responses. Corticosteroids

Neuroendocrine interactions with the immune system

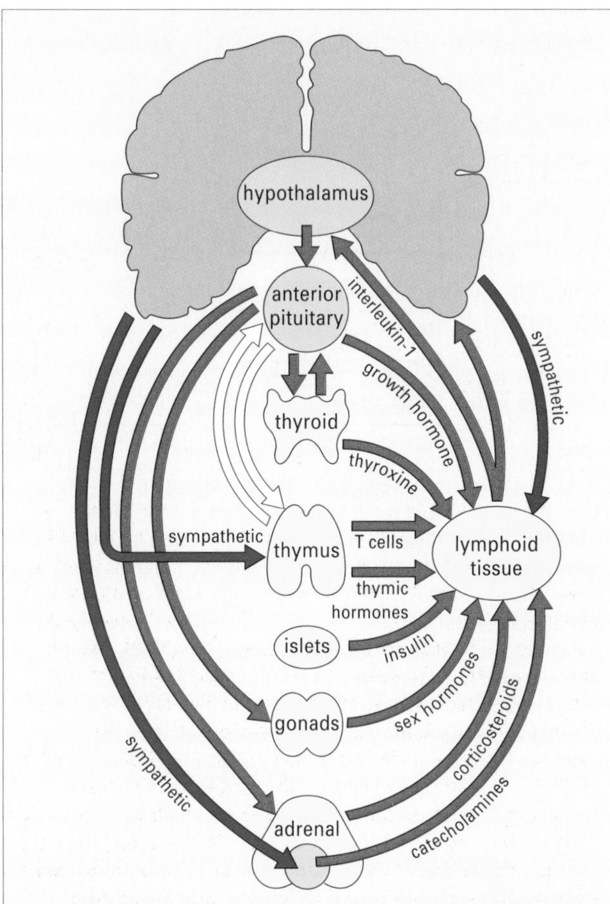

Fig. 11.17 The diagram indicates some of the potential connections between the endocrine, nervous and immune systems. Blue arrows indicate nervous connections, red arrows indicate hormonal interactions, and white arrows indicate postulated connections for which the effector molecules have not been established.

have also been shown to induce the production of TGFβ, which in turn may inhibit the immune response. The low levels of plasma corticosteroids found in Lewis rats are believed to contribute to the susceptibility of this strain to a variety of induced autoimmune conditions: after induction of EAE in this strain, spontaneous recovery is associated with an increase in corticosteroid levels. Moreover, adrenalectomy prevents recovery. The importance of steroids in the overall susceptibility to disease induction is further demonstrated in PVG rats – rats of this strain are normally resistant to EAE, but become susceptible if adrenalectomized.

The interplay between the neuroendocrine system and the immune system is not just unidirectional. Cytokines, in particular IL-1 and IL-6, have been shown to have a role as bidirectional modulators of neuroendocrine–immune communication. These cytokines are potent stimulators of adrenal corticosteroid production through their influence on corticotrophin-releasing hormone (CRH). In addition to the production of IL-1 by macrophages and of IL-6 by T cells, both IL-1 and IL-6 are synthesized by neurons and glial cells and, in addition, by cells in the pituitary and adrenal glands, further emphasizing their potential as bidirectional mediators in response to stress.

GENETIC CONTROL OF IMMUNE RESPONSES

Familial patterns of susceptibility to infectious agents have suggested that resistance or susceptibility might be an inherited characteristic. Such patterns of resistance and susceptibility are also shown with autoimmune diseases. Often many genes are involved in governing susceptibility or resistance to disease and the disease is thus said to be under polygenic control. Considerable advances have been made in mapping and in some cases identifying the genes governing the response to some of the diseases. This has been largely due to the development and use of techniques such as microsatellite mapping and the availability of a large number of DNA samples from susceptible and resistant individuals. In most cases these studies have led to the identification of potential candidate genes but their real role in disease susceptibility remains to be clarified. In other cases single mutations in genes of known function have been found and the mechanism by which they contribute to disease identified.

There are several ways in which genes influence the immune response.

MHC haplotypes influence the ability to respond to an antigen

With the development of inbred mouse strains, it became possible to analyse genetic influences more rigorously and it was conclusively demonstrated that genetic factors have a role in determining immune responsiveness. For example, strains of mice with different MHC haplotypes vary in their ability to mount an antibody response to specific antigens (*Fig. 11.18*). This function depends on MHC class II molecules, and is specific for each antigen – a high-responder strain for some antigens will be a low-responder strain for others. It was shown furthermore that genes within the MHC (see Chapters 5 and 6) play a fundamental part in influencing the response against infectious agents.

MHC-linked immune response genes control all immune responses that involve antigen recognition by T cells

As discussed in previous chapters, the immune response depends upon the activation of clones of lymphocytes. In the case of T cells, these recognize antigen only when it is presented to them as peptide complexed to class I or class II major histocompatibility (MHC) antigens. For example, $CD8^+$ T-cytotoxic (TC) cells will only lyse virally infected target cells derived from an MHC class I-matched mouse strain (see *Fig. 5.19*). Genetic restriction can be tracked to specific MHC molecules from one particular locus. For example, in the cytotoxic response of A.TL mice to LCMV virus, the cytotoxic T cells are principally directed against H–2D locus targets. However, Sendai virus in this strain is presented more effectively by other MHC class I

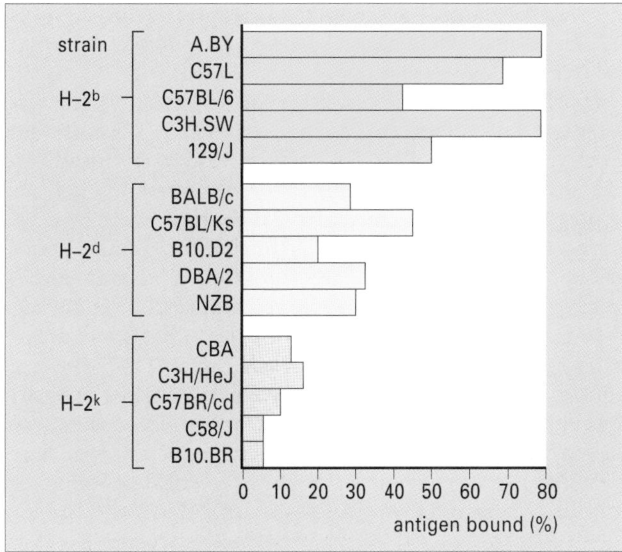

Fig. 11.18 Fifteen strains of mice were given a standard dose of the synthetic antigen (TG)-A-L. Antibody responses are expressed as the antigen-binding capacity of the sera. Animals of the H–2[b] haplotype are high responders, H–2[d] are intermediate and H–2[k] are low responders. However, there is some overlap between the levels of response in different haplotypes, indicating that H-2-linked genes are not the only ones controlling the antibody response.

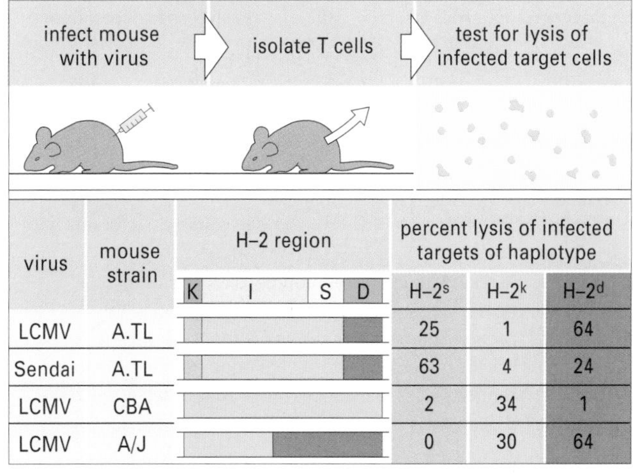

virus	mouse strain	H-2 region (K I S D)	percent lysis of infected targets of haplotype H–2[s]	H–2[k]	H–2[d]
LCMV	A.TL		25	1	64
Sendai	A.TL		63	4	24
LCMV	CBA		2	34	1
LCMV	A/J		0	30	64

Fig. 11.19 The Tc cells of virus-infected adult mice (strains A.TL, CBA and A/J) were tested for their ability to kill virus-infected target cells with haplotypes H–2[k], H–2[s] and H–2[d]. The strain A.TL is H–2K[s], H–2I[k] and H–2D[d], and its cells kill target cells infected with lymphocytic choriomeningitis virus (LCMV) only if the targets share the H–2K[s] or the H–2D[d] haplotypes. This shows that the antiviral cytotoxic T cells are class I-restricted. (Note that the cytotoxicity to LCMV is determined mostly by the H–2D locus). By comparison, in A.TL mice infected with Sendai virus, the cytotoxicity is principally determined by the H–2[k] locus. Infection of CBA mice with LCMV confirms the importance of genetic restriction in these responses. The infection of A/J mice with LCM confirms the finding that cytotoxicity to LCMV is strongest to the H–2[d]-matched infected targets. Different viruses may associate preferentially with particular H–2[k] or H–2[d] MHC molecules to present a target for cytotoxic cells.

molecules (*Fig. 11.19*); MHC restricted recognition is learnt in the thymus during ontogeny (see *Fig. 12.4*).

As will be explained in Chapter 12, T cells are subjected to two selection processes during development in the thymus – positive and negative selection (see *Fig. 12.3*). The peripheral T-cell repertoire is influenced both by the range of self antigens presented in the thymus and in the periphery, and by their ability to bind to the individual's MHC antigens (see *Figs 12.9* and *12.10*). The ability of peptide to bind to MHC is determined by the amino acid sequences in the binding sites of the MHC molecules. We now know that most of the polymorphic residues in MHC molecules reside in the peptide-binding groove. Thus the extensive sequence polymorphism of MHC molecules has a deep impact on peptide binding and, as a consequence, on T-cell activation.

MHC-linked genes control the response to infections

MHC-linked genes have been shown to play a part in the immune response to infectious agents. In some cases the gene involved is the MHC gene itself, but in others it is believed to be a gene that is simply linked to the MHC.

Susceptibility to infection by Trichinella spiralis is affected by the I–E locus in mice

The first observation that genes (*Ts-1* and *Ts-2*) within the MHC could influence the response to parasites involved the susceptibility to *Trichinella spiralis*. (It is interesting that such an effect should be noted with an antigenically complex organism, especially as these parasites express different antigens at different stages in their life cycle, with different APCs being involved in their presentation.) If different recombinant mouse strains are infected with *T. spiralis*, it can be seen that resistance or susceptibility is affected by the I–E locus. Mouse strains that express I–E appear to be susceptible (*Fig. 11.20*). An additional MHC-linked gene has been shown to influence the response to *T. spiralis*; in this case it is not an MHC-encoded gene, but another gene in linkage disequilibrium. This gene, which has been designated *Ts-2*, maps close to the TNF genes.

The I–E locus also influences susceptibility to Leishmania donovani

Using H–2 congenic mice, it was shown that I–E-expressing mice were unable to combat visceral leishmaniasis. Direct involvement of the I–E product in this susceptibility was shown by the ability of anti-I–E antibody, but not the anti-I–A antibody, to enhance parasite clearance. Furthermore, insertion of an I–E transgene into a mouse strain lacking I–E makes them unable to clear parasites from the liver and spleen as effectively as the original strain.

Certain HLA haplotypes confer protection from infection

In humans, a comparison of the HLA haplotypes revealed

Susceptibility to *Trichinella spiralis*

mouse strain	H–2 haplotype	I–E expression	resistance index	resistance phenotype
B10.BR	k	+	0	sus
B10.P	p	+	–22	sus
B10.RIII	r	+	33	sus
B10	b	–	63	res/int
B10.S	s	–	100	res
B10.M	f	–	104	res
B10.Q	q	–	105	res

Fig. 11.20 Association of H–2 haplotype, expression of cell-surface I–E molecules, and susceptibility to infection with *Trichinella spiralis.* The resistance index is measured as number of parasites present after a constant challenge, relative to strains B10.BR (susceptible = 0% resistance) and B10.S (resistant = 100% resistance). B10 shows intermediate resistance.

that certain MHC class I and class II alleles (HLA-B*5301 and DRB1*1302, respectively) were associated with a reduced risk of severe malaria. DRB1*1302 has been shown to bind peptides different from those bound by DRB1*1301, as a result of a single amino acid difference in the β chain. This would clearly influence the response to the malaria parasite. HLA-DRB1*1302 has also been associated with an increased clearance of the hepatitis B virus and hence a decreased risk of chronic liver disease.

In human T-lymphotropic virus-1 (HTLV-1) infection, the MHC class I type, HLA-A*02, is associated with a reduction in the risk of disease development. The viral load was lower in HLA-A*02 positive healthy carriers of HTLV-1 correlating with the presence of high levels of virus-specific cytotoxic T cells. In HIV-1 infection a selective advantage against disease has been noted in individuals expressing maximal HLA heterozygosity of class I loci (A, B and C) and lacking expression of HLA-B*35 and HLA-Cw*04.

Protection is not necessarily related to the class I and II molecules. For example, tumour necrosis factor-α (TNFα) lies within the MHC and polymorphisms in the promoter region of this gene influence its level of expression possibly through altered binding of the transcription factor, OCT-1. One of these polymorphisms, which is commonly associated with cerebral malaria, results in high levels of TNF expression which may lead to upregulation of ICAM-1 on vascular endothelium and to increased adherence of infected erythrocytes and subsequent blockage of blood flow. This polymorphism in the TNFα promoter has also been associated with lepromatous but not tuberculous leprosy and with mucocutaneous leishmaniasis and death from meningococcal disease.

MHC genes have a major influence on susceptibility to autoimmune diseases

Insulin-dependent diabetes mellitus (IDDM), an autoimmune disease in which the beta cells of the pancreas are destroyed by cells of the immune system, is associated with HLA-DR3 and HLA-DR4. The highest risk is in fact seen in HLA-DR3/4 heterozygotes. Because of linkage disequilibrium, although the original associations were seen with DR, they are in reality with DQ. Molecular genetic analysis has permitted the association to be analysed in more detail, and it seems that the primary association in Caucasians is with DQB1*0302. In multiple sclerosis the initial association with HLA-DR2 in Northern Europeans appears to relate to the extended haplotype DQB1*0602–DQA1*0102–DRB1*1501. Interestingly however there are different risk haplotypes in Southern Europeans. This suggests that different environmental risk factors interact with particular MHC molecules in each population. In rheumatoid arthritis, the predominant association is with HLA-DR4 or DR1 in several ethnic groups, but there is little association with HLA-DQ. *Figure 11.21* provides examples of MHC linkages to autoimmune disease. The way in which these MHC associations contribute to disease susceptibility remains unclear, but possible explanations include repertoire differences through positive and negative selection on different class II genes, or preferential binding of disease-inducing epitopes of bacteria or viruses to particular MHC molecules. Analysis of the amino acid sequences of peptide binding grooves of HLA-DR4 and DR1 has supported this hypothesis by demonstrating the presence of differently charged residues in susceptible or resistant subtypes of HLA-DR.

The NOD mouse spontaneously develops IDDM and as in humans the development of this autoimmune disease is under polygenic control, with MHC-linked genes playing a major role in determining resistance or susceptibility.

MHC associations and autoimmune disease

disease	HLA allele	relative risk
Ankylosing spondylitis	B27	90–100
Dermatitis herpetiformis	DR3	56
IDDM	DR3/4 DR3 DR4	25 5 5
Myasthenia gravis	DR3	5
Multiple sclerosis	DR2 DQ6	4 12
Pemphigus vulgaris	DR4	14
Psoriasis	Cw6	13
RA	DR4	4
SLE	DR2/3	5
Sjögren's syndrome	Dw3	6

Fig. 11.21 Relative risk is defined as the probability of a disease developing in individuals with a particular HLA allele(s) versus individuals lacking those HLA alleles and is calculated by dividing the frequency of the HLA allele in the patient population by the frequency in the whole population. Values given are for Caucasian populations – different populations may have different risk genes, and values may vary considerably between different studies.

Effect of MHC encoding transgenes on the development of diabetes

transgene	incidence of IDDM (%)*
none	80
Ead	0
Abg7 asp (Ser → Asp57)	15
Abg7 pro (His → Pro56)	0

Fig. 11.22 The non-obese diabetic (NOD) mouse normally has a high incidence of insulin-dependent diabetes (80%). Insertion of transgenes for the class II molecule H–2EA[d] prevents diabetes. Mutation of the H–2A gene at positions 55 or 56 also drastically reduces disease susceptibility.

TNFα and lupus nephritis

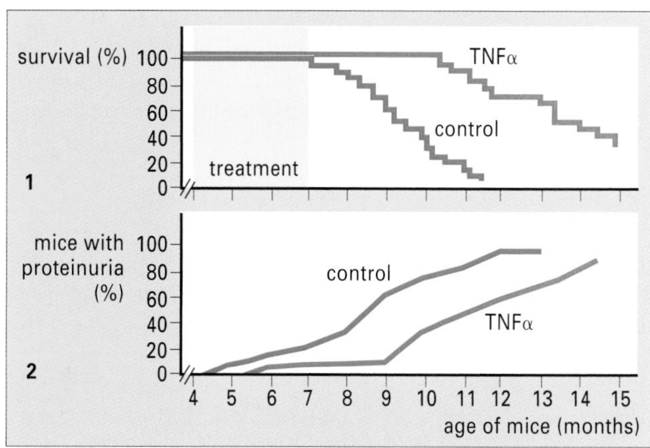

Fig. 11.23 (**1**) Twenty (NZB × NZW) F_1 female mice were treated with recombinant murine TNFα. Their survival is compared with age- and sex-matched F_1 controls. (**2**) Cumulative frequency of significant proteinuria (≥300 mg/dl) in (NZB × NZW) F_1 mice treated with TNFα, and in controls.

This mouse strain does not express an H–2E molecule and expresses an unusual H–2A heterodimer, I-A^{g7}, comprising Aα^{d} and Aβ^{g7}. While most mouse H–2Aβ chains have an aspartate at position 57 and a proline at position 56, the NOD H–2β chain contains a serine and a histidine at these respective positions. Transgenic NOD mice expressing mutated H–2A^{g7} where the *Abg7* gene has been mutated to encode an aspartate at position 57 or a proline at position 56 have markedly reduced incidence of IDDM. Additionally restoration of H–2E expression through transgenesis also prevents IDDM (*Fig. 11.22*). The crystal structure of this diabetes-associated class II molecule has recently been solved. This shows clearly that peptide binding preferences are different between NOD class II molecules and those of many other strains. Such a difference in peptide binding would have profound implications for central tolerance and peripheral T-cell activation.

The ability of H–2E to influence the development of autoimmunity is not just restricted to IDDM. Alterations in levels of H–2E expression either through transgenesis or through use of recombinant mouse strains has been shown to reduce the incidence of SLE-like disease. This effect of H–2E expression has been attributed to an excessive generation of H–2Eα peptides which compete with self peptides for binding to H–2A.

Genes in linkage disequilibrium with MHC influence the development of autoimmunity

NZB × NZW F1 mice spontaneously develop systemic lupus erythematosus (SLE). Disease development is under complex genetic control but one gene has been linked to the H–2^{z} of the NZW parent. It has been clearly demonstrated that this association was not with an MHC gene itself, but with the closely linked *Tnfa* gene. The NZW *Tnfa* allele gives rise to the production of low amounts of TNFα. If the concentration of this cytokine is increased, the mice are protected from the development of lupus nephritis (*Fig. 11.23*).

Associations with genes involved in processing

Other MHC-linked genes have recently been identified which may influence immune responses. These genes are involved in the generation (by proteolysis) and transport of antigen peptide fragments. They are polymorphic, and such polymorphism has functional consequences. For example, in the rat, different allelic forms of the *cim* locus (encoding TAP2 protein) affect peptide loading into the class I MHC, which in turn affects the ability of the class I MHC molecule to be recognized as an alloantigen. It is therefore possible that some of the MHC-linked disease associations that have been identified are attributable to similar genes, involved in proteolysis and transport of antigen peptides to the MHC molecules for presentation to cells of the immune system.

Many non-MHC genes also modulate immune responses

The immune response is also governed by some genes outside the MHC region. However, these genes are generally less polymorphic than MHC genes and they make a lesser contribution to variations in disease susceptibility in a population than do the MHC genes. Nevertheless, their effects have been clearly shown in autoimmune diseases, allergy and infection. For example:

- Individuals with defects in the complement components C1q, C1r, C1s are predisposed to develop SLE and lupus nephritis. Deficiency in C3 leads to an increased susceptibility to bacterial infections and a predisposition to immune-complex disease as does deficiency in C2 and C4, both of which are located within the MHC region. The development of SLE-like symptoms in C1q knockout mice parallels the human situation.
- High IgE production in some allergy-prone families has been shown to associate with the presence of an 'atopy gene' on human chromosome 11q.
- Biozzi generated two lines of mice by selective inbreeding, based on their responsiveness to erythrocyte antigens. These high-responder and low-responder Biozzi mice make quantitatively different amounts of

antibody in response to antigenic challenge. The basis for these differences has in part been attributed to genetic differences in macrophage activity. These high- and low-responder strains also differ markedly in their ability to respond to parasitic infections, and this does not necessarily correlate with the amount of antibody they make.

Non-MHC-linked genes affect susceptibility to infection

Macrophages have a key role in the immune system. Genes regulating their activity may therefore determine the outcome of many immune responses. A good example of such genetic control of macrophage function is provided by the *Lsh/Ity/Bcg* gene. This gene governs the early response to infection with *Leishmania donovani*, *Salmonella typhimurium*, *Mycobacterium bovis*, *M. lepraemurium* and *M. intracellulare*. Its influence is on the early phase of macrophage priming and activation, and it has wide-ranging effects, including:

- Upregulation of the oxidative burst.
- Enhanced tumoricidal activity.
- Enhanced antimicrobial activity.
- Upregulation of MHC class II expression.

Recent congenic studies have identified the natural-resistance-associated macrophage protein 1 (*Nramp1*) as the *bcg* gene. As *Nramp1* encodes a membrane protein with homology to known transport proteins, the suggestion has been made that it may be implicated in the transport of NO_2^- into the phagolysosome, thus facilitating the killing of intracellular organisms. The human homologue (*NRAMP1*) of the mouse gene, *Nramp1*, has been cloned and several different alleles identified. Polymorphisms in this gene may contribute to resistance to tuberculosis in humans although the data thus far is not so convincing as in the mouse.

Polymorphisms in the genes encoding cytokine receptors have been shown to correlate with an increased susceptibility to infection, severe combined immunodeficiency (SCID) or inflammatory conditions. The outcome of the mutation is dependent on the cytokine gene which is affected. For example, humans with mutations in the IL-7R develop a selective deficit in T cells and those with deficiency in the common cytokine receptor γ chain (γc), which is a component of the functional receptors for IL-2, IL-4, IL-7, IL-9 and IL-15 (see *Fig. 7.7*), have reduced numbers of T cells and NK cells and have impaired B-cell function, in part attributable to the lack of T-cell help (*Fig. 11.24*). Further examples are the mutations in the IFN-γR or IL-12R which markedly increase susceptibility to mycobacterial infection. A list of genetic defects which contribute to impaired immune responses are listed in *Figure 11.25*. (See also *Fig. 7.14* for a description of defects in mouse strains lacking particular cytokines or their receptors.)

Mutations in the cytokine promoters have been shown to influence the levels of expression of cytokine. Polymorphisms such as these have been linked to certain autoimmune conditions and also to susceptibility to infections. Susceptibility to severe malaria is under complex genetic control with other genes in addition to MHC playing an important role. Recent studies, for example, have linked the development of cerebral malaria to a polymorphism in the promoter region of the TNFα gene. Other studies have implicated polymorphisms in the promoter region of the inducible NO synthase gene (*NOS2*).

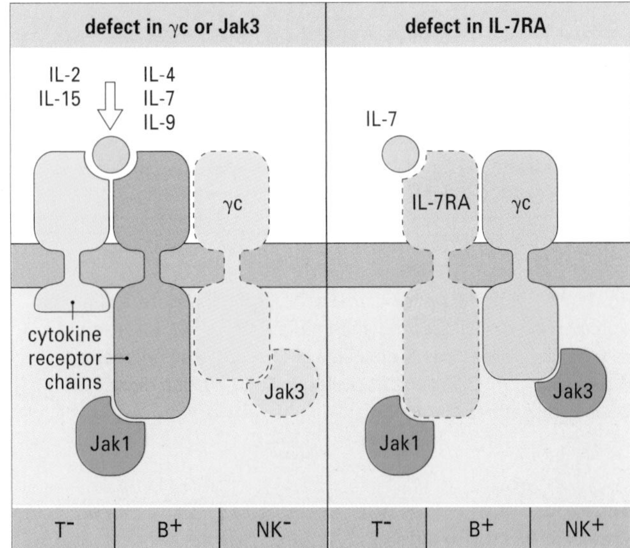

Fig. 11.24 A defect in the common chain (γc) of the cytokine receptors IL-2, IL-15, IL-4, IL-7 and IL-9, leads to a severe combined immune deficiency, with loss of both T cells and NK cells. A similar deficiency results from mutation in the janus kinase (Jak3), which transduces signals from the γc chain (left panel). Note that IL-2 and IL-15 have three chains in their high-affinity receptor, while IL-4, IL-7 and IL-9 have only two chains. Absence of the specific IL-7 receptor chain also produces a severe immunodeficiency, but this primarily affects T-cell development (right panel).

Eosinophils have an important role in the host response to parasitic infection. It has been shown that the degree of eosinophilia following infection is genetically determined, with marked differences seen in different inbred strains of mice. Similar observations have been made in guinea-pigs and sheep, in which a consistent correlation has been found between resistance to nematode infection and the extent of eosinophilia. These observations may relate to polymorphisms which influence relevant cytokine and chemokine levels, including IL-5 and eotaxin.

Some genes involved in immune responses can affect disease susceptibility, but not because they affect immune responsiveness. For example, disease progression to AIDS has been shown to be associated with polymorphisms in the chemokine receptor gene-5 (CCR-5). CCR-5 is a co-receptor which is used in the entry of macrophage-trophic strains of HIV-1 into cells. A mutation which inactivates this receptor is found in some individuals of European origin but is rare in populations of Asian or sub-Saharan African descent. Individuals homozygous for this CCR-5 mutation have been found to be very resistant to HIV-1 infection. In this case resistance is related to the reduced

Genetic defects associated with immune deficiency or abnormalities

condition	defective gene	result
SCID	γc IL-2Rα IL-7Rα Jak3 CD3γ CD3ε ZAP70 ADA RAG1/2	failure of signal transduction by cytokines failure of IL-2 signal in activation and development failure of IL-7 signal in lymphocyte development lack of signal transduction by cytokines no signal transduced from T-cell receptor no signal transduced from T-cell receptor no signal transduced from T-cell receptor T-cell toxicity failure in TCR and BCR gene recombination
T-cell deficiency	PNP	T-cell development failure
class II deficiency	CIITA	failure to express MHC class II molecules
class I deficiency	TAP1/2	failure to load MHC class I molecules
X-linked hyper-IgM	CD40L	no maturation of antibody response
X-linked-agammaglobulinaemia	Btk	failure of B-cell development
X-linked lymphoproliferative syndrome	SH2D1A/SAP	impaired negative signals to B cells
Autoimmune lymphoproliferative syndrome	Fas (CD95) or FasL	extended lymphocyte lifespan due to reduced apoptosis
mycobacterial infection	IFNγR1/2 IL-12R	impaired TH1 responses

Fig. 11.25 Based on a review by Leonard, 2000. ADA = Adenosine deaminase, Btk = Bruton's tyrosine kinase, PNP = purine nucleoside phosphorylase, RAG = recombination activating gene.

primary spread of the virus, rather than an enhanced immune response against it.

Non-MHC-linked genes also affect development of autoimmune disease

Major advances have recently been made in mapping the loci which govern susceptibility to the autoimmune disease, insulin-dependent diabetes mellitus (IDDM). This work has been largely carried out using the NOD mouse strain, which spontaneously develops an autoimmune disease similar to IDDM in humans. At least 18 genetic loci have been identified in the NOD mouse (*Idd-1* to *18*). Only one locus (*Idd-1*) is linked to the mouse MHC on chromosome 17, and is believed to encode MHC class II molecules themselves. The other genes have been mapped to other chromosomes, but their identity and functional roles in determining resistance or susceptibility are not yet known.

When the lymphoproliferative (*lpr*) gene is present in mouse strains, it causes the development of a characteristic clinical syndrome. The mice develop anti-DNA antibodies, rheumatoid factor, circulating immune complexes and glomerulonephritis. There is also a lymphadenopathy in these mice, involving a polyclonal expansion of double negative ($CD4^-CD8^-$) T cells in the periphery. It has been shown that mice with the *lpr* gene have a defect in CD95 (Fas), a transmembrane molecule belonging to the TNF receptor superfamily that interacts with CD95L to induce apoptosis. (CD95L is a member of the tumour necrosis–nerve growth factor family.) The defect in Fas results in the failure of apoptosis but it does not appear to affect negative selection and the generation of a normal repertoire of mature single positive T cells in the thymus. Evidently Fas is only one of the ligands which mediate apoptosis. It is now proposed that the defect leads to the expansion of double-negative T cells in the periphery and an acceleration of an autoimmune syndrome. The defect in apoptosis also affects B cells – autoreactive B cells accumulate in the periphery.

Other studies have shown that the *gld* gene which encodes a defective FasL results in an autoimmune phenotype similar to that seen in mice homozygous for the *lpr* defect. Thus mice which are homozygous for the *gld* mutation do not express a functional ligand, have a defect in apoptosis of peripheral B and T cells, and develop autoimmunity. The *gld* gene is located on chromosome 1 in the mouse and thus provides yet another example of a gene that affects immune function, but which is not MHC linked. Comparable syndromes have been described in humans, which are attributable to defects in Fas activity and function (*Fig. 11.25*). Studies of patients with autoimmune lymphoproliferative syndrome (ALPS) have provided insight into the interactions between Fas and FasL. Some of the patients suffering from ALPS have a dominant mutation in the gene encoding Fas. Detailed analysis of the mechanism by which the mutant allele dominantly interferes with apoptosis suggests that Fas is normally found as a trimeric complex at the cell surface. Trimer formation is dependent on a domain within Fas called the pre-ligand assembly domain (PLAD) and Fas molecules with mutations within this region interfere with trimer formation by normal Fas molecules. This results in defective Fas/FasL mediated apoptosis and the development of an autoimmune syndrome in patients with the dominant Fas mutation.

Another example of polymorphism affecting immune responses is seen in FcγRIIb in mice. Recall that FcγRIIb inhibits B-cell activation when it is co-ligated by antibody bound to a multivalent antigen (*Fig. 11.5*). Polymorphisms have been detected in the FcγRIIb transcriptional regulatory regions of the mouse. One of these polymorphisms which results in diminished expression of FcγRIIb on germinal centre B cells is common in autoimmune prone mouse strains and is associated with elevated levels of Ig consistent with a lack of feedback regulation on the B cell (*Fig. 11.26*). This has led to the suggestion that such polymorphism may contribute to some forms of autoimmune pathology such as SLE and Sjögren's syndrome.

Clearly, many genes involved in immune responses affect susceptibility to infection and autoimmunity. Gene defects often cause serious impairment to the immune system. Functional polymorphism is particularly evident in MHC class I and II genes, but there is increasing evidence for limited polymorphism in gene structure or gene expression of many non-MHC immune response genes. Cumulatively, these variations may well be as important as those in the MHC-linked genes.

Elevated antibody responses in autoimmune mouse strains

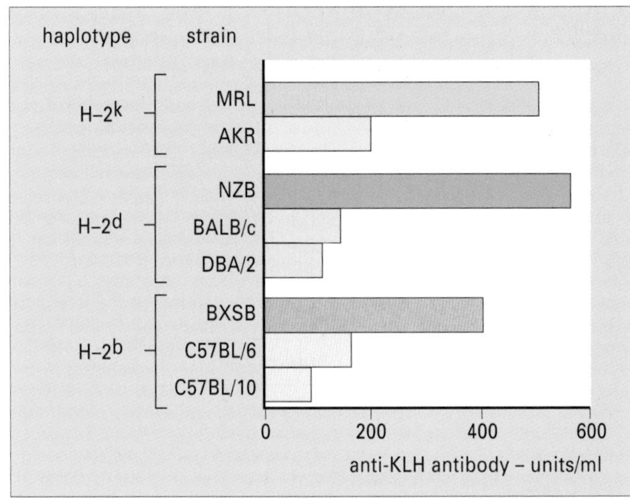

Fig. 11.26 Eight different mouse strains were immunized at 5 and 9 weeks of age with KLH antigen. The sera were assayed for antibodies at 11 weeks. In these secondary antibody responses, the autoimmune-prone strains MRL, NZB and BXSB, all had higher antibody levels to KLH than normal mouse strains with the same MHC haplotype. It is thought that the higher antibody levels are related to a polymorphism in the FcγRIIb gene in the autoimmune-susceptible strains. Based on data of Jiang et al, 2000.

CRITICAL THINKING • Immune response modulation by experimental treatment

(Explanations on p. 456)

In each of the following studies an immune response is modulated by the experimental treatment. Based on the mechanisms described in this chapter, provide explanations for the ways in which each treatment may regulate the immune response.

11.1 Experimental allergic encephalomyelitis (EAE) is induced in Lewis rats by immunization with an encephalitogenic peptide of guinea-pig myelin basic protein. If however this peptide is covalently coupled to anti-IgD antibody, the conjugate does not induce EAE. Moreover if the conjugate is administered at the same time as the isolated peptide, the development of EAE is suppressed. How could the anti-IgD-peptide conjugate prevent the development of disease?
Based on a study by Day *et al. J Exp Med* 1992; **175**: 655–9.

11.2 BALB/c mice infected with *Leishmania* develop a fatal progressive disease, characterized by little IFNγ production, high production of IL-4 and elevated serum IgE. Treatment of the animals with high doses of recombinant IFNγ does not prevent the disease. However, treatment with anti-IL-4 antibody leads to a complete cure in 85% of animals, and an associated increase in the levels of IFNγ in lymph node cells draining the site of infection. Nevertheless treatment with anti-IFNγ in the anti-IL-4 treated mice did not stop them being cured. How could the anti-IL-4 promote recovery from *Leishmania* infection?
Based on a study by Sadick *et al. J Exp Med* 1990; **171**:115–27.

11.3 Mouse lymphocytes were primed by immunization with sheep red blood cells (SRBC) coupled to the hapten trinitrophenyl (TNP). The lymphocytes produce a strong antibody response against TNP and SRBC *in vitro*. If the cultures were also treated with a monoclonal IgG2a antibody against TNP, the specific antibody response to SRBC was suppressed by 98%. However $F(ab')_2$ of the same anti-TNP monoclonal antibody failed to suppress the anti-SRBC response. How can antibody to TNP suppress the response to SRBC, and why does the $F(ab')_2$ not work?
Based on a study by Heyman. *Scand J Immunol* 1990; **5**:601–7.

FURTHER READING

Blalock JE, Bost KL (eds). Shared ligands and receptors as a molecular mechanism for communication between immune and neuroendocrine systems. *Ann NY Acad Sci* 1994;**741**:292–8.

Biron C, Nguyen KB, Pien GC, Cousens LP, Salazar-Mather TP. Natural killer cells in antiviral defense: function and regulation by innate cytokines. *Annu Rev Immunol* 1999;**17**:189–220.

Chambers DA, Schauenstein K. Mindful immunology: neuroimmunomodulation. *Immunol Today* 2000;**21**:168–70.

Groux H, Powrie F. Regulatory T cells in inflammatory bowel disease. *Immunol Today* 1999;**20**:442–5.

Heymann B. Regulation of antibody responses via antibodies, complement, and Fc receptors. *Annu Rev Immunol* 2000;**18**:709–38.

Hill AVS. The immunogenetics of human infectious diseases. *Annu Rev Immunol* 1998;**16**:593–617.

Jiang Y, Hitose S, Abe M, Sonokawa-Akakura, Ohtsugi M et al. Polymorphines in the IgG Fc receptor IIb regulatory regions associated with autoimmune susceptibility. *Immunogenetics* 2000;**51**:429–35.

Lalani AS, Barrett JW, McFadden G. Modulating chemokines: more lessons from viruses. *Immunol Today* 2000;**21**:100–6.

Lenardo M, Chan F K-M, Hornung F, *et al.* Mature T lymphocyte apoptosis–immune regulation in a dynamic and unpredictable antigenic environment. *Annu Rev Immunol* 1999;**17**:221–53.

Leonard WJ. Genetic effects on immunity. *Curr Opin Immunol* 2000;**12**:465–67.

Mahalingam S, Karupiah G. Modulation of chemokines by poxvirus infections. *Curr Opin Immunol* 2000;**12**:409–12.

Mason D, MacPhee I, Antoni F. The role of the neuroendocrine system in determining genetic susceptibility to experimental allergic encephalomyelitis in the rat. *Immunology* 1990;**70**:1–5.

Metzler B, Wraith DC. Inhibition of experimental autoimmune encephalomyelitis by inhalation but not oral administration of the encephalitogenic peptide: influence of MHC binding affinity. *Int Immunol* 1993;**5**:1159–65.

Ridge JP, Fuchs EJ, Matzinger P. Neonatal tolerance revisited: turning on newborn T cells with dendritic cells. *Science* 1996;**271**:1723–6.

Seddon B, Mason D. The third function of the thymus. *Immunol Today* 2000;**21**:95–9.

Vyse TJ, Kotzin BL. Genetic susceptibility to systemic lupus erythematosus. *Annu Rev Immunol* 1998;**16**:261–92.

Wicker LS, Todd JA, Peterson LB. Genetic control of autoimmune diabetes in the NOD mouse. *Annu Rev Immunol* 1995;**13**:179–200.

Wilder RL. Neuroendocrine–immune system interactions and autoimmunity. *Annu Rev Immunol* 1995;**13**:307–38.

Zlotnik A, Yoshie O. Chemokines: a new classification system and their role in immunity. *Immunity* 2000;**12**:121–7.

12 Immunological tolerance

- **Tolerance mechanisms** are needed because the immune system randomly generates a vast diversity of antigen-specific receptors and some of these will be self reactive; tolerance prevents harmful reactivity against the body's own tissues.
- **Central thymic tolerance to self antigens** (autoantigens) results from deletion of differentiating T cells that express antigen-specific receptors with high binding affinity for intrathymic self antigens. Low-affinity self-reactive T cells, and T cells with receptors specific for antigens that are not represented intrathymically, mature and join the peripheral T-cell pool.
- **Post-thymic tolerance to self antigens** has five main mechanisms. Self-reactive T cells in the circulation may ignore self antigens, for example when the antigens are in tissues sequestered from the circulation. Their response to a self antigen may be suppressed if the antigen is present in a privileged site. Self-reactive cells may under certain conditions be deleted or rendered anergic and unable to respond. Finally a state of tolerance to self antigens can also be maintained by immune regulation.
- **B-cell deletion** takes place in both bone marrow and peripheral lymphoid organs. Differentiating B cells that express surface immunoglobulin receptors with high binding affinity for self-membrane-bound antigens will be deleted soon after their generation in the bone marrow. A high proportion of short-lived, low-avidity, autoreactive B cells appear in peripheral lymphoid organs. These cells may be recruited to fight against infection.
- **Tolerance can be induced artificially** by various regimens that may eventually be exploited clinically to prevent rejection of foreign transplants and to manipulate autoimmune and allergic diseases.

INTRODUCTION

Immunological tolerance is a state of unresponsiveness that is specific for a particular antigen; it is induced by prior exposure to that antigen. Active tolerance mechanisms are required to prevent inflammatory responses to the many innocuous air-borne and food antigens that are encountered at mucosal surfaces in the lung and gut. The most important aspect of tolerance, however, is self tolerance, which prevents the body from mounting an immune attack against its own tissues. There is potential for such attack because the immune system randomly generates a vast diversity of antigen-specific receptors, some of which will be self reactive. Cells bearing these receptors therefore must be eliminated, either functionally or physically.

Self reactivity is prevented by processes that occur during development, rather than being genetically preprogrammed. Thus, while homozygous animals of histoincompatible strains A and B reject each other's skin, and their F_1 hybrid offspring (which express the antigens of both the A and B parents) reject neither A skin nor B skin, the ability to reject such skin reappears in homozygotes of the F_2 progeny. Thus it is clear that self–non-self discrimination is learned during development: immunological 'self' must encompass all epitopes (antigenic determinants) encoded by the individual's DNA, all other epitopes being considered as non-self.

However it is not the structure of a molecule per se that determines whether it will be distinguished as self or non-self. Factors other than the structural characteristics of an epitope are also important. Among these are:

- The stage of differentiation when lymphocytes first confront their epitopes.
- The site of the encounter.
- The nature of the cells presenting epitopes.
- The number of lymphocytes responding to the epitopes.

Historical background

Soon after the existence of antibody specificity was established, it was realized that there must be some mechanism to prevent autoantibody formation. As early as the turn of the century, Ehrlich coined the term 'horror autotoxicus', implying the need for a 'regulating contrivance' to stop the production of autoantibodies. In 1938, Traub induced specific tolerance by inoculating mice *in utero* with lymphocytic choriomeningitis virus, producing an infection that was maintained throughout life. Unlike normal mice, these inoculated mice did not produce neutralizing antibodies when challenged with the virus in adult life. In 1945, Owen reported an 'experiment of nature' in non-identical cattle twins which showed that cells carrying self and non-self antigens could develop within a single host. These animals exchanged haemopoietic (stem) cells via their shared placental blood vessels and each animal carried the erythrocyte markers of both calves. They exhibited lifelong tolerance to the otherwise foreign cells, in being unable to mount antibody responses to the relevant erythrocyte antigens. Following this observation, Burnet and Fenner postulated that the age of the animal at the time of first encounter was the critical factor in determining responsiveness, and hence recognition, of non-self antigens. This hypothesis seemed logical, as the immune system is usually confronted with most self components before birth and only later with non-self antigens.

Experimental support came in 1953, when Medawar and his colleagues induced immunological tolerance to skin allografts (grafts that are genetically non-identical, but are from the same species) in mice by neonatal injection of allogeneic cells (*Fig. 12.1*). This phenomenon was easily accommodated in Burnet's clonal selection theory (1957), which states that a particular immunocyte (a particular B or T cell) is selected by antigen and then divides to give rise to a clone of daughter cells, all with the same specificity.

Induction of specific tolerance in mice

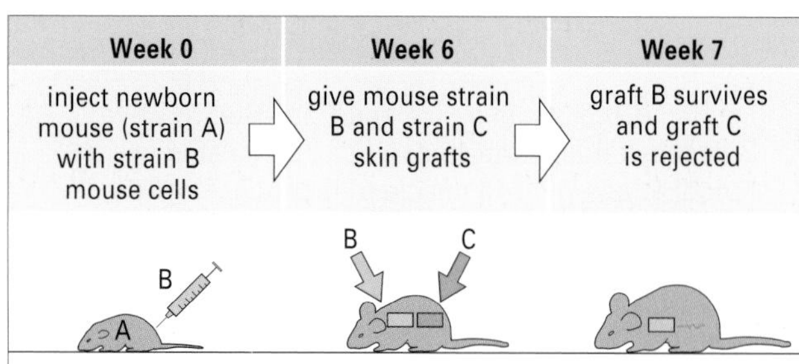

Fig. 12.1 The experiment demonstrates the induction of specific tolerance to grafted skin, induced by neonatal injection of spleen cells from a different strain. Mice of strain A normally reject grafts from strain B. However, if newborn mice of strain A receive cells from strain B, they show tolerance to skin grafts from this donor at 6 weeks of age, but reject grafts from other strains (C). This phenomenon is due to immune deviation.

According to this theory, antigens encountered after birth activate specific clones of lymphocytes, whereas when antigens are encountered before birth the result is the deletion of the clones specific for them, which Burnet termed 'forbidden clones'. Implicit in the theory is the need for the entire immune repertoire to be generated before birth, but in fact lymphocyte differentiation continues long after birth. The key factor in determining responsiveness is thus not the developmental stage of the individual, but rather the state of maturity of the lymphocyte at the time it encounters antigen. This was suggested by Lederberg in 1959, in his modification of the clonal selection theory: immature lymphocytes contacting antigen would be subject to 'clonal abortion', whereas mature cells would be activated. It is now established that the neonate is in fact immunocompetent. The reason that one can induce tolerance to certain antigens in the neonate is simply that the type of immune response to antigen can be functionally different in the neonate compared with that in the adult. Past descriptions of neonatal tolerance may therefore have been early examples of this type of 'immune deviation' (see below).

Key discoveries in the 1960s established the immunological competence of the lymphocyte, the crucial role of the thymus in the development of the immune system, and the existence of two interacting subsets of lymphocytes: T and B cells. This set the scene for a thorough investigation of the cellular mechanisms involved in tolerance.

EXPERIMENTAL INDUCTION OF TOLERANCE

Transgenic technology has allowed the study of tolerance to authentic self antigens

Until recently, only artificially induced tolerance was amenable to experimental study: antigens or foreign cells were inoculated into an animal and the fate of responding T or B cells was investigated under a variety of circumstances. It was not clear, however, to what extent these experimental models resembled natural self tolerance.

Transgenic methods have now made possible the direct investigation of self tolerance. These methods allow one to introduce a specific gene into mice of defined genetic background and to analyse its effects upon the development of the immune system. Furthermore, if the introduced gene is linked to a tissue-specific promoter, its expression can be confined to specific cell types. The protein product encoded by a 'transgene' is treated by the immune system essentially as an authentic self antigen (autoantigen), and its effects can be studied *in vivo* without the trauma and inflammation associated with grafting foreign cells or tissues. In addition, the parent strain and the transgenic strain are ideal for control experiments and lymphocyte transfer studies because they are congenic – that is, they differ at only one locus. One can even create transgenic mice in which all of either their B or T lymphocytes express a single antigen receptor. By so increasing the frequency of antigen-specific precursor cells, one can readily dissect tolerance mechanisms. Finally, the use of targeted mutagenesis has allowed immunologists to 'knock out' specific genes in order to study the role of their gene products in the process of immunological tolerance.

There are five possible ways in which self-reactive lymphocytes may be prevented from responding to self antigens:

1. Self-reactive T cells in the circulation may ignore self antigens, for example when the antigens are in tissues sequestered from the circulation.
2. Their response to a self antigen may be suppressed if the antigen is present in a privileged site.
3. Self-reactive cells may be deleted at certain stages of development, or
4. Self-reactive cells may be rendered anergic and unable to respond.
5. Finally, a state of tolerance to self-antigens can also be maintained by immune regulation.

Which of these fates awaits the self-reactive lymphocyte depends on numerous factors, including: (i) the stage of maturity of the cell being silenced; (ii) the affinity of its receptor for the self antigen; (iii) the nature of this antigen; (iv) its concentration; (v) its tissue distribution; and (vi) its pattern of expression.

CENTRAL THYMIC TOLERANCE TO SELF ANTIGENS

The process of generating new T-cell receptors involves gene rearrangement in addition to N-region modifications. This allows the immune system to generate a vast array of T-cell receptors. Such a broad repertoire is clearly necessary to provide protection against the multitude of different infectious agents that any individual in the species is likely to encounter. T lymphocytes are not, however, simply effector cells of the immune system. They also function as regulators of the system through provision of help for some and suppression of other responses. For effective control, lymphocytes must interact with other cells of the immune system and this is one reason why MHC restriction of T-cell recognition has evolved. Central tolerance among T lymphocytes revolves around a schooling process in which key cells are educated so that they become dependent on self MHC for survival, while at the same time potentially rebellious lymphocytes are identified and eliminated. This process of central tolerance among T lymphocytes takes place during their development within the thymus and depends on a number of check points through which the cells have to pass in order to develop further.

T-cell development involves positive and negative selection and lineage commitment

T lymphocytes develop from precursors in the bone marrow and are derived from a common lymphoid progenitor cell that gives rise to B cells, natural killer (NK) cells and both the αβ and γδ subsets of T lymphocytes (*Fig. 12.2*). Here we will concentrate on the αβ population of T lymphocytes whose function in the maintenance of self tolerance is now well understood.

When immature T cells enter the thymus they express neither CD4 nor CD8 co-receptor molecules (*Fig. 12.3*). These so-called double negative (DN) cells constitute approximately 3% of total thymocytes. At this stage the T-cell receptor (TCR) β chain genes start their recombination. This involves sequential rearrangement of variable (V), diversity (D) and junctional (J) region genes from the multiple copies available in the genome. First diversity and junctional genes rearrange and this is followed by rearrangement of the DJ gene with a variable region gene (see *Fig. 5.3*). The VDJ then combines with a constant region by alternative splicing of RNA to give the complete β chain gene. At this point the α chain genes remain in their genomic configuration but the transcribed and translated β chain nevertheless appears at the cell surface. This is only possible because the β chain can pair with a 'surrogate' α chain and other components of the CD3 signalling complex, in order to migrate from the endoplasmic reticulum to the cell surface. Surface expression of this complex allows double negative cells to switch off their RAG genes, begin to proliferate and mature into CD4 and CD8 double positive (DP) cells (see *Fig. 12.3*). There is no evidence that this 'checkpoint' (the β selection checkpoint) involves recognition of antigen.

Newly formed DP cells reactivate RAG genes allowing rearrangement of the α chain. Like the immunoglobulin light chain, the T-cell receptor α chain has no D segment and the first event is to direct rearrangement of Vα to Jα region genes. Suitable pairing of α and β chains at the α-selection checkpoint allows T cells to proceed to the next selection stage. Evidence shows, however, unlike the β chain that largely permits rearrangement of only one β gene through allelic exclusion, α chain rearrangement can continue to generate a second chain. In fact, up to 30% of mature human T cells express more than one rearranged α chain. This implies that T cells like B cells undergo a degree of 'receptor editing' of the α chain in order to increase the likelihood of positive selection of cells selected to interact with self MHC.

The potential for α–β pairing in combination with TCR gene rearrangement allows for a massive repertoire of TCR structures. Interestingly, however, some 95% of these structures fail to contribute to the T-cell repertoire found in peripheral lymphoid tissues. This is because thymocytes undergo a rigorous education before they exit the thymus. Education requires preliminary selection of cells for survival and their subsequent commitment to a particular lineage (positive selection). This is then followed by death of those cells that interact strongly with MHC (negative selection). In other words, T cells are positively selected for 'usefulness' (MHC restriction) and negatively selected against 'dangerous' autoreactivity. The controlling element in thymic education is the MHC expressed by antigen-presenting cells (APC) in the thymus (*Fig. 12.4*). This is such that T-cell development is blocked at the DP stage in a thymus that does not express MHC. In fact, cells at this stage of development need to be nurtured by cells expressing MHC. Cells whose TCR fails to engage either a class I or class II MHC molecule undergo programmed cell death (death by neglect), while cells that recognize MHC with moderate affinity on cortical epithelial cells survive.

Cells mature from DP cells to the single positive (SP) cells where they express either CD4 or CD8. It is clear that

A common lymphoid progenitor gives rise to B, T and one type of dendritic cell

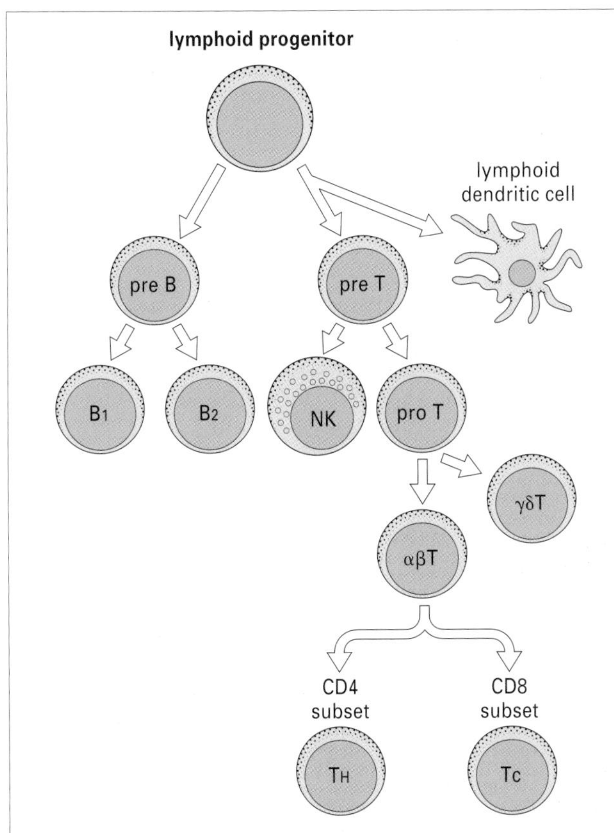

Fig. 12.2 Both B and T lymphocytes develop from a common precursor found in fetal liver or adult bone marrow. T-cell progenitors give rise to both the αβ and γδ lineages as well as NK T cells. Recent studies have shown that early T-cell progenitor cells also give rise to lymphoid dendritic cells in the mouse.

Developmental pathways of murine thymocytes

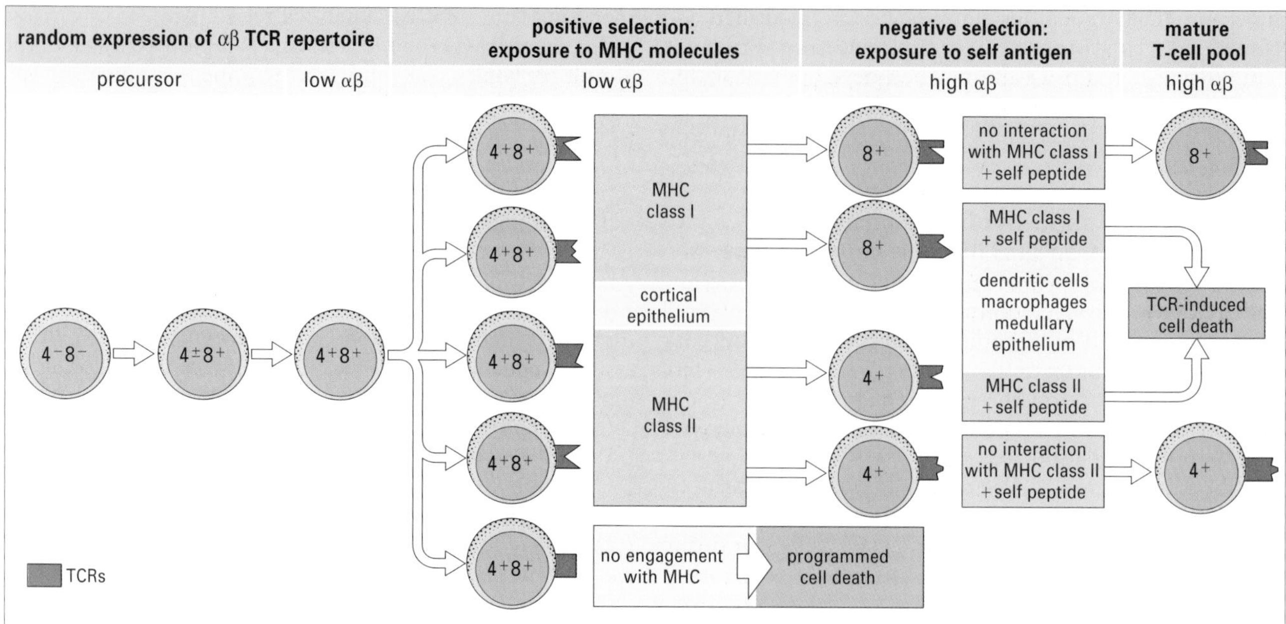

Fig. 12.3 Precursor thymocytes develop into 'double positive' cells expressing low levels of the αβ TCR. These undergo positive selection for interaction with self MHC class I or class II molecules on cortical epithelium. Unselected cells (the majority) undergo programmed cell death by apoptosis. Cells undergoing positive selection lose one or the other of their co-receptor molecules (CD4 or CD8). Finally, self-reactive cells are eliminated by their interaction with self peptides presented on cells at the corticomedullary junction and in the thymic medulla.

T cell–MHC restriction occurs in the thymus

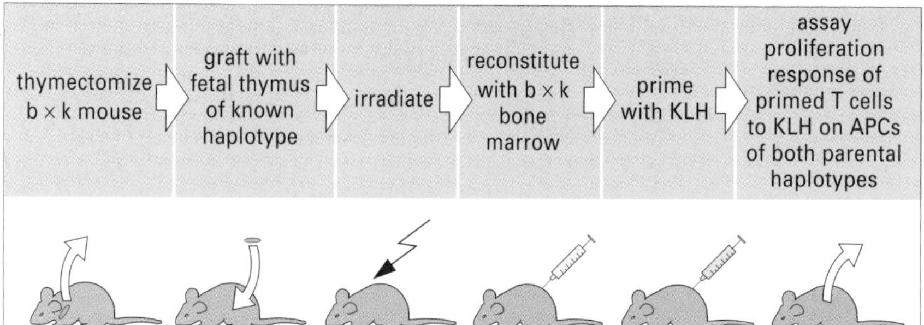

mouse type	engrafted fetal thymus type	proliferation response to APCs from each parental strain	
		H–2^b	H–2^k
b × k	b × k	++	++
b × k	b	++	–
b × k	b(dG-treated)	++	–
b × k	k	–	++
b × k	k(dG-treated)	–	++

Fig. 12.4 Host mice (F1[H-2^b×H-2^k]) were thymectomized, then engrafted with 14-day fetal thymuses of various genotypes. They were subsequently irradiated to remove their resident T-cell populations, then reconstituted with F1 bone marrow to provide stem cells. After priming with antigen (keyhole limpet haemocyanin, KLH), the proliferative response of lymph node T cells to KLH on APCs from each parental strain was evaluated. In some experiments, thymus lobes were incubated before grafting with deoxyguanosine (dG), which destroys intrathymic cells of macrophage/dendritic cell lineage. The results show (i) that the thymic environment is necessary for T cells to learn to recognize MHC and (ii) that bone marrow-derived cells (removed by dG treatment) are not required for this process to occur. (Based on data from Lo D. and Sprent J. *Nature* 1986;**319**:672.)

MHC plays a role in this selection process. Thus mice lacking class I MHC protein in the thymus have few CD8 single positive cells, while mice lacking class II have few CD4 single positive cells. It is likely that evolution has shaped complementarity-determining regions (CDR) 1 and 2 of the TCR, so that the TCR preferentially matches MHC molecules.

Signalling via CD4 and CD8 drives lineage commitment

Why has the immune system evolved two separate types of T cell? Would it not be more economical just to have one double positive cell that could interact with either class I or class II expressing cells? Selection of cells expressing either CD4 or CD8 has evolved just as the need for two pathways of antigen processing has been driven by encounter of vertebrates with increasingly sophisticated pathogens. Class I and class II pathways have evolved to allow the immune system to recognize either cytoplasmic or extracellular/intravacuolar infectious agents respectively. This has then driven evolution of two subsets of T cell equipped with the means to help eradicate these infectious agents. The remaining question is how CD4 and CD8 cells develop from one common precursor?

Until recently there were two theories to explain this process. The instructive model predicts that the co-receptor molecules CD4 and CD8 are involved in signalling. Thus recognition and simultaneous binding of class II MHC by suitable TCR and associated CD4 molecules directs inactivation of CD8 expression. Accordingly, a cell with a class II binding TCR develops into a CD4 cell and a cell bearing a class I binding TCR into a CD8 cell. The alternative hypothesis is that this whole process occurs in a random or stochastic fashion. Recent evidence strongly favours the instructional model.

Logic dictates that a newly rearranged TCR should not necessarily distinguish between class I or II MHC prior to thymic selection. It is therefore reasonable to assume that a signal for lineage commitment might be delivered by co-receptors, CD8 and CD4. These molecules are, after all, known to have an inherent affinity for class I and class II molecules respectively. This belief is supported by the fact that transgenic mice expressing a class I restricted TCR aberrantly generate predominantly CD4 cells when their developing T cells express a hybrid CD8 (extracellular)/ CD4 (intracellular) co-receptor molecule. This suggests that intracellular signalling via the CD4 intracellular domain leads to selective commitment along the CD4 lineage with associated inactivation of CD8 expression.

Recent experiments have revealed the nature of a molecular switch that associates with co-receptor molecules and controls lineage commitment. The src-family kinase Lck plays an important role in this process and is known to associate better with CD4 when compared with CD8 molecules. In DP thymocytes some 25–50% of surface CD4 associates with Lck, compared with only 2% for CD8. Consistent with a role in lineage commitment, it turns out that a constitutively active Lck molecule drives overselection of CD4 cells, whereas a constitutively inactive Lck drives CD8 selection (*Fig. 12.5*). These results show that the intensity of Lck signalling is crucial for the development of lineage commitment.

Further experiments indicate that strength of signalling via the TCR can also influence lineage commitment. Artificially increasing the signal delivered via the TCR during thymocyte development has been shown to encourage the generation of CD4 SP cells even among class I restricted cells. DP cells therefore dictate their own fate depending on the strength of integrated signals delivered via both their cell surface TCR and co-receptor-linked Lck molecules. At low signal strength CD8 selection takes place, while at a higher strength CD4 commitment is observed (*Fig. 12.6*). Co-receptor molecules dictate lineage commitment by virtue of the amount of the src-kinase Lck that they bring to the TCR–MHC synapse during positive selection (see *Figs 6.21* and *6.22*).

Lck directs lineage commitment in developing T lymphocytes

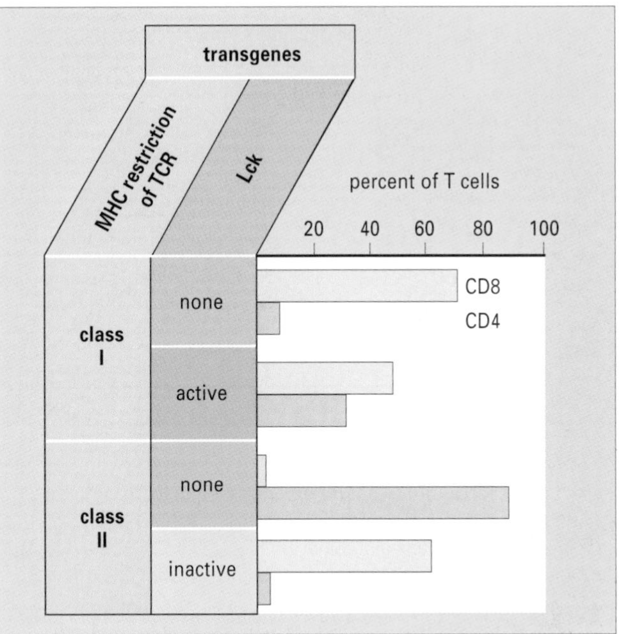

Fig. 12.5 T-cell receptor genes restricted to either class I or class II MHC were introduced into transgenic mice. Double transgenic strains were produced carrying either a constitutively active or inactive src-kinase (Lck). The graph shows the percentages of single positive CD8 (red) or CD4 (blue) single positive (SP) cells in the thymus. Normally class I-restricted TCR will develop into CD8 SP and class II restricted TCR into CD4 SP cells. These results show that thymocytes carrying a class I-restricted TCR can develop into functional CD4 T cells when Lck activity is increased. Conversely, thymocytes carrying a class II restricted TCR can develop into functional CD8 T cells when Lck activity is reduced. This proves that Lck plays a crucial role in regulating lineage commitment. (Based on data of Hernandez-Hoyos *et al. Immunity* 2000;**12**:313.)

Antigen recognition is important for development of the T-cell repertoire

Do T cells need to see antigen for positive selection and if so does this have to be a specific MHC-bound peptide? Mice deficient in the proteins required to transport peptides into the endoplasmic reticulum (TAP proteins) do not allow selection of CD8 cells. This proves that peptide antigen in conjunction with MHC class I is required for CD8 cell differentiation. But how many peptides are required for a completely functional T-cell repertoire. This question has been addressed in the class II system through the creation of transgenic mice in which the vast majority of class II MHC molecules are occupied by a single peptide. These mice produce CD4 SP cells and are able to respond to a number of different antigens. Careful analysis of these mice, however, reveals their T-cell repertoire is far from normal. Although the number of cells present in these mice was only reduced by about 50%, the resulting repertoire was stunted and the single MHC-peptide

Lineage commitment is controlled by the relative balance of signals delivered by the TCR and Lck

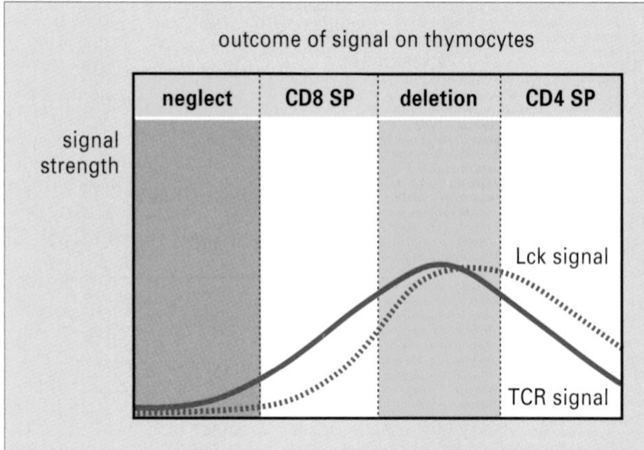

Fig. 12.6 Low signal strength signalling with little Lck activation is sufficient for commitment to the CD8 lineage. Increasing the TCR-dominated signal leads to cell deletion. MHC/antigen stimulation that results in a relatively high Lck to TCR ratio results in commitment to the CD4 lineage. This model explains the following: (i) Why overexpression of either Lck, or the Lck-associated co-receptor CD4, in mice bearing a class I-restricted transgenic TCR leads to differentiation of CD4 cells. (ii) Why class II-restricted TCR transgenic mice expressing either an inactive Lck or lacking CD4 produce CD8 rather than CD4 SP cells. (Based on Basson *et al. J Exp Med* 1998;**187**:1249.)

Thymic cells involved in negative selection

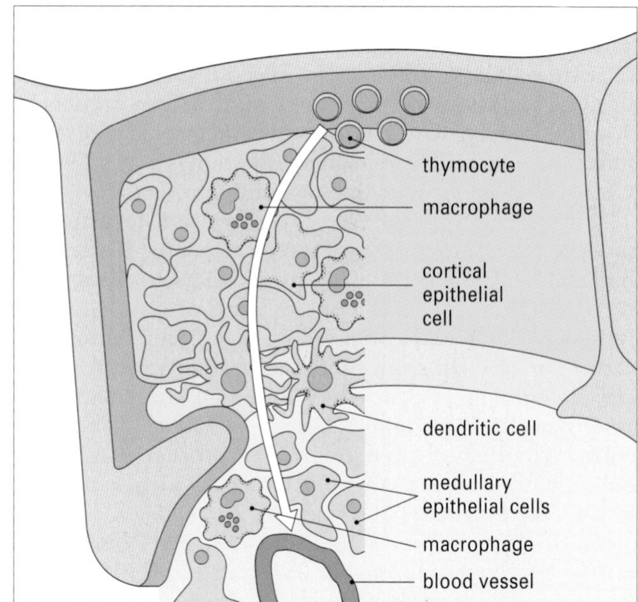

Fig. 12.7 The deleting population includes bone marrow-derived macrophages or dendritic cells, which are located at the corticomedullary junction. Other cells involved in deletion may be the thymocytes themselves, through their veto function, and some types of thymic epithelial cells, possibly in the medulla.

complex was unable to select a number of known TCRs when these were introduced as transgenes.

T-cell selection is compartmentalized in the thymus

The thymus is made up of lobes, each of which is organized into outer cortical and inner medullary regions (*Fig. 12.7*). Immature lymphocytes are found in the cortical region associated with cortical epithelial cells. Cells in the outer cortex are rapidly proliferating immature cells. Cells in the inner cortex are more mature DP cells probably undergoing positive selection. The medulla contains mature SP lymphocytes, medullary epithelial cells and bone marrow-derived macrophages and dendritic cells. It is a matter of hot debate as to whether spatial separation of MHC on different APCs and their isolation in different thymic regions influence positive and negative selection. Clearly haematopoietic cells are restricted to the medulla. Two important considerations are the fact that the thymic cortex is relatively inaccessible to large circulating proteins because of its vascular supply and the observation that cortical epithelial cells are inefficient at presenting exogenous proteins. These cells would thus be predicted to present endogenous antigens only and not antigens carried to the thymus in the blood supply. Cortical epithelial cells definitely play a role in positive selection because mice expressing class II MHC only on these cells show normal levels of positive selection but impaired negative selection. By contrast, bone marrow-derived macrophage and dendritic cells account for the removal of at least 50% of all positively selected cells.

A further question relates to how the thymus could ever possibly express all of the antigens that a T cell might encounter outside of the thymus. There seems little doubt that the thymus does not express all potential self antigens. Nevertheless, there is increasing evidence suggesting that medullary epithelial cells can express antigens such as insulin from the pancreas and proteolipid protein from brain, previously thought to be expressed only in peripheral tissues. Medullary epithelial cells may, therefore, contribute to negative selection either by direct presentation of antigen or possibly by transfer of antigens to myeloid APCs such as dendritic cells (*Fig. 12.8*).

T-cell development includes a series of checkpoints

In conclusion, the architecture of the thymus appears to be designed to compartmentalize thymic selection. Cortical epithelial cells present a wide range of endogenous antigens and contribute to positive selection. Interestingly, it is estimated that a developing thymocyte might only ever interact with a single cortical epithelial cell. The imprint that this leaves on the T cell clearly has a profound effect on the resulting T-cell repertoire. Medullary APCs have access to circulating antigens and are largely responsible for negative selection. It is now also clear that antigens from a wide variety of tissues are expressed at low levels in the thymus, most probably by medullary epithelial cells. These cells may well contribute to negative selection either alone

Tolerance induction by self antigens expressed in the thymus

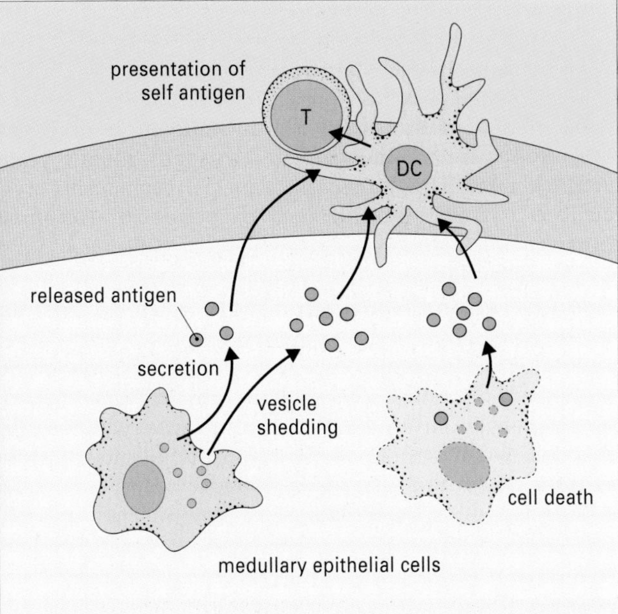

Fig. 12.8 A possible mechanism for tolerance induction by self antigens expressed in rare medullary epithelial cells. Self antigens (blue) are released from the epithelial cells by either secretion, vesicle shedding or cell death. The efficiency of presentation of the released self antigen is a function of the processing capacity of neighbouring APC. Because of their high efficiency in presentation of exogenous antigen, thymic dendritic cells (DC) would be the most likely cell to function as an APC.

The correlation between avidity and thymocyte selection

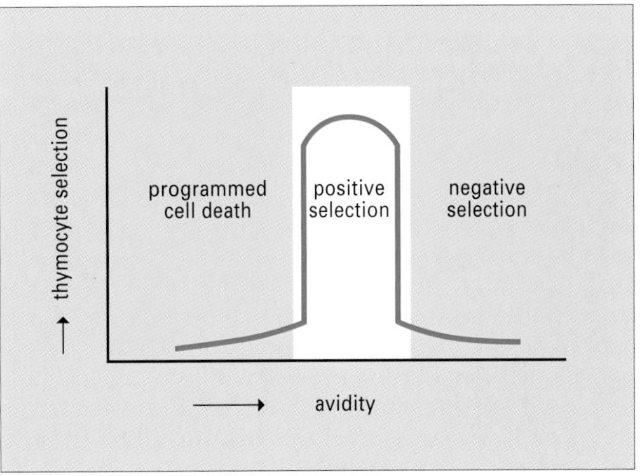

Fig. 12.9 The avidity of a T cell's interaction with antigenic peptide presented by an APC will depend on the level of expression of the MHC–peptide complex [MHC + peptide] on the APC and both the affinity and surface expression of TCR on the T cell. [MHC + peptide] depends on the affinity of peptide for MHC and the stability of the complex once formed.

or in partnership with myeloid cells. Furthermore, there is evidence that antigen recognition in the thymus may contribute to the generation of regulatory T lymphocytes that play such an important role in peripheral tolerance (see below).

Checkpoints in central T-cell tolerance include:

- β-selection checkpoint: only cells with a rearranged β chain mature from double negative to double positive cells. This process is not dependent on MHC proteins.
- α-selection checkpoint: cells expressing an αβ complex must interact with MHC to survive.
- Lineage commitment checkpoint: cells are instructed to repress expression of either CD4 or CD8 and to develop into single positive cells.
- Negative selection checkpoint: cells that interact strongly with MHC and antigen in the thymus are deleted (*Fig. 12.9*).

It is important to consider how a cell with one TCR can receive signals instructing it to survive and undergo lineage commitment without coincidentally receiving a signal to undergo negative selection. The most likely explanation is that this relies on the avidity of the cells' interaction with MHC and peptide. Experiments have shown that the decision to undergo positive and negative selection is directly related to the half-life of TCR binding to the MHC–peptide complex (*Fig. 12.10*). Selection also depends on the architecture of the thymus, the nature of APCs in the cortex versus the medulla of the thymus and the types of antigen that these cells are able to present.

TCR affinity for MHC–peptide complex influences positive selection

nature of peptide	half-life(s)	thymocyte selection	mature T-cell response
agonist	++	negative	++
antagonist	±	positive	±
irrelevant	–	no effect	–

Fig. 12.10 The affinity of a soluble TCR for complexes between various peptides and the appropriate MHC restriction element can be measured by biophysical techniques such as surface plasmon resonance. There is a direct correlation between the half-life of TCR binding to the MHC–peptide complex and the response made by mature T cells expressing the same receptor (i.e. agonist > antagonist > irrelevant peptide). In thymocyte organ cultures, however, addition of the agonist peptide causes deletion of the developing cells (negative selection), whereas the antagonist stimulates positive selection. This demonstrates that low-avidity interaction promotes positive selection, whereas high-avidity interaction leads to negative selection. (Data summarized from Alam *et al. Nature* 1996;**381**:616.)

Peripheral blood cells from a healthy individual respond to the self antigen myelin basic protein

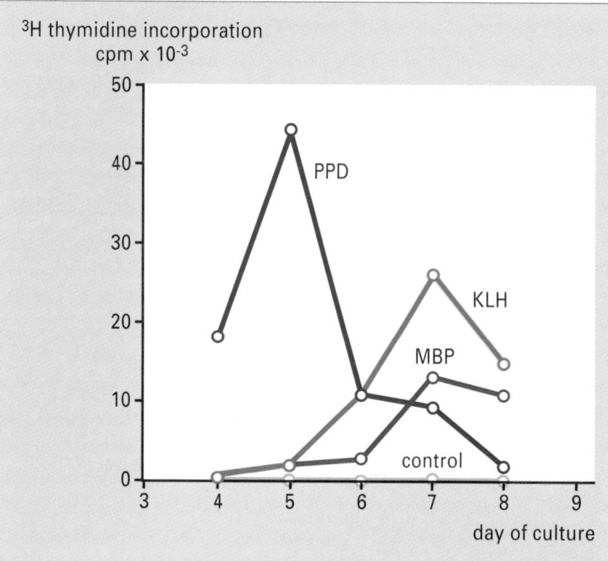

Fig. 12.11 Purified white blood cells can be stimulated in tissue culture with antigens such as purified protein derivative (PPD) from *mycobacterium tuberculosis* or keyhole limpet haemocyanin (KLH). The rate at which the cells respond (measured by incorporation of ^{3}H-thymidine) reflects whether the response is primary/naïve (KLH) or secondary/memory (PPD). Note that blood cells from a healthy individual respond with primary kinetics to purified human myelin basic protein (MBP). This experiment shows how cells that have escaped tolerance induction in the thymus can nevertheless respond to self antigens under artificial conditions. (Reproduced with permission from Drs M. Ponsford and G. Mazza, University of Bristol.)

PERIPHERAL OR POST-THYMIC TOLERANCE TO SELF ANTIGENS

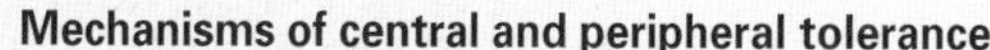

There is no doubt that many potentially autoreactive T cells escape central tolerance. This reflects the fact that many antigens are either not present or are present at insufficiently high levels to induce tolerance in the thymus. Thus, for example, peripheral blood lymphocytes from healthy individuals respond vigorously to purified myelin basic protein, a major constituent of myelin in the brain, following their culture *in vitro* (*Fig. 12.11*). So, how are these cells kept at bay in healthy individuals and why are autoimmune diseases directed to such proteins so incredibly rare? This is because various mechanisms have evolved to maintain tolerance in peripheral lymphoid organs (*Fig. 12.12*).

Sequestration of antigen occurs in some tissues

Both developing and mature lymphocytes may never encounter self antigens. Many of these are sequestered away from the immune system by physical or immunological barriers. In this way, tissue antigens may never be available to T lymphocytes, either because of their location or the fact that they may never be processed by functional APCs.

Privileged sites are protected by regulatory mechanisms

Cells that have escaped tolerance in the thymus can also ignore self antigens if they are expressed in a privileged site. Within these sites pro-inflammatory lymphocytes are controlled either by apoptosis (Fas-ligand expression) or cytokine (transforming growth factor-β/interleukin 10, TGFβ/IL-10) secretion. Well-characterized immunologically privileged sites include the brain, anterior chamber of the eye and testes. These are defined as privileged sites because transplanted tissues have an enhanced chance of survival within them. Immune privilege in the eye is known to result from an active downregulation of systemic and local immunity rather than 'ignorance'. Antigens introduced into the anterior chamber of the eye are collected by APCs and subsequently carried to the spleen. In this case, antigen-specific regulatory T cells are generated in the spleen. Regulatory T cells generated by this process of anterior chamber–associated immune deviation (ACAID)

Mechanisms of central and peripheral tolerance

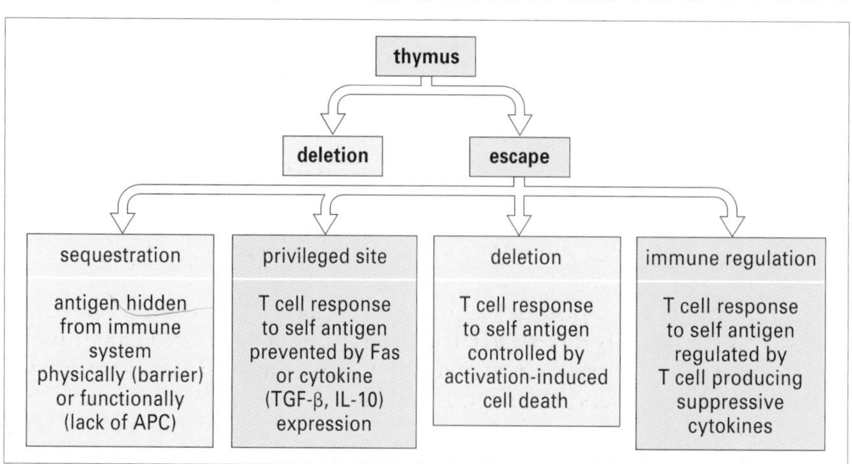

Fig. 12.12 Cells which have escaped negative selection in the thymus are still subject to control in the periphery. Most healthy individuals maintain self tolerance by a variety of mechanisms of peripheral tolerance involving sequestration, expression at a privileged site, deletion or immune regulation. (Based on Anderton *et al. Immunol Rev* 1999;**169**:123.)

can be adoptively transferred to naïve animals where they confer antigen-specific protection against inflammatory responses. A similar process of immune privilege is found in the brain. Here, however, the process depends on presentation of antigen in cervical lymph nodes rather than the spleen. Does immune privilege contribute to self tolerance or is it a phenomenon only seen by the introduction of foreign antigen to the privileged site? Immune privilege is clearly designed to dampen down inflammatory responses in certain vital organs. The same suppressive mechanisms would equally apply to inflammation caused by an immune response to either an infectious or self antigen. Immune privilege does not discriminate and therefore contributes to peripheral tolerance, at least in these particular organs.

T-cell death can be induced by persistent activation or neglect

Apoptotic death of lymphocytes is an extremely important mechanism of immune control and is essential for the maintenance of immune homeostasis in healthy individuals. It contributes both to the deletion of cells with high avidity for antigen and death of lymphocytes when the immune response is no longer required. These functions are fulfilled by two distinct mechanisms, activation-induced cell death (AICD) and passive cell death (PCD). Cells repeatedly stimulated with antigen undergo AICD by mechanisms involving so-called 'death receptors' of the tumour necrosis factor-receptor family. Among these, the most important molecule is Fas that on cross-linking by its ligand (FasL) leads to activation of the caspase cascade via caspase 8 and subsequent apoptopic death of the cell (*Fig. 12.13*). This can occur by cell–cell interactions and there is, in addition, evidence that T lymphocytes can kill themselves through 'fratricidal cell death' following the secretion of soluble FasL (*Fig. 12.14*). In addition, many activated cells die by PCD because their antigen is simply eliminated, as happens, for example, following clearance of an infection. Removal of the antigen then deprives cells of essential survival stimuli including growth factors. Under these conditions mitochondria in the cell respond by releasing cytochrome c. This, in combination with apoptosis activating factor 1, leads to activation of the caspase cascade following cleavage and activation of caspase 9 (*Fig. 12.13*).

Presumably, the survival rate of T cells that cross-react with self antigens, but which are generated during the immune response to infection, will be increased in the absence of AICD. The importance of the Fas pathway for AICD has been revealed by genetic defects in both mouse and man. For example, the lpr mouse has a mutation in Fas while the gld mouse has a mutation in Fas L. Both mutations lead to lymphadenopathy (expanded secondary lymphoid tissue). Importantly this lack of regulation also leads to the generation of autoimmunity, autoantibody production and nephritis with similarities to systemic lupus erythematosus in humans. Note that thymus selection in the lpr mouse is normal, showing that the Fas pathway is not essential for central tolerance but is clearly required for peripheral tolerance.

Recent studies have shown that analogous mutations lead to a similar form of disease known as human auto-

Two distinct mechanisms of lymphocyte apoptosis

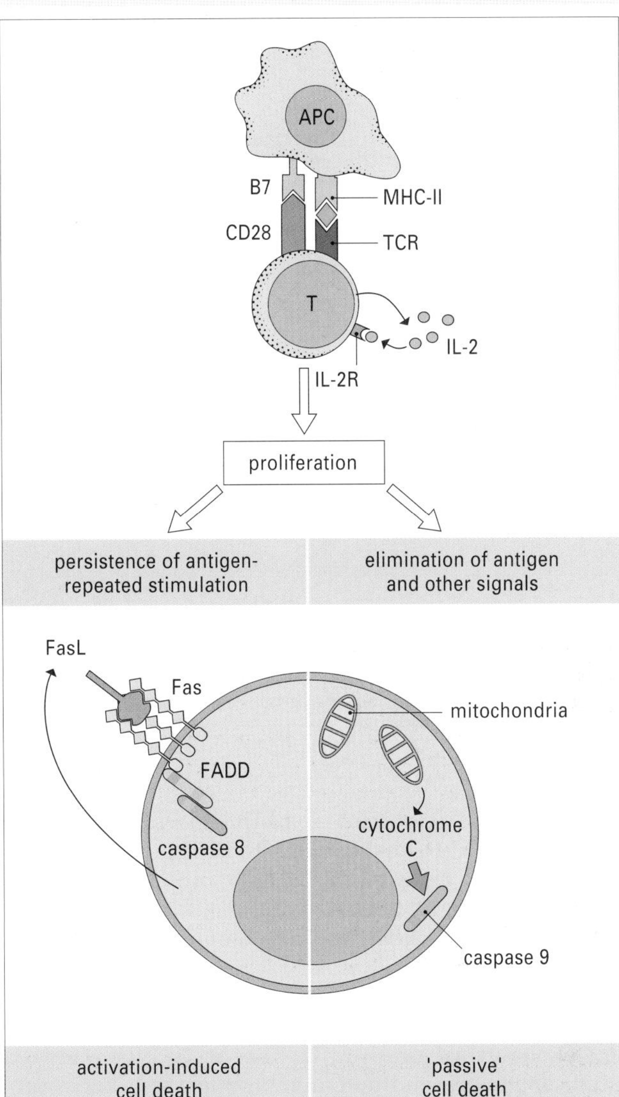

Fig. 12.13 Activated T lymphocytes will die by passive cell death (PCD) when deprived of an antigenic stimulus. This mechanism is designed to maintain homeostasis in the immune system. Activated T lymphocytes will die by activation-induced cell death (AICD) if repeatedly stimulated with antigen. This mechanism is designed to limit hypersensitivity reactions to allergens and autoantigens.

immune lymphoproliferative syndrome (ALPS) characterized by defective lymphocyte apoptosis, lymphocyte accumulation and humoral autoimmunity. The ALPS phenotype is associated with inherited mutations in the Fas gene (ALPS type 1a) or the Fas ligand gene (ALPS type 1b).

Both activation-induced and programmed cell death are tightly regulated and the two apoptopic pathways are under independent regulation. Bcl family members, for example, block PCD, by inhibiting the release of cytochrome c, but do not affect AICD. AICD, on the other hand, is inhibited by proteins binding to the death receptor complex. Of

The role of the Fas system in T-cell death

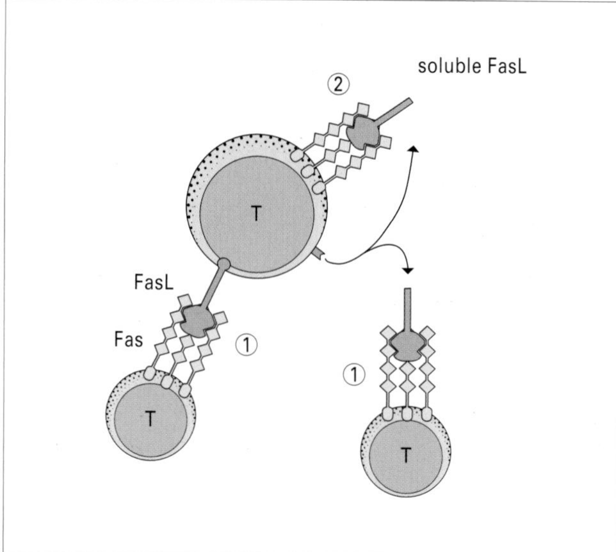

Fig. 12.14 Activated T cells express both Fas (CD95) and the ligand for this molecule (FasL). Fratricide (**1**) can result either from direct cell contact or from cleavage of FasL and the ligation of Fas by soluble FasL. Autocrine suicide (**2**) can result from the interaction of soluble FasL with Fas.

T-cell activation is controlled by co-stimulatory signals

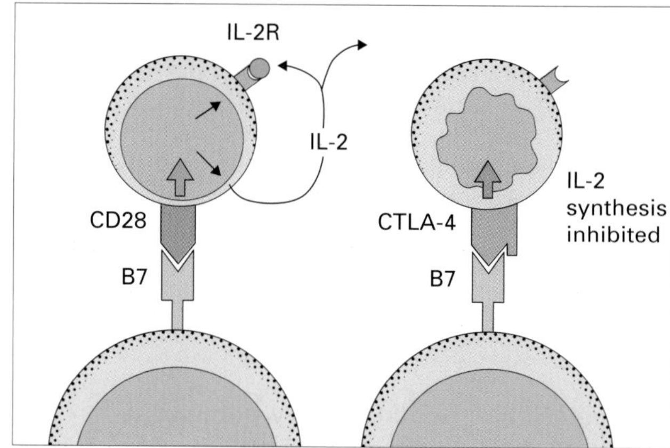

Fig. 12.15 Ligation of CD28 stimulates intracellular signals that lead to IL-2 production, IL-2 receptor expression and cell cycle progression in activated T cells. Ligation of cell-surface CTLA-4 blocks these CD28-dependent responses and causes inhibition of IL-2 synthesis.

these the most important is FLIP (FLICE inhibitory protein where FLICE is the FADD-like IL-1β converting enzyme). FLIP binds to the adaptor protein FADD or a precursor form of caspase-8 and blocks generation of the Fas-associated death receptor complex. AICD is also regulated by IL-2. This cytokine stimulates Fas-mediated AICD by enhancing transcription and expression of Fas L while inhibiting transcription of FLIP. Note that disruption of the genes for IL-2, IL-2Rα or IL-2Rβ leads to lymphadenopathy and autoimmunity in these knockout mice. This is proof of the central role played by IL-2-driven apoptotic death (propriocidal death) in homeostasis and peripheral tolerance.

The balance of co-stimulatory signals affects immune homeostasis and self tolerance

Naïve T lymphocytes require two signals to proliferate and differentiate. The first signal is triggered by TCR recognition of the appropriate peptide–MHC complex. The second signal is delivered by CD80 (B7.1) and CD86 (B7.2) co-stimulatory molecules expressed by APCs. How a T cell interprets co-stimulation depends on which co-stimulation receptor it uses. The CD28 molecule is constitutively expressed on T cells and signalling via CD28 enhances cell survival, prevents anergy induction and enhances CD40L expression. Ligation of CTLA-4 (CD152), however, inhibits T-cell responses. At the molecular level CTLA-4 ligation inhibits early T-cell activation including expression of the IL-2 receptor α chain and secretion of IL-2. The CTLA-4 pathway also inhibits IL-2 messenger RNA accumulation and inhibits upregulation of cyclin-dependent kinases 4 and 6, hence inhibiting progression through the cell cycle. CTLA-4 has a higher avidity (100×) for CD80 and CD86 but is normally isolated to the perinuclear Golgi apparatus. On T-cell contact with an APC, CTLA-4 traffics to the plasma membrane at the TCR–APC interface (*Fig. 12.15*). The role of CTLA-4 in normal homeostasis is revealed in the CTLA-4 knockout mouse. These mice show normal thymus selection but suffer from polyclonal T-cell expansion and die from a fatal lymphoproliferative disease. Interestingly, CTLA-4 influences CD4 cells more than CD8 cells, since depletion of CD4 cells from the CTLA-4 knockout mouse prevents the lymphoproliferative disease in this mouse.

Lymphoid dendritic cells contribute to peripheral tolerance

Lymphocytes do not possess an inherent capacity to distinguish between foreign and self antigens. Once selected, autoreactive cells are controlled by regulatory mechanisms but their activation is not differentially controlled. How then are responses to foreign antigens induced while avoiding autoimmune responses? Foreign antigens encountered by the immune system are predominantly components of infectious agents and the immune system has evolved ways to recognize the inherent adjuvant properties of these infectious agents. It is known that these elements upregulate co-stimulatory molecules but they also control migration of APC into the T-cell zones of secondary lymphoid tissues. Most dendritic cells in the T-cell zones of resting lymph nodes are lymphoid dendritic cells that arise from the same progenitor cells as T and B lymphocytes. Myeloid dendritic cells are normally found outside the T-cell zones but migrate into the zone when they first encounter the types of adjuvants contained in infectious agents (*Fig. 12.16*). In addition, myeloid dendritic cells are functional APCs whereas lymphoid dendritic cells are unable to internalize exogenous antigens. Lymphoid dendritic cells do, however, present endogenous antigens

Characteristics distinguishing myeloid and lymphoid dendritic cells of the mouse

Myeloid dendritic cells	Lymphoid dendritic cells
Precursor shared with macrophages	Precursor shared with T and B cells
Granulocyte–macrophage colony-stimulating factor dependent growth	IL3-dependent growth
Located in non-haematopoietic tissues in immature form and in marginal zones of secondary lymphoid tissue	Located in thymic medulla and T-cell zones of secondary lymphoid tissue
Migration to T zones of secondary lymphoid tissue following interaction with microbial products	Generated *in situ*
Receptor-mediated endocytosis of foreign antigen	Receptor-mediated endocytosis of self antigen
Induce immunity in naïve T cells	Induce tolerance in naïve T cells

Fig. 12.16 Two distinct lineages of dendritic cells exist in mice. These cells regulate immune responses by discriminating between endogenous and exogenous antigens. The control of migration of the myeloid dendritic cell prevents the cell from presenting self antigen until it becomes activated by microbial products. (Adapted from Fazekas de St Groth. *Immunol Today* 1998;**19**:448.)

and recognition of these 'self' antigens presented by lymphoid dendritic cells leads to apoptopic cell death among potential autoreactive T cells. Only when antigen-bearing myeloid dendritic cells migrate into the T-cell zones does the balance swing in favour of immunity to antigen presented by these cells.

In summary, homeostatic balance in the immune system is required to prevent lymphoproliferative responses. Lymphoproliferative disorders are associated with responses to both foreign and self antigens. Lack of homeostatic control leads to autoimmunity and hence the molecules involved in homeostatic control are important regulators of peripheral tolerance. These molecules include:

- CTLA-4 that acts as a brake on the normal immune response to both foreign and self antigens.
- Members of the TNF-R family, particularly Fas and Fas L.
- Components of the caspase cascade.
- IL-2 and the IL-2 receptor that together regulate sensitivity to Fas-mediated apoptosis.

The role of regulatory T lymphocytes in peripheral tolerance

Peripheral tolerance to antigens can be 'infectious'. The experimentally induced tolerance to one antigen can thus maintain tolerance or suppress the immune response to a second antigen as long as the two antigens are structurally or physically associated (e.g. within the same tissue). This implies that mechanisms other than ignorance and cell death must be involved in tolerance. One explanation for such phenomena depends on the existence of two populations of T lymphocytes that produce distinct cytokines. Many inflammatory autoimmune diseases are caused by TH1 cells that produce cytokines such as interferon-γ (IFNγ) and tumour necrosis factor-α (TNF-α). Cytokines derived from TH2 cells (IL-4, IL-5, IL-6, IL-10) support antibody production. A major additional effect of TH2-derived cytokines such as IL-10, however, is down-regulation of macrophage effector functions, including antigen presentation to TH1 and naïve T cells. TH2 cells are thus able to suppress inflammatory (delayed-type hypersensitivity, DTH) responses. TH1-cell-derived IFNγ can prevent the differentiation of TH0 to TH2 cells. This type of immune deviation was defined more than 30 years ago to describe how an individual animal could respond to the same antigen in two completely different ways. Guinea pigs primed with antigen in alum produced high levels of IgG1 antibody, but did not support a DTH response, whereas animals primed with the same antigen in complete Freund's adjuvant developed strong DTH responses. It was subsequently suggested that the ability of the same antigen to induce either 'humoral' or 'cellular' immunity could reflect the distinct activation of two mutually antagonistic arms of the immune system. The results of these experiments were undoubtedly a form of immune deviation resulting from the selective induction of TH2 rather than TH1 cells. Immune deviation can influence hypersensitivity conditions. Diabetes in the NOD mouse is known to be caused by TH1 cells and can be prevented by antigen-primed TH2 cells, whereas allergic disorders can be treated by induction of TH1 cells.

Peripheral T-cell tolerance depends on the genetic make-up of the individual. A transgenic model has been created in which a viral antigen (influenza haemagglutinin, HA) is expressed in the islet cells of the pancreas and a TCR specific for this antigen is expressed on the T cells. These double-transgenic mice are then bred with mice that differ in their non-MHC genes – that is, the mice have different background genes. In one mouse strain (BALB/c background), the HA-reactive T cells produce large amounts of both IL-4 and IFNγ and show no signs of inflammatory disease in the pancreas. In another mouse strain (B10.D2 background), the HA-reactive cells produce only TH1 cytokines and the T cells are able to infiltrate the pancreatic islets and cause diabetes. Immune deviation is clearly controlled by background genes, many of which combine to control the susceptibility of an individual to autoimmune disease.

IL-10 is required for regulation of inflammatory bowel disease mediated by activated T cells

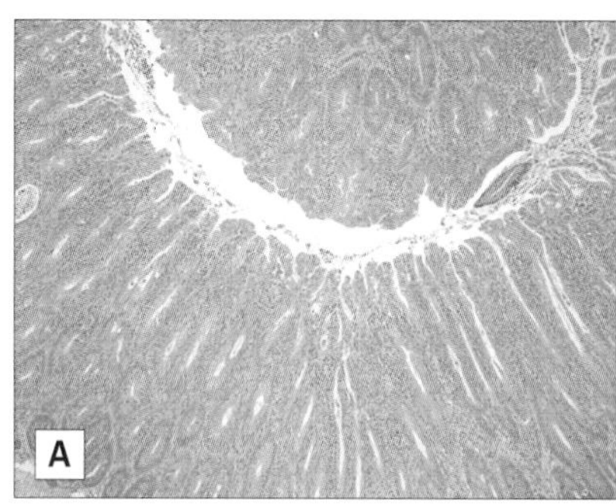

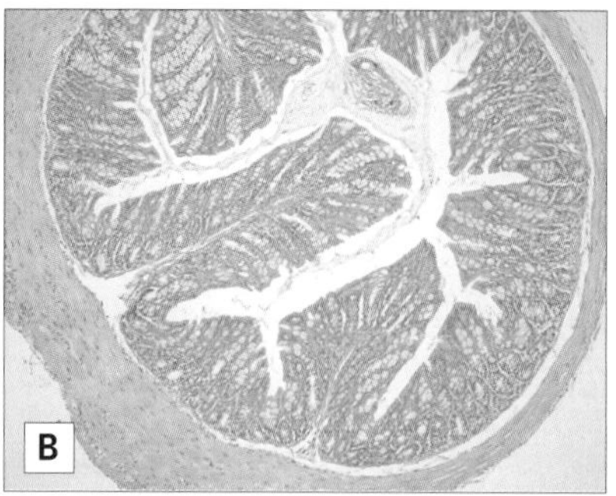

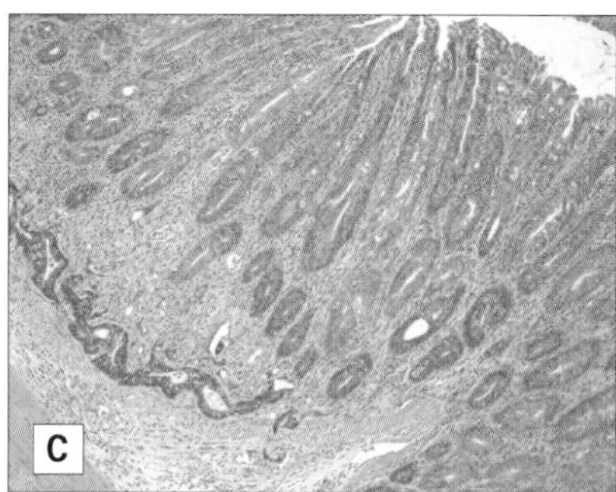

Fig. 12.17 (A) Severe colitis in a mouse injected with CD45RB^{high} CD4$^+$ T cells from normal mice. (B) Normal appearance of the colon in a mouse restored with both CD45RB^{high} and CD45RB^{low} cells. This shows that the CD45RB^{low} population of T cells is able to inhibit inflammation caused by normal CD45RB^{high} cells. (C) Severe colitis in a mouse restored with both CD45RB^{high} and IL-10$^{-/-}$ CD45RB^{low} cells. This experiment demonstrates that CD45RB^{low} cells that cannot produce IL-10 fail to serve as regulators of disease. (Based on Asseman *et al.* Reproduced from *The Journal of Experimental Medicine* 1999;**190**:995 by copyright permission of The Rockefeller University Press.)

T-cell-mediated diseases (such as insulin-dependent diabetes, thyroiditis and gastritis) can be produced in otherwise normal mice by simply eliminating a subpopulation of CD4$^+$ T cells expressing CD5, CD25 or a particular isoform of CD45. This is best illustrated by the transfer of subsets of murine cells isolated from healthy mice into Rag$^{-/-}$ mice that otherwise do not contain T cells of their own. Naïve and activated murine T cells can be distinguished according to the level of cell surface expression of CD45 RB – activated cells have low levels of this isoform and naïve cells have high levels. Activated or naïve populations are then transferred into recipient Rag$^{-/-}$ mice. Transfer of naïve cells leads to inflammatory bowel disease (IBD) in the Rag$^{-/-}$ recipients, but co-transfer of relatively few activated cells prevents disease (*Fig. 12.17*). The activated cells either produce or induce production of the immune suppressive cytokine TGFβ. Another cytokine, IL-10, undoubtedly plays a role in the function of the activated, regulatory cells because transfer of these regulatory cells from an IL-10 knockout mouse fails to suppress the induction of IBD by naïve cells.

A further subset of regulatory lymphocytes is distinguished by expression of the α chain of the IL-2 receptor (CD25). Elimination of these cells from normal mice leads to the generation of various organ-specific autoimmune conditions. These natural regulatory T cells are anergic to TCR-mediated activation but potently suppress the activation of other T cells. In contrast to cells such as the CD45RB^{low} regulators, however, the CD25$^+$ CD4 T cells are probably cytokine independent but suppress other cells by an APC-dependent mechanism involving cognate cellular interactions.

It is now clear that natural regulators play a central role in maintaining self tolerance. How and where are these cells generated? Interestingly not all CD25$^+$ cells serve as regulators. The CD25 marker is upregulated on naïve T cells in response to antigen and yet this is normally associated with an active immune response rather than regulation. It now appears that the thymus plays a crucial role in generation of CD25$^+$ regulators (*Fig. 12.18*). Thymectomy of mice before thymus-derived CD25$^+$ cells have had time to populate peripheral lymphoid organs leads to generation of autoimmune diseases similar to

The role of CD25$^+$,CD4$^+$ cells in maintaining self tolerance

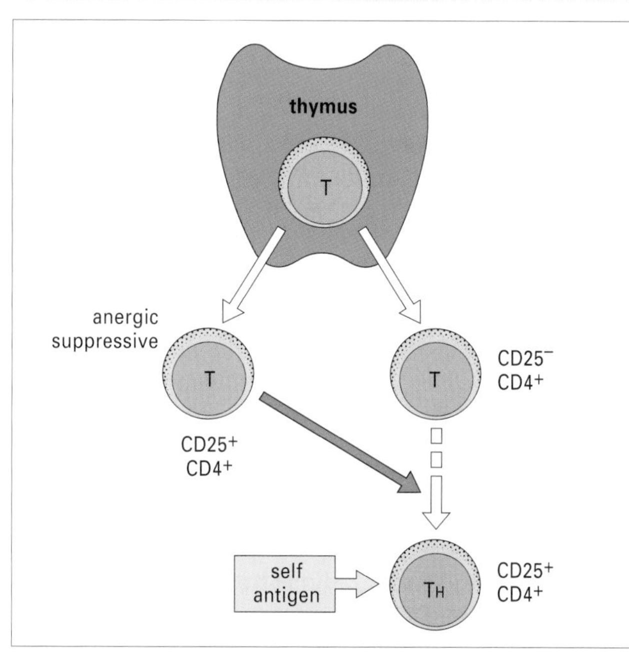

Fig. 12.18 Although the thymus is extremely efficient in deleting self-reactive T lymphocytes from the T-cell repertoire, potentially autoreactive CD25$^-$4$^+$ cells are still produced. The normal thymus also continuously produces anergic and suppressive CD25$^+$4$^+$ T cells that suppress the activation and expansion of autoreactive cells from the CD25$^-$4$^+$ population. When the CD25$^+$4$^+$ T cells are deleted from a normal, healthy animal, the CD25$^-$4$^+$ population expands rapidly, causing widespread autoimmunity. (See Itoh *et al. J Immunol* 1999;**162**:5317.)

those caused by elimination of CD25$^+$ cells from lymphoid organs of the adult mouse. How then does the immune system ever make a response to foreign antigens and infectious antigens if CD25$^+$ cells are such potent regulators? Note that these cells are normally anergic. Both their anergic and regulatory phenotypes can, however, be temporarily reversed by high local levels of cytokines such as IL-2. Thus a strong immune response to an infectious agent would temporarily overcome regulatory activity of the CD25$^+$ cells, thus permitting the localized immune response to the infectious agent to proceed.

It would appear that the active regulatory T cells identified in mice are antigen specific and regulate peripheral tolerance by the production of immune suppressive cytokines such as TGFβ and IL-10. The thymus-derived CD25$^+$ population, on the other hand, appears not to depend on such cytokines and may suppress neighbouring T cells in a contact-dependent fashion. Other subsets of lymphocytes may also contribute to the regulation of immune responses. In certain cases immune suppressive CD8$^+$ T cells have been described. These could in fact be cells of TCR-γδ type, since CD8$^+$ γδ T cells have been shown to both suppress allergic responses and control diabetes in a mouse model of this disease. Diabetes has also been controlled in mice by transfer of thymocytes bearing the NK1 marker that appears to produce the TH2 cytokines IL-4 and IL-10.

In conclusion, regulatory lymphocytes play a crucial role in the control of autoimmune responses. Scientists are only just beginning to reveal the mechanisms by which these cells mediate their suppressive activity. Furthermore we know very little about how these cells are generated in the normal immune repertoire of healthy individuals. There is little doubt that clarification of these questions will help in the control of many hypersensitivity conditions including allergic and autoimmune diseases.

B-CELL TOLERANCE TO SELF ANTIGENS

High-affinity IgG production is T cell dependent. For this reason, and because the threshold of tolerance for T cells is lower than that for B cells, the simplest explanation for non-self reactivity by B cells is a lack of T-cell help.

Until quite recently it was therefore felt that immunological tolerance should be the responsibility of T lymphocytes alone. The logical argument being: Why evolve a complex process of immunological tolerance amongst cells such as B cells when they are then allowed to hypermutate? All nature would have to do would be to evolve a system in which T cells never react with self antigens; a 'perfect' system would delete all self-reactive T cells. The immune system could then allow the B-cell repertoire to expand widely and generate as many autoreactive B cells as possible by random rearrangement. Without help from T cells these B cells would remain harmless. Now we appreciate that the immune system is not allowed to be 'perfect'. If it were, it would almost inevitably develop 'holes' in the immunological repertoire through which faster evolving microorganisms would inevitably break. We now appreciate that autoreactive T cells exist in all of us and that the balance between health and autoimmunity is a fine one, dependent on numerous polymorphisms in regulatory mechanisms. It is now clear that the B lymphocyte pool is subject to analogous but subtly different mechanisms of immunological tolerance to those that apply to the T lymphocyte pool.

There are clearly circumstances in which B cells must be tolerized directly. For example, some microorganisms have cross-reactive antigens that have both foreign T-cell-reactive epitopes and other epitopes that resemble self epitopes and are capable of stimulating B cells. Such antigens could provoke a vigorous antibody response to self antigens (*Fig. 12.19*). Furthermore, in contrast to TCRs, the immunoglobulin receptors on mature, antigenically stimulated B cells can undergo hypermutation and may acquire anti-self reactivities at this late stage. Tolerance thus needs to be imposed on B cells both during their development and after antigenic stimulation in secondary lymphoid tissues.

Self-reactive B cells may be deleted or anergized, depending on the affinity of the B-cell antigen receptor and the nature of the antigen. Tolerance induction by self antigens can lead to one of several results, such as deletion or anergy. The outcome depends on the affinity of the B-cell antigen receptor and on the nature of the antigen it encounters, whether this is an integral membrane protein or a soluble and largely monomeric protein in the circulation. The fate of self-reactive B cells has been determined using transgenic technology (*Figs 12.20* and *12.21*).

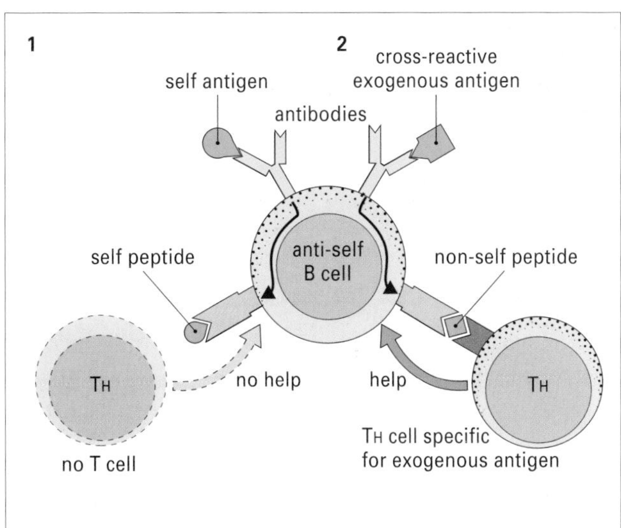

Fig. 12.19 (**1**) If TH cells are not available, either because of a hole in the T-cell repertoire, or because of deletion resulting from self tolerance achieved intrathymically, any B cells that are self-reactive will be unable to mount an anti-self antibody response. (**2**) Autoantibodies can be produced if an anti-self B cell collaborates with an anti-non-self TH cell in response to cross-reactive antigens containing both self and non-self determinants.

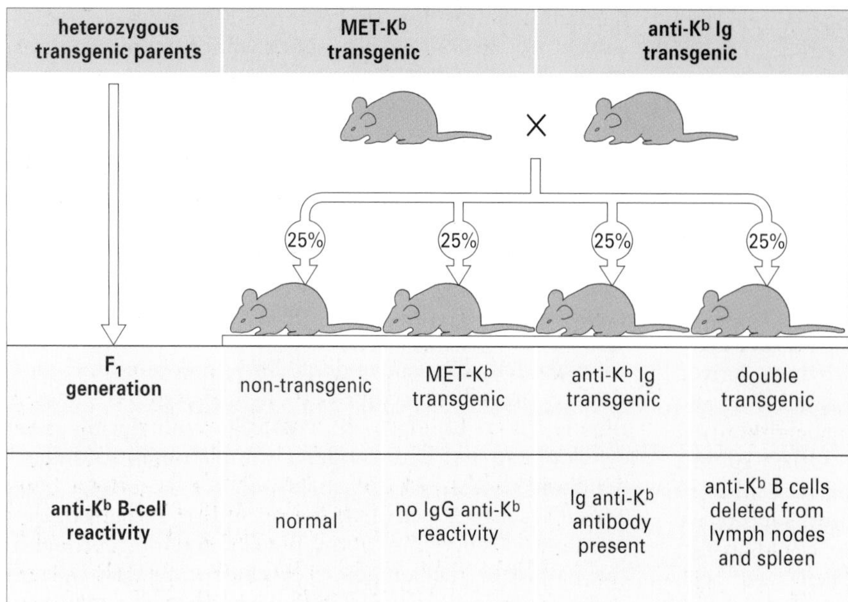

Fig. 12.20 Non-b haplotype mice were given the gene for H-2K^b, which is a foreign MHC class I molecule. The gene was controlled by the metallothionein promotor, specific for such sites as the liver (MET-K^b transgenic). These mice were crossed with other non-b mice which had been given the genes for anti-H-2K^b antibodies (anti-K^b Ig transgenic). Double transgenic offspring expressed H-2K^b in the liver and exported B cells specific for H-2K^b from the bone marrow. However, these self-reactive B cells were partially deleted in the spleen and entirely deleted in the lymph nodes, and thus no autoantibody was produced – no idiotype corresponding to the anti-K^b Ig was detectable.

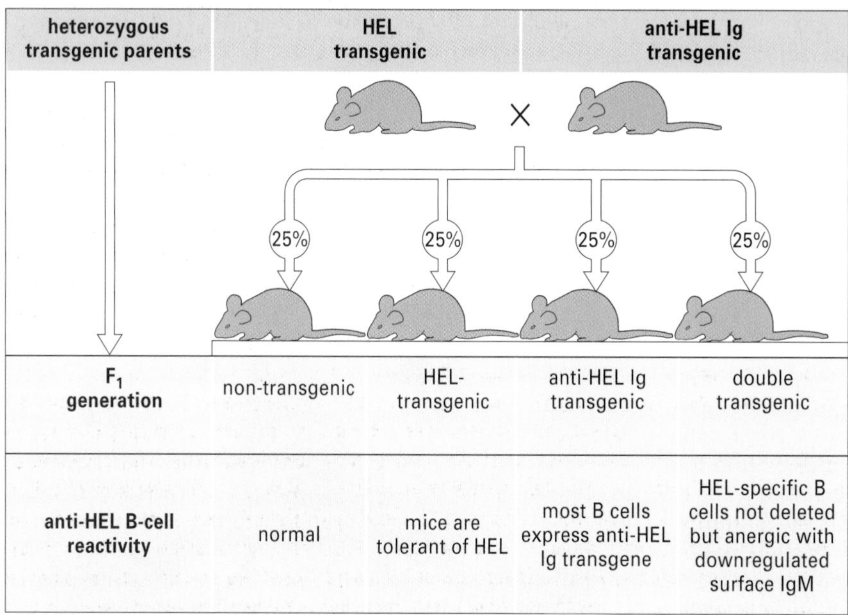

Fig. 12.21 A mouse was given the hen egg lysozyme gene (HEL), linked to a tissue-specific promoter. The (largely soluble) HEL induced B- and T-cell tolerance. A second transgenic line (anti-HEL Ig) carried rearranged heavy and light chain genes encoding a high-affinity HEL antibody. An allotypic marker (IgH^a) distinguished this from endogenous immunoglobulin (IgH^b). The majority of B cells in these transgenics carried IgM and IgD of the 'a' allotype. Double transgenic offspring were highly HEL tolerant, producing neither anti-HEL antibody nor antibody-secreting B cells. HEL-binding (self reactive) B cells were not however deleted, but had downregulated surface IgM, but not IgD receptors. They behaved as anergic cells.

B cells pass through several developmental checkpoints

B-cell development shows similar features to T-cell development but takes place largely in the bone marrow. Development is marked by ordered expression of surrogate receptor molecules. The first notable event takes place at the late pro-B stage when the CD79a and CD79b (Igα and Igβ) molecules appear at the cell surface (see *Figs 8.1* and *8.3*). Progression to the pre-B stage is accompanied by VDJ recombination at the heavy chain locus. The rearranged heavy chain can then appear at the cell surface in combination with both CD79a and b and the VpreB and λ5 molecules that act as surrogate light chains (see *Fig. 8.2*). There are clear analogies with T-cell development here: T cells rearrange the heavy chain genes first and also employ a surrogate light chain. In addition, it appears that expression of the pre-B cell receptor is necessary for successful allelic exclusion at the heavy chain locus. As pre-B cells develop, recombination at the light chain locus proceeds and the cells become immature B cells. At this point the cells are IgD$^-$. B cells then go through a 'transitional' stage in development becoming IgD^{low} as well as IgM$^+$. Mature B cells express IgD at higher levels than IgM.

Checkpoints in B-cell development include:

- Successful expression of CD79a and b in late pro-B cells.
- Successful rearrangement at the heavy chain locus in pre-B cells.
- Successful rearrangement at the light chain locus and receptor editing.

Self tolerance begins when IgM first appears at the surface of the developing cell. Immature cells are resistant to apoptosis, although the development of immature B cells can still be blocked by interaction with self antigen. However, immature B cells can edit their receptor, thus allowing development to progress.

Receptor editing allows potentially self-reactive B cells to continue development

When the IgM receptor on an immature, bone marrow B cell reacts with self antigen further cell differentiation is blocked but light chain rearrangement can continue. If the new IgM receptor does not react with a self antigen in bone marrow, B-cell development can proceed. Interestingly the 'immature' B cell is relatively resistant to apoptotic cell death, whereas the later 'transitional' cell is sensitive. Allowing light chain rearrangement to continue among immature cells permits the B cell to edit its receptor and thus rescue potentially autoreactive cells from inevitable death. This mechanism of altering offending receptors before the B cell becomes sensitive to antigen-mediated cell death clearly allows the immune system to optimize the generation of its repertoire. In fact it looks like mechanisms have evolved to promote receptor editing in B cells. The κ light chain locus can be inactivated by recombination of a recombining sequence (RS). Recombination of the RS element results in deletion of CK and other sequences required for transcription of the κ allele. It is important to appreciate that 40–60% of IgM$^+\lambda^+$ B cells carry a Vκ Jκ rearrangement inactivated by this RS recombination. Receptor editing therefore plays an important role in generation of the normal B-cell repertoire.

Self reactive B cells are usually deleted

As B cells mature through the transitional stage they become poor at reactivating the recombinase activating genes. So, if receptor editing has failed to eliminate autoreactive B cells they are likely to be eliminated by apoptotic death, since they can no longer select a new receptor. Interestingly these transitional IgM^{hi}IgD^{lo} cells can emigrate to the periphery where their high IgM level ensures that apoptotic cell death can still take place.

Peripheral B-cell tolerance

Recent studies have shown that the bone marrow exports a higher proportion of new B cells than the thymus does new T cells. Also, unlike T cells leaving the thymus, B cells leaving the bone marrow are relatively immature. These cells express the heat stable antigen (HSA) and migrate from the bone marrow to the outer T-cell zone of the spleen. It is among these cells that the most significant amount of negative selection takes place. This splenic environment eliminates unwanted B cells as effectively as the thymus removes unwanted T cells (*Fig. 12.22*). Self-reactive B cells are purged by a process that (i) induces anergy; (ii) prevents migration into B-cell follicles; and (iii) rapidly leads to cell death. Self-reactive B cells in the outer T-cell zone are short-lived (1–3 days), whilst cells selected to enter B-cell follicles become long-lived and recirculate from 1 to 4 weeks. Short-lived, autoreactive B cells may, however, contribute to immune responses to foreign antigens. Anergy in such an autoreactive B cell can be overcome by high-avidity antigen. Self-reactive B cells may then be recruited into the functional immune repertoire because their B-cell receptor cross-reacts sufficiently strongly with foreign antigen.

At first sight, allowing B-cell tolerance to self antigen to be overwhelmed by foreign antigen would seem a risky business. Why promote a pluripotent B-cell repertoire at the risk of autoimmunity? This question must be considered a balance between the risk of autoimmunity and protection of the species from infectious pandemics. The immune system has evolved to ensure that among the population there will be individuals equipped to fight almost any infection. Diversity among T cells is generated by rearrangement of their receptors in concert with MHC polymorphism. MHC polymorphism and T-cell receptor selection together provide sufficient diversity across the population to protect against almost any infection. MHC polymorphism has evolved to fill holes in the protective repertoire of the species. Likewise the fact that the B-cell pool permits a proportion of short-lived and potentially autoreactive B cells to emigrate to the periphery provides an additional level of protection from infection. In the absence of an infection these cells die rapidly. This short-lived pool of cells can, however, contribute to broadening the potential B-cell repertoire. Such repertoire diversity and further differences between the repertoires of individuals within the population will ensure that there will always be some individuals ready to mount an effective immune response to infection.

A second window of susceptibility to tolerance occurs transiently during the generation of B-cell memory. Secondary B cells (derived from memory B cells produced by T-cell-dependent stimulation) are highly susceptible to tolerance by epitopes presented multivalently in the absence of T-cell help. Such a tolerance-susceptible stage probably ensures that newly derived memory B cells that have acquired self reactivity (as a result of accumulated somatic mutations) are purged from the repertoire.

ARTIFICIALLY INDUCED TOLERANCE *IN VIVO*

Chimerism is associated with tolerance

Tolerance can be induced by the inoculation of allogeneic cells into hosts that lack immunocompetence, for example neonatal hosts, or adult hosts after immunosuppressive regimens such as total body irradiation, drugs (e.g. cyclosporin) or anti-lymphocytic antibodies (anti-lymphocyte globulin, anti-CD4 antibodies, etc.). For tolerance to be maintained, a certain degree of chimerism – the coexistence of cells from genetically different individuals – must be

Self-reactive B cells die in peripheral lymphoid tissues

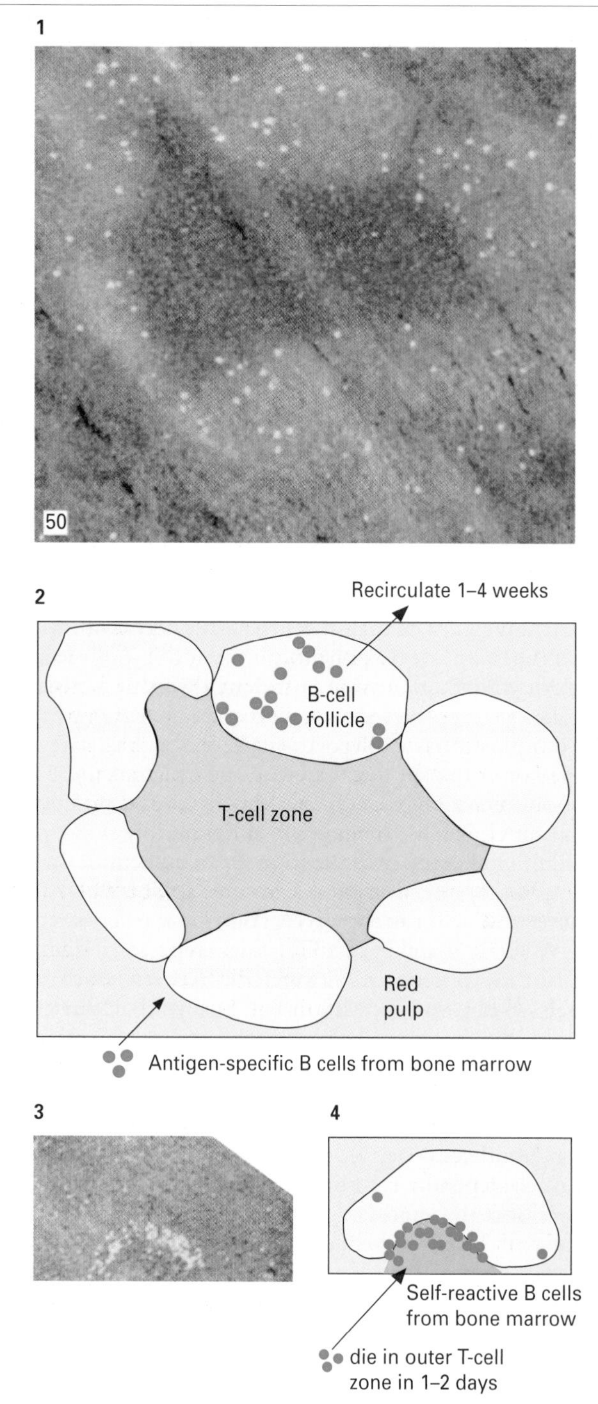

Fig. 12.22 Transgenic B cells expressing a BCR specific for lysozyme were stained green and adoptively transferred into either normal mice (**1**) and (**2**) or mice expressing soluble lysozyme as a self antigen (**3**) and (**4**). In the absence of antigen the B cells migrate to B-cell follicles. In the presence of the self antigen the B cells are excluded from B-cell follicles in the outer T-cell zone where they die in 1–2 days. (From Townsend SE *et al.* *Immunology Today* 1999;**20**:217 with permission from Elsevier Science.)

maintained. This is best achieved if the inoculum contains cells capable of self renewal (e.g. bone-marrow cells).

If mature T cells are present in the injected cell population, they may react against the histocompatibility antigens of their host and induce a severe and often fatal disease known as graft-versus-host disease.

Antibodies to co-receptor and co-stimulatory molecules induce tolerance to transplants

Tolerance of transplanted tissues can be achieved in adult animals by monoclonal antibodies directed against the T-cell molecules, CD4 and CD8 (the antibodies can be either the T-cell-depleting or the non-depleting type). In this situation, tolerance of skin allografts is obtained even in the absence of cellular chimerism.

Another highly promising approach to transplantation tolerance has arisen through the use of agents designed to blockade co-stimulatory molecules. As mentioned above, T cells require co-stimulatory signals for effective priming. CD28 and CD154 both play important roles in co-stimulation. The CD28 pathway of activation can be inhibited by blocking both B7 molecules with a soluble form of CTLA-4 (CTLA-4-Ig). In combination with an antibody to the ligand for CD40 (CD154), CTLA-4-Ig has been shown to block recognition of allografts and allow long-term skin allograft survival in mice. Antibodies to CD154 alone will prolong renal allograft survival in non-human primates. It is thought that anti-CD154 prevents the three-cell interplay between CD4, CD8 and dendritic cells that is required for the maturation of CD8 cells (*Fig. 12.23*).

Soluble antigens readily induce tolerance

Tolerance is inducible in both neonatal and adult animals by administering soluble protein antigens in deaggregated form. T and B cells differ in their susceptibility to tolerization by these antigens. Thus tolerance is achieved in T cells from spleen and thymus after very low antigen doses and within a few hours. Tolerance of spleen B cells requires much more time and higher doses of antigen (*Fig. 12.24*). The antigen levels which will produce B-cell tolerance in neonates are about one-hundredth of those required in adults.

Oral administration of antigens induces tolerance

Orally administered antigens induce tolerance to themselves by a variety of mechanisms. High doses of antigen can cause anergy or deletion; this could be one situation in which the term anergy is being used to describe a state of paralysis preceding cell death. Lower doses of antigen can, however, induce the priming of T cells in the gut. As an effective antibody response in the gut requires class-switching to the IgA isotype, it comes as no surprise that antigen feeding induces T cells that support IgA production. These 'TH3-like' cells produce cytokines including IL-10 and TGFβ and serve to inhibit inflammatory responses mediated by TH1 cells. TGFβ inhibits the proliferation and function of B cells, cytotoxic T cells and NK cells, inhibits cytokine production in lymphocytes and antagonizes the effects of TNF. Although the induction of mucosal TH3 cells is antigen specific, the suppressive

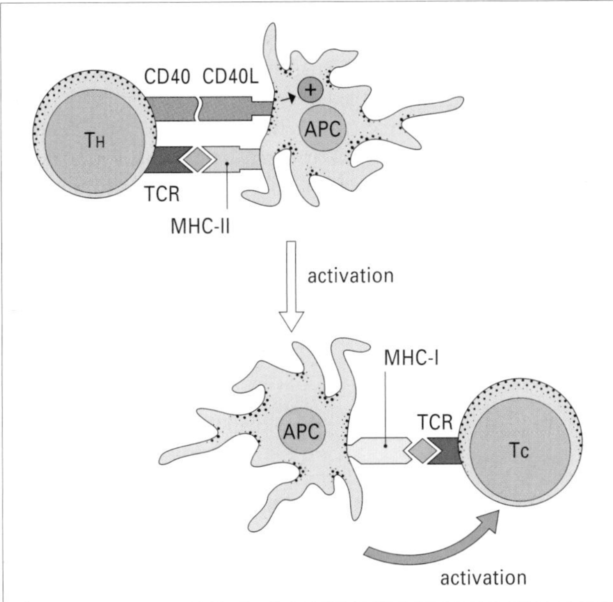

Fig. 12.23 CD8 T killer cells will not respond to resting APC. T-helper cell recognition of antigen is one way that APCs such as dendritic cells can be armed to present antigen to CD8 cells. The molecules responsible for the interaction between CD4 T helper cells and dendritic cells are called CD40L and CD40. Ligation of CD40 on the surface of dendritic cells leads to their activation. Blocking this interaction is one way to prevent the presentation of alloantigens to CD8 cells and hence preventing allograft rejection. (Based on Lanzavecchia A. *Nature* 1998;**393**:413.)

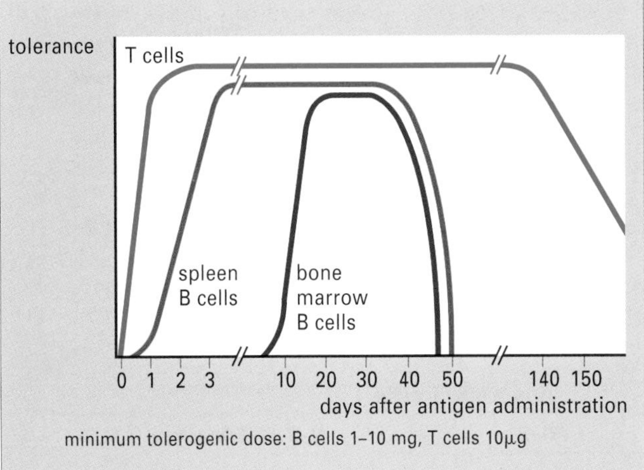

Fig. 12.24 A mouse was given a T-dependent antigen (human γ-globulin) at tolerance-inducing doses, and the duration of tolerance was measured. T-cell tolerance was more rapidly induced and more persistent than B-cell tolerance. Bone marrow B cells may take considerably longer to tolerize than splenic B cells. Typically, much less antigen is needed to tolerize T cells – 10 μg as opposed to 1–10 mg, a 1000-fold difference.

activity of cytokines such as TGFβ is not. Hence, the induction of oral tolerance to one antigen is able to suppress the immune response to a second, associated antigen. The effect of 'bystander suppression' by mucosal TH3 cells allows the suppression of complex organ-specific autoimmune diseases by feeding with a single antigen derived from the affected tissue.

Other mucosal surfaces are proving equally effective as routes for the induction of antigen-specific tolerance. Nasal deposition of class II-restricted peptides has been used to control both 'humoral' and 'cellular' immune responses. In addition, administration of aerosolized antigen to the lung can be used to control either allergic responses to foreign antigens or autoimmune responses to self antigens. The fact that one can inhibit both autoimmune (TH1 type) and allergic (TH2 type) responses argues against immune deviation as a mechanism for tolerance induction in this case. Recent evidence suggests that cells producing IL-10 may be responsible for nasal peptide-induced tolerance. It could be that other cell types, including CD8 cells, are responsible for suppressing the immune response that follows aerosol administration of protein antigens.

Extensive clonal proliferation can lead to exhaustion and tolerance

Tolerance in T cells, and to a lesser extent in B cells, can be due to clonal exhaustion, the end result of a powerful immune response. Repeated antigenic challenge may stimulate all the antigen-responding cells to differentiate into short-lived end cells, leaving no cells that can respond to a subsequent challenge with antigen.

Anti-idiotypic responses can be associated with tolerance

An antibody's combining site may act as an antigen and induce the formation of 'anti-idiotypic antibodies'. By cross-linking immunoglobulin on B cells, these antibodies can block B-cell responsiveness of the cell. Because, in some animals, most of the antibodies produced in response to particular antigens bear a particular idiotype, suppression of this idiotype by anti-idiotypic antibody can significantly alter the response. This type of tolerance will be partial, however, because it affects only those B cells carrying the idiotype.

The idiotype of a T cell is represented by the polymorphic regions of the TCR α and β chains. TCR-specific regulatory cells, induced after vaccination with self-reactive T cells, TCR peptides or even DNA-encoding TCR molecules, have been shown to prevent autoimmunity in animal models.

Tolerance *in vivo* relates to persistence of antigen

Persistence of antigen plays a major part in maintaining a state of tolerance to it *in vivo*: when the antigen concentration decreases below a certain threshold, responsiveness is restored. If the tolerance results from clonal deletion, recovery of responsiveness is related to the time required to generate new lymphocytes from their precursors. This tolerance can be prevented by measures such as thymectomy. If, on the other hand, the tolerance is maintained by a suppressive mechanism resulting, for example, from the induction of regulatory T cells, then the state of tolerance can be relatively long lived.

POTENTIAL THERAPEUTIC APPLICATIONS OF TOLERANCE

A better understanding of tolerogenesis could be valuable in many ways. It could be used to promote tolerance of foreign tissue grafts or to control the damaging immune responses in hypersensitivity states and autoimmune diseases. The various ways of establishing artificial tolerance in adult animals are being investigated for their potential clinical applications. Some success has been obtained in the case of transplants associated with chimerism and performed under the umbrella of immunosuppressive agents. Treatment with monoclonal non-depleting anti-CD4 and anti-CD8 or anti-CD154 antibodies has also been used successfully with foreign tissue or organ transplants. The possibility that tolerance can be induced either by mucosal administration of the target antigen or through the use of peptide drugs awaits extensive clinical trials in humans.

It is also important to learn how to activate T cells that ignore certain antigens, so as to enable the immune system to mount an appropriate active response. This could be exploited to limit the growth of tumours that may express their own unique tumour-specific genes.

CRITICAL THINKING • Tolerance (Explanations on p. 456)

Experimental mouse	CD4 cells	CD8 cells	Experimental mouse	CD4 cells	CD8 cells
AND AND/dLGKR	487 4	8 39	OT-1 OT-1dLGF	6 380	113 37

Data summarized from Hernandez-Hoyos *et al. Immunity* 2000;**12**:313–322.

Lineage commitment in thymocyte development
Thymocytes bearing MHC class I-restricted TCRs differentiate into CD8 T cells, while those recognizing MHC class II become CD4 T cells. It was previously thought that this process might be random or 'stochastic', but it now appears that this is an 'instructive' process.

AND mice express a transgenic TCR specific for a peptide derived from pigeon cytochrome c in the context of I–E^k (class II). Normally the majority of thymocytes in these mice develop into CD4 single positive (SP) cells. OT-1 mice bear a transgenic TCR specific for an ovalbumin peptide that is H-$2K^b$ (class I) restricted. Normally the majority of thymocytes in these mice develop into CD8 SP cells. $TCR^{+/-}$ heterozygotes were crossed with heterozygotes expressing either a constitutively active (dLGF) or catalytically inactive (dLGKR) form of Lck.

Thymocytes from AND, AND/dLGKR, OT-1 or OT-1/dLGF were stained with antibodies specific for CD4 or CD8 and analysed by flow cytometry. The table below shows the absolute number of CD4 and CD8 SP cells obtained from three individual experiments (median values) in which littermates were studied.

12.1 What drives expression of CD4 cells in a mouse expressing a class I-restricted TCR?

12.2 What effect does inhibiting the activity of Lck have on thymocyte development?

12.3 Are the results seen with the four different strains of mice mutually consistent?

The molecular basis of activation-induced cell death (AICD)
The 3A9 transgenic mouse expresses a TCR specific for a peptide derived from hen eggwhite lysozyme. These mice were crossed onto the lpr, gld or TNF-R1 knockout background. Remember that the lpr and gld mice have defective *fas* and *fasL* genes respectively.

Previously activated T cells may undergo AICD on further restimulation *in vitro*. T cells from the 3A9 backcrossed mice were activated *in vitro* and then restimulated with anti-CD3 (to induce AICD), IL-2 or IL-2 with anti-Fas antibody (to induce death via the Fas pathway). The cells were then assayed for apoptosis by propidium iodide staining.

Mice	Apoptotic T cells		
	Anti-CD3	IL-2	IL-2 and Anti-Fas
3A9	++	–	++
3A9.lpr knockout	–	–	–
3A9. TNF-R1 knockout	++	–	++
3A9.gld knockout	–	–	++

Data summarized from Rafaeli *et al. Immunol Rev* 1999;**169**:273–282.

12.4 Is AICD mediated by signalling through the Fas or TNF-R1 pathway?

12.5 What evidence is there to support your choice?

12.6 Why are T cells from the gld mouse susceptible to anti-Fas-mediated death?

12.7 Why has the immune system developed a way of killing off activated T cells?

12.8 If T cells die on reactivation how does immune memory arise?

The role of regulatory T cells in peripheral tolerance
Certain mice are congenitally athymic and do not have mature T lymphocytes. The 'nude' mouse carries a mutation in the gene for the Wnt transcription factor. This results in lack of hair and absence of the thymus. Nude mice can, however, be reconstituted with lymphocytes from normal mice. In the experiment for which results are shown below, either thymocytes or spleen and lymph node (SP/LN) cells from normal mice were treated with various antibodies and complement to deplete cell subsets and then transferred into 'nude' recipients by intravenous injection. The recipient mice were left for 3 months and then examined for histological and serological evidence of autoimmune disease.

12.9 Why do $CD25^-$ lymphocytes cause widespread autoimmunity?

12.10 Where do $CD25^+$ cells arise?

12.11 Why are certain tissues more susceptible to autoimmune disease than others?

	Inoculated cells	Number of mice with autoimmune disease					
		Number of mice	OOP	THR	SIAL	ADR	GN
A	Whole thymocytes	12	0	0	0	0	0
B	$CD25^-$ thymocytes	12	12	4	3	1	3
C	$CD4^+8^-$ thymocytes	5	0	0	0	0	0
D	$CD25^-4^+$ thymocytes	5	5	2	1	2	1
E	Whole SP/LN cells	8	0	0	0	0	0
F	$CD25^-$ SP/LN cells	8	8	5	5	2	2
G	$CD25^-$ thymocytes and $CD4^+$ SP/LN cells	8	0	0	0	0	0

Data summarized from Itoh *et al. J Immunol* 1999;**162**:5317–5326.
OOP = oophoritis, THR = thyroiditis, SIAL = sialoadenitis, ADR = adrenalitis, GN = glomerulonephritis.

FURTHER READING

Benschop RJ, Cambier JC. B cell development: signal transduction by antigen receptors and their surrogates. *Curr Opin Immunol* 1999;**11**:143–51.

Chambers CA, Allison JP. Costimulatory regulation of T cell function. *Curr Opin Immunol* 1999;**11**:203–10.

Goldrath AW, Bevan MJ. Selecting and maintaining a diverse T-cell repertoire. *Nature* 1999;**402**:255–62.

Mason D, Powrie F. Control of immune pathology by regulatory T cells. *Curr Opin Immunol* 1998;**10**:649–55.

Refaeli Y, Parijs LV, Abbas AK. Genetic models of abnormal apoptosis in lymphocytes. *Immunol Rev* 1999;**169**:273–82.

Townsend SE, Weintraub BC, Goodnow CC. Growing up on the streets: why B cell development differs from T cell development. *Immunol Today* 1999;**20**:217–20.

13 Evolution of immunity

- **Phagocytosis and encapsulation** are important in eliminating non-self material in invertebrates, with circulating white blood cells mediating these processes in many species.
- **Recognition of foreign transplants** is evident early in evolution, but there is little evidence for specificity and clonal expansion in invertebrates.
- **Lectins and prophenoloxidase** are centrally involved in recognition of self/non-self in invertebrates.
- **Cytokine-like molecules** effect immunoregulation in many invertebrates.
- **An inducible, broad-spectrum, humoral immunity** is found in some coelomate invertebrates.
- **Rearranging antigen receptors** are absent from all invertebrates and agnathan fishes, although Ig-like domains are found in many invertebrate phyla.
- **B cells and IgM** are universally found in jawed vertebrates. Although additional non-μ heavy chains are found in ectotherms, antibody affinity remains low. Recombinant DNA technology has revealed several patterns of Ig gene organization during vertebrate phylogeny.
- **The major histocompatibility complex (MHC)** has been identified from cartilaginous fish upwards.
- **γδ and αβ T-cell receptors (TCRs)** are considered to have evolved in cartilaginous and bony fish. However other characteristic T-cell markers (e.g. CD3 and CD5) have only been described at the amphibian stage of evolution.
- **Natural killer (NK) cells, phagocytes, complement components and immunoregulatory cytokines** constitute non-adaptive elements of the immune systems of vertebrates.

An evolutionary progression towards the sophisticated mammalian immune system is apparent from detailed studies of a range of vertebrates. However, the phylogenetic origins of the vertebrate adaptive immune system, particularly at the molecular level, remain uncertain despite extensive research into invertebrate immunity. Nevertheless, much can be learned about the origins of vertebrate non-adaptive (innate) immunity (e.g. phagocytosis) from the examination of invertebrates. Because invertebrates comprise over 95% of all animal species – they occur as solitary or colonial animals, with or without body cavities (coelomate/acoelomate), with or without blood systems – there are many suitable experimental subjects.

Figure 13.1 shows a simplified evolutionary tree of the animal kingdom with the coelomate invertebrates divided into two main evolutionary lines, based principally upon embryological differences. One line, leading to the molluscs, annelids and arthropods (the protostomes), diverged early in evolution from the pathway forming the echinoderms, tunicates and vertebrates (the deuterostomes). Research on invertebrate immunity has concentrated on arthropods and molluscs because many of these are pests transmitting diseases or competing for agricultural products. Consequently, work with groups that are phylogenetically relevant to the vertebrates (e.g. tunicates and echinoderms) has been neglected. In addition, because the ancestors of vertebrates are now extinct, attempts to trace the origin of vertebrate immunity within the invertebrates, in groups such as the tunicates (*Fig. 13.2*), are speculative and assume that some living animals are close relatives of the vertebrate ancestor. *Figure 13.1* also shows cellular and humoral immune phenomena discovered in the invertebrates.

Figure 13.3 presents possible steps in the evolution of vertebrate blood cells and immunity. Despite the success of the invertebrates, only vertebrates possessing jaws have lymphocytes with clonally restricted antigen receptors and display a highly specific long-term memory component. What environmental pressures might have led to the increased sophistication of the vertebrate anticipatory (adaptive) immune system? Perhaps the enhanced threat of cancer and of viral infections in these complex, long-lived animals was important, favouring the development of a finely tuned immune system, with circulating effector cells recognizing foreign peptides presented by major histocompatibility complex (MHC) glycoproteins on the surface of infected or mutated cells. As there is an evolutionary link between the presence of jaws and the development of the anticipatory immune system, it has been proposed that masticated particles causing gut damage created the selective pressure to drive development of mucosal-based adaptive immunity.

INVERTEBRATE IMMUNITY

Classification of blood cells in invertebrates

Most invertebrates possess white blood cells (leucocytes), but usually lack red blood cells (erythrocytes). The leucocytes can be fixed, free within blood vessels, or occupy fluid-filled body cavities called the coelom (coelomocytes) or haemocoel (haemocytes).

The first blood cells probably evolved from a free-living, protozoan-like ancestor. In primitive metazoans such as sponges, coelenterates and flatworms, wandering phagocytic amoebocytes not only function in host defence but are also involved in nutrition and excretion. In coelomates (both protostomes and deuterostomes), whose bodies are larger and more complex, a circulatory system is required to transport food and waste substances around the body. The amoebocyte-like cells, no longer required to gather food, probably migrated from the surrounding connective tissue into the circulatory system. Here, an array of cell types evolved, some of which took on specific roles in immune reactivity (*Fig. 13.4*).

Due to the huge diversity of invertebrates, and in contrast to the vertebrates, it is impossible to categorize free

Immunopotentialities of vertebrates and invertebrates

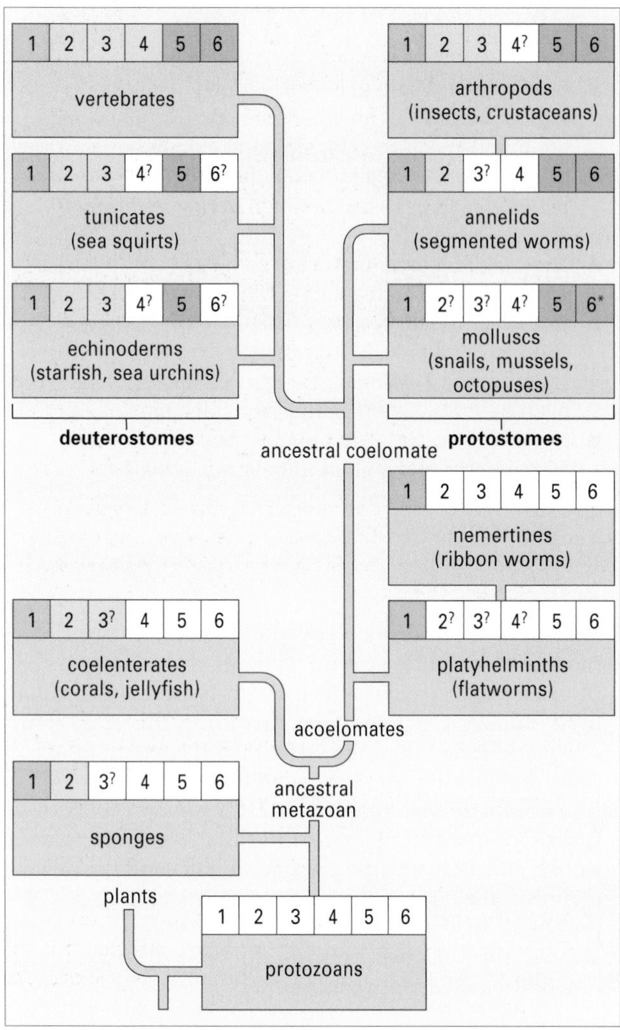

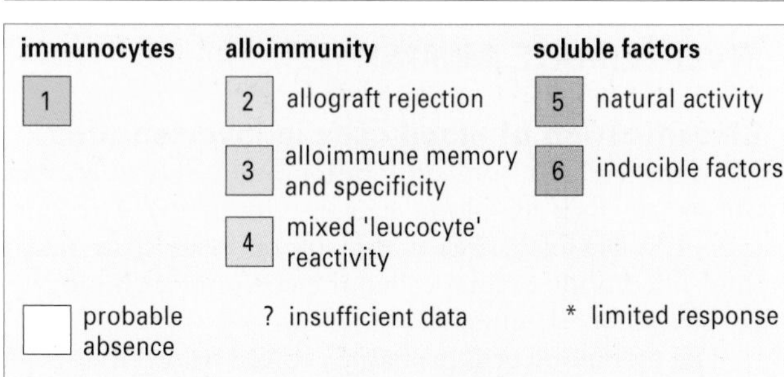

Fig. 13.1 Partial evidence for certain cellular and humoral immune phenomena in diverse invertebrate and vertebrate phyla is shown.

leucocytes into well-defined classes by staining and morphology alone. However, a functional scheme can be devised with five main groups of cells (*Fig. 13.4*):

- **Progenitor cells**, together with a variable array of haemopoietic tissue, may act as stem cells for the other cell types. Superficially, they resemble vertebrate lymphocytes (*Fig. 13.5*) although evidence for true homology is strictly limited.

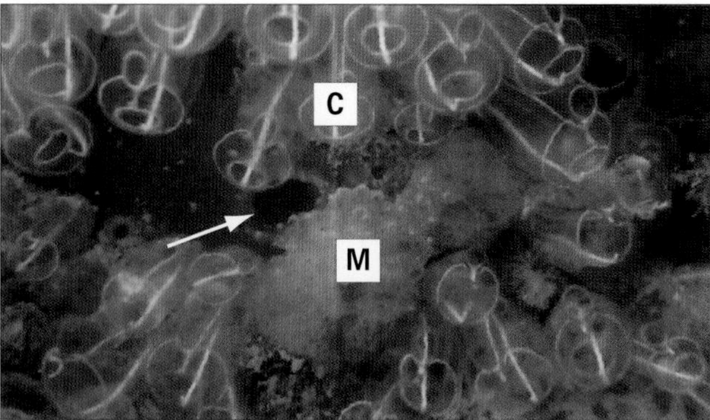

Fig. 13.2 Two colonial sea squirts (tunicates), *Clavelina lepadiformis* (C) and *Morchellium argus* (M), competing for space. The siphon of an underlying solitary tunicate can be seen towards the centre (arrowed). The diameter of an individual *Clavelina* is approximately 4 mm. (Courtesy of Dr P. Dyrynda.)

Evolution of the immune system

evolutionary step or selection pressure	immunological implications
single-celled animals	recognition and discrimination
multicellularity (including colonial forms)	histocompatibility system, allogeneic recognition and short-term memory
mesoderm and circulatory system, nutrition and defence as separate functions	freely circulating and more diverse blood cell types, cellular immunity and erythrocytes
cancer and viral infections associated with increasing complexity and longevity	immunosurveillance of own cells for those that are infected or cancerous
ancestral protovertebrates	increased recognition and discriminatory powers?
cartilaginous and bony fish: increased size, longer lifespan and reduced reproductive potential compared with invertebrates; evolution of jaws	true T and B lymphocytes, lymphoid tissue and antibody production, adaptive immunity with long-term memory
emergence onto land, exposure to irradiation and development of high pressure blood vascular systems	bone marrow, additional antibody classes, lymphoid organs with increased complexity
amniotes (reptiles, birds, mammals) with loss of free-living larval form	advanced differentiation of immunocompetent cells allowing increased diversity and efficiency of immune system
homoiothermy provides a more favourable environment for pathogens	increased efficiency of immune system, integrated cellular and humoral responses, germinal centres in secondary lymphoid organs, lymph nodes
viviparity with maternal–foetal interactions	additional fine-tuning of immune system to avoid rejection by mother

Fig. 13.3 Evolutionary steps of possible significance in the phylogeny of blood cells and the immune system. (Adapted from Rowley AF, Ratcliffe NA, eds. *Vertebrate Blood Cells*. Cambridge: Cambridge University Press, 1988; with permission.)

Cells and tissues of invertebrate immune systems

cells/tissues	role(s) in immunity/physiology
mucus, cuticle, shells, tests and/or gut barrier	physicochemical barriers to invasion
five groups of free and sessile white blood cells	mediate cellular and many of the humoral defence reactions
I progenitor cells	may act as stem cells for other cell types
II phagocytic cells	phagocytosis, encapsulation, clotting, wound healing and killing
III haemostatic cells	plasma gelation and clotting by cell aggregation; non-self recognition, lysozyme and agglutinin production
IV nutritive cells	encapsulation reactions and wound healing? nutritive role?
V pigmented cells	role in defence (if any) unknown; respiratory function
fixed cells such as pericardial cells, nephrocytes or pore cells etc.	pinocytose colloids and small particulates; synthesize lysozyme (pericardial cells) and other antimicrobial factors?
haemopoietic organs – well organized in some invertebrates	haemopoiesis and phagocytosis; synthesize antimicrobial factors in a few animals
fat body (insects), mid-gut and sinus lining cells (molluscs, crustaceans)	synthesize immune proteins and agglutinins (fat body), phagocytosis (mid-gut cells), clearance of foreign particles (sinus lining cells)

Fig. 13.4 Invertebrate immune systems. (Adapted from Ratcliffe NA. *Immunol Lett* 1985;**10**:253–70; Elsevier Science Publications, with permission.)

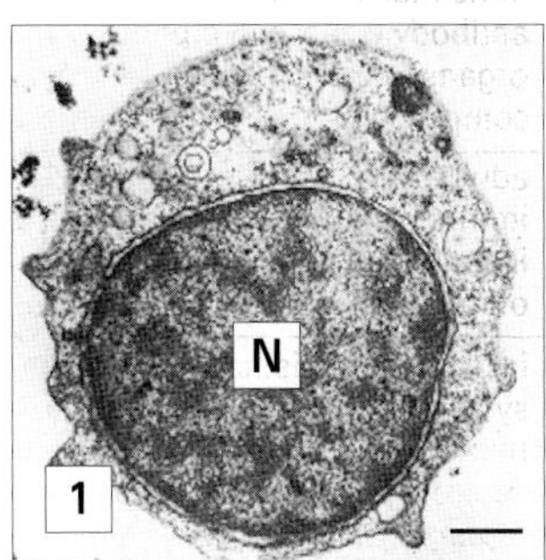

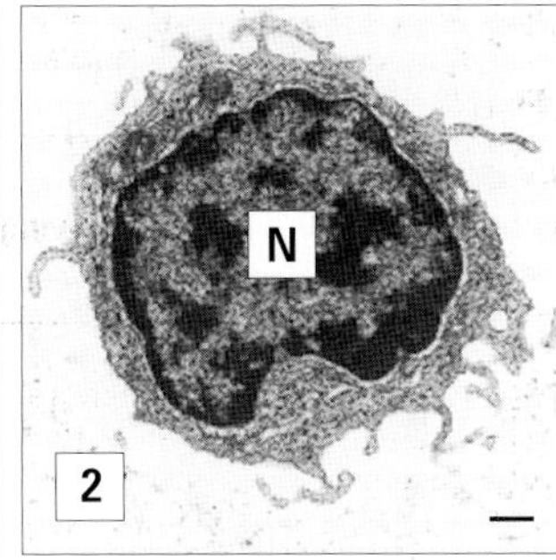

Fig. 13.5 Electron micrographs of a lymphocyte-like cell from the tunicate, *Ciona intestinalis* (1), and a lymphocyte from a fish, the blenny, *Blennius pholis* (2). Note the similarity in morphology; both cells have a large nucleus and a thin rim of undifferentiated cytoplasm. Scale bar = 0.5 μm. (Courtesy of Dr A.F. Rowley, from *Endeavour* (*New Series*) **13**:72–77, with permission. © Maxwell Pergamon Macmillan plc, 1989.)

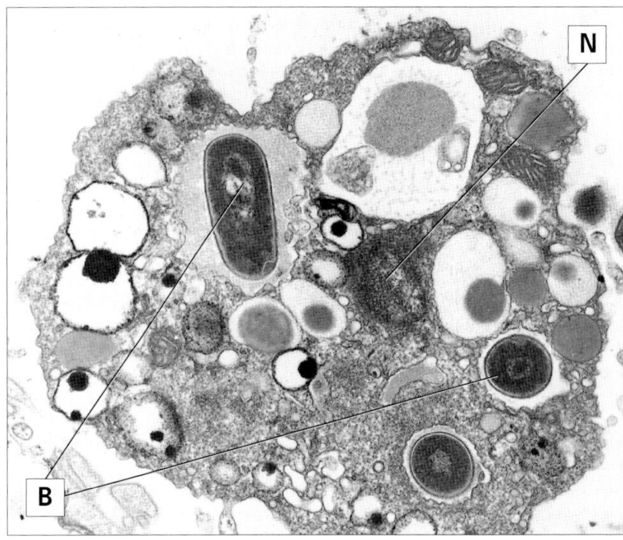

Fig. 13.6 Electron micrograph of a phagocytic cell from the tunicate, *Ciona intestinalis*. Note the ingestion of three bacteria (B) by this cell. N = nucleus. Scale bar = 0.5 μm. (Courtesy of Dr A.F. Rowley.)

- **Phagocytic cells** (*Fig. 13.6*) are probably the only blood cell type present throughout the animal kingdom. They correspond to the mammalian granulocyte or macrophage but have different surface markers.
- **Haemostatic (granular) cells** are involved in coagulation and wound healing, and are important effectors of non-self recognition.
- **Nutritive cells** are present in only a few species.
- **Pigmented cells** are present in many species but in a few species they contain respiratory pigment, thus resembling vertebrate erythrocytes.

Invertebrates lack lymphocytes and antibodies but have very efficient host defence mechanisms

Invertebrate immune systems apparently lack immunoglobulins, interactive lymphocyte subpopulations and lymphoid organs. Nevertheless, the huge numbers and diversity of invertebrates attests to the efficiency of their host defences.

Like vertebrates, invertebrates have extremely effective physicochemical barriers as a first line of defence (*Fig. 13.4*). The mucus that surrounds the body of many coelenterates, annelids, molluscs, and some tunicates entraps and kills potential pathogens (*Fig. 13.7*). Tough external skeletons such as tests or shells form barriers to invasion in some coelenterates and molluscs, echinoderms and arthropods.

Once these barriers are breached, would-be invaders are then exposed to a range of interacting cellular and humoral defence reactions:

- Blood clotting/coagulation and wound healing.
- Phagocytosis.
- Encapsulation responses.
- Natural and inducible antimicrobial factors.

These reactions depend on non-self recognition and

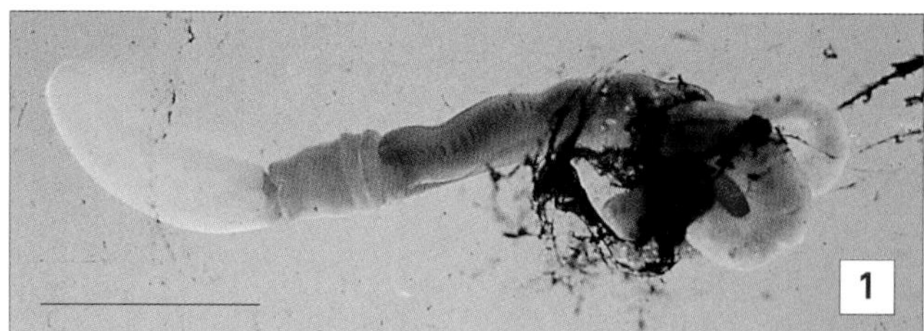

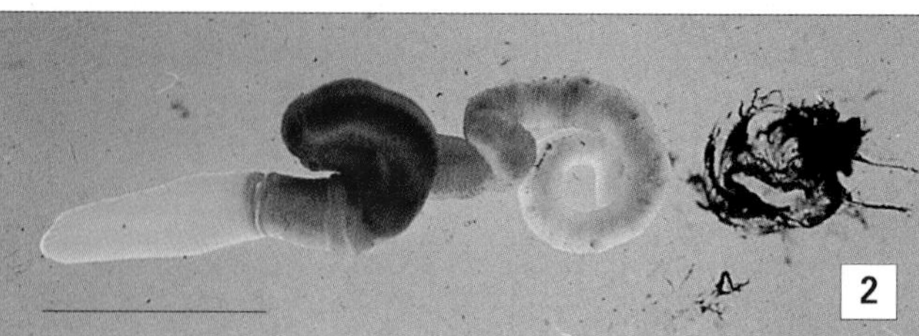

Fig. 13.7 Foreign particle entrapment and removal by the mucous layer surrounding the acorn worm, *Saccoglossus ruber*. A specimen was placed in a suspension of carbon in sea water for 2–3 minutes, then transferred to clean sea water. After 12 minutes large amounts of carbon were still enmeshed in the mucous layer surrounding the animal (**1**). By 15 minutes the carbon was completely removed, wrapped in a ball of mucus (**2**). Trapped microorganisms are probably dealt with in a similar fashion. Acorn worms are in a group of 'higher invertebrates' related to the tunicates. Scale bar = 5 mm. (Courtesy of Dr D.A. Millar.)

receptor molecules present in the blood and on the surfaces of the blood cells.

Wounds are rapidly closed by coagulation of body fluids induced both by haemostatic cells and plasma components

Invertebrates rapidly seal wounds caused by injury or parasitic invasion, and so prevent the fatal loss of body fluids. The wound is closed by the extrusion of the fat body or gut, by muscular contraction, by coagulation of body fluids, by blood cell aggregation and clotting, and/or by melanin deposition. Leucocyte migration to the wound is probably stimulated by cytokine-like factors (see below).

Plasma gelation or coagulation at wound sites occurs mainly in arthropods, although it has also been reported in annelids and echinoderms. Coagulation involves haemostatic cells, which aggregate at the injury and discharge their contents, causing the plasma to gelate and strengthen the cell clot. There is also a contribution from plasma components in many species. The coagulation process, as in mammals, involves a complex enzyme cascade which is activated at the wound site by damaged tissue, microbial components, and changes in Ca^{2+} or pH. It has been likened to the alternative pathway in complement activation. The system is so sensitive that in horseshoe crabs it is elicited by as little as 4 ng/ml of *Escherichia coli* endotoxin. The coagulation process is extremely important, as it forms a highly sensitive method of recognizing foreign invaders through the degranulation of haemostatic cells. Gelation may involve the enzyme prophenoloxidase (PpO) which, upon conversion to phenoloxidase (PO) by a cascade of serine proteases, may generate factors mediating later events in immunity (*Fig. 13.8*). The PpO cascade has recently been shown to be present in other invertebrates, such as annelids and tunicates.

Activation of prophenoloxidase to phenoloxidase in arthropods

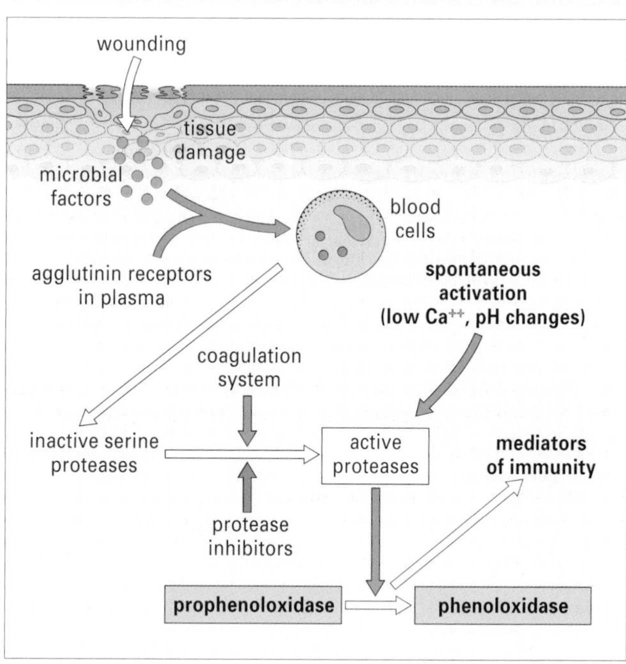

Fig. 13.8 Possible scheme for activation of prophenoloxidase (PpO) to phenoloxidase (PO) in arthropods. Activation is stimulated at the wound site by tissue damage, microorganisms and changes in Ca^{++} and pH, which may lead to plasma coagulation and the generation of factors mediating later events in immunity. Green arrows = activation; red arrow = inhibition; white arrows = production. (Based largely on data from Drs K. Söderhäll, M. Ashida and N.A. Ratcliffe.)

Phagocytic cells ingest microbial invaders whilst larger invaders are enclosed in multicellular capsules

Phagocytic cells occur throughout the invertebrates and, with natural humoral factors (see below), form the first line of defence against microorganisms (*Fig. 13.6*). Chemotaxis, attachment, ingestion and killing phases have all been described, and are similar to those seen in vertebrates. However, recognition of the target is not mediated by Fc receptors, and C3b-like receptors have only been reported on the phagocyte surface in one species. Phagocytosis can occur, as in vertebrates, without opsonic factors. However, it is enhanced in molluscs, arthropods and tunicates by plasma lectins and by components of the prophenoloxidase cascade.

If invading pathogens are too large or too numerous then they are enclosed in multicellular aggregates, termed nodules or capsules, resembling mammalian granulomas (*Fig. 13.9*). Sequestered organisms are thought to be killed by lysosomal enzymes and lysozyme present in leucocytes,

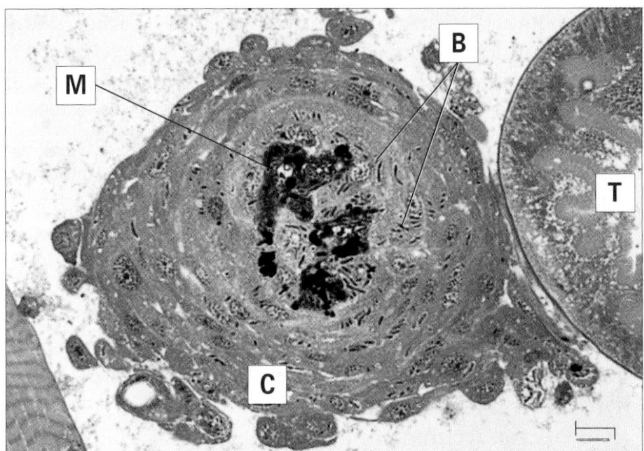

Fig. 13.9 Encapsulation of bacteria by the blood cells of a caterpillar. Final-stage larvae of the butterfly *Pieris brassicae* were injected with bacteria (heat-killed *Bacillus cereus*). After 24 hours, the capsules that had formed around the bacteria were excised and sectioned. Note the dark pigmented core of melanin (M), the multilayered sheath of blood cells (C), rod-shaped bacteria (B) and the attachment of the capsule to the Malpighian tubule (T). Scale bar = 10 μm.

and by peroxidase and reactive oxygen species (recorded in a few annelids, molluscs and arthropods).

Both phagocytosis and encapsulation are dependent on cell cooperation between the haemostatic and phagocytic cells (see below).

The body fluids of invertebrates contain a range of naturally occurring and inducible humoral defence factors

Naturally occurring defence factors

Invertebrates probably lack immunoglobulins but their body fluids contain a range of humoral defence factors. These include agglutinins, lysozyme and other lysins, non-lysozyme bactericidins, lysosomal enzymes and immobilization factors. There is also some evidence for the presence of components of the complement system. For example, sea urchin phagocytes may bear C3b-like receptors, and a humoral lytic system similar to complement has been reported. Furthermore, blood from a caterpillar has been found to react with bound cobra venom factor (cobra C3b) to produce a C3-convertase activity that cleaves bovine C3, generating a molecule similar to C3b. The prophenoloxidase cascade of arthropods has also been compared with the alternative pathway of the complement system, as both are activated directly by microbial components and involve a series of sequentially activated proteases (*Fig. 13.8*). Confirmation that the forerunners of the alternative complement pathways arose in invertebrates awaits detailed molecular analysis.

Inducible humoral defence factors

Although it is known that agglutinin and haemolysin levels can sometimes be enhanced in invertebrates, inducible antimicrobial factors from insects are the only molecules to have been studied in great detail. There is now evidence for their presence in a few other invertebrates but their more widespread detection and characterization may await the correct immunogens and/or immunization schedule. In insects such as moths, flies and bees, up to 15 antibacterial proteins can be induced within a few hours of injection of an antigen (*Fig. 13.10*). Many of these peptides have been purified and sequenced; they have a broad-spectrum activity which only lasts a few days, and are therefore very different from vertebrate immunoglobulins. Recently, similar antibacterial proteins have been found in certain vertebrates and these molecules probably represent ancient, but still important, immune factors. One such factor, a cecropin called P4 or haemolin (*Fig. 13.10*), has homology (38%) with certain immunoglobulin domains. It could represent a primitive form of immunoglobulin, but may have evolved independently in invertebrates. In the American cockroach, a different sort of inducible protein has been detected which is much more like vertebrate immunoglobulin. It has a molecular mass of 700 kDa, is highly specific and lasts weeks rather than days. Again, detailed comparison with vertebrate immunoglobulin awaits molecular characterization. Recently the Toll family of signalling receptors has been shown to play a crucial role in the induction of immune response in *Drosophilia*; this pathway, which recognizes invariant molecular structures of pathogens is also involved in mammalian innate immunity.

Inducible immune proteins of *Hyalophora cecropia*

immune protein	molecular mass	function and properties
P4 (haemolin)	48 000	main immune protein, non-self recognition?
P5 attacins A–F	21–23 000	narrow spectrum antibacterial activity against some Gram-negative bacteria
P7 (lysozyme)	15 000	kills some Gram-positive bacteria
cecropins A–F (6 proteins)	~4000	some have broad spectrum antibacterial activity against both Gram-positive and Gram-negative bacteria

Fig. 13.10 Inducible immune proteins of the moth, *Hyalophora cecropia*, isolated from the blood 10 hours after immunization with bacteria (*Enterobacter cloacae*). (Based on the work of H. Boman, D. Hultmark and colleagues.)

Non-self recognition and cell–cell cooperation are mediated by various factors

Invertebrates can discriminate, often quite specifically, between various foreign substances. Factors present in invertebrate body fluids acting as recognition molecules include agglutinins, components of the prophenoloxidase cascade and haemolin.

Purified agglutinins

From the blood of molluscs, insects and tunicates, these enhance the recognition of test particles *in vitro*, as well as their clearance from the circulation *in vivo*. Such agglutinins also occur on the surface of blood cells to form bridging molecules between the leucocyte and the foreign particle, as in the mammalian immune system.

The prophenoloxidase (PpO) system

In arthropods, this is also a likely source of recognition factors. During conversion of PpO to phenoloxidase (PO) (*Fig. 13.8*) recognition factors are released from haemostatic cells which enhance phagocytosis and encapsulation. An agglutinin, purified from cockroach blood and termed BDL1, has recently been shown to activate the PpO cascade, so that a unifying concept is now available for these two recognition systems. BDL1 also has many structural and functional similarities to the mannose-binding lectins (MBLs) of vertebrates. (The MBLs are essential components of vertebrate non-specific immunity because they can bind to the surface of invading microorganisms, and activate complement-mediated attack.) Like MBLs, BDL1 activates complement and has collagenous and carbohydrate-recognition domains.

Haemolin

In addition to agglutinins and PpO, the blood of insects also contains an immune protein called haemolin. It has four immunoglobulin-like domains that bind to bacterial surfaces, and may be involved in the recognition of non-self molecules.

The process of non-self recognition and subsequent phagocytosis involves cell–cell cooperation between haemostatic cells and phagocytic cells (*Fig. 13.11*). Thus, although invertebrates lack interacting antigen-presenting cells and lymphocyte subpopulations, the various immunocytes cooperate during cell-mediated immunity.

The cellular and humoral defence reactions of vector species also act as determinants of infection by parasites

Evidence is accumulating to suggest that the immune capability of certain invertebrate disease vectors (e.g. mosquitoes, tsetse flies, sandflies, blackflies, kissing bugs and pulmonate snails) is an important determinant of their ability to transmit disease (malaria, sleeping sickness, tropical sores, river blindness, Chagas' disease and blood flukes). For example, in mosquitoes and pulmonate snails encapsulation responses have been reported to effectively

Two hypothetical models for cell–cell cooperation in arthropod immunity

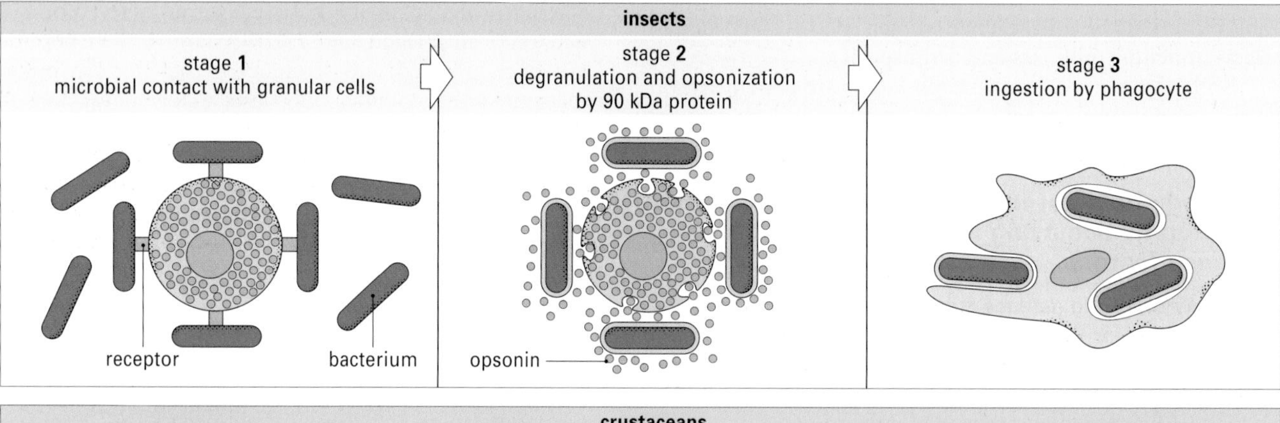

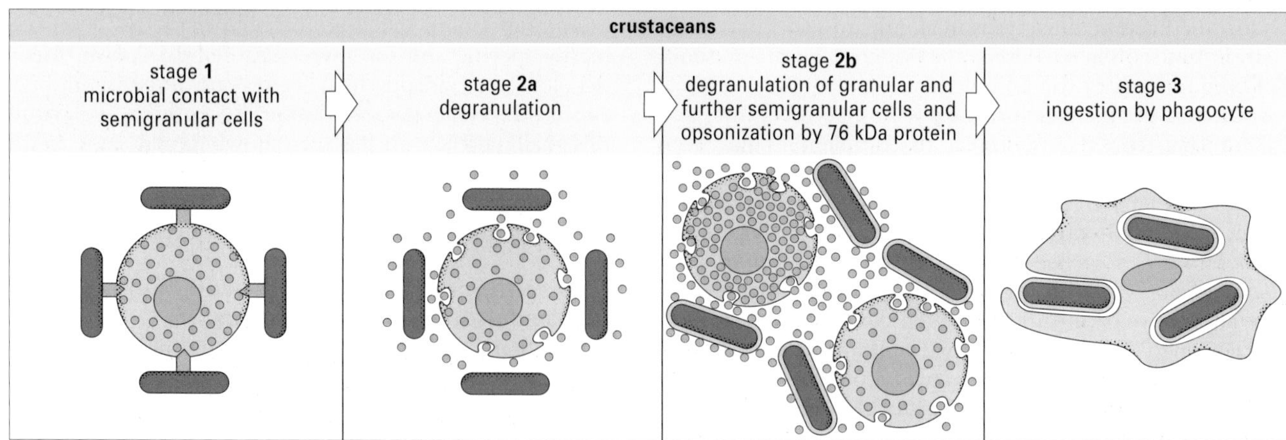

Fig. 13.11 Schemes derived from experiments which observed the reactions of purified blood cell populations to test particles. In insects, non-self recognition (stages **1** and **2**) is carried out by the granular (haemostatic) cells, and ingestion (stage **3**) by the phagocytes. The crustacean model has an extra amplification step at stage **2b**, in which semigranular and granular cells interact to enhance the response. The 90-kDa and 76-kDa proteins detected in insects and crustaceans, respectively, are opsonic (recognition) molecules generated by activation of the prophenoloxidase cascade. (Adapted from Ratcliffe NA. In: Warr GW, Cohen N, eds. *Phylogenesis of Immune Functions*. Oxford: CRC Press, 1991:62. Data on crustaceans from the work of Professor K. Söderhäll and associates.)

sequester and possibly kill the enclosed parasites. In addition, recent research has identified gut-associated agglutinins in mosquitoes, tsetse flies, sandflies and kissing bugs as possibly playing major roles in growth and survival of invading protozoan parasites taken in with a blood meal. In some *Glossina* tsetse flies, for example, the inhibition of the midgut agglutinin with D-glucosamine significantly increases midgut infection rates with *Trypanosoma brucei rhodesiense*. Prophenoloxidase may also be important; female *Glossina morsitans morsitans* tsetse flies show low levels of mature salivary gland infections with *T.b. rhodesiense* compared with male flies, and have much higher levels of PpO than the male flies. The inducible antibacterial peptides present in the blood of *Simulium* blackflies have also been shown to kill immature stages of nematode worm parasites. Much has yet to be learned in this exciting new research field, including the methods adopted by the parasites to evade the vectors' immune defences.

Host defences are regulated by a network of cytokines, some of which resemble vertebrate interleukins

Cytokine-like molecules found in invertebrates may regulate the host defences by a network resembling that seen in vertebrates. The fact that molecules related to cytokines are present in protozoans suggests they are to be found throughout the animal kingdom. For example, a protozoan pheromone, Er-1, has structural and functional similarities to interleukin-2 (IL-2). In addition, molecules with activities resembling those of IL-1α, IL-1β and tumour necrosis factor (TNF) have recently been isolated and characterized from annelids, echinoderms and tunicates. IL-1α and IL-1β were detected using a vertebrate assay system (the murine thymocyte proliferation assay) and were shown to be inhibited by polyclonal antisera to vertebrate IL-1. Invertebrate IL-1 stimulates the 'blood' cells of these primitive animals to aggregate, phagocytose and proliferate. TNF-like activity from invertebrates has been detected with a cytotoxicity assay, normally used for vertebrate TNF.

A range of other molecules with cytokine-like activity has been reported from invertebrates. In insects, these include a plasmatocyte (leucocyte-type) depletion factor, a leucocyte activator (termed haemokinin) and various stimulants for encapsulation and phagocytosis. A factor produced by the leucocytes of echinoderms (the sea-star factor) is mitogenic for mammalian lymphocytes and also induces the accumulation of starfish white blood cells. In addition, an inflammatory cytokine from tunicates has been shown to affect antibody production, phagocytosis and cell-mediated cytotoxicity in vertebrates, and leucocyte phagocytic activity in prawns. Additional molecular characterization of these molecules is awaited. Finally, mention should also be made of research indicating that eicosanoids and opioid peptides are also involved in the immune reactivity of invertebrate blood cells.

Many invertebrates can reject allogeneic and xenogeneic grafts

Vertebrate immunity is characterized by a high degree of specificity and enhanced reactivity (memory, or anamnesis) following a second exposure to antigen. These processes are governed by lymphocytes with clonally distributed antigen receptors and the MHC. To determine levels of specificity and memory in invertebrates, transplantation, implantation and cytotoxicity studies have been undertaken. Such transplantation studies are difficult to perform in invertebrates, due to their tough exoskeletons or delicate outer layers. It can also be difficult to judge whether rejection has occurred. Despite these difficulties, it is now known that most invertebrates destroy xenografts, and allogeneic recognition has been observed in the sponges, coelenterates, annelids, insects, echinoderms and tunicates (*Figs 13.1, 13.12, 13.13*). The apparent lack of allogeneic recognition in the molluscs probably reflects the technical problems in grafting these animals. Not all the groups exhibiting allograft rejection produce reactions characterized by specificity and memory; the reactions are usually strictly limited and short term (*Fig. 13.1*). The great variability in results of grafting may stem from the temperature dependence of the rejection process and the lack of appreciation of this by some workers.

It is not surprising that allogeneic recognition occurs in colonial invertebrates such as the sponges, coelenterates and tunicates, as the integrity of the colony is constantly threatened by overgrowth from adjacent colonies (*Fig. 13.2*). Work with the larvae of tunicate colonies has shown that both allorecognition and fertilization are controlled by a single gene locus with multiple alleles. Thus, there are similarities between this tunicate system and the mammalian histocompatibility genes.

Once again, note that the limited specificity and memory of invertebrate allorecognition and xenorecognition does not seem to hamper their immune system or success. After all, invertebrates rapidly respond to pathogens and parasites and are hugely abundant.

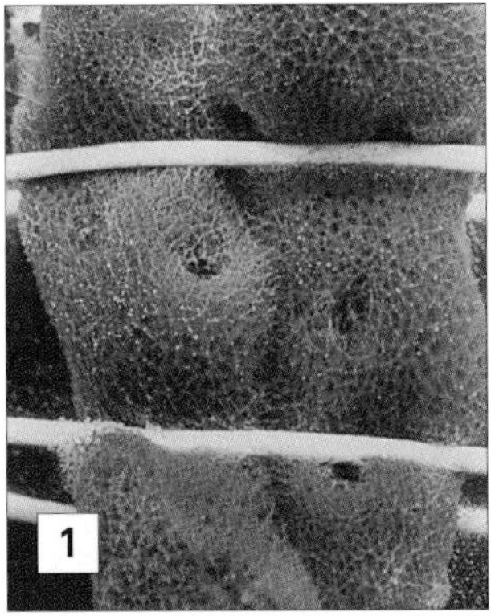

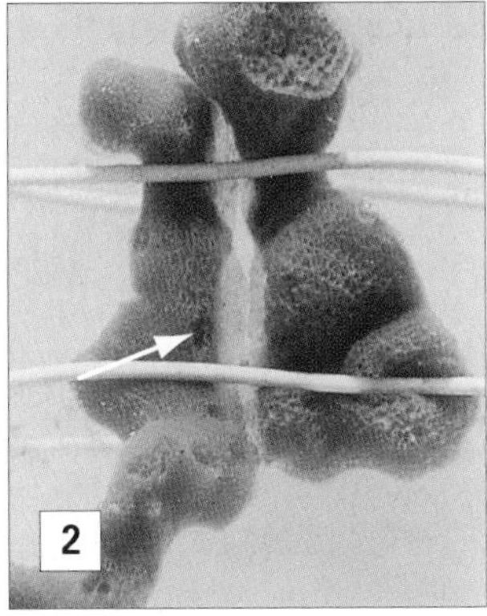

Fig. 13.12 Demonstration of cell-mediated immunity in sponges: allogeneic incompatibility and isogeneic compatibility. Two intact fingers of sponge (*Callyspongia* spp.) from the same colony and two from different colonies are parabiosed (their circulations are fused) by being held together with vinyl-covered wire. (**1**) The interfacial fusion between isogeneic parabionts (intracolony) persists indefinitely. ×0.5. (**2**) Incompatibility between allogeneic parabionts (intercolony) results in a cytotoxic interaction and necrosis (arrow) after 7–9 days (24–27°C). ×0.25. (Courtesy of Dr W.H. Hildemann.)

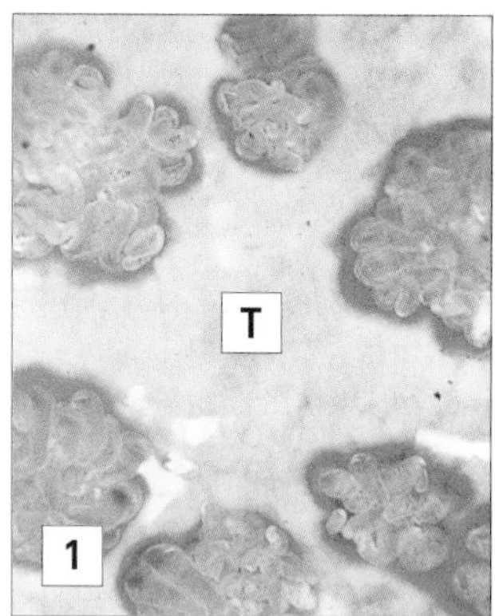

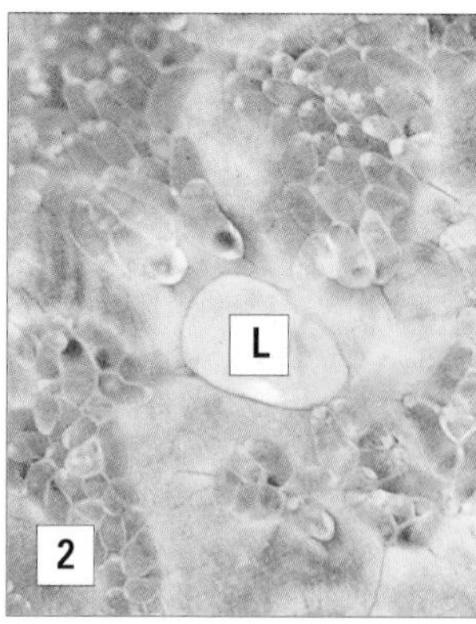

Fig. 13.13 Transplantation immunity in echinoderms: allograft rejection in starfish (*Dermasterias*). **(1)** In spite of the technical difficulties involved, this autograft (T) remains in perfect condition 300 days after transplantation. **(2)** An allograft (L) rejected at 287 days (14–16°C) is blanched and contracted. Rejection involves lymphocyte-like cells and larger phagocytic cells. ×4. (Courtesy of Dr W.H. Hildemann.)

Evidence for evolution of immunoglobulin supergene family molecules in invertebrates?

The presence of allogeneic recognition in many invertebrates indicates that the ancestors of the MHC could be present in these animals. Since invertebrates do not possess immunoglobulins or T-cell receptors, it is possible that the MHC may be ancestral to and separate from the T- and B-cell antigen receptors of vertebrates. On this argument, primitive vertebrates retained MHC and evolved the T-cell receptor (TCR) and immunoglobulin systems separately, to provide a more precise recognition potential in the form of cell-surface receptors and circulating antibodies. With further vertebrate evolution, the MHC, TCR and immunoglobulin systems would have become more closely integrated to provide the high level of control necessary for interacting antigen-presenting cells (APCs) and lymphocytes. The above proposal is, however, hypothetical; there is no evidence, structural or functional, that invertebrate cells express either MHC glycoproteins or dimeric cell receptors for antigens. In addition, invertebrates may lack mixed leucocyte reactivity (*Fig. 13.1*) which is a functional marker of the MHC in vertebrates. This lack of supporting data has led to some counter-hypotheses; some argue that the MHC evolved in vertebrates from heat-shock proteins.

The discovery of β_2-microglobulin-like molecules in earthworms, crustaceans and insects, however, does support the idea that MHC precursors may have arisen in the invertebrates. Although β_2-microglobulin in vertebrates is encoded by a gene not linked to the MHC, it associates with class I MHC molecules and belongs to the immunoglobulin supergene family. Thus MHC molecules may be the descendants of a single domain molecule like β_2-microglobulin that has been expanded by gene rearrangement, gene duplication and natural selection.

Finally, there is a group of molecules including Thy-1 (present in squid brain), and amalgam, fasciclin II, neuroglian and haemolin (all from insects), which also belong to the immunoglobulin superfamily; it has been suggested that these evolved to mediate interactions between cells, and could potentially produce an immune system recognizing 'non-self'. Such a step may have already been made in insects with haemolin (see above). Immunoglobulin superfamily domain found in invertebrates are of the 'V-' or 'C2-' types. The 'C1-' type of domain is restricted to vertebrates that somatically rearrange their antigen receptor genes.

VERTEBRATE IMMUNITY

Origins of the adaptive immune system

Compared with the immense variety of forms seen within the invertebrate phyla, vertebrates possess a fairly uniform basic plan of organization and are members of just one phylum – the Chordata. Although there is considerable evolutionary divergence within vertebrate stock, which includes jawless fish, cartilaginous and bony jawed fish, amphibians, reptiles, birds and mammals, the basic cellular and molecular components of anticipatory (also referred to as 'adaptive' or 'combinatorial') immunity are strikingly conserved throughout extant gnathostome (jawed) species. As rearranging Ig and TCR genes, MHC genes and RAG genes have not been isolated in agnathan fish (e.g. hagfish and lamprey), they are considered to lack the essential elements of an adaptive immune system. T-cell antigen receptors (both $\alpha\beta$ and $\gamma\delta$), Ig receptors (H and L chains) and MHC proteins are found from cartilaginous fish upwards (*Fig. 13.14*). The emergence of the adaptive immune system seems to have occurred in a relatively short period of evolutionary time and is considered as a 'Big Bang' event during the emergence of jawed vertebrates from Ostracoderm ancestors. Evolution of TCRs and Igs is thought to have involved the horizontal transfer of genes involved in DNA recombination, from microbes and/or fungi, thus allowing combinatorial diversity to occur within the V region of an Ig precursor molecule.

Evolution of the MHC

Jawed vertebrates from cartilaginous fish upwards have all been shown to possess an MHC, by functional criteria and/or through molecular and genetic characterization. Functional criteria require that mixed lymphocyte reactivity (MLR) and acute allograft rejection are shown to be controlled by a single polymorphic genetic region, and that phenomena such as T–B cell collaboration, the generation of antigen-specific cytotoxic T lymphocytes (CTLs) and thymic education of T-lineage cells are all under MHC control.

The MHC has been well characterized in the ectothermic vertebrate Xenopus

MHC genes evolved in cartilaginous fish whose ancestors diverged from other vertebrates more than 400 million years ago. However, the best studied ectothermic (cold-blooded) vertebrate with respect to MHC genes and proteins is the clawed frog, *Xenopus*. Its MHC (the XLA) is compared with the avian MHC (B locus) and murine MHC (H–2) in *Figure 13.15*.

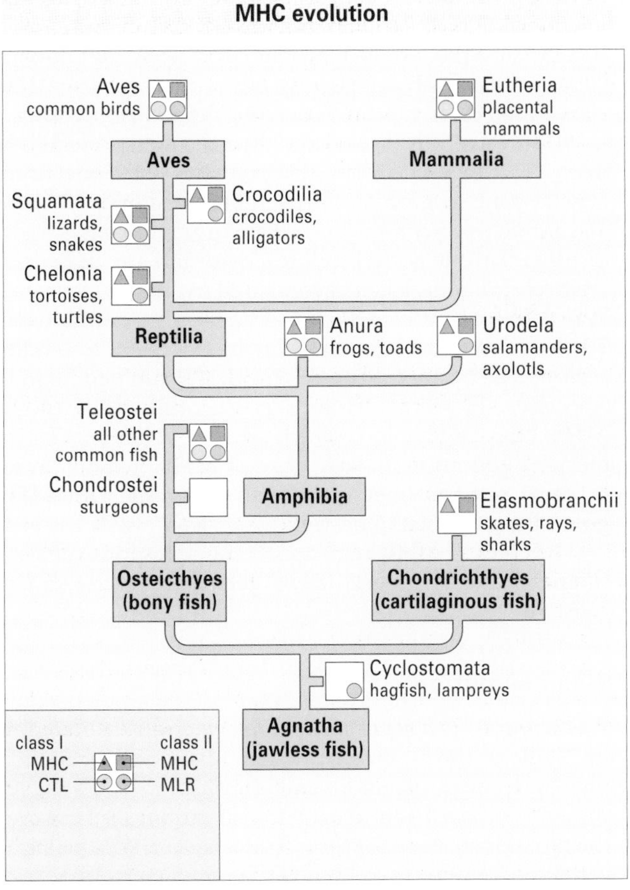

Fig. 13.14 This vertebrate phylogenetic tree illustrates aspects of MHC evolution. Evidence for two functional indications of an MHC (cytotoxic T lymphocytes (CTL) and mixed leucocyte reaction (MLR)) is shown, together with current biochemical and molecular evidence for the expression of class I and II MHC proteins and genes. A blank box indicates insufficient evidence for that characteristic.

Classical MHC (Ia) in Xenopus – *Xenopus* class Ia proteins are polymorphic, with approximately 20 alleles. These proteins are expressed on the surfaces of all adult cells, highest expression being on haemopoietic cells. The class Ia chains of *Xenopus* are 40–44 kDa, with three domains, and are non-covalently bound to β_2-microglobulin. Genes (lmp and TAP) encoding antigen-processing molecules are linked with the *Xenopus* MHC. *Xenopus* class I MHC proteins are unusual in that they are encoded by just one gene locus (contrast with three in humans and mice). *Xenopus* β_2-microglobulin has recently been cloned.

Non-classical MHC (Ib) in Xenopus – The first *Xenopus* class I gene to be identified was one of a large family of monomorphic, 'non-classical' (class Ib) MHC-like molecules. Class Ib genes occur on the same chromosome as the 'classical' (MHC Ia) genes, but separated by a great distance and are minimally polymorphic. Class Ib-encoded molecules have homology with protein-binding regions of the heat-shock protein 70 (Hsp 70) family. It has been suggested that the peptide-binding region of class I MHC molecules evolved from pre-existing Hsps. (Hsps are evolutionarily conserved molecules found in all organisms, which act as 'chaperones' and are involved in protein folding and intracellular transport.) However, recent crystal structure of the peptide-binding region (PBR) of a bacterial Hsp-70 homologue does not indicate its resemblance to the MHC antigen-binding site.

MHC class II in Xenopus – *Xenopus* class II MHC molecules are polymorphic (about 30 alleles) and are expressed constitutively on only a limited range of adult cells, including thymocytes, B and T cells, and various APCs such as putative Langerhans'-like cells of the skin epidermis (*Fig. 13.16*). Class II proteins are composed of MHC-encoded α and β chains, both of which are 30–35-kDa transmembrane glycoproteins. *Xenopus* has three MHC class II β gene loci, and the genes for *Xenopus* MHC class II β chains encode

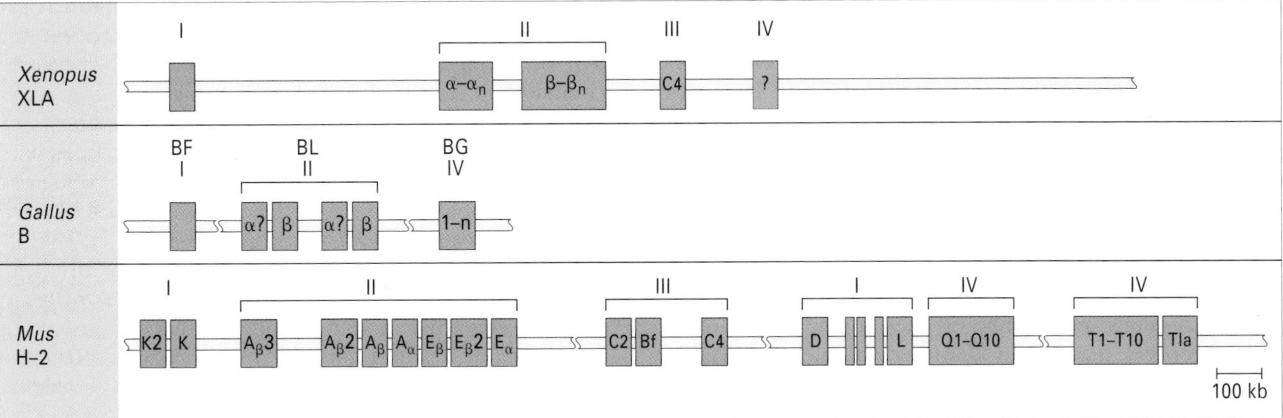

Fig. 13.15 The MHC can be identified in all jawed vertebrates. Speculative organization of MHC loci is here shown for the clawed frog (*Xenopus*) and the chicken (*Gallus*). The architecture of the mouse (*Mus*) H-2 complex is well known. Distances for *Xenopus* and *Gallus* are arbitrary. (Courtesy of Dr L. Du Pasquier.)

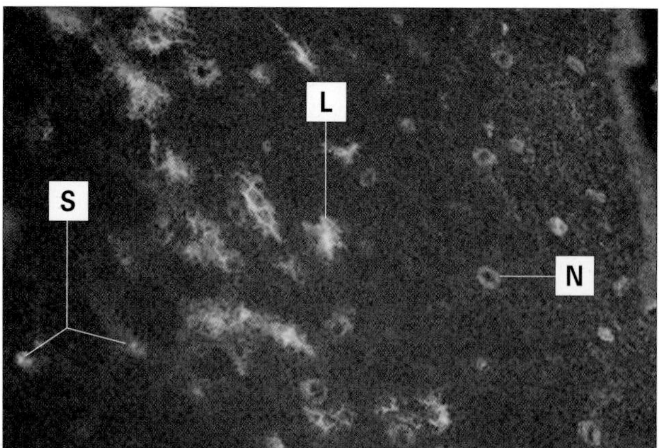

Fig. 13.16 Immunofluorescence showing class II MHC-positive dendritic cells in *Xenopus*. 'Langerhans-like' cells (L) frequent the basal epidermal layer of the skin. Also visible are class II⁺ neck cells of the skin gland opening through the epidermis (N), and skin glands below the epidermis (S). ×100.

polypeptides with nearly 50% homology to mammalian class II β chains. An invariant chain is transiently associated with class II during biosynthesis.

MHC expression in Xenopus varies with each stage of the life cycle

One particularly interesting feature of MHC expression in *Xenopus* is that class Ia MHC molecules are not detectable on most cell surfaces prior to metamorphosis. Recently molecular approaches confirmed that class Ia transcripts are undetectable in tadpole spleen, thymus and skin, but can be found in lung, gill and intestine in late larval life. No mRNA for class Ib is detectable prior to metamorphosis. Therefore, early development and functioning of the larval immune system appears not to require expression of class Ia and Ib MHC proteins. Indeed, if tadpoles expressed class I proteins they could generate MHC-restricted CTL against antigens derived from pathogens, and such cells could theoretically cross-react with the very large number of adult antigens (e.g. adult haemoglobin and keratin) emerging at metamorphosis, thereby eliciting devastating autoimmunity.

Class II-restricted cellular immunity may well play a crucial role during this ontogenetic period. The widespread distribution of class II MHC in tadpoles compared with adults suggests that this pattern might represent the way in which antigen was presented in a more primitive immune system.

MHC in other vertebrates

Class Ia genes are found in all jawed vertebrates examined. Class Ib genes, which may or may not be linked to the MHC proper, have been identified in chicken, *Xenopus*, teleosts and cartilaginous fish. Class Ib proteins have been found associated with epithelial surfaces and may have varying functions; some are thought to recognize the Hsps of pathogens or infected/stressed cells, and subsequently present these conserved peptides to T cells. Class Ia and Ib molecules are invariably heterodimers with H chains of ~350 amino acids non-covalently linked to β_2-microglobulin of ~100 amino acids. β-2M, required for a functional MHC class I protein, has been identified in various teleost fish, supporting the notion that fish MHC class I molecules are translated into functional proteins.

MHC class II α/β genes and their encoded proteins have been described in all jawed vertebrates. In bony fishes, class II gene loci are on different chromosomes to class I and antigen-presenting genes. Among amphibians, axolotls display relatively poor T-cell reactivity and are, in general, relatively immunodeficient compared to other higher vertebrates. In contrast to *Xenopus*, the axolotl has only one class IIb locus with no variability in its polypeptide-binding region, which may explain this urodele's subdued immune responses. However, axolotls possess numerous (6–21) MHC class Ia gene loci, which are very polymorphic. Extensive duplication of class I and II MHC genes is found in some teleosts (e.g. cod). This contrasts with MHC gene-silencing seen in polypoid *Xenopus*.

The chicken MHC regulates immune responsiveness to a variety of antigens and MHC genotype governs disease resistance.

T-cell evolution

T cells and TCRs have been identified in diverse vertebrates

αβ TCRs or their component chains have now been identified in many cartilaginous and bony fish; γδ TCRs are also thought to have evolved early in fish evolution. However, the physiological role of these TCR-like chains in primitive vertebrates awaits experimental analysis. Genes encoding α and β chains of the axolotl TCR have been cloned, as have TCRβ and the CD3 gene complex in *Xenopus*. Despite considerable effort, antibodies to lower vertebrate T-cell receptors have not yet been produced. Anti-*Xenopus* monoclonal antibodies identifying candidate CD5 (71–88 kDa, and expressed on all T cells) and CD8 (35 kDa, and expressed on cytotoxic T cells) are now available. The CD8α gene has been cloned in rainbow trout and CD8β in the axolote. This ectotherm CD8α lacks an associated p56 tyrosine kinase. CD4 has not yet been identified in ectotherms. αβ and γδ TCRs, together with CD3, CD4 and CD8 co-receptor molecules, have been identified in birds.

A novel receptor called CTX (cortical thymocyte antigen of *Xenopus*) has recently been identified on cortical (immature) *Xenopus* thymocytes. This receptor is also expressed by several *Xenopus* thymus lymphoid tumour cell lines, but is not expressed on peripheral T cells. CTX belongs to the Ig superfamily, is a dimeric cell-surface receptor related to the RAGE (receptor involved in recognition of advanced glycosylation end products) family. CTX has a C2 type of constant domain, contrasting the C1 constant domains of Ig, TCR and MHC; the V region of CTX does not undergo somatic rearrangement and the molecule displays limited polymorphism. Receptors homologous to CTX have subsequently been discovered in birds and mammals. CTX appears to control thymocyte proliferation and is thought to play a role in tumorigenesis; it may represent a very early lymphocyte receptor which contributed to the evolution of T and B lymphocytes.

Temperature plays a crucial role in immune responses

in ectotherms. In catfish, low temperatures inhibit T-cell (but not B-cell) proliferation. These effects are due to the lower level in fish T cells of certain saturated fatty acids (e.g. oleic acid) which can fluidify membranes. Diets high in appropriate fatty acids may therefore allow fish to adapt better to low temperatures. Oleic acid can also reverse the suppression of *in vitro* responses of mammalian T cells that occurs at low temperatures, although the precise temperature-sensitive signalling events have not yet been elucidated.

Evolution of B cells and immunoglobulins

Immunoglobulin heavy and light chains have been characterized in diverse vertebrates

Proteins from hagfish initially described as antibodies have now been identified as complement proteins C3–C5. Indeed, no immunoglobulin superfamily molecules have yet been found in the agnathan (jawless) hagfish and lamprey.

All jawed vertebrates make antibodies to a wide range of antigens. However, ectotherm antibodies are of relatively low affinity and B-cell responses display poor immunological memory compared with endothermic (warm-blooded) vertebrates. The structure of antibodies is evolutionarily conserved, with multi-domain, heavy and light immunoglobulin polypeptide chains (see Chapter 4). These immunoglobulins may be expressed on the B-cell surface as antigen receptor or secreted into the circulation by activated B cells.

Polymeric IgM is universally found in jawed vertebrates (*Fig. 13.17*) and is the major serum antibody of fish. Each heavy μ chain comprises four constant domains and one variable domain; disulphide bonds link heavy and light chains. The μ chain family displays considerable phylogenetic diversity; e.g. only 24% amino acid sequence homology exists between catfish and mouse μ chains.

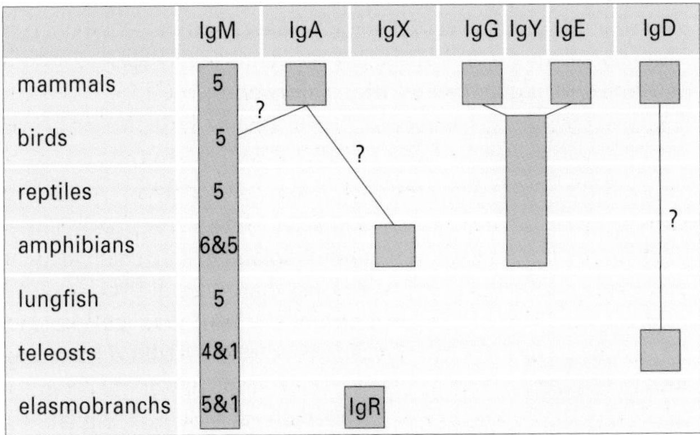

Fig. 13.17 Distribution and possible relationships of immunoglobulins in the vertebrates. Polymeric IgM is found in all jawed vertebrates, but with varying numbers of basic units (2H + 2L chains), as shown. Monomeric IgM is also found in blood of cartilaginous (elasmobranch) and teleost fish. Non-μ heavy chain isotypes are found in diverse groups, but the roles of these immunoglobulin isotopes often remain uncertain. (Adapted from Dr G.W. Warr.)

Non-μ low molecular weight antibodies are found in some cartilaginous fish, such as skates, rays and sharks (*Fig. 13.17*), although the evolutionary relationship of IgR to other heavy chain isotypes is uncertain. Amphibians, reptiles and birds possess a heavy chain isotype called IgY, with four constant domains, believed to be the precursor of mammalian IgG and IgE, with which IgY shares common structural and functional properties. The IgY of axolotls may also be a secretory immunoglobulin, as in the gut this immunoglobulin isotype becomes associated with 'secretory-piece-like' molecules. It is interesting that fish lack IgE, yet teleosts display Type I hypersensitivity reactions which may reflect tissue-bound homocytotropic antibody. An Ig isotype related to IgD has recently been found in teleosts; immortalized B cells from catfish express high levels of this isotype, allowing its function to be analysed. Different redox forms of IgM found in teleosts may have different functions and substitute for lack of Ig isotype diversity. *Xenopus* IgX which, unlike IgY, is thymus independent, is possibly the equivalent of mammalian secretory IgA, since this isotype is mainly found in the gut. IgA first appears in advanced birds.

Light chain diversity also occurs in many ectotherms. Two antigenically distinct types of light chains, one of which is κ-like, have been demonstrated in *Xenopus*, and two exist in catfish, trout and alligators. Both κ- and λ-like light chains are known to exist in sharks, indicating that divergence of the ancestral light chain into isotypes occurred prior to the emergence of cartilaginous fish.

A new immunoglobulin superfamily molecule, possibly the evolutionary forerunner of immunoglobulin and TCR, has been identified in the nurse shark. The molecule (named New Antigen Receptor, NAR) has one variable and five constant domains and is found as a dimer in the serum; it is encoded by a gene locus that undergoes rearrangements and somatic diversification. A novel chimeric antibody class, a composite of IgR and NAR, has also now been identified in cartilaginous fish, casting doubt on the dogma that IgM is the primordial Ig isotype.

Immunoglobulin genes in lower vertebrates are organized in one of four ways

Analysis of the immunoglobulin gene loci in ectotherms using recombinant DNA technology has advanced rapidly in recent years, revealing four patterns of organization.

Amphibians, teleosts and holostean fish – These have a mammalian-type ('translocon') form of IgH organization. For example, in *Xenopus* there are approximately 80–100 *VH*, 15 *DH* and 9 *JH* segments (*Fig. 13.18*). Both framework and complementarity-determining regions are found. Each *Xenopus* heavy chain constant region (IgM, IgX, IgY) is coded for by four CH exons. Amphibians are the first group where Ig class switching occurs. Two separate chromosomes, each with *VL*, *JL* and *CL* segments, code for *Xenopus* light chains. Teleost immunoglobulin light chain genes show the 'multicluster' organization typifying shark immunoglobulin genes (see below). Teleosts are the only group found that has a different configuration of gene loci coding for H and L chains.

Multiple rearrangements of *Xenopus* immunoglobulin

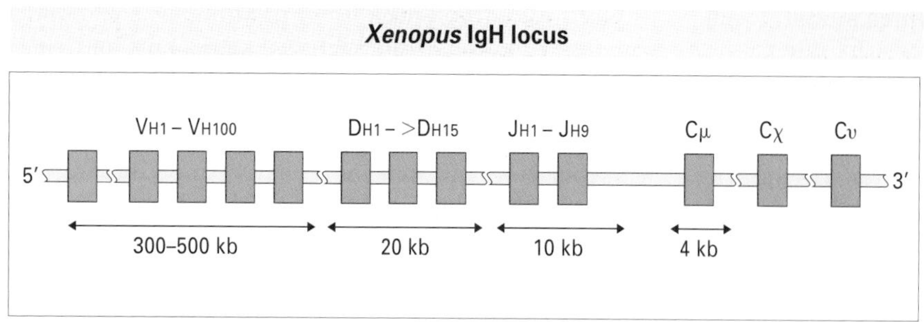

Fig. 13.18 The IgH locus in *Xenopus* is of similar architecture to that seen in teleost fish and resembles that in mammals. Recombination signal sequences adjoin all the gene segments. D segments rearrange first to JH; later, VH genes arrange to D–J. The rearranged V–D–J genes are finally joined to a constant region gene, producing IgM, IgX or IgY. (Based on data from Dr L. Du Pasquier.)

genes, similar to those occurring in mammals, proceed during B-cell development and allelic exclusion exists, resulting in monospecific B lymphocytes. Recombinase-activating genes (involved in immunoglobulin gene rearrangements) are found in *Xenopus*, but antibody (V region) diversity is quite low, there being only some 5×10^5 different antibody molecules in adults. The restricted affinity maturation seen following B-cell activation in *Xenopus* (and in other ectotherms) apparently does not relate to absence of somatic mutations of immunoglobulin genes. Rather it is believed to relate to lack of efficient selection of mutants due to absence of appropriate germinal centres in ectotherm lymphoid organs. Lymph nodes with germinal centres have until recently been considered to be found only in birds and mammals. However, some type of primitive 'germinal centre' may exist in trout spleen, where RAG proteins have been identified in cell clusters. Although *Xenopus* larvae possess all three Ig isotypes found in adults, larval and adult antibody repertoires are different. The adult repertoire is affected by gene rearrangements occurring in a new wave of B-cell development after metamorphosis. The third hypervariable region of the IgH chain in the adult is diversified by random addition of N residues, but this does not occur in larvae.

The generation of antibody diversity in birds – This involves a second pattern of immunoglobulin gene organization and takes place in a unique site, the cloacal bursa of

Primary lymphoid organs in birds

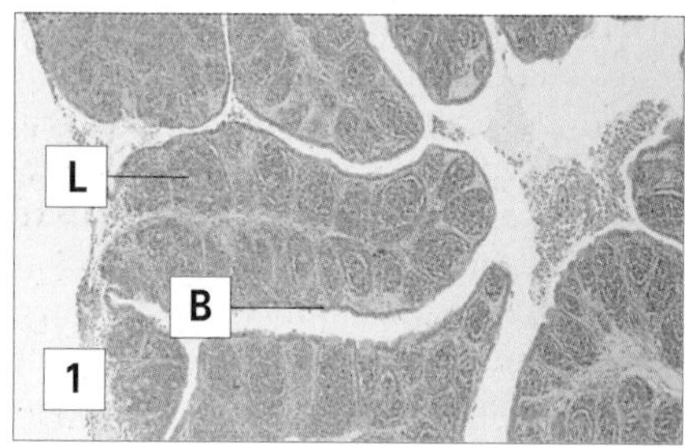

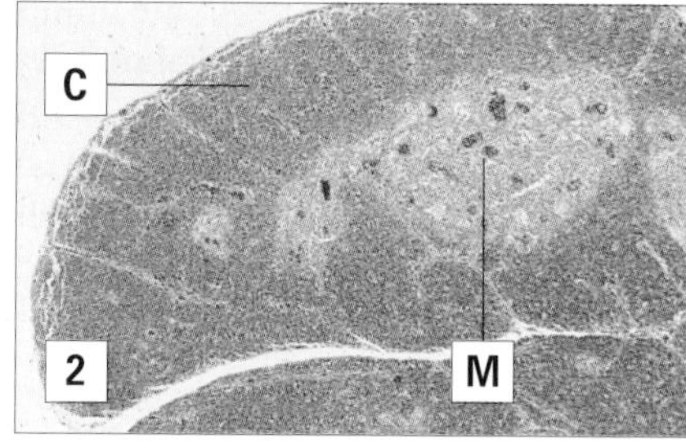

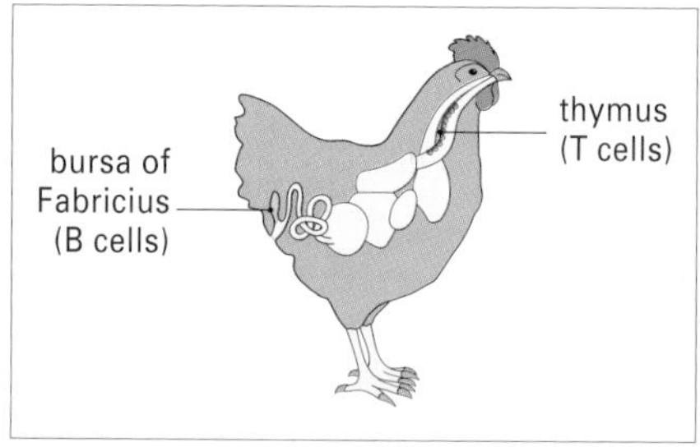

Fig. 13.19 The two central organs in the avian immune system are the bursa of Fabricius (**1**) and the thymus (**2**). Lymphocytes developing in the thymus are termed T cells and those in the bursa, B cells. Lymphoid follicles (L) and bursal lumen (B) are marked, as are the cortex (C) and medulla (M) of the thymus. H&E stain, ×20.

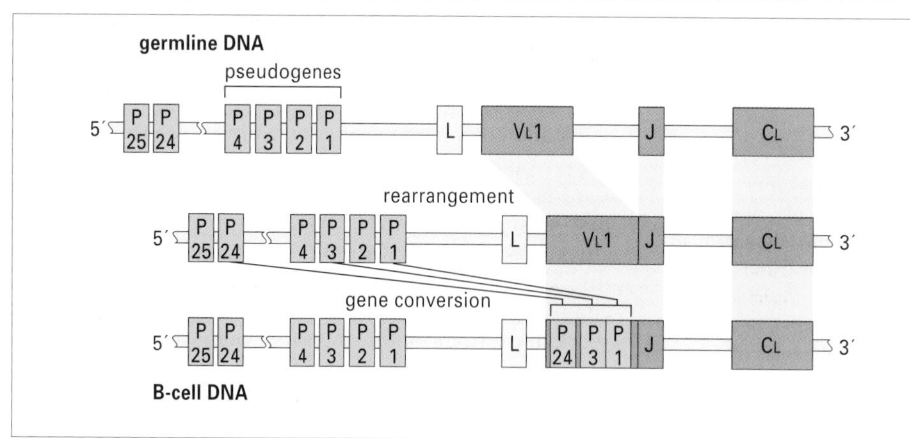

Fig. 13.20 The chicken germ line immunoglobulin light chain locus has less than 30 kb of DNA. A single functional V gene (VL) lies 2 kb upstream from a single J–C unit, with an adjacent cluster of 25 pseudogenes (P) in a 19-kb region. Rearrangement occurs briefly during early B-cell development. Antibody diversity is achieved by gene conversion between P and the rearranged sequence. The arrangement shown (P1, P3 and P24) is illustrative; converted segments do not necessarily lie in order in the V gene segment.

Fabricius (*Fig. 13.19*). The chicken Ig light chain locus has a single V gene which is initially rearranged and joined to a single J–C unit (*Fig. 13.20*). Multiple D region genes also exist in the chicken IgH locus. Rearrangement takes place only for a limited period during early development when stem cells colonize the bursa, whereas in mice and humans immunoglobulin gene rearrangements occur in the B-cell precursors throughout life. Subsequently, in the chicken, stretches of nucleotide sequences from pseudogenes (adjacent to the single V gene) replace 10–120 base-pair segments within the rearranged immunoglobulin gene sequences. This high-frequency gene conversion mechanism (which is also seen in rabbits) operates throughout the time B cells proliferate in the bursa.

A third pattern of Ig gene loci is seen in cartilaginous fish – Here both heavy (μ) and light (κ- and λ-like) immunoglobulin chains are coded for by many small discrete gene clusters (cassettes) (*Fig. 13.21*), within which V, (D), J and C genes are all found. Each immunoglobulin gene cluster differs in DNA sequence from other clusters. These sequences are in germ line configuration. Shark antibodies apparently possess a diverse array (many millions) of binding specificities, but lack inter-individual immunoglobulin variation, because diversity is encoded in the germ line, rather than by somatic mechanisms. The use of somatic gene rearrangements to accomplish immunoglobulin diversity (as in teleosts, amphibians, birds and mammals) is therefore not universal to vertebrates. These cartilaginous fish have a high level of natural antibodies to a diverse set of antigens, similar to the polyspecific (frequently autoreactive) IgM antibodies of mammals, which are secreted by CD5$^+$ B cells early in ontogeny. Whether the cluster arrangement of immunoglobulin gene subunits seen in sharks can achieve B-cell clonal restriction is not certain, although increase in specific antibodies without a general increase in serum Ig is found in sharks, implying that clonal selection is operating.

Shark immunoglobulin VH loci

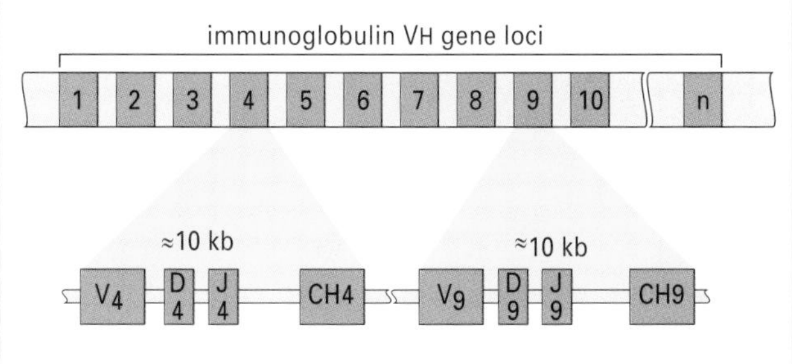

Fig. 13.21 In the shark there is a series of about 200 heavy chain gene clusters, each with a single V, D, J and C gene segment. The fourth and ninth clusters are shown expanded. VH, DH and JH segments are closely linked and occur within approximately 1.3 kb. Together with the CH segment, they occupy only about 10–15 kb. The arrangement of genes within a cluster appears to be encoded in the germ line, rather than by somatic rearrangement mechanisms, which may account for the lack of inter-individual variation associated with the immune response of this species. (Based on data of Dr J.J. Marchalonis and Dr G.W. Litman.)

Novel patterns in coelocanths – Preliminary studies reveal that a novel IgH locus (clusters of V–D genes distributed along the chromosome) may be present in coelocanths, the evolutionary 'relics' found to be alive in the Indian Ocean.

Cells of the non-adaptive immune system

Natural killer (NK) cells occur in most vertebrates

Mammalian NK cells lie at the interface between innate and adaptive immunity, providing non-antigen-specific defence against target cells deficient in MHC class I protein expression (e.g. certain tumours and virally infected cells), which cannot be recognized by MHC-restricted CTL (see Chapter 10). In view of the heterogeneity of antigen recognition molecules found on mammalian NK cells, the identification of NK receptors and also their target antigens that are conserved throughout vertebrate evolution would indicate the fundamental importance of these structures in NK cell function.

NK-like lymphoid cells have been demonstrated in several lower vertebrate groups including birds, reptiles, amphibians and teleost fish. Indeed, non-specific cytotoxic cells have recently been demonstrated in protochordates; these can kill mammalian tumour cell lines. In both cartilaginous and bony fish, macrophages have been shown to display spontaneous cytotoxicity, and antibody-dependent cell-mediated cytotoxic (ADCC) reactions are found in sharks. A monoclonal antibody (5C6) raised against catfish natural cytotoxic cells (NCCs) is able to modulate killing of human transformed lines by both fish and human NK cells, suggesting an evolutionary conservation of antigen-receptor molecules involved. The antigen receptor on catfish cells is called 'NCC receptor protein 1' (NCCRP-1). Catfish also have other types of NK-like cells distinct from NCCs, e.g. those that can kill allogeneic effectors and which, unlike NCCs, are not blocked by mAb 5C6.

NK cells have recently been identified in *Xenopus* spleen, liver and intestine using monoclonal antibodies (e.g. mAb 1F8, *Fig. 13.22*). Following 48-hour culture in cytokine-rich medium, 1F8-purified cells kill *Xenopus* thymus lymphoid tumour cells which are deficient in MHC class Ia and II expression (*Fig. 13.23*). Early-thymectomized *Xenopus* have elevated proportions of NK cells, which presumably play a crucial role in the survival of these T-cell-deficient animals (see below). *Xenopus* NK cells kill by inducing apoptosis of target tumour cells (*Fig. 13.24*). The nature of *Xenopus* NK receptors remains to be elucidated, as does the question of whether NK cells can develop in tadpoles that lack MHC I expression, the normal inhibitory ligands of these cells.

Candidate NK cells, which mediate MHC-unrestricted cytotoxicity, have been identified in the chicken. Avian NK cells resemble mammalian NK cells in being cytoplasmic CD3$^+$ but surface TCR–CD3$^-$, and often express CD8. These features indicate the close relationship of NK cells to T cells. Both avian and mammalian NK cells are, however, extrathymically derived.

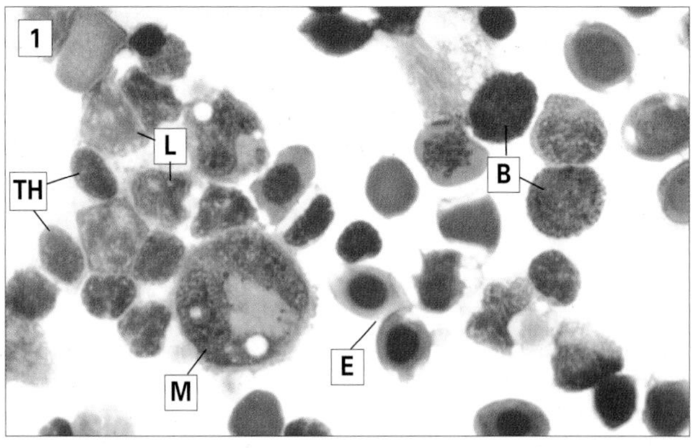

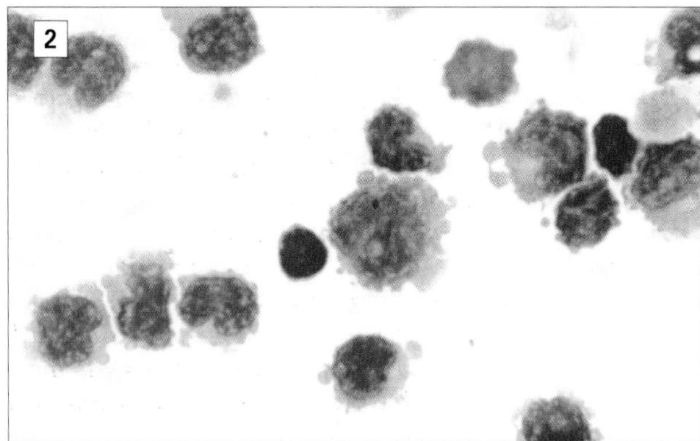

Fig. 13.22 ***Xenopus*** **NK cell morphology.** Wright–Giemsa-stained cytospins of splenocytes reveal that diverse cell types (including lymphocytes (L), basophils (B), macrophages (M), thrombocytes (TH) and erythrocytes (E)) are found in splenocytes depleted of NK cells (**1**), whereas mAb-purified NK cells are large lymphoid cells with distinct pseudopodia (**2**). ×600

Phagocyte activity in fish

There is special interest in promoting disease resistance in fish in aquaculture. In this respect, parameters for enhancing fish phagocyte activity are being considered in some detail. The considerable progress in establishing long-term *in vitro* cultures of fish leucocytes (e.g. from catfish and carp) is fostering work in this area. Enhanced activity of fish phagocytes to bacterial antigens, possibly due to release of macrophage-activating factors, can readily be achieved by injecting killed pathogens and their products. β-glucans (polysaccharides from cell walls of yeasts and fungi) are also being used as enhancers of phagocyte-mediated immunity in fish, and are proving to be good adjuvants for vaccines although their mechanism of action awaits clarification. Cytokines such as fish T-cell-derived 'gamma interferon' and human TNFα, synergize in elevating the respiratory burst pathways of trout macrophages, which leads to production of bactericidal oxygen free radicals (superoxide anion and hydrogen peroxide). Mammalian transforming growth factor-β (TGFβ) can inhibit fish macrophage activation. Chemokine-like factors are found in fish (see below) and these can influence fish phagocyte locomotion. Since stress-induced immunosuppression may well be a problem in fish aquaculture, the recently reported ability of the immunoactive peptide FK-565 to block such immunosuppression is of interest.

Leukotrienes and other lipid mediators (collectively known as eicosanoids) are known to be involved in a variety of inflammatory processes in mammals. There is now evidence that eicosanoids are produced in fish (and amphibians) and play an important role in inflammatory responses in fish. For example, leukotriene-B_4 enhances the migration of rainbow trout leucocytes, and eicosanoids can modulate trout T-cell proliferation. Because dietary lipids can modulate fish eicosanoid production, dietary considerations are crucial in developing fish vaccination, and this is currently an active research area.

Thrombocytes

Fish, amphibian (*Fig. 13.22*) and avian blood contains nucleated thrombocytes that are considered to be the evolutionary forerunners of platelets. Thrombocytes are involved in blood clotting and this process in trout involves putative integrin-like fibrinogen receptors. Thrombocytes are also

NK cell-mediated cytotoxicity

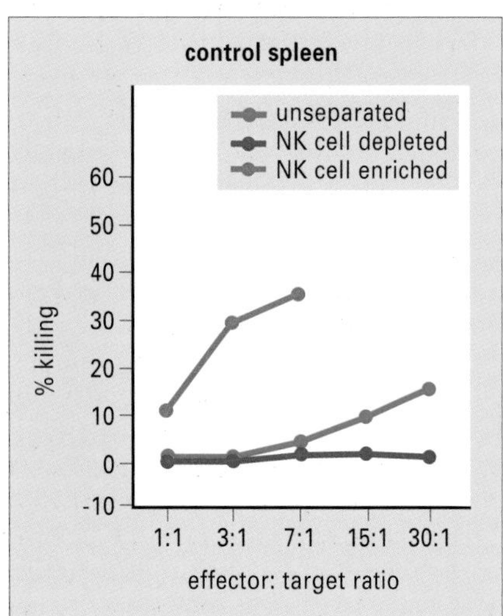

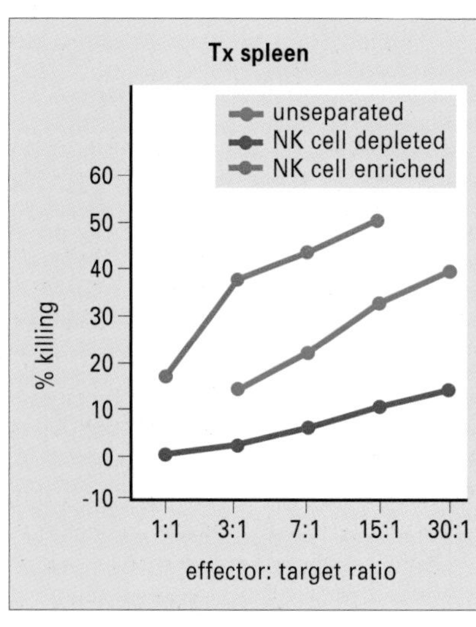

Fig. 13.23 Cytotoxicity towards B_3B_7 *Xenopus* lymphoid tumour targets is mediated by mAb(1F8)-enriched, *Xenopus* NK cells, but not by mAb-depleted splenocytes. The figure compares lymphokine-activated killing mediated by splenocytes from control and early thymectomized (Tx) frogs, and shows % killing of ^{51}Cr-labelled targets at various effector : target (E : T) ratios following 6-hour assay.

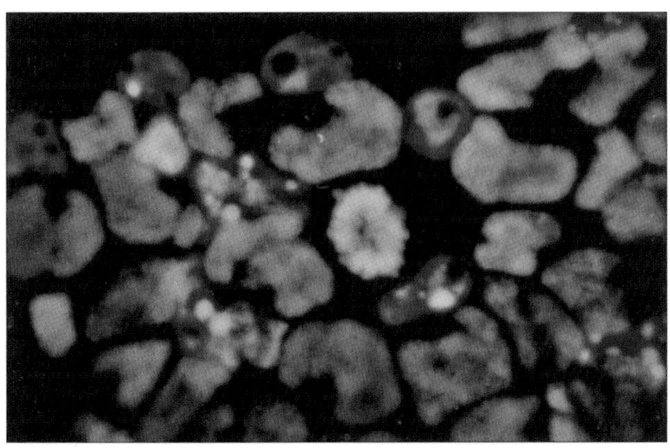

Fig. 13.24 *Xenopus* NK cells kill targets by inducing apoptosis. Cytospin of B_3B_7 *Xenopus* lymphoid tumour cells cultured for 6 hours with purified NK cells; tumour cells subsequently isolated from NK cells and stained for apoptosis-specific protein (ASP) (green fluorescence), and counterstained with propidium iodide (stains DNA orange). After co-culture with NK cells, but not following culture with NK-depleted lymphocytes, tumour cells frequently display fragmented DNA, visible as orange spots, and ASP-rich cytoplasm. Healthy tumour cells have intact nuclei and no green fluorescence. ×700. (Courtesy of Dr R. Stewart.)

known to be phagocytic. Monoclonal antibodies against fish and amphibian thrombocytes have recently been produced.

Non-antigen-specific molecules

Complement classical, alternative and lytic pathways are well developed in vertebrates

Agnathans possess antibody-independent, complement-like proteins. In hagfish these have homology with mammalian C3, C4 and C5, and act as opsonins, for which a 105-kDa receptor has been found on phagocytic leucocytes. Indirect evidence for the existence of terminal lytic components of the complement pathway in agnathans comes from identification of a hagfish homologue of CD59, which in mammals inhibits lysis of autologous cells by preventing formation of the membrane attack complex.

Both the classical (antibody-mediated) and alternative pathways of complement activation have been demonstrated in all vertebrate classes from sharks upwards. Cloning of shark complement genes should help elucidate the evolutionary origins of complement. Complement components C1–C9, together with factors B and D, have all been isolated in carp. Multiple forms of C3 exist in several teleost fish – allowing these fish to expand their innate capacity for immune recognition.

Considerable homology exists between the gene for C3 in *Xenopus* and the gene for mammalian C3. Characterization of other complement components in anurans includes C1q, C4, C5, the membrane attack complex and factor B. Basic properties of mammalian complement (such as thermolability, and requirements for Ca^{2+} and Mg^{2+}) are shared by fish and amphibian complement. Understandably, however, the temperature range over which ectotherm complement remains active is greater, with activity remaining at 4°C. Despite this, heat inactivation can be achieved at a lower temperature; *Xenopus* serum, for example, is entirely stripped of complement activity by treatment at 45°C for 40 minutes. Guinea-pig complement may be used successfully in haemolytic antibody assays *in vitro* using antibody from adult amphibians. For most fish species and larval *Xenopus*, the complement used must be from the same species or a closely related species.

Cytokines functionally similar to those in mammals are found in lower vertebrates

In comparison with the constantly increasing availability of data at the molecular level concerning the evolution of immunoglobulins, TCR and the MHC, research on cytokines, and especially cytokine receptors, of lower vertebrates rather lags behind. Bioassays have, however, revealed that several groups of cytokines do exist in many vertebrate classes. These include interleukins, interferons, tumour necrosis factor, colony-stimulating factors and chemokines.

For example, T-cell growth factors (TCGF), able to promote the proliferation of T-cell lymphoblasts *in vitro*, have now been identified from culture supernatants of stimulated T lymphocytes taken from bony fish, urodele and anuran amphibians, snakes and chickens. The purification of *Xenopus* TCGF indicates a protein of molecular mass 16 kDa, with biochemical and functional similarity to mammalian IL-2. The 'IL-2' gene and receptors for *Xenopus* 'IL-2' have not yet been identified.

'IL-1-like' activity has been detected in the macrophages of bony fish, amphibians and birds. The IL-1β gene has been cloned in rainbow trout and very recently in *Xenopus*. 'Interferon-like' factors, with macrophage-activating and antiviral function, have also been discovered in ectotherms (e.g. in farmed fish where viral diseases can decimate fish stocks). Interferon-inducible proteins are found in fish and are important components of the antiviral response. Oligonucleotide probes based on conserved sequences of mammalian cytokines have recently been successful in identifying ectotherm cytokine genes. These genes include fibroblast growth factor in amphibians, TGFβ (TGFβ5 in *Xenopus*, where it can inhibit T-cell proliferation, and TGFβ4 in chickens) and flatfish IL-2. At least two different TGFβ isoforms have been identified in cloning studies on teleost fish. Evolutionary conservation of TNF receptors is indicated, because the activating effects of human TNFβ on rainbow trout macrophages can be blocked by pre-incubating these phagocytes with anti-human TNF (p55) receptor antibodies. Two trout chemokine receptors have been isolated that have homology with CXCR4 and CCR7.

Anti-microbial peptides

Anti-microbial peptides, structurally related to invertebrate antibacterial proteins (described earlier), are also important immune factors of the vertebrate immune system. Thus, cecropins have been discovered in pig intestine, and defensins are found in mammalian phagocytes and certain intestinal cells, where they control microbial growth. Another family of peptides, called magainins, are secreted by granular glands in the skin and gut of *Xenopus*. Magainins have broad-range biocidal activity against Gram-negative and Gram-positive bacteria, fungi and protozoa. Moreover, they have also been shown to be cytotoxic for various human malignant cells. Several magainins have now been synthesized in the laboratory and are being considered as potential therapeutic agents in humans. Squalamine, a steroid that acts as a systemic antibiotic in sharks, has similarly become a candidate for human drug development.

LYMPHOMYELOID TISSUES IN LOWER VERTEBRATES

The lymphomyeloid system produces and stores lymphocytes, granulocytes and other blood cells, and provides the anatomical framework to allow appropriate immunocyte–antigen interaction, as in members of the *ikaros* family of transcription factors, that are crucial to mammalian lymphopoiesis.

Fish lymphomyeloid tissues

The agnathan hagfish possesses neither thymus nor spleen, its lymphocytes developing in the head, kidney or gut. A primitive spleen and bone marrow-like tissue are found in the lamprey.

Jawed fish lack lymphoid bone marrow, lymph nodes and nodular gut-associated lymphoid tissue (GALT) (*Fig. 13.25*). However, they have a well-developed thymus and spleen, diffuse GALT and lymphomyeloid tissue associated with kidney and liver (*Fig. 13.26*). The epigonal organ is a primary lymphoid tissue, equivalent to bone marrow. One notable feature of fish lymphomyeloid tissue is the abundance of melano-macrophage centres within the liver of 'primitive' forms and also within the spleen and kidney of teleost fish (*Fig. 13.27*). These centres are heavily laden with pigments, for example haemosiderin, ceroid, melanin and, in particular, lipofuscin. Pigment accumulation in the fish 'macrophage aggregates' may be partly related to the animals' high levels of unsaturated fats, which maintain membrane fluidity at low temperatures; these fats are particularly prone to peroxidation and formation of lipofuscin.

Evolution of lymphomyeloid tissues in vertebrates

vertebrate group	lymphomyeloid tissue: thymus	spleen	bone marrow	lymph nodes	GALT-associated	kidney/liver
mammals	presence/homology	presence/homology	presence/homology	presence/homology	presence/homology	presence/homology
birds	presence/homology	presence/homology	presence/homology	presence/homology	presence/homology	presence/homology
reptiles	presence/homology	presence/homology	presence/homology	partial evidence	presence/homology	presence/homology
frogs/toads	presence/homology	presence/homology	presence/homology	partial evidence	presence/homology	presence/homology
salamanders/newts	presence/homology	presence/homology	probable absence	probable absence	partial evidence	presence/homology
lungfish	presence/homology	presence/homology	probable absence	probable absence	partial evidence	presence/homology
teleost fish	presence/homology	presence/homology	probable absence	probable absence	partial evidence	presence/homology
sharks/rays	presence/homology	presence/homology	probable absence	probable absence	partial evidence	presence/homology
jawless fish	probable absence	partial evidence	probable absence	probable absence	partial evidence	presence/homology

Key: presence/homology; partial evidence; probable absence

Fig. 13.25 Lymphoid and myeloid compartments are intermingled in fishes and amphibians.

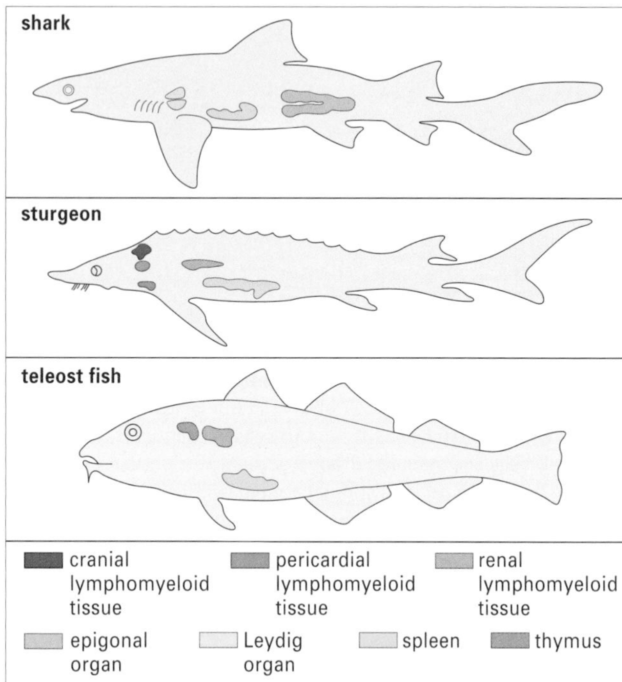

Fig. 13.26 Note that the intestines of sharks and sturgeons are also rich in lymphomyeloid tissue (in the spiral valve). (Courtesy of Dr R. Fänge.)

Amphibian lymphomyeloid tissues

The thymus

The adult *Xenopus* thymus lies just under the skin, behind the middle ear. Detachment of the thymus from the pharyngeal epithelium occurs early in development, as it does in most other vertebrates except teleost fish. The thymus is differentiated into an outer cortex and a central (paler-staining) medulla. The rapidly proliferating cortical lymphocytes are particularly sensitive to irradiation (*Fig. 13.28*). Apoptosis in the *Xenopus* thymus is enhanced by *in vitro* glucocorticoid treatment. Elevated *in vivo* levels of corticosteroids can induce thymic atrophy in *Rana*.

There is considerable evidence that the ectotherm thymus, like its counterpart in endotherms, produces lymphocytes with T-cell functions. The ultrastructure of thymic lymphocytes and neighbouring epithelial cells is shown in *Figure 13.29*. Several other stromal cell types are found within the amphibian thymus, including large dendritic (interdigitating) cells, macrophages, cysts and granular cells. Myoid cells are also found, as they are in the reptilian and mammalian thymus (*Fig. 13.29*). Myoid cells may be involved in promoting circulation of tissue fluids within the thymus and may also act as a source of macrophage-stimulating factors. Thymic epithelial cells,

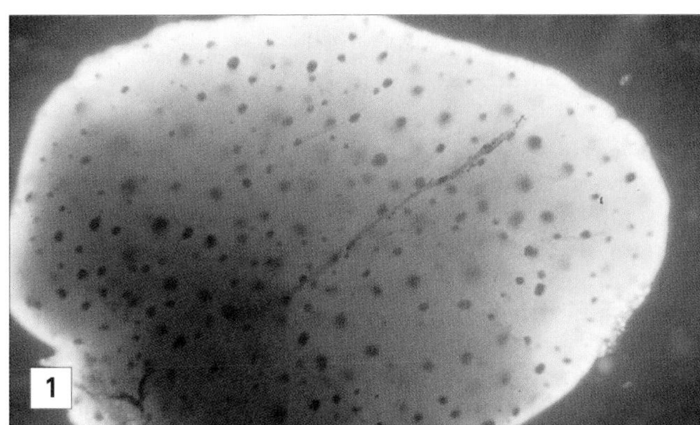

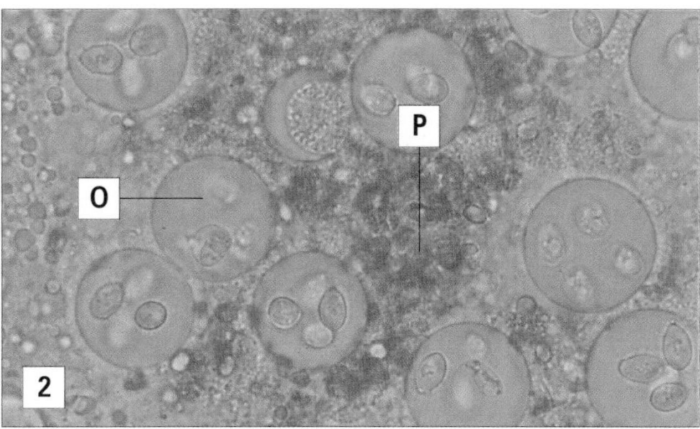

Fig. 13.27 Melano-macrophage centres (MMCs) in fish liver. Gross and microscopic views of liver of a cyptinodontid fish (*Rivulus marmoratus*) experimentally infected with the coccidian parasite *Calyptospora funduli*. At 60 days post-infection, distinct MMCs have appeared (**1**, ×60). The squash preparation (**2**, ×600) shows that these MMCs consist of degenerating oocysts (O) of the parasite and associated host pigment (P). The mononuclear phagocytes play a dominant role in MMC formation. (Courtesy of Dr W.K. Vogelbein.)

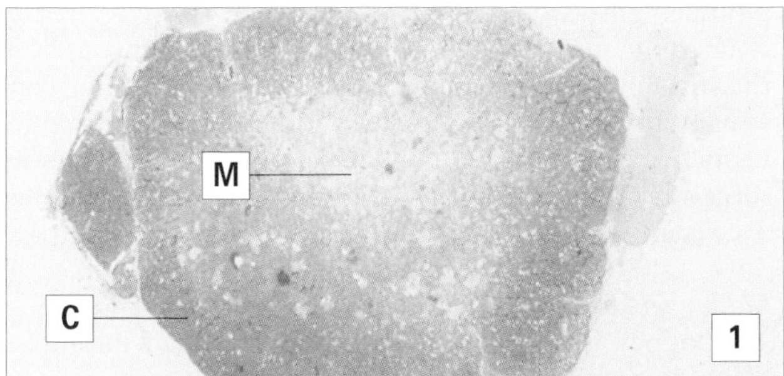

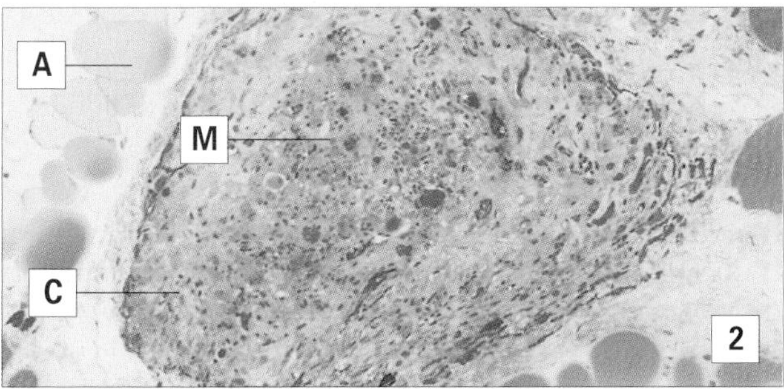

Fig. 13.28 Thymus of young adult *Xenopus*: effect of irradiation. Normal thymus (**1**, ×35) has an extremely lymphoid cortex (C) and a paler-staining, less cellular medulla (M). Gamma-irradiated thymus (9 days after 30 Gy (3000 rad) irradiation) is shown (**2**) (×90). Note the dramatic loss of lymphocytes from the cortex (C) following irradiation, but retention of some lymphocytes in the medulla (M). The irradiated thymus is reduced in size. Adipose tissue (A) surrounds the thymus. Toluidine blue stain.

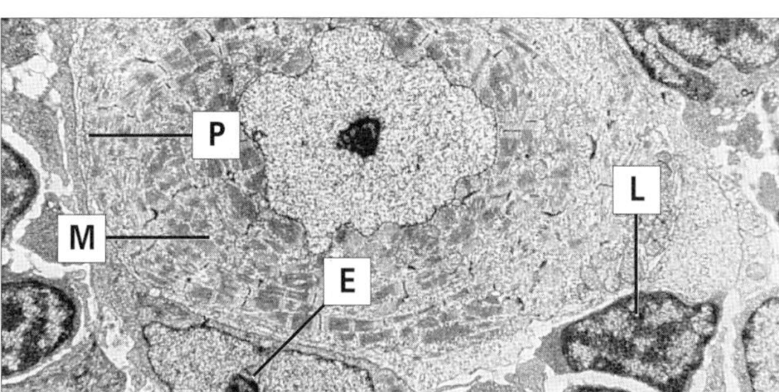

Fig. 13.29 Electron micrograph of thymus medulla of larval *Xenopus*. The myoid cell nucleus is surrounded by concentric rings of striated myofibrils (M) resembling those of skeletal muscle. The nuclear chromatin of the small lymphocytes (L) is organized into a series of electron-dense zones; the cytoplasm is scant with few organelles. The epithelial cell nuclei (E) have evenly dispersed chromatin and prominent nucleoli; the cytoplasm is extensive and projections (P) extend in an interdigitating fashion between lymphocytes and other cell types to form a supportive network. ×700. (Courtesy of Dr J.J. Rimmer.)

which express MHC class II antigens early in development, appear to be involved in 'educating' T-lineage cells (see below). Nurse cell-like complexes of stromal cells and enclosed thymocytes have been found in the frog thymus and may represent sites of T-cell education. B cells have also been found in the thymus of diverse vertebrate species, including amphibians, though this organ is not involved with their production. High endothelial venules have been described in the *Rana* thymus, which may promote cell immigration.

The spleen

The spleen is a major peripheral lymphoid organ in all jawed vertebrates. Together with the 'lymph nodes' and kidneys, it traps antigen, houses proliferating lymphocytes after their stimulation by antigen, and provides for the appropriate release of these cells and their products. Thymus-dependent and -independent lymphoid zones within the spleen have been demonstrated in *Xenopus* (*Fig. 13.30*). The white pulp follicles are rich in B cells (*Fig. 13.31*), shown by selective staining of this region with anti-immunoglobulin monoclonal antibodies. Splenic T cells, found especially in the perifollicular (marginal zone) regions, lack surface immunoglobulin, but a population will bind with anti-T-cell monoclonal antibodies (*Fig. 13.31*).

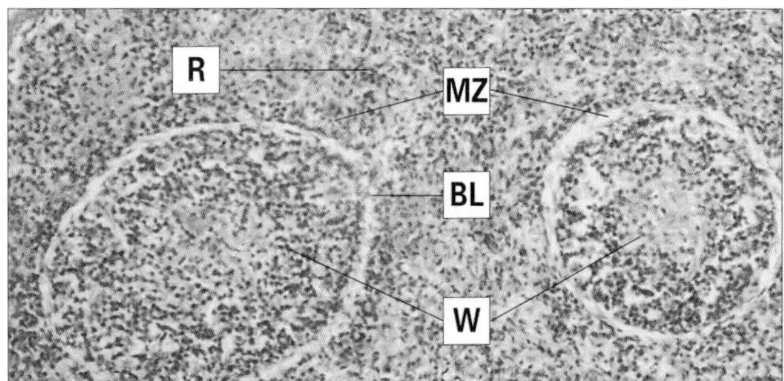

Fig. 13.30 Spleen section of adult *Xenopus*. Thymus-dependent (perifollicular red pulp or marginal zone (MZ)) and thymus-independent (white pulp) areas are shown. In *Xenopus* (unlike many other ectotherms) the white pulp (W) is clearly separated from the surrounding red pulp (R) by lightly staining boundary layer cells (BL). Concentrations of lymphocytes are also seen in the red pulp. H&E stain, ×80.

Blood vessels enter the spleen through the white pulp central arteriole, which is in close association with noradrenergic sympathetic nerve fibres. This nerve innervates the spleen and plays an immunomodulatory role. Capillaries leave the central arteriole and empty into the surrounding red pulp marginal zone; capillary walls contribute to the boundary layer. Experimental studies with India ink-stained and fluoresceinated antigens reveal that it is the red pulp that initially receives material circulating in the blood. Circulating antigens are later trapped within the white pulp follicles, that is they are closely associated with potential antibody-producing cells. Antigen is held on the surfaces of large dendritic cells, whose cytoplasmic processes extend pseudopods through the boundary layer and into the marginal zone, which is rich in T cells. The overall arrangement of the amphibian spleen is similar to that of the mammalian spleen, although germinal centres have not been identified in the former. The spleen of amphibians plays an important role in B-cell development in both the larva (along with the liver) and in the adult, where it constitutes the main site of B-cell differentiation.

Surprisingly, B lymphocytes of *Xenopus* do not constitutively express CD5, the marker found on 'primitive' natural antibody-producing B1 cells of mammals.

The lymphomyeloid nodes

Lymphomyeloid nodes, bearing a superficial functional resemblance to the lymph nodes of endothermic vertebrates, are seen for the first time in vertebrate evolution in 'advanced' amphibians such as the ranid and bufid frogs and toads, but not in urodeles or in *Xenopus*. The lymphomyeloid nodes of anurans are different from their mammalian counterparts in being mainly blood-filtering organs, although they can also trap material from surrounding lymph. Although a major site of antibody-producing cells, the anuran lymphomyeloid nodes do not have the clearly defined architecture of mammalian lymph nodes and germinal centres are not seen. In the adult frog, 'lymph nodes' are found in the neck and axillary regions; the lymph gland of the larva is structurally similar (*Fig. 13.32*).

Gut-associated lymphoid tissue

Nodular gut-associated lymphoid tissue (GALT), analogous to the mammalian GALT system, occurs throughout the small intestine in amphibians. In *Xenopus*, GALT contains both IgM and IgX-secreting plasma cells. Immunohistochemistry with anti-T-cell monoclonal antibodies reveals both nodular (lamina propria) and intra-epithelial T cells in *Xenopus* intestine (*Fig. 13.33*).

Kidney and liver

The kidney is a major lymphomyeloid organ in amphibians, as it is in fish, but this function wanes in the kidneys of reptiles, birds and mammals. In anurans, B-cell development in ontogeny begins in the kidney and/or liver. These organs are, in fact, intimately involved with the early differentiation of erythroid, lymphoid and myeloid cells in diverse vertebrates.

Bone marrow

Bone marrow is found in amphibians, but its immunological role awaits clarification. In adult *Rana pipiens*,

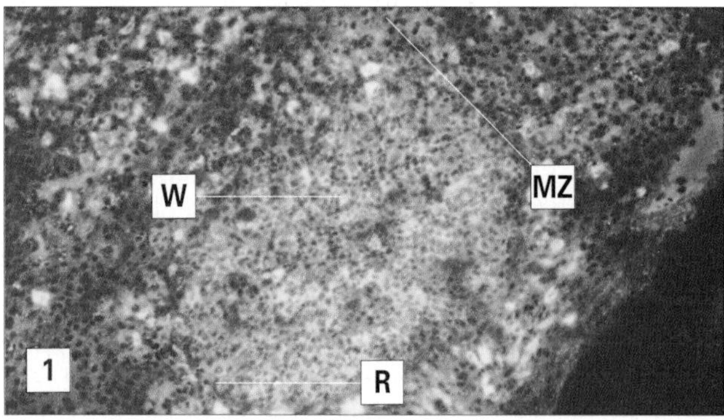

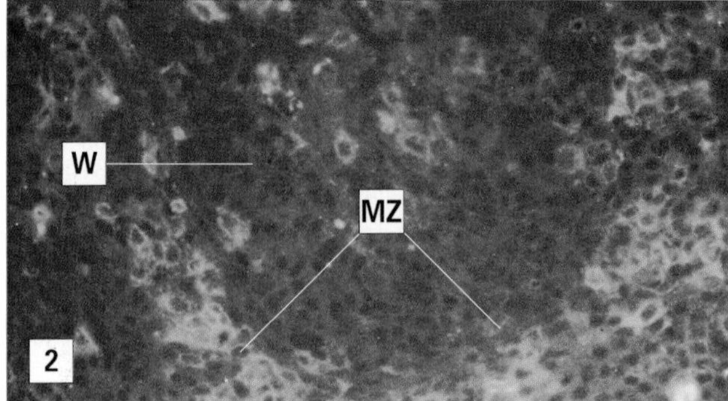

Fig. 13.31 Adult *Xenopus* spleen, showing B- and T-cell-rich zones. (**1**) B cells frequent the white pulp follicle (W); they are also seen in the marginal zone (MZ) and red pulp (R), mainly as densely staining plasma cells. Anti-B-cell (anti-IgM) mAb stain, ×100. (**2**) T cells are seen concentrated in the marginal zone, just outside the white pulp follicle (W). They are seen especially in the perifollicular (marginal) zone (MZ) and lack surface immunoglobulin. Anti-T-cell stain, ×200.

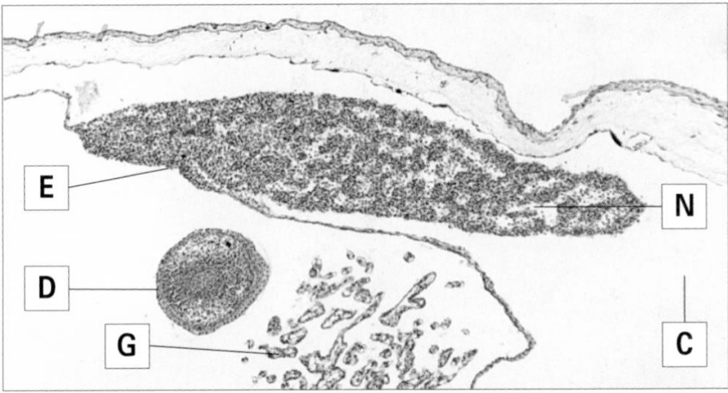

Fig. 13.32 Lymph gland section of larval *Rana*. The elongated (paired) lymphomyeloid node (N) is seen attached ventrally to the epithelium (E) of the gill chamber and projects into a large lymphatic channel (C). Gills (G), and a digit (D) of the anterior limb lying in the gill chamber, are seen medially; the larval skin lies above. The lymph gland consists of an extensive lymphoid parenchyma with phagocytes and intervening sinusoids (pale-staining). The lymph gland is mainly a blood-filtering organ. H&E stain, ×25.

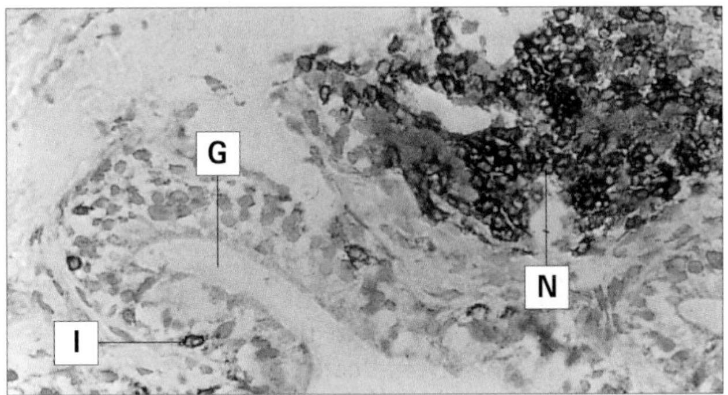

Fig. 13.33 Cryostat section of *Xenopus* small intestine stained with anti-CD5 (a pan T cell) monoclonal antibody and visualized by immunoperoxidase staining. Intraepithelial T cells (I) and nodular collections of T cells (N) in lamina propria can be seen, as can the gut lumen (G). T cells from both locations are lost after early thymectomy. ×300.

bone-marrow lymphomyeloid tissue is readily evident (*Fig. 13.34*) and is an important source of antibody-producing cells. In *Xenopus*, on the other hand, bone marrow appears to be more rudimentary and is mainly a site for the differentiation of neutrophilic granulocytes (*Fig. 13.34*).

AMPHIBIAN MODELS FOR STUDYING ONTOGENY OF IMMUNITY

In recent years, several isogeneic and inbred families of *Xenopus* have become available for immunological research. Different *Xenopus* families, that are either MHC compatible or possess one or two MHC haplotype differences, are proving invaluable for investigating the ontogeny of the immune system.

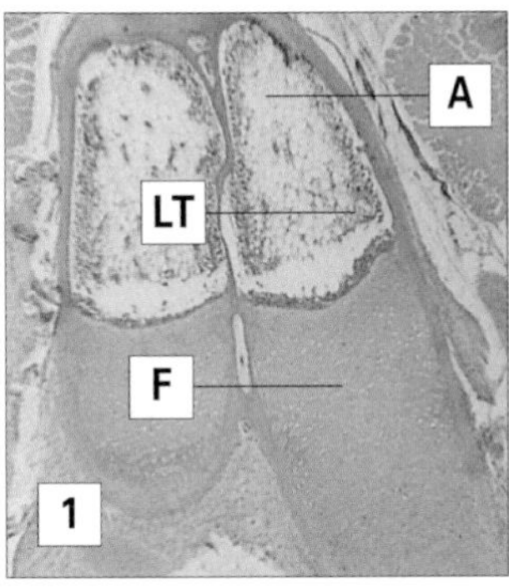

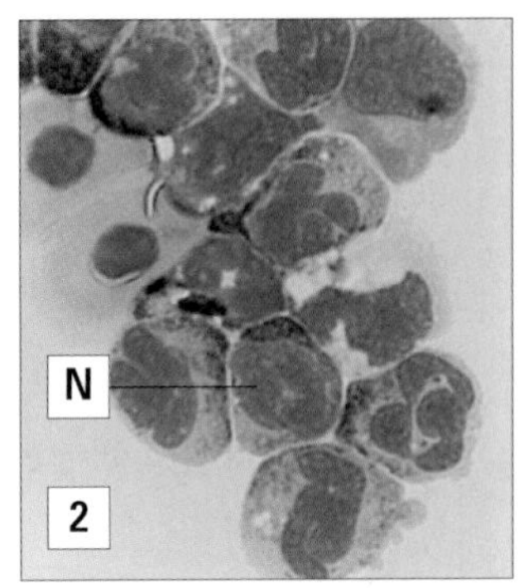

Fig. 13.34 Bone marrow. (**1**) Lymphomyeloid tissue (LT), an important source of antibody-producing cells, in bone marrow from *Rana*. Femur (F) and adipose tissue (A) are also marked. H&E stain, ×20. (**2**) A bone marrow cytocentrifuge preparation from *Xenopus*, showing peroxidase-positive neutrophilic granulocytes (N). ×700. (Cytocentrifuge preparation, courtesy of Dr I. Hadji-Azimi.)

The development of the thymus

Thymus development and thymectomy experiments

Xenopus is ideally suited for investigating the role of the thymus in immune system development, because the free-living larva can be thymectomized very early in life when the thymus is still immature (*Figs 13.35, 13.36*). In *Xenopus* the paired thymus develops from the dorsal epithelium of the second pharyngeal pouches. Experimental studies reveal that lymphoid precursor cells first enter the thymic epithelial rudiments at 3–4 days of age. RAG expression begins at day 3.5 and fully rearranged TCRβ transcripts can be detected by 5 days. A T-cell differentiation antigen, the XTLA-1 marker (120 kDa), recognized by anti-thymocyte mouse monoclonal antibody XT-1, begins to appear on the thymic lymphoid cell population at 7 days. Cell-surface expression of the cortical thymocyte antigen CTX is first detectable on thymocytes at 8 days. A majority of thymocytes express T-cell-surface antigens by 10 days of age, when candidate T cells are first identified in the periphery. Larval lymphocytes are very sensitive to corticosteroids and are destroyed by apoptosis due to increased levels of these hormones that occur in the absence of serum binding factors at metamorphosis. Larval immune cells may be removed to avoid autoimmunity to adult-specific antigens appearing at metamorphosis. After thymus involution at metamorphosis a new wave of colonization by stem cells occurs; following metamorphosis, thymocyte numbers increase, reaching maximal levels at 15–16 months. Recent evidence suggests that larval and adult *Xenopus* express different TCRβ repertoires.

Early thymectomy of *Xenopus* (at 4–8 days of age) has clearly demonstrated the existence of T-dependent (T_{dep}) and T-independent (T_{ind}) components of immunity. Following this early thymectomy, cells expressing high levels of T-cell markers (e.g. CD5 and CD8) are no longer found in larval and adult lymphoid organs, whereas surface-IgM$^+$ B cells are plentiful (*Fig. 13.37*). Although a proportion of lymphoid cells in liver and gut of thymectomized *Xenopus* continue to express low levels of CD5 and CD8,

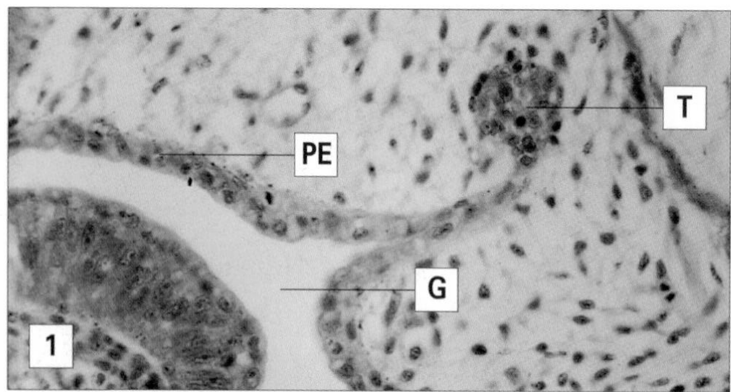

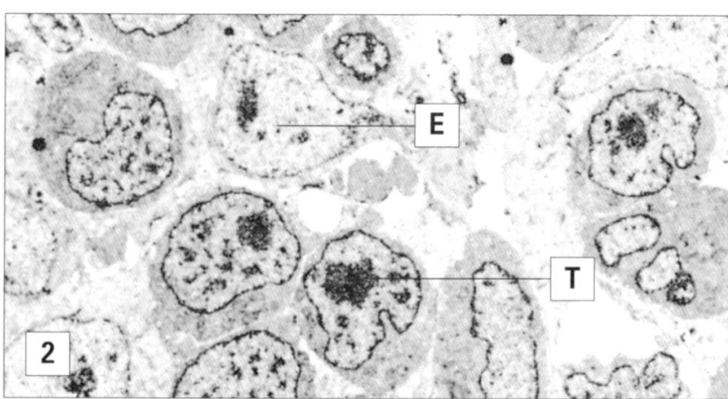

Fig. 13.35 *Xenopus* thymus at 3 days and 7 days. (**1**) At 3 days, developing thymus (T) is still attached to the pharyngeal epithelium (PE) and composed mostly of epithelial cells. A gill pouch (G) is also shown. H&E stain, ×100. (**2**) At 7 days, the thymus consists of less than 1000 cells of two major types. The epithelial cells (E) have a prominent nucleolus, dispersed chromatin and pale-staining cytoplasm. Lymphoid cells (L) possess large amounts of densely staining cytoplasm with an abundance of free ribosomes and mitochondria. At 7 days, the XT-1 marker begins to appear on the thymic lymphoid cell population, and MHC class II proteins are first expressed on epithelial cells. Electron micrograph, ×500.

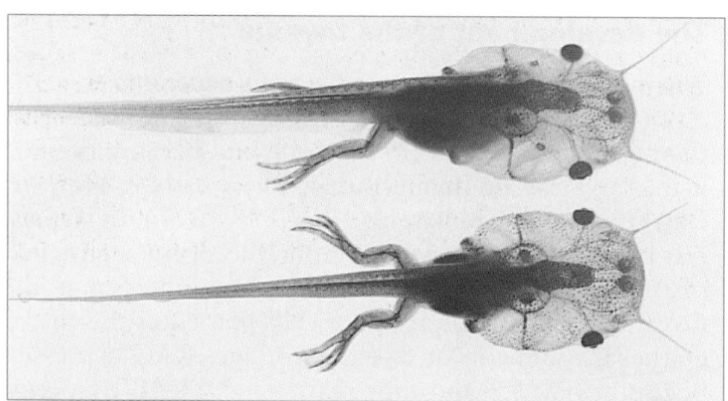

Fig. 13.36 *Xenopus* thymus at 38 days. The pigmented paired thymus lies behind the eyes (upper); its absence is readily apparent in the sibling thymectomized at 7 days (lower).

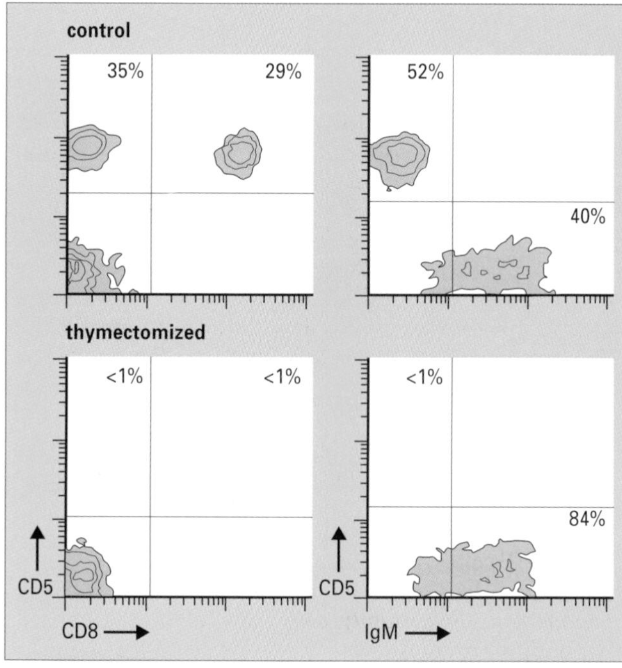

Fig. 13.37 Dual colour flow cytometric analysis of mAb-stained splenocytes from control and thymectomized adult *Xenopus*. Splenocytes were stained sequently with anti-CD8 (FITC) and then anti-CD5 (PE) mAbs, or with anti-IgM (FITC) followed by anti-CD5 (PE) and surface fluorescence evaluated by flow cytometry. Percentages of CD5+ve/CD8–ve lymphocytes (putative helper T cells), CD5+ve/CD8+ve lymphocytes (cytotoxic T cells) and CD5–ve/IgM+ve B cells are indicated. Quadrants were set to exclude 98% cells stained with control reagents from positive analysis.

TCRβ expression is always minimal following thymectomy. The thymus therefore appears to be critical for T-cell maturation at this level of evolution.

Thymectomy of larvae at various time points during development suggests that different T-cell functions require the presence of the thymus for varying periods in order to become established in the periphery. Studies in intact animals reveal that alloimmune reactivity (*in vivo* and *in vitro*), together with the ability of splenocytes to respond to T-cell mitogens, develops early in the tadpole's larval life, whereas good IgY antibody responses are only seen in the froglet, which expresses appropriate T-cell helper function.

Thymic education in Xenopus involves positive selection and limited negative selection

Foreign thymus, grafted into early-thymectomized *Xenopus*, can promote the differentiation of host precursor cells along a T-cell pathway. The *in vivo* development of thymuses, with epithelial and lymphoid compartments expressing different MHC markers, can readily be achieved by a different surgical approach. This involves joining the anterior part of one 24-hour embryo, containing the thymic epithelial buds, to the posterior portion of an MHC-incompatible embryo, from which the haemopoietic stem cells, including lymphocytes, arise (*Fig. 13.38*).

These two experimental systems have been used to

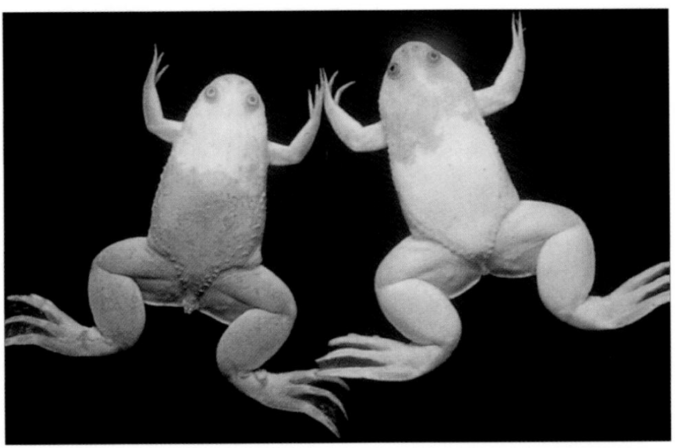

Fig. 13.38 Chimeric toads. Chimeric *Xenopus* were made by exchanging the anterior and posterior regions of two embryos 24 hours after fertilization. At this stage, the thymic anlage (e.g. thymic epithelium) is in the anterior region; all the lymphocyte precursors are in the posterior. One embryo was from an albino variant with white skin and red eyes, the other embryo was from a normal *Xenopus*. These chimeras are useful for studying thymic education. (Courtesy of Dr M. Flajnik and Dr L. Du Pasquier.)

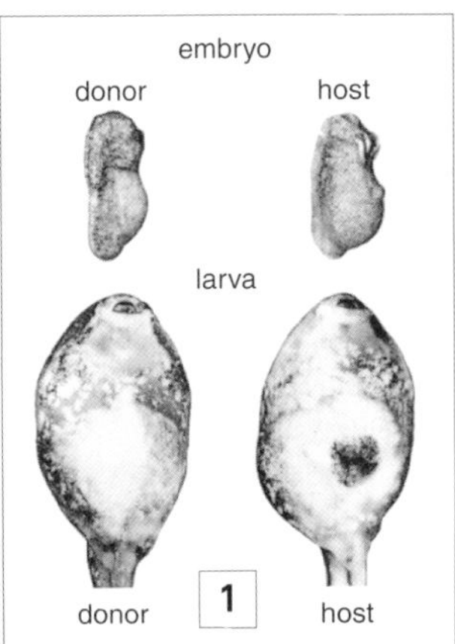

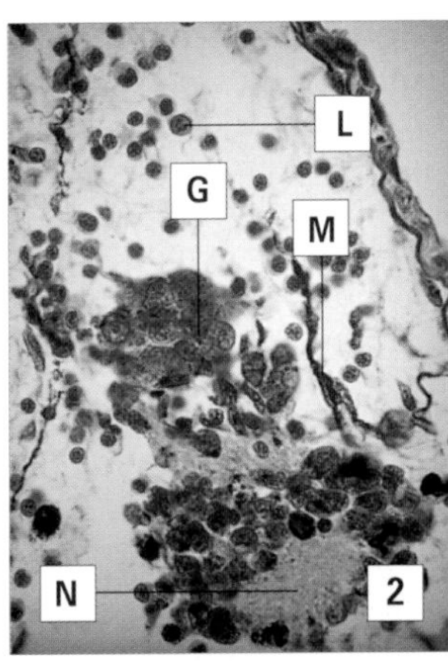

Fig. 13.39 Transplantation of embryonic tissue in *Rana* – ontogeny of alloimmunity. (**1**) A piece of neural fold removed from one embryo (tail-bud stage) is transplanted to the mid-ventral surface of another embryo (host). Intimately associated with the neural folds are the neural crest elements which are precursors of diverse cell types, including pigment cells. The pigment cells that differentiate are an externally visible means of following the progress of the embryonic transplant. The host larva has developed a distinctive mass of graft-derived pigment cells. (**2**) The section shows differentiated graft elements, large ganglion cells (G) with prominent nucleoli, other nervous tissue (N) and melanin (M), 15 days after transplantation. Despite the earliness of the transplantation, lymphocytes and granulocytes are invading the graft (L = leucocyte invading). H&E stain, ×100. (Courtesy of Dr E.P. Volpe.)

explore the role played by thymic stromal cells in thymic education. This involves negative selection (establishing tolerance of T cells to self antigens) and positive selection (restricting the MHC-antigen specificities with which helper and effector T-cell populations preferentially interact). These experiments on *Xenopus* have indicated involvement of the foreign thymus epithelium in positive selection and in inducing tolerance towards skin grafts of thymus MHC type, although interestingly this tolerance does not appear to prevent a mixed lymphocyte reaction towards thymus donor cells. Similar findings have been made with bird and mammal embryos. However, in mammals the view persists that thymic interdigitating (dendritic) cells, which are a stromal population of extrinsic origin, rather than thymic epithelial cells, play a crucial role in negative selection by deleting T cells with high affinity for self MHC.

Ontogeny of alloimmunity, self- and allotolerance and antibody production

Onset of alloimmunity (to MHC antigens) and specific antibody responses in tadpoles correlates with the appearance of the necessary T- and B-cell populations in the periphery (*Fig. 13.39*) and can occur when the lymphoid system contains less than a million lymphocytes. Immunological memory can be transferred over metamorphosis, but whether this reflects transfer of memory cells or is due to antigen persistence is unknown. The presence of 'self' eye lens proteins during early development has been shown to be crucial for establishment and maintenance of tolerance of frogs to their own eye tissue. Immunocompetent larvae (but not adults) can readily be rendered tolerant to allogeneic skin; such allotolerance induction is particularly easy at metamorphosis (*Fig. 13.40*). The size of grafts applied and the degree of histoincompatibility appear to be critical. Those that are only slightly incompatible are always tolerated by larval and peri-metamorphic *Xenopus*. Tolerance induced by grafting foreign skin and lymphoid tissues in larval life is seldom 'complete', as signs of anti-donor reactivity (such as an MLR) can still be demonstrated before or after metamorphosis. There is evidence that larvally induced transplantation tolerance is mediated by 'suppressor' T cells.

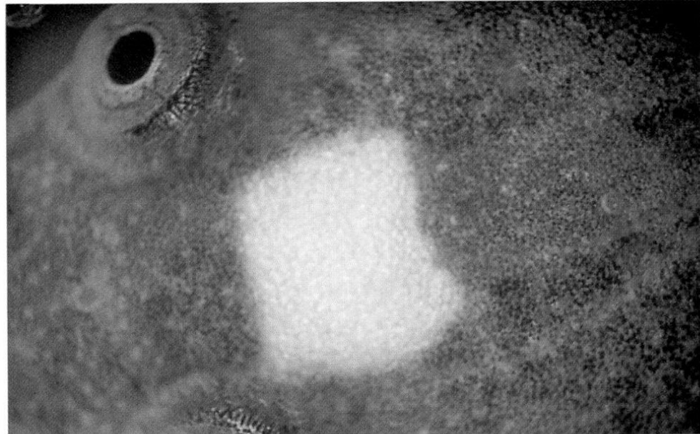

Fig. 13.40 Skin graft tolerance in *Xenopus*. Allogeneic skin, even from an MHC-disparate donor, may be tolerated by a larval or metamorphosing recipient. Subsequent skin grafts (here a piece of white belly skin) from the same donor are similarly retained by the adult frog. However, skin from a different donor is rejected within 3 weeks at 25°C.

Models for the study of lymphoid cell origins

Amphibian (and avian) embryos have contributed greatly to our knowledge of the origins of haematopoietic cells. It has been established that definitive haematopoiesis involves different stem cell populations. For example, in *Xenopus*, lymphoid precursor cells destined for the thymus have been shown to arise from ventrolateral plate mesoderm (ventral blood islands) and dorsolateral plate mesoderm of the embryo. Two waves of stem cell entry into the thymus occur in young *Xenopus*, one during early larval life, the other during metamorphosis, which presumably allows the adult T cells to be educated in an environment where adult-specific antigens are expressed.

A region near the dorsal aorta gives rise to definitive haematopoietic precursors in teleost fish. Lymphoid-specific transcription factors (e.g. *ikaros*) and enzymes (e.g. RAG 1 and 2) delineate primary lymphoid tissues. Together with mutants developed in the zebrafish system, these molecular markers are beginning to provide a comprehensive view of haematopoiesis in lower vertebrates.

Metamorphosis presents a problem for the immune system

Immunologists are intrigued to know how amphibians escape the risk of dying from an autoimmune disease at metamorphosis, as adult-specific cell markers are first expressed at this time. The significance of MHC class I first being expressed at metamorphosis remains to be elucidated. On the one hand, the involvement of suppressor functions seems likely. On the other hand, high plasma corticosteroid levels and increased expression of corticosteroid receptors on lymphocytes are found during the metamorphic climax. Such hormonal alterations may directly impair cell-mediated immunity, possibly by inhibiting IL-2 production. Amphibian metamorphosis is a fascinating period for probing the interplay between neuroendocrine and immune systems, which will undoubtedly have significance outside purely phylogenetic considerations. It has recently been speculated that the worldwide disappearance of amphibians may relate to environmental changes that cause habitat defects; such defects may exacerbate the increased lymphocyte loss that occurs at metamorphosis, resulting in greater risk of infection and death.

CRITICAL THINKING • The evolution of immunity (Explanations on pp 456–457)

Cloning and sequencing studies in the 1990s have shown that the crucial genetic components of adaptive immunity (namely T-cell receptor and immunoglobulin genes together with the MHC gene complex) are present in all ectothermic vertebrates from cartilaginous fish through to anuran amphibians, but are absent in invertebrates and agnathan fish. However, this chapter has highlighted several gaps in our knowledge concerning the evolution of immune system molecules and cells. A recent review on comparative immunology identified a 'top 10' set of questions which are currently outstanding in this field.

13.1 What 10 issues in the field of comparative vertebrate immunology do you consider remain unanswered and warrant further investigation in order to provide a more complete understanding of immunoevolution?

FURTHER READING

Andemon KA. Toll signalling pathways in the innate immune response. *Curr Opin Immunol* 2000;**12**:13–19.

Chretien I, Marcuz A, Courtet M, *et al.* CTX, a *Xenopus* thymocyte receptor, defines a molecular family conserved throughout vertebrates. *Eur J Immunol* 1998;**28**:4094–104.

Clem LW, Warr G (ed). Proceedings of the 7th Congress of Developmental & Comparative Immunology. *Devel Comp Immunol* 1997;**21**:77–252.

Cooper EL (ed). Invertebrate immune responses: cells and molecular products. *Adv Comp Environ Physiol* 1996:**23**.

Du Pasquier L. The phylogenetic origin of antigen-specific receptors. In origin and evaluation of the vertebrate immune system. *Curr Topics in Microbiology and Immunology* 2000;159–85.

Du Pasquier L, Wilson M, Robert J. The immune system of *Xenopus*: with special reference to B cell development and immunoglobulin genes. In: Tinsley RC, Kobel HR (ed). *The Biology of Xenopus*. Oxford: Clarendon Press; 1996:301–13.

Flajnik MF. Primitive vertebrate immunity: what is the evolutionary derivation of molecules that define the adaptive immune system? In: *Antimicrobial Peptides*. CIBA Foundation Symposium. Chichester: Wiley. 1994;**186**:224–32.

Greenberg AS, Avila D, Hughes M, *et al.* A novel antigen receptor gene family that undergoes rearrangement and extensive somatic diversification in sharks. *Nature* 1995;**374**:168–73.

Greenberg AS, Hughes AL, Guo J, *et al.* A novel chimeric antibody class in cartilagenous fish: IgM may not be the primordial immunoglobulin. *Eur J Immunol* 1996;**26**:1123–9.

Hansen JD, Zapata AG. Lymphocyte development in fish and amphibians. *Immunol Rev* 1998;**166**:199–220.

Horton JD. Amphibians. In: Turner RJ (ed). *Immunology: A Comparative Approach*. Chichester: Wiley; 1994:101–36.

Horton JD, Horton TL, Ritchie P. Immune system of *Xenopus*: T cell biology. In: Tinsley RC, Kobel HR (eds). *The Biology of Xenopus*. Oxford: Clarendon Press; 1996:279–99.

Horton JD, Milner A, Horton TL, *et al.* Apoptotis specific protein (ASP) identified in apoptotic *Xenopus* thymus tumor cells. *Devel Immunol* 1998;**5**:333–48.

Horton TL, Minter R, Stewart R, *et al.* *Xenopus* NK cells identified by novel monoclonal antibodies. *Eur J Immunol* 2000;**30**: in press.

Humphreys T, Reinherz EL. Invertebrate immune recognition, natural immunity and the evolution of positive selection. *Immunol Today* 1994;**15**:316–20.

Kasahara M (ed). *Major Histocompatibility Complex: Evolution, Structure and Function.* London: Springer-Verlag, 2000

Lackie AM (ed). *Immune Mechanisms in Invertebrate Vectors. Zoological Society of London Symposia,* Vol 56. Oxford: Oxford University Press, 1986.

Marsh J, Goode JA (eds). *Antimicrobial Peptides. Ciba Foundation Symposium.* Chichester: Wiley 1995:186.

Parham P (ed). Immune systems of ectothermic vertebrates. *Immunol Rev* 1998;**166**:5–384.

Pastoret P, Griebel P, Bazin H, *et al.* (eds). *Handbook of Vertebrate Immunology.* London: Academic Press, 1998.

Raftos DA, Raison R (eds). *Developmental and Comparative Immunology.* Oxford: Pergamon Press 2000;**24**:S1–S105, Proceedings of the 8th Congress of Developmental and Comparative Immunology.

Rast JP, Anderson MK, Strong SJ, *et al.* α,β,γ, and δ T cell antigen receptor genes arose early in vertebrate phylogeny. *Immunity* 1997;**6**:1–11.

Ratcliffe NA, Rowley AF (eds). *Invertebrate Blood Cells,* Vols 1, 2. London: Academic Press, 1981.

Ratcliffe NA, Rowley AF, Fitzgerald SW, *et al.* Invertebrate immunity: basic concepts and recent advances. *Int Rev Cytol* 1985;**97**:183–350.

Robert J, Cohen N. Evolution of immune surveillance and tumor immunity: studies in *Xenopus. Immunol Rev* 1998;**166**:231–43.

Robert J, Guiet C, Du Pasquier L. Lymphoid tumors of *Xenopus laevis* with different capacities for growth in larvae and adults. *Devel Immunol* 1994;**3**:297–307.

Rowley AF, Ratcliffe NA (eds). *Vertebrate Blood Cells.* Cambridge: Cambridge University Press, 1988.

Schluter SF, Bernstein RM, Marchalonis JJ. Molecular origins and evolution of immunoglobulin heavy-chain genes of jawed vertebrates. *Immunol Today* 1997;**18**:543–9.

Secombes CJ. The phylogeny of cytokines. In: Thomson AW (ed). *The Cytokine Handbook.* London: Academic Press; 1991:387–412.

Soderhall K (ed). Invertebrate Immunity. *Devel Comp Immunol* 1999;**23**:263–442.

Soderhall K, Iwanga S, Vasta GR (eds). *New Directions in Invertebrate Immunology.* Fair Haven: SOS Publications; 1996:1–494.

Stolen JS, Fletcher TC, Bayne CJ (eds). *Modulators of Immune Responses, The Evolutionary Trail.* Fair Haven: SOS Publications; 1996:1–600.

Turner RJ (ed). *Immunology: A Comparative Approach.* Chichester: Wiley, 1994.

Turpen JB. Induction and early development of the haemopoietic and immune sytems in *Xenopus. Devel Comp Immunol* 1998;**22**:265–78.

Warr G. The immunoglobulin genes of fish. *Devel Comp Immunol* 1995;**19**:1–12.

14 Immunity to viruses

- **Viruses are obligate intracellular parasites.** They vary in their complexity and replication strategies. Some produce acute infection and are eliminated from the host, whereas others persist indefinitely producing late disease.
- **Innate immune mechanisms** restrict the early stages of infection and delay spread of virus. These defences include interferon and NK cells.
- **Antibody restricts the spread of virus** to neighbouring cells and tissues by neutralizing virus infectivity. This is an important defence mechanism in preventing reinfection.
- **Cytotoxic T cells** recognize virus infected cells. They are able to destroy infected cells early in the virus replication cycle before new viral progeny appear.
- **Viruses have evolved strategies to avoid recognition by the host.** These include latency, antigenic variation and the production of decoy proteins that interfere with the host's antiviral defences.
- **Viruses may directly disrupt the function of the immune system** by initiating immunosuppression and immunodeficiency disorders, and by triggering autoimmune disease.

MODES OF VIRUS INFECTION

Viruses are obligate intracellular parasites, and require the host cell's biochemical machinery to drive protein synthesis and metabolize sugars. They are extremely diverse in terms of their structure and genetic complexities – some have RNA genomes encoding only a few genes, and others have DNA genomes encoding up to 200 genes. Structurally, a virus is little more than a bag of protein and nucleic acid. However, life-forms even simpler than this have been identified:

- **Viroids** are infectious agents of plants which consist of nucleic acid alone, encoding no protein.
- **Prions** are essentially 'infectious proteins' associated with degenerative neurological diseases of animals and man, including scrapie, bovine spongiform encephalopathies (BSE) and Creutzfeldt–Jakob disease (CJD). The infectious prion proteins (PrPsc) are thought to catalyse changes in normal prion protein (PrPc), resulting in the formation of protein complexes in neurons called fibrils, leading to neuropathology.

A typical virus infection of a cell is shown in *Figure 14.1.* Viruses bind to host cells via specific receptors. This specificity identifies in part the tropism of a virus for a particular host or cell. Examples of cellular receptors used by viruses are shown in *Figure 14.2.* Following entry the virus uncoats, nucleic acid is released, and transcription occurs followed by the production of viral proteins. The viral genome is replicated and new 'progeny' virus particles (virions) are assembled and released to infect neighbouring cells and tissues. The details of this process depend on the particular virus and on the metabolic state of the host cell. For example, picornaviruses (small RNA viruses) take around

Infection and replication of viruses

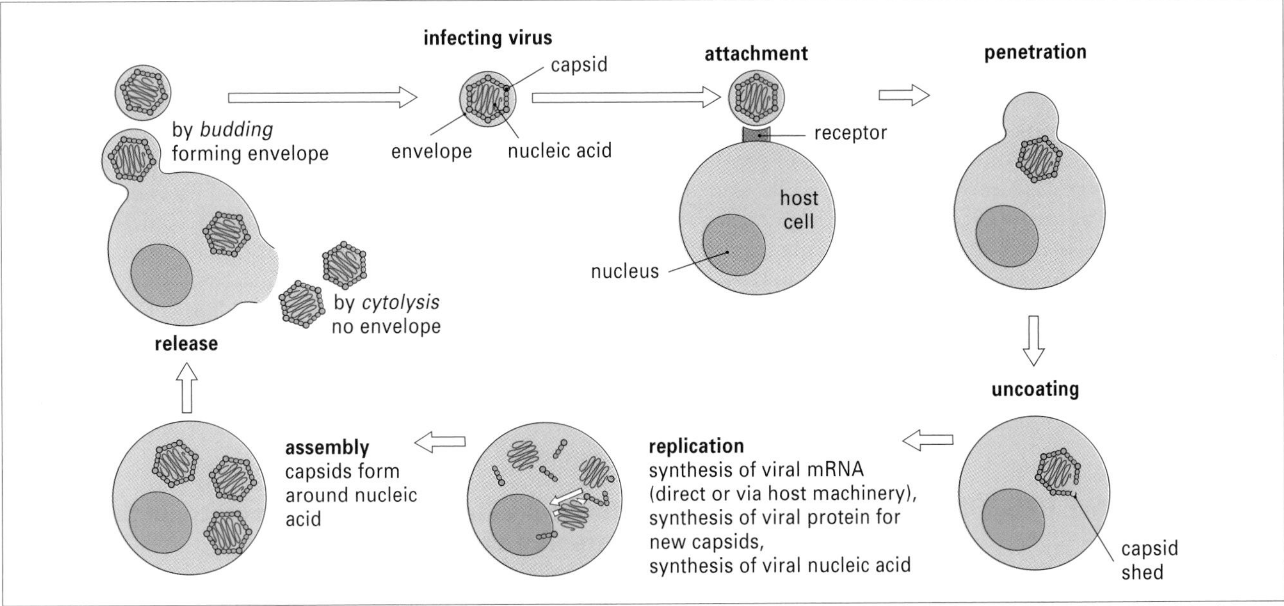

Fig. 14.1 Viruses must infect a host cell before they can replicate.

Virus receptors on host cells

virus	receptor	cell type infected
human immunodeficiency virus (HIV)	CD4	TH cells
Epstein–Barr virus	CR2 (complement receptor type 2)	B cells
influenza A virus	glycophorin A	many cell types
transmissible gastroenteritis virus	aminopeptidase N CD13	enterocytes
rhinovirus	ICAM-1	many cell types
polio virus	polio virus receptor (immunoglobulin superfamily)	neurons
measles virus	CD46	many cell types
human herpes virus 6	CD46	many cell types

Fig. 14.2 Viruses attach to cells via specific receptors and this partly determines which cell types become infected.

8 hours to produce new virions, whereas human cytomegalovirus (a DNA virus) may take up to 48 hours.

Viruses are extremely diverse in their ability to infect, persist and initiate disease in a host. Entry is commonly at mucosal surfaces; puncturing skin (e.g. by insect bites or needles) is another very efficient means of introducing virus directly into the blood stream. Replication usually occurs at epithelial surfaces, followed in some cases by viraemia (blood-borne spread) to infect other tissues. Recovery from the infection can involve the elimination of the virus from the host. Some viruses however (e.g. herpes virus) persist in a latent (non-infectious) form after the acute infection is resolved, and can reactivate to produce new infectious virions. Other viruses can persist in an infectious form despite the presence of the immune response (e.g. hepatitis B virus and lymphocytic choriomeningitis virus). In scrapie and CJD there is no acute stage; these agents persist as a slow infection, producing disease after many years. Unlike viruses, prions do not provoke an immune response nor is interferon produced following infection. However, dendritic cells can be infected by these agents and constitute an important step in the pathogenesis of infection, by transporting the agents from tissue sites (e.g. gut, skin) to the lymphoid system, where an amplification of prions takes place. Therefore, through subsequent lymphocyte trafficking, the lymphoid system serves to aid in the transmission of the agent to the nervous system. A summary of the different forms of infection is shown in *Figure 14.3.*

Different types of virus infection

initial infection	consequences	example
acute	recovery and elimination of virus	influenza virus, rotavirus
acute	latency (non-infectious virus); on reactivation, new viruses are shed	varicella zoster virus, herpes simplex virus
acute	persistence with continuance or intermittent shedding	hepatitis B virus, Epstein–Barr virus
not acute	persistent slow infection	Creutzfeldt–Jakob disease, scrapie

Fig. 14.3 Virus infections can be acute or non-acute, and produce a variety of consequences.

INNATE IMMUNE RESPONSE TO VIRUSES

The early stage of an infection is often a race between the virus and the host's defence system. The initial defence against virus invasion is the integrity of the body surface. Once breached, early 'non-specific' or innate immune defences such as interferon, natural killer (NK) cells and macrophages become active.

Interferon (IFN) stimulates inhibition of viral replication

There are three types of interferon:

- IFNα (leucocyte interferon) is encoded by a family of some 20 genes on chromosome 9.
- IFNβ (fibroblast interferon) is encoded by a single gene on chromosome 9.
- IFNγ (immune interferon) is encoded by a single gene on chromosome 12.

Virus infection of a cell leads to the production of IFNα/β, which activates antiviral mechanisms in neighbouring cells enabling them to resist virus infection (*Fig. 14.4*). Interferons activate a number of genes, including two with direct antiviral activity: a 67 kDa protein kinase which inhibits the phosphorylation of eIF-2 and blocks translation of proteins; and a 2′,5′-oligoadenylate synthetase which activates a latent endonuclease (RNaseL) involved in degrading viral RNA.

Other antiviral mechanisms exist which have a more specific action. The Mx proteins inhibit viral transcription of a range of RNA viruses, but have little effect on DNA viruses. In addition to the direct inhibition of virus replication, IFNγ and IFNα/β enhance the efficiency of the adaptive immune response by stimulating increased expression of MHC class I and II, and both these interferons serve to activate macrophages and NK cells, promoting their antiviral activity (see below).

The importance of interferons *in vivo* is underlined by the increased susceptibility of mice to virus infection following the depletion of interferons by specific antibody treatment.

Natural killer (NK) cells are cytotoxic for virally infected cells

Active NK cells are detected within 2 days of a virus infection. They have been identified as major effector cells against herpes viruses, and, in particular, cytomegalovirus (CMV). An absence or reduction of NK cell activity,

The molecular basis of interferon action

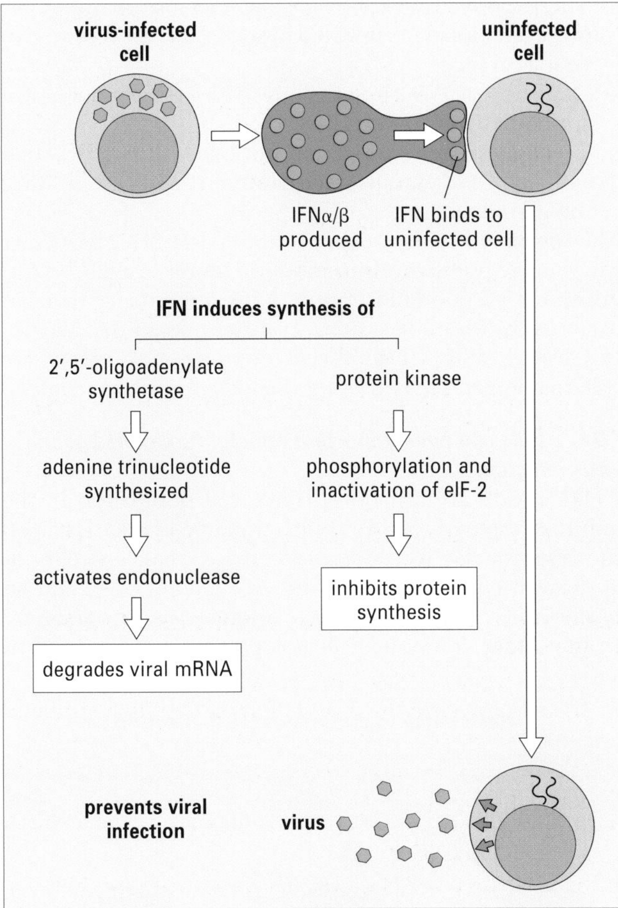

Fig. 14.4 The antiviral state develops within a few hours of interferon stimulation and lasts for 1–2 days.

as seen in Chediak–Higashi syndrome and beige mutant mice, correlates with an increased susceptibility to CMV infection. It is still unclear which molecules the NK cells recognize on the surface of virus infected cells. However, there is an inverse correlation between MHC class I expression and NK cell killing. This is an interesting feature since a number of viruses are now known to downregulate MHC class I expression; this is presumably a strategy to evade T-cell recognition. Interferon-γ activates NK cell function and provides an important mechanism for focusing and activating cells at sites of infection. NK cells are also one of the main mediators of antibody-dependent cellular cytotoxicity (ADCC).

HOST DEFENCE INVOLVING B AND T CELLS

An absence of T cells renders the host highly susceptible to virus attack. For example, cutaneous infection of congenital athymic 'nude' mice (which lack mature T cells) with herpes simplex virus (HSV) results in a spreading lesion; the virus eventually travels to the central nervous system, resulting in the death of the animal. The transfer of HSV-specific T cells shortly after infection is sufficient to protect the mice. The significance of T and B cells countering viral infections will now be discussed.

Antibodies and complement can limit viral spread or reinfection

Antibodies can neutralize the infectivity of viruses

As the infection proceeds, the adaptive (specific) immune response unfolds, with the appearance of cytotoxic T cells, helper T cells and antiviral antibodies. Antibodies provide a major barrier to virus spread between cells and tissues and are particularly important in restricting virus spread in the blood stream. IgA production becomes focused at mucosal surfaces where it serves to prevent reinfection.

Antibodies may be generated against any viral protein in the infected cell, although only those directed against glycoproteins that are expressed on the virion envelope or on the infected cell membrane are of importance in controlling infection. Antibody-mediated immunity can be achieved in a number of ways, involving quite diverse mechanisms.

Defence against free virus particles involves neutralization of infectivity, which can occur in various ways (*Fig. 14.5*). Such mechanisms are likely to operate *in vivo*, since injection of neutralizing monoclonal antibodies is highly effective at inhibiting virus replication. Clearly the presence of circulating virus-neutralizing antibodies is an important factor in the prevention of reinfection.

Complement is involved in the neutralization of some free viruses

Complement can also damage the virion envelope, a process known as virolysis. Some viruses can directly activate the classical and alternative complement pathways. However, complement is not considered to be a major factor in the defence against viruses since individuals with complement deficiencies are not predisposed to severe viral infection.

Antiviral effects of antibody

target	agent	mechanism
free virus	antibody alone	blocks binding to cell blocks entry into cell blocks uncoating of virus
	antibody + complement	damage to virus envelope blockade of virus receptor
virus-infected cells	antibody + complement	lysis of infected cell opsonization of coated virus or infected cells for phagocytosis
	antibody bound to infected cells	antibody-dependent cellular cytotoxicity by NK cells, macrophages and neutrophils

Fig. 14.5 Antibody acts to neutralize virus or kill virally infected cells.

Antibodies mobilize complement and/or effector cells to destroy virus-infected cells

Antibodies are also effective in mediating the destruction of virus-infected cells. This can occur by antibody-mediated activation of the complement system, leading to the assembly of the membrane attack complex and lysis of the infected cell (see Chapter 3). This process requires a high density of viral antigens on the membrane (about 5×10^6/cell) to be effective. In contrast, ADCC mediated by NK cells can recognize as few as 10^3 IgG molecules in order to bind and kill the infected cell. The IgG coated cells are bound using the FcγRIII (CD16), and are rapidly destroyed by a perforin-dependent killing mechanism (see Chapter 10). Just how important these mechanisms are *in vivo* is difficult to resolve. The best evidence in favour of ADCC comes from studying the protective effect of non-neutralizing monoclonal antibodies in mice. Although these antibodies fail to neutralize virus *in vitro*, they can protect C5-deficient mice from a high-dose virus challenge. (C5-deficient mice are used in this study to eliminate the role of the late complement components.)

T cells mediate viral immunity in several ways

T cells exhibit a variety of functions in antiviral immunity. Most of the antibody response is thymus dependent, requiring the presence of $CD4^+$ T cells for class switching and affinity maturation. $CD4^+$ T cells also help in the induction of $CD8^+$ cytotoxic T cells and in the recruitment and activation of macrophages at sites of virus infection. CD8 T cells are also effective in prevention of re-infection (following vaccination) by viruses such as influenza virus and respiratory syncytial virus. However, even memory T cells need time to evolve a response to a re-infecting virus, and therefore antibodies assume a more dominant role by neutralizing incoming virus and containing the infection by preventing spread to other tissues (see above).

$CD8^+$ cytotoxic T cells

The principal T-cell surveillance system operating against viruses is highly efficient and selective. MHC class I restricted, cytotoxic $CD8^+$ T cells focus at the site of virus replication and destroy virus-infected cells. Virtually all cells in the body express MHC class I molecules, making this an important mechanism for identifying and eliminating virus-infected cells.

Processing and presentation of virus proteins

Virtually any viral protein can be processed in the cytoplasm to generate peptides, which are then transported to the endoplasmic reticulum and are associated with MHC class I molecules. This has particular advantages for the host, since viral proteins expressed early in the replication cycle can be targeted, enabling T-cell recognition to occur long before new viral progeny are produced. For example, T-cell-mediated immunity against murine CMV is mediated by immediate early protein pp89. The epitope has been identified as a nonamer peptide presented by the MHC class I molecule L^d. Immunization of mice with a recombinant vaccinia containing pp89 is sufficient to confer complete protection from murine CMV-induced disease; deletion of the DNA sequence encoding the nonapeptide abolishes the protective effect of the protein.

The importance of T-cell mechanisms *in vivo* have been identified using various techniques:

- The adoptive transfer of specific T-cell subpopulations or T-cell clones to infected animals and monitoring of viral clearance.
- Depletion of T-cell populations *in vivo* using monoclonal antibodies to CD4 or CD8.
- Creation of 'gene knockout' mice, in which genes such as CD4, CD8, and β_2 microglobulin are removed from the germline.

The continued ability of knockout mice that lack particular lymphocyte populations to mount a response against virus infections is a good illustration of the redundancy that can occur in the immune system. For example, in the absence of $CD8^+$ T cells, $CD4^+$ T cells or other mechanisms are able to compensate and bring the infection under control.

$CD4^+$ T cells can have important effector functions against virus infections

$CD4^+$ T cells are a major effector cell population in the immune response to HSV-1 infection of epithelial surfaces. In this instance recruitment of macrophages occurs as in delayed-type hypersensitivity (see Chapter 24) and an accelerated clearance of virus results. Macrophages are an important component in this process, inhibiting virus

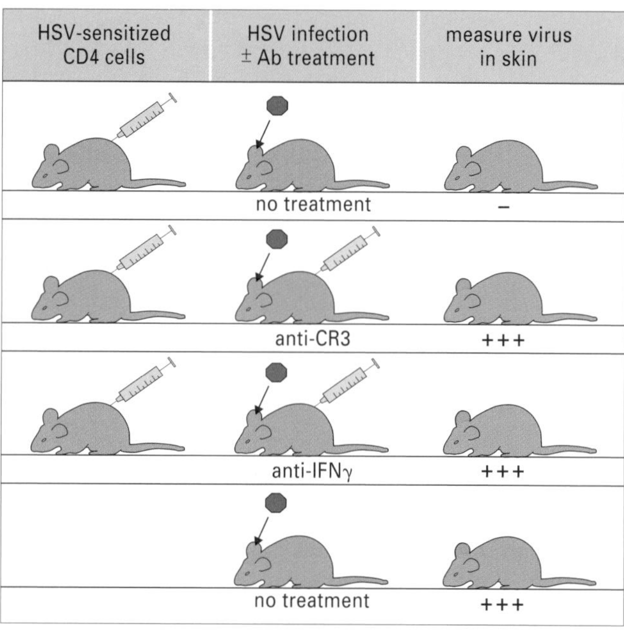

Fig. 14.6 $CD4^+$ T cells, macrophages and IFNγ all have a protective role in cutaneous infections with HSV. $CD4^+$ T cells were obtained from mice infected with HSV 8 days previously. The cells were transferred to syngeneic mice infected with HSV in the skin. These mice were treated with anti-CR3 (to block macrophage migration to the site of infection), or anti-IFNγ (to block the activation of macrophages) or were untreated. An additional control group was infected but did not receive $CD4^+$ T cells. The amount of infectious virus remaining after 5 days was then determined. The results demonstrate that the protective effects of $CD4^+$ T cells are mediated by macrophages and IFNγ.

infection probably through the generation and action of nitric oxide (*Fig. 14.6*). Key cytokines in this response include IFNγ, important in the activation of monocytes, and tumour necrosis factor (TNFα). TNFα has several antiviral activities, including the induction of intracellular interferon defence mechanisms and apoptotic cell death following interaction with the apoptotic TNF receptor.

$CD4^+$ cytotoxic T cells

In measles virus infection, cytotoxic $CD4^+$ T cells are generated which recognize and kill MHC class II positive cells infected with the virus. This suggests that measles virus peptides are generated by normal pathways of antigen presentation (i.e. following phagocytosis and degradation – see Chapter 6). However, other pathways have been implicated in which some measles proteins/peptides enter class II vesicles from the cytosol by an unknown mechanism.

A summary of antiviral defence mechanisms is illustrated in *Figure 14.7*, and the kinetics of their induction is shown in *Figure 14.8*.

STRATEGIES FOR EVADING IMMUNE DEFENCES

Viruses have evolved various strategies to evade recognition by antibody and T cells. Antigenic variation is the most effective ploy. It involves mutating regions on proteins that are normally targeted by antibody and T cells. Antigenic variation is seen in HIV and in foot and mouth disease virus, and is responsible for the antigenic shift and drift seen with influenza virus (*Fig. 14.9*). Humoral immunity to such diseases lasts only until the new virus strain emerges, making effective, long-lasting vaccinations difficult to produce. In HIV infection, sequence changes (mutations) can arise in those viral peptides that bind to MHC class I molecules to which the initial T-cell response arose. This results in a failure of T-cell surveillance and the emergence of new pathogenic variant viruses.

Antibody can remove viral antigens from the plasma membrane by capping. This may possibly be a mechanism for forcing some viruses into a persistent intracellular infection. The herpesviruses (HSV and human CMV) encode glycoproteins with IgG-Fc receptor binding activity. This viral strategy could interfere with complement activation and block the action of antiviral antibodies.

Some viruses (e.g. Epstein–Barr virus and adenovirus) produce their own defences against the actions of interferon, synthesizing short stretches of RNA that compete for the protein kinase and somehow inhibit the activation of the enzyme. Other viruses (e.g. adenovirus and CMV) encode proteins that are able to inhibit the transport of MHC class I molecules to the cell membrane. This strategy can give the virus a distinct advantage, helping it to avoid cytotoxic T-cell recognition. However, as indicated above, a loss of MHC class I expression favours NK cell recognition and killing. Both human and mouse cytomegalovirus can counter this deficiency of MHC class I expression by producing their own version of the MHC class I molecule on the infected cell membrane, thereby thwarting the attentions of NK cells.

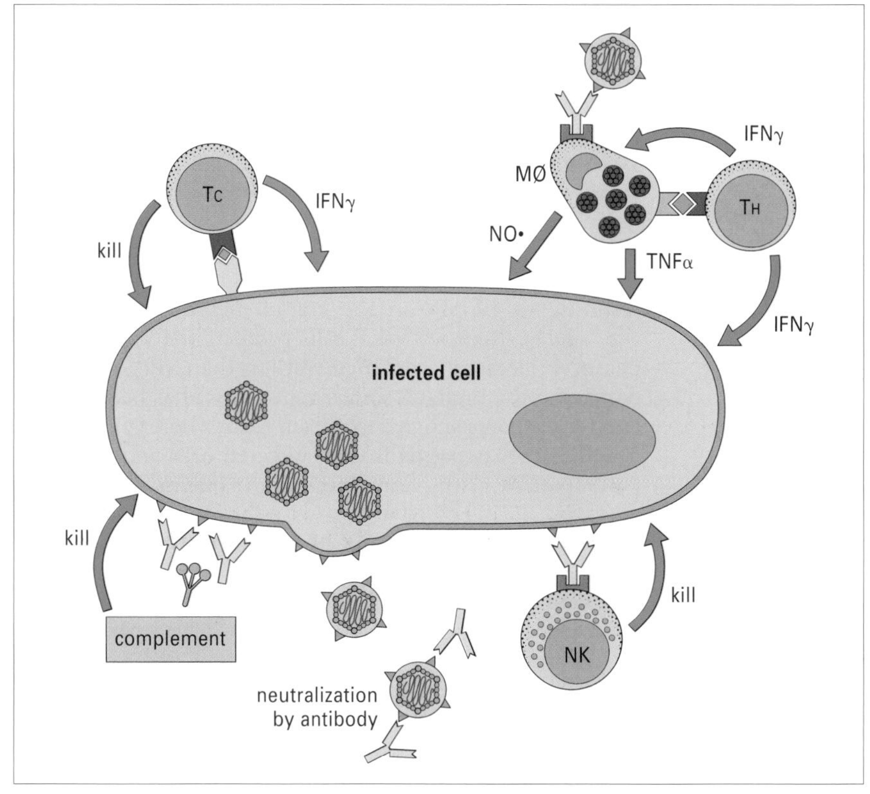

Fig. 14.7 Entry of virus at mucosal surfaces is inhibited by IgA. Following the initial infection, the virus may spread to other tissues via the blood stream. Interferons produced by the innate (IFNα and IFNβ) and adaptive (IFNγ) immune responses make neighbouring cells resistant to infection by spreading virus. Antibodies are important in controlling free virus, whereas T cells and NK cells are effective at killing infected cells.

Response to a typical acute virus infection

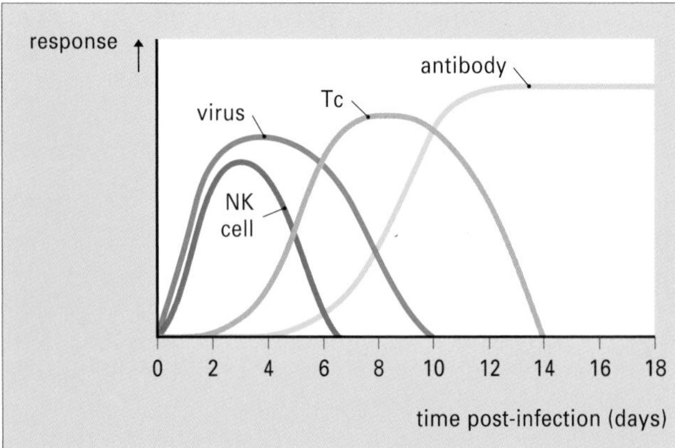

Fig. 14.8 Kinetics of host defences in response to a typical acute virus infection. Following an acute virus infection, for example by influenza or herpes virus, NK cells and interferon are detected in the blood stream and locally in infected tissues. Cytotoxic T cells (Tc) then become activated in local lymph nodes or spleen, followed by the appearance of serum in neutralizing antibodies. Although activated T cells are absent by the second to third week, T-cell memory is established and lasts for many years.

Antigenic shift and drift in influenza virus

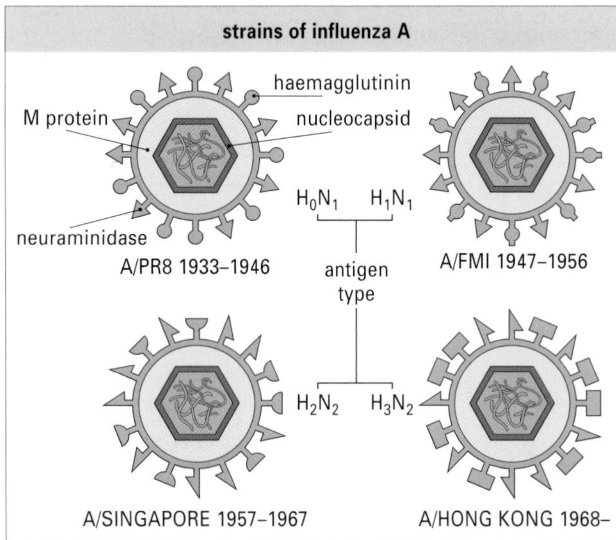

Fig. 14.9 The major surface antigens of influenza virus are haemagglutinin and neuraminidase. Haemagglutinin is involved in attachment to cells, and antibodies to haemagglutinin are protective. Antibodies to neuraminidase are much less effective. The influenza virus can change its surface slightly (antigenic drift) or radically (antigenic shift). Alterations in the structure of the haemagglutinin antigen render earlier antibodies ineffective and thus new virus epidemics break out. The diagram shows strains that have emerged by antigenic shift since 1933. The official influenza antigen nomenclature is based on the type of haemagglutinin (H_0, H_1 etc.) and neuraminidase (N_1, N_2 etc.) expressed on the surface of the virion. Note that although new strains replace old strains, the internal antigens remain unchanged.

Some virus genes encode homologues of cytokine receptors or even cytokines. Soluble forms of the IL-1β, TNF and IFNγ receptors are secreted from poxvirus-infected cells and may subvert local cytokine activity. Poxviruses and murine gammaherpesvirus also secrete novel chemokine binding proteins, which are thought to interfere with the recruitment of inflammatory cells to sites of infection. Epstein–Barr virus encodes an IL-10 homologue which mimics mammalian IL-10 activity *in vitro* and Kaposi's sarcoma herpesvirus (KSHV) encodes viral equivalents of IL-6, MIP-1α and MIP-1β. The full significance of these virus gene products *in vivo* has still to be elucidated.

Examples of virus encoded homologues of the host defence system are shown in *Figure 14.10.*

IMMUNOPATHOLOGY

Responses to viral antigens can cause tissue damage

Damage due to the formation of immune complexes

Immune complexes may arise in body fluids or on cell surfaces and are most common during persistent or chronic infections, for example with LCMV or hepatitis B virus. Antibody is ineffective (non-neutralizing) in the presence of large amounts of the viral antigen; instead, immune complexes form and are deposited in the kidney or in blood vessels, where they evoke inflammatory responses leading to tissue damage, for example as glomerulonephritis (see Chapter 23).

An unusual pathological consequence of some virus non-neutralizing antibody interactions is the Fc receptor-mediated uptake of the complex by macrophages and subsequent enhancement of virus infectivity. This is seen in Dengue virus infection and is implicated as the underlying mechanism of Dengue haemorrhagic fever and Dengue shock syndrome, which involves hyperactivation of the complement system.

T-cell-mediated tissue damage

In any virus infection some tissue damage is likely to arise from the activity of T cells. However, in some situations this damage may be considerable, resulting in the death of the animal. The best example of this is the cytotoxic T-cell response to LCMV in the central nervous system (see *Fig. 14.11*). Removal of T cells protects the animal from death, indicating that they, rather than the virus, are damaging the brain. A similar mechanism has been postulated for chronic active hepatitis in man, whereby cytotoxic T cells target hepatitis B virus infected cells and may also participate in a non-viral autoimmune disease.

Viruses can infect cells of the immune system

Some viruses (e.g. HIV) directly infect lymphocytes or macrophages, resulting in pathogenic effects. Immunocompetent cells are also favoured sites of virus persistence. In the resting state, leucocytes harbour the virus in a non-infectious form; on activation of the infected cells, the virus may also be reactivated to produce infectious virus particles. Examples of viruses infecting B cells, T cells and macrophages are shown in *Figure 14.12.*

Examples of viral products that interfere with host defences

host defence affected	virus	virus product	mechanism
interferon	EBV	EBERS (small RNAs)	blocks protein kinase activation
	vaccinia	eIF-2α homologue	prevents phosphorylation of eIF-2α by protein kinase
complement	vaccinia	homologues of complement control proteins	blocks complement activation
	HSV-1	gE/gI	binds Fcγ and blocks function
cytokines	myxoma	IFNγ receptor homologue	competes for IFNγ, blocks function
	shope fibroma virus	TNF receptor homologue	competes for TNF, blocks function
	EBV	IL-10 homologue	reduces IFNγ function
MHC class I	murine cytomegalovirus	early protein	prevents transport of peptide-loaded MHC
	adenovirus	E3	blocks transport of MHC to surface

Fig. 14.10 Viruses use a great variety of ingenious strategies to outwit the host defences.

Lymphocytic choriomeningitis virus (LCM) in mice

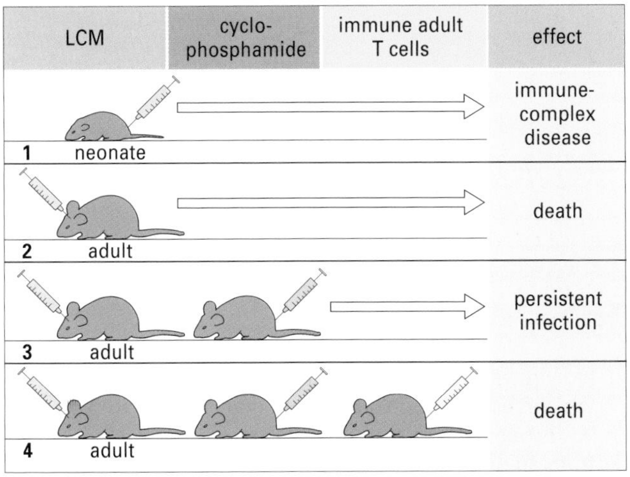

LCM	cyclo-phosphamide	immune adult T cells	effect
1 neonate			immune-complex disease
2 adult			death
3 adult			persistent infection
4 adult			death

Fig. 14.11 The different effects of LCMV are related to differences in immune status. Infection of neonatal mice (**1**) produces chronic virus shedding and immune-complex disease, manifesting itself as glomerulonephritis and vasculitis. Intracerebral infection of adult mice (**2**) results in death. This is due to a T-cell reaction, since suppression of immunity with cyclophosphamide (**3**) leads to persistent infection, but prevents death. This 'protective' effect produced by cyclophosphamide can be reversed by T cells from an immune animal (**4**).

Virus infection of immunocompetent cells

B lymphocytes	Epstein–Barr virus murine gamma herpes virus infectious bursal disease virus
T lymphocytes	human T-lymphotropic virus Types 1 and 2 HIV measles virus herpes virus Saimiri human herpesvirus 6
macrophages	Visna virus HIV lactate dehydrogenase virus cytomegalovirus

Fig. 14.12 Some viruses persist indefinitely in immunocompetent cells. Periodically, this infection may lead to pathological consequences, involving the death of the cell (HIV) or transformation leading to neoplasia (Epstein–Barr virus, HTLV–1).

Human immunodeficiency virus (HIV) infects CD4⁺ cells

Many of the points raised in previous sections are illustrated by HIV, the retrovirus that causes AIDS. Infection with HIV is characterized by prolonged clinical latency, ineffective immunity, continuous virus mutation, neuropathology, and a tendency to infect bone marrow-derived cells and lymphocytes (see Chapter 19).

HIV is taken up by T cells and macrophages following binding of a viral glycoprotein (gp120) to CD4 and certain chemokine receptors (CXCR4 and CCR5). It also enters other APCs by this route. However, entry into cells bearing Fc receptors can be enhanced by antibody, suggesting that this provides an alternative route into phagocytic cells, or enhances entry when CD4 is scarce.

There is a long but variable period of clinical latency; in about 50% of patients, progression to AIDS does not occur for 10 years. During this latent period, HIV can exist as a provirus, integrated within the host's genomic DNA, without any transcription occurring. Numerous factors can lead to the activation of transcription. *In vitro* both TNF and IL-6 cause increased production of infectious virus from latently infected T-cell lines. This may be important *in vivo*, because monocytes from individuals carrying HIV tend to release abnormally large quantities of these cytokines; it is possible that there is a cycle of TNF and IL-6 release, leading to enhanced virus transcription (*Fig. 14.13*). This could lead to infection of further cells, and release of more cytokine. Production is increased *in vitro* by other cytokines and lymphokines, and by mitogens and phorbol esters. Elimination of the virus does not occur for a variety of reasons, including latency, viral mutation (giving rapid antigenic drift) and progressive immunodeficiency.

Viral infection may provoke autoimmunity

Viruses may trigger autoimmune disease in a number of ways.

Virus induced damage – During the course of some virus infections tissues become damaged, provoking an inflammatory response during which 'hidden' antigens become exposed and can be processed and presented to the immune system. Examples of this include Theiler's virus (a murine picornavirus) and murine hepatitis virus infection of the nervous system, in which the constituents of myelin (the insulating material of axons) become targets for antibody and T cells.

Molecular mimicry – A sequence in a viral protein that is homologous to a 'self' protein can become recognized, leading to a breakdown in immunological tolerance to cryptic self antigens in the consequent attack on host tissues by the immune system (see Chapter 26). Although experimental systems can be contrived to illustrate this mechanism, there is currently little evidence to suggest that it operates in natural virus infection.

Infection of lymphocytes and macrophages by HIV

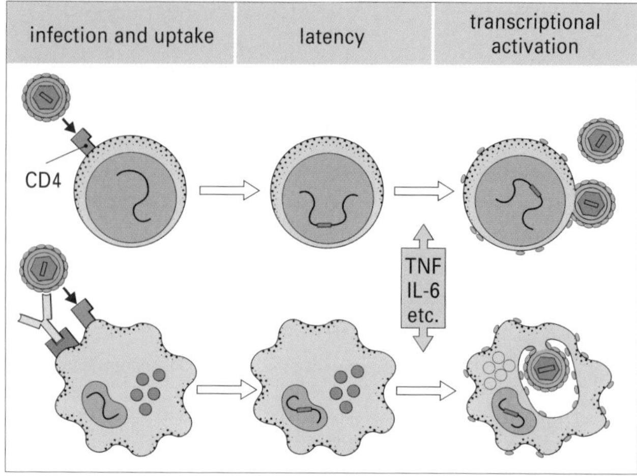

Fig. 14.13 The gp120 on the surface of HIV virions binds to CD4 and chemokine receptors on the lymphocyte membrane, and this triggers uptake. The virus can enter macrophages which express relatively low levels of CD4, but this may be assisted by binding through antibody to Fc receptors. The virus remains latent, integrated in the host cell's genomic DNA, until some stimulus (e.g. cytokines) causes transcriptional activation. Assembled viruses bud from the outer membrane of T cells, or into intracytoplasmic vacuoles of macrophages, where a large reservoir of potentially infectious particles can accumulate.

CRITICAL THINKING • Virus–immune system interactions (Explanations on p. 457)

14.1 What are the features of a virus that enable it to evade host defence mechanisms?

14.2 A series of IgG monoclonal antibodies were developed against glycoprotein D of herpes simplex virus. When tested *in vitro* for virus neutralizing activity the antibodies could be divided into two groups: those capable of neutralizing virus infectivity and non-neutralizing antibodies. However, when individual neutralizing or non-neutralizing antibodies were injected into mice infected with herpes simplex virus, both sets of antibodies protected the animals from an overwhelming infection.

i. How do you explain the protection achieved by the non-neutralizing monoclonal antibodies?
ii. What experiments would you propose to support some of your conclusions?

FURTHER READING

Biron CA, Nguyen KB, Pien GC, Cousens LP, Salazar-Mather TP. Natural killer cells in antiviral defence: function and regulation by innate cytokines. *Annu Rev Immunol* 1999;**17**:189–220.

Chisari FV, Ferrari C. Hepatitis B virus immunopathogenesis. *Annu Rev Immunol* 1995;**13**:29–60.

Clements JE, Gidovin SL, Montelaro RC, *et al.* Antigenic variation in lentiviral disease. *Annu Rev Immunol* 1988;**6**:139–59.

Dimmock NJ. Neutralization of animal viruses. *Curr Topics Microbiol Immunol* 1993;**183**:1–149.

Doherty PC, Allan W, Eichelberger M, *et al.* Roles of α/β and γ/δ T cell subsets in viral immunity. *Annu Rev Immunol* 1992;**10**:123–51.

Levy JA. Pathogenesis of human immunodeficiency virus infection. *Microbiol Rev* 1993;**57**:183–289.

McMichael A. How viruses hide from T cells. *Trends Microbiol* 1997;**5**:211–14.

McMichael A. HIV. *Curr Opin Immunol* 2000;**12**:367–86

Miller DM, Sedmak DD. Viral effects on antigen processing. *Curr Opin Immunol* 1999;**11**:94–9.

Mims CA. Interactions of viruses with the immune system. *Clin Exp Immunol* 1986;**66**:1–16.

Nash AA, Cambouropoulos P. The immune response to herpes simplex virus. *Semin Virol* 1993;**4**:181–6.

Oldstone MBA. Molecular mimicry and autoimmune disease. *Cell* 1987;**50**:819–20.

Ramsay AJ. A case for cytokines as effector molecules in the resolution of virus infection. *Immunol Today* 1993;**14**:155.

Smith GA. Virus strategies for evasion of the host response to infection. *Trends Microbiol* 1994;**2**:81–8.

Smith GA, Symons JA, Khanna A, Vanderplasschen A, Alcami A. Vaccinia virus immune evasion. *Immunol Rev* 1997;**159**:137–54.

Vilcek J, Sen GC. Interferons and other cytokines. In: Fields BN, Knipe DN, Hawley PM, *et al.* (eds) *Fields Virology*, 3rd edn. Philadelphia: Lippincott-Raven, 1996;375–99.

15 Immunity to bacteria and fungi

- **Mechanisms of protection** from a bacterial species can be deduced from the structure of the organism, particularly its cell wall, and its mode of pathogenicity.
- **Neutralizing antibody** may be all that is needed for protection if the organism is pathogenic only because of a single toxin or adhesion molecule.
- **Non-specific, phylogenetically ancient recognition pathways** for conserved bacterial structures, trigger phagocytosis, the alternative complement pathway and release of cytokines.
- **Complement** can kill some bacteria, particularly those with an exposed outer lipid bilayer such as Gram-negative bacteria.
- **Phagocytes kill the majority of bacteria** following a multistage process of chemotaxis, attachment, uptake and killing.
- **Successful pathogens** have evolved a startling diversity of mechanisms for avoiding the effects of complement, avoiding phagocyte function, or misdirecting the T-cell-dependent activation of phagocyte killing mechanisms.
- **Excessive release of cytokines** caused by microorganisms can result in immunopathological syndromes, such as endotoxin shock and the Shwartzman reaction.
- **Chronic tissue-damaging immunopathology** (as in tuberculosis) probably results from an imbalance of cytokine release patterns, leading to inappropriate effector functions.
- **Immunity to fungi** is poorly understood but is apparently cell-mediated and similar to immunity to bacteria.

IMMUNITY TO BACTERIA

The defence mechanisms appropriate for a particular bacterial infection are related to the structure of the invading bacteria, and hence the immunological mechanisms to which they are susceptible, and to the mechanism of their pathogenicity.

Mechanisms of immunity are related to bacterial surface structure

There are four main types of bacterial cell wall (*Fig. 15.1*) belonging to the following groups.

- Gram-positive bacteria.
- Gram-negative bacteria.
- Mycobacteria.
- Spirochaetes.

The outer lipid bilayer of Gram-negative organisms is of particular importance because it is often susceptible to mechanisms that can lyse membranes, such as complement and certain cytotoxic cells. In contrast, killing of the other types of bacteria usually requires uptake by phagocytes.

The outer surface of the bacterium may also contain fimbriae or flagellae, or it may be covered by a protective capsule. These can impede the functions of phagocytes or complement, but they also act as targets for the antibody response, the role of which is discussed later (see p. 253).

Mechanisms of immunity are related to bacterial mechanisms of pathogenicity

The two extreme patterns of pathogenicity are:

- Toxicity without invasiveness.
- Invasiveness without toxicity (*Fig. 15.2*).

However, most bacteria are intermediate between these extremes, having some invasiveness assisted by some locally acting toxins and spreading factors (tissue-degrading enzymes).

Corynebacterium diphtheriae and *Vibrio cholerae* are examples of organisms that are toxic but not invasive. Since their pathogenicity depends almost entirely on toxin production, neutralizing antibody to the toxin is probably sufficient for immunity, although antibody, binding to the bacteria and so blocking their adhesion to the epithelium, could also be important.

In contrast, however, the pathogenicity of most invasive organisms does not rely so heavily on a single toxin, so immunity requires killing of the organisms themselves.

The first lines of defence are antibacterial mechanisms that do not depend on antigen recognition

The body's first line of defence against pathogenic bacteria consists of simple barriers to the entry or establishment of the infection. Thus, the skin and exposed epithelial surfaces have non-specific or innate protective systems which limit the entry of potentially invasive organisms (see *Fig. 1.1*). Intact skin is impenetrable to most bacteria. Additionally, fatty acids produced by the skin are toxic to many organisms. Indeed, the pathogenicity of some strains correlates with their ability to survive on the skin. Epithelial surfaces are cleansed, for example, by ciliary action in the trachea or by flushing of the urinary tract. Many bacteria are destroyed by pH changes in the stomach and vagina, both of which provide an acidic environment. In the vagina, the epithelium secretes glycogen, which is metabolized by particular species of commensal bacteria, producing lactic acid. More generally, commensals can limit pathogen invasion through production of anti-bacterial proteins termed colicins. Thus commensals may occupy an ecological niche that would otherwise be occupied by something more unpleasant. When the normal flora are disturbed by antibiotics, infections by *Candida* or *Clostridium difficile* can occur, and the latter is a major cause of antibiotic-induced colitis and diarrhoea. Several

Bacterial cell walls

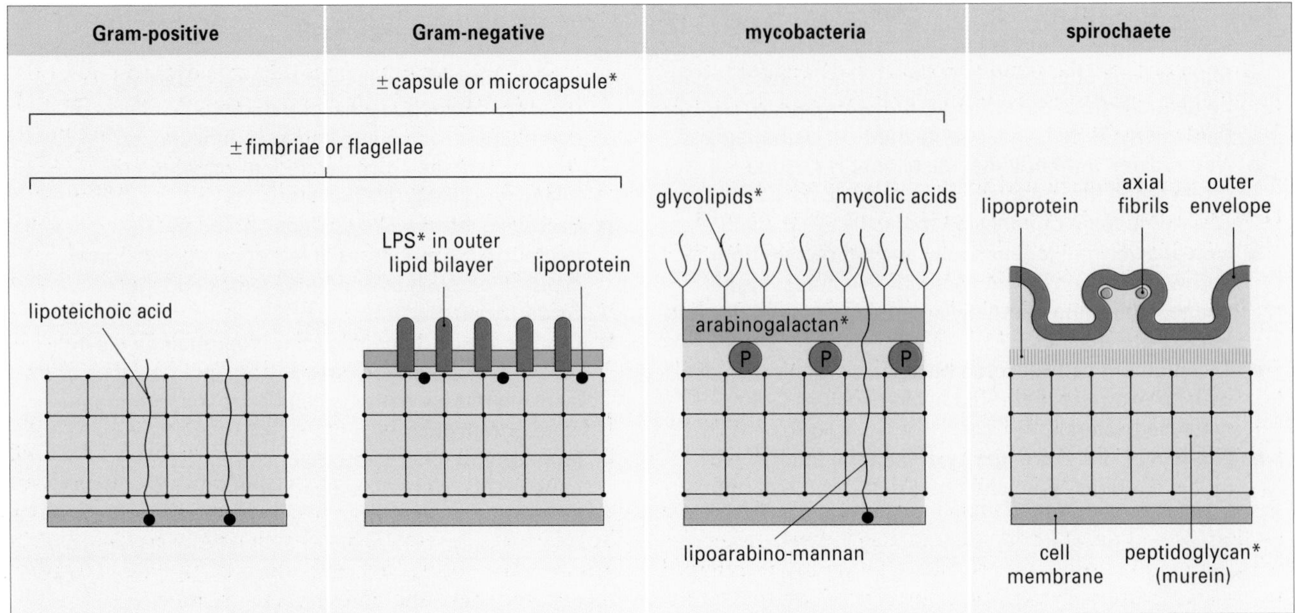

Fig. 15.1 Different immunological mechanisms have evolved to destroy the cell-wall structure of the different groups of bacteria. All types have an inner cell membrane and a peptidoglycan wall. Gram-negative bacteria also have an outer lipid bilayer in which lipopolysaccharide (LPS) is embedded. Lysosomal enzymes and lysozyme are active against the peptidoglycan layer, while cationic proteins and complement are effective against the outer lipid bilayer of the Gram-negative bacteria. The compound cell wall of mycobacteria is extremely resistant to breakdown, and it is likely that this can only be achieved with the assistance of the bacterial enzymes working from within. Some bacteria also have fimbriae or flagellae, which can provide targets for the antibody response. Others have an outer capsule which renders the organisms more resistant to phagocytosis, or to complement. The components indicated with an asterisk (*) all have adjuvant properties; that is, they are recognized by the immune system as a non-specific 'danger' signal that selectively boosts some aspects of immune activity. (Gram-staining is a method which exploits the fact that crystal violet and iodine form a complex which is more abundant on Gram-positive bacteria. The complex easily elutes from Gram-negative bacteria.)

Mechanisms of immunopathogenicity

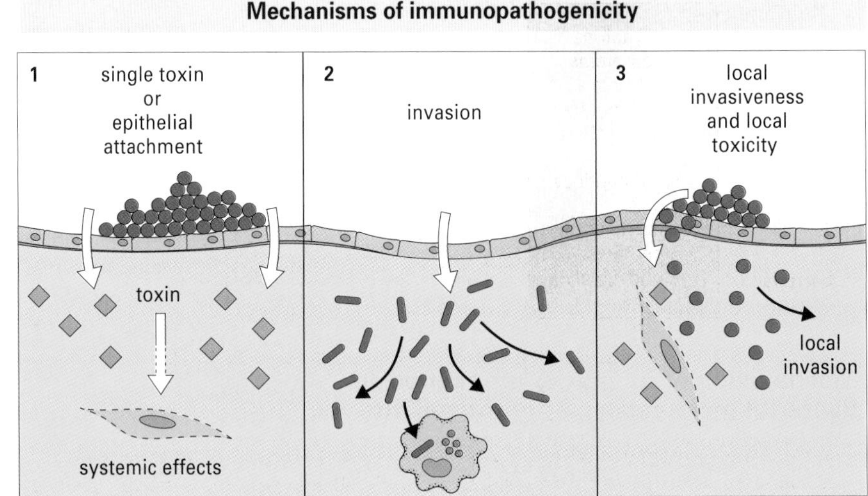

Fig. 15.2 (**1**) Some bacteria cause disease only because of a single toxin (e.g. *Corynebacterium diphtheriae, Clostridium tetani*) or because of an ability to attach to epithelial surfaces, without invading the host's tissues (e.g. in group A streptococcal sore throat). Immunity to such organisms may require only antibody to neutralize this critical function. (**2**) At the other extreme there are organisms which are not toxic, and cause disease by invasion of tissues and sometimes cells, where damage results mostly from the bulk of organisms, or from immunopathology (e.g. lepromatous leprosy). Where organisms invade cells, they must be destroyed and degraded by the cell-mediated immune response. (**3**) Most organisms fall between the two extremes, with some local invasiveness assisted by local toxicity and enzymes which degrade extracellular matrix (e.g. *Staphylococcus aureus, Clostridium perfringens*). Antibody and cell-mediated responses are both involved in resistance.

studies suggest that the re-introduction of non-pathogenic 'probiotic' organisms such as lactobacilli into the intestinal tract can alleviate the symptoms, presumably by replacing those killed by the antibiotics.

In practice, only a minute proportion of the potentially pathogenic organisms around us ever succeed in gaining access to the tissues.

The second line of defence is mediated via recognition of common bacterial components

If the organisms do enter the tissues, they can be combated initially by further elements of the innate immune system. Numerous bacterial components are recognized in ways which do not rely on the antigen-specific receptors of either B cells or T cells. These types of recognition are phylogenetically ancient 'broad-spectrum' mechanisms that evolved before antigen-specific T cells and immunoglobulins, allowing protective responses to be triggered by common microbial components bearing so-called 'pathogen-associated molecular patterns' (PAMPs) such as lipopolysaccharide and mannan. The host molecules which recognize these microbial components are referred to as the 'pattern recognition molecules' of the innate immune system. Many organisms, such as non-pathogenic cocci, are probably removed from the tissues as a consequence of these pathways, without the need for a specific adaptive immune reaction. *Figure 15.3* shows some of the microbial components involved, and the host responses which are triggered. It is interesting to note that the 'Limulus assay', which is used to detect contaminating lipopolysaccharide (LPS) in preparations for use in humans is based on one such recognition pathway found in an invertebrate species. In *Limulus polyphemus* (the horseshoe crab), tiny quantities of LPS trigger formation of fibrin which walls off the LPS-bearing infectious agent. Many bacterial PAMPs activate cells via Toll-like receptors (TLR). These are homologues of a receptor mediating antifungal immune responses in the fruit fly *Drosophila*.

Mechanism of action of LPS – There is a complex pathway that neutralizes LPS, and also passes it on to cell-membrane-associated receptors on leucocytes and probably endothelial cells so that appropriate effector functions can be activated. These events are illustrated in *Figure 15.4.* Some other conserved microbial components may be recognized and handled in a similar manner.

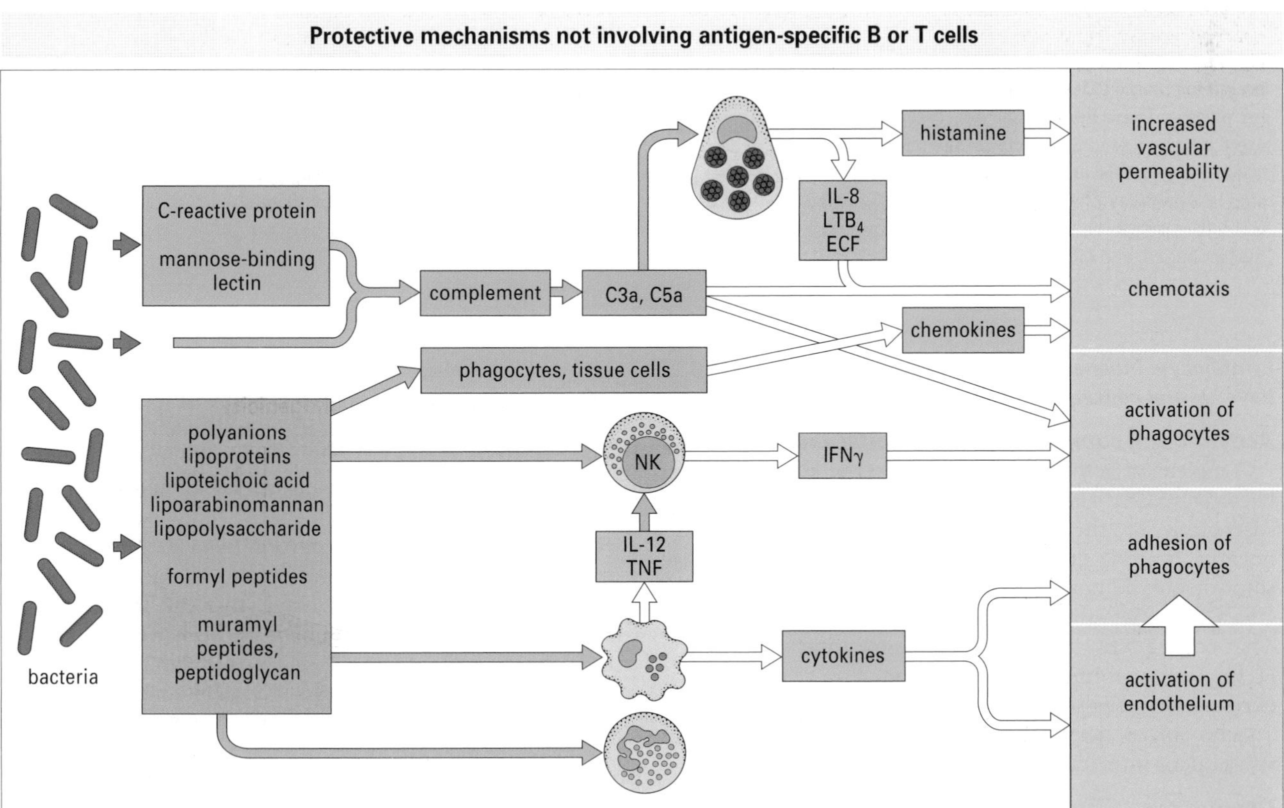

Fig. 15.3 Several common bacterial PAMPs are recognized by molecules present in serum, and by receptors on cells. These recognition pathways result in activation of the alternative complement pathway (Factors C3, B, D, P), with consequent release of C3a and C5a; activation of neutrophils, macrophages and NK cells; triggering of cytokine and chemokine release; mast-cell degranulation, leading to increased blood flow in the local capillary network; increased adhesion of cells and fibrin to endothelial cells. These mechanisms, plus tissue injury caused by the bacteria, may activate the clotting system and fibrin formation, which limit bacterial spread.

Effects of LPS

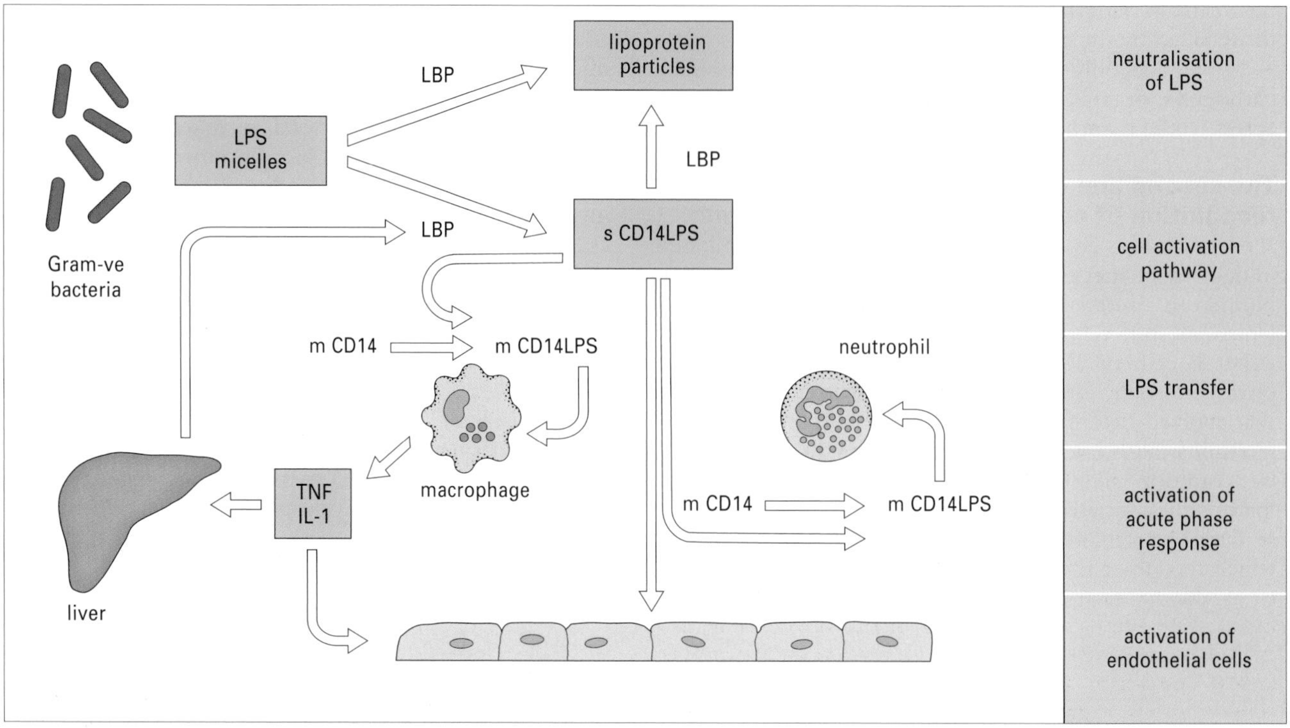

Fig. 15.4 LPS released from Gram-negative bacteria becomes bound to soluble CD14 (sCD14) and to lipoprotein particles in the plasma. These interactions are catalysed by a lipid transfer protein known as LPS-binding protein, or LBP. Binding to the lipoprotein particle neutralizes LPS, but binding to sCD14 is a step in a pathway of cell activation. Thus CD14 also exists as a GPI-linked membrane protein (mCD14) on neutrophils and macrophages, and LPS is transferred from the sCD14–LPS complex to this membrane-bound form. Then the mCD14–LPS complex, in association with other membrane-bound factors such as the Toll-like receptor 2 (TLR2) transduces signals that cause increased expression of integrins (adhesion molecules) and increased release of TNFα and IL-1. These in turn activate endothelial cells and drive the acute phase response in the liver. One product of the acute phase response is further LBP.

Lymphocyte-independent bacterial recognition pathways have several consequences

Activation of complement via the alternative pathway – Complement activation may result in the killing of some bacteria, particularly those with an outer lipid bilayer susceptible to the lytic complex (C5b–9), i.e. Gram-negative bacteria. It also releases C3a and C5a which cause smooth-muscle contraction and mast-cell degranulation. C5a also attracts and activates neutrophils (see Chapter 3). The consequent release of histamine and leukotriene (LTB_4) contributes to further increases in vascular permeability (*Fig. 15.3*). Opsonization of the bacteria, by attachment of cleaved derivatives of C3, is important in subsequent interactions with phagocytes.

Chemotaxis – This attracts more phagocytes to the site of infection. It may be due both to complement activation and to direct chemotactic effects of bacterial products and to the release of chemokines triggered by bacterial PAMPs.

Release of cytokines from macrophages – The rapid release of cytokines such as tumour necrosis factor (TNF) and interleukin-1 (IL-1) from macrophages leads to systemic activation of phagocytic cells, and their increased adhesion to endothelium, facilitating passage into inflamed tissue. There is also a consequent release of chemokines such as MCP-1 and MIP-1α, which enhance the specific motility of leukocyte populations (see Chapter 3).

Release of cytokines from natural killer (NK) cells – When murine NK cells are stimulated by IL-12 or TNF, they can release interferon-γ (IFNγ). This in turn can activate macrophages. This T-cell-independent pathway helps to explain the unexpected resistance of mice with SCID (severe combined immunodeficiency, a defect in lymphocyte maturation) to infections such as *Listeria monocytogenes.*

Adjuvant effects – 'Adjuvant' is derived from the Latin adiuvare, to help. When given experimentally, soluble antigens evoke stronger T- and B-cell-mediated responses if they are mixed with bacterial components that act as adjuvants. Components with this property are indicated in *Figure 15.1.* The best known adjuvant in laboratory use, known as complete Freund's adjuvant, consists of killed *Mycobacterium tuberculosis* suspended in oil, which is then emulsified with the aqueous antigen solution. This effect probably reflects the fact that, when the antigen-specific immune response evolved, it did so in a tisssue environment that already contained these pharmacologically active bacterial components. The response to a pure bacterial antigen, injected without adjuvant-active bacterial components, can be regarded as an artificial situation that does not occur in nature.

Selection of the appropriate lymphocyte-mediated response – 'Adjuvant' components of bacteria, and the early release of cytokines, play an important role in this. Different bacteria exert optimal adjuvant effects on different parameters of the immune system by interacting with different pattern recognition molecules. This may reflect the need for the immune response to 'perform' some elementary 'taxonomy' on the infecting organisms, so that it can activate the appropriate effector functions. Cytokine release triggered by bacteria may also assist in this decision-making step, which is described in greater detail in Chapter 7.

Selection of inappropriate responses – Some microorganisms may exploit adjuvanticity to direct the immune response towards inappropriate mechanisms. Adjuvanticity is clearly an adaptation of the host. However, some microorganisms may exploit it to disturb immunoregulation, and so activate an inappropriate subset of helper T (TH) cells. This has been most clearly demonstrated in a model of infection of mice with the protozoan parasite *Leishmania major*. In this model, activation of TH2 cells leads to fatal disease, whereas activation of TH1 cells is fully protective (see Chapter 16).

Shock syndromes – If cytokine release is sudden and massive, several acute tissue-damaging syndromes can result and these are potentially fatal (explained in detail on p. 253).

Antibody provides an antigen-specific protective mechanism

The relevance to protection of interactions of bacteria with antibody depends on the mechanism of pathogenicity. Antibody clearly plays a crucial role in dealing with bacterial toxins. It neutralizes diphtheria toxin by blocking the attachment of the binding portion of the molecule to its target cells. Similarly it may block locally acting toxins or extracellular matrix-degrading enzymes which act as spreading factors, and it can interfere with motility by binding to flagellae.

An important function on external and mucosal surfaces, often performed by secretory IgA (sIgA – see Chapter 4), is to stop bacteria binding to epithelial cells. For instance, antibody to the M proteins of group A streptococci gives type-specific immunity to streptococcal sore throats. It is also likely that some antibodies to the bacterial surface can block functional requirements of the organism such as binding of iron-chelating compounds or intake of nutrients (*Fig. 15.5*).

However, the most important role of antibody in immunity to non-toxigenic bacteria is the more efficient targeting of complement. With the aid of antibodies, even organisms that resist the alternative (i.e. innate) pathway (see below) are damaged by complement, or become coated with C3 products, which then enhance the binding and uptake by phagocytes (*Figs 15.6* and *15.7*). The most efficient complement-fixing antibodies in man are IgG1, IgG3 and IgM. IgG1 and IgG3 are also the subclasses with the highest affinity for Fc receptors. Pathogenic bacteria may avoid the effects of antibody. *Neisseria gonorrhoeae* is an example which uses several strategies shown in *Figure 15.8*.

The antibacterial roles of antibody

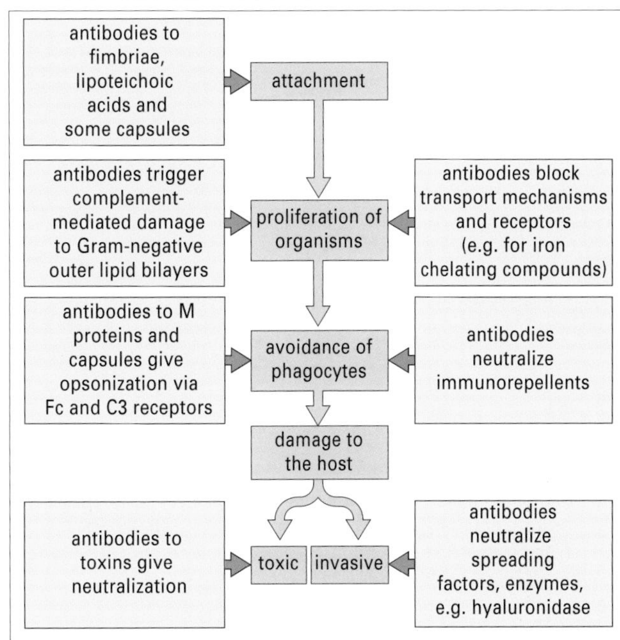

Fig. 15.5 This diagram lists the stages of bacterial invasion (blue) and indicates the antibacterial effects of antibody (yellow) that operate at the different stages. Antibodies to fimbriae, lipoteichoic acid and some capsules block attachment of the bacterium to the host-cell membrane. Antibody triggers complement-mediated damage to Gram-negative outer lipid bilayers. Antibody directly blocks bacterial surface proteins that pick up useful molecules from the environment and transport them across the membrane. Antibody to M proteins and capsules opsonizes the bacteria via Fc and C3 receptors for phagocytosis. Bacterial factors that interfere with normal chemotaxis or phagocytosis, are neutralized. Bacterial toxins may be neutralized by antibody, as may bacterial spreading factors that facilitate invasion (e.g. by the destruction of connective tissue or fibrin).

Pathogenic bacteria can avoid the detrimental effects of complement

Some bacterial capsules are very poor activators of the alternative pathway (*Fig. 15.9*). Alternatively, long side-chains (O antigens) on bacterial LPS may fix C3b at a distance from the otherwise vulnerable lipid bilayer. Similarly, smooth-surfaced Gram-negative organisms (*Escherichia coli*, *Salmonella* spp., *Pseudomonas* spp.) may fix but then rapidly shed the C5b–C9 membrane lytic complex.

Other organisms exploit the physiological mechanisms that block destruction of host cells by complement. When C3b has attached to a surface it can either interact with Factor B leading to further C3b amplification, or it can

Effect of antibody and complement on rate of clearance of virulent bacteria from the blood

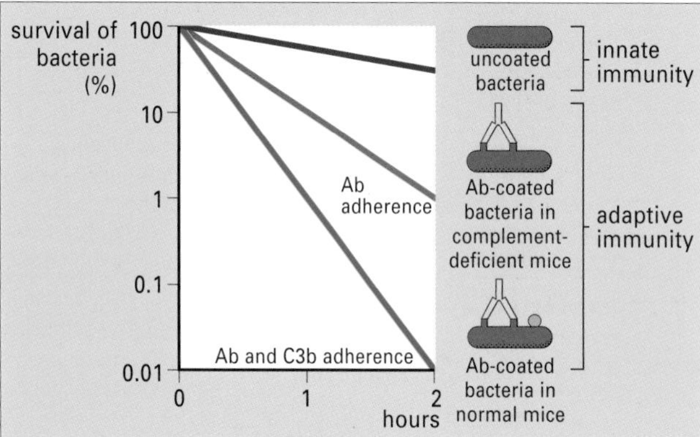

Fig. 15.6 Uncoated bacteria are phagocytosed rather slowly (unless the alternative pathway is activated by the strain of bacterium); on coating with antibody, adherence to phagocytes is increased many-fold. The adherence is somewhat less effective in animals temporarily depleted of complement.

The interaction between bacteria and phagocytic cells

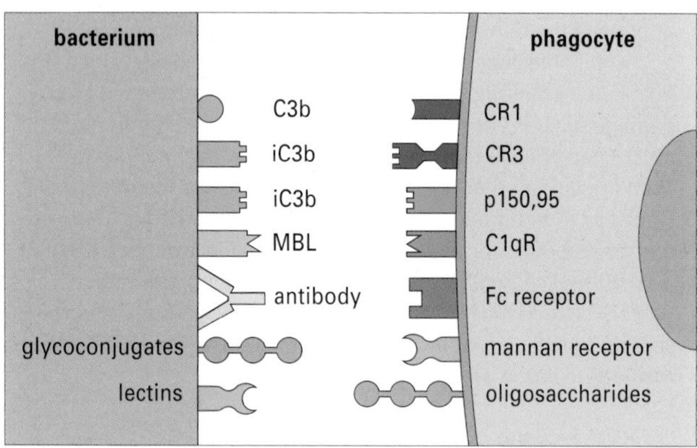

Fig. 15.7 A variety of molecules facilitate the binding of the organisms to the phagocyte membrane. The precise nature of the interaction may determine whether uptake occurs, and whether appropriate killing mechanisms are triggered. Note that apart from complement, antibody and mannose-binding lectin (MBL) which bind to the bacterial surface, the other components are constitutive bacterial molecules.

Mechanisms used by *Neisseria gonorrhoeae* to avoid the effects of antibody

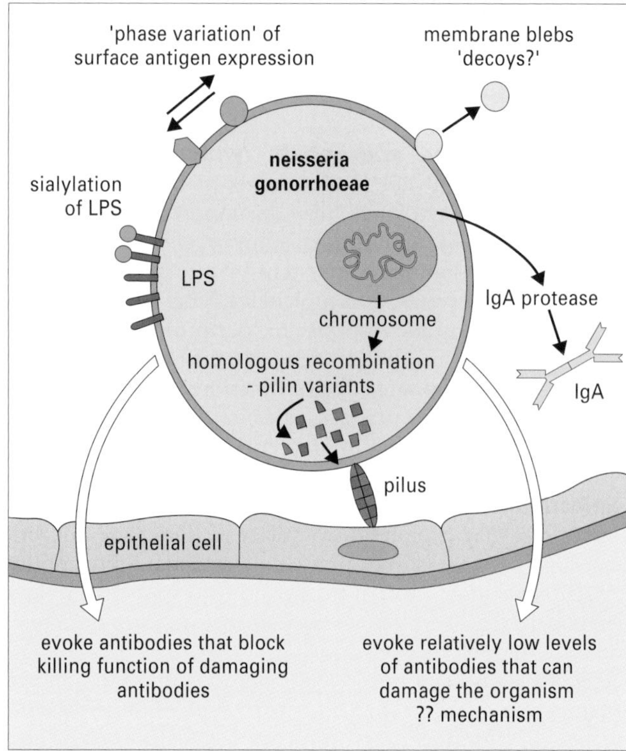

Fig. 15.8 *Neisseria gonorrhoeae* is an example of a bacterium that uses several strategies to avoid the damaging effects of antibody. First, it fails to evoke a large antibody response, and the antibody that does form tends to block the function of damaging antibodies. Secondly the organism secretes an IgA protease to destroy antibody. Thirdly blebs of membrane are released, and these appear to adsorb and so deplete local antibody levels. Finally, the organism uses three strategies to alter its antigenic composition (i) the LPS may be sialylated, so that it more closely resembles mammalian oligosaccharides and promotes rapid removal of complement; (ii) the organism can undergo phase variation, so that it expresses an alternative set of surface molecules (iii) the gene encoding pilin, the subunits of the pilus, undergoes homologous recombination to generate variants.

become inactivated by Factors H and I. Capsules rich in sialic acid (as host-cell membranes are) seem to promote this interaction with H and I. *Neisseria meningitidis*, *E. coli K1*, and group B streptococci all resist complement attachment in this way. The M protein of group A streptococci acts as an acceptor for Factor H, thus potentiating C3bB dissociation. These bacteria also have a gene for a C5a protease.

Ultimately most bacteria are killed by phagocytes

A few, mostly Gram-negative, bacteria are directly killed by complement, as stated earlier. There are also reports that some organisms, particularly Gram-negative bacteria, can be killed by mere contact with NK cells, or even cytotoxic T (Tc) cells. This probably involves the membrane-lysing mechanism of these cells (see Chapter 10), acting on the outer lipid bilayer that is characteristic of Gram-negative organisms.

However, most bacteria are killed by phagocytes. This process involves several steps (see *Fig. 15.9*).

Chemotaxis – Bacterial components such as f-Met-Leu-Phe (which is chemotactic for leucocytes), complement products such as C5a, and locally released chemokines and cytokines attract the phagocytes (see Chapter 3).

Attachment of the phagocyte to the organism – This is an important interaction which may determine whether

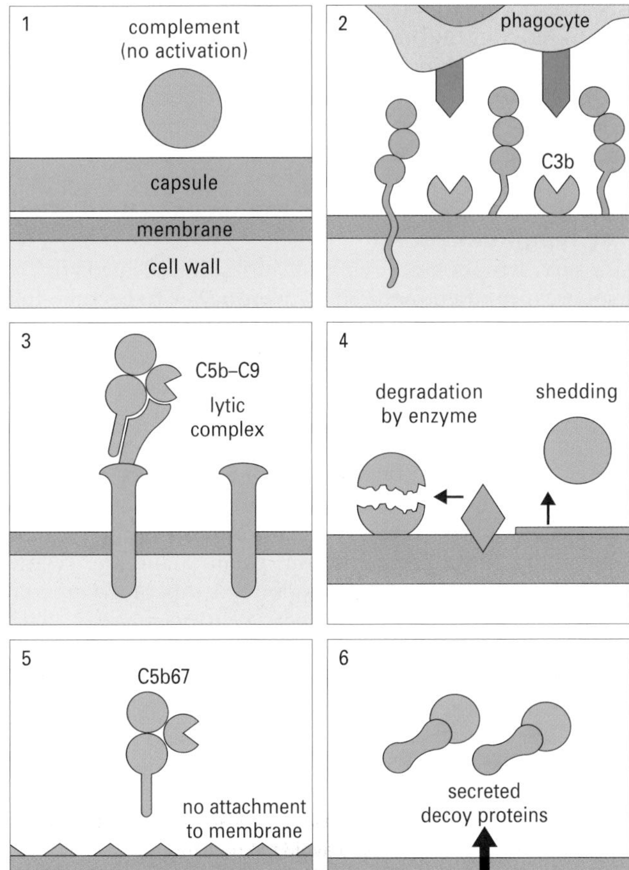

Fig. 15.9 Bacteria avoid complement-mediated damage by a variety of strategies. **(1)** An outer capsule or coat prevents complement activation. **(2)** An outer surface can be configured so that complement receptors on phagocytes cannot obtain access to fixed C3b. **(3)** Surface structures can be expressed which divert attachment of the lytic complex (MAC) from the cell membrane. **(4)** Membrane-bound enzyme can degrade fixed complement or cause it to be shed. **(5)** The outer membrane can resist the insertion of the lytic complex. **(6)** Secreted decoy proteins can cause complement to be deposited on them and not on the bacterium itself.

uptake subsequently occurs, and whether killing mechanisms are triggered during uptake. The binding can be mediated by the following entities.

- **Lectins on the organism**, for example the mannose-binding lectin on the fimbriae of *E. coli*.
- **Lectins on the phagocyte**. Of particular interest in this respect are the complement receptors CR3 and p150,95 and the related molecule LFA-1 (leucocyte functional antigen-1 – a mediator of intercellular adhesion), which have multiple binding sites specific for different carbohydrate moieties. They can bind to β-glucans and to the LPS endotoxin of Gram-negative bacteria. The mannan receptor targets glycoconjugates on the bacterial surface.
- Complement deposited on the organism via the alternative or classic pathways. It has recently been discovered that complement can also be fixed by mannose-binding lectins present in serum, which can itself bind to C1q receptors.
- Fc receptors on the phagocyte, which link to antibody bound to the bacteria (*Fig. 15.7*).

Triggering of uptake – The binding of an organism to a receptor on the macrophage membrane does not always lead to its uptake. For example, zymosan particles (derived from yeast) bind via the glucan-recognizing lectin-like site on the CR3 of the macrophage and are taken up, whereas erythrocytes coated with iC3b are not, even though the iC3b also binds to CR3.

Triggering of microbicidal activity – Just as the binding of an organism to membrane receptors does not guarantee uptake, so uptake does not guarantee the triggering of killing mechanisms. For example, *Yersinia pseudotuberculosis* induces its own uptake, but it also releases a gene product that modulates the uptake signal so that killing is not triggered.

Phagocytic cells have many killing methods

The killing pathways can be oxygen dependent and oxygen independent. The former are discussed in detail in Chapter 9. Briefly one oxygen-dependent pathway involves the reduction of oxygen to superoxide anion (which is molecular oxygen to which a single unpaired electron has been added). This then interacts with numerous other molecules to give rise to a series of free radicals and other toxic derivatives. A second oxygen-dependent pathway involves the creation of nitric oxide (NO•) from the guanidino nitrogen of L-arginine. This in turn leads to further toxic substances such as the peroxynitrites, which result from interactions of NO• with the products of the oxygen reduction pathway.

Oxygen-independent killing mechanisms may be important

These mechanisms may be more important than was previously thought. Many organisms can be killed by cells from patients with chronic granulomatous disease, which cannot produce reactive oxygen intermediates, or from patients with myeloperoxidase deficiency, which cannot produce hypohalous acids. Some of this killing may be due to NO•, but many organisms can be killed anaerobically, so other mechanisms must exist. Some have been identified.

Cationic proteins with antibiotic-like properties – The defensins are cysteine- and arginine-rich cationic peptides of 30–33 amino acids, found in rabbit macrophages and human neutrophil polymorphs, where they comprise 30–50% of the granule proteins. They evolved early in evolution and similar molecules are found in insects. They form ion-permeable channels in lipid bilayers and probably act early after phagolysosome formation, before acidification takes place. Defensins can kill organisms as diverse as *Staphylococcus aureus*, *Pseudomonas aeruginosa*, *E. coli*, *Cryptococcus neoformans* and the enveloped virus *Herpes* *simplex*. There are also cationic proteins with different pH optima, including cathepsin G and azurocidin, both of which are related to elastase but which have activity against Gram-negative bacteria; this is unrelated to their enzyme activity.

Other antimicrobial mechanisms – Following lysosome fusion there is a transient rise in pH before acidification (a fall in pH) of the phagolysosome takes place. This occurs within 10–15 minutes. Killing of some organisms may be due to the acidification itself, though it is more likely to be related to the low pH optima of lysosomal enzymes. Certain Gram-positive organisms may be killed by lysozyme, which is active against their readily exposed peptidoglycan layer. A variety of other substances, such as lactoferrin (produced by neutrophil polymorphs), have also been implicated in killing. Lactoferrin can bind iron and render it unavailable to bacteria even at an acid pH (thus, the ability of polymorphs to kill some bacteria is lost if they are loaded with iron). These mechanisms may all require phagolysosome fusion (*Fig. 15.10*).

Resting macrophages can kill, but killing can be enhanced, and new mechanisms can be expressed on activation

Activation occurs through exposure to microbial products, and to lymphokines derived from T cells. Similarly, the decline that usually occurs if the cells are kept in culture for a week can be reversed by treatment with suitable activating stimuli.

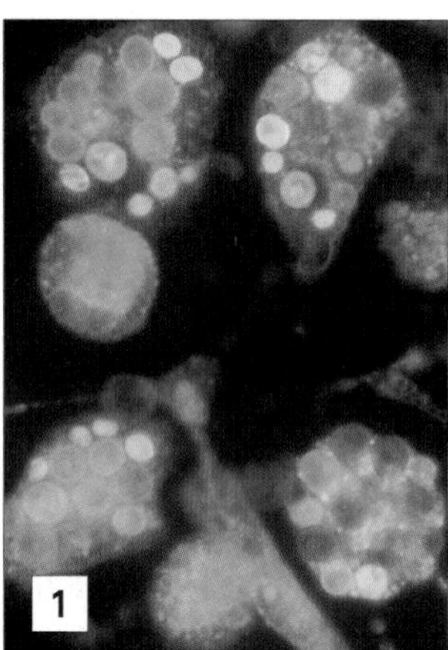

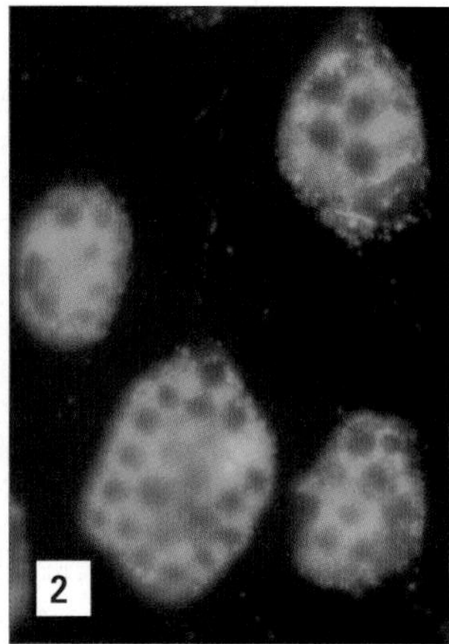

Fig. 15.10 Inhibition of fusion of secondary lysosomes with yeast-containing phagosomes by the addition of ammonium chloride. Mouse peritoneal macrophages were incubated in acridine orange, which concentrates in secondary lysosomes. Live baker's yeast was then added – these assume the appearance of 'holes' in the cell. Normally, the secondary lysosomes fuse with the phagosomes, and the acridine orange enters them, fluorescing green, yellow or orange depending on the concentration (**1**). However, in the presence of ammonium chloride, fusion does not occur and the 'holes' remain dark (**2**). Such blocking of lysosomal fusion may be employed by *M. tuberculosis* and some leishmania, which secrete ammonia. Some polyanions, such as polyglutamic acid or suramin, may also do this. (Courtesy of Mr R. Young and Dr P. D. Hart.)

Some microbial products can activate macrophages in the absence of lymphocyte recognition

A number of microbial products cause direct activation of monocytes and macrophages, or indirect activation by triggering cytokine release from them or from NK cells. The cytokines then activate the phagocytes. This was discussed earlier in relation to the non-lymphocyte-dependent recognition of bacteria.

Further activation of macrophages is mediated by lymphokines

In vivo, lymphokines released during T-cell-mediated responses are often required for phagocytes to become fully activated. The lymphokine most often implicated is IFNγ, which enhances both oxygen-dependent and oxygen-independent killing mechanisms. There are also reports implicating IL-2, granulocyte–macrophage colony stimulating factor (GM–CSF), TNF, and other cytokines. As discussed in greater detail in Chapter 7, activation of some functions requires combinations of cytokines.

Lymphokines *in vivo* have two effects on phagocytes – attracting them and activating them – and the relative importance of these two components differs for different organisms. Thus for immunity to *L. monocytogenes*, which can be killed by the baseline levels of oxygen-dependent mechanisms in both monocytes and neutrophils, it is the attraction of the cells to the lesion which is most important. In contrast, for *M. tuberculosis*, which thrives inside neutrophils and monocytes, it is the activation of the cells which is critical.

Human and murine macrophages are different

This is important because much experimental work is based on murine macrophages. Mycobacteria illustrate the complexity of this topic. IFNγ can activate murine macrophages to destroy mycobacteria completely. This appears to be due to the nitric oxide pathway. However, IFNγ acting on human macrophages causes, at best, feeble inhibition of *M. tuberculosis* or, at worst, significantly increased growth. This may relate to species differences in NO• production.

On the other hand, human cells do something which has not been reported in murine cells. IFNγ causes human macrophages to express a 1-hydroxylase enzyme that converts the circulating inactive form of 25-hydroxycholecalciferol (vitamin D_3) into an active metabolite, 1,25-dihydroxycholecalciferol. This metabolite activates antimycobacterial mechanisms in the macrophages rather more efficiently than IFNγ itself, though the mechanism of the enhanced antimicrobial effect is not known.

Successful pathogens have evolved mechanisms for the avoidance of phagocyte-mediated killing

Since most organisms are ultimately killed by phagocytes, it is not surprising that successful pathogens have evolved an array of mechanisms to counteract this risk (*Fig. 15.11*).

Intracellular pathogens may 'hide' in cells that have little antimicrobial potential

Infected cells can be killed by Tc cells

Some organisms may thrive inside damaged or metaboli-

Evasion mechanisms of bacteria

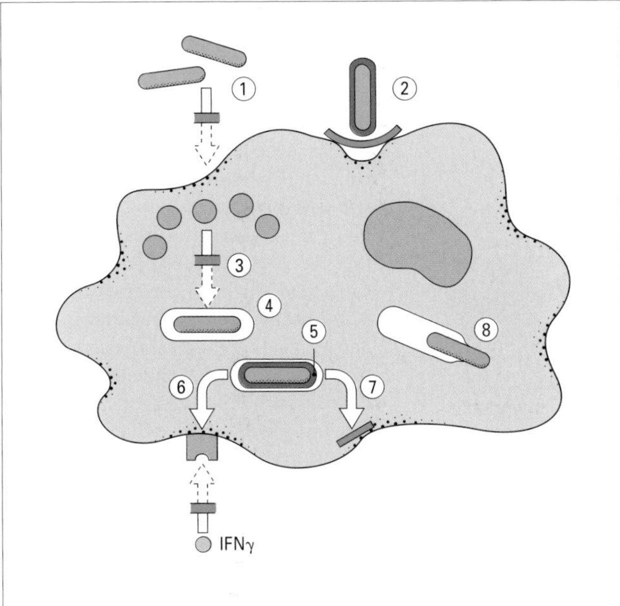

Fig. 15.11 Bacteria, particularly those which are successful intracellular parasites, have evolved the ability to evade different aspects of phagocyte-mediated killing. **(1)** Some can secrete repellents or toxins that inhibit chemotaxis. **(2)** Others have capsules or outer coats which inhibit attachment by the phagocyte. **(3)** Others permit uptake but release factors that block subsequent triggering of killing mechanisms. Once ingested, some, such as *M. tuberculosis*, secrete molecules which inhibit lysosome fusion with the phagosome. They also inhibit the proton pump which acidifies the phagosome so the pH does not fall. **(4)** They may also secrete catalase which breaks down hydrogen peroxide. **(5)** Organisms such as *M. leprae* have highly resistant outer coats. *M. leprae* surrounds itself with a phenolic glycolipid which scavenges free radicals. **(6)** Mycobacteria also release a lipoarabinomannan, which blocks the ability of macrophages to respond to the activating effects of IFNγ. **(7)** Infected cells may also lose their efficacy as antigen-presenting cells. **(8)** Several organisms (e.g. *M. leprae*), can escape from the phagosome to multiply in the cytoplasm. Finally, the organism (e.g. *M. tuberculosis*) may kill the phagocyte.

cally deranged host phagocytes, or escape killing by moving out of phagosomes into the cytoplasm. *Listeria monocytogenes* achieves this by releasing enzymes that lyse the phagosome membrane. This organism also illustrates the point that bacteria are not just inert particles. They have evolved strategies for taking control of functions of the host cell (*Fig. 15.12*). Other organisms, such as *Mycobacterium leprae*, can cause themselves to be taken up by cells that are not normally considered phagocytic, and have little antibacterial potential. Before they can be taken up by activated phagocytes, or exposed to other killing mechanisms, the organisms may need to be released from such cells. Tc cells may perform this function by killing the infected cell. For instance mice become strikingly susceptible to *M. tuberculosis* if the β_2-microglobulin gene is

Invasion of cells by *Listeria monocytogenes*

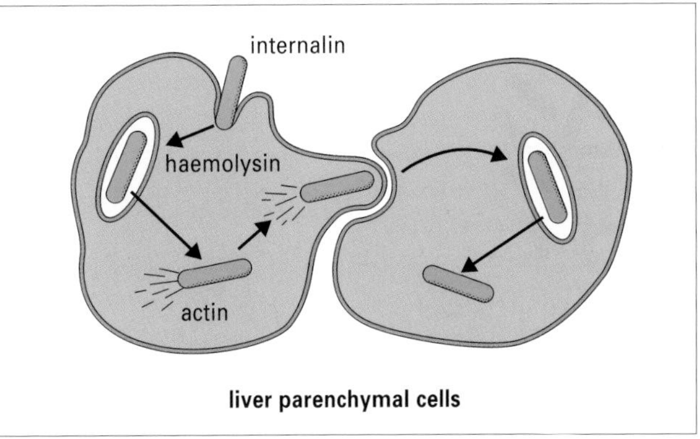

Fig. 15.12 Internalin (encoded by *inlA*) stimulates the uptake of *Listeria* by liver parenchymal cells; its haemolysin (so-called because this was how it was discovered) enables it to escape from the phagosome into the cytoplasm. There it interacts with actin filaments which act like a motor driving it into a neighbouring cell, where it will initially be surrounded by two membranes, both of which are then lysed by the haemolysin.

knocked out so that Class I MHC cannot be recognized by the Tc cells. This is consistent with an essential role for cytotoxic T cells.

γδ T cells are usually cytotoxic, and may kill infected cells

A large proportion of T cells bearing γδ receptors seem to proliferate in response to bacterial antigens. Some subsets of these cells home to epithelial surfaces (see Chapter 2). Thus it seems likely that they have a role in infection, but this is not yet understood. In general they are cytotoxic, so they may destroy parasitized cells.

Some tissue cells can express antimicrobial mechanisms

Tissue cells which are not components of the immune system can also harbour bacteria such as *M. leprae*, invasive *Shigella* and *Salmonella* species, or *Rickettsia* and *Chlamydia*. As mentioned earlier, these infected cells may be sacrificed by Tc. On the other hand, activation of fibroblasts by IFNγ can inhibit growth of intracellular organisms, probably via the NO• pathway, which is not confined to phagocytic cells.

The response to bacteria can result in immunological tissue damage

Excessive cytokine release can lead to endotoxin shock

Endotoxin (septicaemic) shock occurs when there is massive production of cytokines, usually caused by bacterial products released during septicaemic episodes. Endotoxin (LPS) from Gram-negative bacteria is usually responsible, though Gram-positive septicaemia can cause a similar syndrome. There can be life-threatening fever, circulatory collapse, diffuse intravascular coagulation, and haemorrhagic necrosis, leading eventually to multiple organ failure (*Fig. 15.13*).

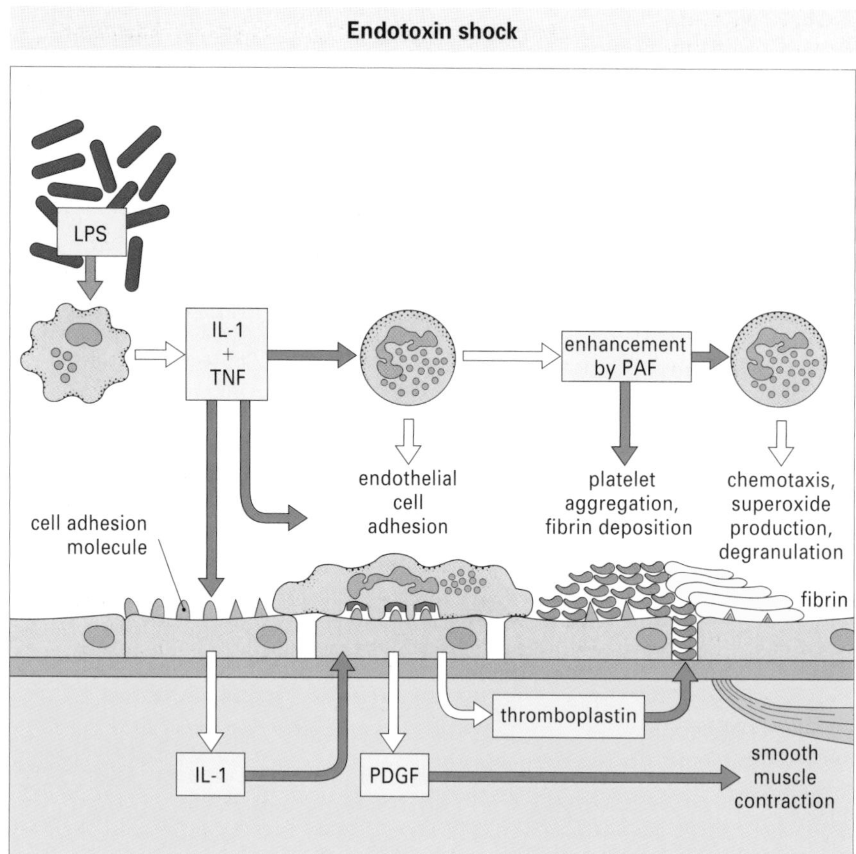

Fig. 15.13 Excessive release of cytokines, often triggered by the endotoxin (LPS) of Gram-negative bacteria, can lead to diffuse intravascular coagulation with consequent defective clotting, changes in vascular permeability, loss of fluid into the tissues, a fall in blood pressure, circulatory collapse, and haemorrhagic necrosis, particularly in the gut. This figure illustrates some important parts of this pathway at the cellular level. The cytokines TNF and IL-1 cause endothelial cells to express cell adhesion molecules and tissue thromboplastin. These promote adhesion of circulating cells and deposition of fibrin, respectively. Platelet activating factor (PAF) enhances these effects. In experimental models, shock can be blocked by neutralizing antibodies to TNF, and greatly diminished by antibodies to tissue thromboplastin, or by inhibitors of PAF or of nitric oxide production. Gram-positive bacteria can induce shock, for example by massive release of cytokines mediated by superantigens (see opposite). (PDGF = platelet-derived growth factor, produced by both platelets and endothelium.)

The Schwartzman reaction is a form of cytokine-dependent tissue damage occurring in inflammatory sites without a significant T-cell component

Schwartzman observed that if Gram-negative organisms were injected into the skin of rabbits, followed by a second dose given intravenously 24 hours later, haemorrhagic necrosis occurred at the prepared skin site. This is known as the Schwartzman reaction (*Fig. 15.14*). He also noted that two intravenous injections 24 hours apart caused a systemic reaction, commonly involving circulatory collapse and bilateral necrosis of the renal cortex. Sanarelli had made similar observations and this is now known as the systemic Schwartzman, or Sanarelli–Schwartzman, reaction. These reactions can also be accompanied by necrosis in the pancreas, pituitary, adrenals and gut. There is marked diffuse intravascular coagulation and thrombosis.

Many other organisms are now known to 'prepare' the skin in the same way, including streptococci, mycobac-

The Schwartzman reaction

induction in rabbit	human clinical equivalent
endotoxin injected into skin	a minor septicaemic episode results in dissemination of meningococci to the skin
24 hrs later endotoxin given intravenously	24 hrs later a further larger septicaemic episode results in systemic release of cytokines and activation of leukocytes
haemorrhagic necrosis in the 'prepared' skin site	this results in necrosis in the sites where bacteria lodged after the first episode

Fig. 15.14 The Schwartzman reaction: cytokine mediated tissue damage in a site of previous inflammation. This phenomenon is fundamental to several clinical situations in man. The first injection into the skin prepares the site by inducing inflammation and upregulating cytokine receptors which are now the target for systemic cytokines released by the later intravenous injection of endotoxin (LPS).

teria, *Haemophilus* spp., corynebacteria and vaccinia virus. Endotoxin (LPS) is the active component of the intravenous 'triggering' injection. Early work implicated endothelial changes, fibrin deposition, neutrophil accumulation and degranulation, and platelets as mediating the damage. This is correct, but it is now clear that TNFα, IFNγ, IL-12 and IL-1 are the critical mediators. Direct injection of TNFα into sites of inflammation (evoked by a previous injection of bacteria) causes a similar type of necrosis; the injected TNFα may be doing the same work as the TNFα that arrives via the circulation after an intravenous dose of LPS.

This phenomenon explains the characteristic haemorrhagic rash seen in children with meningococcal meningitis. A first episode of septicaemia results in widespread inflammatory sites which are small and subclinical at the time, but which remain exquisitely cytokine-sensitive. A second, larger septicaemic episode triggers enough cytokine release to cause necrosis in those sites.

The Koch phenomenon is necrosis occurring in T-cell-mediated mycobacterial lesions and skin-test sites

This is a necrotic response to antigens of *M. tuberculosis*, originally demonstrated by Robert Koch in tuberculous guinea pigs (*Fig. 15.15*). It may be related to the necrosis, which also occurs in the lesions in this disease. It is at least partly due to the release of cytokines into a T-cell-mediated inflammatory site (delayed hypersensitivity site – see Chapter 24). Such sites can be extremely sensitive to the tissue-damaging effects of cytokines, as seen in the Schwartzman reaction, particularly when there is mixed TH1 and TH2 activity.

The Koch phenomenon

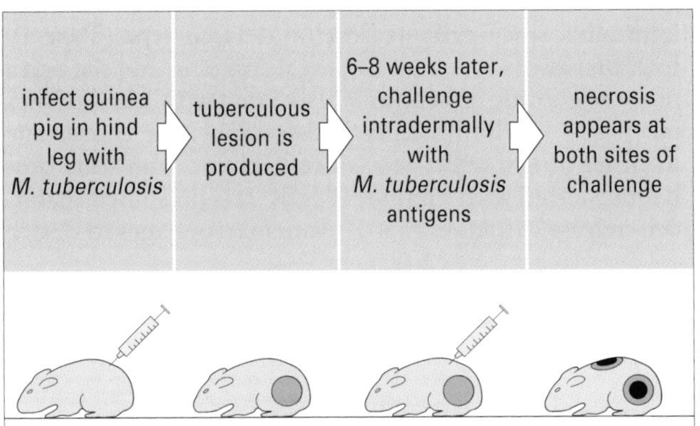

Fig. 15.15 Robert Koch observed that injection of *Mycobacterium tuberculosis*, or soluble antigens from *M. tuberculosis*, into the skin of tuberculous guinea-pigs resulted in a necrotizing reaction both at the challenge site, and in the original tuberculous lesion. This is at least partly due to the fact that the delayed hypersensitivity reaction to mycobacterial antigens can, like the LPS-injected site in the Schwartzman reaction, be very sensitive to the toxicity of cytokines. These may be released locally in the skin-test site. A similar reaction is seen in humans who have, or have had, tuberculosis. Responses to the same antigen, in individuals who are skin-test positive as a result of BCG vaccination, do not usually show necrosis.

Immunity in some important bacterial infections

infection	pathogenesis	major defence mechanisms
Corynebacterium diphtheriae	non-invasive pharyngitis – toxin	neutralizing antibody
Vibrio cholerae	non-invasive enteritis – toxin	neutralizing and adhesion-blocking antibodies
Neisseria meningitidis (Gram-negative)	nasopharynx →bacteraemia →meningitis →endotoxaemia	killed by antibody and lytic complement; opsonized and phagocytosed
Staphylococcus aureus (Gram-positive)	locally invasive and toxic in skin etc.	osponized by antibody and complement; killed by phagocytes
Mycobacterium tuberculosis	invasive, evokes immunopathology, ? toxic	? macrophage activation by cytokines from T cells
Mycobacterium leprae	invasive, space-occupying and/or immunopathology	

Fig. 15.16 This table provides examples of how a knowledge of the organism, and the mechanism of disease, can lead to a prediction of the relevant protective mechanism.

Figure 15.16 uses examples to illustrate the relationship between the nature of the organism, the disease and immunopathology caused, and the mechanism of immune response which leads to protection.

Further topics in bacterial immunology

Superantigens bypass antigen processing and presentation

These recently recognized bacterial components are so named because they bind directly (i.e. unprocessed) to the variable regions of β chains (Vβ) of antigen receptors on certain subsets of T cells, and cross-link them to the MHC of antigen-presenting cells (APCs) (see *Fig. 6.22*). As a result, all T cells bearing the relevant Vβ gene product are activated, without the processing and presentation of the antigen as peptides in the cleft of the MHC that is normally required for T-cell activation. Such superantigens have been found in staphylococci, streptococci, mycoplasmas and other species. The full biological significance of this bacterial adaptation is not yet clear, but one obvious effect can be the toxicity of the massive cytokine/lymphokine release that results from the simultaneous stimulation of a large subset of T cells. The staphylococcal toxins responsible for the toxic shock syndrome (TSST-1, etc.) appear to operate in this way.

Heat-shock proteins (stress proteins) are highly conserved and prominent targets of immune responses

These proteins are found in all eukaryotic and prokaryotic cells, where they have essential roles in the assembly, folding and transport of other molecules. Cells exposed to abnormally elevated temperatures (or to other stresses) express higher levels of these proteins, which reflects their role in the stabilization of protein structure. Their amino acid sequences are very highly conserved and there is currently much speculation that, because bacterial heat-shock proteins are so similar to human ones, they may be involved in the initiation of autoimmunity. Paradoxically, in spite of their similarity to host proteins, they seem to be target antigens in the protective response against many infectious organisms. This makes sense from an evolutionary point of view, because if the host possesses T cells that recognize a range of conserved heat-shock protein epitopes, these T cells are likely to recognize any pathogen encountered.

Thus peptides derived from microbial heat-shock proteins (hsp) and presented in the conventional manner by antigen-presenting cells, can be targets of $CD4^+$ T cells or of $CD8^+$ cytotoxic T cells. Infection can also stress a host cell, so that it 'flags' its distress by overexpressing its own hsp. There is some evidence that peptides derived from host hsp can under these circumstances be T-cell targets, so that the infected cell is sacrificed. There is also evidence that host hsp may become associated with the cell membrane and act as signalling molecules that alert the system to 'danger'.

The 'hygiene hypothesis'

Several groups of diseases, all characterized by defects in the regulation of the immune system, are becoming more common, particularly in developed countries. These diseases include allergies, inflammatory bowel diseases (Crohn's disease and ulcerative colitis) and autoimmune problems such as multiple sclerosis. In Europe increased incidences are seen first in the more developed northern states, and in western Europe rather than in the old communist block. Epidemiological data are compatible with the hypothesis that *increasing* immunological dysregulation correlates with *decreasing* exposure to harmless environmental bacteria. Decreased exposure could be due to hygiene, vaccines and antibiotic use. The hypothesis is rational because environmental inputs that have always been present throughout evolution may have become genetically encoded necessities to the developing immune system. If proved correct the solution will clearly not be the abandonment of the most important achievements of medicine (hygiene, vaccines, antibiotics) but rather the identification of the environmental factors that are lacking from the modern lifestyle, so they can be replaced as vaccines or probiotics. Probiotics are harmless organisms added to food ('functional foods') or even to the environment in order to exert a therapeutic effect. There is now also talk of 'prebiotics' which are dietary components intended to influence the bowel flora. Whatever their nature, effective products will need to regulate the balance of TH1/TH2 response, and promote the maturation of the regulatory T-cell circuits that control autoimmunity to host antigens such as heat-shock proteins. There are experimental and clinical trial data to suggest that some bacterial vaccines can achieve both objectives.

IMMUNITY TO FUNGI

Fungal infection is a growing problem because of the markedly increased numbers of immunologically compromised hosts. Thus it is regularly seen in HIV-infected patients, and in cancer patients undergoing chemotherapy, in transplant patients on immunosuppressive agents and in some patients taking long term corticosteroids.

There are four categories of fungal infection

Little is known of the precise mechanisms involved in immunity to fungal infections, but it is thought they are essentially similar to those involved in resistance to bacterial infections. The fungal infections of humans fall into four major categories.

- **Superficial mycoses:** these are caused by fungi known as dermatophytes, and are usually restricted to the non-living keratinized components of skin, hair and nails.
- **Subcutaneous mycoses:** saprophytic fungi can cause chronic nodules or ulcers in subcutaneous tissues following trauma, for example chromomycosis, sporotrichosis and mycetoma.
- **Respiratory mycoses:** soil saprophytes produce subclinical or acute lung infections (rarely disseminated), or granulomatous lesions, e.g. histoplasmosis and coccidioido-mycosis.
- **Candidiasis:** *Candida albicans* (a ubiquitous commensal) causes superficial (rarely systemic) infections of skin and mucous membranes.

Cell-mediated immunity is apparently the basis of resistance

Cutaneous fungal infections are usually self-limiting and recovery is associated with a certain limited resistance to reinfection. Resistance is apparently based on cell-mediated immunity, since patients develop delayed-type (Type IV) hypersensitivity reactions to fungal antigens, and the occurrence of chronic infections is associated with a lack of these reactions. T-cell immunity is also implicated in resistance to other fungal infections, since resistance can sometimes be transferred with immune T cells. It is presumed that TH cells release cytokines that activate macrophages to destroy

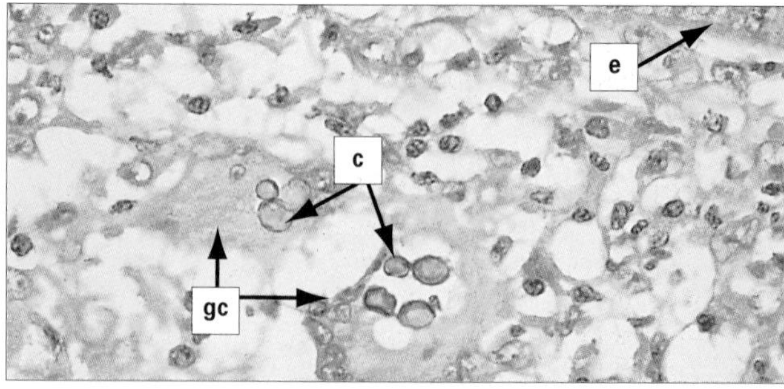

Fig. 15.17 Evidence for T-cell immunity in chromomycosis. The pigmented fungal cells of chromomycosis (a subcutaneous mycosis) (c) are visible inside giant cells (gc) in the dermis of a patient. The area is surrounded by a predominantly mononuclear cell infiltrate. The basal layer of epidermis (e) is visible at the top of the frame. H&E stain, ×400. (Courtesy of Prof R. J. Hay.)

the fungi (*Fig. 15.17*). In respiratory mycoses, spectra of disease activity somewhat similar to the spectrum of activity in leprosy can be seen. Disturbance of normal physiology by immunosuppressive drugs, or of normal flora by antibiotics, can predispose to invasion by *Candida*. *Candida* infections are also common in immuno-deficiency diseases (severe combined immunodeficiency, thymic aplasia, AIDS, etc.), implying that the immune system is involved in confining the fungus to its normal commensal sites.

Moreover in leukaemia patients, the proportion of infections with fungi other than Candida has increased more than five fold in the last decade. Infections are seen with *Malassezia furfur*, *Trichosporon* spp., *Blastoschizomyces capitatus, Rhodotorula rubra, Saccharomyces cerevisiae, Clavispora lusitaniae, Cryptococcus laurentii* and *Hansenula anomala*, but immunological data are sparse.

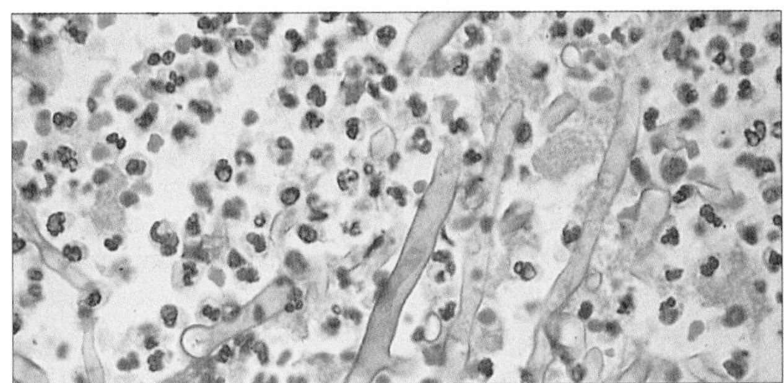

Fig. 15.18 Evidence for neutrophil-mediated immunity to mucormycosis. This is a section of a lung of a patient suffering from mucormycosis – an opportunistic infection in an immunosuppressed subject. The inflammatory reaction consists almost entirely of neutrophil polymorphs around the fungal hyphae. The disease is particularly associated with neutropenia (lack of neutrophils). Silver stain, ×400. (Courtesy of Professor R. J. Hay.)

Monocyte/macrophage killing of fungi

organism	source of monocytes/macrophages		
	normal	chronic granulomatous disease	myeloperoxidase deficiency
Candida albicans	killed	sometimes killed	sometimes killed
Candida parapsilosis	killed	not killed	unknown
Cryptococcus neoformans	killed	unknown	killed
Aspergillus fumigatus conidia	killed	killed	unknown
Aspergillus fumigatus hyphae	killed	killed	unknown

Fig. 15.19 Many fungi are killed by monocytes or macrophages. Cells from patients with chronic granulomatous disease and individuals with myeloperoxidase deficiency can also effect killing, showing that non-oxygen-dependent mechanisms are important.

There is also evidence for neutrophil polymorph involvement in immunity to some respiratory mycoses such as mucormycosis (*Fig. 15.18*). It is possible that the cationic proteins (defensins – see p. 251) are important for protection from fungi, since phagocytes from patients with defective oxygen reduction pathways nevertheless kill yeast and hyphae with near normal efficiency (*Fig. 15.19*). However, the nitric oxide pathway is effective against *Cryptococcus*, and this mechanism may turn out to be important for many fungi.

CRITICAL THINKING • Immuno-endocrine interactions in the response to infection
(Explanations on p. 457)

Humans subclinically infected with tuberculosis (about one-third of the world's population) may harbour live organisms for the rest of their lives. Similarly tuberculosis can establish a latent non-progressive infection in mice.

If animals with such latent infection are subjected to a period of restraint stress (placed in a tube that limits movement) each day for several days, the infection may reactivate. This also happens if cattle with latent disease are transported in trucks. Similarly tuberculosis increases in human populations in war zones, probably due to reactivation of latent disease.

15.1 What is the physiology of this reactivation?

When American military trainees were subjected to an extremely stressful training schedule their serum IgE levels rose, and they lost their previously positive delayed hypersensitivity skin-test responses. The levels of mRNA encoding IFNγ in the peripheral blood mononuclear cells of medical students were lower during the examination period than at other times of the year.

15.2 Do these observations suggest changes in cytokine profile? If so, why did it happen?

FURTHER READING

General

Roitt IM, Delves PJ, (ed). *Encyclopedia of Immunology.* London: Academic Press, 1992. (See numerous entries under names of individual fungi and bacteria.)

Bacteria

Cohen IR, Young DB. Autoimmunity, microbial immunity and the immunological homunculus. *Immunol Today* 1991;**12**:105–10.

Falkow S, Isberg RR, Portnoy DA. The interaction of bacteria with mammalian cells. *Annu Rev Cell Biol* 1992;**8**:333–63.

Heeg K, Miethke T, Wagner H. Superantigen-mediated lethal shock: the functional state of ligand-reactive T cells. *Curr Top Microbiol Immunol* 1996;**216**:83–100.

Henderson B, Poole S, Wilson M. Bacterial modulins: a novel class of virulence factors which cause host tissue pathology by inducing cytokine synthesis. *Microbiol Rev* 1996;**60**:316–41.

Hoffmann JA, Kafatos FC, Janeway CA, Ezekowitz RA. Phylogenetic perspectives in innate immunity. *Science* 1999;**284**:1313–8.

Jones B, Pascopella L, Falkow S. Entry of microbes into the host: using M cells to break the mucosal barrier. *Curr Opin Immunol* 1995;**7**:474–8.

Kaufmann SH. Immunity to intracellular bacteria. *Annu Rev Immunol* 1993;**11**:129–63.

Levy O. Antibiotic proteins of polymorphonuclear leukocytes. *Eur J Haematol* 1996;**56**:263–77.

Matricardi PM, Rosmini F, Riondino S, *et al.* Exposure to foodborne and orofecal microbes versus airborne viruses in relation to atopy and allergic asthma; epidemiological study. *Br Med J* 2000;**320**:412–17.

Moffitt MC, Frank MM. Complement resistance in microbes. *Springer Semin Immunopathol* 1994;**15**:327–44.

Moors MA, Portnoy DA. Identification of bacterial genes that contribute to survival and growth in an intracellular environment. *Trends Microbiol* 1995;**3**:83–5.

Ofek I, Goldhar J, Keisari Y, *et al.* Nonopsonic Phagocytosis of microorganisms. *Annu Rev Microbiol* 1995;**49**:239–76.

Orme I, Flynn JL, Bloom BR. The role of CD8$^+$ T cells in immunity to tuberculosis. *Trends Microbiol* 1993;**1**(3):77–8.

Rietschel ET, Brade H, Holst O, *et al.* Bacterial endotoxin: chemical constitution, biological recognition, host response, and immunological detoxification. *Curr Top Microbiol Immunol* 1996;**216**:39–81.

Rook GAW, Hernandez-Pando R. The pathogenesis of tuberculosis. *Annu Rev Microbiol* 1996;**50**:259–84.

Rothstein JL, Schreiber H. Synergy between tumour necrosis factor and bacterial products causes haemorrhagic necrosis and lethal shock in normal mice. *Proc Natl Acad Sci USA* 1988;**85**:607–11.

Russell MW, Hedges SR, Wu HY, Hook E, Mestecky J. Mucosal immunity in the genital tract: prospects for vaccines against sexually transmitted diseases – a review. *Am J Reprod Immunol* 1999;**42**:58–63.

Takeuchi O, Hoshino K, Kawai T, *et al.* Differential roles of TLR2 and TLR4 in recognition of gram-negative and gram-positive bacterial cell wall components. *Immunity* 1999;**11**:443–51.

Thiel S. Mannan-binding protein, a complement activating animal lectin. *Immunopharmacology* 1992;**24**:91–9.

Yamamura M, Uyemura K, Deans RJ, *et al.* Defining protective responses to pathogens: cytokine profiles in leprosy lesions. *Science* 1991;**254**:277–9.

Yu B, Wright SD. Catalytic properties of lipopolysaccharide (LPS) binding protein. Transfer of LPS to soluble CD14. *J Biol Chem* 1996;**271**:4100–5.

Zevering Y, Jacob L, Meyer TF. Naturally acquired human immune responses against *Helicobacter pylori* and implications for vaccine development. *Gut* 1999;**45**:465–74.

Fungi

Jones HE. Immune response and host resistance of humans to dermatophyte infection. *J Am Acad Dermatol* 1993;**28**:S12–18.

Leibovici V, Evron R, Axelrod O, *et al.* Imbalance of immune responses in patients with chronic and widespread fungal skin infection. *Clin Exp Dermatol* 1995;**20**:390–4.

Levitz SM. Overview of host defenses in fungal infections. *Clin Infect Dis* 1992;**14**:S37–42.

Murphy JW. Mechanisms of natural resistance to human pathogenic fungi. *Annu Rev Microbiol* 1991;**45**:509–38.

Romani L. The T cell response against fungal infections. *Curr Opin Immunol* 1997;**9**:484–90.

16 Immunity to protozoa and worms

- **Parasites infect many millions of people.** They are generally host specific and most cause chronic infections. Many are spread by invertebrate vectors and have complicated life cycles. Their antigens are stage specific.
- **Host resistance** depends upon a number of mechanisms. Effector cells such as macrophages, neutrophils, eosinophils and platelets can kill both protozoa and worms. They secrete cytotoxic molecules such as reactive oxygen radicals and nitric oxide. All are more effective when activated by cytokines.
- **T cells are fundamental** to the development of immunity. Antibody, alone or with complement, is effective against extracellular parasites. It enhances the phagocytic and cytotoxic potential of effector cells, and can prevent the invasion of new host cells.
- **Evasion of the host's immune response** by parasites occurs in various ways. Some exploit the host response for their own development. Most interfere with it.
- **Worm infections** are characteristically associated with an increase in eosinophil number and circulating IgE. T-1 and T-2 helper responses both play a role in immunity. TH2 cells are necessary for the elimination of intestinal worms.
- **Both $CD4^+$ and $CD8^+$ T cells** can be necessary for protection. TH1 cells provide protection against intracellular protozoa by secreting interferon-γ (IFNγ), which activates macrophages.
- **Parasitic infections** are associated with large amounts of non-specific antibody, splenomegaly and hepatomegaly. Much immunopathology may be T-cell mediated.

Parasitic infections typically stimulate a number of immunological defence mechanisms, both antibody- and cell-mediated, and the responses that are most effective depend upon the particular parasite and the stage of infection. The general principles of immunity to parasitic diseases are considered in this chapter, with special reference to some of the more important infections of man, which affect the host in diverse ways (*Fig. 16.1*).

Parasitic protozoa may live in the gut (e.g. amoebae), in the blood (e.g. African trypanosomes), within erythrocytes (e.g. *Plasmodium* spp.), in macrophages (e.g. *Leishmania* spp., *Toxoplasma gondii*), including those of the liver and spleen (e.g. *Leishmania* spp.), or in muscle (e.g. *Trypanosoma cruzi*). Parasitic worms that infect man include trematodes or flukes (e.g. schistosomes), cestodes (e.g. tapeworms) and nematodes or roundworms (e.g. *Trichinella spiralis*, hookworms, pinworms, *Ascaris* spp. and the filarial worms). Tapeworms and adult hookworms inhabit the gut, adult schistosomes live in blood vessels, and some filarial worms, for example, live in the lymphatics (*Fig. 16.2*). It is clear that there is widespread potential for damaging pathological reactions.

Many parasitic worms pass through complicated life cycles, including migration through various parts of the host's body. Hookworms and schistosome larvae invade their hosts directly by penetrating the skin; tapeworms, pinworms and roundworms are ingested; and filarial worms depend upon an intermediate insect host or vector to transmit them from person to person. Most protozoa rely upon an insect vector apart from *Toxoplasma, Giardia* and amoebae, which are transmitted by ingestion. Thus, malarial parasites are spread by mosquitoes, trypanosomes by tsetse flies, *T. cruzi* by Triatomid bugs, and *Leishmania* by sandflies.

FEATURES OF PARASITIC INFECTIONS

Parasites infect very large numbers of people

Parasitic infections present a major medical problem, especially in tropical countries (*Fig. 16.1*). Malaria, for example, kills 1–2 million people every year. Intestinal worms infect a third of the world's population; the severity of disease depends upon the worm burden, but in children even moderate intensities of infection may be associated with stunted growth and slow mental development. Anaemia and malnutrition are also associated with parasitic disease.

Parasitic infections have some common features

Protozoan parasites and worms are considerably larger than bacteria and viruses (*Fig. 16.3*), and consequently contain a greater variety and a greater quantity of antigens. Some species can also change their surface antigens, a process known as antigenic variation. Parasites that have complicated life histories may express certain antigens only at a particular stage of development, giving rise to a stage-specific response. Thus, the protein coat of the sporozoite (the infective stage of the malarial parasite transmitted by the mosquito) induces the production of antibodies that do not react with the erythrocytic stage; the different stages of the worm *T. spiralis* also display different surface antigens.

Protozoa that are small enough to live inside human cells have evolved a special mode of entry. The merozoite, the invasive form of the blood stage of the malarial parasite, binds to certain receptors on the surface of the erythrocyte and uses a specialized organelle, the rhoptry, to enter the cell. *Leishmania* spp. parasites, which inhabit macrophages, use complement receptors to encourage the cells to engulf them. These parasites can also gain entry to the cell by using the mannose–fucose receptor on the macrophage surface.

Most parasites are host specific

Over millions of years of evolution, parasites have become well adapted to their hosts and show marked host specificity. For example, the malarial parasites of birds, rodents or man can each multiply only in their own particular kind of host. There are some exceptions to this general rule: for

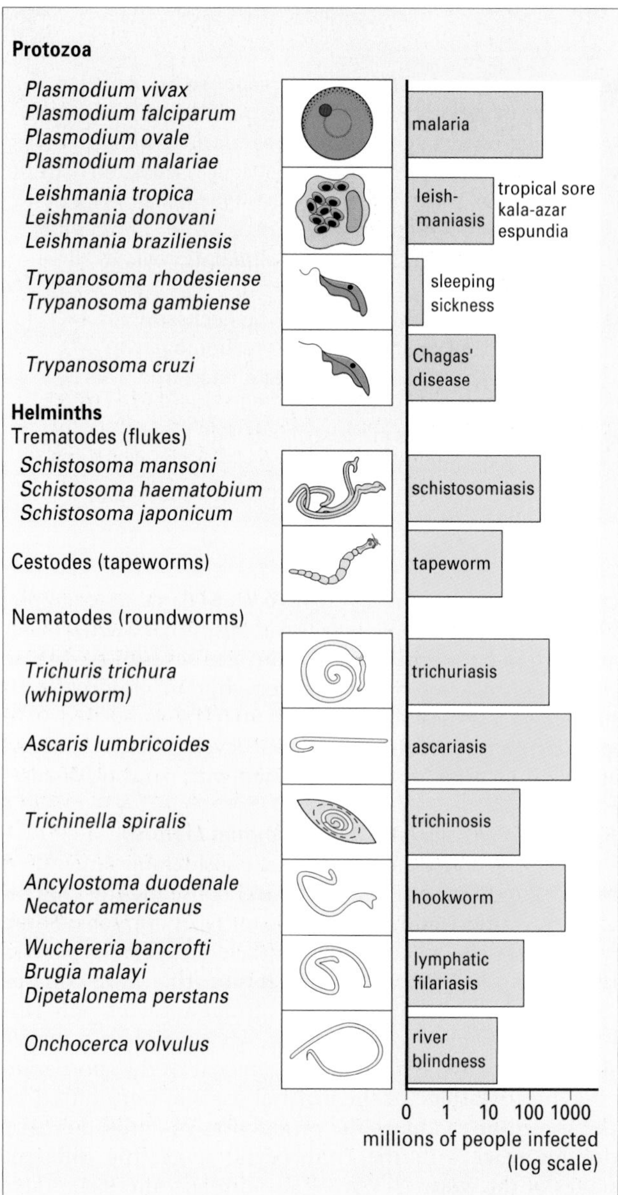

Fig. 16.1 Including data from the World Health Organization (1993).

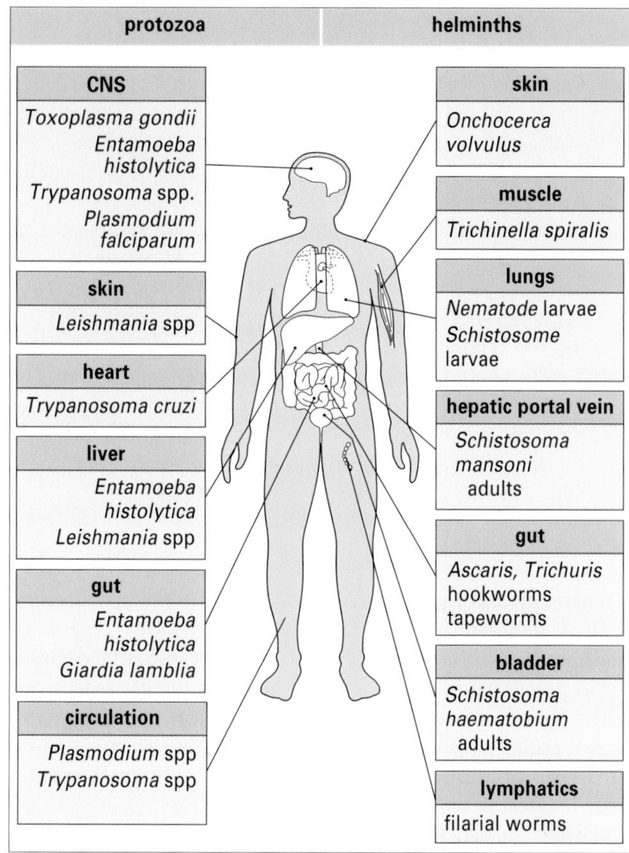

Fig. 16.2 Sites of infection of medically important parasites.

example, the protozoan parasite *T. gondii* is not only able to invade and multiply in all nucleated mammalian cells, but can also infect immature mammalian erythrocytes, insect cell cultures, and the nucleated erythrocytes of birds and fish. Similarly, the tapeworm of the pig can also infect humans.

Host resistance to parasite infection may be genetic

The resistance of individual hosts to infection varies, and may be controlled by a number of immune response genes. Strains of mice – and some people – carrying certain MHC genes are less able to make antibody to one of the peptides of the malarial sporozoite coat because their T cells do not become sensitized. Similarly, the possession of certain HLA antigens, widespread in native West Africans but rare in Caucasians, appears to correlate with protection against severe malaria.

Non-MHC genes can also be important:

- The susceptibility of mice to infection by *Leishmania donovani* and several other intramacrophage pathogens is determined by a single dominant gene Nramp1 which is known to be an iron transporter protein and has effects on macrophage activation (see chapter 9).
- Merozoites of the malarial parasite *Plasmodium vivax* use a particular blood group substance on the erythrocyte surface, the Duffy antigen, as a receptor to effect their entry into the cell. Certain African populations lack this antigen – presumably from the pressures of natural selection – and are totally resistant to infection by the parasite.

In most helminth infections a heavy worm burden occurs in comparatively few individuals, but it should not be assumed that this is necessarily due to genetic differences in resistance. Studies of human behaviour suggest that even in a small community people may vary greatly in their risk of infection through differences in their exposure to the invasive parasite.

Comparative size of various parasites

scale	size	parasite	group
naked eye	1m	tapeworm, guinea worm	worms
	10^{-2}	adult schistosome	worms
		adult filaria	worms
	10^{-3}	larval filaria	worms
light microscope		schistosome larva	worms
		amoeba, *Leishmania*, trypanosome	protozoa
		Plasmodium	protozoa
	10^{-5}	*Staphylococcus*	bacteria
		pox virus	viruses
electron microscope		influenza virus	viruses
	10^{-8}	polio virus	viruses
metres			

Fig. 16.3 Comparative size of various parasites.

Many parasitic infections are chronic

It is not in the interest of a parasite to kill its host, at least not until transmission to another host has been ensured. During the course of a chronic infection the type of immune response may change and immunosuppression and immunopathological effects are common.

Host defence depends upon a number of immunological effector mechanisms

The development of immunity is a complex process arising from the interactions of many different kinds of cells over a period of time. Effects are often local and many cell types secreting several different mediators may be present at sites of immune rejection. Moreover, the processes involved in controlling the multiplication of a parasite within an infected individual may differ from those responsible for the ultimate development of resistance to further infection. In some helminth infections a process of 'concomitant immunity' occurs, whereby an initial infection is not eliminated but becomes established, and the host then acquires resistance to invasion by new worms of the same species.

In very general terms, humoral responses are necessary to eliminate extracellular parasites such as those that live in blood (*Fig. 16.4*), body fluids, or the gut. However, the type of response conferring most protection varies with the parasite. For example, antibody, alone or with complement, can damage some extracellular parasites, but is better when acting with an effector cell. As emphasized above, within a single infection different effector mechanisms act against different developmental stages of parasites. Thus in malaria, antibody against extracellular forms blocks their capacity to invade new cells but cell-mediated responses prevent the development of the liver stage within hepatocytes. Protective immunity to malaria does not correlate simply with antibody levels and can even be induced in the absence of antibody. This was shown in mice immunized with genetically engineered *Salmonella typhimurium* carrying a gene coding for a malaria sporozoite surface antigen and then challenged with sporozoites. Although the mice did not make specific antibody, they developed immunity to the parasite.

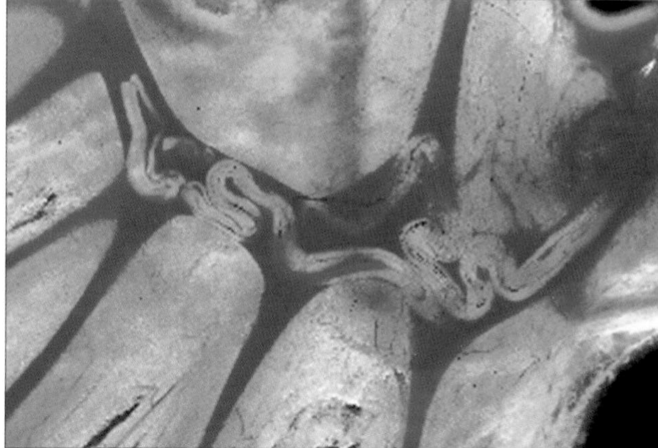

Fig. 16.4 Adult schistosome worm pairs in mesenteric blood vessels. Although very exposed to immune effectors, they are highly resistant. Adult schistosomes can persist for an average of 3–5 years. (Courtesy of Dr Alison Agnew.)

EFFECTOR MECHANISMS

Before a parasite succeeds in establishing itself within a new host and before specific immunity has been initiated or achieved, the parasite must overcome the host's pre-existing defence mechanisms. Complement plays a role here, as several types of parasite, including the adult worms and infective larvae of *T. spiralis* and the schistosomules of *Schistosoma mansoni,* carry molecules in their surface coats that activate the alternative pathway.

Macrophages, neutrophils, eosinophils and platelets form the first line of defence

Antibody and cytokines produced specifically in response to parasite antigens enhance the anti-parasitic activities of all these effector cells. However, tissue macrophages, monocytes and granulocytes all have some intrinsic activity, even before enhancement. The point of entry of the parasite is obviously important, for example:

- The cercariae of *S. mansoni* enter through the skin – experimental depletion of macrophages, neutrophils and eosinophils from the skin of mice increases their susceptibility to infection.

- Trypanosomes and malarial parasites entering the blood are removed from the circulation by phagocytic cells in the spleen and liver
- Comparison of strains of mice with various immunological defects for their resistance to infection by *Trypanosoma rhodesiense* shows that the African trypanosomes are destroyed by macrophages. Later in infection, when opsonized with antibodies and complement C3b, they are taken up by macrophages in the liver more quickly still.

Before acting as antigen-presenting cells initiating an immune response macrophages act as effector cells to inhibit the multiplication of parasites or even to destroy them. They also secrete molecules which regulate the inflammatory response. Some – IL-1, IL-12, tumour necrosis factor-α (TNFα) and the colony-stimulating factors (CSFs) – enhance immunity by activating other cells or stimulating their proliferation. Others, like IL-10, prostaglandins and transforming growth factor-β (TGFβ) may be anti-inflammatory and immunosuppressive.

Macrophages can kill extracellular parasites

Phagocytosis by macrophages provides an important defence against the smaller parasites; however, these cells also secrete many cytotoxic factors, enabling them to kill parasites without ingesting them. When activated by cytokines, macrophages can kill both relatively small extracellular parasites, such as the erythrocytic stages of malaria, and also larger ones, such as the larval stages of the schistosome.

Macrophages also act as killer cells through antibody-dependent cell-mediated cytotoxicity (ADCC); specific IgG and IgE, for instance, enhance their ability to kill schistosomules. They also secrete cytokines, such as TNFα and IL-1, that interact with other types of cell, for example, rendering hepatocytes resistant to malarial parasites.

Reactive oxygen intermediates (ROIs) are generated by macrophages and granulocytes following phagocytosis of *T. cruzi, T. gondii, Leishmania* spp. and malarial parasites, for instance; filarial worms and schistosomes also stimulate the respiratory burst. When activated by cytokines, macrophages release more superoxide and hydrogen peroxide than normal resident macrophages, and their O_2-independent killing mechanisms are similarly enhanced.

Nitric oxide (NO), a product of L-arginine metabolism, is one of the potent O_2-independent toxins. Its synthesis by macrophages in mouse experimental systems is induced by the cytokines IFNγ and TNFα and is greatly increased when they act together. Nitric oxide can also be produced by endothelial cells. It contributes to host resistance in leishmaniasis, schistosomiasis and malaria, and is probably important in the control of most parasitic infections (*Fig. 16.5*). For instance, the innate resistance to infection by *T. gondii* that is lost in immunocompromised individuals appears to be due to the inhibition of parasite mutiplication by such an O_2-independent mechanism.

Activation of macrophages is a general feature of the early stages of infection

All macrophage effector functions are enhanced soon after infection. Although their specific activation is by cytokines secreted by T cells (e.g. IFNγ, GM-CSF, IL-3 and IL-4), they can also be activated by T-cell-independent mechanisms, for example:

- NK cells secrete IFNγ when stimulated by IL-12 produced by macrophages.
- Macrophages secrete TNFα in response to some parasite products (e.g. phospholipid-containing antigens of malarial parasites and some *T. brucei* antigens); this TNFα then activates other macrophages.

Although TNFα may be secreted by several other cell types, activated macrophages are the most important source of this molecule, which is necessary for protective responses to several species of protozoa (e.g. *Leishmania* spp.) and helminths. Thus TNFα activates macrophages, eosinophils and platelets to kill the larval form of *S. mansoni*, its effects being enhanced by IFNγ.

Note that TNFα may have harmful as well as beneficial effects on the infected host, depending upon the amount produced and whether it is free in the circulation or locally confined. Thus serum concentrations in falciparum malaria correlate with the severity of the disease. Administration of TNFα cures a susceptible strain of mice infected with the rodent malarial parasite *P. chabaudi*, but kills a genetically resistant strain. Presumably the latter can already make enough TNFα to control parasite replication, and any more has toxic effects.

Toxic effect of NO on *Leishmania in vitro*

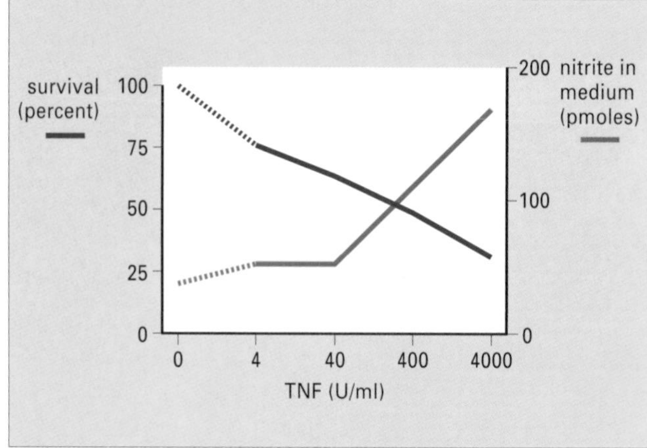

Fig. 16.5 Evidence that the killing of *Leishmania major* by activated macrophages is correlated with the release of nitric oxide. Mouse macrophages in culture are activated by recombinant TNFα in a dose-related fashion, the highest doses decreasing parasite survival to about a third of that in control cultures. At the same time, the amount of NO released, measured as nitrite present in the culture medium, increases. Interference with NO production allows parasites to survive. (Based on data from Liew *et al. Immunol* 1990;**71**:556.)

Neutrophils can kill large and small parasites

The effector properties displayed by macrophages are also seen in neutrophils. Neutrophils are phagocytic and can kill by both O_2-dependent and O_2-independent mechanisms, including nitric oxide. They produce a more intense respiratory burst than macrophages and their secretory granules contain highly cytotoxic proteins (see Chapter 2). They can be activated by cytokines, such as IFNγ, TNFα, and granulocyte-macrophage–colony-stimulating factor (GM–CSF). Extracellular destruction by neutrophils is mediated by H_2O_2, whereas granular components are involved in intracellular destruction of ingested organisms. Neutrophils are present in parasite-infected inflammatory lesions and probably act to clear parasites from bursting cells. Like macrophages, neutrophils bear Fc receptors and complement receptors and can participate in antibody-dependent cytotoxic reactions, to kill the larvae of *S. mansoni* for example. In this mode, they can be more destructive than eosinophils against several species of nematode, including *T. spiralis,* although the relative effectiveness of the two types of cell may depend upon the isotype and specificity of antibody.

Eosinophils are characteristically associated with worm infections

It has been suggested that the eosinophil evolved specifically as a defence against the tissue stages of parasites that are too large to be phagocytosed, and that the IgE-dependent mast-cell reaction has evolved primarily to localize eosinophils near the parasite and enhance their anti-parasitic functions.

The importance of these effector cells *in vivo* has been shown by experiments using antiserum against eosinophils. Mice infected with *T. spiralis* and treated with the anti-serum develop more cysts in their muscles than the controls: without the protection offered by eosinophils, the mice cannot eliminate the worms and so encyst the parasites to minimize damage.

However, recent work has shown that although eosinophils can help the host to control a worm infection, particularly by limiting migration through the tissues, they do not always do so. For instance, their removal does not abolish the immunity of mice infected with *S. mansoni,* nor does this increase the parasite load in a tapeworm infection.

Eosinophils can kill helminths by both O_2-dependent and O_2-independent mechanisms

Eosinophils are less phagocytic than neutrophils. They degranulate in response to perturbation of their surface membrane and their activities are enhanced by cytokines such as TNFα and GM–CSF. Most of their activities, however, are controlled by antigen-specific mechanisms. Thus their binding *in vitro* to the larvae of worms coated with IgE or IgG (e.g. *S. mansoni* and *T. spiralis*) increases the release of their granular contents onto the surface of the worms. Damage to schistosomules can be caused by the major basic protein (MBP) of the eosinophil crystalloid core. MBP is not specific for any particular target, but since it is confined to a small space between the eosinophil and the schistosome, there is little damage to nearby host cells. Eosinophils and mast cells can act together. For example, the killing of *S. mansoni* larvae by eosinophils is enhanced by mast cell products, and when studied *in vitro,* eosinophils from patients with schistosomiasis are found to be more effective than those from normal subjects. The antigens released cause local IgE-dependent degranulation of mast cells and the release of mediators. These selectively attract eosinophils to the site and further enhance their activity. Other products of eosinophils later block the mast cell reactions. That these effector mechanisms may function *in vivo* has been shown in monkeys, where schistosome killing is associated with eosinophil accumulation (*Fig. 16.6*).

Platelets can kill many types of parasite

Potential targets for platelets include the larval stage of flukes, *T. gondii* and *T. cruzi.* Like other effector cells, their cytotoxic activity is enhanced by treatment with cytokines (e.g. IFNγ and TNFα). In rats infected with *S. mansoni,* platelets become larvicidal when acute-phase reactants appear in the serum but before antibody can be detected. Incubation of normal platelets in such serum can cause their activation. Platelets, like macrophages and the other effector cells, also bear Fcε receptors on their surface membrane,

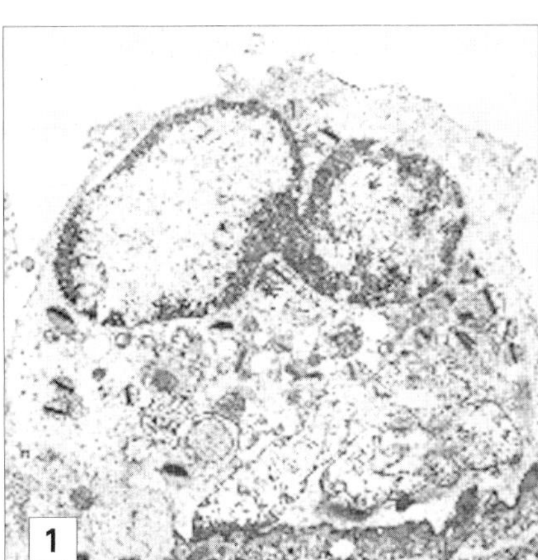

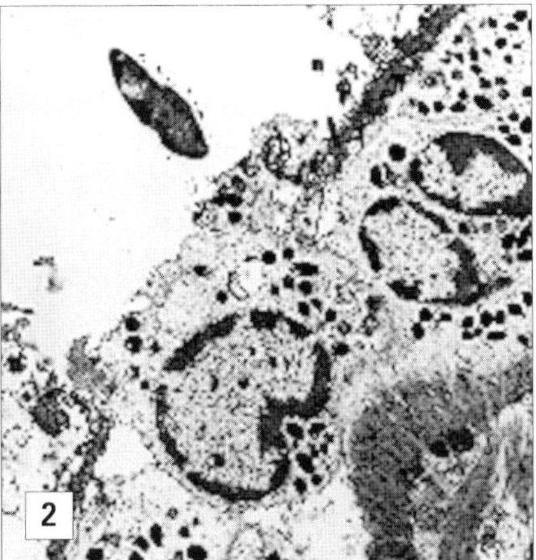

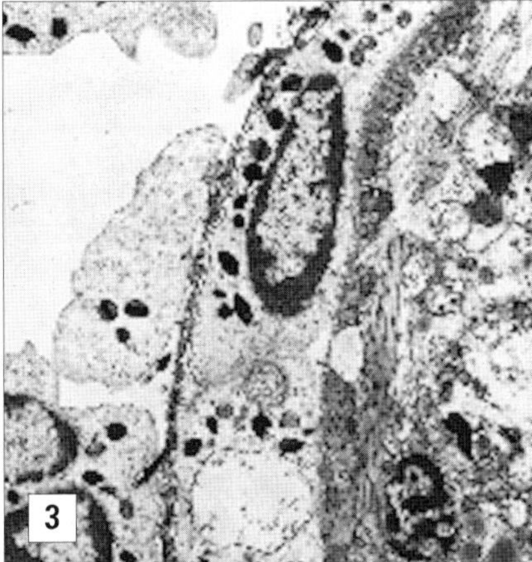

Fig. 16.6 Killing of schistosome larvae by eosinophils. Eosinophils can adhere to schistosomules and kill them. The damage is associated with degranulation of the eosinophils and the release of the contents of the granules onto the surface of the worm. This series of electron micrographs shows adherence of the eosinophils and degranulation onto the surface of the worm larva (**1**), and stages in the breakup of the worm tegument and migration of eosinophils through the lesions (**2** and **3**). (Courtesy of Dr D. McLaren.)

by which they mediate antibody-dependent cytotoxicity associated with IgE.

PIVOTAL ROLE OF T CELLS IN THE DEVELOPMENT OF IMMUNITY

In most parasitic infections, protection can be conferred experimentally on normal animals by the transfer of spleen cells, especially T cells, from immune animals. The T-cell requirement is also demonstrable by the way in which nude (athymic) or T-deprived mice fail to clear otherwise non-lethal infections of protozoa such as *T. cruzi* or *P. yoelii*, and by the way T-deprived rats fail to expel the intestinal worm *Nippostrongylus brasiliensis* (*Fig. 16.7*). However, it should be noted that in some cases transfer of T cells from acutely infected animals can suppress the protective response and cause the death of the recipients. This is because these T cells secrete IL-4 and IL-10, which inhibit the production and activity of the IFNγ required to activate macrophages and eliminate the parasite.

The role of cytokines in parasitic infections has been elucidated by administering the cytokine to infected animals, or eliminating it either with monoclonal antibodies or from the analysis of mice made transgenic for a particular cytokine, and from mice in which the cytokine gene has been inactivated (*'knockout' mice*). We now know that many cytokines not only act on effector cells to enhance their cytotoxic or cytostatic capabilities but also act as growth factors to increase cell numbers. Thus in malaria, the monocytosis and the characteristic enlargement of the spleen, caused by an enormous increase in cell numbers, are T-cell dependent. Other examples include the accumulation of macrophages in the granulomas that develop in the liver in schistosomiasis, the eosinophilia characteristic of helminth infections, and the recruitment of eosinophils and mast cells into the gut mucosa that occurs in worm infections of the gastrointestinal tract. Mucosal mast cells and eosinophils, both important in determining the outcome of some helminth infections, proliferate in response to the products of T cells: IL-3 and GM–CSF, and IL-5, respectively.

However, an increase in cell number can itself harm the host. Thus administration of IL-3 to mice infected with *Leishmania major* can exacerbate the local infection and increase the dissemination of the parasites, probably through the proliferation of bone marrow precursors of the cells the parasites inhabit.

Both CD4⁺ and CD8⁺ T cells are needed for protection against some parasites

The type of T cell responsible for controlling an infection varies with the parasite and the stage of infection, and depends upon the kinds of cytokine they produce. For example, $CD4^+$ and $CD8^+$ T cells protect against different phases of *Plasmodium* infection: $CD4^+$ T cells mediate immunity against blood stage *P. yoelii* while $CD8^+$ cells protect against the liver stage of *P. berghei*. The action of $CD8^+$ cells is twofold: they secrete IFNγ, which inhibits the multiplication of the parasites within hepatocytes, and they destroy infected hepatocytes. The hepatocytes express MHC class I but not MHC class II, so $CD4^+$ T cells do not recognize them and are not stimulated to secrete IFNγ. Similarly, $CD8^+$ cells do not affect the blood stage parasites because erythrocytes do not express MHC class I.

The immune response against *T. cruzi* depends not only upon $CD4^+$ and $CD8^+$ T cells, but also on NK cells and antibody production; the same is true for the immune response against *T. gondii*. In experiments, $CD8^+$ cells confer protection in mice depleted of $CD4^+$ T cells, both

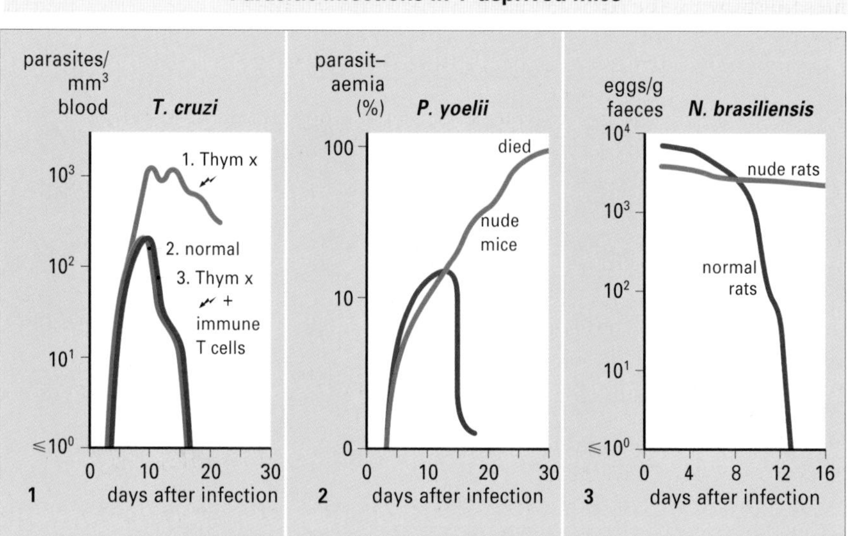

Fig. 16.7 The first two graphs plot the increase in number of blood-borne protozoa (parasitaemia) following infection. **(1)** *Trypanosoma cruzi* multiplies faster (and gives fatal parasitaemia) in mice that have been thymectomized and irradiated to destroy T cells (Thym x). In normal mice, parasites are cleared from the blood by day 16. Reconstitution of T-deprived mice with T cells from immune mice (immune-T) restores their ability to control the parasitaemia. In these experiments both thymectomized groups were given fetal liver cells to restore vital haematopoietic function. **(2)** *Plasmodium yoelii* causes a self-limiting infection in normal mice and the parasites are cleared from the blood by day 20. In nude mice the parasites continue to multiply, killing the mice after about 30 days. **(3)** This graph illustrates the time course of the elimination of the intestinal nematode *Nippostrongylus brasiliensis* from the gut of rats. In normal rats the worms are all expelled by day 13, as determined by the number of worm eggs present in the rats' faeces. T cells are necessary for this expulsion to occur, as shown by the establishment of a chronic infection in the gut of nude rats.

through their production of IFNγ and because they are cytotoxic for infected macrophages. NK cells, stimulated by IL-12 secreted by the macrophages, are another source of IFNγ. Chronic infections are associated with reduced production of IFNγ. These observations probably underlie the high incidence of toxoplasmosis in AIDS patients, who are short of CD4⁺ T cells.

The cytokines produced by CD4⁺ T cells can be important in determining the outcome of *infection*.

T-helper cells have been phenotypically divided into TH1 and TH2 subsets (see Chapter 7) based on the cytokines produced. As TH1 and TH2 cells have contrasting and cross-regulating cytokines profiles, the role of TH1 or TH2 cells in determining the outcomes of parasitic infections have been extensively investigated. As a result of early studies, predominantly in mouse infections, certain dogmas have arisen suggesting that TH1 responses mediate killing of intracellular pathogens and that TH2 responses eliminate extracellular ones. However, this is very much an oversimplication of the true picture. Although the TH1/TH2 paradigm may be a useful tool in some situations it is probably more realistic to consider that TH1 and TH2 phenotypes represent the extremes of a continuum of cytokine profiles and that perhaps it may be more accurate to look at the role of the cytokines themselves in the resolution of infectious disease. Examples of the role of TH1/TH2 cells and the cytokines produced in various parasitic infections will be given. (For a discussion of the cytokines produced by these subsets and the effector mechanisms induced, see Chapters 7–9).

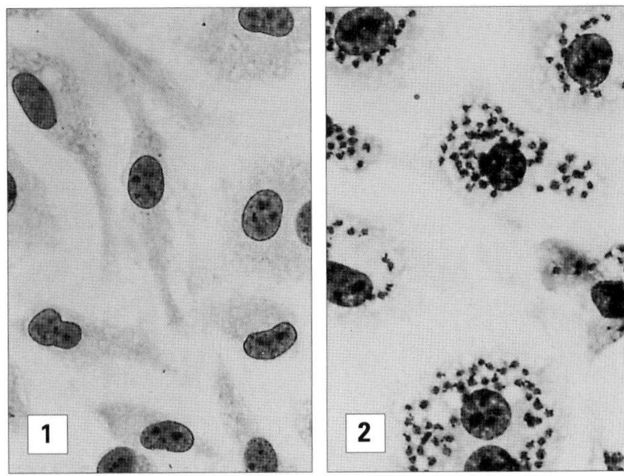

Fig. 16.8 Inhibition of parasite multiplication in macrophages treated with cytokines. Peritoneal macrophages from BALB/c mice, infected 72 hours previously with 10^7 amastigotes of *Leishmania donovani,* were treated with either a supernatant from activated T cells (containing cytokines) or a control supernatant. Cells treated with cytokines do not contain any parasites following culture (**1**), whereas untreated macrophages contain many parasites (**2**). Subsequent studies using recombinant IFNγ and monoclonal antibody against IFNγ showed that the inhibition was mediated by this cytokine. (Courtesy of Dr H. Murray, with permission from *J Immunol* 1982;**129**:344–357, © American Association of Immunologists.)

Cytokines produced by TH1 cells enhance protective immunity against some intracellular protozoa

The TH1/TH2 paradigm can be useful in describing the roles of particular T cells in some infections. The effects of IFNγ (produced by TH1 cells) are clearly illustrated by studies on *Leishmania donovani* where resistant strains of mice are shown to control the development of cutaneous lesions through their production of IFNγ (*Fig. 16.8*). In susceptible mice, which develop progressive disease, the role of IL-4 (a TH2 cytokine) is clearly demonstrated by administration of anti-IL-4 antibodies which cures the infection. Since IL-4 downregulates the production of IFNγ the removal of IL-4 allows the expansion of IFNγ-producing cells. Administration of IFNγ to susceptible mice was not in itself able to effect a cure, however, IL-12 (produced by macrophages and B cells) which induces IFNγ production and suppresses IL-4 production was able to effect a cure in the susceptible mice.

In people, diffuse cutaneous leishmaniasis and progressive visceral leishmaniasis are characterized by deficient IFNγ and increased expression of IL-10 (which downregulates TH1 cells). *In vitro,* IL-4 inhibits the IFNγ-induced activity of human monocytes against *L. donovani* (*Fig. 16.9*).

The dependence on IFNγ for protection against other intracellular parasites can also be profound. Experiments where IFNγ was administered to mice with acute *T. cruzi* infection were able to prevent death (*Fig. 16.10*). The IFNγ is not necessarily produced by TH1 cells, however. In *Toxoplasma gondii* infection, the administration of IL-12

Action of TH1 and TH2 cells in *Leishmania* infection

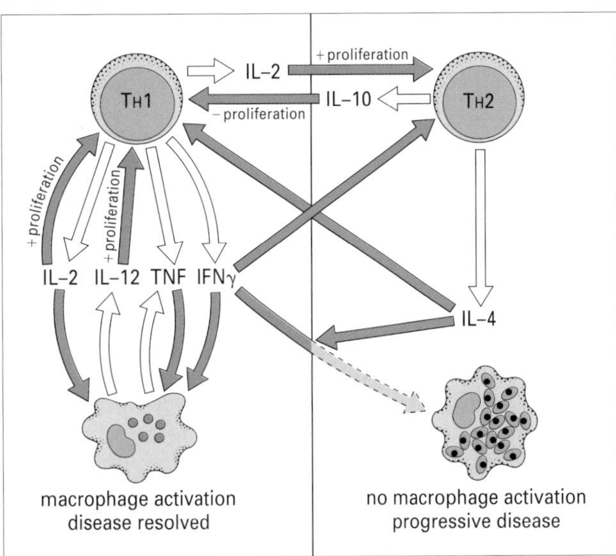

Fig. 16.9 Development of the immune response to *Leishmania* infection illustrating the cytokines secreted by the different subsets of T cells and their effect on the resolution of the disease. Note that IL-12, which is also produced by B cells, promotes the growth of NK cells as well as TH1 cells, and these cells are also a source of IFNγ, the cytokine which is essential for elimination of the parasite.

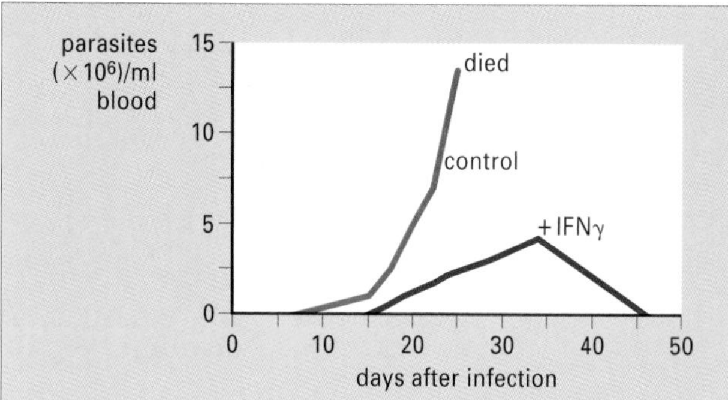

Fig. 16.10 The effect of administration of the T-cell cytokine IFNγ on acute infection caused by *Trypanosoma cruzi.* In this strain of mice, the parasites multiply to kill their host in about 3 weeks. Administration of recombinant mouse IFNγ controls their multiplication which is followed ultimately by their elimination.

to severe combined immunodeficiency mice (SCID) is able to effect a cure and in this situation the IL-12 induces IFNγ by natural killer (NK) cells.

Malaria infection is controlled by multiple cell types

The TH1/TH2 paradigm does not work particularly well in determining the control of effector mechanisms against malaria as it seems different mechanisms are required against different life cycle stages. Infection of liver cells by sporozoites can be prevented by IL-12 and IFNγ and the same cytokines can limit the development of the parasite within the Kupffer cells. In order to eliminate the blood stage parasites, although *P. chabaudi* infection in mice requires TH1 cells to control the peak of parasitaemia, antibodies produced with the help of TH2 cells are critical for the clearance of parasites.

Both TH1 and TH2 responses are important in helminth infections

IgE and eosinophilia are the hallmarks of the immune response to worm infections, and depend upon cytokines secreted by TH2 cells. However, the relative contribution of the TH1 and TH2 subsets in the development of immunity to these parasites is still uncertain. To complicate matters further, responses in mice and rats and people differ, in schistosomiasis at least: in humans, resistance to reinfection after drug treatment is correlated with the production of IgE dependent on TH2 cytokines. In the mouse, IFNγ is needed for vaccine-induced protection and TH2 cells are associated with egg-related immunopathology. The switch to TH2 is triggered by egg antigens.

The pattern of cytokine production in infected hosts may be different from that in vaccinated hosts. For example, in mice infected with *S. mansoni*, IL-5 producing TH2 cells predominate. In mice that have been immunized, IgE levels and eosinophil numbers are low and TH1 cells predominate. IFNγ activates effector cells that destroy lung stage larvae, via the production of nitric oxide. However, when adult worms start to produce eggs, a soluble egg antigen is released that has an effect only in susceptible mice. The antigen reduces levels of IFNγ and increases production of IL-5.

In some parasitic infections, the immune system cannot completely eliminate the parasite, but reacts by isolating the organism with inflammatory cells. The host reacts to locally released antigen which stimulates the release of cytokines that recruit cells to the region. An example of this has been shown in mice vaccinated with radiation-attenuated schistosome cercariae, Infiltrating cells, which are mostly TH1 type lymphocytes, surround the lung-stage larvae as early as 24 hours after intravenous challenge infection (*Fig. 16.11*). This prevents subsequent migration to the site necessary for development into the adult parasite. The schistosome egg granuloma in the liver is another example of the host reacting by 'walling off' the parasite. This reaction is a chronic cell-mediated response to soluble antigens released by eggs that have become trapped in the liver. Macrophages accumulate and release fibrogenic factors that stimulate the formation of granulomatous tissue and, ultimately, fibrosis. Although this reaction may benefit the host, in that it insulates the liver cells from toxins secreted by the worm eggs, it is also the major source of pathology, causing irreversible changes in the liver and the loss of liver function. In the absence of T cells, there is no granuloma formation and no subsequent fibrous encapsulation.

Different mechanisms may affect the worms that inhabit different anatomical sites, such as the gut (e.g. *Trichuris frichura*) or the tissues (e.g. *Onchocerca volvulus*), and at different stages of the life cycle (e.g. schistosome larvae in the lungs and adult worms in the veins).

TH2 cells are clearly necessary for elimination of intestinal worms

Experiments have shown that TH2 controlled effector mechanisms are important in intestinal worm infections. For example, mice normally resistant to infection by a murine whipworm develop persistent infection if IL-4 is neutralized. Conversely, susceptible mice expel the worms if IL-4 activity is promoted by administration of neutralizing antibody against IFNγ. Similarly, administration of IL-12 to rats soon after infection with the intestinal worm *N. brasiliensis* stimulates IFNγ production, and delays expulsion of the worms. IL-12 acts by inhibiting the production of TH2 cytokines, in particular IL-4 and IL-5, and thus prevents the production of IgE and the hypertrophy of intestinal mast cells, mediated by IL-4, and the development of the eosinophilia, which is mediated by IL-5.

What is clear from a number of studies is that there is no single mechanism by which a TH2 response mediates expulsion of all intestinal worms. The species of worm, its anatomical position within the gut and the immune status of the host are all factors likely to influence whether a particular immune mechanism will be effective at promoting worm loss. For example, in the case of *Trichinella spiralis* there is good evidence to suggest the involvement of mucosal mast cells. Mast cells contain a number of lipid mediators, such as prostaglandins (see Chapter 21), proteases and histamine. In addition, they also represent a source of

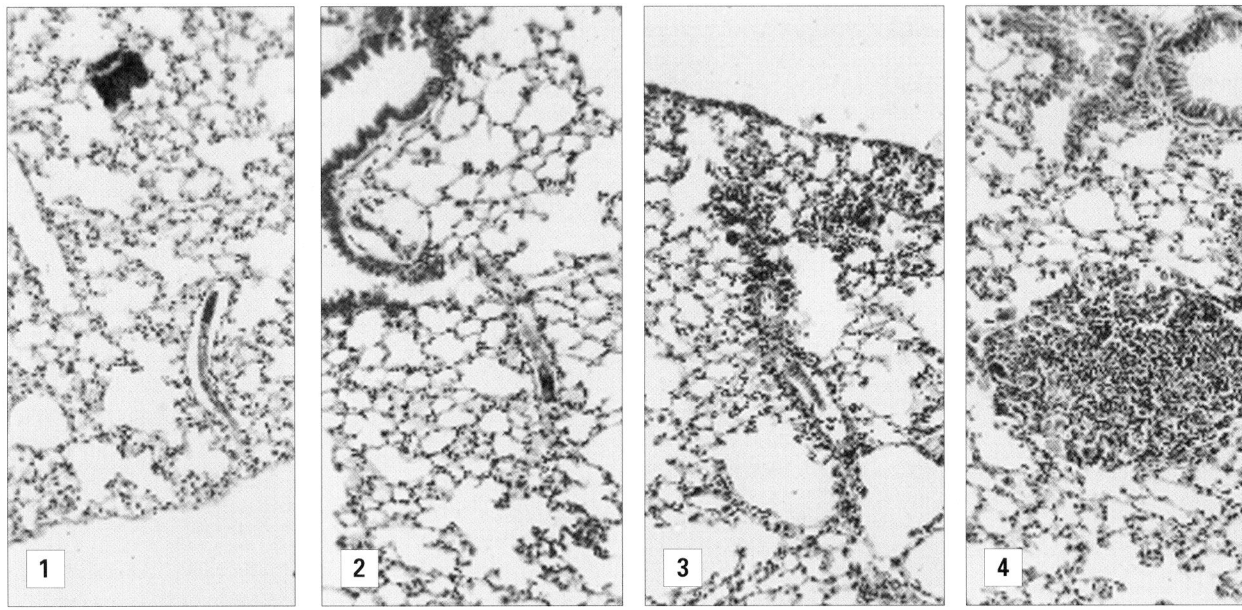

Fig. 16.11 Photomicrographs of mouse lung tissue showing pulmonary foci around migrating schistosomula of *Schistosoma mansoni*. Lung schistosomula were administered intravenously; panel (**1**) shows a challenge larva in the naive mouse at 24 h. In mice protected by vaccination with radiation-attenuated cercariae, infiltrating cells appear as early as 24 h (**2**). Panels (**3**) and (**4**) show the development of foci 2 and 12 days post-challenge. Bronchoalveolar sampling and immunocytochemistry have revealed that CD4 T lymphocytes are a major component of the pulmonary infiltrates. IFNγ is the dominant cytokine produced by these cells in culture and mRNA for IFNγ is induced in whole lung tissue, from which it can be inferred that the protective response is mediated by TH1 cells. (Courtesy of Dr Lesley Smythies with permission from *Parasite Immunol* 1996;**18**:359–69.)

cytokines such as IL-3, IL-4, IL-5, GM–CSF and TNFα. Consequently, following mast cell activation their contents are released resulting in changes to the permeability of the intestinal epithelium and ultimately an environment which appears hostile for continued *T. spiralis* survival. By contrast, expulsion of *N. brasiliensis* still proceeds normally following depression of mastocytosis, suggesting that the mast cell is not the major effector cell type. Therefore although TH2 cytokines are critical for the elimination of worms from the gut, the exact effector mechanism operating may vary (*Fig. 16.12*).

Parasites induce non-specific and specific antibody production

Many parasitic infections provoke a non-specific hypergammaglobulinaemia, much of which is probably due to substances released from the parasites acting as B-cell mitogens. Level of total immunoglobulins are raised: IgM in trypanosomiasis and malaria, IgG in malaria and visceral leishmaniasis. The relative importance of antibody-dependent and antibody-independent responses varies with the infection (*Fig. 16.13*). The mechanisms by which specific antibody can control parasitic infections and its effects are summarized in *Figure 16.14* and are as follows:

- Antibody can act directly on protozoa to damage them, either by itself or by activating the complement system (*Fig. 16.15*).
- Antibody can neutralize a parasite directly by blocking its attachment to a new host cell, as with *Plasmodium* spp., whose merozoites enter red blood cells through a special receptor: their entry is inhibited by specific antibody (*Fig. 16.16*). Antibody may also act to prevent spread, for example in the acute phase of infection by *T. cruzi*.
- Antibody can enhance phagocytosis by macrophages. Phagocytosis is increased even more by the addition of complement. These effects are mediated by Fc and C3 receptors on the macrophages, which may increase in number as a result of macrophage activation.
- Antibody is also involved in antibody-dependent cell-mediated cytotoxicity, for example, in infections caused by *T. cruzi, T. spiralis, S. mansoni* and filarial worms. Cytotoxic cells such as macrophages, neutrophils and eosinophils adhere to antibody-coated worms by means of their Fc and C3 receptors and exocytose in apposition to the parasite.

Different antibody isotypes may have different effects. As mentioned previously, in individuals infected with schistosomes parasite-specific IgE is associated with resistance to infection and there is an inverse relationship between the amount of IgE in their blood and reinfection. IgG4 appears to block the action of IgE; reinfection is more likely in children who have high levels of IgG4. The development of immunity seems to depend upon a switch from IgG4 to IgE that occurs with age; infection rates are highest in 10- to 14-year-olds, when IgG4 levels are also at their highest.

In many infections it is difficult to distinguish between cell-mediated and antibody-mediated responses, since both act in concert against the parasite. This is illustrated in

Processes involved in expulsion of nematodes from the gut

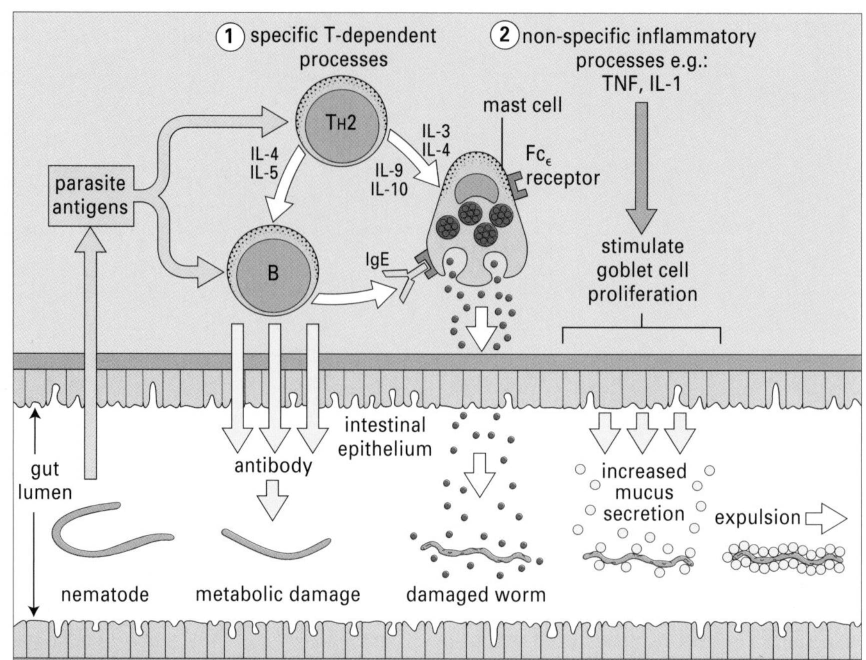

Fig. 16.12 The expulsion of some intestinal nematodes occurs spontaneously a few weeks after primary infection. There seem to be two stages in the expulsion, which is achieved by a combination of T-dependent and T-independent mechanisms. (**1**) T cells (predominantly TH2 cells) respond to parasite antigens and induce (a) the production of antibody by B cells that have proliferated in response to IL-4 and IL-5, (b) the proliferation of mucosal mast cells, in response to IL-3, IL-4, IL-9 and IL-10, and (c) hyperplasia of mucus-secreting goblet cells in the intestinal epithelium. The worms are damaged by antibody together with products of IgE-sensitized mast cells which degranulate following contact with antigen, and so release histamine which increases the permeability of the intestinal epithelium. These processes are not sufficient to eliminate the worms. (**2**) Non-specific inflammatory molecules secreted by macrophages, including TNF and IL-1, contribute to goblet cell proliferation and cause increased secretion of mucus. The mucus coats the worms and leads to their expulsion. The numbers of goblet cells in the jejunal epithelium and the secretion of mucus increase in proportion to the worm burden. The antigen-specific effector T cells are generated early in infection and the rate-limiting step is the onset of antibody damage. The relative importance of these various processes varies with the infecting nematode.

Relative importance of antibody-dependent and -independent responses in protozoal infections

parasite and habitat	antibody-dependent			antibody-independent	
	importance	mechanism	means of evasion	importance	mechanism
T. brucei free in blood	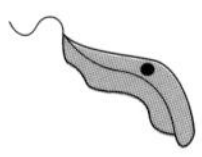 + + + +	lysis with complement which also opsonizes for phagocytosis	antigenic variation	–	
Plasmodium inside red cell	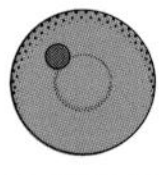 + + +	blocks invasion, opsonizes for phagocytosis	intracellular; antigenic variation	liver stage + + + blood stage + + +	cytokines macrophage activation
T. cruzi inside macrophage	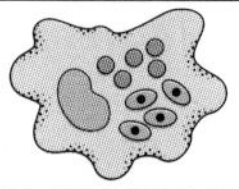 + +	limits spread in acute infection, sensitizes for ADCC	intracellular	+ + + (chronic phase)	macrophage activation by IFNγ and TNFα, and killing by NO and metabolites of O_2
Leishmania inside macrophage	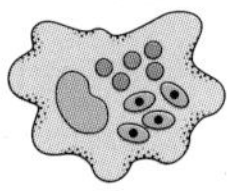 +	limits spread	intracellular	+ + + +	

Fig. 16.13 This table summarizes the relative importance of the two immune responses, the mechanisms involved and, for antibody, the means by which the protozoan can evade damage by antibody. Antibody is the most important part of the immune response against those parasites that live in the bloodstream, such as African trypanosomes and malarial parasites, whereas cell-mediated immunity is active against those like *Leishmania* that live in the tissues. Antibody can damage parasites directly, enhance their clearance by phagocytosis, activate complement or block their entry into their host cell and so limit the spread of infection. Once inside, the parasite is safe from its effects. *Trypanosoma cruzi* and *Leishmania* are both susceptible to the action of oxygen metabolites release by the respiratory burst of macrophages, and to nitric oxide. Treating macrophages with cytokines enhances release of these products and diminishes entry and survival of the parasites. Malarial parasites within the red cell may be destroyed by some secreted products of activated macrophages, including hydrogen peroxide and other cytotoxic factors.

Mechanisms by which specific antibody controls some parasitic infections

parasite	*Plasmodium* sporozoite, intestinal worms, trypanosome	*Plasmodium* sporozoite and merozoite, *Trypanosoma cruzi, Toxoplasma gondii*	*Plasmodium*, trypanosome	schistosomes, *Trichinella spiralis*, filarial worm larvae
mechanism	1 complement protein 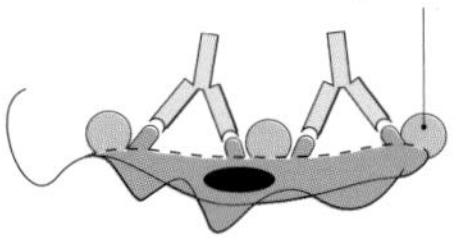	2 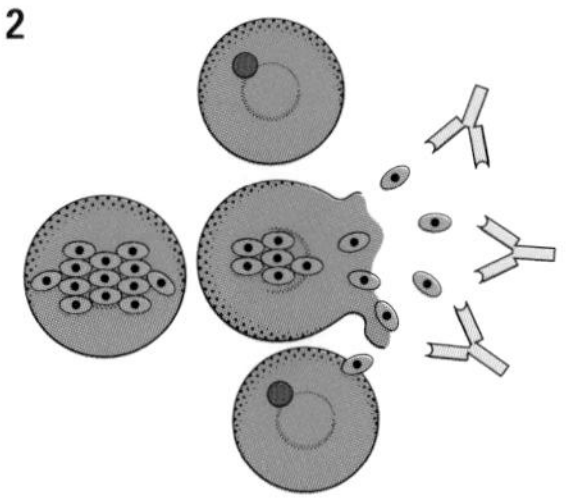	3 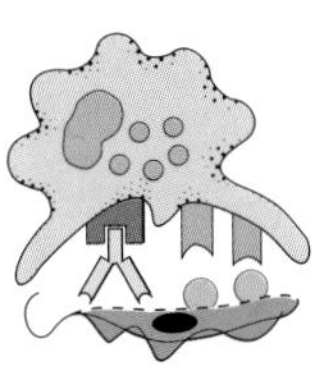	4 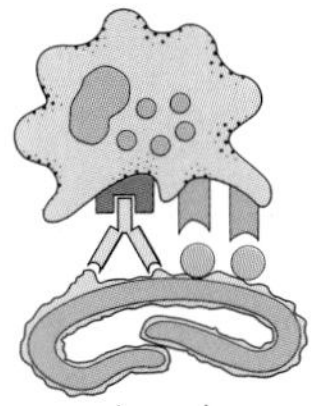 larval worm
effect	direct damage or complement-mediated lysis	prevents spread by neutralizing attachment site, prevents escape from lysosomal vacuole, prevents inhibition of lysosomal fusion	enhancement of phagocytosis	antibody-dependent cell-mediated cytotoxicity (ADCC)

Fig. 16.14 (**1**) Direct damage. Antibody activates the classical complement pathway, causing damage to the parasite membrane and increasing susceptibility to other mediators.
(**2**) Neutralization. Parasites such as *Plasmodium* spp. spread to new cells by specific receptor attachment; blocking the merozoite binding site with antibody prevents attachment to the receptors on the erythrocyte surface and hence prevents further multiplication.
(**3**) Enhancement of phagocytosis. Complement C3b deposited on parasite membrane opsonizes it for phagocytosis by cells with C3b receptors (for example macrophages). Macrophages also have Fc receptors.
(**4**) Eosinophils, neutrophils, platelets and macrophages may be cytotoxic for some parasites when they recognize the parasite via specific antibody (ADCC). The reaction is enhanced by complement.

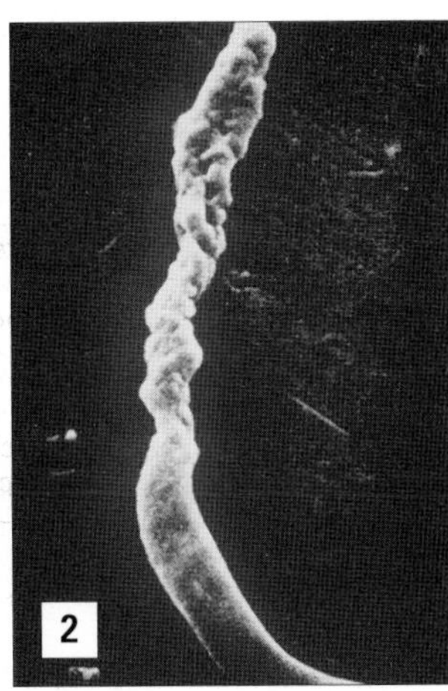

Fig. 16.15 Direct effect of specific antibody on sporozoites of malaria parasites. These scanning electron micrographs show a sporozoite of *Plasmodium berghei*, which causes malaria in rodents, before (**1**) and after (**2**) incubation in immune serum. The surface of the sporozoite is damaged by the antibody which perturbs the outer membrane, causing leakage of fluid. Specific antibody protects against infection with *Plasmodium* spp. at several of the extracellular stages of the life cycle. The antibody is stage specific in each case. (Courtesy of Dr R. Nussenzweig.)

Effect of antibody on malarial parasites

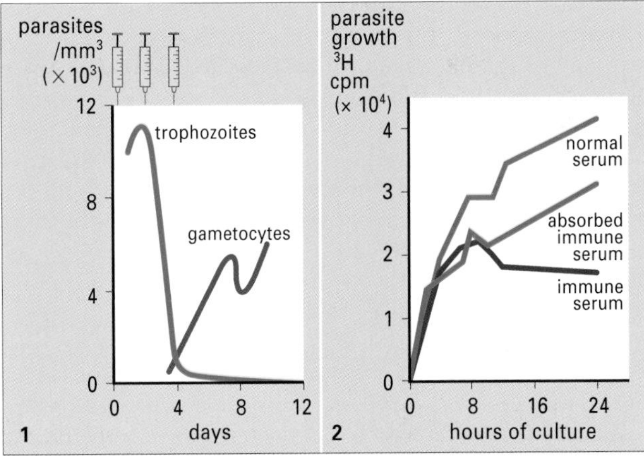

Fig. 16.16 (**1**) Transfer of γ-globulin from immune adults to a child infected with *Plasmodium falciparum* caused a sharp drop in parasitaemia. Specific antibody acts at the merozoite stage in the life of the parasite and prevents the initiation of further cycles of multiplication in the blood. The development of gametocytes from existing intracellular forms is unaffected.
(**2**) In culture, the presence of immune serum blocks the continued increase in number of *P. knowlesi* (a malarial parasite of monkeys), as measured by incorporation of ^{3}H-leucine. It stops multiplication at the stage after schizont rupture by preventing the released merozoites from invading fresh red blood cells. The inhibitory activity of the immune serum can be reduced by prior absorption of the specific antibody with free schizonts.

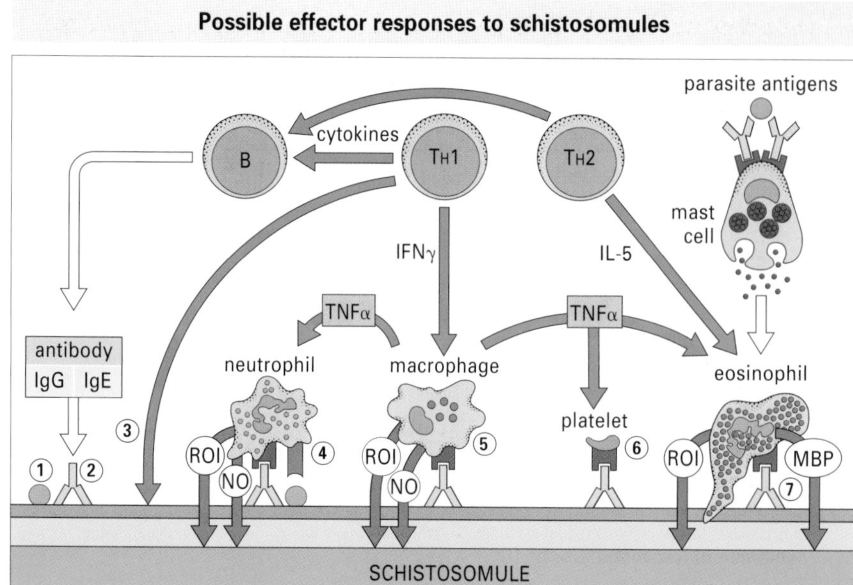

Fig. 16.17 This diagram illustrates the various effector mechanisms that have been shown to damage schistosomes *in vitro*. Complement alone damages worms (**1**) and also does so in combination with antibody (**2**). TH1 cells may act directly inhibiting the degree of larvae in the lungs (**3**). Antibody sensitizes neutrophils (**4**), macrophages (**5**), platelets (**6**) and eosinophils (**7**) for antibody-dependent cell-mediated cytotoxicity. Neutrophils and macrophages probably act by releasing toxic oxygen and nitrogen metabolites, whereas eosinophils damage the worm tegument by release of major basic protein plus reactive oxygen intermediates. The response is potentiated by cytokines (e.g. TNFα). IgE antibody is important both in sensitizing eosinophils and local mast cells, which release a variety of mediators, including those that activate the eosinophils.

Figure 16.17 which summarizes the immune reaction that can be mounted against schistosome larvae.

ESCAPE MECHANISMS

It is a necessary characteristic of all succesful parasitic infections that they can evade the full effects of their host's immune responses; parasites have developed many different ways of doing this. Some even exploit cells and molecules of the immune system to their own advantage: *Leishmania* parasites, by using complement receptors to effect their entry into macrophages, avoid triggering the oxidative burst and thus destruction by its toxic products.

Despite their protective role in the immune response to many different parasites, host TNFα actually stimulates egg production by adult worms of *S. mansoni*, while IFNγ is used as a growth factor by *T. brucei.*

Parasites can resist destruction by complement

In the case of *Leishmania*, such resistance correlates with virulence. *L. tropica*, which is easily killed by complement, causes a localized self-healing infection in the skin, whereas *L. donovani*, which is ten times more resistant to complement, becomes disseminated throughout the viscera, causing a disease that is often fatal.

The mechanisms whereby parasites can resist the effect of complement differ. The lipophosphoglycan surface coat of *L. major* activates complement, but the complex is then shed so the parasite avoids lysis. The trypomastigotes of *T. cruzi* bear a surface glycoprotein which has activity resembling the decay accelerating factor (DAF) that limits the complement reaction (see Chapter 3). The resistance schistosomules acquire as they mature is also correlated with the appearance of a surface molecule similar to DAF.

Intracellular parasites avoid destruction by various means

Those that live inside macrophages have evolved different ways of avoiding being killed by oxygen metabolites and lysosomal enzymes (*Figs 16.18 and 16.19*). *T. gondii* penetrates the macrophage by a non-phagocytic pathway (*Fig. 16.19*) and so avoids triggering the oxidative burst; *Leishmania* spp. can enter by binding to complement receptors – another way of avoiding the respiratory burst. *Leishmania* organisms also possess enzymes such as superoxide dismutase which protects them against the action of oxygen radicals. It can be demonstrated that the vacuole in which *Leishmania* organisms survive is lyosomal in nature (*Fig. 16.20*) but the parasites have evolved mechanisms which protect it against enzymatic attack. The lipophosphoglycan surface coat not only acts as a scavenger of oxygen metabolites and affords protection against enzymatic attack, but a glycoprotein, Gp63 (*Fig. 16.21*), inhibits the action of the macrophage's lysosomal enzymes. *Leishmania* spp. can also downregulate the expression of MHC class II on the macrophages they inhabit, thus reducing their capacity to stimulate TH cells. These escape mechanisms, however, are less efficient in the immune host.

Parasites can disguise themselves

Parasites that are vulnerable to specific antibody have evolved different methods of evading its effects. The African trypanosome undergoes antigenic variation: the molecule that forms its surface coat, the variable surface glycoprotein (VSG) changes to protect the underlying surface membrane from the host's defence mechanisms. New populations of parasites are antigenically distinct from previous ones (*Figs 16.22 and 16.23*). Several antigens of malarial parasites also undergo antigenic variation.

Other parasites, such as schistosomes, acquire a surface

The different means by which protozoa that multiply within macrophages escape digestion by lysosomal enzymes

Toxoplasma gondii	*Trypanosoma cruzi*	*Leishmania*
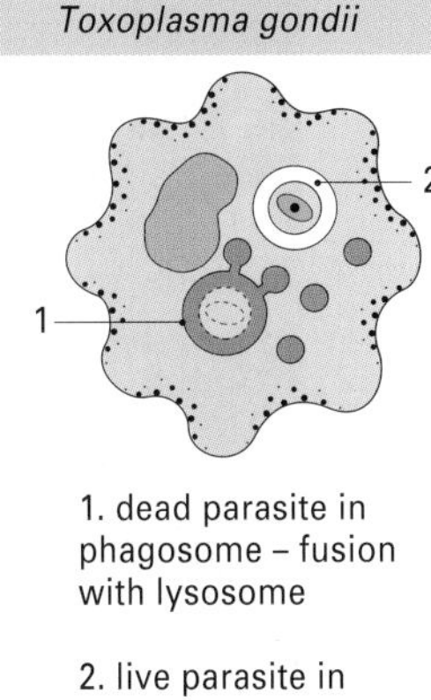	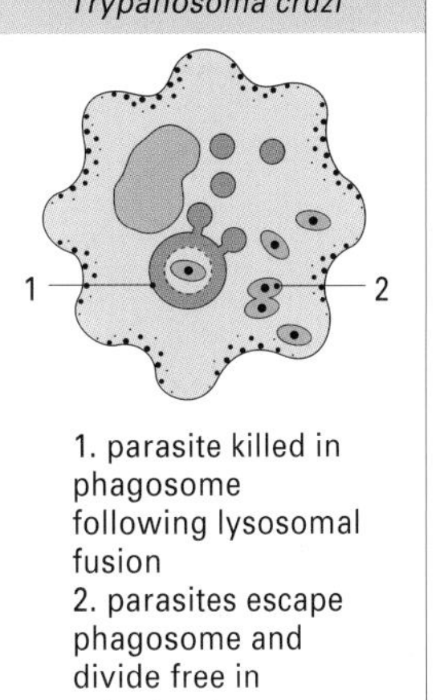	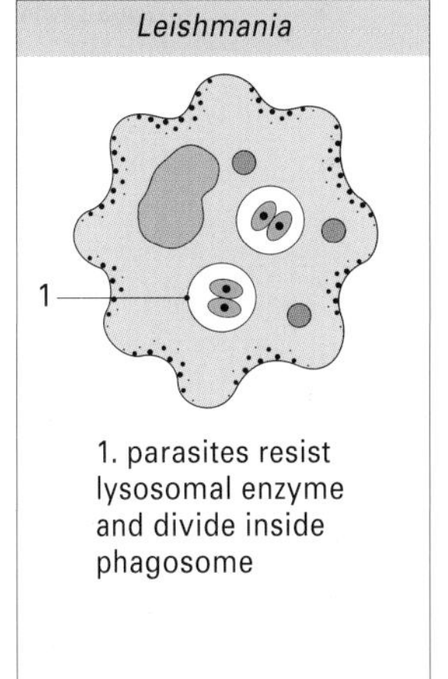
1. dead parasite in phagosome – fusion with lysosome 2. live parasite in endosome – no fusion with lysosome	1. parasite killed in phagosome following lysosomal fusion 2. parasites escape phagosome and divide free in cytoplasm	1. parasites resist lysosomal enzyme and divide inside phagosome

Fig. 16.18 *Toxoplasma gondii.* Live parasites enter the cell actively into a membrane-bound vacuole. They are not attacked by enzymes because lysosomes do not fuse with this vacuole. Dead parasites, however, are taken up by normal phagocytosis into a phagosome (by interaction with the Fc receptors on the macrophage if they are coated with antibody) and they are then destroyed by the enzymes of the lysosomes which fuse with it.
Trypanosoma cruzi. Survival of these parasites depends upon their stage of development; trypomastigotes escape from the phagosome and divide in the cytoplasm whereas epimastigotes do not escape and are killed. The proportion of parasites found in the cytoplasm is decreased if the macrophages are activated.
Leishmania spp. These parasites multiply within the phagosome and the presence of a surface protease helps them resist digestion. If the macrophages are first activated by cytokines the number of parasites entering the cell and the number that replicate diminish.

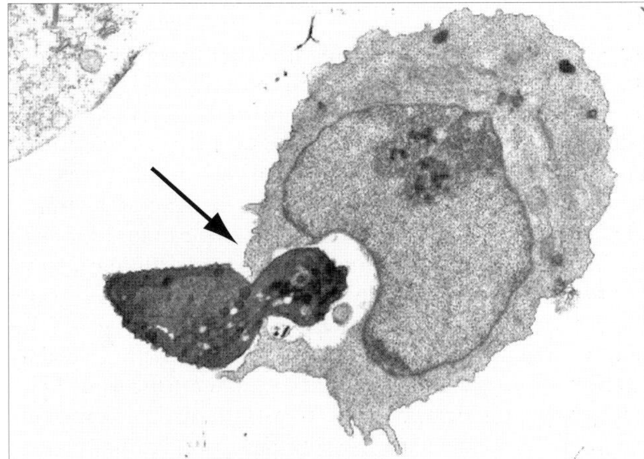

Fig. 16.19 Electron micrograph of *Toxoplasma gondii* actively invading the host cell. During invasion the parasite forms a tight junction with the host cell membrane (arrowed) and modifies the newly formed phagosome to inhibit subsequent lysosomal fusion. (Courtesy of Dr Judith Smith.)

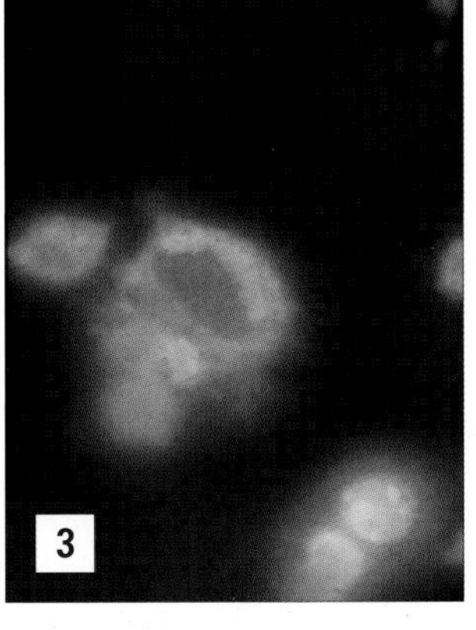

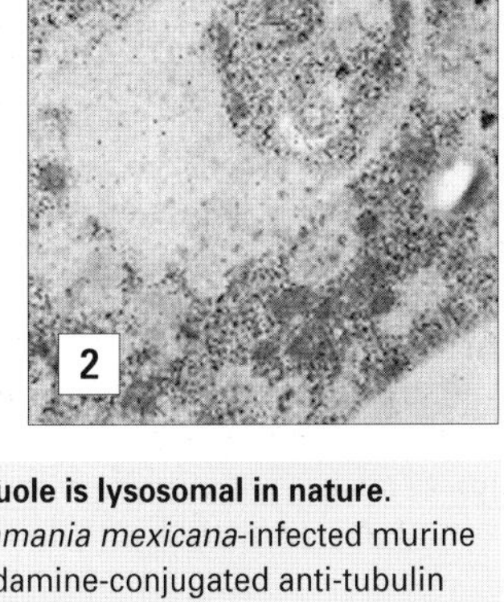

Fig. 16.20 The Leishmanial vacuole is lysosomal in nature. (**1**) Immunofluorescence of *Leishmania mexicana*-infected murine macrophages probed with a rhodamine-conjugated anti-tubulin antibody to illustrate the parasite (stained yellow/red) and a fluorescein-conjugated monoclonal antibody which reacts with the late endosomal/lysosomal marker LAMP-1 (stained green). (**2**) Immunoelectron micrograph of *L. mexicana*-infected murine macrophage probed with gold-labelled anti-cathepsin D demonstrating the lysosomal aspartic proteinase in the leishmanial vacuole. (Courtesy of Dr David Russell.)

layer of host antigens, so that the host does not distinguish them from 'self'. Schistosomules cultured in medium containing human serum and red blood cells can acquire surface molecules containing A, B and H blood-group determinants. They can also acquire MHC molecules. However, schistosomules maintained in medium devoid of host molecules also become resistant to attack by antibody and complement, as mentioned before.

Some extracellular parasites hide from immune attack

Some species of protozoa (e.g. *Entamoeba histolytica*) and of helminths (e.g. *T. spiralis*) form protective cysts, while adult worms of *O. volvulus* in the skin induce the host to surround them with collagenous nodules. Intestinal nematodes and tapeworms are preserved from many host responses simply because they are in the gut.

Two surface antigens of *Leishmania*

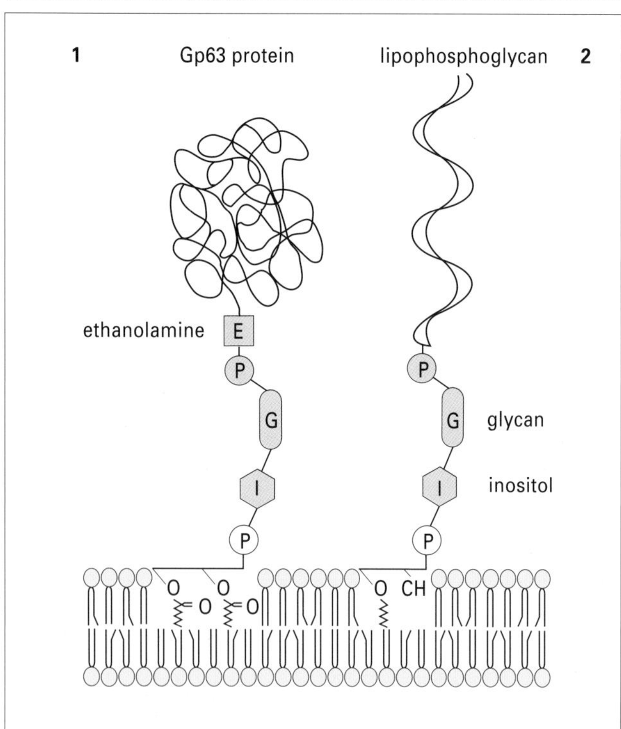

Fig. 16.21 Schematic representation of two surface antigens of *Leishmania* that are anchored to the membrane by phosphatidylinositol tails (GPI anchors).
(**1**) This protein antigen, Gp63, has protease activity. That of *L. mexicana,* together with a lipophosphoglycan (LPG), binds complement. This enables the promastigote to enter the macrophage through the C3 complement receptor.
(**2**) This glycolipid antigen, a lipophosphoglycan, imparts resistance to complement-mediated lysis. That of *L. major* binds C3b, the third component of complement, enabling the promastigote to enter through the CR1 complement receptor. Antibodies to both antigens confer protection against murine cutaneous leishmaniasis.
Note that many coat proteins of parasites, such as the variable surface glycoprotein (VSG) of *T. brucei,* are now known to be bound to the surface membrane by a GPI anchor.

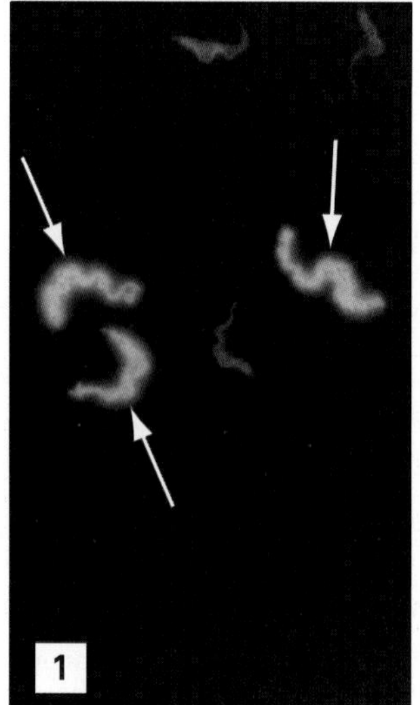

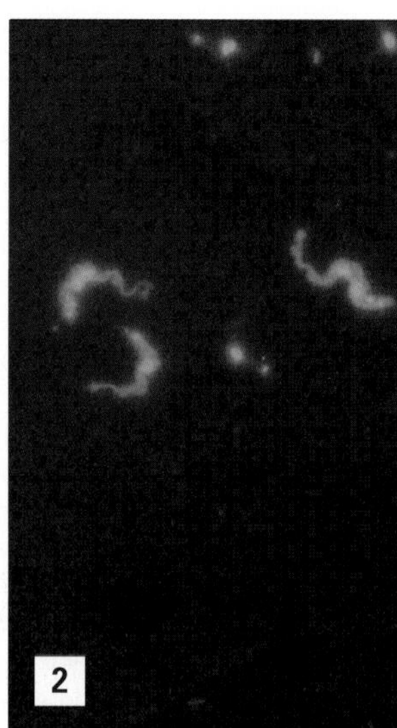

Fig. 16.22 Antigenic variation in trypanosomes. Immunofluorescent labelling of trypanosomes with a variant antigen-type specific monoclonal antibody (**1**). Panel (**2**) shows the same field of view where the nuclei and kinetoplasts of all the parasites are stained with a dye that binds to DNA. Only some of the parasites express a given antigen variant (arrowed). (Courtesy of Dr Mike Turner.)

Some extracellular parasites can withstand immune attack

There are numerous examples of simple, physical, protective strategies in parasites: nematodes have a thick extracellular cuticle which protects them from toxic onslaught (*Fig. 16.24*); the tegument of schistosomes thickens during maturation to offer similar protection; the loose surface coat of many nematodes may slough off under immune attack; tapeworms actually prevent attack by secreting an elastase inhibitor, which stops them attracting neutrophils.

Many parasitic worms have evolved methods of resisting the oxidative burst. For instance, schistosomes have surface-associated glutathione S-transferases, and *Onchocerca* can secrete superoxide dismutase. Some nematodes and trematodes have evolved an elegant method of disabling antibodies by secreting proteases which cleave immunoglobulins, removing the Fc portion.

Most parasites interfere with the immune response

Immunosuppression is a universal feature of parasite infection (*Fig. 16.25*) and has been demonstrated for both antibody- and cell-mediated responses. Although some parasites can cause disruption of lymphoid cells directly (e.g. newly hatched larvae of *T. spiralis*, which release a soluble lymphotoxic factor), much of the suppression may be due to interference with macrophage function. Work using implanted infections of *B. malayi* into the peritoneal cavity of mice has shown that a macrophage population can be induced which suppresses T-cell proliferation even though antigen-specific cytokine production continues in these cells. There is also considerable evidence that parasites affect antigen presentation; thus macrophages from schistosome- and African trypanosome-infected mice are defective at presenting antigen.

Parasites produce molecules which interfere with host immune function

Phosphorylcholine (PC) containing molecules are commonly found in infectious organisms and experiments using a nematode PC-bearing glycoconjugate have shown that proliferation by both T cells and B cells can be inhibited. This molecule causes a decreases in the level of protein kinase-C and can render both B and T cells anergic. Parasites also produce cytokine-like molecules mimicking TGFβ, migration inhibition factor (MIF) and a histamine-releasing factor. Genes encoding possible cytokine homologues are being found as part of the genome sequencing

Antigenic variation in African trypanosomes

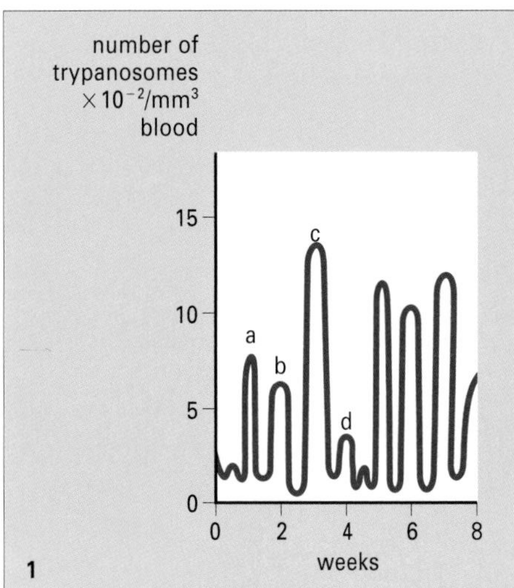

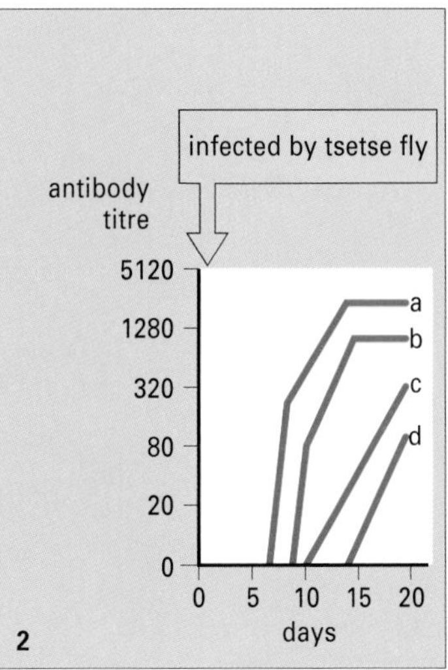

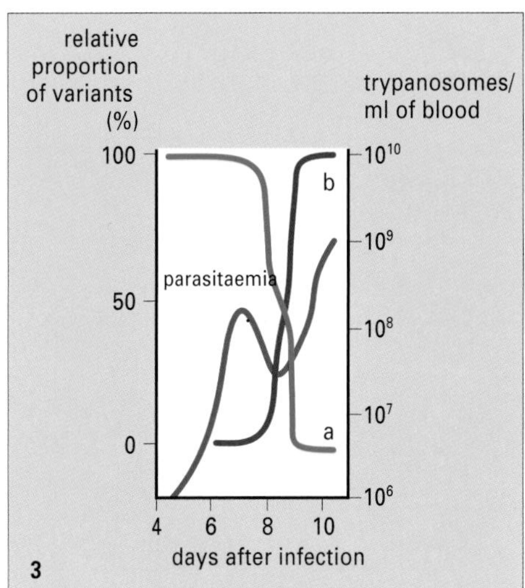

Fig. 16.23 Trypanosome infections may run for several months giving rise to successive waves of parasitaemia.
Graph (**1**) shows a chart of the fluctuation in parasitaemia in a patient with sleeping sickness. Although infection was initiated by a single parasite, each wave is caused by an immunologically distinct population of parasites (a,b,c,d); protection is not afforded by antibody against any of the preceding variants. There is a strong tendency for new variants to appear in the same order in different hosts. Variation does not occur in immunologically compromised animals (that is, animals treated to deprive them of some aspect of immune function).
Graph (**2**) shows the time-course of production of antibody against four variants in a rabbit bitten by a tsetse fly carrying *Trypanosoma brucei*. Antibody to successive variants appears shortly after the appearance of each variant and rises to a plateau. The appearance of antibody drives the parasite towards another variant type.
Graph (**3**) shows the kinetics of one cycle of antigenic variation. A rat was infected with a homogeneous population of one variant (a) of *T. brucei*. The second wave of parasitaemia develops as the new variant (b) emerges and predominates.

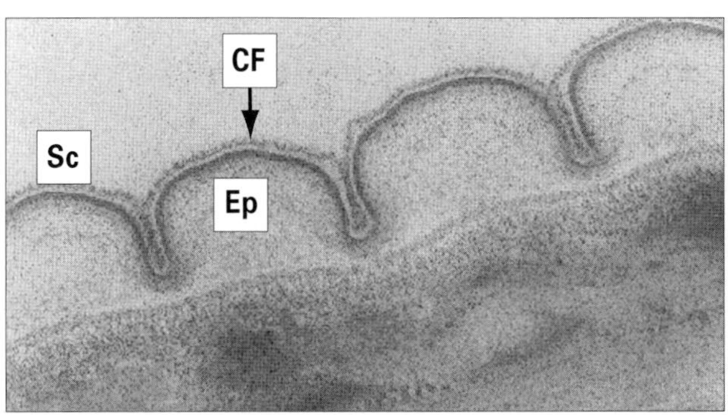

Fig. 16.24 Electron micrograph of an infective larva of *Toxocara canis* illustrating the surface coat (Sc) bound with cationized ferritin (CF) overlying the epicuticle (Ep). Larvae were fixed with glutaraldehyde and osmium tetroxide before processing for electron micrography. (Courtesy of Professor Rick Maizels with permission from *Exp Parasitol* 1992;**75**:72–86.)

projects that are underway for many parasites. Although the sequences are related to cytokines or cytokine receptors their functions remain to be established. Filarial worms secrete a protease inhibitor which has been shown to affect the proteases that are critical in the processing of proteins to peptides and is thus causative in the reduction of class II presentation in this infection.

Soluble parasite antigens released in huge quantities may impair the host's response by a process termed immune distraction. Thus the soluble antigens (S- or heat-stable antigens) of *P. falciparum* are thought to mop up circulating antibody, providing a 'smokescreen' and diverting the antibody from the body of the parasite. Many of the surface antigens that are shed are soluble forms of molecules inserted into the parasite membrane by a GPI anchor, including the VSG of *T. brucei*, the LPG or 'excreted factor' of *Leishmania* (*Fig. 16.21*) and several surface antigens of schistosomules. These are released by endogenous phosphatidylinositol-specific phospholipases.

Antigen-specific suppression also occurs by affecting the balance of cytokines produced by CD4$^+$ T cells to the parasite's advantage. Thus in leishmaniasis, T cells from patients infected with *L. donovani* when cultured with specific antigen do not secrete IL-2 or IFNγ. Their production of IL-1 and expression of MHC class II is also decreased, whereas secretion of prostaglandins is increased. IL-2, characteristic of TH1 responses, is also deficient in other protozoal infections including malaria, African trypanosomiasis and Chagas' disease. In mice infected with *T. cruzi*, a parasite product appears to interfere with expression of the IL-2 receptor. Helminth infections are characterized by the host having TH2-dominated responses involving IL-4, IL-5, IL-9 and IL-13 production and high levels of IgG4 which block protective IgE responses. The ability of helminths to drive TH2 type responses remains to be explained but there are a number of possibilities. The antigen-presenting cell, in particular the dendritic cell which presents antigen to the T cell appears to play a

Interference with host's immune response by free antigens released by protozoa or worms

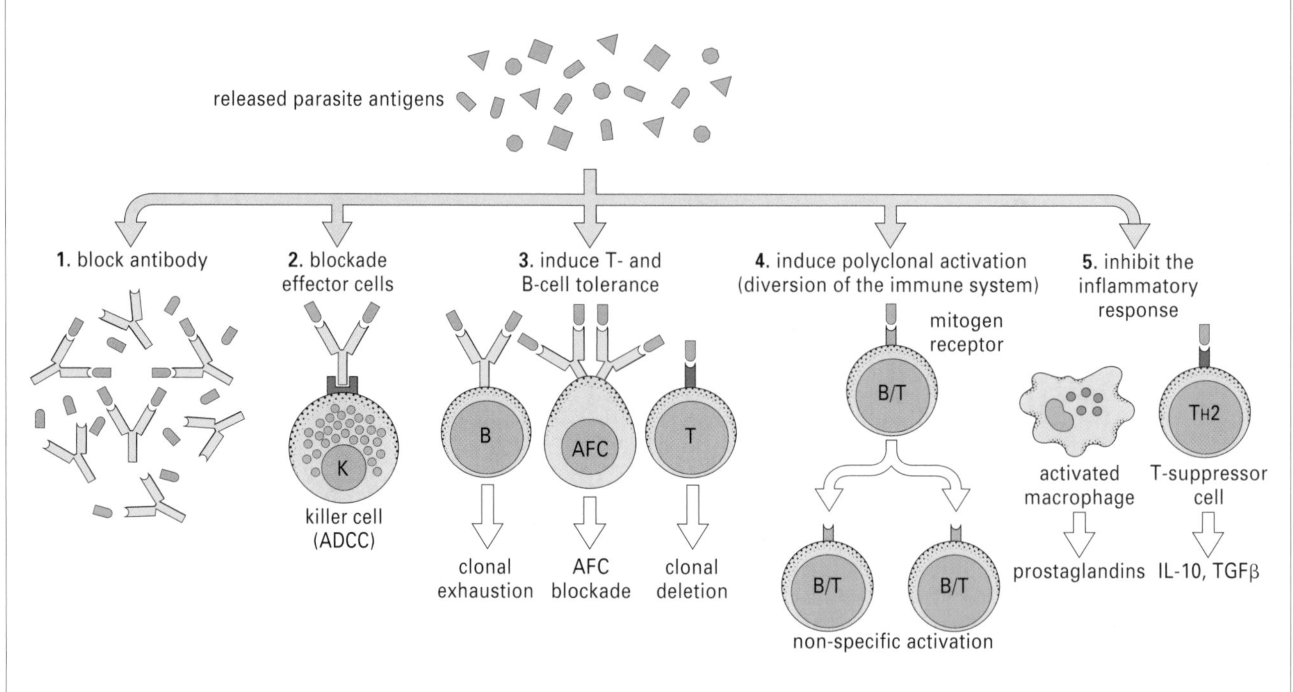

Fig. 16.25 Free antigens can:
(**1**) Combine with antibody and divert it from the parasite. The variant surface glycoprotein of *Trypanosoma brucei* and the soluble antigens of *Plasmodium falciparum,* which are also polymorphic and contain repetitive sequences of amino acids, are thought to act in this way as a smokescreen or decoy.
(**2**) Blockade effector cells, either directly or as immune complexes. Circulating complexes, for example, are able to inhibit the action of cytotoxic cells active against *Schistosoma mansoni.*
(**3**) Induce T- or B-cell tolerance, presumably by blockage of antibody-forming cells (AFC) or by depletion of the mature antigen-specific lymphocytes through clonal exhaustion or by induction of anergy.
(**4**) Cause polyclonal activation. Many parasite products are mitogenic to B or T cells, and the high serum concentrations of non-specific IgM (and IgG) commonly found in parasitic infections probably result from this polyclonal stimulation. Its continuation is believed to lead to impairment of B-cell function, the progressive depletion of antigen-reactive B lymphocytes and thus immunosuppression.
(**5**) Activate T cells, especially TH2 cells, or macrophages, or both, to release immunosuppressive molecules.

pivotal role in determining the final response phenotype. There is also evidence that certain parasite antigens have the ability to induce TH2 cytokines or IgE in isolation from the infection when injected as a soluble preparation.

Some of the escape mechanisms discussed above are summarized in *Figure 16.26*, p. 17.

IMMUNOPATHOLOGICAL CONSEQUENCES OF PARASITIC INFECTIONS

Apart from the directly destructive effects of some parasites and their products on host tissues, many immune responses themselves have pathological effects. In malaria, African trypanosomiasis and visceral leishmaniasis, the increased number and heightened activity of macrophages and lymphocytes in the liver and spleen lead to enlargement of those organs. In schistosomiasis much of the pathology results from the T-cell-dependent granulomas forming around eggs in the liver. The gross changes occurring in individuals with elephantiasis are probably caused by immunopathological responses to adult filariae in the lymphatics. The formation of immune complexes is common; they may be deposited in the kidney, as in the nephrotic syndrome of quartan malaria, and may give rise to many other pathological changes. For example, tissue-bound immunoglobulins have been found in the muscles of mice infected with African trypanosomes and in the choroid plexus of mice with malaria.

The IgE of worm infections can have severe effects on the host due to release of mast-cell mediators. Anaphylactic shock may occur when a hydatid cyst ruptures. Asthma-like reactions occur in *Toxocara canis* infections, and in tropical pulmonary eosinophilia when filarial worms migrate through the lungs.

Autoantibodies, which probably arise as a result of polyclonal activation, have been detected against red blood cells, lymphocytes and DNA (e.g. in trypanosomiasis and in malaria). Antibodies against the parasite may cross-react with host tissues. For example, the chronic cardiomyopathy, enlarged oesophagus and megacolon that occur in Chagas' disease are thought to result from the autoimmune effects

Some mechanisms by which parasites avoid host defences

parasite	habitat	main host effector mechanism	method of avoidance
Trypanosoma brucei	bloodstream	antibody + complement	antigenic variation
Plasmodium spp.	hepatocyte blood cell	CD8+ cells, antibody, cytokines	intracellular, antigenic variation
Toxoplasma gondii	macrophage	O_2 metabolites, NO, lysosomal enzymes	failure to trigger, inhibits fusion of lysosomes
Trypanosoma cruzi	many cells	O_2 metabolites, NO, lysosomal enzymes	escapes into cytoplasm, so avoiding digestion
Leishmania	macrophage	O_2 metabolites, NO, lysosomal enzymes	O_2 burst impaired and products scavenged, avoids digestion
Trichinella spiralis	gut, blood, muscle	myeloid cells, antibody + complement	encystment in muscle development of DAF
Schistosoma mansoni	skin, blood, lungs, portal vein	myeloid cells, antibody + complement	acquisition of host antigens, blockade by antibody, soluble antigens and immune complexes, antioxidants
Wuchereria bancrofti	lymphatics	myeloid cells, antibody + complement	thick extracellular cuticle, antioxidants

Fig. 16.26 A summary of the various methods which parasites have evolved to avoid host defence mechanisms. DAF = decay accelerating factor (see Chapter 3).

on nerve ganglia of antibody and of cytotoxic T cells that cross-react with *T. cruzi*. Similarly *O. volvulus*, the cause of river blindness, possesses an antigen which cross-reacts with a protein in the retina.

Excessive production of some cytokines may contribute to some of the manifestations of disease. Thus the fever, anaemia, diarrhoea and pulmonary changes of acute malaria closely resemble the symptoms of endotoxaemia and are probably caused by TNFα. The severe wasting of cattle with trypanosomiasis may also be mediated by TNFα. Several immunological mechanisms may combine in producing pathological effects, as is likely in the anaemia of malaria (*Fig. 16.27*).

Lastly, the non-specific immunosuppression that is so widespread probably explains why people with parasitic infections are especially susceptible to bacterial and viral infections (e.g. measles). It may also account for the association of Burkitt's lymphoma with malaria.

Possible causes of development of anaemia in malaria

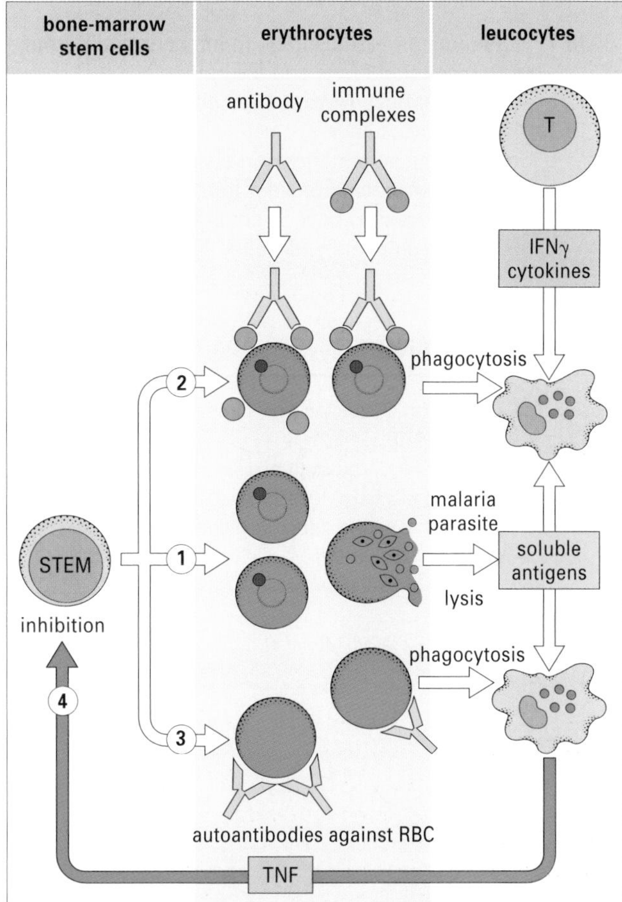

Fig. 16.27 There is more destruction of erythrocytes in malaria than can be accounted for by the number infected by parasites. In addition to those lost by lysis when the schizont ruptures (**1**), immunopathological mechanisms probably contribute to the anaemia. Parasite antigens, or immune complexes containing parasite antigens, may bind to unparasitized erythrocytes and accelerate their clearance by cells of the macrophage/monocyte lineage in the spleen and liver (**2**). There is also some autoantibody produced against normal erythrocytes which again accelerates their removal (**3**). TNFα released in response to infection inhibits red blood cell development from bone marrow stem cells and alters the kinetics of red cell turnover (**4**).

VACCINES

Some vaccines that are composed of attenuated living parasites have proved successful in veterinary practice. However, so far there are none in use against human parasites, although much effort has been directed towards the development of subunit vaccines against malarial parasites and schistosomes in particular. Some clinical trials of vaccines against malaria, based on combinations of putatively protective peptides are in progress. For further details, see Chapter 17.

CRITICAL THINKING • Immunity to protozoa and helminths (Explanations on pp 457–458)

16.1 In general, protozoa and helminths adopt different strategies for survival and for transmission to the subsequent host. How do they differ?

16.2 Many parasites have evolved to live in host cells. Consider the advantages and disadvantages to this mode of existence. Consider the different cell types and how parasites have to adapt this environment to their advantage. In particular *Toxoplasma gondii, Trypanosoma cruzi and Leishmania* sp. have adapted to live in the macrophage and can escape destruction by lysosomal enzymes, but the way in which they do this is different. How have these adaptations helped parasite survival?

16.3 Extracellular parasites must have evolved sophisticated mechanisms to avoid the immune response. Consider examples of how they do this.

FURTHER READING

Allen JE, Maizels RM. TH1–TH2: reliable paradigm or dangerous dogma? *Immunol Today* 1997;**18**:387–92.

Bogdan C, Rollinghoff M. How do protozoan parasites survive inside macrophages? *Parasitol Today* 1999:**15**:22–8.

Butterworth AE. Human Immunity to schistosomes: some questions. *Parasitol Today* 1994;**10**:378–9.

Clark IA, Rockett KA. Nitric oxide and parasitic disease. *Adv Parasitol* 1996;**37**:1–58.

Maizels RM, Bundy DAP, Selkirk ME, *et al.* Immunological modulation and evasion by helminth parasites in human populations. *Nature* 1993;**365**:797–804.

Reiner SL, Locksley RM. The regulation of immunity of *Leishmania major*. *Annu Rev Immunol* 1995;**13**:51–177.

Internet addresses: There are various newsgroups on the Net, although not all dedicated to immunology. They can be accessed by exploring keywords. There are several discussion groups operating through the bionet, e.g, http:/www/bio.net. Parasitology Mail Newsgroup.

17 Vaccination

- **Adaptive immunity** and the ability of lymphocytes to develop memory for a pathogen's antigens underlie vaccination.
- **Active immunization** is known as vaccination.
- **A wide range of antigen preparations** are in use as vaccines, from whole organisms to simple peptides and sugars.
- **Living and non-living vaccines** have important differences, living vaccines being generally more effective.
- **Recombinant DNA technology** will probably be the basis for the next generation of vaccines.
- **Non-specific immunization**, for example by cytokines, may be of use in selected conditions when it is desirable to boost general immune activity.
- **Adjuvants**, substances that enhance antibody production, are usually required with non-living vaccines.
- **Passive immunization,** the direct administration of antibodies, still has a role to play in certain circumstances, for example when tetanus toxin is already in the circulation.

Vaccination is the best known and the most successful application of immunological principles to human health. The first vaccine was named after vaccinia, the cowpox virus. Jenner pioneered its use 200 years ago. It was the first deliberate scientific attempt to prevent an infectious disease (smallpox), but it was done in complete ignorance of viruses (or indeed any kind of microbe) and immunology.

It was not until the work of Pasteur 100 years later that the general principle governing vaccination emerged: altered preparations of microbes could be used to generate enhanced immunity against the fully virulent organism. Thus Pasteur's dried rabies-infected rabbit spinal cords and heated anthrax bacilli were the true forerunners of today's vaccines, while Jenner's animal-derived (i.e. 'heterologous') vaccinia virus has had no real successors.

Even Pasteur did not have a proper understanding of immunological memory or the functions of the lymphocyte, which had to wait another half century. Finally, with Burnet's clonal selection theory (1957) and the discovery of T and B lymphocytes (1965), the key mechanism became clear. The antigen(s) of a vaccine must induce clonal expansion in specific T and/or B cells, leaving behind a population of memory cells. These enable the next encounter with the same antigen(s) to induce a secondary response which is more rapid and effective than the normal primary response. The primary response is often too slow to prevent serious disease (see *Fig. 1.19*).

Vaccination, therefore, involves *adaptive* immunity, the art of vaccination being to produce antigenic preparations from the pathogen that:

- Are safe to administer.
- Induce the right sort of immunity.
- Are affordable by the population at which they are aimed.

For many diseases, this has been achieved with brilliant success, but for others there is no vaccine whatsoever. This chapter is mainly concerned with the reasons for this disparity.

ANTIGENS USED AS VACCINES

The type of antigen used in a vaccine depends on many factors. In general, the more antigens of the microbe retained in the vaccine, the better, and living organisms tend to be more effective than killed ones (see later). Exceptions to this rule are diseases where a toxin is responsible for the pathology. In this case the vaccine can be based on the toxin alone. Another example is a vaccine in which microbial antigens are expressed in another type of cell, which acts as a vector.

Figure 17.1 lists the main antigenic preparations currently available.

The main antigenic preparations

type of antigen		vaccine examples
living organisms	natural	vaccinia (for smallpox) vole bacillus (for TB; historical)
	attenuated	*polio (Sabin; oral polio vaccine) *measles.*mumps.*rubella yellow fever 17D varicella-zoster (human herpes virus 3) *BCG (for TB)
intact but non-living organisms	viruses	*polio (Salk), rabies, influenza, hepatitis A, typhus
	bacteria	*pertussis, typhoid, cholera, plague
subcellular fragments	capsular polysaccharides	pneumococcus meningococcus *Haemophilus influenzae*
	surface antigen	*hepatitis B
toxoids		*tetanus, *diphtheria
recombinant DNA-based	gene cloned and expressed	*hepatitis B (yeast-derived)
	genes expressed in vectors	experimental
	naked DNA	experimental
anti-idiotype		experimental
* Standard in most countries		

Fig. 17.1 A wide range of antigenic preparations are used as vaccines.

Live vaccines can be natural or attenuated organisms

Natural live vaccines have rarely been used

Apart from vaccinia, no other completely natural organism has ever come into standard use. However, bovine and simian rotaviruses have been tried in children, the vole tubercle bacillus was once popular against tuberculosis (TB), and in the Middle East and Russia *Leishmania* infection from mild cases is reputed to induce immunity. It is possible that another good heterologous vaccine will be found, but the safety problems will be considerable.

Attenuated live vaccines have been highly successful

The preferred strategy has been to *attenuate* a human pathogen, with the aim of diminishing its virulence while retaining the desired antigens. This was first done successfully by Calmette and Guérin with a bovine strain (*M. bovis*) of *Mycobacterium tuberculosis*, which during 13 years (1908–1921) of culture *in vitro* changed to the much less virulent form now known as BCG (bacille Calmette–Guérin), which has at least some protective effect against TB. The real successes have been with viruses, starting with the 17D strain of yellow fever virus obtained by passage in mice and chicken embryos (1937), and followed by a roughly similar approach with polio, measles, mumps and rubella (*Fig. 17.2*). Just how successful the latter vaccines are is shown by the decline in these four diseases in the last two to three decades (*Fig. 17.3*).

Effects of attenuation – Attenuation 'changes' microorganisms to make them less able to grow and cause disease in their natural host. In early attenuated organisms 'changed' meant a purely random set of mutations induced by adverse conditions of growth. Vaccine candidates were selected by constantly monitoring for retention of antigenicity and loss of virulence, a tedious process. When viral gene sequencing became possible it emerged that the results of attenuation were widely divergent. An example is the divergence between the three types of live (Sabin) polio vaccine. Type 1 polio has 57 mutations and has almost never reverted to wild type while Type 2 and 3 vaccines depend for their safety and virulence on only two key mutations. Frequent reversion to wild type has occurred, in some cases leading to outbreaks of paralytic poliomyelitis.

Vaccinia virus is not an attenuated smallpox virus, present-day vaccinia virus strains being most closely related to rodent pox viruses; nor is vaccination against smallpox carried out. However, vaccinia virus is returning to use as a vector for antigens of other microorganisms such as HIV and malaria and is yielding very interesting information on the effects of attenuation. Pox viruses contain approximately 200 genes of which about two thirds are essential for growth in mammalian cells *in vitro*. The modified vaccinia Ankara strain (MVA) was grown for a prolonged period in avian cells and has deleted genes required to complete the replicative cycle in mammalian cells but it can still infect them and is a safe and immunogenic smallpox vaccine. Those genes not essential for replication of the virus are mostly concerned with evasion of host responses

Live attenuated vaccines

	disease	remarks
viruses	polio	Types 2, 3 may revert; also killed vaccine
	measles	80% effective
	mumps	
	rubella	now given to both sexes
	yellow fever	stable since 1937
	varicella-zoster	mainly in leukaemia
	hepatitis A	also killed vaccine
bacteria	tuberculosis	stable since 1921; also some protection against leprosy

Fig. 17.2 Attenuated vaccines are available for many, but not all, infections. In general it has proved easier to attenuate viruses than bacteria.

Effect of vaccination on the incidence of viral disease

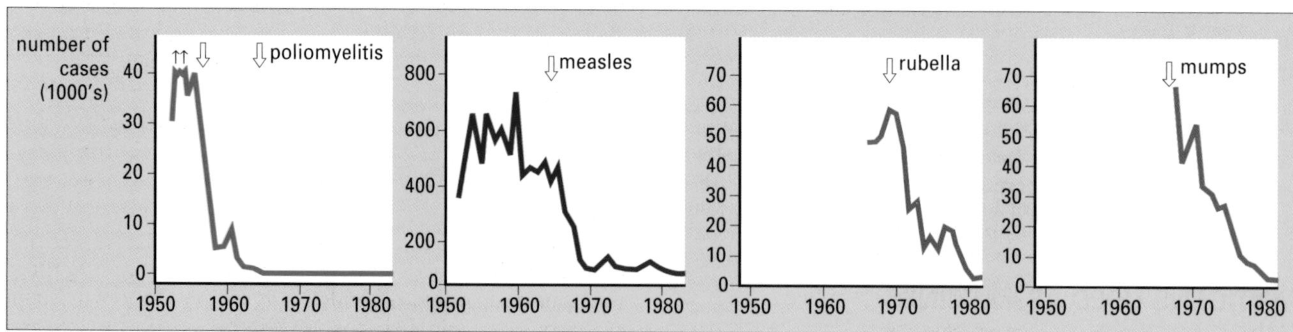

Fig. 17.3 The effect of vaccination on the incidence of various viral diseases in the USA has been that most infections have shown a dramatic downward trend after the introduction of a vaccine (arrows).

and virulence and pox viruses contain a battery of genes that mimic or interfere with cytokine and chemokine function. Some of these have sequence homology to their mammalian counterparts and others do not. Most vaccinia strains lack some of these genes while smallpox virus itself contains almost all of them.

In the future it should be possible to use recombinant DNA technology to remove virulence genes completely or to introduce site-directed mutations to inactivate them.

Killed vaccines are intact but non-living organisms

These are the successors of Pasteur's killed vaccines mentioned earlier. Some are very effective (rabies and the Salk polio vaccine), some moderately so (typhoid, cholera and influenza), some are of debatable value (plague and typhus) and some are controversial on the grounds of toxicity (pertussis). *Figure 17.4* lists the main killed vaccines in use today. Some of these will undoubtedly be replaced by attenuated or subunit vaccines. Acellular pertussis vaccine consisting of a small number of proteins purified from the bacteria is available and has been shown to be effective and less toxic. They are more expensive than the conventional killed vaccine so that initially their use is likely to be restricted to the developed world.

Inactivated toxins and toxoids are the most successful bacterial vaccines

The most successful of all bacterial vaccines – tetanus and diphtheria (*Fig. 17.5*) – are based on inactivated exotoxins (*Fig. 17.6*), and in principle the same approach can be used for several other infections.

Subunit vaccines and carriers

Aside from the toxin-based vaccines which are subunits of their respective microorganisms, a number of other vaccines are in use which make use of antigens either purified from microorganisms or produced by recombinant DNA technology (*Fig. 17.7*). While hepatitis B surface antigen is immunogenic when given with alum adjuvant (see 'Adjuvants', p. 284), the bacterial capsular polysaccharides of *Neisseria meningitidis*, *Streptococcus pneumoniae* and *Haemophilus influenzae* B are relatively poorly immunogenic and often do not induce IgG responses or long-lasting protection because helper T cells are not activated by polysaccharides alone. A significant improvement in the efficacy of these vaccines has been obtained by conjugating the purified polysaccharides to carrier proteins such as tetanus or diphtheria toxoid. These protein carriers are presumed to recruit helper T cells and the conjugates induce IgG antibody responses and more effective protection.

Killed (whole-organism) vaccines

disease		remarks
viruses	polio	preferred in Scandinavia; safe in immunocompromised
	rabies	can be given post-exposure, with passive antiserum
	influenza	strain-specific
	hepatitis A	also attenuated vaccine
bacteria	pertussis	potential to cause brain damage (controversial)
	typhoid	about 70% protection
	cholera	protection dubious; may be combined with toxin subunit
	plague	short-term protection only
	Q fever	good protection

Fig. 17.4 The principal using killed whole-organisms.

Success of immunization against diphtheria

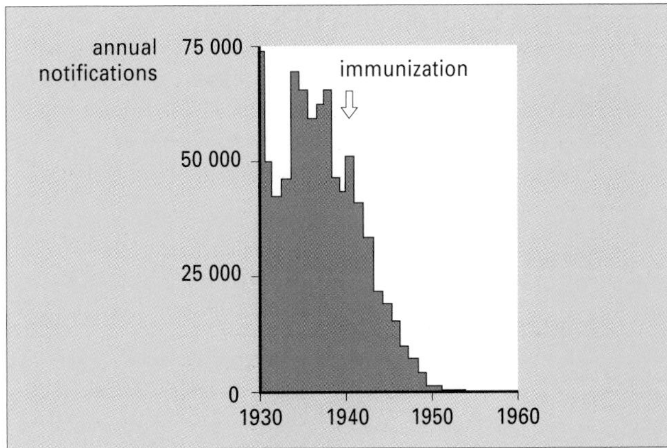

Fig. 17.5 Annual notifications of diphtheria demonstrate the great success of vaccines based on inactivated toxin: the number of cases dropped dramatically after vaccination was introduced in 1940. (Courtesy of Professor J. R. Pattison, Ch. 26 in Brostoff J. *et al.*, eds. *Clinical Immunology*, London: Mosby, 1991.)

Toxin-based vaccines

organism	vaccine	remarks
Clostridium tetani	inactivated toxin (formalin)	3 doses, alum-precipitated; boost every 10 years
Corynebacterium diphtheriae	inactivated toxin (formalin)	usually given with tetanus
Vibrio cholerae	toxin, B subunit	sometimes combined with whole killed organisms
Clostridium perfringens	inactivated toxin (formalin)	for newborn lambs

Fig. 17.6 The principal toxin-based vaccines. Note that there are no vaccines against the numerous staphylococcal and streptococcal exotoxins, or against bacterial endotoxins such as lipopolysaccharides.

Subunit vaccines

	organism	remarks
virus	hepatitis B virus	surface antigen can be purified from blood of carriers or produced in yeast by recombinant DNA technology
	Neisseria meningitidis	capsular polysaccharides or conjugates of group A and C are effective; group B is non-immunogenic
bacteria	*Steptococcus pneumoniae*	84 serotypes; capsular polysaccharide vaccines contain 23 serotypes; conjugates with 5 or 7 serotypes are being tested
	Haemophilus influenzae B	good conjugate vaccines now available

Fig. 17.7 Conjugate vaccines are replacing pure polysaccharides. *N. meningitidis* type B is non-immunogenic in man as the capsular polysaccharide cross-reacts with host carbohydrates.

Small antigens can be made synthetically or by gene cloning

Where it can be shown that a small peptide is protective, which is by no means always the case, it may be more convenient to make it synthetically or by cloning its gene into a suitable expression vector. This approach has been highly successful with the HBs antigen, cloned into yeast and now replacing the first-generation HBs vaccine which was laboriously purified from the blood of HB carriers; it has also brought down the cost of the vaccine.

An attractive feature of this approach is that further sequences can be added – for example selected B- and T-cell epitopes can be combined in various ways to optimize the resulting immune response. It is important to remember that, whereas B cells respond to the 3-dimensional *shape* of antigens, T cells recognize *linear sequences* of amino acids (see Chapter 5). Thus peptides can function well as T-cell epitopes but cannot readily mimic the discontinuous B-cell epitope. Even where a B-cell determinant is linear, antibodies raised against the free flexible peptide do not bind optimally to the sequence in the way that they do when it is present as a more rigid structure within the native protein molecule.

Future vaccines will use genes and vectors to deliver antigens

A development of the use of gene cloning is to insert the desired gene into a vector which can then be injected into the patient, allowed to replicate, express the gene and produce large amounts of the antigen *in situ* (*Fig. 17.8*). Vaccinia is a convenient vector that is large enough to carry several antigens. Modified vaccinia Ankara may be particularly safe because it does not replicate in human cells (see above). Because immunization against smallpox ceased some years ago, the problem of pre-existing immunity is also decreasing. A number of experimental vaccines using recombinant vaccinia have been tested, though none are

Generation of recombinant vaccinia virus for expression of a foreign gene

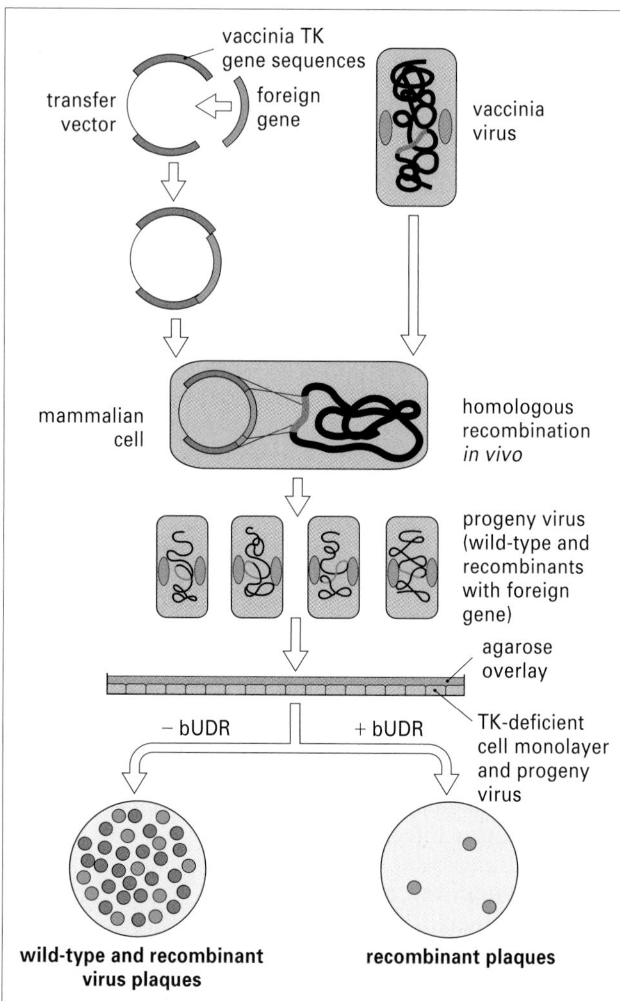

Fig. 17.8 Recombinant vaccinia virus can be generated to express a foreign gene. The foreign gene is inserted into vaccinia's thymidine kinase (TK) gene so that recombinant virus plaques can be distinguished from wild type. TK is used by virus to take up thymidine from the culture medium or intracellular pool for DNA synthesis: the recombinant virus cannot produce TK, because the gene has been interrupted and so must use the separate pathway for *de novo* synthesis of thymidine. In the presence of bromodeoxyuridine (bUDR), a thymidine analogue that blocks DNA synthesis when it is incorporated into DNA, wild-type virus replication is blocked by bUDR but recombinant virus replication continues, using *de novo* synthesis of thymidine. The cell monolayer must be TK deficient so that recombinant virus cannot use the cells' TK to take up bUDR. (Courtesy of Dr D. J. Rowlands, Ch. 26 in Brostoff J. *et al.*, eds. *Clinical Immunology*, London: Mosby, 1991.)

yet in routine use. Many other viruses have also been proposed and tested experimentally as vaccine vectors.

Attenuated bacteria have the advantage that they have genomes large enough to incorporate many genes from other organisms. BCG and salmonellae have been favoured organisms for experimental recombinant bacterial vaccines. Mutant salmonellae can be given by mouth and immunize the gut-associated lymphoid tissue before being eliminated – a very useful property as diarrhoea is one of the world's major killers in infancy. The mutant bacteria are also capable of inducing systemic immunity. However, as yet no bacterial recombinant vaccines are routinely used.

An even more innovative approach is to construct transgenic plants expressing vaccine antigens. Mice have been successfully immunized by eating genetically engineered raw potatoes. Many problems with this approach need to be overcome. Protein antigens may be rapidly degraded in the digestive tract and consistency and dosage will be difficult to control. Finally antigens administered orally often tolerize rather than immunize and oral adjuvants may need to be incorporated into the plants.

Even if edible plant vaccines present problems, however, recombinant plants may provide a cheap and convenient way of producing vaccine antigens, which may be purified from the leaves or fruit of the plant and used in conventional subunit vaccines.

A recent development is the use of 'naked' DNA. Genes of interest coupled with a suitable promoter are injected directly into muscle or coated on to gold microparticles and 'shot' into the skin by pressurized gas – the gene gun. Surprisingly this can induce long-lasting cellular and humoral immunity in experimental animals. The mechanism appears to be through uptake and expression of the DNA in antigen-presenting cells. The method has the advantage that immunomodulatory genes (cytokines or co-stimuli) can be incorporated into the DNA construct along with the genes coding for antigens, to generate and amplify the desired immune response. It has also been found that bacterial CpG DNA sequences have adjuvant properties and these can be included in the plasmids used to produce the DNA.

Although DNA immunization appears promising in experimental animals, initial trials in man have not been overwhelmingly successful and the long-term safety of administering DNA has yet to be established. At present DNA immunization is largely being tested in life-threatening situations (tumours, HIV) rather than routine vaccination of infants. Priming with DNA and boosting with recombinant vaccinia virus is significantly more effective than DNA alone, at least in animals. Clinical trials have been initiated.

Anti-idiotype vaccines could be used when the original antigen is unsuitable

This is the only type of vaccine for which immunological thinking has been entirely responsible. The idea is to use monoclonal antibody (mAb) technology to make large amounts of anti-idiotype (anti-Id) against the V region (idiotype) of an antibody of proven protective value. The anti-Id, if properly selected, would then have a three-dimensional shape similar to the original immunizing antigen and could be used in place of it (*Fig. 17.9*). Though often dismissed as 'armchair immunology', this strategy could have real value where the original antigen is not itself suitable, i.e. is not immunogenic. Polysaccharides are one example, and the lipid A region of bacterial endotoxin (LPS) is another. The advantage of the mAb would be that since it is a protein it should induce memory, which polysaccharides and lipids normally do not.

Anti-idiotype antibodies as vaccines

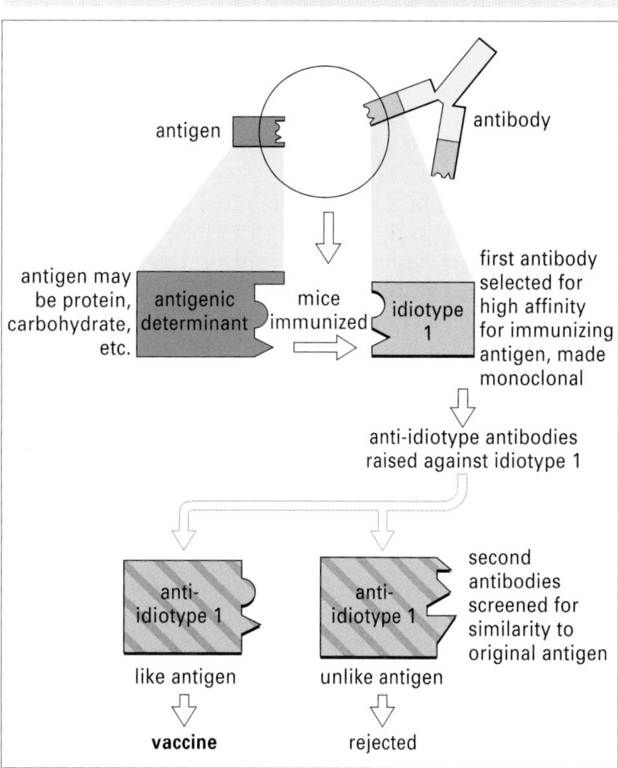

Fig. 17.9 Monoclonal antibody technology and the discovery of the 'idiotype network' (see Chapter 11) has meant that immunoglobulins can now be used as 'surrogate' antigens. In the case of a carbohydrate or lipid antigen, this allows a protein 'copy' to be made, which may have some advantages as a vaccine.

EFFECTIVENESS OF VACCINES

To be introduced and approved, a vaccine must obviously be effective, and the efficacy of all vaccines is reviewed from time to time. Many factors affect it. An effective vaccine must:

- **Induce the right sort of immunity:** antibody for toxins and extracellular organisms such as *Streptococcus pneumoniae*; cell-mediated immunity for intracellular organisms such as the tubercle bacillus. Where the ideal type of response is not clear (as in malaria, for instance), designing an effective vaccine becomes correspondingly more difficult.
- **Be stable on storage:** this is particularly important for living vaccines, which normally require to be kept cold,

i.e. a complete 'cold chain' from manufacturer to clinic, by no means always easy to maintain.

- **Have sufficient immunogenicity:** with non-living vaccines it is often necessary to boost their immunogenicity with an *adjuvant* (see later).

Live vaccines are generally more effective than killed ones

Induction of appropriate immunity depends on the properties of the antigen. Living vaccines have the great advantage of providing an increasing antigenic challenge that lasts days or weeks, and inducing it in the right site – which in practice is most important where mucosal immunity is concerned (*Fig. 17.10*). Live vaccines are likely to contain the greatest number of microbial antigens. Killed vaccines may suffer from two other inconveniences: T-cell independence and major histocompatibility complex (MHC) restriction (see Chapter 6). Polysaccharides are typically thymus independent, since they do not bind to MHC and so do not immunize T cells. The present strategy for inducing memory is to couple them either to a standard protein carrier such as tetanus toxoid or to a protein from the immunizing organism such as the outer membrane protein of pneumococci, *Haemophilus*, etc. MHC restriction affects small peptides in the 10–20 amino acid range, and shows up as 'genetic unresponsiveness' because the peptides bind only to certain MHC molecules. This is probably more hypothetical than real, since most candidate vaccines are considerably larger than this. Nevertheless, even the most effective vaccines often fail to immunize every individual; for example, about 5% fail to seroconvert after the full course of hepatitis B vaccine.

Antibody responses to live and killed polio vaccine

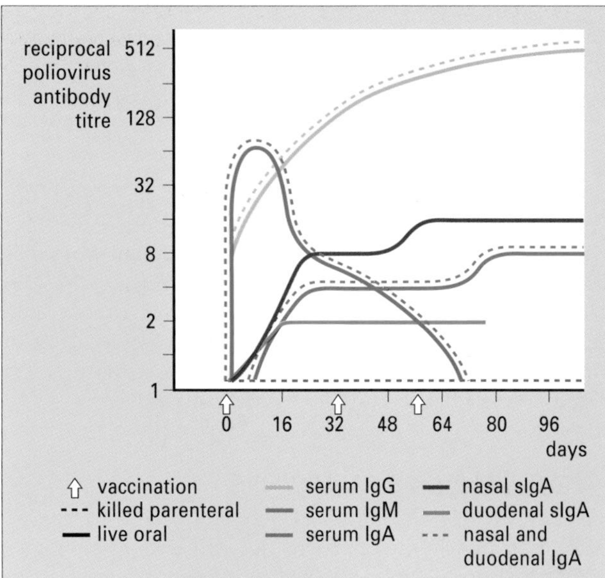

Fig. 17.10 The antibody response to orally administered live-attenuated polio vaccine (solid lines) and intramuscularly administered killed polio vaccine (broken lines). The live vaccine induces production of secretory IgA (sIgA) in addition to serum antibodies. As sIgA is the immunoglobulin of the mucosa-associated lymphoid tissue (MALT) system (see Chapter 2), the live vaccine confers protection at the portal of entry of the virus, the gastrointestinal mucosa. (Courtesy of Professor J. R. Pattison, Ch. 26 in Brostoff J. *et al.*, eds. *Clinical Immunology*, London: Mosby, 1991.)

VACCINE SAFETY

Having been somewhat ignored in the early days, safety has now become an overriding consideration. It is of course a relative term, minor local pain or swelling at the injection site, and even mild fever, being generally acceptable, although the public is becoming increasingly aware of the possibilities of profitable litigation. This is not surprising when one remembers that, unlike antibiotics, etc., most vaccinations are given to people who have previously been perfectly well.

Some of the more serious complications may stem from the vaccine or from the patient (*Fig. 17.11*). Vaccines may be contaminated with unwanted proteins or toxins, or even live viruses. Supposedly killed vaccines may not have been properly killed; attenuated vaccines may revert to the wild type. The patient may be hypersensitive to minute amounts of contaminating protein, or immunocompromised, in which case any living vaccine is usually contraindicated.

COST OF VACCINATION

Although vaccination can safely be considered the most cost-effective treatment for infectious disease, new vaccines may be very expensive. The initial high cost is necessary

Safety problems with vaccines

type of vaccine	potential safety problems	examples
attenuated vaccines	reversion to wild type	especially polio Types 2 and 3
	severe disease in immunodeficient patients	vaccinia, BCG, measles
	persistent infection	varicella-zoster
	hypersensitivity to viral antigens	measles
	hypersensitivity to egg antigens	measles, mumps
killed vaccines	vaccine not killed	polio accidents in the past
	yeast contaminant	hepatitis B
	contamination with animal viruses	polio
	contamination with endotoxin	pertussis

Fig. 17.11 The potential safety problems encountered with vaccines emphasize the need for continuous monitoring of both production and administration.

to recoup the enormous development costs (US$100–200 million). A good example is the recombinant hepatitis B vaccine. This was initially marketed in 1986 at US$150 for three doses and although the cost has decreased greatly, even $1 is beyond the health budget of many of the world's poorer nations. By contrast, the cost of the six vaccines included in the World Health Organization Expanded Programme on Immunization (diphtheria, tetanus, whooping cough, polio, measles and tuberculosis) is less than $1, although the actual cost of immunizing a child is several times greater than this as it includes the cost of laboratories, transport, the cold chain, personnel and research. The Children's Vaccine Initiative, set up in 1990, is a global forum that aims to bring together development agencies, governments, donors, commercial and public sector vaccine manufacturers, vaccine researchers and national immunization manufacturers to seek means of delivering vaccines to the world's poorest populations who most need them.

CURRENT VACCINES

Vaccines in general use have variable success rates

Figure 17.12 lists the vaccines in standard use worldwide. Four of them – polio, measles, mumps and rubella – are so successful that these diseases are earmarked for eradication early in the 21st century. If this happens, it will be an extraordinary achievement, because mathematical modelling suggests that they are all more 'difficult' targets for eradication than smallpox was. In the case of polio where reversion to virulence of Types 2 and 3 can occur, it has been suggested that it will be necessary to switch to the use of killed virus vaccine for some years, so that virulent virus shed by live-virus-vaccinated individuals is no longer produced. For a number of reasons, other vaccines are less likely to lead to eradication of disease:

- **The carrier state:** eradication of hepatitis B would be a major triumph, but it will require the breaking of the carrier state, especially in the Far East, where mother to child is the normal route of infection.
- **Suboptimal effectiveness:** effectiveness of BCG varies markedly from country to country (tuberculosis is on the increase, especially in patients with immune deficiency syndrome, or AIDS), and the pertussis vaccine is only about 70% effective.
- **Side-effects:** the pertussis vaccine is suspected of having side-effects, reducing the public's willingness to be vaccinated.
- **Free-living forms and animal hosts:** the free-living form of tetanus will presumably survive indefinitely, and it will not be possible to eradicate diseases that also have an animal host, such as yellow fever.

One of the future problems is going to be maintaining awareness of the need for vaccination against diseases that seem to be disappearing. Another problem is that as the reservoir of infection diminishes, cases tend to occur at a later age, which with measles and rubella could actually lead to worse clinical consequences.

Some vaccines are reserved for special groups only

In the developed world BCG and hepatitis B fall into this category, but some vaccines will probably always be confined to selected populations – travellers, nurses, the elderly, etc. (*Fig. 17.13*). In some cases this is because of geographical restrictions (e.g. yellow fever) or the rarity of exposure (e.g. rabies), while in others it is due to problems in producing sufficient vaccine in time to meet the demand. For example, each influenza epidemic is caused by a different strain, requiring a new vaccine. A vaccine effective against all strains of influenza would be of tremendous value; unfortunately, however, both the haemagglutinin and neuraminidase antigens, which together make up the outer layer of the virus and are the

Vaccines in general use

disease	vaccine	remarks
tetanus	toxoid	given together in 3 doses between 2 and 6 months; tetanus and diphtheria boosted every 10 years
diphtheria	toxoid	
pertussis	killed whole	
polio	killed (Salk) or attenuated (Sabin)	
measles	attenuated	given together ('MMR') at 12–18 months
mumps		
rubella		
Haemophilus	polysaccharide	new; may be added to above

Fig. 17.12 Vaccines that are currently given, as far as is possible, to all individuals.

Vaccines restricted to certain groups

disease	vaccine	eligible groups
tuberculosis	BCG	tropics: at birth UK: 10–14 years USA: at-risk only
hepatitis B	surface antigen	at-risk (medical, nursing staff, etc.) drug addicts; male homosexuals known contacts of carriers
rabies	killed	at-risk (animal workers) post-exposure
meningitis yellow fever typhoid, cholera hepatitis A	polysaccharide attenuated killed or mutant killed or attenuated	travellers
influenza	killed	at-risk; elderly
pneumococcal pneumonia	polysaccharide	elderly
varicella-zoster	attenuated	leukaemic children

Fig. 17.13 Vaccines that are currently restricted to certain groups.

antigens of importance in the vaccine, are subject to variation.

For parasitic and some other infections, there are only experimental vaccines

Some of the most intensely researched vaccines are those for the major tropical protozoal and worm infections. However, none has come into standard use, and some have argued that none will, since none of these diseases induces effective immunity and 'you cannot improve on nature'. Nevertheless, extensive work in laboratory animals has shown that vaccines against malaria, leishmaniasis and schistosomiasis are perfectly feasible, and there is a moderately effective vaccine against babesia in dogs. In cattle an irradiated vaccine against the lungworm has been in veterinary use for decades.

It remains possible, however, that the parasitic diseases of humans are uniquely difficult to treat, partly because of the polymorphic and rapidly changing nature of many parasitic antigens. For example, none of the small animal models of malaria shows such extensive antigenic variation as does *Plasmodium falciparum*, the protozoan causing malignant tertian malaria in humans. Similarly, rats appear to be much easier to immunize against schistosomiasis than other animals, including possibly humans. Part of the problem is that these parasites are usually not in their natural host in the laboratory.

Several trials of clinical malaria vaccine have been published, using antigens derived from either the liver or the blood stage, with only very moderate success. Malaria is unusual in that its life cycle offers a variety of possible targets for vaccination (*Fig. 17.14*). A trial of killed leishmania parasites combined with BCG gave no less than 90% protection in Venezuela.

A problem with these chronic parasitic diseases is that of immunopathology. For example, the symptoms of *Trypanosoma cruzi* infection (Chagas' disease) are largely due to the immune system, i.e. autoimmunity. A bacterial parallel is leprosy, where the symptoms are due to the (apparent) over-reactivity of TH1 or TH2 cells. A vaccine that boosted immunity without clearing the pathogen could make these conditions worse. Another example of this unpleasant possibility is with dengue, where certain antibodies enhance the infection by allowing the virus to enter cells via Fc receptors. Enhancing antibodies have also been reported in an experimental model of a transmission-blocking anti-malarial vaccine.

Other experimental vaccines

Some other viral and bacterial vaccines are also in the experimental category (cholera toxin, attenuated shigella, Epstein–Barr virus surface glycoprotein). A rotavirus vaccine has undergone trials in the USA. Unfortunately although effective, the vaccine was associated with an unacceptable risk of intussusception (a form of intestinal obstruction) and has been withdrawn.

For many diseases there is no vaccine available

There remains a long list of serious infectious diseases where no vaccine is currently available (*Fig. 17.15*). Headed by human immunodeficiency virus (HIV), these represent the major challenge for research and development in the coming decade.

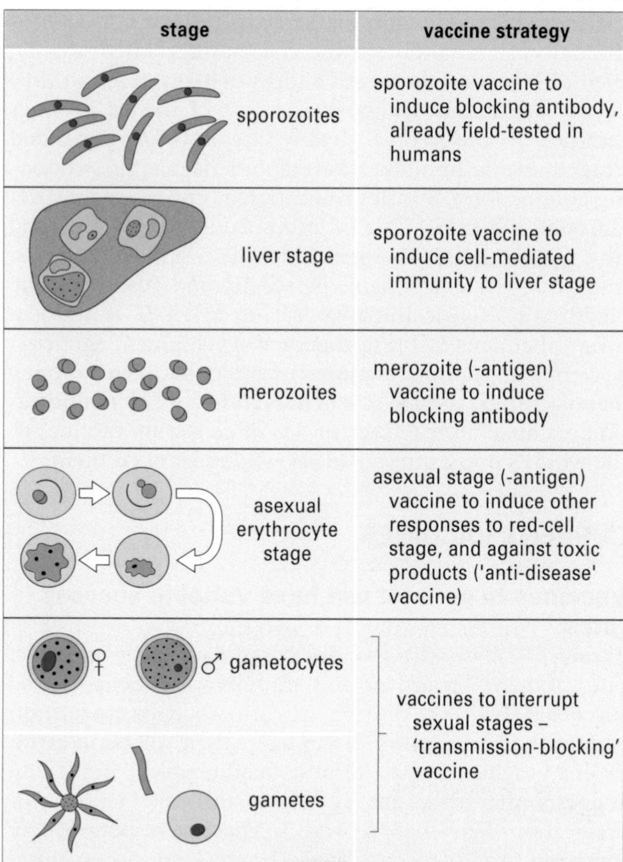

Fig. 17.14 A number of different approaches to malaria vaccines are being investigated, reflecting the complexity of both the life cycle of malaria and immunity to it.

ADJUVANTS

During work in the 1920s on the production of animal sera for human therapy, it was discovered that certain substances, notably aluminium salts, added to or emulsified with an antigen, greatly enhance antibody production; that is, they act as *adjuvants*. Aluminium hydroxide is still widely used with, for example, diphtheria and tetanus toxoids. With modern understanding of the processes leading to lymphocyte triggering and the development of memory, considerable efforts have been made to produce better adjuvants, particularly for T-cell-mediated responses. *Figure 17.16* gives a list of these, but it should be stressed that none of the new adjuvants is yet accepted for routine human use.

Adjuvants either concentrate antigen at appropriate sites or induce cytokines

It appears that the effect of adjuvants is due mainly to two activities: the concentration of antigen in a site where lymphocytes are exposed to it (the 'depot' effect) and the

Major diseases for which no vaccines are available

disease		problems
viruses	HIV	antigenic variation; immunosuppression?
	herpes viruses	risk of reactivation? (but varicella-zoster appears safe)
	adenoviruses, rhinoviruses	multiple serotypes
bacteria	staphylococci	early vaccines ineffective (antibiotics originally better)
	group A streptococci	
	Mycobacterium leprae	(BCG gives some protection)
	Treponema pallidum (syphilis)	ignorance of effective immunity
	Chlamydia	early vaccines ineffective
fungi	*Candida*	ignorance of effective immunity
	Pneumocystis	
protozoa	malaria	antigenic variation
	trypanosomiasis: sleeping sickness Chagas' disease	extreme antigenic variation immunopathology; autoimmunity trials encouraging
	leishmaniasis	
worms	schistosomiasis	(trials in animals encouraging)
	onchocerciasis	ignorance of effective immunity

Fig. 17.15 For some serious diseases there is currently no effective vaccine. The predominant problem is the lack of understanding of how to induce effective immunity.

Adjuvants

adjuvant type	routinely used in man	experimental* or too toxic for human use†
inorganic salts	aluminium hydroxide (alhydrogel)	
	aluminium phosphate	beryllium hydroxide
	calcium phosphate	
delivery systems		liposomes*
		ISCOMS*
		block polymers
		slow release formulations*
bacterial products		BCG
	Bordetella pertussis (with diphtheria, tetanus toxoids)	*Mycobacterium bovis* and oil† (complete Freund's adjuvant)
		muramyl dipeptide (MDP†)
natural mediators (cytokines)		IL-1 IL-2 IL-12 IFNγ

Fig. 17.16 A variety of foreign and endogenous substances can act as adjuvants, but only aluminium and calcium salts and pertussis are routinely used in clinical practice.

induction of cytokines which regulate lymphocyte function. Aluminium salts probably have a predominantly depot function, inducing small granulomas in which antigen is retained. Newer devices such as liposomes and immune-stimulating complexes (ISCOMs) achieve the same purpose by ensuring that antigens trapped in them are delivered to antigen-presenting cells. Bacterial products such as mycobacterial cell walls, endotoxin, etc., probably act mainly by stimulating the formation of the appropriate cytokines. This theory is supported by the fact that cytokines themselves have been shown to be effective adjuvants, particularly when coupled directly to the antigen. Cytokines may be particularly useful in immunocompromised patients (see *Fig. 17.18*), who often fail to respond to normal vaccines. It is hoped that they might also be useful in directing the immune response in the desired direction – for example in diseases where only TH1 (or TH2) cell memory is wanted.

PASSIVE IMMUNIZATION

Driven from use by the advent of antibiotics, the idea of injecting preformed antibody to treat infection is still valid for certain situations (*Fig. 17.17*). It can be life-saving where

Passive immunization

disease	source of antibody	indication
diphtheria	human, horse	prophylaxis, treatment
tetanus		
varicella-zoster	human	treatment in immunodeficiencies
gas gangrene	horse	post-exposure
botulism		
snake bite scorpion sting		
rabies	human	post-exposure (plus vaccine)
hepatitis B	human	post-exposure
hepatitis A	pooled human immunoglobulin	prophylaxis (travel)
measles		post-exposure

Fig. 17.17 Although not so commonly used as 50 years ago, injections of specific antibody can still be a life-saving treatment in specific clinical conditions.

toxins are already circulating (e.g. in tetanus, diphtheria and snake-bite), and where high-titre specific antibody is required, generally made in horses but occasionally obtained from recovered patients. At the opposite end of the scale, normal pooled human immunoglobulin contains enough antibody against common infections for a dose of 100–400 mg of IgG to protect hypogammaglobulinaemic patients for a month. Over 1000 donors are used for each pool, and the sera must be screened for HIV and hepatitis B and C.

The use of specific monoclonal antibodies, though theoretically attractive, has not yet proved to be an improvement on traditional methods, and their chief application to infectious disease at present remains in diagnosis. This may change as human monoclonal antibodies become more readily available (and less expensive) either through cell culture or protein engineering (see Chapter 27).

NON-SPECIFIC IMMUNOTHERAPY

Many of the same compounds that act as adjuvants for vaccines have also been used on their own in an attempt to boost the general level of immune activity (*Fig. 17.18*). The best results have been obtained with cytokines, and among these interferon-α (IFNα) is the most widely used, mainly for its antiviral properties (but also for certain tumours – see below and Chapter 18). Perhaps the most striking clinical effect of a cytokine has been that of granulocyte–colony-stimulating factor (G–CSF) in restoring bone-marrow function after anti-cancer therapy, with benefit to both bleeding and infection.

Finally cytokine inhibitors can be used for severe or chronic inflammatory conditions. Various ways of inhibiting tumour necrosis factor (TNF) and interleukin-1 (IL-1) have proved valuable in rheumatoid arthritis and, more controversially, in septic (Gram-negative) shock and severe malaria. In a few years, one would expect the clinical pharmacology of cytokines and cytokine inhibitors to be clarified so that these communication molecules of the immune system can be fully exploited, in the same way as vaccination has exploited the properties of the lymphocyte.

Non-specific immunotherapy

source		remarks
microbial	filtered bacterial cultures	used by Coley (1909) against tumours
	BCG	some activity against tumours
cytokines	IFNα	effective in chronic: hepatitis B hepatitis C herpes zoster wart virus prophylactic against common cold (also some tumours)
	IFNγ	effective in some cases of: chronic granulomatous disease lepromatous leprosy leishmaniasis (cutaneous)
	IL-2	leishmaniasis (cutaneous)
	G–CSF	bone-marrow restoration after cytotoxic drugs
cytokine inhibitors	TNF antagonists	septic shock
	IL-1 antagonists	severe (cerebral) malaria?
	IL-10	

Fig. 17.18 Non-specific stimulation or inhibition of particular components of the immune system may sometimes be of benefit.

VACCINATING AGAINST CANCER

The idea of non-specifically stimulating the immune system to reject tumours goes back almost a century to the work of Coley, who used bacterial filtrates with considerable success, possibly through the induction of cytokines such as TNF and IFN. However, attempts to equal his results with purified cytokines or immunostimulants (e.g. BCG) have been successful only in a restricted range of tumours, and current efforts are mainly directed at the induction of *specific* immunity – just as for infectious microbes – encouraged by the evidence that tumours may sometimes be spontaneously rejected as if they were foreign grafts. This subject is dealt with more fully in Chapter 18.

FUTURE VACCINES

In principle, conception and implantation can be interrupted by inducing immunity against a wide range of pregnancy hormones. The target of the most successful experimental trials has been human chorionic gonadotrophin (hCG), the embryo-specific hormone responsible for maintaining the corpus luteum. Vaccines based on the β chain of hCG, coupled to tetanus or diphtheria toxoid, have been extremely successful in preventing conception in baboons and, more recently, humans. In the human trial, infertility was only temporary, and no serious side-effects were observed. Clearly this represents a powerful new means of safely limiting family size, though there are of course cultural and ethical aspects to consider too.

Another use of immunization that is being explored is the treatment of drug dependency. It is possible to neutralize the effect of a drug by pre-immunization with the drug coupled to a suitable carrier (the 'hapten–carrier' effect).

CRITICAL THINKING • Vaccination (Explanations on p. 458)

17.1 Why have attenuated vaccines not been developed for all viruses and bacteria?

17.2 'A vaccine cannot improve on nature.' Is this unduly pessimistic?

17.3 'The smallpox success story is unlikely to be repeated.' Is this true?

17.4 Will vaccines eventually replace antibiotics?

17.5 BCG: vaccine, adjuvant, or non-specific stimulant?

17.6 Why could an anti-worm vaccine do more harm than good?

17.7 By what means, other than their reaction with antibodies, might you identify antigens that could be used as vaccines?

FURTHER READING

HMSO. *Immunisation against Infectious Disease.* London; 1996.

Naz RK. Vaccine for contraception targetting sperm. *Immunol Rev* 1999; **171**:193–202.

Ramsay AJ, Kent SJ, Strugnell RA, Suhrbier A, Thomson SA, Ramshaw IA. Genetic vaccination strategies for enhanced cellular, humoral and mucosal immunity. *Immunol Rev* 1999;**171**:27–44.

WHO and UNICEF. *State of the World's Vaccines and Immunisation.* Geneva; 1996.

18 Tumour immunology

- **Immune surveillance** is a concept that envisages prevention of the development of most tumours through early destruction of abnormal cells by the host's immune system.
- **Surveillance probably acts against viruses not tumours.** The evidence for this is that although there is an increased incidence of tumours in immunosuppressed indivduals, the most dramatic increase is in tumours associated with oncogenic viruses.
- **Cellular responses to tumour-associated antigens occur;** the antigens may be virus coded, or they may be altered or overexpressed host gene products.
- **Differentiation antigens** expressed on tumours can be detected by monoclonal antibodies or patients' sera. Although the antigens are not restricted to tumour cells, they are useful for diagnosis and may be targets for antibody-mediated therapy.
- **Passive immunotherapy with monoclonal antibodies** is promising when single cells are targeted or the problem of poor penetration into tumour masses can be circumvented.
- **Immunotherapy by active immunization** or by passive transfer of cells is still largely experimental, because of tumour escape mechanisms. Cytokines are active against a few tumour types.

THE TUMOUR AS A TISSUE GRAFT

The idea that there might be immune responses to tumours is an old one. At the turn of the century, Paul Ehrlich suggested that in humans there was a high frequency of 'aberrant germs' (tumours), which if not kept in check by the immune system would overwhelm us. Thus tumours came to be regarded as similar to grafted tissue recognizable by the immune system. This, in turn, led to attempts to stimulate the immune system to reject them. Occasional regressions following treatment with bacterial vaccines (Coley's toxin), or occurring spontaneously, were taken as evidence of an effective immune response.

Early in the century, experimentalists began to investigate tumour immunity and noted that transplanted tumours usually regressed. Although much of this work fell into disrepute when it was realized that the immune response was directed against foreign major histocompatibility complex (MHC) antigens, it did establish that the immune system can reject a large tumour mass when there is an antigenic disparity between tumour and host. Only in the post Second World War period, when genetically homogeneous inbred rodents became available, did it become possible to investigate the immune response of animals bearing a tumour expressing identical MHC antigens. An added impetus to these studies was provided by Burnett and Thomas, who developed Ehrlich's idea of immune responses to 'aberrant germs', elaborating it into the theory of immune surveillance.

IMMUNE SURVEILLANCE

Surveillance is most effective against viruses not tumour cells

Burnett and Thomas' idea was that the immune system continually surveyed the body for the presence of abnormal cells, which were destroyed when recognized. The immune response to a tumour was therefore thought to be an early event, leading to the destruction of the majority of tumours before they became clinically apparent. It was also proposed that the immune system played an important role in delaying the growth, or causing regression of established tumours. A variety of evidence was adduced to support these ideas:

- Postmortem data suggest that there may be more tumours than become clinically apparent.
- Many tumours contain lymphoid infiltrates and in some tumours this may be a favourable sign.
- Spontaneous regression of tumours occurs.
- Tumours occur more frequently in the neonatal period and in old age, when the immune system functions less effectively.
- Tumours arise frequently in immunosuppressed individuals.

Although at first sight this appears impressive evidence in favour of the theory, on closer examination the strongest point, the association between immunosuppression and increased tumour incidence, is less conclusive. The largest body of data comes from the study of kidney transplant recipients, many of whom have been followed for over 20 years. The frequency of many tumour types is increased in this population (*Fig. 18.1*), and in several of these there is strong evidence that a virus may be involved (*Fig. 18.2*). There is also a slight but definite increased risk for many other cancers in which viruses are not known to play a role. This suggests that the immune response may be most important in preventing the spread of potentially oncogenic viruses and that surveillance against other non-viral tumours is relatively ineffective. Certainly, normal humans who become infected with EBV carry the virus for life and make strong cellular and humoral responses to the virus. Increased virus replication and shedding of viral particles in secretions, occurs in immunodeficient individuals, so that it is clear that the immune response limits virus replication under normal circumstances (*Fig. 18.3*).

Animal experimental data support the view that immune surveillance is largely directed towards viruses rather than tumours. Studies of athymic nude mice or mice immunosuppressed with anti-lymphocyte serum, did not show a general increase in tumour frequency. However, a high proportion of the mice developed tumours caused by viruses

Relative risk of tumours in immunosuppressed kidney transplant recipients

Tumour type	Approximate relative risk
Kaposi's sarcoma	50–100
Non-Hodgkin lymphoma	25–45
Carcinoma of the liver	20–35
Carcinoma of the skin	20–50
Carcinoma of the cervix	2.5–10
Melanoma	2.5–10
Lung	1–2

Fig. 18.1 In all forms of immunodeficiency the relative risk of developing tumours in which viruses are known to play a role is greatly increased. This is the case for all those listed except cancer of the lung. The relative risks vary in different studies according to the length of follow up and the presence of cofactors such as sunlight for skin cancer.

Tumour viruses and immunodeficiency

cause of immunodeficiency	common tumour types	viruses involved
inherited immunodeficiency	lymphoma	EBV
immunosuppression for organ transplants or due to AIDS	lymphoma cervical cancer skin cancer liver cancer Kaposi's sarcoma	EBV papilloma viruses probably papilloma viruses hepatitis B and C viruses human herpes virus 8
malaria	Burkitt's lymphoma	EBV
autoimmunity	lymphoma	EBV

Fig. 18.2 In organ transplant recipients cancer of the skin is the most common form of tumour in absolute numbers. In other forms of immunodeficiency tumours of the immune system dominate. Most normal adults carry both EBV and many papilloma viruses throughout life with no ill effects because they have anti-viral immunity.

(introduced in the anti-lymphocyte serum), which seldom cause tumours in normal animals. When tumours were induced by the carcinogen methyl cholanthrene in SCID (Severe Combined Immunodeficiency) and normal mice, there was no difference in tumour incidence, but the tumours arising in SCID mice were more immunogenic. These data suggest that a functional immune system prevents oncogenesis by viruses but not the development of non-viral tumours. Once a tumour has arisen, less immunogenic variant cells may be selected by an anti-tumour immune response.

Role of EBV in tumorigenesis

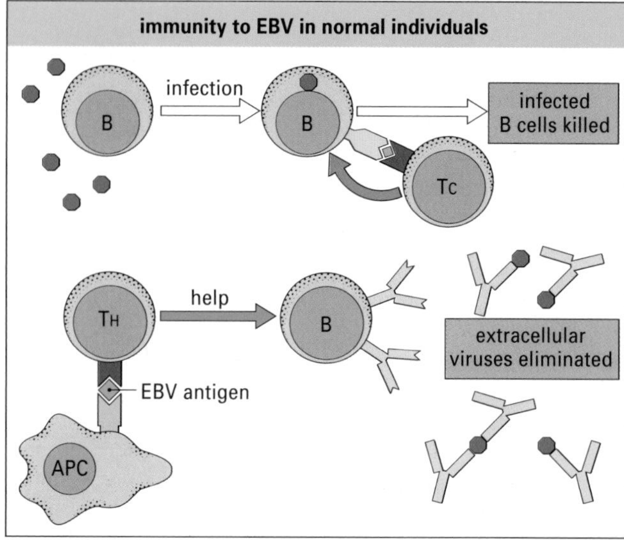

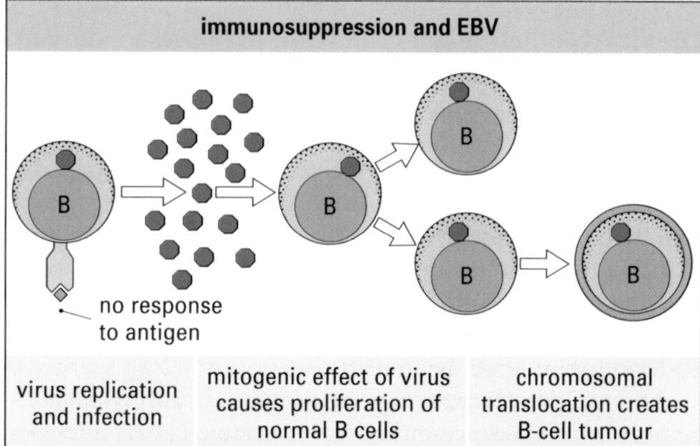

Fig. 18.3 In normal individuals EBV infects B lymphocytes but spread of infection is prevented by Tc cells and antibody, which eliminate infected cells and virus. In immunosuppressed individuals, and in some patients receiving the immunosuppressant cyclosporin, the virus replicates and infects more B cells. The virus is also mitogenic for B cells, so in an immunosuppressed individual infected B cells tend to proliferate more rapidly. A chromosomal translocation in an infected B cell can then lead to malignant transformation.

How important are microorganisms for human cancer?

In man relatively few tumour types are known to be caused by viruses (*Fig. 18.4*), but liver and cervical cancer cause over a million deaths worldwide, implying that hepatitis and papillomaviruses must be able to evade immune surveillance in normal individuals. A recent addition to the list of microorganisms associated with tumours is the bacterium *Helicobacter pylori* in stomach cancer. Interestingly, stomach cancer does not show a great increase in immunosuppressed individuals. Unlike oncogenic viruses, *H. pylori* is not an intracellular pathogen and cannot directly transform cells so that the relationship between the pathogen, epithelial cells that are potential targets for transformation,

Micro-organisms and human tumours

Tumour	Organism
Adult T-cell leukaemia	Human T leukaemia virus I (HTLV I)
Burkitt's lymphoma and lymphoma in immunosuppression	EBV
Cervical cancer	Human papilloma viruses (HPV 16 and 18 and others)
Liver cancer	Hepatitis B and C
Nasopharyngeal cancer	EBV
Skin cancer	Probably human papilloma viruses
Stomach cancer	*Helicobacter pylori*

Fig. 18.4 EBV causes Burkitt's lymphoma in endemic malaria areas of Africa and nasopharyngeal carcinoma in China, suggesting that cofactors, either genetic or environmental, are required for tumour development. *Helicobacter* is the only bacterium so far known to be involved in the aetiology of a human cancer.

the host response and other genetic and dietary factors is likely to be complex.

TUMOUR ANTIGENS

Tumour antigens may be detected by immune cells or antibodies

Viral antigens may be targets for cellular and humoral immune responses but there is also abundant evidence of genetic alterations (mutation, gene amplification, chromosomal deletion or translocation) in most, if not all, tumours. Some of these lead to the expression of altered molecules in tumour cells and others to overexpression of normal molecules. These changes may be demonstrated either by detecting the host immune response or experimentally by deliberately immunizing other species with tumour.

Tumour-associated antigens detected by immune cells

Tumour antigens were first demonstrated by transplantation tests. When a tumour was grafted onto an animal previously immunized with inactivated cells of the same tumour, resistance to the graft was seen. Tumour resistance, subsequently shown to be mediated by immune cells, was directed at tumour-associated transplantation antigens (TATAs) of two types. The first are antigens that are shared by many tumours (T antigens), even though these may not even be of the same tissue of origin. The second are antigens that are specific to an individual tumour (tumour-specific transplantation antigens – TSTAs). Tumours may express both specific and shared antigens.

Shared tumour antigens are of viral origin

These antigens are found on tumours induced by viruses such as the small DNA polyoma and SV40 viruses, which can cause tumours in experimental animals, and the papillomaviruses, which are implicated in human cervical cancer. These viruses code for T (tumour) antigens that are shared by other viruses of the same group. T antigens are nuclear proteins, which play a role in the maintenance of the transformed (cancerous) state. Herpes viruses cause tumours in many species including man in the case of EBV.

In animals, infectious RNA oncogenic viruses cause leukaemias and sarcomas, and at least one human leukaemia virus (HTLV I) has been discovered (*Fig. 18.4*). These viruses bud from the cell membrane of infected cells, and the viral envelope's glycoprotein can be detected at the host cell membrane. There are strong humoral and cell-mediated responses to antigens of DNA- and RNA-tumour viruses (*Fig. 18.3*), which can protect against tumour challenge. Because tumours produced by a given oncogenic virus all share the same antigen, mice immunized, say, with SV40 virus-induced tumour cells reject a different SV40-induced tumour but are susceptible to one induced by polyoma virus.

In some strains of mice, activation of endogenous RNA tumour viruses occurs regularly, leading to leukaemia. In others, when carcinogenic chemicals are given, the resulting tumours may express viral antigens and produce infectious mouse leukaemia virus (MuLV). Such tumours express common tumour-associated antigens as well as the tumour-specific transplantation antigens (TSTAs) discussed below. Host immune responses to endogenous RNA viruses are weak, perhaps because of immunological tolerance (see Chapter 12).

Tumour-specific transplantation antigens are due to alterations in tumour genes or gene expression

TSTAs are antigens which can induce tumour rejection, but the animal must have been previously immunized with the same tumour (*Fig. 18.5*). These antigens were first detected using tumours from inbred mice that had been induced by chemical carcinogens and their nature has now been elucidated, as described below.

A transplantable (therefore poorly immunogenic) tumour of inbred DBA2 strain mice was exposed *in vitro* to a powerful mutagen. This produced mutant subclones, some of which would no longer grow *in vivo*, unless very large numbers of tumour cells were implanted. The mutants had clearly become more immunogenic than the parent tumour. One of these tumour- (tum-) variant clones was used to immunize syngeneic mice. This generated T-cytotoxic (Tc) cells, which would kill only the immunizing tumour and not the parental tumour line or other tum- variants (*Fig. 18.6*). The Tc cells were then used as probes to identify the presence of the mutated tumour antigen during molecular cloning of the tumour antigen gene. Ultimately the mutant gene coding for the tumour antigen (the tum- gene) was identified and sequenced. Comparison of this gene with the homologous gene from the parental tumour showed a single amino acid difference. Formal proof that this mutation could generate the immunogenic antigen recognized by the Tc cells was then obtained: parental tumour cells incubated with a ten-amino-acid peptide having the tum- sequence could be killed, while if they were incubated with the homologous peptide from

Demonstration of tumour-specific antigens of chemically induced tumours

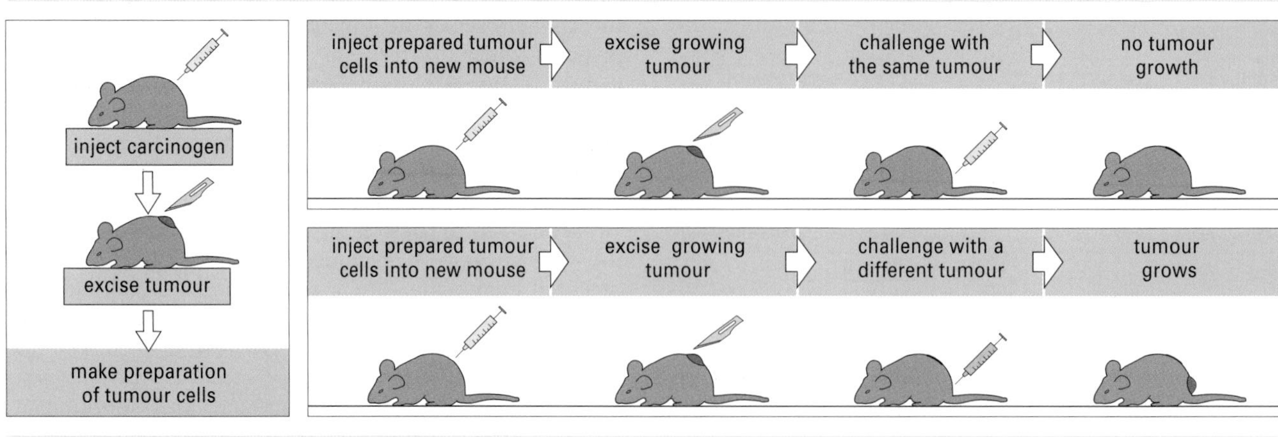

Fig. 18.5 Mice were induced to produce tumours by the injection of a chemical carcinogen (methyl/cholanthrene). Tumour cells from these mice were then injected subcutaneously into genetically identical mice. Later, the growing tumours were removed surgically. Mice challenged with the same tumour were able to reject it, but those challenged with a different tumour (induced with the same carcinogen) were not. The ability to reject the tumour could be transferred with lymphoid cells.

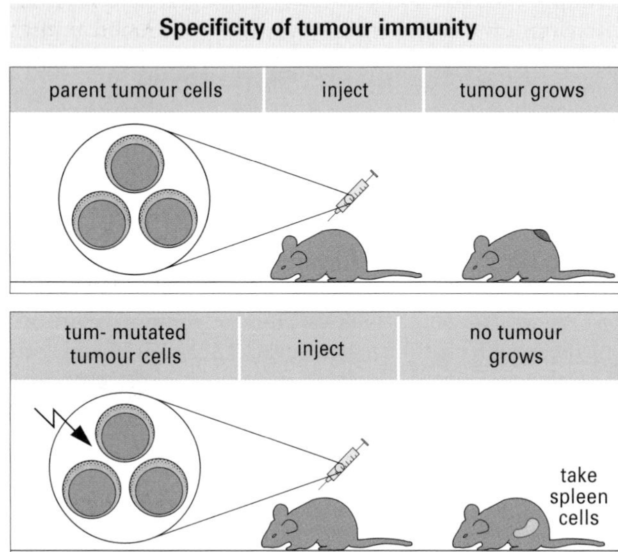

tumour cell type	effect of spleen cells on tumour
parent tumour	no effect
tum− variant	cytotoxic

Fig. 18.6 The production of a highly immunogenic (tum− variant) tumour in DBA2 mice and Tc cells specific for it are shown. After inducing mutations in the parent tumour cells, subclones were obtained, some of which would no longer grow in DBA2 mice. Spleen Tc cells from mice injected with these tum− cells could kill tum− cells, but not the parent tumour, *in vitro.*

Specificity of Tc cells for a tumour antigen peptide

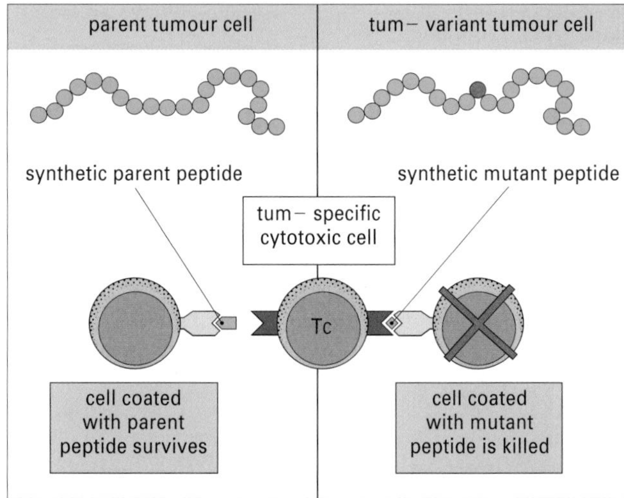

Fig. 18.7 Tc cells were taken from a mouse immunized with a tum− variant tumour. *In vitro,* they killed tumour cells coated with a peptide from the tum− gene sequence, but not cells coated with the homologous peptide from the parental tumour. The two peptides differ by a single amino acid.

parental cells they were not (*Fig. 18.7*). As Tc cells are MHC class I restricted, it is clear that the tumour-specific protein is processed within the cell to generate a peptide that becomes associated with MHC class I and is transported to the cell surface (see *Fig. 6.12*).

In contrast to the first tum- antigen, antigen genes cloned from other tum- variants were sometimes identical to the parental gene. In these tum- variants, the difference from the parent tumour was that the antigen was over-expressed in the cells.

There is good evidence that there are T-helper (TH) cell responses to tumours, but much less is known about the antigens recognized in association with MHC class II. This is because these antigens are normally recognized by TH cells on antigen-presenting cells rather than the tumour cell itself. This creates additional difficulties in cloning the genes coding for the antigens.

HUMAN TUMOUR-ASSOCIATED ANTIGENS DETECTED BY IMMUNE CELLS

Mixed lymphocyte–tumour cultures reveal anti-tumour responses *in vitro*

The realization that responses of antigen-primed TH and Tc cells could be revealed by re-stimulating them with specific antigen *in vitro* led to experiments in which lymphocytes from patients were cultured with inactivated tumour cells in mixed lymphocyte–tumour culture (MLTC) (*Fig. 18.8*). The lymphocytes might be taken from peripheral blood, from tumour-draining lymph nodes or from the tumour itself (the latter are known as tumour-infiltrating lymphocytes or TILs).

MLTC may stimulate CD4 TH cells, which proliferate and secrete effector cytokines, and CD8 Tc. The latter can be assayed by measuring their cytotoxic activity in a ^{51}Cr-release assay (see Chapter 27). Tc cells can also be obtained from TILs by culturing them in IL-2 to expand any effector cells generated *in vivo*. Tc clones obtained by these means have been used to identify human TSTA genes by similar molecular expression cloning techniques to those used for tum- variant genes in the mouse.

Melanoma appears to be particularly immunogenic and melanoma-specific CTL clones were therefore produced and used to screen a melanoma cDNA library. The first human tumour antigen identified, MAGE 1 (melanoma antigen 1), was an overexpressed unaltered antigen (*Fig. 18.9*). More remarkably the antigen belongs to a large previously undiscovered gene family of cancer testis antigens, which are widely expressed in tumours and seldom in normal tissues. Subsequently several other melanoma antigens as well as antigens of other tumours have been cloned. The majority of antigens identified by this methodology are unaltered. Many are differentiation antigens, normal molecules that are expressed in a tissue-specific fashion and play a role in the function of the normal cellular counterpart of the tumour cell, in the case of melanoma, the melanocyte. However, mutations and genetic rearrangements creating new sequences are common in tumours (*Fig. 18.10*) and some tumour patients can respond to peptides of mutant *ras* oncogene or the HER2/*neu* oncogene product. Computer analysis indicates that many of the new sequences formed by genetic alterations in tumours could bind to common HLA alleles, such as HLA-A2, and may therefore be potential tumour target antigens. These studies have also established the principle that most tumour antigens do not differ from other antigens recognized by T cells; they are short peptides presented by MHC molecules.

Mixed lymphocyte–tumour culture

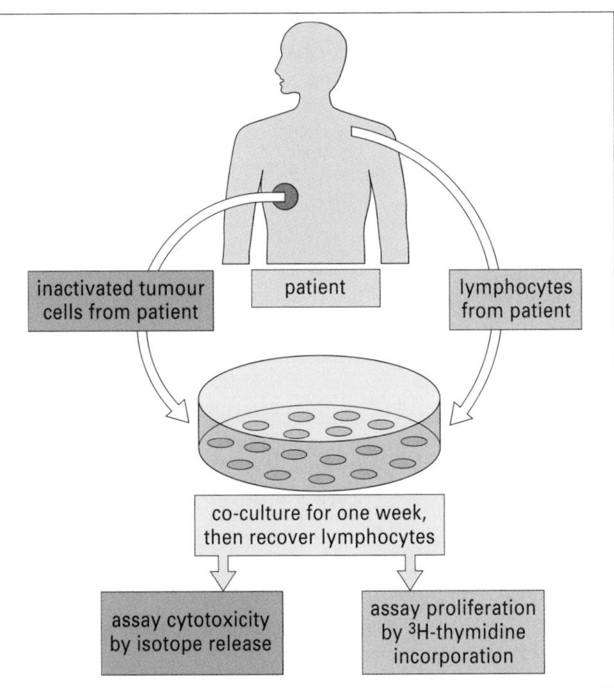

Fig. 18.8 Lymphocytes taken from blood, draining lymph nodes or directly from tumour tissue, are co-cultured with autologous tumour cells, which have been inactivated by X-irradiation or treatment with mitomycin-C. After a suitable period of culture, the lymphocytes can be assayed for proliferation by incorporation of ^{3}H-thymidine (from the culture medium). Their effector function can be assessed by measuring cytokines released into the culture medium, or by their ability to lyse target cells in isotope release assays.

Human tumour-associated antigens recognized by T lymphocytes

Antigen name(s)	Tumour types	Normal tissue distribution
Cancer/testis antigens MAGE 1 MAGE 3 BAGE GAGE	Some melanomas and other tumour types	Testis
Melanocyte differentiation antigens MelanA/MART-1 Tyrosinase gp100/Pmel 17 gp75/TRP-1	Melanoma	Normal melanocytes
Differentiation antigens of other tissues Prostate specific antigen (PSA)	Prostate	Prostate
Carcinoembryonic antigen (CEA)	Colon and other carcinomas	Colon
Mutated antigens Mutated ras	Many carcinomas	Not present
Her-2/neu	Breast and ovary	Not present

Fig. 18.9 An unexpected finding to emerge from the cloning of these antigens is the large number of antigens expressed only in tumours and the testis in adults. Antigens recognized by T cells may be found in all locations within the cell or may even be secreted antigens.

Genetic alterations in human tumours producing new protein sequences

Alteration	Function of protein	Tumour type
Point mutations		
ERB B2	Growth factor receptor	Breast carcinoma
FMS	CSF-1 receptor	AML, myelodysplasia
ras	GTP-binding protein	Carcinomas and others
p53	Tumour suppressor cell cycle control	Many including bladder, colon, lung
RB1	Tumour suppressor cell cycle control	Retinoblastoma, osteosarcoma, pancreatic carcinoma
Chromosomal translocations		
BCR-ABL	Tyrosine kinase	CML, ALL
EZA-PRL	Transcription factor	Pre-B cell ALL
H4-RET	Growth factor receptor/tyrosine kinase	Thyroid carcinoma
TPR-MET	Growth factor receptor/tyrosine kinase	Gastric carcinoma
L MYC-RLF	Transcription factor	Small cell lung carcinoma
NPM/ALK	Tyrosine kinase	Lymphoma
Deletion mutations		
ERB-B	Growth factor receptor	Gliomas

Fig. 18.10 Genetic alterations occur during the development of most tumours. Because they are only present in tumours, mutated antigens appear ideal targets for immunotherapy but the mutation is not the same in every tumour and the altered peptide epitope may not be well displayed by self MHC molecules. The mutated antigen may therefore be poorly immunogenic. In addition there may be positive selection for cells which have downregulated their MHC.

TUMOUR-ASSOCIATED ANTIGENS DETECTED BY ANTIBODIES

Few antigens are unique to tumours

There have been many attempts to detect antigens unique to tumours, using either sera from animals deliberately immunized with tumour material (heterologous typing) or sera from tumour-bearing animals or patients (autologous typing). In recent years heterologous typing has relied on monoclonal antibodies (mAbs) and although few molecules uniquely expressed in tumours have been detected, several types of antigen associated with tumours have been identified (*Fig. 18.11*).

Tumours may express normal differentiation antigens that have a restricted distribution in normal cells

Most tumour cells represent the clonal progeny of a single cell, and cells of that type may be relatively rare. The tumour cells may therefore express antigens present on

Antigens identified by monoclonal antibodies

Tumour-specific antigens	Tumour type	Normal tissue distribution
Idiotypes of the TCR and immunoglobulin	B- and T-cell lymphomas and leukaemias	None
Oncofoetal differentiation antigens		
carcinoembryonic antigen (CEA)	Colon and many other carcinomas	High expression in fetal intestine and low in normal adult tissues
α-fetoprotein (AFP)	Liver carcinoma	Fetal liver, low in normal adult tissue
Differentiation antigens		
common acute lymphoblastic leukaemia antigen (CALLA)	Acute lymphoblastic leukaemia	Subset of immature B cells
17-1A Epithelial antigen	Colon cancer	Colonic and other normal epithelia
Altered differentiation antigens		
MUC-1 (mucin)	Breast and other carcinomas	Some epitopes expressed equally on tumours and normal epithelium, others equally on tumours and lactating breast
Overexpressed differentiation antigens		
Prostate specific antigen (PSA)	Prostate carcinoma	Low level in normal prostate

Fig. 18.11 Many monoclonal antibodies have been produced by immunizing rodents with human tumours. The majority of these recognize molecules present both on tumours and normal cells. Nevertheless because the antigen is expressed at a higher level in tumours, is only expressed on a small number of normal cells or in fetal but not adult tissues, many of these may be useful for immunodiagnosis or immunotherapy.

Expression of CALLA in normal cells and *leukaemias*

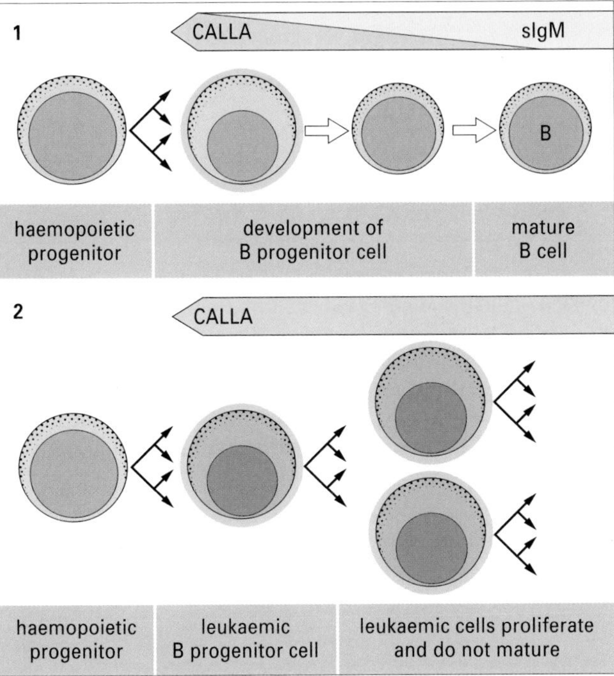

Fig. 18.12 (1) CALLA is normally expressed only on B-cell progenitors or lymphoblasts, which make up <1% of normal bone marrow cells. (2) CALLA becomes much more abundant in the commonest form of childhood leukaemia.

only a few normal cells. The Common Acute Lymphoblastic Leukaemia Antigen (CALLA or CD10) is an example (*Fig. 18.12*). Oncofetal antigens are differentiation antigens expressed during fetal development but normally not expressed, or expressed at very low levels, in adult life. Examples are α-fetoprotein (AFP), which is produced by liver cancer cells, and carcinoembryonic antigen (CEA) produced by colon cancer cells and other epithelial tumours.

Normal antigens expressed in tumours may be altered by glycosylation

Glycosylation is altered in many tumours. This may give rise to the expression of new carbohydrate epitopes, such as the Thomsen–Friedenreich antigen, a disaccharide which is usually hidden on normal cells. Aberrant blood groups can also be created in this way. Alterations in glycosylation may also reveal epitopes on the protein backbone that are rarely detected in normal cells. For example, polymorphic epithelial mucins are produced by many normal epithelial cells. They are high-molecular-weight glycoproteins with a repeating core peptide carrying the carbohydrate side chains. In epithelial tumours, new peptide epitopes can be detected in the repeating core structure of polymorphic epithelial mucin 1 (MUC 1), but these new epitopes are also detectable in the lactating breast (*Fig. 18.11*).

Sera from patients with tumours detect widely distributed antigens

Until recently autologous typing was extremely difficult because most human sera are complex and contain many antibodies capable of reacting to tumour cells including anti-HLA, anti-blood group and anti-carbohydrate antibodies. Many antibodies are IgM and of low affinity. Generation of human monoclonal antibodies has been technically difficult and the resulting hybridoma antibodies often detect widely distributed autoantigens, perhaps because they are derived from the pool of natural autoantibody-producing B1 cells. The importance of these antibodies in the host response to tumours is unclear.

Serological analysis of human tumour antigens by recombinant cDNA expression cloning (SEREX)

More recently SEREX has been developed. Sera from patients are used to screen cDNA expression libraries from fresh tumour material. Isolation of antigens detected only by high titre IgG or IgA antibodies ensures that the method does not detect IgM natural antibodies. The SEREX method has the disadvantage that it may not detect all conformational epitopes of a protein and does not identify carbohydrate antigens because the bacteria used to express the antigens do not glycosylate them. Nevertheless, over 900 sequences of genes cloned using the SEREX method have already been deposited in a data base set up for this purpose. These include known TSTAs such as MAGE-1 and tyrosinase, sequences identical (or nearly identical) to known genes not previously known to elicit an autoantibody response (e.g. kinectin a transporter asociated with Golgi vesicles), and a large group of previously unknown genes (*Fig. 18.13*). A complete description of the expression patterns of 900 genes in normal and tumour tissue, let alone analysis of their functions, is a major undertaking, but will eventually identify many new targets for immunotherapy.

Antigens identified by SEREX

Name	Source cDNA library
Cancer testis antigens	
HOM-Mel-40	Melanoma
NY-ESO-1	Melanoma
MAGE 1	Melanoma
Differentiation antigens	
Tyrosinase	Melanoma
Galectin-9	Hodgkin's disease
Carbonic anhydrase	Renal carcinoma
Housekeeping genes	
Proliferating cell nuclear antigen (PCNA)	Melanoma
Endogenous retroviral genes	
HERV-K10	Renal carcinoma
Mutated antigens	
p53 (mutated)	Colon carcinoma

Fig. 18.13 The SEREX methodology depends on the use of IgG antibodies from tumour patient sera. It is allowing for the first time molecular definition of antigens to which tumour-bearing patients make a T cell-dependent antibody response. A surprisingly broad range of antigens are recognized.

IMMUNODIAGNOSIS

Antigens need not be tumour specific to be used for diagnosis

Although there are few molecules which are exclusive to tumour cells, antibodies to tumour-associated molecules can be very useful in tumour diagnosis, by either detecting increased amounts of an antigen or the presence of an antigen in an abnormal site.

In vivo

Radiolabelled antibodies against tumour-associated molecules have been used for the detection of tumours (*Fig. 18.14*), but the method is seldom more sensitive than modern methods of computerized tomography or nuclear magnetic resonance imaging. In addition, immunoscintigraphy has the disadvantage that antibodies need to be freshly labelled for each patient, and different antibodies are optimal for different tumour types. The development of recombinant multivalent fragments of high-affinity antibodies may improve the sensitivity of immunoscintigraphy in the future.

In vitro

Antibodies are useful for identifying the cell of origin of undifferentiated tumours (*Fig. 18.15*) and for the detection of micrometastases in bone marrow, cerebrospinal fluid, lymphoid organs or elsewhere (*Fig. 18.16*). There are also immunoassays available for several tumour-associated molecules which can be detected in the serum. These include CEA, AFP and PSA. Raised levels of CEA or AFP may be useful for diagnosis but CEA may be raised in association with several tumour types and both CEA and AFP in some non-malignant conditions so that they are generally more useful in following the course of treatment (*Fig. 18.17*).

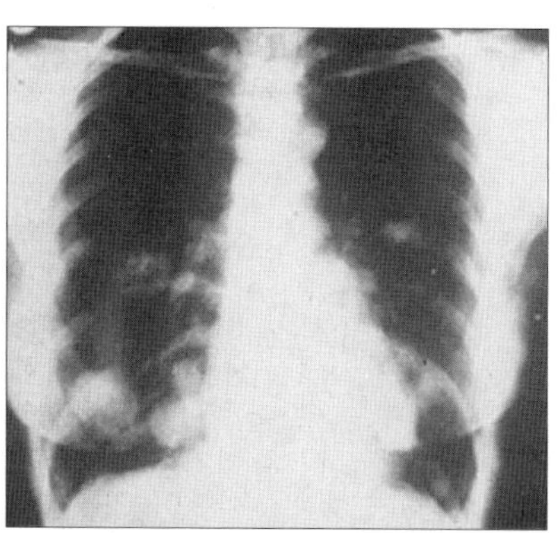

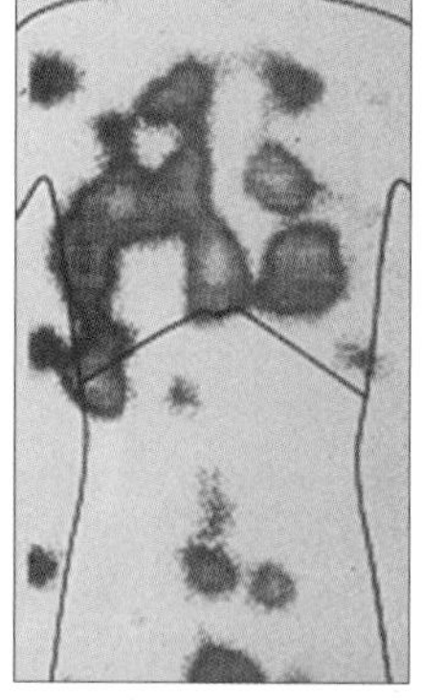

Fig. 18.14 Chest radiograph and immunoscintigraphy scan of a patient with carcinoma of the colon who has lung and liver metastases. The monoclonal antibody YPC2/12.1, raised against human colorectal cancer, binds to CEA. (It reacts with a glycoprotein of 180 kDa.) The antibody was radiolabelled with ^{131}I and administered intravenously. Scintigrams were obtained after 48 hours. The image is that obtained after a subtraction procedure to eliminate background blood-borne antibody. (Courtesy of Professor K. Sikora.)

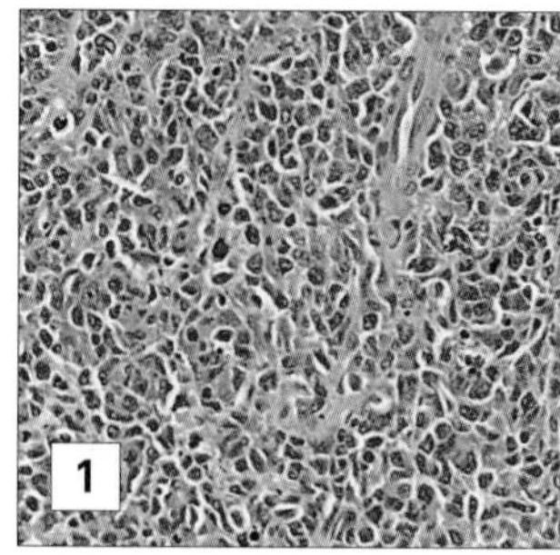

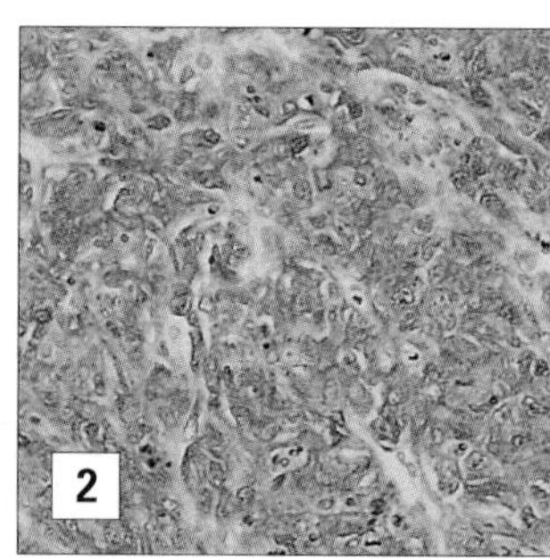

Fig. 18.15 Identification of the cell of origin of an undifferentiated tumour. Conventional histology of a biopsy of this tumour (**1**) showed a sheet of undifferentiated tumour cells which could not be identified. When the tumour was stained by the indirect immunoperoxidase method (**2**) with an antibody against CD45 (the leucocyte common antigen), it was found to be strongly positive (brown colour), identifying it as a lymphoma.

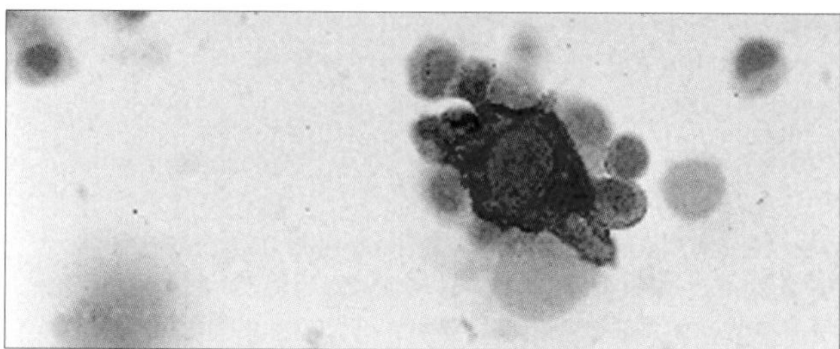

Fig. 18.16 Detection of micrometastases using a monoclonal antibody. The figure shows an imprint of cells from a lymph node draining a tumour site in a cancer patient. The slide is stained by the immunoalkaline phosphatase method with an antibody against a cytokeratin. Carcinoma cells express cytokeratins and a large pink-stained tumour cell is clearly seen. Rare tumour cells, as in this lymph node sample, are easily missed by conventional cytological examination.

Monitoring serum CEA level in colon carcinoma

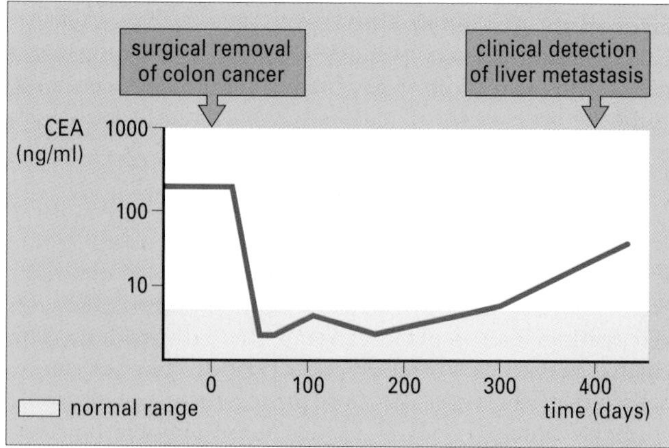

Fig. 18.17 The relationship of serum CEA level to clinical course in a patient with carcinoma of the colon is shown. At presentation there is a high CEA level, which falls following surgery. A rise is found well before the clinical detection of metastatic tumour.

Immunotherapy of tumours

Active	non-specific	BCG, *Corynebacterium parvum*, levamisole, cytokines
	specific	Therapeutic vaccines of tumour cells, cell extracts, purified or recombinant antigens, peptides, heat shock proteins or DNA antigen-pulsed dendritic cells
Passive	non-specific	LAK cells
	specific	Antibodies alone or coupled to drugs, pro-drugs, toxins or radioisotope, bi-specific antibodies T cells
	Combined	LAK cells and bi-specific antibody

Fig. 18.18 Non-specific agents boost specific and non-specific immune mechanisms probably via release of cytokines. Cytokines themselves induce release of further cytokines *in vivo*. Alternatively non-specific LAK cells may be given alone or with cytokines or targeted to tumours with bi-specific antibody to mimic the effects of specific cells.

IMMUNOTHERAPY

Immunotherapy has a limited role at present

Immunotherapy has a long history but is only now becoming established as a reliable form of therapy for some forms of cancer, while most immunotherapeutic strategies remain experimental. Intervention may be active or passive, specific or non-specific. *Figure 18.18* summarizes the possibilities.

Specific active immunotherapy – the mechanisms of activation

Specific active immunization with inactivated tumour cells has shown some success in animal models where immunization is performed before tumour challenge. Attempts to induce regression of established tumours have been much less successful. While much effort has been expended in designing means of making tumour cells more immunogenic, for example by infecting the cells with viruses or coupling chemical groups to the cell surface, most of these have been empirical. More recently it has become clear that induction of immune responses depends on two signals. Signal 1 is delivered through the T-cell receptor (TCR) when it interacts with MHC–peptide complexes and the second essential signal for activation (Signal 2) is delivered by several costimuli. These may be both cell surface molecules on antigen-presenting cells (APC) and soluble cytokines (see *Fig. 6.19*). There is good evidence that T cells may be inactivated if one signal is delivered without the other.

Immunization with tumour antigens

Increased understanding of the mechanisms of T-cell activation has led to more rational strategies to improve the immunogenicity of tumour cells. Transfection of the genes for CD80 (B7) or cytokines such as interleukin-2 (IL-2), IL-4, interferon-γ (IFN-γ) or granulocyte-macrophage–colony-stimulating factor (GM–CSF) into tumour cells has been shown to increase greatly their immunogenicity in animal tumour protection experiments. Similarly, immunization with defined peptide epitopes in novel adjuvants can induce cytotoxic T lymphocyte (CTL) able to cause rejection of experimental tumours. DNA constructs coding for tumour antigens and co-stimuli can also be used directly to immunize animals. Heat-shock proteins extracted from tumour cells have also been used. It is thought that these molecules act as chaperonins during the assembly of MHC–peptide complexes, carrying peptides produced during antigen processing. While all these methods can protect animals against subsequent tumour challenge, they are much less successful in treating established tumours.

Immunization with dendritic cells

A logical extension of attempts to make tumour cells more immunogenic by transfection of co-stimuli is, instead, to use the most effective APCs known. These are dendritic cells, which can be grown from the bone marrow of mice or peripheral blood of man. An additional advantage of this method is that it is thought that even co-stimulus-transfected tumour cells seldom present antigen effectively to resting T cells. Rather, dead or dying tumour cells are more usually taken up by APCs and carried to the draining lymph nodes, where activation of T cells takes place. Antigens can be introduced into dendritic cells *in vitro* as whole (irradiated) tumour cells or as proteins, peptides, DNA, or in recombinant viruses. The cells are then re-introduced into the tumour-bearing animal or patient (*Fig. 18.19*). At least in experimental animals this method, though cumbersome, is showing promising results in tumour therapy experiments.

Active immunization in man

Although no form of active specific immunization has yet become a first-line treatment for any cancer, many clinical trials are currently underway (*Fig. 18.20*). As both TH and Tc cells have been shown to contribute to tumour protection in animal experiments, not all the immunization procedures are aimed at the induction of cytotoxic T cells; for example, the use of oligosaccharides or lipids conjugated to carrier molecules such as Keyhole Limpet Haemocyanin (KLH) would be expected to induce TH and antibody production, but not Tc.

In most trials, prolonged survival has been observed in some patients following immunization and in most cases side effects have been mild. Most trials to date have been in patients who have relapsed after initial treatment by surgery, radiotherapy and chemotherapy. These patients would not be expected to be ideal subjects for immunotherapy as they have a high tumour burden, the tumour will have had time to develop escape mechanisms (see below) and radiotherapy and chemotherapy are immunosuppressive. Future trials will need to be carried out at an earlier stage of disease to test whether immunotherapy is a useful adjunct to standard treatments which have first eliminated the main tumour burden.

Non-specific stimulation of immune responses

A variety of agents have been used to stimulate the immune response non-specifically (*Fig. 18.21*). Most attempts at

Immunization via dendritic cells

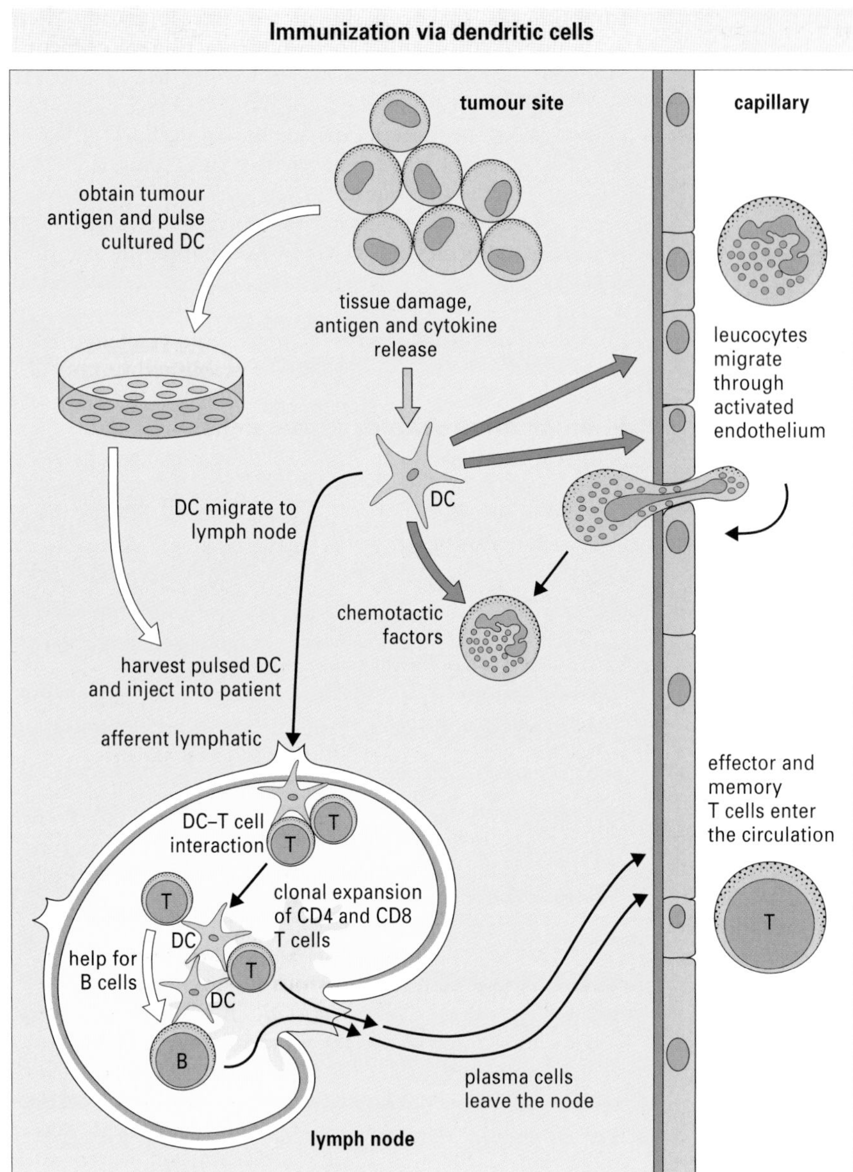

Fig. 18.19 An illustration of how tissue damage caused by a growing tumour may lead to cytokine release, loading of dendritic cells (DC) with antigen, and migration of DC to the draining lymph node to induce an immune response. Local tissue damage also promotes entry of effector leucocytes into the tumour site. Therapy with DC attempts to mimic the natural process of immunization, by loading the DC with tumour antigen, providing them with maturation signals *in vitro* and returning them to the patient.

Clinical trials of active immunization in man

Tumour	Target antigen	Immunization
Breast	MUC 1	Sialyl TN antigen-KLH conjugate with adjuvant Recombinant Vaccinia-MUC 1 virus with IL-2
Cervix	HPV E6/E7	Recombinant Vaccinia HPV E6/E7 Recombinant E6/E7 protein Synthetic peptides in adjuvant
Lymphoma	Immunoglobulin idiotype	Recombinant protein Idiotype single chain Fv-tetanus toxoid DNA construct DC pulsed with idiotypic protein
Melanoma	Various	Allogeneic whole cells, cells transduced with cytokines, peptides, DC pulsed with peptides or tumour lysate
Prostate	Prostate specific antigen (PSA) Globo H hexasaccharide	Liposome encapsulated PSA, DC pulsed with peptides Synthetic antigen-KLH conjugate with QS21adjuvant

Fig. 18.20 A large number of trials of immunotherapy are being undertaken. Most of these are phase 1 trials testing safety and toxicity and they are carried out in patients with advanced cancer and a large burden of tumour. For ethical reasons, very few trials have been carried out in the more favourable situation of minimal residual disease that is often reached after primary treatment with surgery, radiotherapy or chemotherapy.

Non-specific active immunotherapy: biological response modifiers (BRMs)

type of BRM	examples	major effect
bacterial products	BCG, *C. parvum*, muramyl dipeptide, trehalose dimycolate	activate macrophages and NK cells
synthetic molecules	pyran copolymer, MVE, poly I:C, pyrimidines	induce IFN production
cytokines	IFNα, IFNβ, IFNγ, IL-2, TNF	activate macrophages and NK cells
hormones	thymosin, thymulin, thymopoietin	modulate T-cell function

Fig. 18.21 Biological response modifiers (BRMs) are used to enhance immune responses to tumours and fall into four major groups. Broadly speaking, bacterial products have adjuvant effects on macrophages (see Chapters 15 and 17); a variety of synthetic polymers, nucleotides and polynucleotides induce IFN production and release; the cytokines administered directly act on macrophages and NK cells, and a variety of hormones including the thymic hormones can be used to enhance T-cell function. (MVE = maleic anhydride divinyl ether; TNF = tumour necrosis factor; poly I : C = polyinosinic–polycytidylic acid.)

Cytokine therapy for tumours

cytokine	tumour type and results	cytokine effects and possible anti-tumour mechanisms
IFNα	prolonged remissions of hairy-cell leukaemia	possible cytostatic effect on tumour
	weak effects on some carcinomas	increased expression of MHC class I, cytostasis
IFNγ	ineffective systemically, remissions of peritoneal carcinoma of the ovary	increased MHC class I and II macrophage activation, Tc activation, cytostasis
IL-2	remissions in renal cancer and melanoma	T-cell activation and proliferation, NK-cell activation
TNFα	can reduce malignant ascites	?increased tumour cell adhesion, macrophage and lymphocyte activation

Fig. 18.22 Most cytokines have been given systemically in high doses. The mechanism of the anti-tumour effect is uncertain in most cases. *In vitro*, IFNα and TNFα are cytostatic for some tumour cells, but *in vivo* any effects seen may be indirect because many cytokines induce production of other cytokines (the cytokine cascade). The fact that some patients treated with IL-2 suffer transient autoimmune thyroiditis provides some evidence that cytokine administration does potentiate immune responses.

systemic therapy in man have not been conspicuously successful, but intralesional BCG can cause regression of melanoma and non-specific local immunization with BCG is effective against bladder tumours.

Immunotherapy with cytokine can cause tumour regression

Many cytokines have been cloned, expressed and used for tumour therapy. *Figure 18.22* gives information on those that have been most thoroughly investigated to date. Successes have so far been few and far between, though IFNα can induce prolonged remission of the rare hairy-cell leukaemia and IL-2 is effective in a proportion of melanomas and renal carcinomas. There are also encouraging results in the treatment of intraperitoneal ovarian tumours with IFNγ and tumour necrosis factor-α (TNFα). Some cytokines are finding a useful role in supportive therapy. Colony-stimulating factors can shorten the period of aplasia after bone marrow transplantation or cytotoxic therapy, and erythropoietin can relieve the anaemia.

Immunization against oncogenic viruses

Because there is increasing evidence for a role of viruses in some human cancers, the most promising avenue for active immunization may be in preventing infection with potentially oncogenic agents. Successful mass immunization against hepatitis B virus is already decreasing the incidence of primary hepatoma in endemic areas. It may be possible eventually to vaccinate at-risk populations against papillomaviruses, HTLV-1 or EBV.

PASSIVE IMMUNOTHERAPY

Therapy with lymphokine-activated killer cells

When human peripheral blood mononuclear cells are cultured *in vitro* with IL-2, they become highly cytotoxic to a wide variety of tumour targets, many of which are resistant to freshly isolated natural killer (NK) cells. Initial animal and human experiments, in which these lymphokine-activated killer (LAK) cells were re-infused, gave some good results, especially when IL-2 was given at the same time. However, controlled trials have given less encouraging results and the therapy, involving high-dose IL-2, has significant toxicity. It seems likely that few LAK cells localize in tumours, and this may contribute to the poor results. To overcome this, bi-specific mAbs have been used. In these, one antibody is directed against a tumour molecule and the other against lymphocyte surface markers. In theory these antibodies should help to localize the LAK cells on the tumour. While such strategies certainly work *in vitro*, their effectiveness *in vivo* remains to be established.

Immunotherapy with T cells

T cells extracted from tumour sites can also be expanded *in vitro* using IL-2 and eventually re-infused. In a proportion of cases the cultured T cells show relative specificity for the tumour from which they were derived. In animal model systems there is no doubt that tumour-specific cytotoxic T cells can cause dramatic regression of tumour. The tumour toxicity of such TILs may be increased by transfecting into them genes coding for cytokine production. In humans large numbers of EBV-specific Tc cells have been grown *in vitro* using IL-2 and infused into patients who have developed lymphoma following bone marrow transplantation. Remission of tumour occurred. In this case the strong viral antigens of EBV are the target but although these results are encouraging, the efficacy of this strategy against common epithelial malignancies remains to be tested.

The efficacy of anti-tumour lymphocytes is also shown by the graft-versus-leukaemia effect. Following allogeneic bone marrow transplantation for leukaemia, it was noticed that patients who developed graft-versus-host disease (see Chapter 25) had a better prognosis than those who did not. This led to the use of leucocyte transfusions from the donor of the bone marrow, in addition to the bone marrow transplant itself. This has been shown to be effective in chronic myeloid leukaemia. Attempts are being made to separate cells mediating the graft-versus-leukaemia effect from those causing graft-versus-host disease. The possibility of using allogeneic cells for treatment of other forms of cancer is being explored.

Therapy with antibodies

Early attempts at passive immunotherapy with polyclonal antisera were limited because of the difficulty of achieving high titre and specificity. The advent of monoclonal antibodies overcame these difficulties. Although, with the exception of B-cell and T-cell idiotypes on lymphomas, surface antigens unique to tumours have not been discovered, some antigens show increased expression on certain tumour cells and in other cases, damage to normal body cells carrying the same antigen may be unimportant or tolerable. Monoclonal antibodies may be used either alone, or coupled to drugs, pro-drugs, toxins, cytokines or isotopes (*Fig. 18.23*). There are however, a number of limitations to antibody therapy:

- Antibody penetration into large tumour masses is often poor. In principle this might be overcome by smaller molecules that retain specific antigen binding, e.g. F(ab′) fragments, or by engineered single-domain antibodies. Alternatively, it may be possible to target therapy to the endothelium of tumour blood vessels.
- Antibodies are bound by any normal cells expressing the target antigen, and non-specifically by cells bearing Fc receptors or receptors for immunoglobulin carbohydrates. Chemical modification or genetic engineering of the antibody molecules may partially overcome these difficulties. Better discrimination between tumour and normal cells might be obtained with bi-specific antibodies against two different antigens which are both present on the tumour cells but only found separately on normal cells.
- Antibodies are immunogenic and may therefore be attacked by the immune system. Even chimeric or humanized antibodies may induce an immune response to their idiotype. The use of different mAbs for successive courses of therapy might solve this problem.

In spite of these difficulties there have been some encouraging results. In a randomized study the 17-1A monoclonal antibody has been used to treat colon cancer following surgery to remove the primary tumour. Here the aim was to target micrometastases, avoiding the problem of poor penetration into large tumour masses. The treated group showed significantly improved survival. An antibody to the HER2/neu growth factor receptor has been licensed in the USA for treatment of breast cancers expressing the receptor. In this case the most promising results appear to be obtained in combination with chemotherapy. A monoclonal antibody to the CD20 B-lymphocyte differentiation antigen has also received a licence for treatment of lymphoma.

Therapeutic modification of monoclonal antibodies

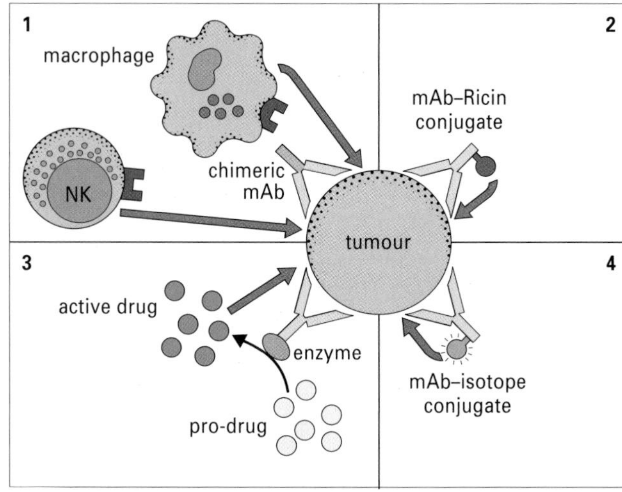

Fig. 18.23 **(1)** Genetically engineered chimeric antibodies with a human Fc portion attached to a mouse F(ab)′2 reduce the risk of an immune response to the mAb. Human Fc will also recruit human effector mechanisms. Alternatively, various molecules can be coupled to mAbs for targeting to tumour cells. Theses include toxins **(2)**, cytotoxic drugs or enzymes capable of activating pro-drugs **(3)** or radioactive isotopes **(4)**.

Radiolabelled anti-B-cell antibodies also show promise against lymphomas resistant to conventional therapy and a labelled monoclonal against the MUC-1 antigen appears to prolong survival (compared to historical controls), when administered intraperitoneally to patients with ovarian cancer.

Antibodies may also be used *in vitro* either to purge tumour cells from bone marrow for autografting (*Fig. 18.24*) or to remove T cells for prevention of graft-versus-host disease in allotransplants.

IMMUNE ESCAPE MECHANISMS

Tumours show multiple mechanisms for evading immune responses

Because spontaneous tumours grow and kill the host, many tumours must escape the host immune response. Many mechanisms have been proposed. The most obvious is that the tumour is non-immunogenic. This might be because potential tumour antigens are lacking but, as described earlier, increasing numbers of antigens recognized by cells or antibodies of tumour bearers are now being identified.

***In vitro* purging of tumour-infiltrated bone marrow**

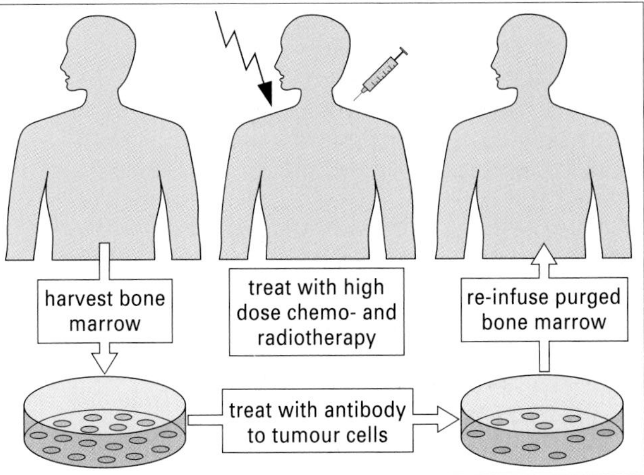

Fig. 18.24 Bone marrow containing tumour cells can be purged using mAbs and complement, antibody–toxin conjugates or antibodies coupled to magnetic beads. The purged marrow is stored while the patient is given high-dose chemo- and radiotherapy. The purged marrow is then returned to the patient. This therapy has given encouraging results in some leukaemia and lymphoma patients who were not helped by their conventional therapy.

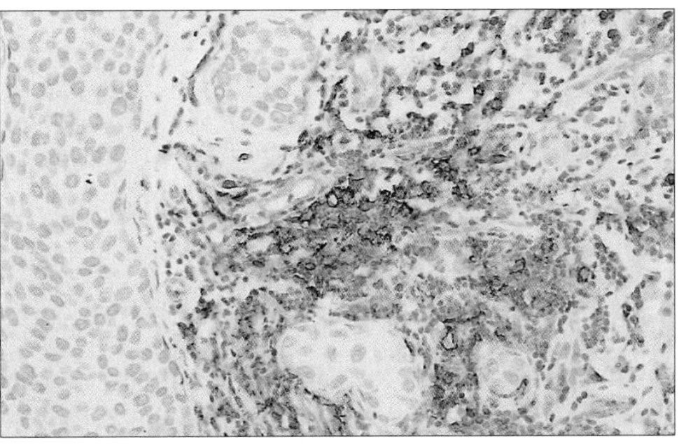

Fig. 18.25 Breast cancer tissue reactive with a monoclonal antibody to a monomorphic determinant of HLA class I antigens. Only stromal cells are stained (brown colour), as malignant epithelial cells fail to express normal MHC class I antigens. Some 50% of primary human cancers fall into this category. Aberrant class II expression may also occur on some tumours. (Indirect immunoperoxidase technique, counterstained with haematoxylin.)

More likely the weak response to tumours is because they are poor antigen-presenting cells. Even if effector cells are generated, these may recognize (and kill) the tumour cells with difficulty.

A particularly important escape mechanism is loss of MHC antigens leading to inability to present tumour antigen peptides. More than 50% of tumours may lose one or more MHC class I alleles and sometimes all class I (*Fig. 18.25*). A variety of molecular mechanisms has been identified, including mutations in β-2 microglobulin and peptide transporters. The common occurrence of MHC loss in tumours strongly suggests that there is selection for it, presumably by cytotoxic T cells.

Induction of immune responses requires co-stimuli, as does optimal function of effector cells. The CD80 (B7) and CD40 molecules, present on specialized APC, are now known to be key co-stimuli acting via their counter-receptors CD28 and CD40L on the T-cell surface. Experimentally, presentation of MHC–peptide antigen complexes to the T-cell receptor in the absence of CD80 co-stimulation may lead to anergy, and there is evidence that TILs may sometimes be anergic. This effect may be part of a more general defect in immune responsiveness in cancer patients, because even peripheral blood T cells of tumour patients frequently show defective T-cell receptor signalling *in vitro*.

Tumour cells may also lack other molecules required for adhesion of lymphocytes such as LFA-1, LFA-3 or ICAM-1, or they may express molecules such as mucins, which can be anti-adhesive. They may also secrete immunosuppressive cytokines such as transforming growth factor-β (TGFβ) and vascular endothelial growth factor (VEGF).

CRITICAL THINKING • The host immune response to tumours (Explanations on p. 458)

18.1 There is evidence that there is a host immune response to tumour-associated antigens in many patients. Nevertheless, if they are not treated, most cancers grow and eventually kill their host. How can this paradox be accounted for?

18.2 Immunotherapy for cancer has been attempted over the last 100 years. Why has success been limited so far and what is the likelihood of greater success in the future?

18.3 Tumour immunology is often discussed as almost a separate subject. Are there special features of immune responses to tumours which set them apart?

18.4 Prophylactic immunization against infectious disease has been highly effective. Will this be the greatest contribution of immunology to oncology?

FURTHER READING

Agrawal S, Marquet J, Delfau-Larue MH, *et al.* CD3 hyporesponsiveness and in vitro apoptosis are features of T cells from both malignant and nonmalignant secondary lymphoid organs. *J Clin Invest* 1998;**102**:1715–23.

Boon T. Tumor antigens and perspectives for cancer immunotherapy. *Immunologist* 1995;**3**:262–3.

Franks LM, Teich N. *Introduction to the Cellular and Molecular Biology of Cancer.* Oxford: Oxford University Press, 1991.

Girolomoni G, Ricciardi-Castagnoli P. Dendritic cells hold promise for immunotherapy. *Immunol Today* 1997;**18**:102–4.

Link BK, Weiner GJ. Monoclonal antibodies in the treatment of human B-cell malignancies. *Leuk Lymphoma* 1998;**31**:237–49.

Pardoll DM. Cancer vaccines. *Nat Med* 1998;**4**:525–31.

Riethmuller G, Holz E, Sclimok G, *et al.* Monclonal antibody therapy for resected Dukes' C colorectal cancer: seven-year outcome of a multicenter randomized trial. *J Clin Oncol* 1998;**16**:1788–94.

Scott AM, Welt S. Antibody-based immunological therapies. *Curr Opin Immunol* 1997;**9**:717–22.

Sheil AG. Patterns of malignancies following renal transplantation. *Transplant Proc* 1999;**31**:1263–5.

19 Primary immunodeficiency

- **Defective antibody responses** result in increased susceptibility to pyogenic infections and are due to failure of B-cell function, such as occurs in X-linked agammaglobulinaemia, or from failure of proper T-cell signals to B cells such as occurs in hyper-IgM syndrome, common variable immunodeficiency (CVID) and transient hypogammaglobulinaemia of infancy.
- **Defective cell-mediated immunity** results in increased susceptibility to opportunistic infections and is due to failure of T-cell function such as occurs in severe combined immunodeficiency (SCID), MHC class II deficiency, ataxia-telangiectasia, the Wiskott–Aldrich syndrome and the DiGeorge anomaly.
- **Hereditary complement component defects** are found in a number of clinical syndromes, the most common of which is that of the C1 inhibitor, which results in hereditary angioedema.
- **Hereditary complement deficiencies** of the terminal complement components (C5, C6, C7 and C8) and the alternative pathway proteins (Factor H, Factor I and properdin) lead to extraordinary susceptibility to infections with the two *Neisseria* species, *N. gonorrhoeae* and *N. meningitidis.*
- **Defects in the oxygen reduction pathway of phagocytes,** so that the phagocytes cannot assemble NADPH oxidase and produce the hydrogen peroxide and oxygen radicals that kill bacteria, are the basis of chronic granulomatous disease. The resulting persistence of bacterial products in phagocytes leads to abscesses or granulomas depending on the pathogen.
- **Leucocyte adhesion deficiency** is associated with a persistent leucocytosis because phagocytic cells with defective integrin molecules cannot migrate through the vascular endothelium from the blood stream into the tissues.

Immunodeficiency disease results from the absence, or failure of normal function, of one or more elements of the immune system. Specific immunodeficiency diseases involve abnormalities of T or B cells, the cells of the adaptive immune system. Non-specific immunodeficiency diseases involve abnormalities of elements such as complement or phagocytes, which act non-specifically in immunity. Primary immunodeficiency diseases are due to intrinsic defects in cells of the immune system and are for the most part genetically determined.

Immunodeficiency diseases cause increased susceptibility to infection in patients. The infections encountered in immunodeficient patients fall, broadly speaking, into two categories. Patients with defects in immunoglobulins, complement proteins or phagocytes are very susceptible to recurrent infections with encapsulated bacteria such as *Haemophilus influenzae*, *Streptococcus pneumoniae* and *Staphylococcus aureus.* These are called pyogenic infections, because the bacteria give rise to pus formation. On the other hand, patients with defects in cell-mediated immunity, i.e. in T cells, are susceptible to overwhelming, even lethal, infections with microorganisms that are ubiquitous in the environment and to which normal people rapidly develop resistance. For this reason, these are called opportunistic infections; opportunistic microorganisms include yeast and common viruses such as chickenpox.

B-CELL DEFICIENCIES

Patients with common defects in B-cell function (*Fig. 19.1*) have recurrent pyogenic infections such as pneumonia, otitis media and sinusitis. If untreated, they develop severe obstructive lung disease (bronchiectasis) from recurrent pneumonia, which destroys the elasticity of the airways.

Primary B-cell deficiencies
X-linked agammaglobulinaemia
IgA deficiency
IgG subclass deficiency
immunodeficiency with increased IgM
common variable immunodeficiency
transient hypogammaglobulinaemia of infancy

Fig. 19.1 The range of B-cell deficiencies varies from a delayed maturation of normal immunoglobulin production, through single isotype deficiencies to X-linked agammaglobulinaemia, where affected male children have no B cells and no serum immunoglobulins.

In X-linked agammaglobulinaemia (X-LA) early B-cell maturation fails

The model B-cell deficiency is X-linked agammaglobulinaemia. It was the first immunodeficiency disease to be understood in detail, the underlying deficiency being discovered in 1952. Affected males have few or no B cells in their blood or lymphoid tissue; consequently their lymph nodes are very small and their tonsils are absent. Their serum usually contains no IgA, IgM, IgD or IgE, and only small amounts of IgG (less than 100 mg/dl). For the first 6–12 months of life, they are protected from infection by the maternal IgG that crossed the placenta into the fetus. As this supply of IgG is exhausted, affected males develop recurrent pyogenic infections. If they are infused intravenously with large doses of gammaglobulin they remain healthy.

The X-linked immunodeficiencies

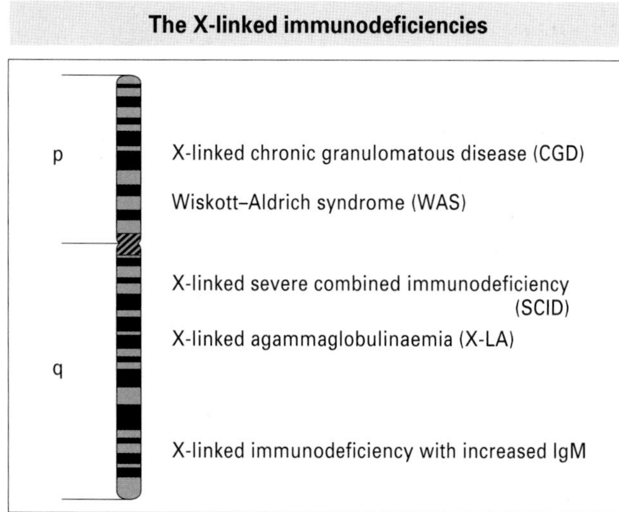

Fig. 19.2 The genes for many immunodeficiency diseases are located on the X-chromosome. The genetic defects have been identified for all these diseases. (Adapted from Schwaber J, Rosen FS. X chromosome linked immunodeficiency. *Immunodefic Rev* 1990;2:233–51.)

The X-LA gene lies on the long arm of the X-chromosome (*Fig. 19.2*). This is the site of many other hereditary immunodeficiency diseases, and the localization of these genes facilitates prenatal diagnosis. The gene that is defective in X-LA has recently been identified as a B-cell cytoplasmic tyrosine kinase (*btk*) belonging to the *src* oncogene family. Its role in B-cell maturation is not yet understood, but it is obviously vital for the process of B-cell maturation. Bone marrow of males with X-LA contains normal numbers of pre-B cells but, as a result of mutations in the *btk* gene, they cannot mature into B cells (*Fig. 19.3*).

In IgA and IgG subclass deficiency terminal differentiation of B cells fails

IgA deficiency is the most common immunodeficiency. One in 700 Caucasians have the defect, but it is not found, or is found only rarely, in other ethnic groups. People with IgA deficiency tend to develop immune-complex disease (Type III hypersensitivity). About 20% of IgA-deficient individuals also lack IgG2 and IgG4, and so are very susceptible to pyogenic infections. In humans, most antibodies to the capsular polysaccharides of pyogenic bacteria are in the IgG2 subclass; a deficiency in IgG2 alone therefore also results in recurrent pyogenic infections. Individuals with deficiency of only IgG2 are also susceptible to recurrent infections. These class and subclass deficiencies result from failure in terminal differentiation of B cells (see *Fig. 19.3*).

In immunodeficiency with increased IgM (HIgM) isotype switching does not occur

A peculiar immunodeficiency results in patients who are IgG- and IgA-deficient but synthesize large amounts (more than 200 mg/dl) of polyclonal IgM. They are susceptible to pyogenic infections and should be treated with intravenous gammaglobulin. They tend to form IgM autoantibodies to neutrophils, platelets and other elements of the blood, as well as to tissue antigens, thereby adding the complexities of autoimmune disease to the immunodeficiency. The tissues, particularly of the gastrointestinal tract, become infiltrated with IgM-producing cells (*Fig. 19.4*). In HIgM the B cells cannot make the switch from IgM to IgG, IgA and IgE synthesis that normally occurs in B-cell maturation. For example, in normal B cells, this switch to IgE is induced by two factors: IL-4 must bind to the B-cell receptor for IL-4, and the CD40 molecule on the B-cell surface must bind to the CD40 ligand on activated T cells. In 70% of cases HIgM is inherited as an X-linked recessive that results from mutations in the CD40 ligand, whose gene maps to precisely the same location on the long arm of the X-chromosome as HIgM.

In common variable immunodeficiency (CVID) there are defects in T-cell signalling to B cells

Individuals with CVID have acquired agammaglobulinaemia in the second or third decade of life, or later. Both males and females are equally affected and the cause is generally not known, but may follow infection with viruses such as Epstein–Barr virus (EBV). Patients with CVID, like males with X-LA, are very susceptible to pyogenic organisms and to the intestinal protozoan, *Giardia lamblia* (*Fig. 19.5*), which cause severe diarrhoea. Most patients (80%) with CVID have B cells that do not function properly and are immature. The B cells are not defective; instead, they fail to receive proper signals from the T cells. However, the T-cell defects have not been defined well in CVID. Patients with CVID should be treated with intravenous gammaglobulin as it provides protection against recurrent pyogenic infections. Many patients develop autoimmune diseases, most prominently pernicious anaemia, and the reason for this is not known. CVID is not hereditary, but is commonly associated with the MHC haplotypes HLA-B8 and HLA-DR3.

IgG production is delayed in transient hypogammaglobulinaemia of infancy

As mentioned above, infants are protected initially by their mother's IgG. The maternal IgG is catabolized, with a half-life of approximately 30 days. By 3 months of age, normal infants begin to synthesize their own IgG, although formation of antibody to bacterial capsular polysaccharides does not commence in earnest until the second year of life. In some infants, the onset of normal IgG synthesis can be delayed for as long as 36 months and, until then, such infants are susceptible to pyogenic infections. The B cells of these infants are normal but they appear to lack help from $CD4^+$ T cells in synthesizing antibodies.

T-CELL DEFICIENCIES

The major T-cell deficiencies are shown in *Figure 19.6*. Patients with no T cells, or poor T-cell function, are susceptible to opportunistic infections. Since B-cell function in humans is largely T-cell dependent, T-cell deficiency also

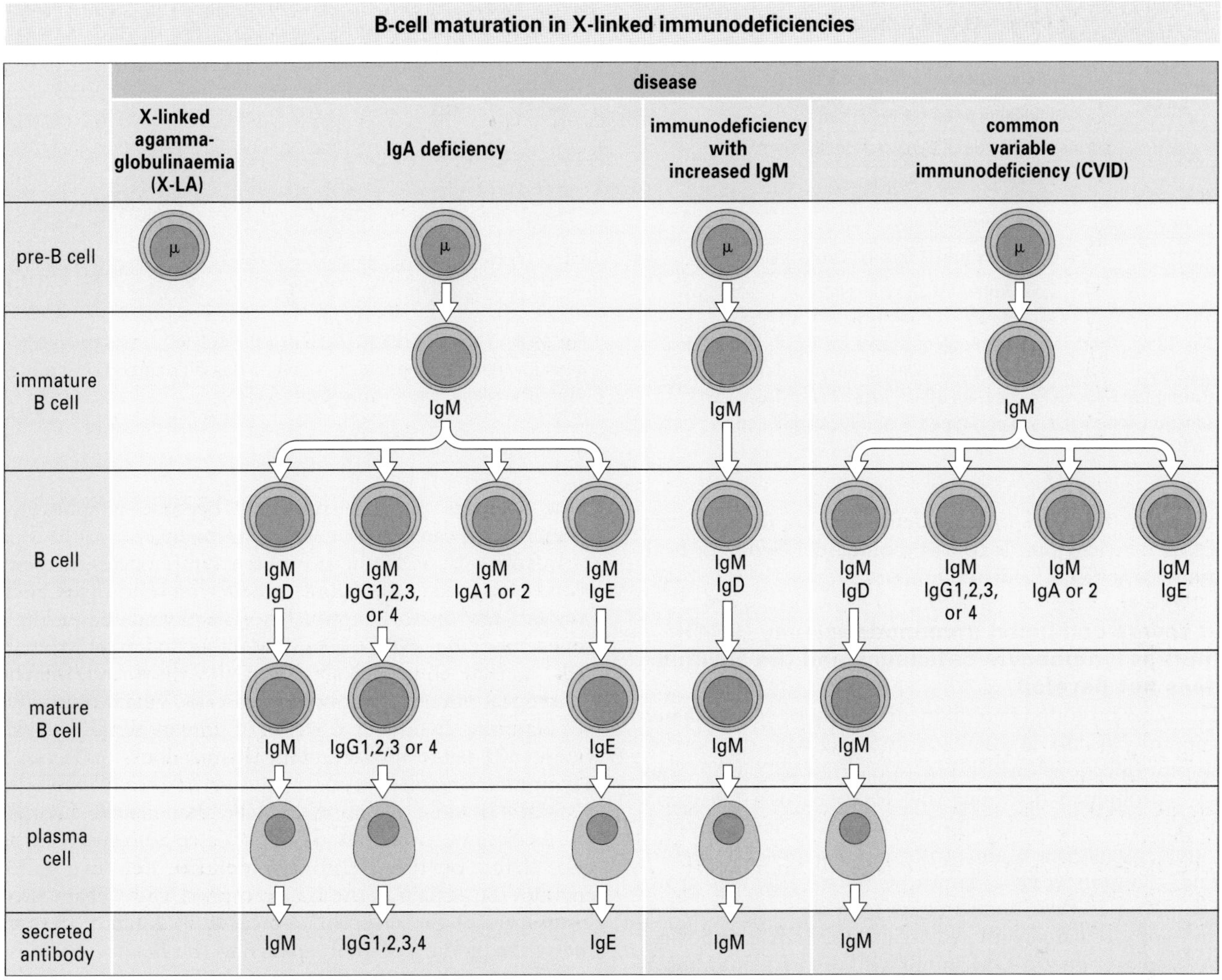

B-cell maturation in X-linked immunodeficiencies

	disease									
	X-linked agammaglobulinaemia (X-LA)	IgA deficiency				immunodeficiency with increased IgM	common variable immunodeficiency (CVID)			
pre-B cell	μ	μ				μ	μ			
immature B cell		IgM				IgM	IgM			
B cell		IgM IgD	IgM IgG1,2,3, or 4	IgM IgA1 or 2	IgM IgE	IgM IgD	IgM IgD	IgM IgG1,2,3, or 4	IgM IgA or 2	IgM IgE
mature B cell		IgM	IgG1,2,3 or 4		IgE	IgM	IgM			
plasma cell										
secreted antibody		IgM	IgG1,2,3,4		IgE	IgM	IgM			

Fig. 19.3 In X-LA, affected male infants have no B cells and no serum immunoglobulins, except for small amounts of maternal IgG. In IgA deficiency, IgA-bearing B cells and in some cases IgG2- and IgG4-bearing B cells, are unable to differentiate into plasma cells. People with immunodeficiency with increased IgM lack IgG and IgA. In CVID, B cells of most isotypes are unable to differentiate into plasma cells.

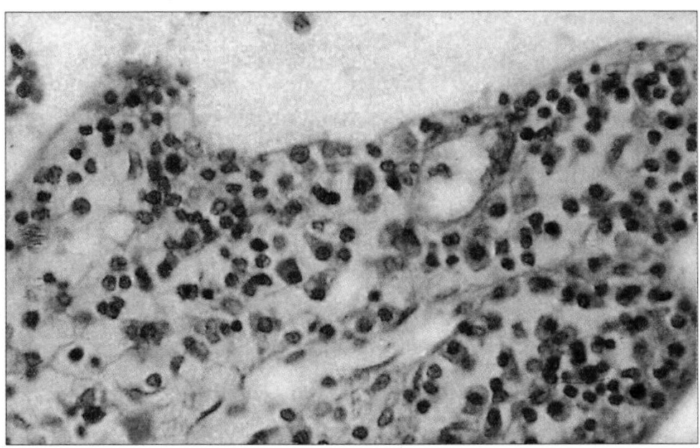

Fig. 19.4 Gall bladder from a patient with immunodeficiency with increased IgM. The submucosa is filled with cells with pink-staining cytoplasm and eccentric nuclei. The cells are synthesizing and secreting IgM.

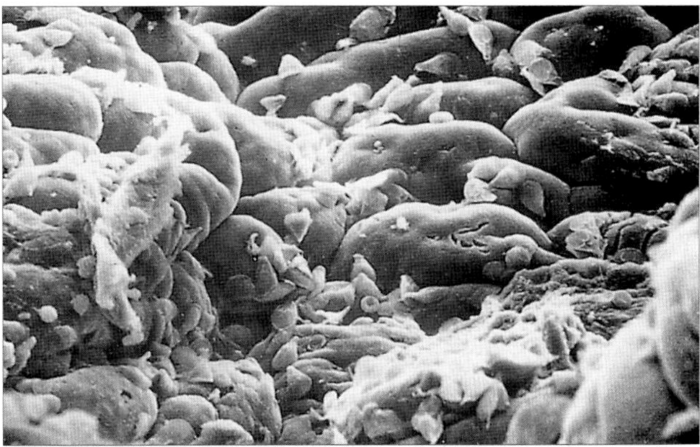

Fig. 19.5 *Giardia lamblia.* Innumerable *Giardia* parasites can be seen swarming over the mucosa of the jejunum of a patient with CVID.

Primary T-cell deficiencies
severe combined immunodeficiency
adenosine deaminase deficiency
purine nucleoside phosphorylase deficiency
MHC class II deficiency
DiGeorge anomaly
hereditary ataxia telangiectasia
Wiskott–Aldrich syndrome

Fig. 19.6 There is a wide range of causes for T-cell deficiencies, ranging from absence of lymphocytes, to enzyme deficiency, through to MHC deficiency. All affect the ability of T cells to function, which leads to combined T- and B-cell deficiency.

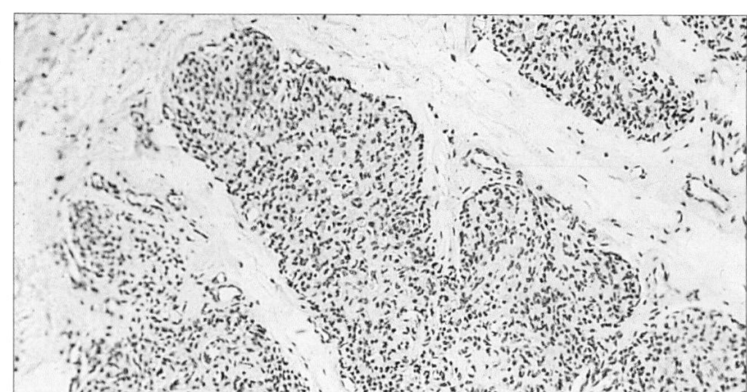

Fig. 19.8 Thymus of SCID. Note that the thymic stroma has not been invaded by lymphoid cells and no Hassall's corpuscles are seen. The gland has a fetal appearance.

results in humoral immunodeficiency; in other words, T-cell deficiency leads to a combined deficiency of both humoral and cell-mediated immunity.

In severe combined immunodeficiency (SCID) there is lymphocyte deficiency and the thymus does not develop

The most profound hereditary deficiency of cell-mediated immunity occurs in infants with SCID who develop recurrent infections early in life (in contrast to X-LA). They have prolonged diarrhoea due to rotavirus or bacterial infection of the gastrointestinal tract and develop pneumonia, usually due to the protozoan, *Pneumocystis carinii*. The common yeast organism *Candida albicans* grows luxuriantly in their mouth or on their skin (*Fig. 19.7*). If they are vaccinated with live organisms, such as poliovirus or bacille Calmette–Guérin (BCG) (used for immunization against tuberculosis), they die of progressive infection from these ordinarily benign organisms. SCID is incompatible with life and affected infants usually die within the first 2 years unless they are rescued with transplants of bone marrow. In this case they become lymphocyte chimeras and can survive and live normally.

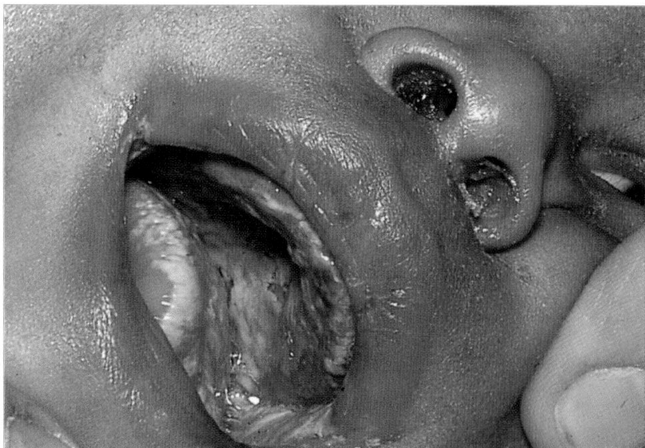

Fig. 19.7 *Candida albicans* in the mouth, in a patient with SCID. This organism grows luxuriantly in the mouth and on the skin of SCID patients.

Infants with SCID have very few lymphocytes in their blood (fewer than 3000/ml). Their lymphoid tissue also contains few or no lymphocytes. The thymus has a fetal appearance (*Fig. 19.8*), containing the endodermal stromal cells derived embryonically from the third and fourth pharyngeal pouch. Lymphoid stem cells, which normally populate the thymus by 6 weeks of human gestation (see Chapter 2), fail to appear and the thymus does not become a lymphoid organ.

SCID is more common in male than female infants (3 : 1) because over 50% of SCID cases are caused by a gene defect on the X-chromosome. The defective gene encodes the γ chain of the IL-2 receptor. This γ chain also forms part of the receptors for IL-4, 7, 11 and 15. Of these, the binding of interleukin-7 to the IL-7 receptor is most important for T-cell maturation. Thus, the lymphoid stem cells are incapable of receiving a number of signals for growth and maturation. The remaining cases of SCID are due to recessive genes on other chromosomes. Of these, half have a genetic deficiency of adenosine deaminase (ADA) or purine nucleoside phosphorylase (PNP). Deficiency of these purine degradation enzymes results in the accumulation of metabolites that are toxic to lymphoid stem cells, namely dATP and dGTP (*Fig. 19.9*). These metabolites inhibit the enzyme ribonucleotide reductase, which is required for DNA synthesis and, therefore, for cell replication. Since ADA and PNP are found in all mammalian cells, why should these defects only affect lymphocytes? The explanation appears to lie in the relative deficiency of 5′ nucleotidase in lymphoid cells; in other cells, this enzyme compensates for defective ADA or PNP by preventing dAMP and dGMP accumulation.

The two recombinase activation genes, Rag-1 and Rag-2, are absolutely required for cleaving double-stranded DNA prior to recombination of DNA to form the immunoglobulin genes and the genes encoding the T-cell receptor. If these gene rearrangements do not occur, B and T lymphocytes do not develop; an autosomal recessive form of SCID results from a mutation in either of the genes encoding Rag-1 or Rag-2.

The optimal treatment for SCID is a bone-marrow

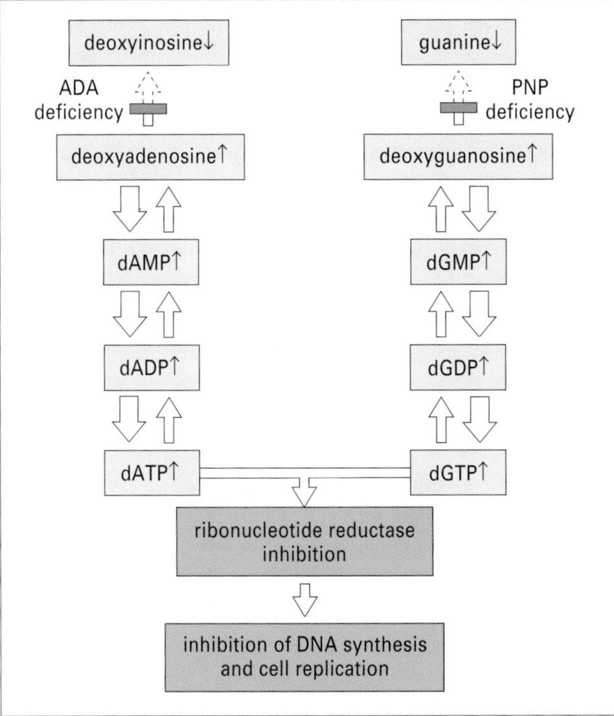

Fig. 19.9 It is thought that deficiencies of ADA and PNP lead to accumulations of dATP and dGTP respectively. Both of these metabolites are powerful inhibitors of ribonucleotide reductase, an essential enzyme for DNA synthesis.

transplant from a completely histocompatible donor, usually a normal sibling. About 70% of patients do not have a histocompatible sibling, in which case parental marrow, which would have one haplotype identical, has been transplanted successfully. Recently a retroviral vector, into which the ADA gene had been inserted, has been used to transfect the lymphocytes of children who are ADA deficient. This was the first example of successful 'gene therapy'.

In MHC class II deficiency TH-cell deficiency results

The failure to express class II MHC molecules on antigen-presenting cells (macrophages and B cells) is inherited as an autosomal recessive characteristic, which is not linked to the MHC locus on the short arm of chromosome 6. Affected infants have recurrent infections, particularly of the gastrointestinal tract. Because the development of CD4⁺ TH cells (T-helper cells) depends on positive selection by MHC class II molecules in the thymus (see Chapter 2), MHC class II deficient infants have a deficiency of CD4⁺ T cells. This lack of TH cells leads to a deficiency in antibodies as well. The MHC class II deficiency results from defects in promoter proteins that bind to the 5′ untranslated region of the class II genes.

The destruction of intracellular microorganisms that flourish in macrophages depends on the activation of microbicidal activity in macrophages by interferon-γ. When microorganisms are taken up by macrophages these cells secrete interleukin-12 (IL-12). IL-12 binds to the IL-12 receptor on T cells and this provokes T cells to secrete interferon-γ. Children with genetic defects in the genes encoding IL-12, the IL-12 receptor or the interferon-γ receptor sustain recurrent infection with non-pathogenic mycobacteria and, to a lesser extent, with salmonella. These various defects are inherited as autosomal recessive traits. The defects can be fatal unless treatment with interferon-γ is undertaken.

The DiGeorge anomaly arises from a defect in thymus embryogenesis

As previously mentioned, the thymic epithelium is derived from the third and fourth pharyngeal pouches by the sixth week of human gestation. Subsequently the endodermal anlage is invaded by lymphoid stem cells that undergo development into T cells. The parathyroid glands are also derived from the same embryonic origin. A congenital defect in the organs derived from the third and fourth pharyngeal pouches results in the DiGeorge anomaly. The T-cell deficiency is variable, depending on how badly the thymus is affected. Affected infants have distinctive facial features (*Fig. 19.10*) in that their eyes are widely separated (hypertelorism), the ears are low set, and the philtrum of the upper lip is shortened. They also have congenital malformations of the heart or aortic arch and neonatal tetany from the hypoplasia or aplasia of the parathyroid glands.

X-linked proliferative syndrome (XLP)

This results from a failure to control the normal proliferation of cytotoxic T cells following an infection with Epstein–Barr virus (EBV), which causes infectious mononucleosis. Affected males appear normal until they encounter EBV, when they develop either fatal infectious mononucleosis, or have complete destruction of their B cells so that agammaglobulinaemia ensues, or develop a fatal lymphoid malignancy or aplastic anaemia. The defective gene on the

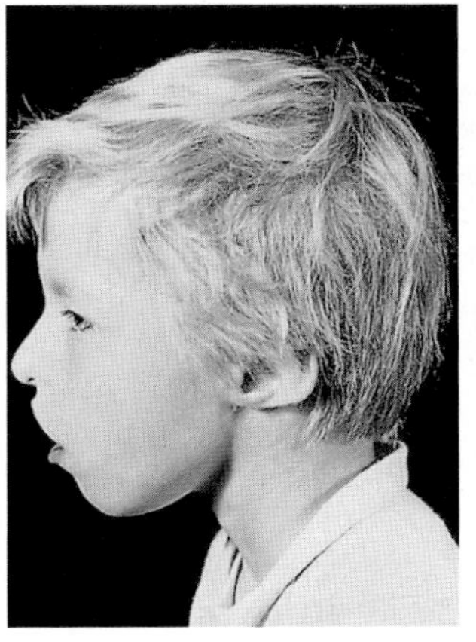
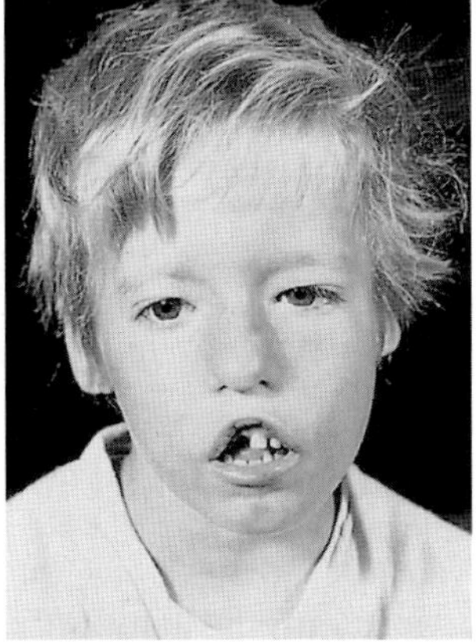

Fig. 19.10 DiGeorge anomaly. Note the wide-set eyes, low-set ears and shortened philtrum of upper lip. Congenital malformations of the cardiovascular system may also occur.

X-chromosome encodes an adapter protein of T and B cells called SAP or the SLAM associated protein. SLAM is expressed on the surface of T and B cells. Its intracellular tail interacts with the adapter protein, SAP. By a mechanism that is not understood, SAP controls the limitless proliferation of cytotoxic T cells. A genetic defect in SAP results in the destruction of lymphoid and other haematopoietic tissue by uncontrolled proliferation of cytotoxic T cells and maternal killer cells.

In hereditary ataxia–telangiectasia (AT) chromosomal breaks occur in TCR and immunoglobulin genes

AT is inherited as an autosomal recessive trait. Affected infants develop a wobbly gait (ataxia) at about 18 months. Dilated capillaries (telangiectasia) appear in the eyes and on the skin by 6 years of age. AT is accompanied by a variable T-cell deficiency. About 70% of AT patients are also IgA deficient and some also have IgG2 and IgG4 deficiency. The number and function of circulating T cells are greatly diminished, so that cell-mediated function is depressed. They develop severe sinus and lung infections. Their cells exhibit chromosomal breaks, usually in chromosome 7 and chromosome 14, at the sites of the T-cell receptor (TCR) genes and the genes encoding the heavy chains of immunoglobulins. The cells of AT patients, as well as those from AT patients *in vitro*, are very susceptible to ionizing irradiation. The defective gene in AT encodes a protein involved in repair of double-strand breaks in DNA.

In Wiskott–Aldrich syndrome (WAS) there are T-cell defects and abnormal Ig levels

WAS is an X-linked immunodeficiency disease. Affected males have small and profoundly abnormal platelets, which are also few in number (thrombocytopenia). Boys with WAS develop severe eczema as well as pyogenic and opportunistic infections. Their serum contains increased amounts of IgA and IgE, normal levels of IgG and decreased amounts of IgM. Their T cells are defective in function and this malfunction of cell-mediated immunity gets progressively worse. The T cells have a uniquely abnormal appearance, as shown by scanning electron microscopy, reflecting a cytoskeletal defect. They have fewer microvilli on the cell surface than do normal T cells. During collaboration of T and B cells in antibody formation, the cytoskeleton of the T cells reorientates itself or becomes polarized towards the B cells. This fails to occur in the Wiskott–Aldrich syndrome, with the result that collaboration among immune cells is faulty.

DEFECTS IN COMPLEMENT PROTEINS

The proteins of the complement system and their interactions with the immune system are discussed in Chapter 3. Genetic deficiencies of almost all the complement proteins have been found in human beings (*Fig. 19.11*) and these deficiencies reveal much about the normal function of the complement system.

Genetic deficiencies of human complement

group	type	deficiency	heredity		
			AR	AD	XL
I	immune-complex deficiency	C1q	•		
		C1s, or C1r + C1s	•		
		C2	•		
		C4	•		
II	angioedema	C1 inhibitor		•	
III	recurrent pyogenic infections	C3	•		
		Factor H	•		
		Factor I	•		
IV	recurrent *Neisseria* infections	C5	•		
		C6	•		
		C7	•		
		C8	•		
		properdin			•
		Factor D	•		
V	asymptomatic	C9	•		

Fig. 19.11 Genetic deficiencies of human complement. (AR = phenotypically autosomal recessive; AD = autosomal dominant; XL = X-linked recessive.)

Clearance of immune complexes, inflammation, phagocytosis and bacteriolysis can be affected

Deficiencies of the classical pathway components,C1q, C1r and C1s, C4 or C2, result in a propensity to develop immune-complex diseases such as systemic lupus erythematosus. This correlates with the known function of the classical pathway in the dissolution of immune complexes. Deficiencies of C3, Factor H or Factor I result in increased susceptibility to pyogenic infections; this correlates with the important role of C3 in opsonization of pyogenic bacteria. Deficiencies of the terminal components, C5, C6, C7 and C8, and of the alternative pathway components, Factor D and properdin, result in remarkable susceptibility to infection with the two pathogenic species of the *Neisseria* genus: *N. gonorrhoeae* and *N. meningitidis*. This clearly demonstrates the importance of the alternative pathway and the macromolecular attack complex in the bacteriolysis of this genus of bacteria.

All these genetic complement component deficiencies are inherited as autosomal recessive traits, except for properdin deficiency, which is inherited as an X-linked recessive, and C1 inhibitor deficiency, which is inherited as an autosomal dominant.

Hereditary angioneurotic oedema (HAE) is due to C1 inhibitor deficiency

Clinically, the most important deficiency of the complement system is that of the C1 inhibitor. This molecule is responsible for dissociation of activated C1, by binding

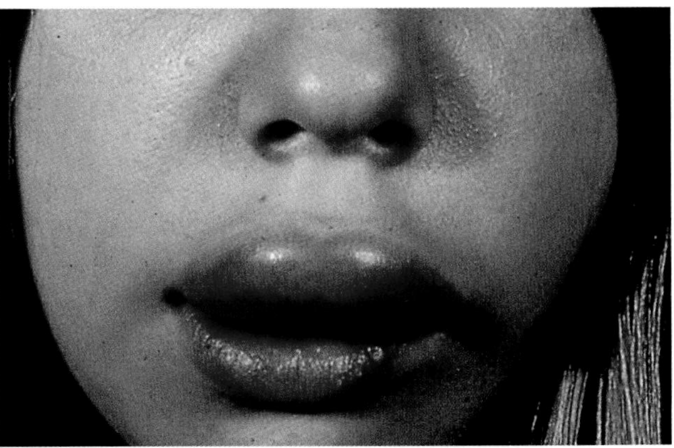

Fig. 19.12 Hereditary angioneurotic oedema. This clinical photograph shows the transient localized swelling which occurs in this condition.

to $\overline{C1r_2C1s_2}$. The deficiency results in the well-known disease, hereditary angioneurotic oedema (HAE) (*Fig. 19.12*). This disease is inherited as an autosomal dominant trait. Patients with HAE have recurrent episodes of circumscribed swelling of various parts of the body (angioedema). When the oedema involves the intestine, excruciating abdominal pains and cramps results, with severe vomiting. When the oedema involves the upper airway, the patients may choke to death from respiratory obstruction. Angioedema of the upper airway therefore presents a medical emergency, which requires rapid action to restore normal breathing.

C1 inhibitor not only inhibits the classical pathway of complement but also joint elements of the kinin, plasmin and clotting systems. The oedema is mediated by two peptides generated by uninhibited activation of the complement and contact systems: a peptide derived from the activation of C2, called C2 kinin, and bradykinin derived from the activation of the contact system (*Fig. 19.13*). The effect of these peptides is on the postcapillary venule, where they cause endothelial cells to retract, forming gaps that allow leakage of plasma (see Chapter 3).

There are two genetically determined forms of HAE. In Type I, the C1 inhibitor gene is defective and no transcripts are formed. In Type II, there are point mutations in the C1 inhibitor gene with the consequence that defective molecules are synthesized. This distinction is important because the diagnosis of Type II disease cannot be made by quantitative measurement of serum C1 inhibitor alone. Simultaneous measurements of C4 must also be done. C4 is always decreased in the serum of HAE patients, because of its destruction by uninhibited, activated C1.

C1 inhibitor deficiency may be acquired later in life. In some cases an autoantibody to C1 inhibitor is found. In others, there is a monoclonal B-cell proliferation such as occurs in chronic lymphocytic leukaemia, multiple myeloma or B-cell lymphoma. Such patients make an anti-idiotype to their over-produced immunoglobulin; the idiotype–anti-idiotype interaction, for unknown reasons, causes consumption of C1, C4 and C2 and of C1 inhibitor without formation of an effective C3 convertase (which

Pathogenesis of hereditary angioneurotic oedema

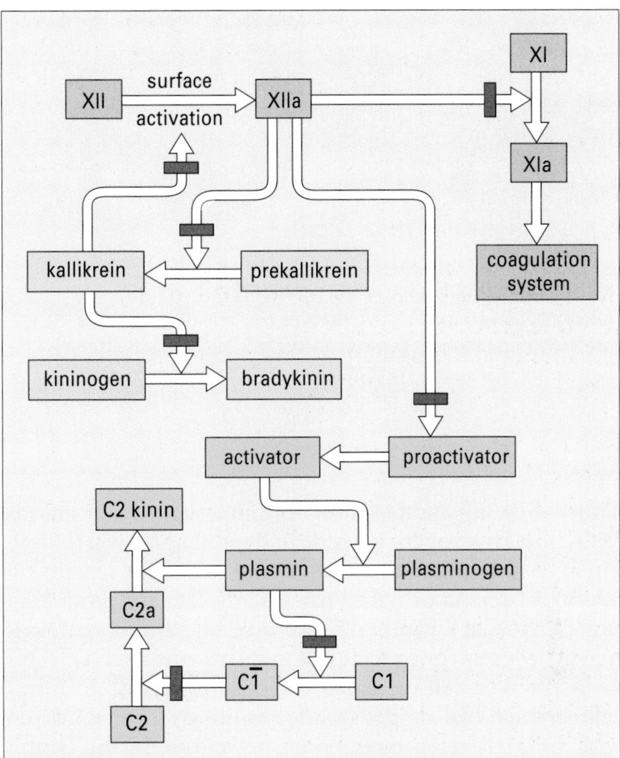

Fig. 19.13 C1 inhibitor is involved in inactivation of elements of the clotting, kinin, plasmin and complement systems, which may be activated following the surface dependent activation of Factor XII (Hageman factor). The points at which C1 inhibitor acts are shown in red. Uncontrolled activation of these pathways results in the formation of bradykinin and C2 kinin, which induce oedema formation.

would cause C3 deposition and removal of the complement complex).

DEFECTS IN PHAGOCYTES

Phagocytic cells – polymorphonuclear leucocytes and cells of the monocyte/macrophage lineage – are important in host defence against pyogenic bacteria and other intracellular microorganisms. A severe deficiency of polymorphonuclear leucocytes (neutropenia) can result in overwhelming bacterial infection. Two genetic defects of phagocytes are clinically important in that they result in susceptibility to severe infections and are often fatal: chronic granulomatous disease and the leucocyte adhesion deficiency.

Chronic granulomatous disease (CGD) is due to a defect in the oxygen reduction pathway

Patients with CGD have defective NADPH oxidase which catalyses the reduction of O_2 to $\bullet O_2^-$ by the reaction:

$$NADPH + 2O_2 \rightarrow NADP^+ + 2\bullet O_2^- + H^+$$

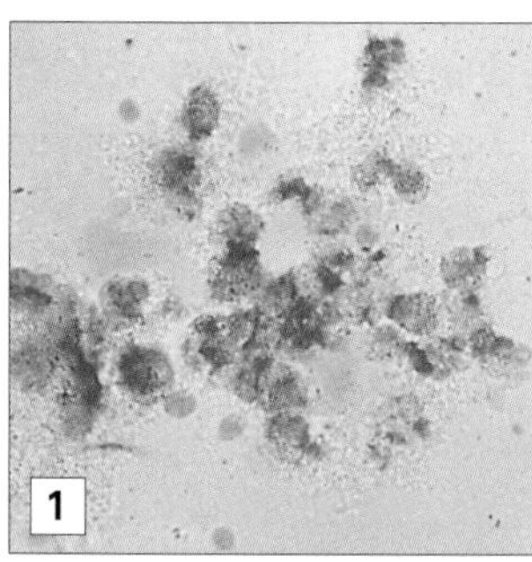

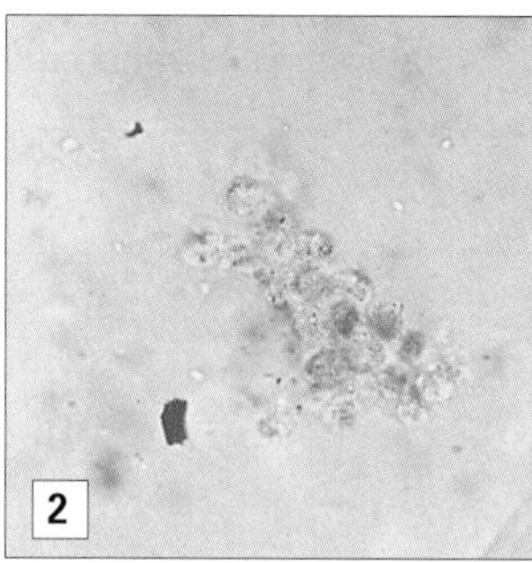

Fig. 19.14 Nitroblue tetrazolium (NBT) test. In normal polymorphs and monocytes, reactive oxygen intermediates (ROIs) are activated by phagocytosis, and yellow NBT is converted to purple-blue formazan (**1**). Patients with CGD cannot form ROIs and so the dye stays yellow (**2**). (Courtesy of Professor A. R. Hayward.)

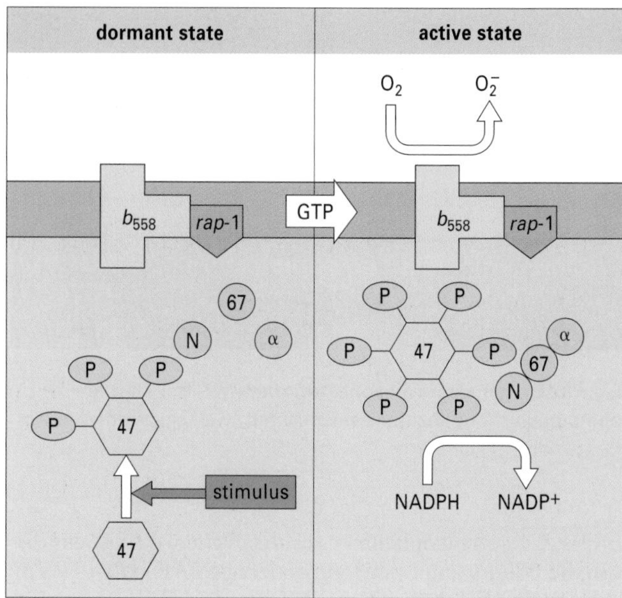

Fig. 19.15 Prevailing knowledge of the NADPH oxidase suggests that, in its dormant state, some of its component parts are in the membrane (cytochrome b_{558} and possibly *rap-1*) while others are in the cytosol (p47^{phox}, p67^{phox}, the NADPH-binding component, N, and a putative fourth component, α). After the stimulus provided phagocytosis, the cytosolic components associate and move to the membrane, an event possibly mediated by phosphorylation (P) of p47^{phox}. Once the cytosol components are associated with the membrane components, the oxidase becomes catalytically active and p47^{phox} is phosphorylated further. In the different forms of CGD, there are defects in the genes for different components of the oxidase. (Adapted from Smith RM, Curnutte JT. Molecular basis of chronic granulomatous disease. *Blood* 1997;**77(4)**:673–86, with permission.)

Thus, they are incapable of forming superoxide anions ($\bullet O_2^-$) and hydrogen peroxide in their phagocytes, following ingestion of microorganisms and so cannot readily kill ingested bacteria or fungi, particularly catalase-producing organisms (see Chapter 15). As a result, microorganisms remain alive in phagocytes of patients with CGD. This gives rise to a cell-mediated response to persistent intracellular microbial antigens, and granulomas form. Children with CGD develop pneumonia, infections in the lymph nodes (lymphadenitis), and abscesses in the skin, liver and other viscera.

The diagnosis of CGD is made by the inability of phagocytes to reduce nitroblue tetrazolium (NBT) dye after a phagocytic stimulus. NBT, a pale, clear, yellow dye, is taken up by phagocytes when they are ingesting a particle. When NBT accepts H and is reduced, as a result of NADPH oxidation, it forms a deep purple precipitate inside the phagocytes; precipitation does not occur in the phagocytes of CGD patients (*Fig. 19.14*).

The NADPH oxidase reaction is complicated and the enzyme complex has many subunits. In resting phagocytes the membrane contains a phagocyte-specific cytochrome, cytochrome b_{558}. This cytochrome is composed of two chains, one of 91 kDa, encoded by a gene on the short arm of the X-chromosome, and one of 22 kDa, encoded by a gene on chromosome 16. When phagocytosis occurs, several proteins from the cytosol become phosphorylated, move to the membrane and bind to cytochrome b_{558}. The complex that is formed acts as an enzyme, NADPH oxidase, catalysing the NADPH oxidation reaction and thereby activating oxygen radical production (*Fig. 19.15*). The most common form of CGD is X-linked and involves a defect in the 91 kDa chain of cytochrome b_{558}. Three types of CGD are autosomal recessive and result from defects in the 22 kDa chain of the cytochrome b_{558}, or from defects in one or other of two proteins, called p47^{phox} or p67^{phox} (*phox* is an abbreviation for phagocytic oxidase).

Leucocyte adhesion deficiency (LAD) is due to integrin gene defects

The receptor in the phagocyte membrane that binds to C3bi on opsonized microorganisms is critical for the ingestion of bacteria by phagocytes. This receptor, an integrin called complement receptor 3 (CR3), is deficient in patients with LAD and consequently they develop severe bacterial infections, particularly of the mouth and gastrointestinal tract.

CR3 is composed of two polypeptide chains: an α chain of 165 kDa (CD11b), and a β chain of 95 kDa (CD18). In LAD, there is a genetic defect of the β chain, encoded by a gene on chromosome 21. Two other integrin proteins share the same β chain, namely lymphocyte function associated antigen (LFA-1) and p150,95 (see Chapter 3). Although they have unique α chains (CD11a and CD11c, respectively), these proteins are also defective in LAD. LFA-1 is important in cell adhesion and interacts with intercellular adhesion molecule-1 (ICAM-1) on endothelial cell surfaces and other cell membranes. Because of the defect in LFA-1, phagocytes from patients with LAD cannot adhere to vascular endothelium and thus cannot migrate out of blood vessels into areas of infection. Thus patients with LAD cannot form pus efficiently; this allows the rapid spread of bacterial invaders.

When leucocytes in the circulation enter an area of

inflammation their speed of movement is greatly retarded by the interaction of selectins that are expressed on the surface of the leucocytes with ligands that are expressed on the surface of the endothelium in areas of inflammation. The leucocytes start to roll on the endothelial surface prior to the interaction of the leucocyte integrins with adhesion molecules such as intracellular adhesion molecule-1 (ICAM-1). The ligands with which the selectins interact are glycoproteins that contain fucosylated sugars such as the blood group sialyl Lewis^x. A genetic defect in the conversion of mannose to fucose results in the failure of normal synthesis in these selectin ligands. Consequently the leucocytes of such patients cannot roll on the endothelium. This causes a second form of LAD, called LAD type 2.

CASE STUDY • Hyper IgM immunodeficiency (Explanations on pp 458–459)

A 6-month-old male infant was brought to the emergency room because of fever and rapid respiration. He had been well up to this time and had received routine immunizations without complications. The family history was uninformative. He had one sibling, a 3-year-old sister, who was in good health.

A chest X-ray resulted in a diagnosis of interstitial pneumonia. Routine Gram stains of a sputum sample revealed normal bacterial flora. However, a silver stain was positive for *Pneumocystis carinii*. The infant was treated with pentamidine.

Investigations

Haemoglobin and white cell counts were in the normal range. Serum IgM was 375 mg/dl, IgG 30 mg/dl, IgA undetectable, IgE undetectable. Antibody to tetanus toxoid: undetectable. Blood typing: A positive, anti-B 1 : 256.

19.1 What clinical and laboratory facts lead to the suspicion that this male infant has hyper IgM immunodeficiency?

19.2 What further laboratory testing should be done to establish the diagnosis?

19.3 In addition to pentamidine to treat the *P. carinii* infection what other therapy should be started?

19.4 How do you explain that this baby had no response to his tetanus immunization and yet has a high titre for this age of antibody to blood group substance B?

19.5 If the mother of this baby were to be tested for random X-chromosome inactivation what results would you expect?

19.6 What would you tell the parents about this child's prognosis?

FURTHER READING

Buckley R. Primary immunodeficiencies. *New Engl J Med.* In press.

Conley ME. Molecular approaches to analysis of X-linked immunodeficiencies. *Ann Rev Immunol* 1992;**10**:215.

Curnutte JT, Orkin SH, Dinauer MC. Genetic disorders of phagocyte function. In: Stamatoyannopoulos G, Nienhuis AW, Majerus PW, Varmus H (eds). *The Molecular Basis of Blood Diseases.* Philadelphia: PA Saunders;1994:443.

Lekstrom-Wimes JA, Gallin JI. Molecular basis of phagocyte immunodeficiencies. *New Engl J Med.* In press.

Rosen FS, Cooper MD, Wedgwood RJP. The primary immunodeficiencies. *New Engl J Med* 1995;**333**:43.

Rosen FS, Seligman M (eds). *Immunodeficiencies.* Switzerland: Harwood Academic Publishers GmbH, 1993.

Snapper SB, Rosen FS. The Wiskott–Aldrich syndrome protein (WASP): roles in signalling and cyto-skeletal organization: *Annu Rev Immunol* 1999;**17**:905–29.

Von Andrian UH, Berger EM, Chambers JD, *et al. In vivo* behaviour of neutrophils from two patients with distinct inherited leukocyte adhesion deficiency syndromes. *J Clin Invest* 1993;**91**:2893.

20 Secondary immunodeficiency

- **Immunomodulatory drugs** can severely depress immune functions.
- **Steroids** affect cell traffic, induce leucocytopenia and inhibit cytokine synthesis.
- **Cyclophosphamide, azathioprine and mycophenolate mofetil** act directly on DNA or its synthesis.
- **Severe protein–energy malnutrition (PEM)** reduces the efficacy of the immune system. Malnutrition increases the risk of infant mortality from infection through reduction in cell-mediated immunity, reduced CD4 helper cells, reduced T-cell help and a reduction of secretory IgA.
- **Trace elements, iron, selenium, copper and zinc** are important in immunity. Lack of these elements can lead to diminished neutrophil killing of bacteria and fungi, susceptibility to viral infections and diminished antibody responses.
- **Vitamins A, B6, C, E** and also folic acid are important in overall resistance to infection. Carotenoids are antioxidants like vitamin C and E and can enhance NK cell activity, stimulate the production of cytokines and increase the activity of phagocytic cells.
- **Diet and nutrition** are powerful innovative tools to reduce illness and death caused by infection.
- **AIDS** is caused by human immunodeficiency virus (HIV), which is a double-stranded RNA retrovirus that binds to CD4 and depletes $CD4^+$ T cells.
- **Severe CD4 depletion** results from a variety of mechanisms, with drastic functional impairment of cell-mediated immunity and death from opportunistic infections.
- **Combination therapy** for AIDS with reverse transcriptase and protease inhibitors is reasonably successful, but costly.
- **Successful vaccines** for HIV have not yet been identified.

IMMUNODEFICIENCY CAUSED BY DRUGS

There have been substantial advances over the past decade in understanding how the immune system is regulated and how drugs may selectively alter function, producing not only immunodeficiency but also, in some circumstances, immune enhancement. This chapter examines the most important agents commonly used for systemic immunotherapy.

Corticosteroids are powerful immune modulators

The immune system is regulated by at least four fundamental mechanisms: hormonal (e.g. glucocorticoids), the cytokine system (including interleukins and interferons), network connectivity (through idiotypic–anti-idiotypic responses) and antigens. Glucocorticoids are the most powerful naturally occurring modulators of the immune response and have profound effects at most levels and on most components. In addition to their direct hormonal action on immune cell traffic and function, steroids have a substantial influence on cytokine synthesis, thereby also exerting a powerful indirect effect.

Significant changes in cell traffic are produced

Administration of steroids causes striking changes in circulating leucocyte populations, even when quite small quantities are used – for example, to produce physiological concentrations in previously adrenalectomized patients. These effects vary between cell types (*Fig. 20.1*).

Steroid treatment causes circulating *lymphocytopenia*, maximal at 4–6 hours and returning to normal by 24 hours. T cells are affected more than B cells and, within the T-cell subsets, CD4 cells are more depleted than CD8 cells. Experimental studies suggest these cells are redistributed to marrow and spleen.

Monocytopenia occurs after steroid treatment, is most evident at 2 hours and recovers by 24 hours but, unlike

Effects of glucocorticoids on circulating leucocytes

cell type	hours after injection		
	0	6	24
neutrophils	4000	10 000	4000
lymphocytes	2000	500	2000
eosinophils	400	100	400
monocytes	300	50	300
basophils	100	0	100

Fig. 20.1 Effect of a dose of glucocorticoid (40 mg/kg), given once at time 0, on circulating human leucocyte numbers (per mm^3).

effects on lymphocyte traffic, further repeated daily dosage does not cause subsequent cycles of depletion.

Neutrophilia is a feature of steroid treatment, due partly to release of mature stored cells from bone marrow and partly to reduction in cells leaving the circulation. However, rapid and prolonged decrease in circulating eosinophils and basophils after steroid treatment occurs in normal individuals, which contrasts markedly with the neutrophilia seen at the same time.

T-cell activation and B-cell maturation are inhibited

T-cell activation and proliferation are inhibited by steroids, which make them unresponsive to IL-1 and therefore unable to synthesize IL-2. Steroids inhibit the earliest stages of B-cell maturation, by blocking monocyte and T-cell involvement, but have little effect on mature B cells. However, after prolonged high dosage there is a modest decrease in each immunoglobulin isotype.

Steroids inhibit production of IL-1 and TNF by monocytes (see below), but do not block the effect of cytokines on phagocytosis; indeed, they can promote it. Thus the binding of IFNγ and subsequent expression of HLA-DR molecules and Fc receptors may be increased by low-dose steroids. However, the function of polymorphs is resistant to levels of steroids achievable pharmacologically, as judged by chemotaxis, phagocytosis and cytotoxicity.

Cytokine synthesis is inhibited

Studies *in vitro* have shown that physiological and pharmacological concentrations of steroids inhibit synthesis of cytokines but have little effect on their function. More impressively, after *in vivo* administration, reduced production of IL-1, -2, -4, -6 and -10, TNFα and IFNγ has been demonstrated. Several different mechanisms may be involved: (1) attachment to potential glucocorticoid response elements in the promoter region of the cytokine genes (IL-4, -6 and -10), (2) direct binding, which antagonizes transcription-activating factors for IL-2, IL-8 and TNFα, or (3) accelerating breakdown of mRNA (IL-1 and -3). The major consequences of this are inhibition of T-cell activation, both TH1 and TH2 cells of the CD4 subpopulation being similarly affected, and inhibition of cells of the monocyte/macrophage system.

Cyclophosphamide acts by covalent alkylation

Together with chlorambucil, cyclophosphamide belongs to the group of immunomodulatory drugs which act by covalent alkylation of other molecules. Cyclophosphamide has no alkylating ability itself, but many of its metabolites are active, each having two active sites to effect the cross-linking of DNA strands, thereby interfering with strand separation during replication. The main side-effect is marrow toxicity, and so leucopenia must be monitored.

Both T- and B-cell functions are affected

Cyclophosphamide mainly affects lymphocyte numbers and function, particularly after low-dose daily oral therapy. Polymorphonuclear cell numbers may remain relatively unchanged. Low-dose oral therapy may have greater impact on cell-mediated responses, and bolus intermittent treatment more effect on antibody production. In both humans and experimental animals, after a low-dose bolus (600 mg/m^2 body surface area), numbers of B lymphocytes are reduced more than T cells and, among T-cell subsets, CD8 more than CD4; however, with higher dosage, all cell types are reduced similarly. Experimental studies have shown that this differential effect of low-dose depletion of CD8 cells allows a paradoxical increase in some CD4-controlled functions, such as antibody production. Evidence that low-dose cyclophosphamide has corresponding clinical relevance in humans remains equivocal.

As cyclophosphamide interferes with both B- and T-cell function, it is effective in controlling both antibody-mediated and cell-mediated immune responses in experimental animals and humans, and thus has a major role in the management of both autoantibody-mediated disease and allograft rejection.

Azathioprine

This drug, which is converted rapidly and non-enzymatically to 6-mercaptopurine *in vivo*, exerts its effect, after metabolism to thioinosinic acid, by competitive inhibition of purine metabolism and by incorporation into DNA as a fraudulent base. Its main effects are thus on DNA synthesis. Unlike cyclophosphamide, which is cytotoxic, azathioprine is cytostatic and is active only on dividing cells, exerting maximal effect if given soon after antigenic challenge. Allopurinol, which inhibits xanthine oxidase, increases the effective dose of azathioprine fourfold, and so if allopurinol is otherwise clinically essential, for example to treat gout, the dose of azathioprine should be reduced by 25%.

T- and B-cell numbers are reduced

Azathioprine is moderately immunosuppressive and produces modest reductions in both T and B cells after prolonged oral therapy at 2–3 mg/kg/day. Both K and NK cell activity appear to be specifically suppressed after its use. Humoral immunity and delayed hypersensitivity are not affected at doses given clinically, although there is a reduction in mitogenic responses to pokeweed mitogen in lymphocytes taken from patients receiving the drug.

Mycophenolate mofetil

This drug was developed to target selectively the final stage of purine synthesis, along a pathway used specifically by lymphocytes proliferating in response to antigenic challenge. Thus, unlike nucleoside analogues such as azathioprine, it does not inhibit DNA repair enzymes or incorporate fraudulent purine analogues into DNA. Mycophenolate is rapidly hydrolysed *in vivo* to the active metabolite, mycophenolic acid.

Lymphocyte proliferation is blocked

Mycophenolate blocks both T- and B-cell proliferative responses in doses that appear to have no effects on other cell types. It also inhibits glycosylation of adhesion molecules involved in leucocyte traffic to endothelial cells, thus restricting amplification of inflammatory injury.

Methotrexate

A structural analogue of folic acid, this blocks folic-acid-dependent synthetic pathways essential for DNA synthesis.

Immunoglobulin synthesis is reduced after prolonged treatment

Several reports note reduction in immunoglobulin synthesis, with significantly lowered levels of all isotypes after three months of treatment. No consistent change has been noted in T-cell subsets, in either the short or long term, or the function of the monocyte/macrophage system. However, inhibition of dihydrofolate reductase involved in purine synthesis releases adenosine, which is a powerful inhibitor of activated polymorphonuclear leucocytes; hence methotrexate is anti-inflammatory. Other effects of methotrexate on inflammation may be mediated by its inhibitory effect on arachidonic acid metabolism. More anti-inflammatory actions are indicated by the rapid decrease in indices of inflammatory activity such as C-reative protein (CRP) and erythrocyte sedimentation rate (ESR), without affecting immune cell function or immunoglobulin synthesis.

Cyclosporin, tacrolimus (FK506) and rapamycin

These three drugs have complicated effects on T-cell signalling and hence T-cell function. They all bind to a class of cytoplasmic proteins (named immunophilins) having peptidyl prolyl isomerase (rotamase) activity, which they inhibit. Immunophilins are believed to have a critical role in transducing signals from cell surface to cell nucleus.

Cyclosporin binds to one family of immunophilins, cyclophilins, whereas tacrolimus and rapamycin bind to the FK binding proteins. The cyclosporin–cyclophilin complex targets a serine threonine phosphatase called calcineurin, as does the tacrolimus–FK binding protein complex. Both inhibit signal transduction pathways which characteristically produce an increase in intracellular free calcium, and inhibit transcriptional activation of cytokines and other genes essential for T-cell proliferation and function. Rapamycin on the other hand, blocks T-cell proliferation by a different mechanism, through inhibition of IL-2-dependent signal transduction pathways which function independently of calcium concentration and do not affect cytokine gene transcription (*Fig. 20.2*).

T-cell proliferation is inhibited

Cyclosporin has a marked inhibitory effect on early events of T-cell proliferation induced by mixed lymphocyte reactions, concanavalin A or phytohaemagglutinin. It has a specific effect on B cells, inhibiting antiglobulin-driven proliferative responses but not those due to stimulation with lipopolysaccharide. Antigen-presentation by monocytes and Langerhans' cells is also affected. Thus the effect of cyclosporin, while profound on T cells, extends to other cells of the immune system. It is believed that tacrolimus has a mode of action similar to that of cyclosporin, albeit by attachment to a different immunophilin. However, rapamycin also affects cells of non-haemopoietic origin; for example, it inhibits proliferation of vascular smooth muscle cells after balloon catheter injury and may then be useful in preventing restenosis after angioplasty. Also, because it inhibits T-lymphocyte proliferation at a later stage than cyclosporin or tacrolimus, it may be used synergistically with these agents, or as an alternative, in conditions refractory to the use of one or the other.

Cyclosporin, tacrolimus and rapamycin

	cyclosporin	tacrolimus	rapamycin
lymphokine secretion (IL-2, -3, -4, -6, GM–CSF, IFNγ)	↓	↓	– or ↑
IL-2 receptor expression	↓	↓	–
inhibition of response to IL-2	–	–	+

Fig. 20.2 Differential effects of cyclosporin, tacrolimus and rapamycin immunophilins on cytokine activity.

NUTRITION AND IMMUNE RESPONSES

The relationship between nutrition and resistance to infection has been suggested by historical accounts of famine and pestilence, clinical observations, and epidemiological data. Generally, nutrient deficiencies are associated with impaired immune responses. The five aspects of immunity most consistently affected by malnutrition are cell-mediated immunity, phagocyte function, the complement system, secretory antibody, and cytokine production. Worldwide, undernutrition is the commonest cause of immunodeficiency.

Economically underprivileged countries have a high prevalence of nutritional deficiencies, as do poor segments of society in many industrialized countries. In addition, many individuals show a nutrition problem secondary to another primary systemic disorder: patients with cancer, chronic renal disease, burns, multiple trauma and chronic infection show a high prevalence of malnutrition. Paradoxically, obesity and excess intake of nutrients are also associated with reduced immune responses.

Malnutrition and infection

Infection and malnutrition usually aggravate each other. However, nutrition does not affect all infections equally: the clinical course and final outcome of pneumonia, diarrhoea, measles and tuberculosis are affected adversely by nutritional deficiency; for some infections (e.g. tetanus and viral encephalitis), the effect of nutritional deficiency is minimal; for others (e.g. influenza virus and human immunodeficiency virus), nutrition exerts a moderate influence.

There are many factors that predispose to development of infection in the malnourished individual, including poor sanitation, contaminated food and water, lack of nutritional and health knowledge, illiteracy and overcrowding.

Lymphoid tissues

Lymphoid tissues are very vulnerable to the damaging effects of malnutrition. The extent and severity of lymphoid dysfunction caused by nutrient deficiencies depend upon several factors, including the rate of cell proliferation, the amount and rate of protein synthesis and the role of individual nutrients in critical metabolic pathways. Numerous enzymes with key roles in immune processes require zinc, iron, vitamin B_6 and other micronutrients in order to function.

Lymphoid atrophy is a prominent morphological feature of malnutrition. The thymus in particular, is a sensitive barometer in young children and the profound reduction in weight and size of the organ in several malnourished subjects has been termed 'nutritional thymectomy'. Histologically, the lobular architecture is ill-defined, there is a loss of corticomedullary demarcation, and there are fewer lymphoid cells. Hassall's corpuscles are enlarged and degenerate; some may be calcified. Atrophy is observed in the thymus-dependent periarteriolar areas of the spleen and in the paracortical section of the lymph nodes.

Protein–energy malnutrition (PEM)

Moderate/severe malnutrition is associated with a significant reduction in cell-mediated immunity, indicated by

Lymphocyte subsets

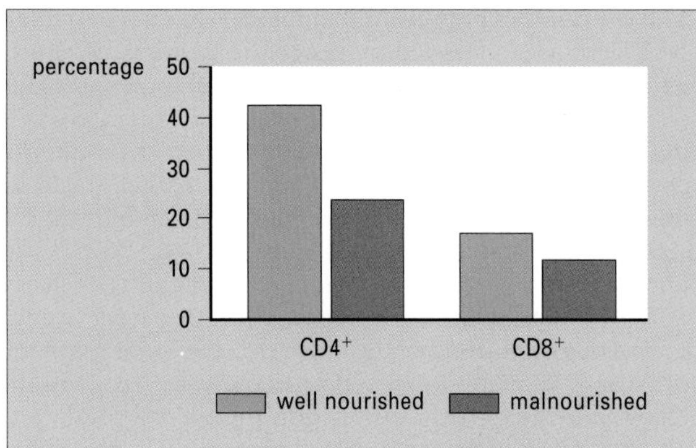

Fig. 20.3 Lymphocyte subsets in children with protein–energy malnutrition and in well-nourished controls. (From Chandra RK. *Clin Exp Immunol* 1983;**51**:126–131, with permission.)

a reduced number of $CD4^+$ T-helper cells, and a lower $CD4^+/CD8^+$ ratio (*Fig. 20.3*). Co-culture experiments indicate a reduction in T-cell help available to B lymphocytes. Lymphocyte proliferative responses to mitogen are decreased. The immaturity of circulating T cells is reflected in increased leucocyte deoxynucleotidyl transferase activity. Reduced thymulin activity may underlie these changes in T-cell number and function. There is a reduction in the secretory IgA antibody response to common vaccine antigens, which may contribute to a higher incidence of mucosal infections.

Phagocytosis is affected in PEM. Opsonization is decreased, largely because of a reduction in levels of various complement components: C3, C5 and Factor B. Whereas ingestion of microorganisms is intact in PEM, the ability of phagocytes to kill intracellular organisms is impaired. The production of certain cytokines, such as IL-2 and TNF, is decreased.

Some innate mechanisms of immunity are also affected by nutrition. The production of lysozyme is slightly decreased. A larger number of bacteria bind to epithelial cells of malnourished subjects; wound healing is impaired. There are very few data on the quality and quantity of mucus produced in PEM.

Individual nutrients

The profound effect of *zinc* deprivation on immune responses has been documented extensively. There is a reduction in delayed cutaneous hypersensitivity, lower $CD4^+/CD8^+$ ratios and T-cell dysfunction. A striking and pathognomonic feature of zinc deficiency is reduction in the activity of serum thymulin, (a nonapeptide that contains zinc as an integral part of its molecule) and lymphoid atrophy.

Intergeneration effect of zinc on immunity: an even more surprising finding is the effect in mice of zinc deficiency in pregnancy. Even the third generation progeny have impaired antibody responses as shown by diminished plaque-forming cells (PFC) and lower levels of IgM (*Fig. 20.4*).

Intergeneration effects of Zn deficiency on immunity

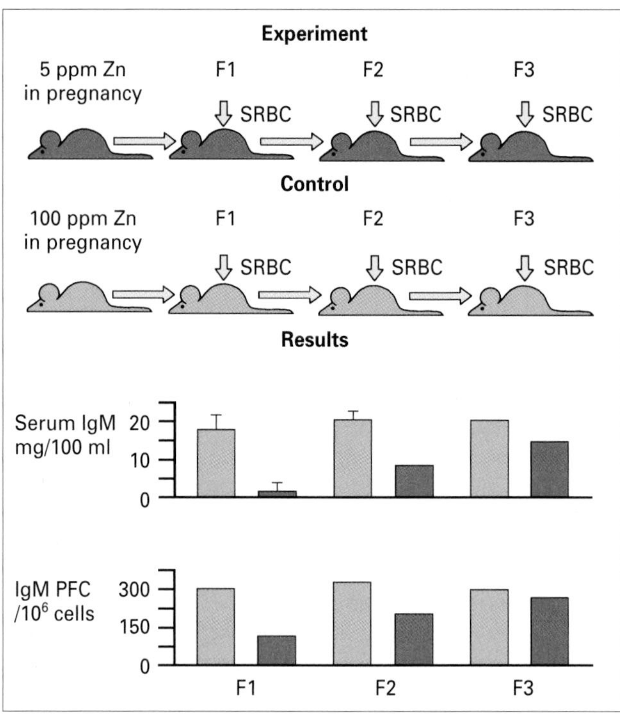

Fig. 20.4 An experimental group of animals was fed a Zn-deficient diet (5 ppm Zn) during the later two-thirds of pregnancy and a control group was fed a Zn-adequate diet (100 ppm Zn) during the same period. The former regime reduced serum Zn to 60–70% of control values. F1, F2 and F3 generations were fed sufficient Zn throughout. Both the PFC response and serum concentration of IgM were assessed at 6 weeks. Results showed that both were low in at least three generations of offspring.

Iron is a double-edged sword: it is required by most microorganisms for their growth, while iron-dependent enzymes have crucial roles in lymphocyte and phagocyte function. Thus iron deficiency is generally associated with reduced ability of neutrophils to kill bacteria and fungi, decreased lymphocyte response to mitogens and antigens, and impaired NK cell activity.

Selenium and *copper* are also important for immune responses. An exciting recent observation indicated that viruses can mutate and show altered virulence in malnourished hosts they infect. Coxsackie virus recovered from selenium-deficient mice produced heightened myocardial damage; there were six nucleotide changes between the avirulent input virus strain and the virulent virus recovered from selenium-deficient animals.

The clinical counterpart of Coxsackie myocarditis and nutritional deficiency is Keshan disease, which was endemic in some parts of China. Selenium supplementation has virtually eradicated this condition.

Vitamin A deficiency alters epithelial structure, leading to metaplasia and increased binding of bacteria. There is a reduction in the numbers of certain lymphocyte subsets and in the response to mitogen.

Vitamin supplementation is of value in preventing complications of severe measles and reducing mortality from this disease.

Vitamin B_6 and *folate* deficiencies reduce cell-mediated immunity, particularly lymphocyte proliferation responses, and also impair antibody production.

Obesity and excessive intake of nutrients

Obese subjects and animals show alteration in various immune responses, including cytotoxicity, NK activity and the ability of phagocytes to kill ingested bacteria and fungi. Altered levels of some micronutrients, lipids and hormones may explain these immunological changes.

Some nutrients given in moderate excess enhance selected aspects of immune responses, particularly cell-mediated immunity. These include vitamin E, vitamin A, zinc and selenium. However, for most nutrients, there is an upper limit of intake beyond which immune responses are impaired.

Clinical implications

There are exciting new possibilities for nutritional intervention for both primary and secondary prevention of infection in high-risk groups. Hospital inpatients who are malnourished are at high risk of complicated opportunistic infection. Nutrient-enriched feeding formulas enhance immunity and reduce the risk of complications such as sepsis and poor wound-healing. In the elderly, respiratory infection is a common cause of illness; modest amounts of micronutrient supplements improve immune responses and, more significantly, reduce the incidence of respiratory infections and antibiotic usage. Furthermore, post-vaccination immune responses are higher in subjects given nutritional supplements than in untreated controls.

Probiotics: in both clinical and veterinary medicine, the value of probiotics is being recognized. These 'desirable' bacteria such as *Lactobacillus acidophilus, L. casei*, cocci such as *Enterococcus faecium* and bifidobacteria are given orally to replace or increase their presence in the gut microflora.

Benefits to health and immunity come from the 'barrier effect' in the gut, production of bacteriocidins and by altering the local immune response via a change in cytokine profile in the gut mucosa and increased antibody production.

It is still an open question as to how the immunological changes translate into improved health but the effect has been shown quite clearly in children with AIDS.

AIDS

Human immunodeficiency virus (HIV) causes AIDS and is transmitted sexually, in blood or blood products, and perinatally. There are two main variants, HIV-1 and HIV-2. HIV-2 is endemic in West Africa and appears to be less pathogenic.

More than 80% of people infected with HIV live in developing countries and spread is 80% by the sexual route (70% vaginal; 10% anal). The World Health Organization (WHO) estimate that, by the year 2000, the cumulative total infected will reach 30 million, with 99% of all infections in developing countries and 2 million people dying of AIDS each year.

The virus

HIV is a single stranded diploid RNA virus 100–120 nm in diameter (*Fig. 20.5*). Its basic gene structure has *gag* (core protein), *pol* (polymerase/reverse transcriptase) and *env* (envelope protein) genes. Additional genes regulate viral protein synthesis. CD4 antigen is the receptor for the virus; it is present on $CD4^+$ T lymphocytes and cells of the monocyte/macrophage lineage. Viral gp120 binds to CD4, but chemokine receptors are involved in the subsequent gp41-mediated fusion and internalization.

Immune dysfunction

There is wide immune dysfunction, with immune depression within a milieu of immune activation, resulting from direct effects of HIV and from the depletion and functional impairment of the $CD4^+$ T-cell subset over time. How HIV kills its target cells is not well understood; several different mechanisms have been proposed, including accumulation of RNA and unintegrated DNA in the cell cytoplasm, and intracellular binding of CD4 and gp120. Infected cells may bind to uninfected cells by gp120–CD4 linkages, with multinucleate giant cell and syncytium formation. gp120 bound to the surface of uninfected $CD4^+$ T cells also makes them vulnerable to antibody-dependent cell-mediated cytotoxicity (ADCC), while infected cells may be killed by gp120-specific cytotoxic T cells. HIV proteins may act as superantigens, resulting in vast expansion and then exhaustive depletion of cells. In addition, HIV may induce T-cell apoptosis and viral budding may lead to cell-membrane weakening and lysis.

The spectrum of immune dysfunction is characterized by depletion of the $CD4^+$ T-cell subset and decreased responses to antigens, mitogens, alloantigens and anti-CD3 antibody, associated with decreased IL-2 production and other changes in cytokine production. Eventually, there is loss of HIV-specific cytotoxic T-cell responses and certain antigen-presenting cell functions. There is an increase in activated and unresponsive $CD8^+$ T cells, increased β_2-microglobulin and neopterin in serum, polyclonal B-cell activation with B cells refractory to T-cell-independent B-cell activators, and an increase in autoantibodies and immune complexes.

Modelling of the plasma virus and $CD4^+$ T-cell responses to antiviral therapy suggests that the average half-life of the virus and infected cells in the circulation is less than two days. 10^9–10^{10} viruses are released from infected cells and similar numbers of new cells are infected and die daily.

Natural history

Primary infection with HIV may be accompanied by transient illness similar to glandular fever, with malaise, muscle pains, swollen lymph nodes, sore throat and rash. There is transient depletion of peripheral $CD4^+$ T cells, expansion of $CD8^+$ T cells and high plasma levels of HIV (*Fig. 20.6*). In 2–6 weeks, antibodies to core and surface proteins can be detected by enzyme-linked immunoassays. A chronic infection ensues without illness, but about 33% of patients have swollen lymph nodes. Fifty per cent of those infected develop AIDS within 9–10 years.

Human immunodeficiency virus and its life cycle

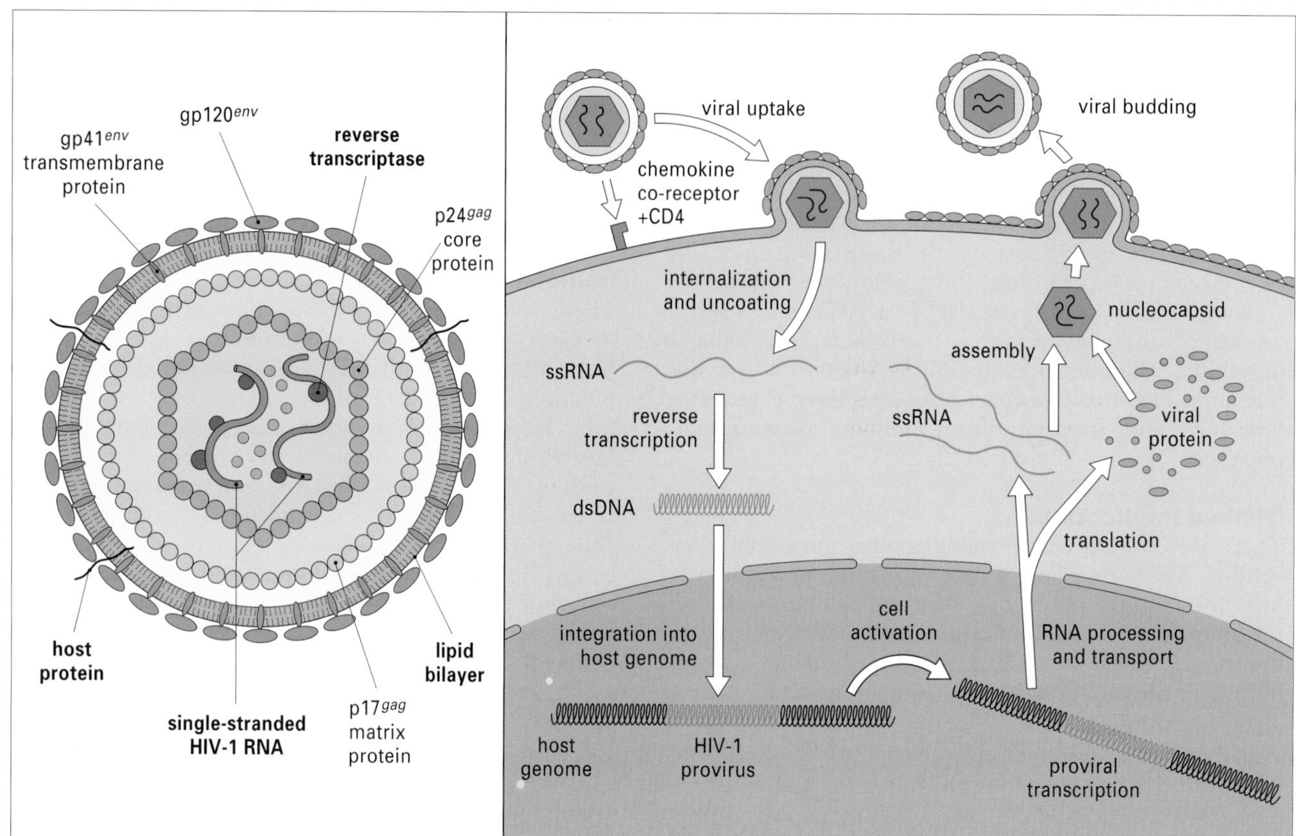

Fig. 20.5 After uncoating, reverse transcription of viral RNA results in the production of double-stranded DNA. This is inserted into the host genome as the HIV provirus, by a virally coded integrase enzyme. Cell activation leads to transcription and the production of viral mRNAs. Structural proteins are produced and assembled. Free HIV viruses are produced by viral budding from the host cell, after which further internal assembly occurs with the cleavage of a large precursor core protein into the small core protein components by a virally coded protease enzyme, producing mature virus particles.

Later in infection, non-specific constitutional symptoms such as fevers, night sweats, diarrhoea and weight loss occur, together with 'minor' conditions that largely affect the mucous membranes and skin: for example, oral candidiasis (thrush), shingles, recurrent anogenital herpes simplex and a variety of skin infections. These conditions often signal the development of serious opportunistic infections and tumours, which constitute AIDS when the $CD4^+$ T-cell count is, usually, below 200/μl (*Fig. 20.6*).

Kaposi's sarcoma, a multifocal tumour of endothelial cells (*Fig. 20.7*), is the commonest tumour. Widespread skin, mucus-membrane, visceral (gut and lungs) and lymph-node disease occurs. Infection with human herpes virus 8 (HHV8) is associated with the development of the tumour. B-cell lymphomas also occur, affecting the brain, gut and bone marrow.

Most of the opportunistic infections are due to reactivation of latent organisms in the host or, in some cases, ubiquitous organisms to which we are continually exposed. They are difficult to diagnose and treatment often suppresses rather than eradicates them. Relapses are common and continuous suppressive or maintenance treatment is necessary, using drugs that cause side-effects.

Three main organ systems are affected: the respiratory system, gastrointestinal tract and nervous system. Pneumonia is common and *Pneumocystis carinii* is the commonest infection (*Fig. 20.7*), but bacterial infections, including *Mycobacterium tuberculosis*, and fungal infections also occur. Discomfort on swallowing is usually caused by candidiasis (thrush), but cytomegalovirus can cause oesophageal ulceration. Protozoa (*cryptosporidium* and microsporidia) are the commonest pathogens isolated in patients with diarrhoea and weight loss (*Fig. 20.7*), but enteric bacteria such as *Salmonella* and *Campylobacter* may also be found.

Neurological complications in AIDS are due to direct effects of HIV infection, opportunistic infections or lymphoma. AIDS-related dementia once affected between 10% and 40% of patients with other manifestations of AIDS, but, with more effective antiviral treatment, has become less common. Spinal cord and peripheral nerve disease also occur. Toxoplasmosis, a protozoal infection, causes cysts in the brain and neurological deficit (*Fig. 20.7*). *Cryptococcus*

Natural history of HIV

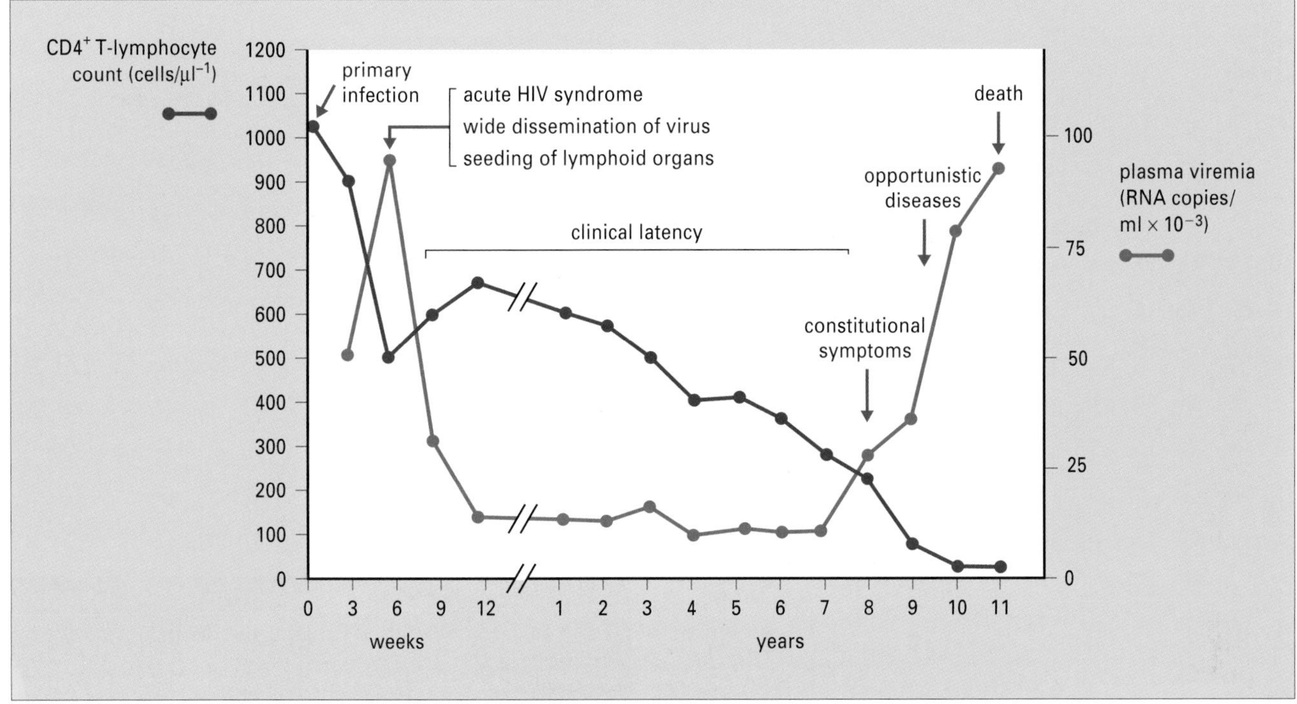

Fig. 20.6 A typical course of HIV infection, courtesy of Dr A. S. Fauci. (Modified with permission from Pantaleo G, Graziosi C. *N Engl J Med* 1993;**328**:327–35.)

neoformans is a fungus which causes meningitis. Cytomegalovirus may cause inflammation of the retinae, brain and spinal cord and its nerve roots, and a polyomavirus (JC virus) which infects oligodendrocytes in the brain produces a rapidly fatal demyelinating disease – progressive multifocal leucoencephalopathy.

Antiviral treatments

In 1987, zidovudine (AZT) was licensed as the first nucleoside analogue reverse transcriptase inhibitor (NRTI), to be used in HIV infection. There have been considerable advances since then, with the development of other NRTIs and non-nucleoside reverse transcriptase inhibitors (NNRTIs) and protease inhibitors (*Fig. 20.5*).

Zidovudine monotherapy in patients with advanced disease reduces the short-term mortality and progression of disease. Early in infection, clinical benefit is small and transient, with no improvement in survival. As a result, combinations of two or more drugs have been used, with the aims of enhancing efficacy through additive or synergistic effects and delaying the emergence of resistance by slowing the rate of mutation of the RT gene or by conferring mutations that might reverse resistance or lead to less competent viruses. Combination of two NRTIs reduces the rate of progression to AIDS and death by approximately 40% over 1–3 years compared with monotherapy. Combinations of NRTIs and protease inhibitors have also been clinically effective. The use of other multiple combinations of NRTIs, NNRTIs and protease inhibitors produces promising antiviral effects, together with impressive short-term $CD4^+$ T-cell increases, which may provide additional clinical benefits.

The optimal time to start therapy remains unclear, but most physicians act on a repeatedly low CD4 count of 200–400 cells/µl^{-1} and in all patients who are symptomatic. Serum HIV RNA levels also influence this decision. The cost even of monotherapy is prohibitive for most developing countries. As no cure or vaccine is currently available, our main weapon is prevention through health education and control of infection.

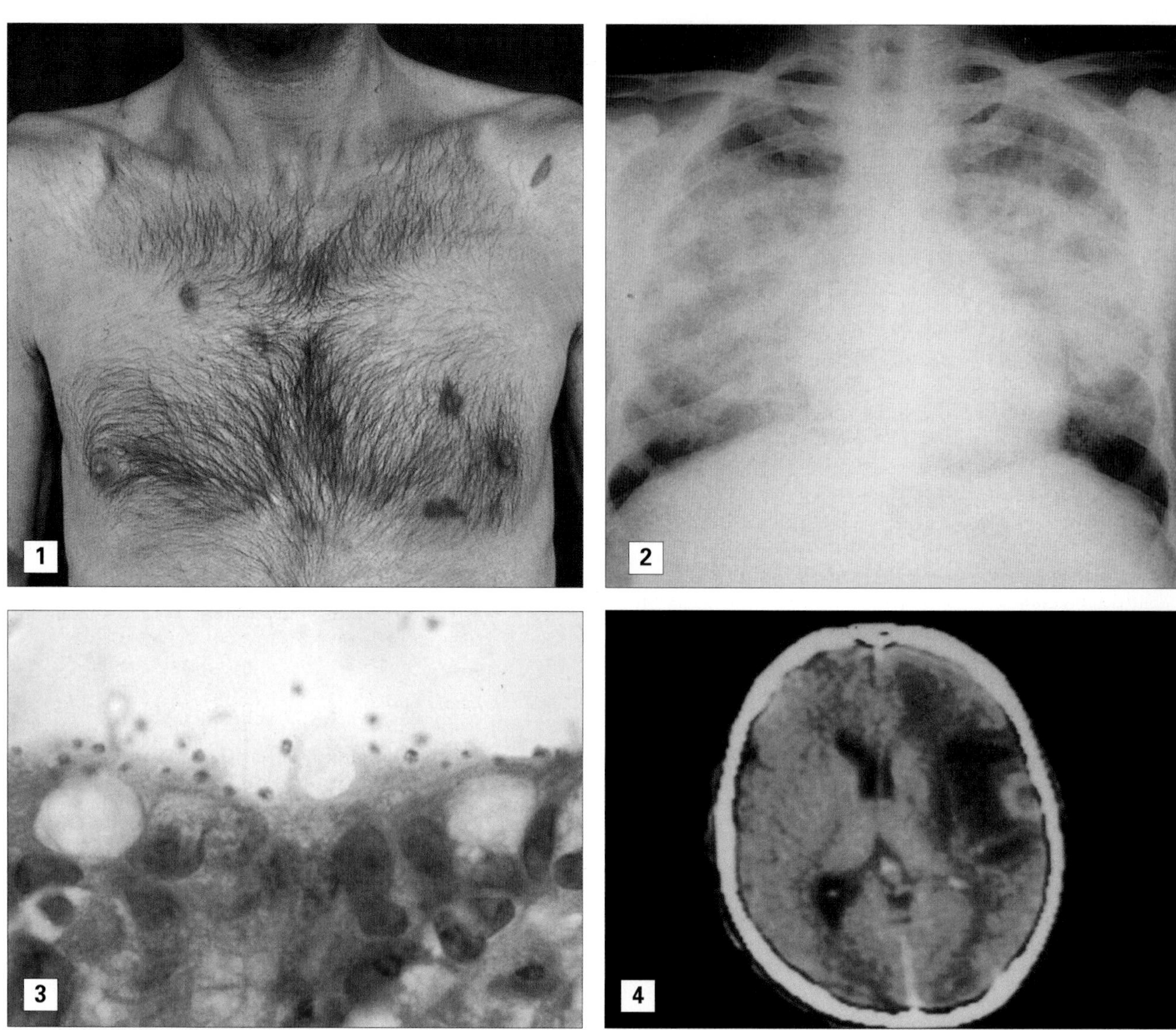

Fig. 20.7 Common features of AIDS. (**1**) Multiple Kaposi's sarcoma lesions on the chest and abdomen. (**2**) Chest radiograph of a patient with *Pneumocystis carinii* pneumonia, showing bilateral interstitial shadowing. (**3**) Small bowel biopsy from a patient with diarrhoea caused by *Cryptosporidium*, showing intermediate forms of cryptosporidia (small pink dots) on the surface of the mucosa. (**4**) Computed tomography (CT) scan of the head of a patient with cerebral toxoplasmosis. The patient presented with a history of fits and weakness of the left arm and leg. Injection of contrast revealed a ring-enhancing lesion in the right hemisphere, with surrounding oedema (dark area).

CRITICAL THINKING • Secondary immunodeficiency (Explanations on pp 459–460)

A 52-year-old record producer developed a severe cough with increasing shortness of breath and cough. He also had a fever, chest pain and malaise. For the past week he complained of pain on swallowing which he attributed to a sore throat. Past medical history included gonorrhoea and genital herpes within the last 3 years. Over the previous 2 months he had suffered from persistent diarrhoea and lost 9 kg in weight from a baseline of 68 kg. He had lived with his male partner with whom he had been having unprotected intercourse for several years. There was no history of intravenous drug abuse.

On examination he was underweight, had enlarged lymph nodes in the neck, axillae and groin. Plaques of *Candida albicans* were visible in his throat. There were abnormal breath sounds in his lungs. The results of the blood tests are shown in *Figure 20.8.*

Because of his sexual history the patient was counselled regarding a human immunodeficiency virus (HIV) test and consented. An enzyme-linked immunosorbent assay (ELISA) was positive for anti-HIV antibodies and a polymerase chain reaction (PCR) test directly demonstrated HIV-1. A clear diagnosis of acquired immunodeficiency syndrome (AIDS) was made and the patient's *Pneumocystis carinii* pneumonia was treated with oxygen by mask and parenteral co trimoxazole. He was discharged from hospital taking oral co-trimoxazole.

Within 3 months he was seen again in accident and emergency with blurred vision and 'flashing lights' in his eyes. He was shown to have an infection of his retina with cytomegalovirus and was treated with injections of ganciclovir. A CD4 count at this time was 0.04×10^9/l. Whilst receiving this treatment the patient became increasingly unwell and became semiconscious. Investigations at this time are shown in *Figure 20.9.*

A diagnosis of cryptococcal meningitis was made and intravenous amphotericin was started. The patient did not respond to treatment and died shortly afterwards. At post mortem, *P. carinii* were isolated from his lungs and evidence of early cerebral lymphoma was noted.

20.1 What diagnostic tests are available for HIV infection?

20.2 Which of these tests should be used if HIV infection is suspected in a mother and her child, infected vertically?

20.3 What serological and cellular indices can be used to monitor the course of HIV infection?

Investigation	Result *(normal range)*
Haemoglobin *(g/dl)*	12.8 *(13.5–18.0)*
Platelet count *(× 10^9/l)*	128 *(150–400)*
White cell count *(× 10^9/l)*	6.2 *(4.0–11.0)*
Neutrophils *(× 10^9/l)*	5.4 *(2.0–7.5)*
Eosinophils *(× 10^9/l)*	0.24 *(0.4–0.44)*
Total lymphocytes *(× 10^9/l)*	0.75 *(1.6–3.5)*
T lymphocytes CD4$^+$ *(× 10^9/l)*	0.12 *(0.7–1.1)*
CD8$^+$ *(× 10^9/l)*	0.42 *(0.5–0.9)*
B lymphocytes *(× 10^9/l)*	0.11 *(0.2–0.5)*
Arterial blood gases	
Pa_{O_2} *(kPa)*	7.8 *(>10.6)*
Pa_{CO_2} *(kPa)*	5.52 *(4.7–6.0)*
pH	7.39 *(7.35–7.45)*
HCO_3^-	25.6
Base excess	–0.9
ECG	Normal
Chest X-ray	Bilateral diffuse interstitial shadowing
Bronchoscopy with bronchoalveolar lavage	Positive for *Pneumocystis carinii*

Fig. 20.8 Results of investigations.

Investigation	Result *(normal range)*
Haemoglobin *(g/dl)*	10.4 *(13.5–18.0)*
Platelet count *(× 10^9/l)*	104 *(150–400)*
White cell count *(× 10^9/l)*	4.1 *(4.0–11.0)*
Neutrophils *(× 10^9/l)*	4.2 *(2.0–7.5)*
Eosinophils *(× 10^9/l)*	0.24 *(0.4–0.44)*
Total lymphocytes *(× 10^9/l)*	0.62 *(1.6–3.5)*
T lymphocytes CD4$^+$ *(× 10^9/l)*	0.03 *(0.7–1.1)*
CD8$^+$ *(× 10^9/l)*	0.40 *(0.5–0.9)*
B lymphocytes *(× 10^9/l)*	0.09 *(0.2–0.5)*
Chest X-ray	Minimal areas of diffuse shadowing
Blood culture	Negative
Blood glucose *(mmol/l)*	7.6 *(<10.0)*
CSF from lumbar puncture	
Appearance	Turbid
White cells *(polymorphs/mm^3)*	2500
Protein *(g/l)*	4.2 *(0.15–0.45)*
Glucose *(mmol/l)*	4.5 *(>60% blood glucose)*
Indian ink stain	Positive for cryptococcus

Fig. 20.9 Results of investigation 3 months later.

FURTHER READING

Chandra RK (ed). *Nutrition and Immunology.* St John's, NF, Canada: ARTS Biomedical; 1992.

Chandra RK. Nutrition, immunity and infection. *Proc Natl Acad Sci USA* 1996;**93**:14304–7.

Chandra RK. Graying of the immune system. Can nutrient supplements improve immunity in the elderly? *JAMA* 1997;**277**:1898–9.

Cunningham-Rundles S, *et al.* Probiotics and immune response. *Am J Gastroenterology* 2000;**95**:522–25.

Gershwin ME, Beach RS, Hurley LS. *Nutrition and Immunity.* New York: Academic Press; 1984.

21 Hypersensitivity – Type I

- **Production of IgE in genetically predisposed, i.e. atopic, individuals** occurs in response to repeated low-dose exposure to inhaled allergens such as dust mite, cat dander or grass pollen.
- **IgE antibodies bind to a specific receptor, FcεRI, on mast cells and basophils.** When bound IgE is cross-linked by specific allergen, mediators including histamine, leukotrienes and cytokines are released.
- **Allergic diseases include anaphylaxis, seasonal hayfever, atopic dermatitis and allergic asthma.** Therapy includes antihistamines, adrenaline, bronchodilators, corticosteroids, reducing exposure to allergens and specific allergen immunotherapy.
- **The severity of symptoms depends on IgE antibodies, the quantity of allergen, and also a variety of factors that can enhance the response** including viral infections and environmental pollutants.
- **Multiple genetic loci influence the production of IgE, the inflammatory response to allergen exposure and the response to treatment.** Polymorphisms have been identified in the genes, in promoter regions and in the receptors for IgE, cytokines, leukotrienes and the β_2-receptors.
- **The biological role of immediate hypersensitivity** is to control helminth infections such as schistosomiasis, hookworm or *Ascaris*. However, it is likely to be a combination of effector TH2 cells, basophils and eosinophils, as well as IgE antibodies on mast cells that control these worms.

The adaptive immune response provides specific protection against infection with bacteria, viruses, parasites and fungi. In particular, it is able to provide rapid protection against a repeated challenge with the same or a similar foreign organism or toxin. By contrast, some immune responses can give rise to an excessive or inappropriate reaction; this is usually referred to as hypersensitivity. Hypersensitivity may occur as an exaggerated form of an appropriate response, for example to a virus, or from a response to an antigen that has no toxic potential, for example asthma with inhaled cat dander or eczematous response of the skin to jewellery containing nickel. Typical examples of hypersensitivity include contact sensitivity, antibody-mediated responses against self antigens, and immune complex deposition in the kidneys, joints or skin. However, the most common forms of hypersensitivity are allergic responses characterized by wheal and flare skin responses to the relevant antigen, which are mediated by IgE antibodies binding to mast cells. Coombs and Gell classified hypersensitivity reactions into four forms, Types I–IV. The classification is a useful guide to understanding the different forms of response. However, some conditions do not fit easily into the classification and only the terms Type I and Type IV are used routinely (*Fig. 21.1*).

Type I or immediate hypersensitivity is characterized by the production of IgE antibodies against foreign proteins

Four types of hypersensitivity reaction

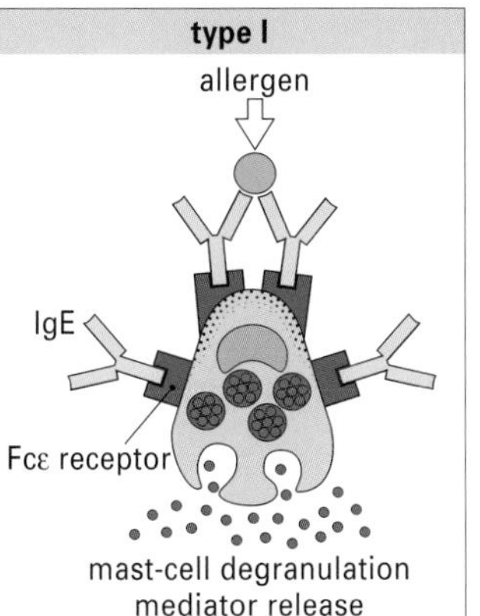

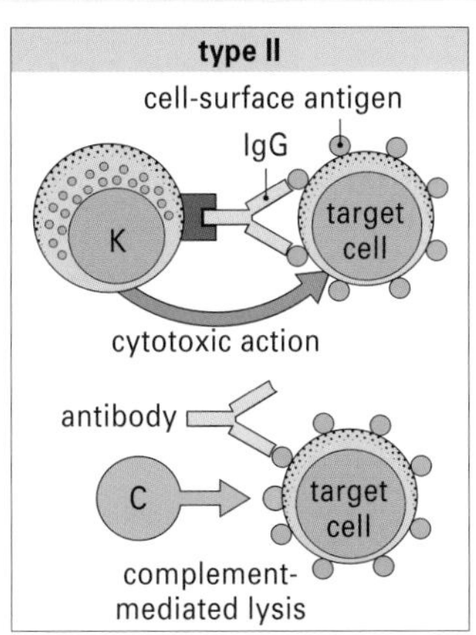

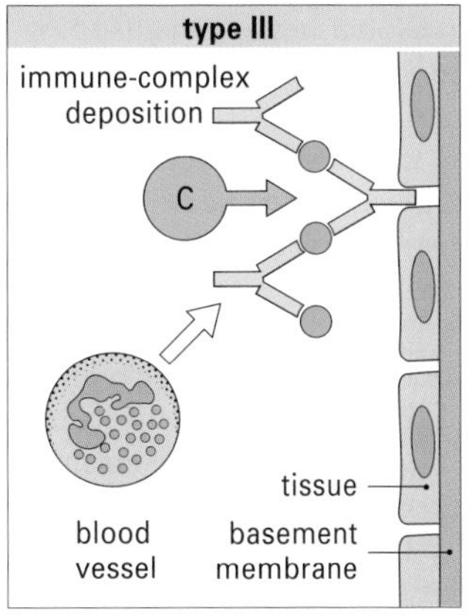

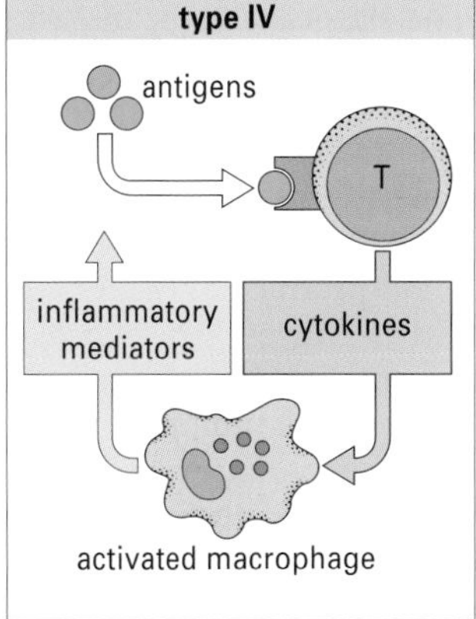

Fig. 21.1 There are four types of hypersensitivity reaction. Type I mast cells bind IgE via their Fc receptors. On encountering allergen the IgE becomes cross-linked, inducing degranulation and release of mediators that produce allergic reactions. Type II antibody is directed against antigen on an individual's own cells (target cell) or foreign antigen, such as transfused red blood cells. This may lead to cytotoxic action by K cells, or complement-mediated lysis. Type III immune complexes are deposited in the tissue. Complement is activated and polymorphs are attracted to the site of deposition, causing local tissue damage and inflammation. Type IV antigen-sensitized T cells release lymphokines following a secondary contact with the same antigen. Cytokines induce inflammatory reactions and activate and attract macrophages, which release inflammatory mediators.

that are commonly present in the environment, for example pollens, animal danders or dust mites. These antibodies bind specifically to a high-affinity receptor on mast cells and basophils, which are the only human cells that contain histamine. Subsequent exposure to the same antigen will lead to rapid release of histamine, and more gradual release of other mediators including leukotrienes and cytokines. The conditions that are associated with Type I hypersensitivity include hayfever, asthma, atopic dermatitis and anaphylaxis. Type II or antibody-mediated food allergy reactions occur when antibodies, either of the IgG or IgM isotypes, are produced against surface antigens present on cells of the body. These antibodies can trigger cytotoxic reactions either by activating complement (C) (e.g. autoimmune haemolytic anaemia) or by facilitating the binding of natural killer cells (NK) (see Chapter 22). Type III or immune complex disease occurs when excess complexes are formed in the circulation that cannot be cleared by macrophages or other cells in the reticuloendothelial system. The formation of immune complexes requires significant quantities of antibodies *and* antigen (typically μg quantities of each). The local accumulation of complexes can trigger either a complement or a cell-mediated local reaction. The classical diseases in which immune complexes are thought to be involved are systemic lupus erythematosus (SLE) and serum sickness. Finally, Type IV or cell-mediated reactions are those in which specific T cells are the primary effector cells. The simplest examples of T cells causing unwanted responses are contact sensitivity (e.g. to nickel or poison ivy) and graft rejection. However, specifically sensitized T cells also play a role in the chronic hypersensitivity skin responses of leprosy or tuberculosis, and are an important part of the exaggerated response to viral infections such as measles.

IMMEDIATE HYPERSENSITIVITY

Historical introduction

The classical allergic disease is seasonal hayfever caused by pollen grains entering the nose (rhinitis) and eyes (conjunctivitis). In severe cases patients may also get seasonal asthma and seasonal dermatitis. Charles Blackley in 1873 demonstrated that pollen grains placed into the nose could induce rhinitis. He also demonstrated that pollen extract could produce a wheal and flare skin response in patients with hayfever. The wheal and flare skin response is an extremely sensitive method of detecting specific IgE antibodies. The timing and form of the skin response is indistinguishable from the local reaction to injected histamine. Furthermore, the immediate skin response can be effectively blocked with antihistamines. In 1903 Portier and Richet discovered that immunization of guinea-pigs with a toxin from the jellyfish *Physalia* could sensitize them so that a subsequent injection of the same protein would cause rapid onset of breathing difficulty, influx of fluid into the lungs, and death. They coined the term anaphylaxis (from the Greek *ana*=non, and *phylaxos*=protection) and speculated about the relationship to other hypersensitivity diseases. They noted that human anaphylaxis had no familial characteristics (unlike most of the other allergic diseases) and that natural exposure to inhaled allergens did not cause anaphylaxis or urticaria. Subsequently, it became clear that injection of any protein into an individual with immediate hypersensitivity to that protein can induce anaphylaxis. Thus, anaphylaxis occurs when a patient with immediate hypersensitivity is exposed to a relevant allergen in such a way that antigen enters the circulation rapidly; this can occur after a bee sting, an injection of penicillin, eating an allergen such as peanut or shellfish, or following a therapeutic allergen injection for hyposensitization (*Fig. 21.2*). The term allergen was first used by von Pirquet to cover all foreign substances that could produce an immune response. He included those substances that could induce 'supersensitivity', the word they used for allergy. Subsequently, the word 'allergen' came to be used selectively for the proteins that cause 'supersensitivity'. Thus, an allergen is an antigen that gives rise to immediate hypersensitivity.

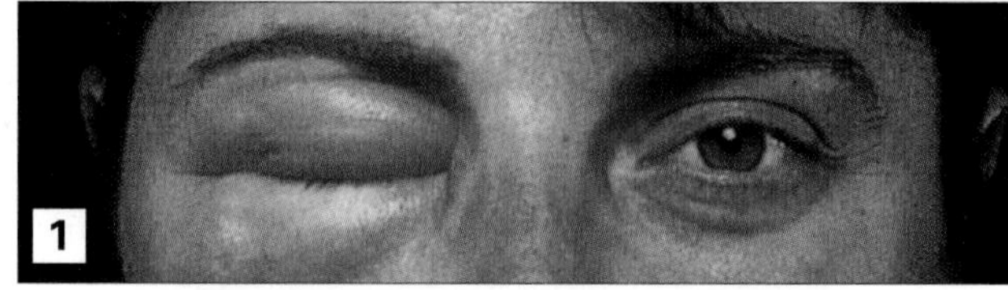

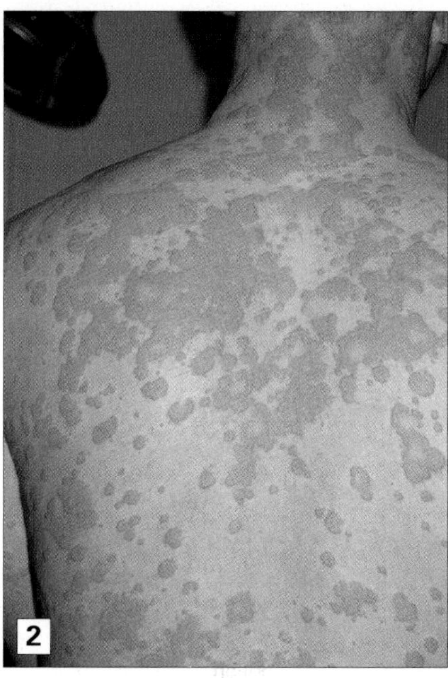

Fig. 21.2 Anaphylaxis and urticaria. **(1)** The anaphylactic response to bee venom in a patient who has IgE antibodies to the venom protein, Phospholipase A. The immediate reaction occurs within 20 minutes and is mediated by the release of histamine and other mediators from mast cells. The patient shown had been stung on the face, but the reaction can become generalized, leading to a fall in blood pressure, generalized urticaria and/or bronchospasm (i.e. anaphylaxis). **(2)** Diffuse urticaria on a patient with severe chronic urticaria. The lesions have a raised edge and come up within minutes or hours. The lesions almost always resolve within 12 hours leaving no trace on the skin.

Characteristics of allergens

Substances that can give rise to wheal and flare responses in the skin and to the symptoms of allergic disease are derived from many different sources. When purified they are almost all found to be proteins and their size ranges in molecular weight from 10 000 to 40 000 Daltons. These proteins are all freely soluble in aqueous solution but have many different biological functions including digestive enzymes, carrier proteins, calycins and pollen recognition proteins. Any allergen can be described or classified by its source, route of exposure and the nature of the specific protein (*Fig. 21.3*). Extracts used for skin testing or *in vitro* measurement of IgE antibodies are made from the whole material which contains multiple different proteins, any of which can be an allergen. Indeed, it is clear that individual patients can react selectively to one or more different proteins within an extract. Estimates of exposure can be made either by visual identification of particles (e.g. pollen grains or fungal spores) or by immunoassay of the major allergens (e.g. Fel d 1 or Der p 1).

IMMUNOGLOBULIN E

In 1921 Küstner, who was allergic to fish, injected his own serum into the skin of Prauznitz, who was allergic to grass pollen but not fish, and demonstrated that it was possible to passively transfer immediate hypersensitivity (the Prausnitz–Küstner or P–K test). Over the next 30 years it was established that P–K activity was a general property of immediate hypersensitivity, and that it was allergen specific, i.e. behaved like an antibody. In 1967 Ishizaka and his colleagues purified the P–K activity from a patient with ragweed hayfever and proved that this was a novel isotype of immunoglobulin: IgE. However, it was obvious that the concentration of this immunoglobulin isotype in serum was very low. The initial antisera to IgE made it possible to identify a patient with multiple myeloma whose serum contained a very high concentration of IgE (~10 mg/ml). Purification of this myeloma protein led to the full structure of IgE and also to the production of potent antisera. Antisera to IgE are used in the radioallergosorbent test (RAST) to measure IgE antibodies in serum, as well as for measuring total serum IgE. IgE is distinct from the other dimeric immunoglobulins because it has an extra constant region domain, a different structure to the hinge region, and binding sites for both high- and low-affinity IgE receptors, FcεRI and FcεRII, respectively (*Fig. 21.4*). The primary cells that bear FcεRI are mast cells and basophils which are the only cells in the human that contain significant amounts of histamine.

The properties of IgE can be separated into three areas: the characteristics of the molecule including its half-life and binding to IgE receptors; the control of IgE and (IgG4) antibody production by T cells; and the consequences of allergen cross-linking IgE on the surface of mast cells or basophils.

Half-life of IgE

The concentration of IgE in the serum of normal individuals is very low compared to all the other immunoglobulin isotypes. Values range from <10 to 10 000 IU/ml, and the international unit (IU) is equivalent to 2.4 ng. Most sera contain less than 1 μg IgE/ml. The reasons why

Properties of allergens

source	airborne particles	Dimension of airborne particle (μm)	allergen		
			name	MW (kDa)	function/homologies
dust mite *D. pteronyssinus*	faeces	10–40	Der p 1 Der p 2	25 13	cysteine protease (epididymal protein)
cats *Felis domesticus*	dander particles	2–15	Fel d 1	36	uteroglobin
German cockroach *Blattella germanica*	frass saliva	≥5	Bla g 2 Bla g 4 Bla g 5	36 21 23	aspartic protease calycin glutathione-*S*-transferase
rat *Rattus norvegicus*	urine on bedding?	2–20	Rat n 1	19	pheromone binding protein
grass	pollen	30	Lol p 1	29	not known
fungi:					
Alternaria alternata	spores	14 × 10	Alt a 1		not known
Aspergillus fumigatus	spores	2	Asp f 1		mitogillin

Fig. 21.3 When a patient becomes 'allergic' to one of the well-recognized sources of allergens, they have actually produced an IgE antibody response to one or more of the proteins that are produced by mites, trees, grass, cats or fungi. The proteins are predominantly water soluble with a molecular weight (MW) ranging from 10 000 to 40 000 kDa. In many cases the function of the proteins is known, but it is not clear whether function such as enzymic activity alters the ability of these proteins to induce an allergic response. The properties of the particles carrying these allergens are very important because they influence both how much becomes airborne, and also where the allergen is deposited in the respiratory tract. The dimensions of the particles airborne vary from ≤2 μm for *Aspergillus* or *Penicillium* spores to ≥20 μm for mite faecal pellets and some pollen grains (sizes are given as diameter in micrometres).

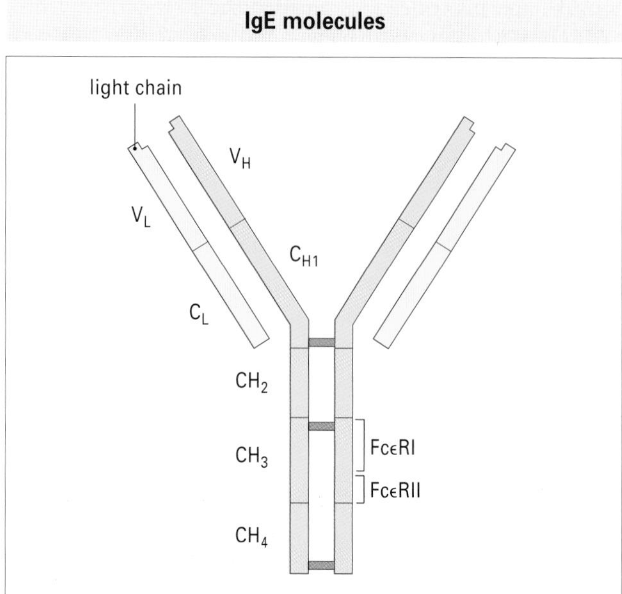

Fig. 21.4 The IgE molecule has four heavy chain constant regions. The binding sites for the high-affinity IgE receptor FcεRI, and for the low-affinity receptor FcεRII, or CD-23 are shown. Monoclonal antibodies to the binding site for FcεRI also block FcεRII.

serum IgE is so low include: (i) serum IgE has a much shorter half-life than other isotypes, ~2 days compared with 21–23 days for IgG; (ii) IgE is produced in small quantities and is only produced in response to a select group of antigens (allergens and parasites); and (iii) IgE antibodies are sequestered on the high-affinity receptor on mast cells and basophils. The half-life of IgE in the serum has been measured both by injecting radiolabelled IgE and by infusing plasma from allergic patients into normal and immune-deficient patients. The half-life of IgE in serum is less than 2 days; by contrast, IgE bound to mast cells in the skin has a half life of ~10 days. However, the low quantities of IgE in the serum must reflect a more rapid breakdown of IgE, as well as removal from the circulation by binding onto mast cells. The most important site of breakdown of IgE being thought to be within endosomes where the low pH facilitates breakdown of free immunoglobulin by cathepsin. Serum is constantly being taken up by endocytosis. Most macromolecules including IgE degrade in the endosome. One major exception is IgG, which is protected by binding to the neonatal Fc gamma receptor, FcγRn (*Fig. 21.5*).

Placental transfer of antibodies

In cord blood the concentration of IgE is very low indeed, generally less than 1 IU/ml (i.e. <2 ng/ml). Thus, there appears to be almost no transfer across the placenta. By contrast, IgG including IgG4 antibodies to allergens such as those from dust mite or cat are very efficiently transferred across the placenta. This process also involves endocytosis and receptor-mediated transport. Passive transfer of IgE to the fetus may be blocked because IgE is broken down in the endosomes or because an Fc receptor is essential for transport, and there is no receptor for IgE on the cells that comprise the placental tissues.

ROLE OF T CELLS IN THE IMMUNE RESPONSE TO INHALANT ALLERGENS

Experiments in animals have established that the production of IgE is completely dependent on T cells. It is also clear that T cells can suppress IgE production. The T cells which can suppress IgE production act predominantly by producing interferon-γ (IFNγ), and are produced when the animal, for example mouse, rat or rabbit, is primed in the presence of Freund's complete adjuvant. This adjuvant, which includes bacterial cell walls and probably bacterial

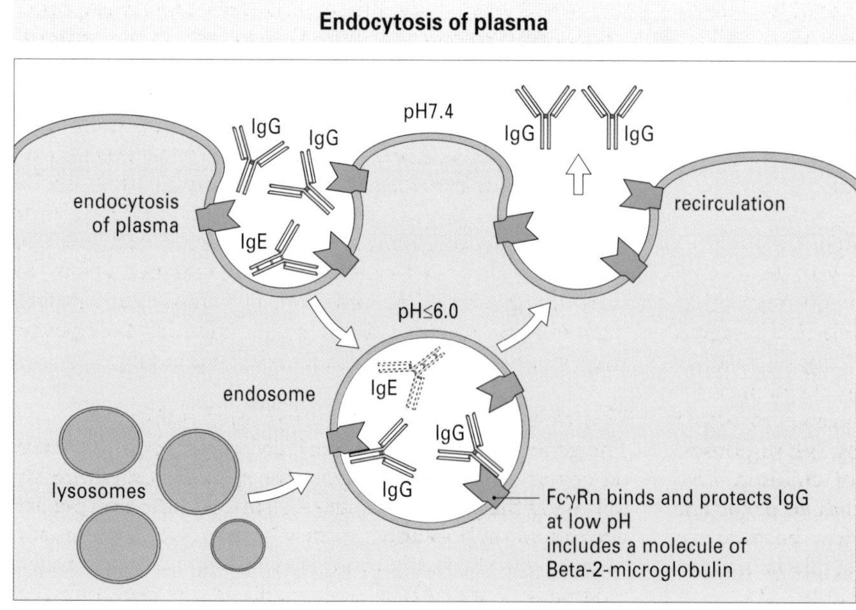

Fig. 21.5 Endocytosis of plasma contributes to the short half-life of IgE, as plasma proteins are taken up and the pH falls because of lysosomes combining with the endosome. At low pH IgG including IgG4 molecules bind to the neonatal Fc gamma receptor (FcγRn). By contrast, IgE molecules do not bind to FcγRn so they are not protected and are digested by cathepsin. As the endosomes recirculate, the pH rises to 7.4 and the undamaged IgG molecules are released into the circulation. The FcγRn includes a molecule of β_2-microglobulin. In keeping with this model the half-life of IgG is shorter than normal in mice that have had the gene for β_2-microglobulin removed (or knocked out).

T-cell differentiation during human immune responses

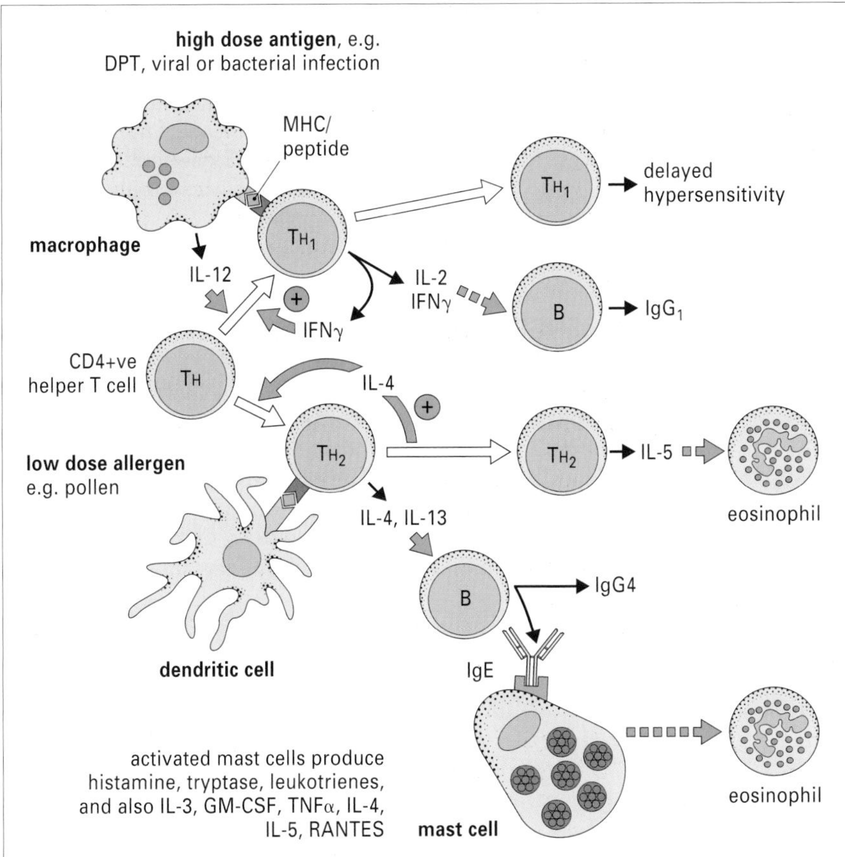

Fig. 21.6 The differentiation of TH cells depends on the antigen source, the quantity of allergen and the cytokines produced. Bacterial antigens or a high dose of antigen will induce IL-12 from macrophages. In addition, the developing TH1 cells produce IFNγ which further enhances the production of TH1 cells. Low dose antigen without adjuvant will induce TH2 cells, which produce both IL-4 and IL-5. IL-4 plays a role in: (**1**) enhancing the growth of TH2 cells; (**2**) the expression of the gene for IgE. In turn IgE binds to the high-affinity receptor for IgE (FcεRI) on mast cells.

DNA, is a very potent activator of macrophages. With the discovery of TH1 and TH2 cells, it became clear that IgE production is dependent on TH2 cells and that any priming that generates a TH1 response will inhibit IgE production. The main cytokines that are specifically relevant to a TH1 response include interleukin-12 (IL-12) produced by macrophages and IFNγ produced by T cells. By contrast, the primary cytokines relevant to a TH2 response are IL-4 (IL-13), IL-5 and IL-10 (*Fig. 21.6*). It is clear from experiments in mice and humans that the expression of the gene for IgE is dependent on IL-4. Thus, if immature human B cells are cultured with anti-CD40 and IL-4, they will produce IgE antibodies.

Cytokine regulation of IgE production

In humans IgE antibodies are the dominant feature of the response to a select group of antigens and most other immune responses do not include IgE. The classical allergens are inhaled in very small quantities (5–20 ng/day) either perennially indoors or over a period of weeks or months outdoors. Immunization of mice with repeated low-dose antigen is a very effective method of inducing IgE responses. By contrast, the routine immunization of children with diphtheria and tetanus toxoid does not induce persistent production of IgE antibodies. This is clear because we do not routinely take precautions against anaphylaxis when administering a booster injection of tetanus. The main factors that influence the development of T cells into the TH1 or TH2 pathways are the cytokines produced at the time of priming, in particular IL-12 and IL-4. IL-12 can be produced by macrophages or dendritic cells and is directly involved in the enhancement of IFNγ production and the associated differentiation towards the TH1 phenotype. As T cells differentiate, TH1 cells express the functional IL-12 receptor with the IL-12 β2 chain; by contrast, TH2 cells express only part of the IL-12 receptor and this part is non-functional. IL-4 is important in the differentiation of TH2 cells and is also a growth factor for these cells. Since IL-4 is produced by TH2 cells, it is at least in part acting in an autocrine fashion. The interaction of IL-4 with T cells can be blocked either with an antibody to IL-4 or with a soluble form of the IL-4 receptor. The release of soluble IL-4R from T cells may be a natural mechanism for controlling T-cell differentiation. It follows that inhaling recombinant soluble IL-4R is a potential therapeutic strategy to control allergic responses in the lung.

The relationship between IgE and IgG4

The genes for immunoglobulin heavy chains are in sequence on chromosome 14. The gene for epsilon occurs directly following the gene for gamma-4. Both of these isotypes are dependent on IL-4 and they may be expressed sequentially (*Fig. 21.7*). The mechanisms by which IgG4 is controlled separately from IgE are not well understood but this

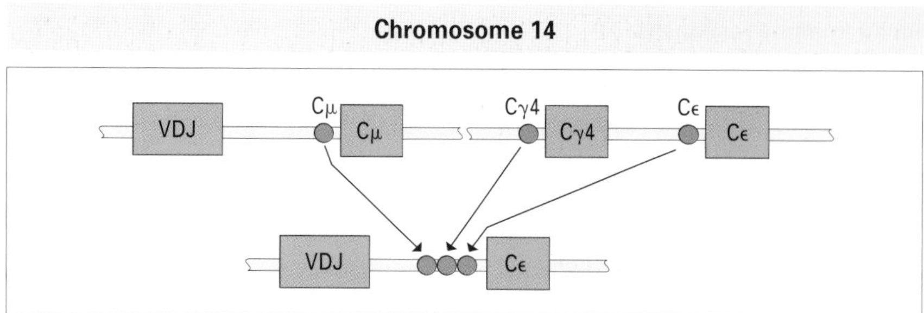

Fig. 21.7 Switch regions and heavy-chain genes for immunoglobulin are arranged sequentially on chromosome 14. Both Cγ4 and Cε expression are dependent on IL-4 produced by T cells. The switch region of IgE often includes elements from Sγ4 indicating that the switching occurs sequentially. However, IgG4 responses can occur without IgE antibody responses.

may include a role for IL-10. Thus, immunotherapy for patients with anaphylactic sensitivity to honey bee venom will induce IL-10 production by T cells, decreased IgE and increased IgG4 antibodies to venom antigens. Recently, it has been shown that children raised in a house with a cat can produce an IgG including an IgG4 antibody response without becoming allergic. Thus, a modified TH2 response (increased IgG4 and decreased IgE) represents an important mechanism of tolerance to allergens (*Fig. 21.8*).

ALLERGENS: THE ANTIGENS THAT GIVE RISE TO IMMEDIATE HYPERSENSITIVITY

Properties of the proteins

In mice a wide range of proteins can be used to induce an IgE antibody response. The primary factors that influence the response are the strain of mouse, the dose and adjuvants used. Thus, repeated low-dose immunization with alum or pertussis (but not complete Freund's adjuvant) will

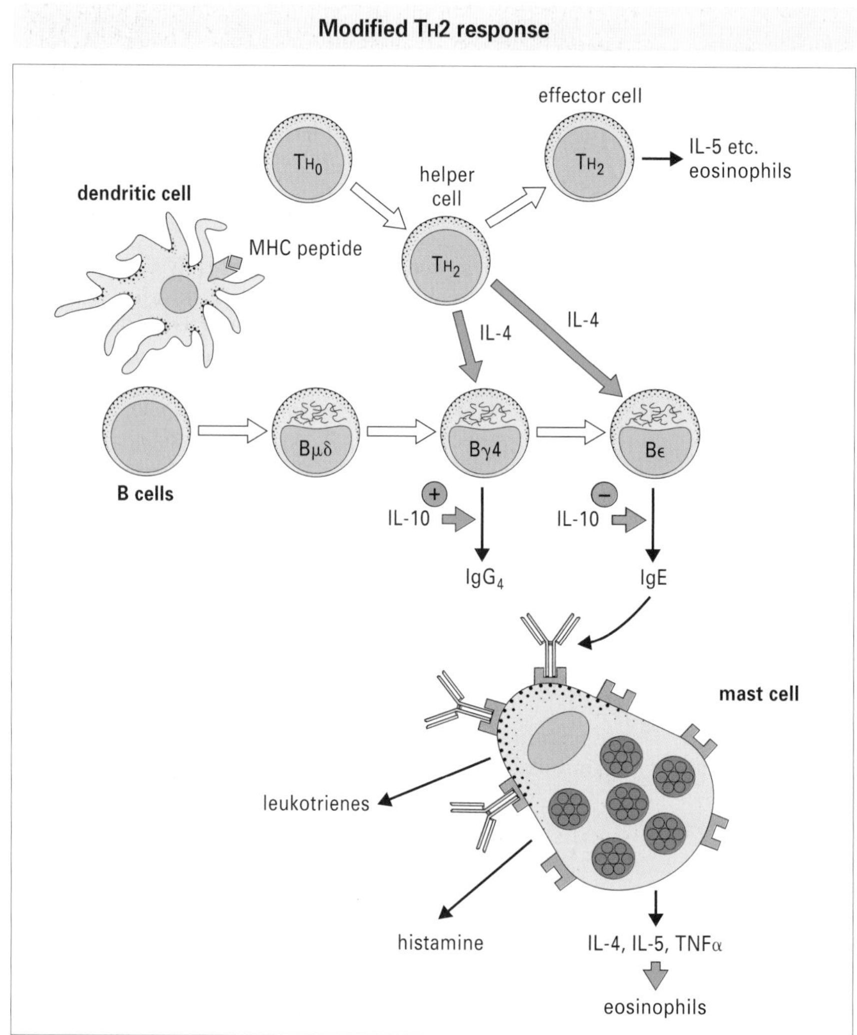

Fig. 21.8 The 'TH2 response' includes: T effector cells, as well as help for IgE and IgG4 antibody production. In turn IgE plays a major role in triggering of mast cells. However, increasing evidence shows that higher doses of allergen, e.g. bee venom, cat dander or rat urine, can induce a modified or tolerant TH2 response. This response includes IgG4 antibodies, but not IgE. The cytokine IL-10 may well play a role in enhancing IgG4 antibody while suppressing production of IgE.

produce IgE responses. However, the dose necessary to induce a response varies greatly from one strain to another.

The allergens that have been defined have similar physical properties (i.e. freely soluble in aqueous solution with a molecular weight between 10 000 and 40 000 Da), but are very diverse biologically. Cloning has revealed sequence homology between allergens and diverse proteins including calycins, pheromone binding proteins, enzymes and pollen recognition proteins. Although many of the allergens have homology with known enzymes, this is not surprising since enzymic activity is an important property of proteins in general. However, some important allergens, for example Der p 2 from mites, Fel d 1 from cats and Amb a 5 from ragweed pollen, have neither enzymic activity nor homology with known enzymes. Thus, enzymic activity is not essential for immunogenicity. Nevertheless, the Group I allergens of dust mites are cysteine proteases and in several model situations it has been shown that this enzymic activity influences the immunogenicity of the protein. Thus cleavage of CD23 or CD25 on lymphocytes by Der p 1 can enhance immune responses. Alternatively, it has been shown that Der p 1 can disrupt epithelial junctions and alter the entry of proteins through the epithelial layer. The interest in this property is increased because many different mite allergens are inhaled together in the faecal particle so that the enzymic activity of one protein (i.e. Der p 1) could facilitate either the physical entry or the response to other mite proteins. However, the lungs contain many different naturally occurring proteinases (as well as anti-proteases) which are just as potent as these allergens.

The primary characterization of allergens relates to their route of exposure. This includes inhaled allergens, foods, drugs, antigens from fungi growing on the body (e.g. *Aspergillus*) and venoms. The routes are important because they define the ways in which the antigens are presented to the immune system. Since antigen presentation may well be the site at which genetic influences play the biggest role, the properties of the different groups need to be considered separately.

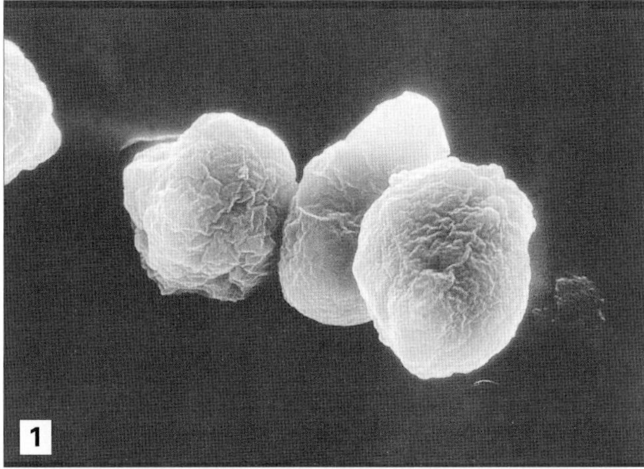

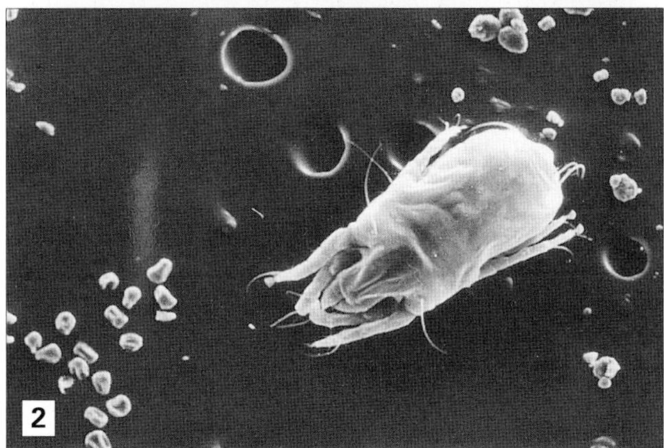

Fig. 21.9 Particles carrying airborne allergens: mite faecal pellets and pollen grains. The dust mite is the most important source of allergen in house dust: largely as faecal particles (**1**). A mite is shown in (**2**) with pollen grains lower left and faecal particles upper right. The mite is ~300 μm in length (i.e. just visible but not small enough to become airborne). Mite faecal particles are ~10–40 μm in diameter and become airborne during domestic disturbance. Pollen grains are similar in size to mite faecal particles (i.e. ~30 μm in diameter). The important allergic sources of pollen (i.e. grass, ragweed and trees) are wind pollinated and the grains are designed to travel in the air for long distances.

Inhalant allergens

The inhalant allergens are the primary causal agents in hayfever, chronic rhinitis and asthma among school age children or young adults; they also play an important role in atopic dermatitis. Almost all the evidence about the genetics of allergic disease relates to inhalant allergens. Allergens can only become airborne in sufficient quantity to cause an immune response or symptoms when they are carried on particles. Pollen grains, mite faecal particles, particles of fungal hyphae or spores and animal dander are the best defined forms in which allergens are inhaled (*Fig. 21.9*). In each case it is possible to define the approximate particle size and the quantity of protein on the particle as well as the speed with which the proteins in the particle dissolve in aqueous solution (*Fig. 21.3*). Thus, for grass pollen, mite faecal pellets and cat dander, the relevant allergens are present in high concentrations (up to 10 mg/cm^3), the particles are 'large' (i.e. 3–30 μm diameter) and the allergens elute rapidly in aqueous solution. The allergens within these particles will be delivered to the nasal epithelium because a large proportion of particles of this size will impact on the mucous membrane during passage of inhaled air through the nose.

Quantities inhaled

Estimates of the quantity of mite or pollen-derived proteins inhaled vary from 5 to 50 ng/day. Thus exposure to some allergens may be as little as 1 μg/year. This is very important because it probably explains why the immune response is consistently of this one kind, i.e. immediate hypersensitivity, and also why no respiratory diseases, other than asthma, have been associated with these allergens. The quantities inhaled also seriously restrict the models about how allergens contribute to asthma. Inhaling between 10 and 100 particles per day will produce localized areas of inflammation in the lungs but would not be expected to induce acute bronchospasm. Equally, the quantities inhaled severely restrict the quantity that enters the blood stream and make it extremely unlikely that the fetus is sensitized or primed to inhalant allergens *in utero*.

Food allergens

While a very large number of food proteins can occasionally give rise to IgE responses, only a small number are common causes of allergic responses. These include egg, milk, peanut, soy, chicken and shellfish. In contrast to inhaled allergens, these proteins are often eaten in very large quantities (i.e. ~10–100 g/day). In general only a small fraction of the food proteins are absorbed. However, small peptides can be freely absorbed and may be recognized by T cells and even by IgE antibodies in a minority of individuals. Nevertheless, the bulk of the allergic and anaphylactic responses to foods are thought to be related to food proteins that have not been digested, either triggering mast cells in the intestine or entering the circulation.

Tertiary structure of modified allergens and peptides

Many different allergens have been cloned, and for a few the tertiary structure is now known either from X-ray crystallography (e.g. Bet v 1), by nuclear magnetic resonance (NMR) (e.g. Der p 2) or by modelling relationships to known homologues (*Fig. 21.10*). Knowledge of the tertiary structure makes it possible to predict surface residues and to define IgE binding sites using site-directed mutagenesis. This approach has the potential to design molecules which have decreased IgE binding properties but with preserved T-cell epitopes. Given the importance of T cells to the control of IgE antibody production and their potential role in the recruitment of inflammatory cells, it is logical to try to use molecules that will directly 'desensitize' T cells. The approach used has been to produce peptides of different lengths. Therapeutic trials have been carried out with peptides from ragweed pollen antigens and the cat allergen Fel d 1. The results show that peptide recognition is restricted by the HLA-DR type of the patient, which means that a wide range of peptides are necessary for treatment. In addition, there is clear evidence that peptides can produce a significant response in the lungs (*Fig. 21.11*). This is the clearest evidence yet that T cells in the lung can contribute to an asthmatic response.

Tertiary structure of two important allergens: Der p 2 and Bla g 2

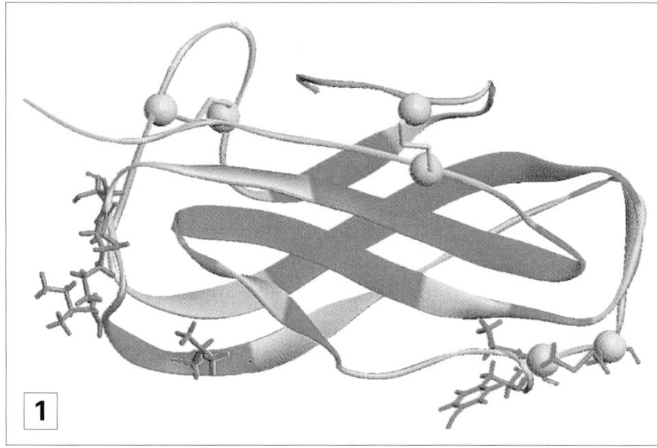

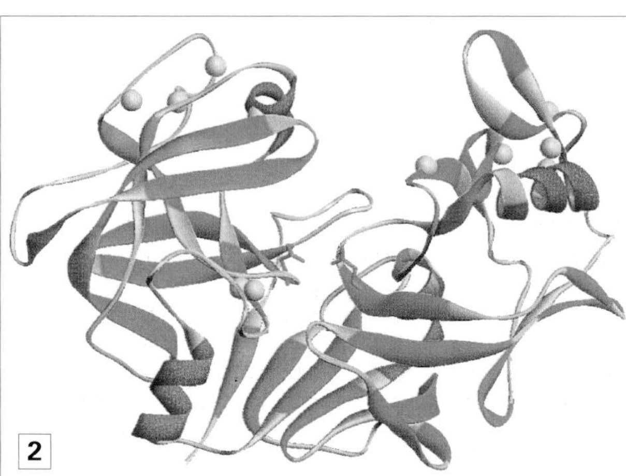

Fig. 21.10 The tertiary structure of the dust mite allergen, Der p 2 (**1**), was derived by nuclear magnetic resonance. This protein has no known function, and the structure shows no enzymic sites. On this structure the amino acids that are part of the binding sites for two monoclonal antibodies are shown (DPX green and 7A1 red). Knowledge of the structure makes it possible to alter the antibody binding sites using site-directed mutagenesis. (Courtesy of Drs Alisa Smith and Geoffrey Mueller.)

The tertiary structure of a cockroach allergen, Bla g 2 (**2**), shows the enzymic cleft and three residues that are considered to form the active site of an aspartic protease. However, the molecule has no enzymic activity due to other changes in the primary amino acid sequence. Some allergens (e.g. Der p 1 and Bla g 5) are active enzymes, but it remains an open question whether this activity contributes to their activity as allergens. (Courtesy of Drs A. Pomes and M. Chapman.) On each structure the beta sheets are shown as green bands, the alpha helical structures in Bla g 2 are shown in red. In addition, cysteines are shown as yellow spheres.

MAST CELLS AND BASOPHILS

The only human cell types that contain histamine are mast cells and basophils. In addition, these are the only cells that express the high-affinity receptor for IgE FcεRI under resting conditions. Under most circumstances the primary and most rapid consequence of allergen exposure in an allergic individual is cross-linking of IgE receptors on these two cell types. Basophils are circulating polymorphs which are not present in normal tissue but can be recruited to a local site by cytokines released from either T cells or mast cells. By contrast, mast cells cannot be identified in the circulation but are present in connective tissue and mucosal surfaces throughout the body (*Fig. 21.12*). Mast cells in different tissues are morphologically and cytogenetically distinct. Both the cells contain histamine and the biology of these cells may be very different in other species. For example, in the rabbit the histamine content of the peripheral blood is almost all in platelets, in the mouse there are few if any circulating basophils and in rats the degranulation of mast cells appears to be one granule at a time (*Fig. 21.12*). By contrast, human granules tend to fuse and release their contents together (*Fig. 21.13*).

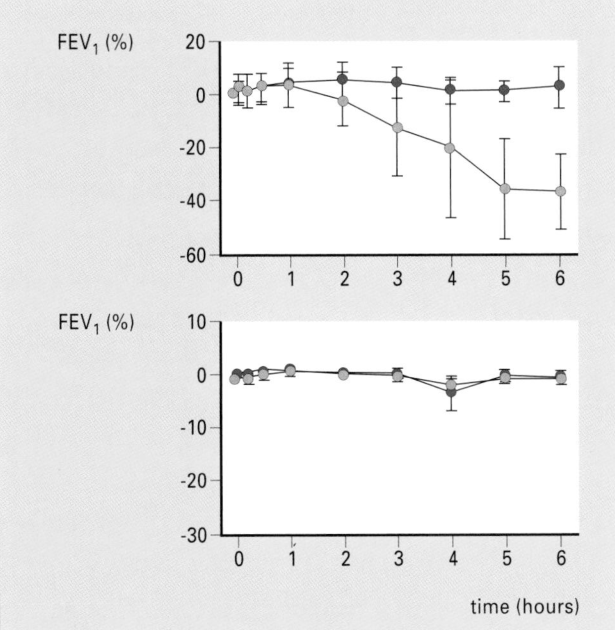

Fig. 21.11 Late asthmatic reactions induced in cat allergic patients by the intradermal injection of peptides derived from the cat allergen, Fel d 1. The nine responders show a mean fall in FEV_1 of ~30%. The response to the peptides is major histocompatibility restricted and correlated with the ability of the patients' T cells to respond to these peptides *in vitro*. Data are shown for challenge days (•) and control days (•) for nine responders (above) and 31 non-responders (below). (Courtesy of Dr M. Larché from *J Exp Med* 1999;**189**:1885.)

Connective tissue and mucosal mast cells

Mast cells were originally identified by Ehrlich who named them (Mast = well fed, or fattening, in German) because of the distinctive, tightly packed granules. Mast cells in different tissues can be distinguished by staining for proteases, and the content of these enzymes may be relevant to their role in allergic diseases. The granule proteases of mast cells have been cloned and sequenced and are distinct for two types of mast cells (*Fig. 21.14*). Mucosal mast cells are characterized by the presence of tryptase without chymase. By contrast, connective tissue mast cells contain both chymase and tryptase. These enzymes may play a direct role in the lung inflammation of asthma, either by breaking down mediators or in the case of tryptase by acting as a fibroblast growth factor. Basophils contain very little of either of these proteases. Staining of basophils in tissue sections requires special fixation and staining. Without this staining the granules in basophils cannot be identified and the cells appear as neutrophils (i.e. polymorphs without special granules).

Local accumulation of mast cells and basophils

Although mast cells are present in normal non-inflamed tissue, their numbers are increased in response to inflammation. It is assumed that this accumulation is T-cell dependent, since in rats infected with *Nippostrongylus brasiliensis* accumulation of mast cells in the gut is dependent on T cells and can be suppressed by corticosteroids. In guinea-pigs the immune response to tick bites includes a large local accumulation of basophils. Indeed, the tick is thought to be killed by basophils that it ingests. In allergic individuals mast cell recruitment has been demonstrated both in the skin in response to repeated allergen exposure and in the nose during the pollen season. In both situations basophils are also recruited. In the nose the recruitment of cells represents a shift so that mast cells move from the subepithelium into the epithelium while basophils appear in the nasal mucus. This process, which brings histamine-containing cells closer to the site of entry of allergen, is one of the ways in which allergic individuals become more sensitive. It is likely but less well established that equivalent processes occur in the human lung and gut.

Degranulation of mast cells and basophils

The process of degranulation in human mast cells and basophils involves fusing of the membrane of the granules containing histamine with the exterior cell membrane (*Fig. 21.13*). The granule membrane becomes part of the cell membrane; the granule contents rapidly dissolve and are secreted, leaving behind a viable degranulated or partially degranulated cell. This process is initiated in most cases by cross-linking of two specific IgE molecules by

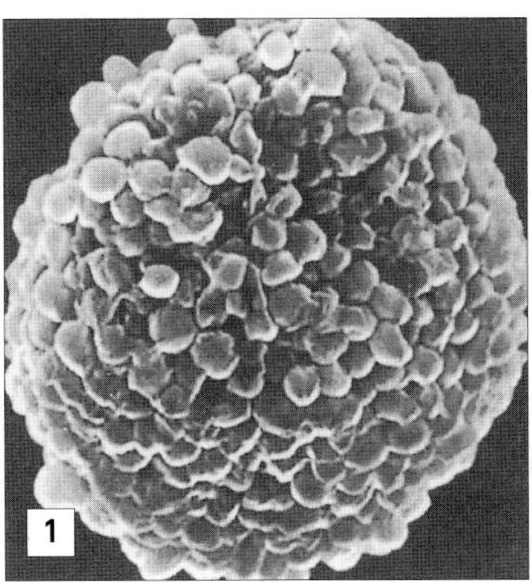

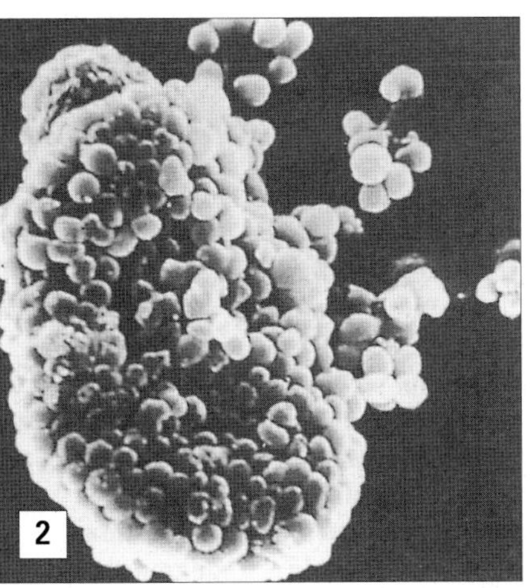

Fig. 21.12 Rat peritoneal mast cells. Scanning electron micrograph of rat peritoneal mast cells. (**1**) An intact mast cell with the cell membrane shrunk onto the granules (see *Fig. 2.14*). (**2**) A rat peritoneal mast cell degranulating following incubation with anti-IgE for 30 seconds. SEM, ×1500. (Courtesy of Dr T.S.C. Orr.)

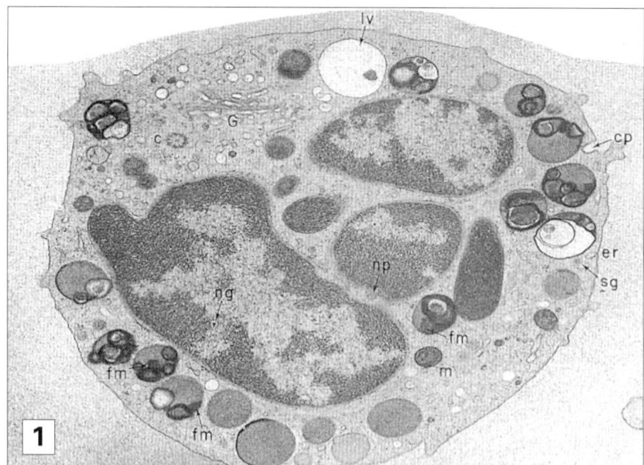

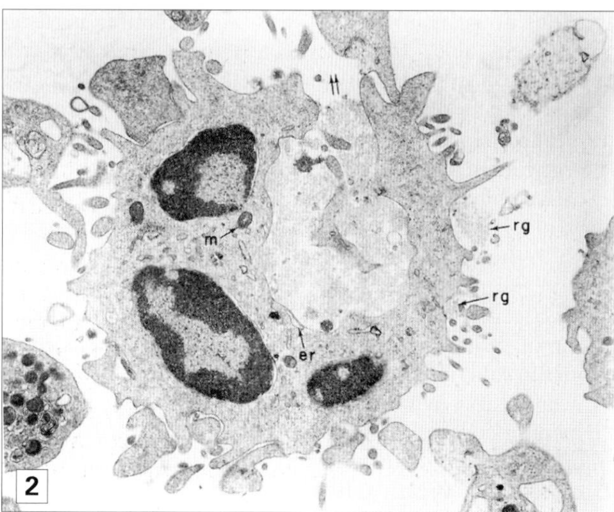

Fig. 21.13 Human basophils. Basophils are circulating mononuclear cells that have multilobed nuclei and distinctive granules that stain with metachromatic stains (**1**). Basophils can be recruited into local tissues such as the skin, nose, lungs or gut by allergic and other immune responses. (**2**) A basophil degranulating 4 minutes after adding allergen. The degranulation that releases histamine occurs by fusion of the granule membrane with the external membrane of the cell (arrows = connection between granule and the exterior of the cell). (Courtesy of Robin Hastie.) c = centriole; cp = coated pit; er = endoplasmic reticulum; np = nuclear pore; G = Golgi apparatus; lv = lucent vesicle; m = mitochondria; ng = perichromatinic granule; rg = residual material from granules; sg = small granules.

their relevant allergen. When two IgE receptors (FcεR1) are cross-linked, signal transduction occurring through the gamma chains of the receptor (see Chapter 10) leads to influx of calcium, which initiates both degranulation and the synthesis of newly formed mediators (*Fig. 21.15*).

Cross-linking of IgE antibodies on FcεR1 by allergens is the primary method by which mediators are released from basophils and mast cells; however, other mechanisms can be involved. Experimentally, degranulation can be triggered through FcεR1 by using lectins such as phytohaemagglutinin (PHA) or concanavalin A (Con A), or with antibodies to the α chain of the receptor. Histamine release

Differences between mast-cell populations – I

	mucosal mast cell	connective tissue mast cell
location *in vivo*	gut and lung	ubiquitous
lifespan	<40 days (?)	>40 days (?)
T-cell-dependent	+	–
number of Fcε receptors	25×10^5	3×10^4
histamine content	+	+ +
cytoplasmic IgE	+	–
major AA metabolite LTC4 : PGD2 ratio	25 : 1	1 : 40
DSCG/theophylline inhibits histamine release	–	+
major proteoglycan	chondroitin sulphate	heparin

Differences between mast-cell populations – II

cell type	location	amount per cell (pg)	
		tryptase	chymase
MC_T (MMC)	lung and nasal cavity, intestinal mucosa	10	<0.04
MC_{TC} (CTMC)	skin, blood vessels, intestinal submucosa	35	4.5
basophil	circulation	0.04	<0.04

Fig. 21.14 There are at least two subpopulations of mast cells, the mucosal mast cells (MMCs) and the connective tissue mast cells (CTMCs). The differences in their morphology and pharmacology suggest different functional roles *in vivo*. MMCs are associated with parasitic worm infections and, possibly, allergic reactions. In contrast to the CTMC, the MMC is smaller, shorter lived, T-cell dependent, has more Fcε receptors and contains intracytoplasmic IgE. Both cells contain histamine and serotonin in their granules; the higher histamine content of the CTMC may be accounted for by the greater number of granules. Major arachidonic acid (AA) metabolites (prostaglandins and leukotrienes) are produced by both mast-cell types, but in different amounts. For example, the ratios of production of the leukotriene LTC_4 to the prostaglandin PGD2 are 25 : 1 in the MMC and 1 : 40 in the CTMC. The effect of drugs on degranulation is different between the two cell types. Sodium cromoglycate (DSCG) and theophylline both inhibit histamine release from the CTMC but not from the MMC. (This may have important implications in the treatment of asthma.) Note that many of these data come from rodent studies and may not apply to humans. Tryptase is a tetramer of 134 kDa which may comprise as much as 25% of the mast-cell protein. Chymase is a monomer of 30 kDa. The relative proportions of these proteases in mast cells define MC_T and MC_{TC} populations, which have different distributions in human tissues. Basophils have very low amounts of both proteases. (The suffixes T and TC represent tryptase and chymase present in the respective cells.)

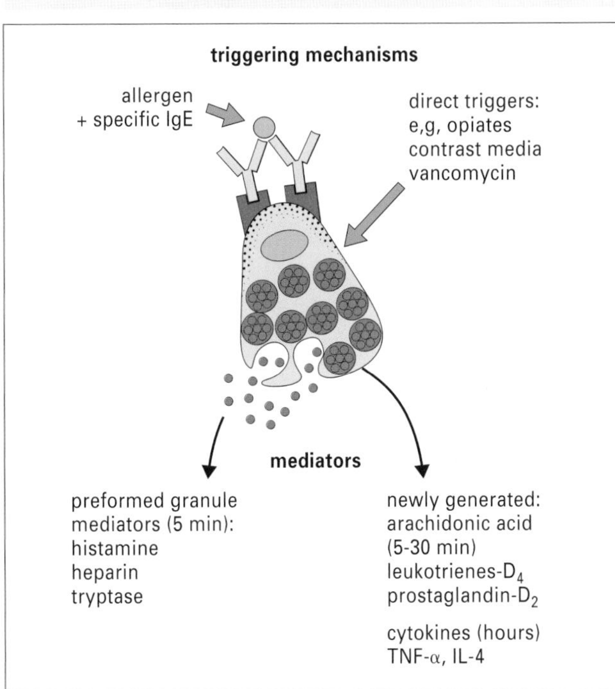

Fig. 21.15 Mast cells release mediators after cross-linking of the IgE receptors on their surface. Preformed mediators are released rapidly while arachidonic acid metabolites such as leukotriene D_4 and prostaglandin D_2 are released more slowly. Mast cells can also be triggered by opiates, contrast media, vancomycin and the complement components C3a and C5a. The mediators which are also released by basophils include histamine, TNFα and IL-4. Histamine released by mast cells can be measured in serum following anaphylaxis or extensive urticaria, but it has a half-life in minutes. By contrast, tryptase can be measured in serum for many hours after an anaphylactic reaction.

can also be triggered by agents that act on other receptorson of the cell surface. Typical examples include the complement components C5a and C3a; drugs such as codeine or morphine; the antibiotic vancomycin; and contrast media used for imaging the kidneys. Acute reactions to these agents which are not thought to involve IgE antibodies are referred to as anaphylactoid.

GENETICS OF ALLERGIC DISEASE

Hayfever and asthma are strongly hereditary

Children with one allergic parent have a 30% chance of developing allergic disease while those who have two allergic parents have as high as a 50% chance. Systematic studies of allergic diseases are difficult because the phenotypes for diseases, such as hayfever and asthma, are not well defined and depend on the approach used to make the diagnosis (*Fig. 21.16*). Thus, asthma defined by a patient questionnaire is less specific than asthma defined by testing of specific or non-specific bronchial hyper-reactivity. Furthermore, studies on asthma are complicated because both IgE antibody responses and bronchial reactivity are genetically controlled. Indeed, it is important not to

IgE levels and atopic disease

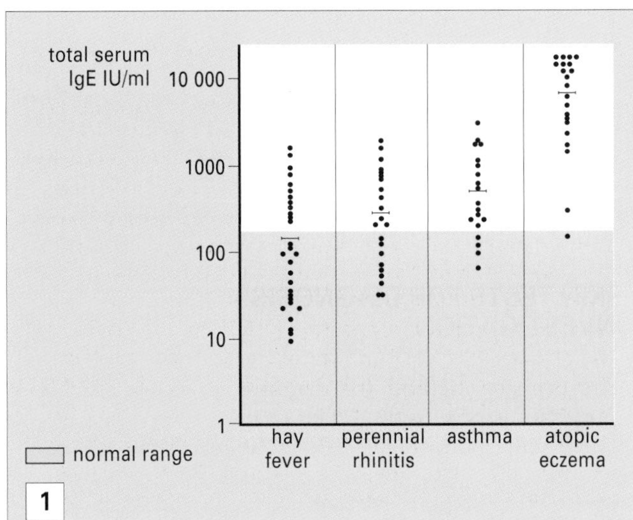

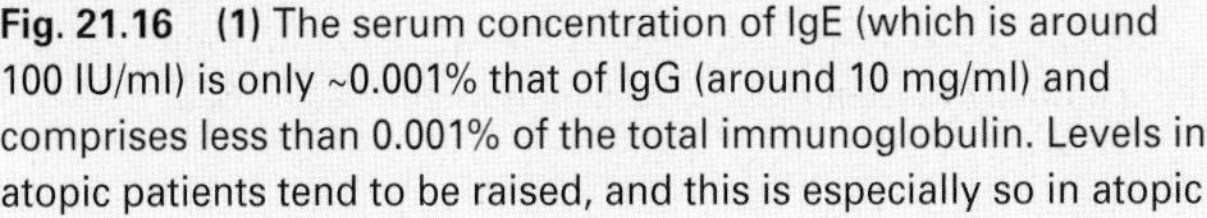

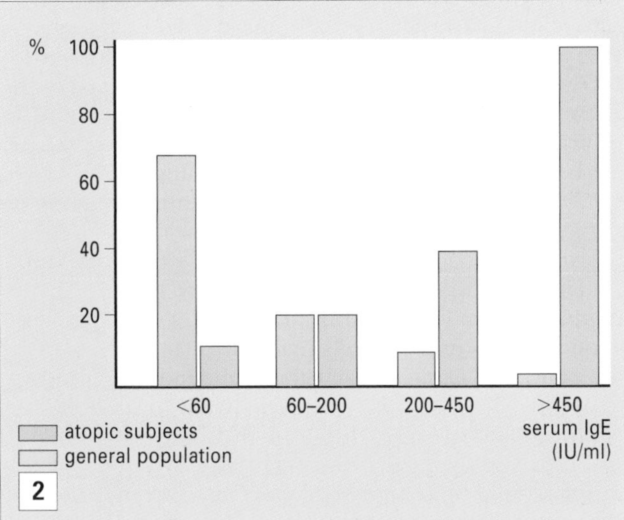

Fig. 21.16 **(1)** The serum concentration of IgE (which is around 100 IU/ml) is only ~0.001% that of IgG (around 10 mg/ml) and comprises less than 0.001% of the total immunoglobulin. Levels in atopic patients tend to be raised, and this is especially so in atopic eczema (1 IU = 2.4 ng). **(2)** The higher the level of IgE the smaller the percentage of the population affected, but the greater the likelihood of atopy. Where the level is greater than 450 IU/ml the majority of subjects are atopic.

Allergens and HLA associations

systematic name	old name	mol.wt (daltons)	primary association	*p* value
Ambrosia (Ragweed) spp.				
Amb a I	AgE	37 800	none	–
Amb a III	Ra3	12 300	A2	0.01
Amb a VI	Ra6	11 500	DR5	$<10^{-7}$
Amb a V	Ra5	5000	DR2/Dw2	$<10^{-9}$
Amb t V	Ra5G	4400	DR2/Dw2	$<10^{-3}$
Lolium (ryegrass) spp.				
Lol p I	Rye I	27 000	DR3/Dw3	$<10^{-3}$
Lol p II	Rye II	11 000	DR3/Dw3	$<10^{-3}$
Lol p III	Rye III	11 000	DR3/Dw3	$<10^{-4}$

Fig. 21.17 HLA association of IgE responses to allergens from ragweed and ryegrass. (Courtesy of Dr D. Marsh.)

confuse simple genetic diseases like cystic fibrosis or haemophilia with complex traits such as asthma or Type II diabetes. Thus, it is not at all surprising that multiple genes have been associated with asthma in different populations. A further major problem in genetic analyses of allergic disease comes from the progressive increase in asthma between 1960 and 2000. Clearly this increase cannot be attributed to genetic change and implies that some of the genes identified would only influence asthma in the presence of other changes influencing the environment or lifestyle. This is referred to as a gene : environment interaction.

Multiple genes or genetic regions are associated with asthma. Analyses of the genetics of immediate hypersensitivity have identified both allergen-specific and non-specific influences. Thus, there are HLA associations with atopy in general and also with sensitization to specific allergens. However, these genetic studies have given the clearest associations when fully purified allergens are used to test sensitization (*Fig. 21.17*). The genetics of asthma has been studied both by genomic screening and by using candidate genes. Genomic screening identifies regions of the genome which link to asthma so that this region can be examined to identify specific genes. If a candidate gene is identified, it is possible to examine the gene for polymorphisms that link to asthma. However, a brief consideration of the possible targets makes it clear how complex the analysis of asthma is likely to be, and indeed is proving to be (*Fig. 21.18*). Typical examples include polymorphisms of the promoter region for IL-4 and polymorphisms of the gene for IL-5, either of which could directly influence the inflammatory response to allergens. Alternatively, a series of polymorphisms have been identified that influence the response of asthma to treatment. These include variants of the β_2-adrenergic receptor α chain, and genetic differences that influence the efficacy of leukotriene antagonists. In the last 10 years multiple 'genes' or genetic regions associated with asthma have been identified. At

Genetic influences over asthma and allergic disease

Allergen specific HLA related
IgE total production FcεRI FcεRII
Cytokines IL-4 promoter and receptor IL-5 IL-10 IFNγ TGFβ promoter IL-11 IL-13 and receptor
Leukotriene pathway Five lipoxygenase activating protein (FLAP) Lipoxygenase LTC_4 synthase Leukotriene receptors LTRI LTRII
β_2-adrenergic receptor polymorphisms
Chemokines CCR3 receptor

Fig. 21.18 Allergic diseases run in families, however the inheritance is not simple. Population-based studies have established that the inheritance of allergic diseases is influenced by multiple genes. Some of these, such as HLA-linked control of the response to pollen antigens or genes controlling total IgE, are related to the immune response. However, many others are related to the mechanisms of inflammation, e.g. IL-4 and IL-5 gene polymorphisms, or to the response to treatment, e.g. leukotriene receptor genes or polymorphisms of the β_2-adrenergic receptor.

present, it appears that the overall effects are too complex to be of any practical significance. Certainly it is most unlikely that gene transfer will ever be of significance. However, as genetic screening becomes easier, pharmacogenetics may well become an important method for identifying the best drugs for individual patients in the management of chronic diseases such as asthma.

SKIN TESTS FOR DIAGNOSIS AND INVESTIGATION

The primary method for diagnosing immediate hypersensitivity is skin testing. The characteristic response is a wheal and flare (*Fig. 21.19*). The wheal is caused by extravasation of serum from capillaries in the skin which results from a direct effect of histamine. This is accompanied by pruritus (also a direct effect of histamine) and a larger erythematous flare which is mediated by an axon reflex. This skin response takes 5–15 minutes to develop and may persist for 30 minutes or more. Techniques for skin testing include a prick test, in which a 25 gauge needle or a lancette is used to introduce 0.1 μl of extract

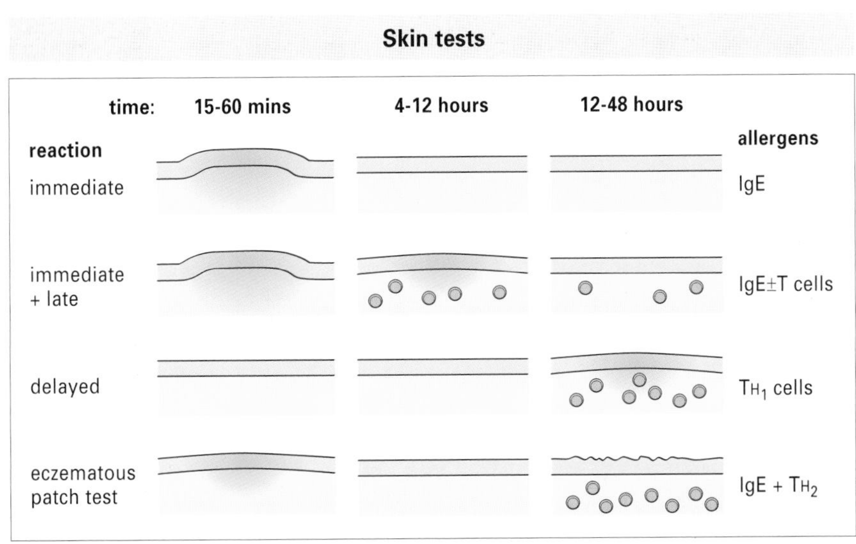

Fig. 21.19 Skin tests are carried out by introducing 0.02 ml of extract intradermally. With allergens such as pollen, cat or dust mite, the positive reaction is an immediate (i.e. within 20 min) wheal, which in some cases is followed by an indurated response occurring late (i.e. at 4–12 hours). Non-allergic individuals make no discernable reaction to testing with these allergens. A delayed skin response is the commonest form of positive response to tuberculin, tetanus and mumps, or to fungi such as *Trichophyton* and *Candida*. The skin typically shows no reaction up to 12 hours and then gradually develops an erythematous indurated, delayed hypersensitivity response, which is maximum at 24–48 hours. Patch tests are performed by applying a gauze pad with allergen to a patch of skin which has been mildly abraided. This procedure may give an immediate wheal response, but this is followed at 24–48 hours by an indurated, erythematous response, which has many of the features of eczema. The patch test is not a diagnostic test but has provided extensive information about the role of allergens in atopic dermatitis.

into the dermis. Alternatively, an intradermal injection of 0.02–0.03 ml is used. All allergen injections have the potential to cause anaphylaxis but the intradermal test which introduces ~200 times more extract should always be preceded by a prick test.

Skin tests are evaluated by the size of the wheal compared to a positive (histamine) and negative (saline) control; in general, a 3×3 mm wheal in children and a 4×4 mm wheal in adults can be considered a positive response to a prick test. A positive skin test indicates that the patient has specific IgE antibodies on the mast cells in their skin. In turn this implies that bronchial or nasal challenge would also be positive if sufficient antigen was administered. In most cases (i.e. ≈80%) where the skin test is positive, IgE antibody will be detectable in the serum. However, blood tests for IgE antibody are generally less sensitive than skin tests.

Relevance of a positive skin test (or IgE antibody assay)

Epidemiologically, sensitization to a relevant inhalant allergen is a 'risk factor' for allergic disease. Thus, an individual with a positive skin test to grass pollen is up to ten times more likely to have hayfever during the grass pollen season (odds ratio ≥10) than a skin test negative individual. Equally an individual with a positive skin test to dust mite or cat allergen is more likely to have asthma (odds ratios 2–6). It is assumed that allergen exposure contributes to the risk, but that relationship is not simple. However, positive skin tests are common, and in individual cases they may not be relevant. This may be because the patient is not exposed to the allergen, i.e. rhinitis symptoms occurring at a time of year when pollen is not present. Alternatively, up to one-third of skin test positive patients do not experience symptoms even when they are exposed.

Late and delayed skin responses

Late reactions can occur following an immediate response to allergen either in the skin or the lungs. A late skin response is only common following a large immediate response, i.e. wheal size 10×10 mm. This response, which is diffuse, erythematous and indurated, generally starts 2–3 hours after the wheal and may last up to 24 hours. The late reaction is considered to be a model of the events that lead to persistent inflammation in the nose, lungs or skin.

Late reactions probably include several different events: (i) the direct effects of prostaglandins, leukotrienes and cytokines released by mast cells following the initial release of histamine; (ii) infiltration of lymphocytes, eosinophils, basophils and neutrophils into the local site mediated by chemokines and other cytokines released from mast cells; (iii) release of products from the infiltrating cells. In general, these different events are occurring in parallel over a period of hours.

Eczematous patch test (atopy patch test)

The infiltration of cells into the skin that occurs in the 24 hours after an allergen is applied can be studied in several ways: by local intradermal injections; by applying a patch of allergen on gauze that stays on the skin for 2 days; or by fixing a chamber containing allergen over a denuded area of skin. The skin chamber allows repeated sampling while the other two techniques require biopsy of the skin. In the patch test 10 μg allergen is applied on a gauze pad 2.5 cm^2, and the biopsy is carried out at 24 or 48 hours. A positive patch response induces macroscopic eczema, spongiosis of the epidermis (a hallmark of eczema) and an infiltrate of cells into the dermis (*Fig. 21.20*). The cellular infiltrate includes eosinophils, basophils and lymphocytes. With persistent allergen at a site, i.e. 6 days, the eosinophils degranulate locally. This is in keeping with the evidence

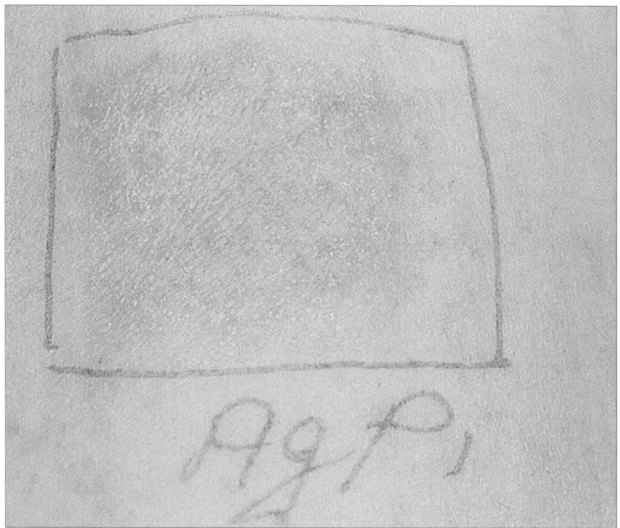

Fig. 21.20 Eczema induced by patch test with mite allergen. An erythematous and eczematous skin response 48 hours after the application of 5 μg of the mite allergen Der p 1 to the skin of a patient with atopic dermatitis who had 56 IU/ml of IgE antibody to the dust mite *Dermatophagoides pteronyssinus.* Biopsy of the patch site revealed an infiltrate of eosinophils, basophils and lymphocytes.

that the skin of patients with eczema has large quantities of the eosinophil granule major basic protein (MBP), even though very few whole eosinophils are visible (*Fig. 21.21*).

Biopsy of patch tests also yields T cells that are specific for the allergen, for example dust mite, thus establishing that antigen-specific T cells are present in the skin after antigen challenge. Some groups have succeeded in cloning allergen-specific T cells from the skin of eczema patients without a preceding patch. This is never possible from normal individuals or allergic patients without eczema. Answering whether allergen-specific T cells are present at local sites is important because T cells could play a role both as effector cells and in the recruitment of other cells. Establishing whether T cells play an effector role is relevant to the nose in rhinitis, the lungs in asthma, the conjunctiva in hayfever, as well as to the skin in atopic dermatitis.

Biopsy of patch test sites has also established that the Langerhans' cells in the skin of patients with eczema express FcεR1. Thus, these antigen-presenting cells use IgE antibodies to help capture allergens and to increase the efficiency of antigen presentation.

Passive transfer of patch test response – Following injection of serum from a patient with atopic dermatitis into the skin of a non-allergic individual, a patch test can be carried out. Biopsy of this passively transferred response reveals large numbers of eosinophils. Thus, at least part of the eczematous response can be passively transferred. The mechanisms for this response are thought to be: (i) passive sensitization of IgE antibodies onto mast cells in the dermis; (ii) triggering of the local mast cells with allergen to release histamine, leukotrienes and cytokines; (iii) recruitment of eosinophils by IL-5 as well as by chemokines such as RANTES or eotaxin.

FACTORS THAT INFLUENCE THE SYMPTOMS OF ALLERGIC DISEASE

The diagnosis of allergy is made by skin tests or by serum assays of IgE antibodies. These antibodies form part of an immune response which also includes antibodies of other isotypes (IgG1, IgG4 and IgA), as well as T cells that are characteristically TH2. The release of histamine within 15 minutes after allergen exposure can only explain a small proportion of allergic disease. In particular, the chronic inflammation in the lungs of patients with asthma and in the skin of patients with atopic dermatitis has many

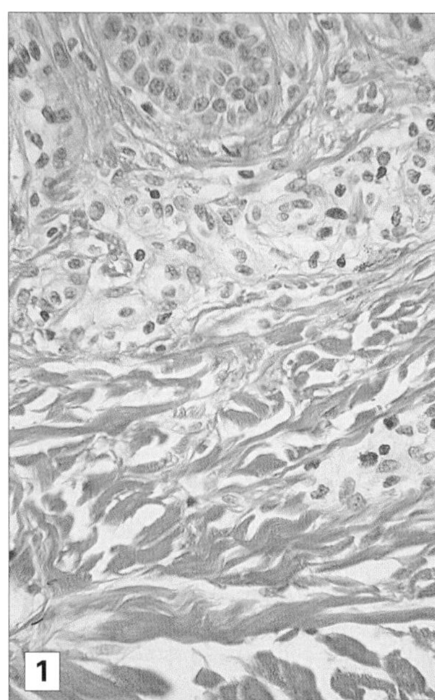

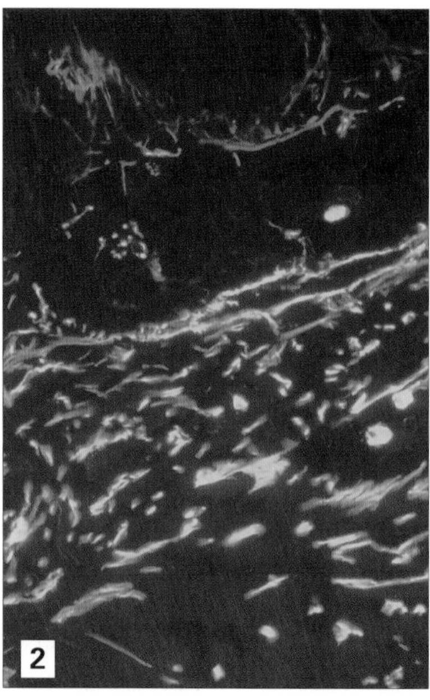

Fig. 21.21 Eosinophil major basic protein in the skin of atopic dermatitis. Skin biopsy from a patient with severe atopic dermatitis. The hematoxylin and eosin stain (**1**) shows an inflammatory infiltrate but very few intact eosinophils are present. The same section stained with antibodies to eosinophil major basic protein (MBP) (**2**) shows extensive deposition of MBP in the dermis, demonstrating that eosinophils had degranulated in the skin. (Courtesy of Dr K. Lieferman.)

Inflammatory response in asthmatic bronchi

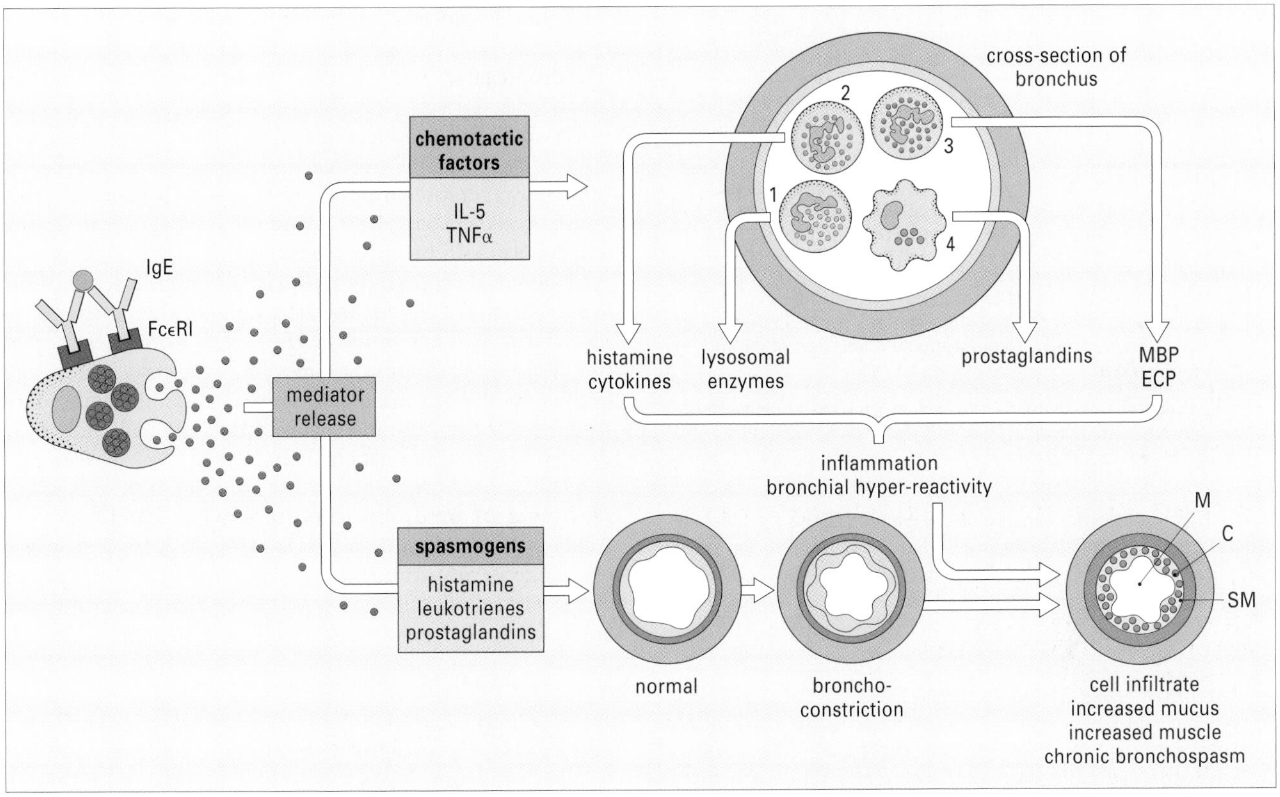

Fig. 21.22 Mast cells release factors that can induce immediate bronchospasm, e.g. histamine and LTD_4, but also release chemotactic factors such as LTB4, IL-5 and TNFα. The spasmogens can induce oedema, increased mucus and smooth muscle constriction resulting in immediate decrease in airway conductance and a fall in the forced expiratory volume at 1 second (FEV_1). By contrast, chemotactic factors recruit cells out of the circulation including eosinophils, neutrophils, lymphocytes and macrophages. These cells can chronically modify the lung with goblet cell hyperplasia, collagen deposition below the basement membrane and possibly smooth muscle hyperplasia. In addition, these cells and their products produce non-specific bronchial hyper-reactivity (BHR). Thus, chronic bronchospasm includes elements of hypersecretion, inflammatory infiltrate thickening the walls of the small bronchi and bronchial smooth muscle spasm. Evidence for this inflammatory response can be obtained from increased exhaled nitric oxide (eNO); increased eosinophils or ECP in induced sputum; and experimentally from biopsies of the lung. neutrophils = 1; basophils = 2; eosinophils = 3; monocytes = 4.

features that cannot be explained by histamine. First, the time course is too long; secondly, there is a cellular infiltrate in these tissues; and third, there are major differences in disease between patients who have apparently similar IgE antibodies in their serum and skin (*Fig. 21.22*).

Several different pathways contribute to chronic symptoms and can alter the severity of allergic disease:

1. Local recruitment of mast cells and basophils, combined with increased 'releasability' of these cells, allows increased response to the same allergen challenge. This mechanism plays a major role in the increased symptoms in the nose during the pollen season.
2. Release of leukotrienes, chemokines and cytokines from mast cells or basophils. The mediators can have direct effects on blood vessels and smooth muscles. IL-5, tumour necrosis factor (TNF) and chemokines are each thought to contribute to the recruitment of inflammatory cells.
3. The action of T effector cells: T cells release a wide range of cytokines which can have direct inflammatory effects.

Separating out the different factors influencing chronic allergic symptoms is difficult. Information may be obtained from: (i) the effects of different drugs, particularly disodium cromoglycate, leukotriene antagonists and anti-IgE; and (ii) passive transfer experiments. The fact that cromoglycate can inhibit both the immediate and the late response of the lung to allergen challenge has been taken as evidence that the late reaction is also dependent on mast cell triggering. However, it clear that cromoglycate can only control part of the chronic inflammation. By contrast, steroids, which are an effective treatment for most of the inflammation in asthma, act selectively on the late response. However, the response to steroid treatment cannot be used to distinguish the delayed effects of mast cell triggering from the direct effects of T cells, since steroids can inhibit both of these mechanisms (*Fig. 21.23*).

Local or systemic injection of IgE antibodies can passively transfer the wheal and flare skin response. However, passive transfer of serum from an allergic patient (i.e. containing IgE antibodies) into the skin of a non-allergic individual, can also transfer some aspects of the delayed

Actions of steroids in allergic disease

• Steroids act primarily on the delayed or chronic effects of allergen exposure and are seen as anti-inflammatory
• In challenge situations steroids block the delayed or late response in the lungs and in particular inhibit the influx of eosinophils, basophils and lymphocytes into local sites
• Following systemic steroids circulating eosinophils decrease rapidly because of margination; in addition, steroids prevent eosinophil production in the bone marrow
• Steroids bind to a receptor which leads to inhibition of the transcription of the genes for many cytokines, including IL-5, TNFα and also some chemokines. Steroids are thought to have limited effects on leukotriene production and do not inhibit histamine release
• The effect of steroids on T cells is clear from the clinical effect on contact sensitivity and from the blockade of delayed hypersensitivity skin tests

Fig. 21.23 Locally active steroids are widely used in seasonal rhinitis, perennial rhinitis, asthma and atopic dermatitis. In addition, courses of systemic steroids are used for the treatment of exacerbations of asthma.

or cellular response. Both late reactions following an intradermal injection of allergen and the patch test response at 48 hours can be passively transferred. This experiment demonstrates that cross-linking of IgE antibody on mast cells in the tissue of a non-allergic individual can lead to local recruitment of eosinophils in the absence of antigen-specific T cells. Thus, in any analysis of the factors influencing the severity of allergic disease, for example response to pharmacological treatment or response to immunotherapy, it is necessary to consider the relevance of both mast cells *and* effector T cells.

ASTHMA AND BRONCHIAL REACTIONS TO INHALED ANTIGENS

Evidence that allergens contribute to asthma

The causal role of bee venom in anaphylaxis or grass pollen in seasonal hayfever is obvious because these diseases occur in individuals who have positive skin tests and the symptoms are directly related to increased exposure. By contrast, the role of inhaled allergens in chronic asthma is less obvious because exposure is perennial, the patients are often not aware of the relationship and only a proportion of skin test positive individuals develop asthma. The evidence that allergens derived from dust mites, cats, dogs, the German cockroach or the fungus *Alternaria* contribute to asthma comes from several different lines of evidence:

1. The epidemiological evidence that positive skin tests or serum IgE antibodies are a major risk factor for asthma.
2. Bronchial challenge with nebulized extracts can produce both rapid bronchospasm, within 20 minutes, and a late reaction, in 4–8 hours, which is characterized by renewed mediator production and a cellular infiltrate.
3. Reduced exposure to allergens can lead to decreased symptoms and decreased non-specific bronchial reactivity. This avoidance can be achieved either by moving patients to an allergen-free unit or by controlling exposure in the home.

The bronchial walls of patients with asthma are characterized by increased mast cells, lymphocytes of the TH2 type, eosinophils and products of eosinophils. In addition, there is increased mucous production secondary to goblet cell hyperplasia, epithelial desquamation and collagen deposition below the basement membrane. These changes are a reflection of chronic inflammation, and it is generally considered that eosinophils play a major role in these events (*Fig. 21.22*). However, recent evidence that anti-IL-5 treatment has limited effects on asthma, although it decreases circulating eosinophils, suggests that other cells may play an important role. Thus, basophils, mast cells, effector T cells and macrophages may all contribute to the non-specific bronchial reactivity.

Analysis of bronchoalveolar lavage (BAL)

Analysis of bronchoalveolar lavage (BAL) after an allergen challenge demonstrates the presence of products derived from mast cells (histamine, prostaglandins and leukotrienes) and eosinophils (major basic protein and eosinophil cationic protein). Furthermore, MBP is present in biopsies of the lungs and can produce epithelial change typical of asthma *in vitro* (*Fig. 21.24*). The subepithelial collagen deposition present in many patients with asthma is probably a reflection of fibroblast responses to local inflammation. Although it has been suggested that these changes, which are referred to as 'remodelling', can lead to progressive decreases in lung function, the evidence for this view is not clear. In particular, progressive loss of lung function is unusual in asthma and there are no studies showing a correlation between the extent of collagen deposition and changes in lung function. None the less, inhaled steroids which can block many different aspects of inflammation are an effective treatment for asthma.

Bronchial hyper-reactivity

Non-specific bronchial hyper-reactivity (BHR) is present in patients with asthma and is a major feature of the disease. Thus, airway obstruction, induced by cold air or exercise, and nocturnal asthma all correlate with non-specific bronchial reactivity. BHR can be demonstrated by challenging the lungs with histamine, methacholine or cold air. The mechanism by which exercise or cold air induces a bronchial response is thought to be evaporation of water with associated cooling of the epithelium. However, it is unclear whether this process triggers nerve endings directly or by causing local mediator release.

Markers of inflammation in patients with asthma

Bronchoscopy is not possible in patients with asthma except as a research procedure. Therefore the only evidence for inflammation of the lungs that can be obtained routinely is indirect. Peripheral blood or nasal smear eosinophils are increased in most patients presenting with an acute episode of asthma (*Fig. 21.25*). In addition, nasal secretions may have increased eosinophil cationic protein (ECP) and IL-8. Additional evidence about inflammation in the lungs

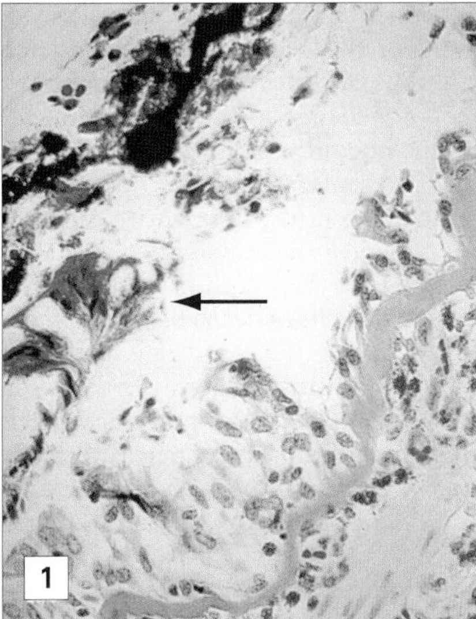
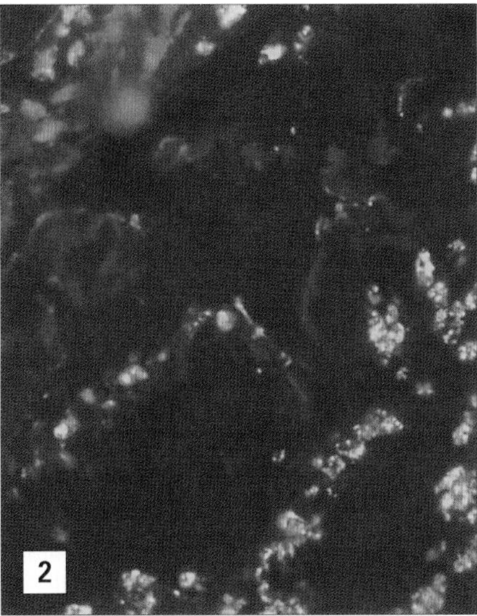
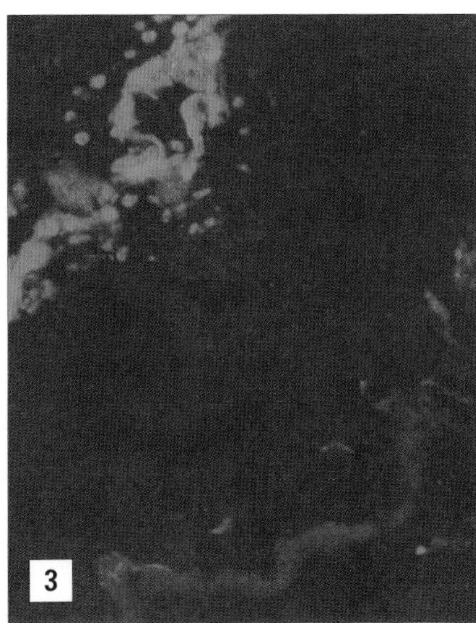

Fig. 21.24 Localization of MBP in the lung of a severe asthmatic. **(1)** Respiratory epithelium showing striking submucosal eosinophil infiltration and a cluster of desquamated epithelial cells in the bronchial lumen (arrowed) next to a 'stringy' deposit of soot. H&E stain. **(2)** The same section stained for major basic protein (MBP) showing immunofluorescent localization in infiltrating eosinophils. MBP deposits are also seen on desquamated epithelial cells on the luminal surface. **(3)** A control section stained with normal rabbit serum does not stain eosinophils or bronchial tissue but does show some non-specific staining of the sooty deposit. (Courtesy of Dr G. Gleich, from *J Allergy Clin Immunol* 1982;**70**:160–9, with permission.)

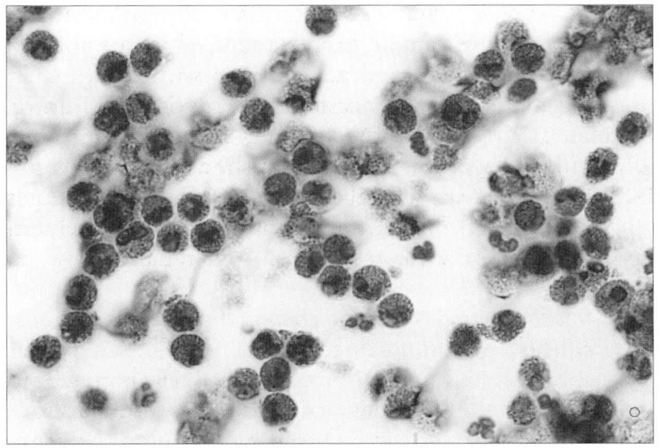

Fig. 21.25 Nasal eosinophils. Nasal smear from an 8-year-old boy presenting with acute asthma. The majority of the cells are eosinophils, polymorphonuclear cells with a cytoplasm that stains red using H&E stain. He was known to be allergic to dust mites and had recently had a rhinovirus infection as judged by PCR on nasal secretions.

can be obtained either from exhaled air or condensates for exhaled air. Nitric oxide gas is increased, i.e. ≥10 ppb, in patients with asthma, and this decreases following systemic or local steroid treatment. In addition, the pH of the condensate decreases during acute episodes. The increased exhaled nitric oxide may reflect upregulation of the enzyme nitric oxide synthase. Alternatively, the nitric oxide gas could also increase acutely as a consequence of the fall in pH which is due to decreased ammonia production in the lung epithelium.

In adults further information about the inflammation in the respiratory tract can be obtained from computerized tomography (CT) of the nasal sinuses. Extensive opacification of the sinuses is present in approximately one-third of patients presenting with acute asthma. This reflects both chronic sinusitis, which is a major feature of late-onset asthma, and also sinus inflammation secondary to acute rhinovirus infection. Whether the changes in the sinuses are a reflection of similar effects occurring in the lungs or a source of mediators or T cells that contribute to lung inflammation, is not clear.

IMMUNOTHERAPY WITH ALLERGEN EXTRACTS

Immunotherapy (or hyposensitization) with allergen extracts was introduced in 1911 by Noon and Freeman. At that time they were trying to establish immunity against pollen toxin. The treatment requires regular injections of allergen over a period of months. It is an established treatment for seasonal hayfever and for anaphylactic sensitivity to bees, wasps and hornets. In addition, immunotherapy is an effective treatment for selected cases of other allergic diseases including asthma. The dose is increased progressively, starting with between 1 and 10 ng and increasing up to ~10 μg allergen per dose. The response to treatment includes an increase in serum IgG antibodies, a striking decrease in the response of peripheral blood T cells to antigen *in vitro*, and a marked decrease in late reactions in the skin. Over a longer period of time there is a progressive decrease in IgE antibodies in the serum (*Fig. 21.26*). The change in antibodies, lymphocyte responses and symptoms could all be secondary to changes

Effects of immunotherapy on allergic rhinitis

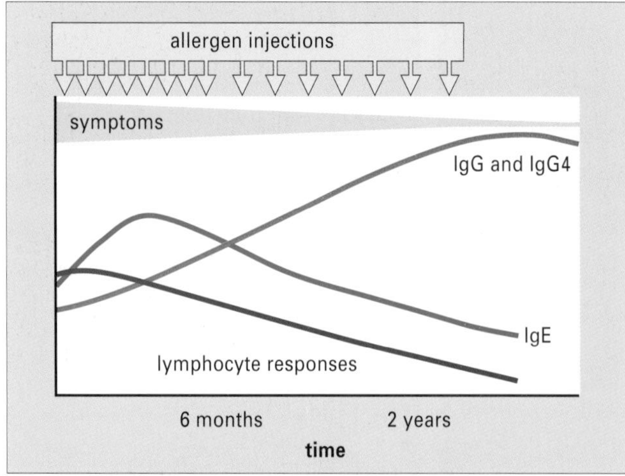

Fig. 21.26 During desensitization or immunotherapy the allergic patient receives regular subcutaneous injections of the relevant allergen. The immunological changes that occur include an initial increase in IgE antibodies followed by a gradual decline, which in pollen-allergic patients is largely due to a blunting of the seasonal increase. Antibodies of the IgG and specifically IgG4 isotype increase progressively and may reach concentrations of ten times those present prior to treatment. Symptoms decline starting as early as 3 months but generally not maximally until 2 years. Changes in T cells are less well defined but include decreased *in vitro* response to allergens and increased production of IL-10.

in T cells. Given the known mechanisms of allergic inflammation a response of T cells to allergen injections could influence symptoms in several ways:

- Decreased local recruitment of mast cells and basophils.
- Decreased recruitment of eosinophils to the nose or lungs.
- Increased IgG including IgG4 antibodies with progressive decreases in IgE. The IgG antibodies may act as blocking antibodies by binding allergen before it cross-links IgE on mast cells.

Some studies of cytokine RNA have suggested that immunotherapy produces a shift in T cell from a TH2 profile (i.e. IL-4 and IL-5) towards a profile that is more typical of TH1 (i.e. IFNγ). Although this could explain decreased help for IgE, and decreased eosinophil recruitment, this would not explain the production of IgG4. The expression of the gene for IgG4 is dependent on IL-4, and may also require the cytokine IL-10. Thus, the response to immunotherapy is better seen as a modification of the TH2 response.

NEW TREATMENTS FOR ALLERGIC DISEASE

New approaches to allergen specific immunotherapy

Peptides from the primary sequence of an allergen can stimulate T cells in vitro

These peptides, usually ~20 amino acids in length, stimulate T cells *in vitro*. In theory, peptides provide a mechanism for stimulating or desensitizing T cells without the risk of anaphylaxis that is always present with traditional allergens. Whether incomplete stimulation of T cells by peptides can lead to 'tolerance' or a change in the cytokine profile is not clear. Problems include surprisingly severe reactions in the lung and the fact that multiple peptides are necessary to allow presentation of antigen to patients with different HLA types.

Modified recombinant allergens have decreased binding to IgE

Genetically modified recombinant allergens that have decreased binding to IgE antibodies can be produced. The advantage of these is that the primary sequence with the T-cell epitopes is preserved. Even if the molecule is extensively modified, any full-length protein has the potential to induce anaphylaxis in allergic individuals. Thus, the use of genetically modified molecules would always require precautions similar to those for traditional immunotherapy. A potential but unlikely problem is that patients would develop IgE antibodies against new epitopes.

Adjuvants can shift the immune response to TH1

Adjuvants 'attached' to allergen molecules have been designed to shift the immune response from TH2 towards TH1. Possible co-molecules that act like an adjuvant include the cytokine IL-12 or immunostimulatory sequences (ISS). ISS are DNA sequences such as cytosine phosphoguanidine (CpG), that are common in bacterial DNA, and which have a profound effect on the mammalian immune system. In mice combining an antigen with two or three molecules of CpG can induce a TH1 response or down-regulate IgE responses. Combining CpG with allergen not only influences the response but also reduces the reactivity of the allergen with IgE. Thus immunization with allergen and CpG may produce a greater immune response with less potential for an acute allergic reaction.

DNA vaccines are designed to change the immune response

The concept of immunizing with the gene for an antigen is well established, i.e. DNA vaccines. This approach has potential for the treatment of allergy because the DNA vector can be designed to change the immune response. Prokaryotic DNA includes CpG motifs so that as the antigen is expressed, it will induce a TH1 response. Experiments with DNA vaccines have been very successful in mice, both in inducing a TH1 response initially and in controlling an existing IgE antibody response. However, the consequences of expressing an allergen within the tissue of an allergic individual are not known. Equally, it is not clear whether inducing a TH1 response to a ubiquitous allergen such as cat would give rise to other forms of inflammatory disease.

New approaches to non-specific therapy

Humanized monoclonal anti-IgE treatment may reduce sensitivity – Antibodies directed against the binding site for FcεRI on IgE can bind to IgE in the circulation but *not* when it is attached to mast cells or basophils. Thus an antibody of this kind can remove IgE from the circulation but will not induce anaphylaxis. Starting with a mouse monoclonal antibody to IgE, the molecule has been chimerized with human IgG1 and then progressively humanized so that less than 10% of the molecule is derived from the original mouse sequence. This molecule can be safely injected into patients and will bind IgE with very high affinity. In clinical trials treatment with anti-IgE antibodies has reduced the symptoms of both asthma and hayfever. In addition, continued treatment which controls free IgE below 10 ng/ml leads to a progressive decrease in the number of IgE receptors on mast cells. Thus, the treatment may achieve a secondary effect further decreasing the sensitivity of histamine-containing cells to allergen. The role of anti-IgE in treating food allergy, atopic dermatitis and drug allergy remains to be established.

Recombinant soluble IL-4 receptor can block biological activity of IL-4 – Given the central role of IL-4 in the TH2 response, it is not surprising that several efforts have been made to block its action. These include a mutated IL-4, (Y124D), antibodies to IL-4 and recombinant soluble IL-4 receptor. The soluble IL-4 receptor (sIL-4R) has proved effective in clinical trials of allergic asthma. The mechanism is that sIL-4R binds to IL-4 before it can react with the receptor on T cells or B cells, and thus blocks its biological activity. However, it is less clear which of the many actions of IL-4 is relevant to the clinical effects. Blocking the action of IL-4 on B cells may reduce IgE production but would probably require several weeks to produce a clinical effect. However, the autocrine effect of IL-4 on TH2 cells may be an essential growth factor. The efficacy of sIL-4R provides further evidence for the role of T cells in allergic disease.

Humanized monoclonal anti-IL-5 decreases circulating eosinophils – Anti-IL-5 (like anti-IgE) is a humanized mouse monoclonal antibody. Following successful studies in baboons, anti-IL-5 has been shown to decrease circulating eosinophils in patients. Thus, it is assumed that binding IL-5 produced by T cells (or mast cells) can decrease the production of eosinophils in the bone marrow. However, the results do not answer whether the treatment acts on IL-5 in the circulation or on IL-5 produced by T cells (or mast cells) locally in the bone marrow and/or the respiratory tract.

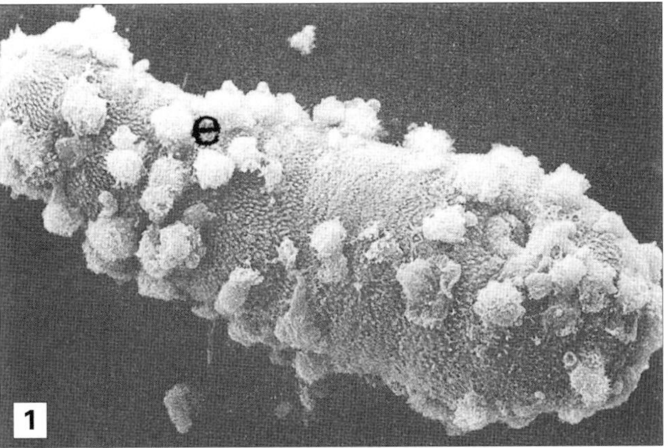

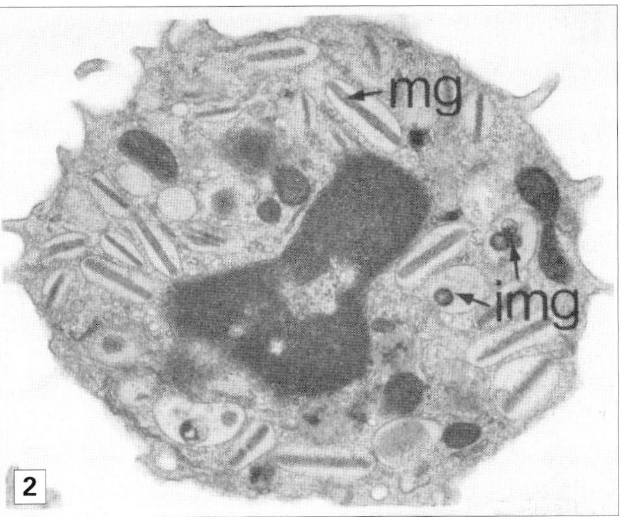

Fig. 21.27 (1) Schistomosomule being killed by eosinophils. A schistomosomule being killed by eosinophils which had been cultured from mouse bone marrow in the presence of IL-5. The larval helminth had been first treated with IgG antibodies and the eosinophils adhere by means of their Fcγ receptors. (Courtesy of Dr C. Sanderson.) **(2) Electron micrograph of eosinophil.** Transmission EM of an eosinophil. Degranulation of eosinophils usually leads to death of the cells. The mediators released include major basic protein (MBP) eosinophil cationic protein (ECP), eosinophil peroxidase (EPO) and eosinophil derived neurotoxin (EDN). In addition, eosinophils can produce leukotrienes and the cytokines IL-5, granulocyte macrophage colony-stimulating factor (GM–CSF) and TGFα. img = immature granules; mg = mature granules with crystalline core. The scale bar is 1 μm. (Courtesy of Dr C. Sanderson.)

THE BIOLOGICAL ROLE OF IgE

The biological role of IgE has been studied both in relation to human disease and using animal models. In tropical countries total serum IgE is usually much higher than in the West. Typical mean serum IgE levels among rural populations in tropical countries are 1000–2000 IU/ml compared to ~100–200 IU/ml. The best established cause of increased IgE is infection with helminths, for example ascaris, hookworm or schistosomiasis. Elevated serum IgE is not a feature of protozoal infections such as malaria and trypanosomiasis, or of bacterial infections such as tuberculosis or leprosy. The hypothesis is that IgE antibodies play a critical role in the defence against helminths, primarily by acting as a gate keeper. A good example is to consider the possible role of immediate skin sensitivity in the protection against schistosomiasis. As the schistosomules enter through the skin of a sensitized individual, they will trigger mast cell degranulation with release of histamine, leukotrienes and cytokines.

These mediators lead to the local accumulation of serum (which contains IgG antibodies) and eosinophils. IgG antibodies bound to schistosomules interact with FcγR on eosinophils leading to degranulation on the surface of the worm which kills it (*Fig. 21.27*). Another important protective mechanism against helminths is the expulsion of worms from the gut. This involves increased mucus production, activated peristalsis, as well as a role for eosinophils and mast cells. Whether IgE and IgE antibodies are essential for this expulsion is not clear. However, the best analysis is that protection against worm infection is a primary role of the TH2 system. This includes roles for effector T cells, mast cells, basophils and IgE antibodies. Furthermore, the primary mechanisms are focused on preventing entry of new worms. Given that one third of the world's population is infested with helminths, it is clear that a protective system could have sufficient survival advantage to explain the presence of an effective TH2 system. Perhaps as a consequence of living in the West without helminth infection, a large proportion of the population generates a TH2-based allergic response against irrelevant antigens such as those on pollen grains, cat dander or mite faecal particles.

CRITICAL THINKING • Severe anaphylactic shock (Explanations on pp 460–461)

Sixty-two-year-old Mrs Young was stung by a bee from a hive in her back garden. Harvesting the honey had left her with several stings during the course of the summer. Several minutes after the recent sting she complained of an itching sensation in her hands, feet and groin accompanied by cramping abdominal pain. Shortly afterwards she felt faint and acutely short of breath. Moments later she collapsed and lost consciousness. Her husband, a doctor, noticed that her breathing was rapid and wheezy and that she had swollen eyelids and lips. She was pale and had patchy erythema across her neck and arms.

On examination her apex beat could be felt but her radial pulse was weak. Her husband immediately administered 0.5 ml of 1/1000 adrenaline intramuscularly and 10 mg of chlorpheniramine (an H_1-receptor antihistamine) intravenously with 100 mg of hydrocortisone. She regained consciousness and her respiratory rate dropped. By the following day she had recovered completely. Results of investigations at this time are shown in the figure.

Mrs Young had no previous history of adverse reactions to bee venom, foods or antibiotics. In addition there was no history of asthma, allergic rhinitis, food allergy or atopic dermatitis. A diagnosis of anaphylactic shock due to bee venom sensitivity was made based on the history and investigations and a decision taken to commence desensitization therapy.

She was made aware of the possible risk of the procedure and consented to it. She was injected subcutaneously with gradually increasing doses of bee venom, the procedures being performed in hospital with access to resuscitation apparatus. No further allergic reactions occurred and she was maintained on a dose of bee venom at 1-month intervals for the next 2 years. She was stung by a bee the following summer and had no adverse reaction.

Investigation	Result (*normal range*)
Haemoglobin (*g/dl*)	14.2 (*11.5–16.0*)
White cell count (× *10^9/l*)	7.5 (*4.0–11.0*)
Neutrophils (× *10^9/l*)	4.4 (*2.0–7.5*)
Eosinophils (× *10^9/l*)	0.40 (*0.4–0.44*)
Total lymphocytes (× *10^9/l*)	2.4 (*1.6–3.5*)
Platelet count (× *10^9/l*)	296 (*150–400*)
Serum immunoglobulins	
IgG (*g/l*)	10.2 (*5.4–16.1*)
IgM (*g/l*)	0.9 (*0.5–1.9*)
IgA (*g/l*)	2.1 (*0.8–2.8*)
IgE (*IU/ml*)	320 (*3–150*)
RAST	
Bee venom	Class 4
Wasp venom	Class 0
Skin prick tests	Grade (*0–5*)
Bee venom (*10 μg/ml*)	3+

21.1 What mechanisms are involved in anaphylaxis?

21.2 What are the clinical features and management of acute anaphylaxis?

21.3 How may such sensitivity be detected and what can be done to desensitize patients?

FURTHER READING

Akdis CA, Blaser K. IL-10-induced anergy in peripheral T cell and reactivation by microenvironmental cytokines: two key steps in specific immunotherapy. *FASEB J* 1999;**13**:603–9.

Beaven MA, Metzger H. Signal transduction by Fc receptors: the FcεRI case. *Immunol Today* 1993;**14**:222–6.

Borish L, Rosenwasser L. TH1/TH2 lymphocytes: doubt some more (editorial). *J Allergy Clin Immunol* 1997;**99**:161–4.

Bruynzeel-Koomen C, Wichen D, Toonstra J, *et al.* The presence of IgE molecules on epidermal Langerhans' cells in patients with atopic dermatitis. *Arch Dermatol Res* 1986;**278**:199–205.

Coca AF, Cooke RA. On the classification of the phenomenon of hypersensitiveness. *J Immunol* 1923;**8**:163.

Coyle AJ, Wagner K, Bertrand C, Tsuyaki S, Bews J, Heusser C. Central role of immunoglobulin (Ig) E in the induction of lung eosinophil infiltration and T helper 2 cell cytokine production: inhibition by a non-anaphylactogenic anti-IgE antibody. *J Exp Med* 1996;**183**:1303–10.

Galli SJ. New concepts about the mast cell. *N Engl J Med* 1993;**328**:257–65.

Geha RF. Regulation of IgE synthesis in humans. *J Allergy Clin Immunol* 1992;**90**:143–50.

Haselden BM, Kay AB, Larch M. Immunoglobulin E-independent major histocompatibility complex-restricted T cell peptide epitope-induced late asthmatic reactions. *J Exp Med* 1999;**189**:1885–94.

Holt PG, Macaubus C, Stumbles PA, Sly PD. The role of allergy in the development of asthma. *Nature* 1999;**402**(6760 suppl):B12–B17.

Marsh DG, Neely JD, Breezeale DR, *et al.* Linkage analysis of IL-4 and other chromosome 5q31.1 markers and total serum immunoglobulin E concentrations. *Science* 1994;**264**:1152–6.

Miller JS, Schwartz LB. Human mast cell proteases and mast cell heterogeneity. *Curr Opin Immunol* 1989;**1**:637–42.

Montford S, Robinson HC, Holgate ST. The bronchial epithelium as a target for inflammatory attack in asthma. *Clin Exp Immunol* 1992;**22**:511–20.

Platts-Mills TAE, Vervloet D, Thomas WR, Aalberse RC, Chapman MD. Indoor allergens and asthma: report of the Third International Workshop [review]. *J Allergy Clin Immunol* 1997;**100**:S2–S24.

Platts-Mills TAE, Woodfolk J, Sporik R et al. Decreased risk of sensitization and asthma in children with high exposure to cat allergen is ameliorated with a modified TH2 response. *Lancet* 2001: In press.

Prausnitz C, Kustner H. In: Gell PGH, Coombes RRA (eds) *Clinical Aspects of Immunology.* Oxford: Blackwell Scientific Publications, 1962:808–16.

Sedgwick JD, Holt PG. Induction of IgE-secreting cells in the lymphatic drainage of the lungs of rats following passive antigen inhalation. *Int Arch Allergy Appl Immunol* 1986;**79**:323–31.

Sporik R, Holgate ST, Platts-Mills TAE, Cogswell JJ. Exposure to house-dust mite allergen (Der p I) and the development of asthma in childhood. A prospective study. *N Engl J Med* 1990;**323**:502–7.

Spry CJF, Kay AB, Gleich GJ. Eosinophils 1992. *Immunol Today* 1992;**13**:384–7.

Wan H, Winton HL, Soeller C, *et al.* Der p 1 facilitates transepithelial allergen delivery by disruption of tight junctions. *J Clin Invest* 1999;**104**:123–33.

Wide L, Bennich H, Johansson SGO. Diagnosis of allergy by an *in vitro* test for allergen antibodies. *Lancet* 1967;**ii**:1105.

22 Hypersensitivity – Type II

- **Type II hypersensitivity reactions** are caused by IgG or IgM antibodies against cell surface and extracellular matrix antigens. Antibodies to intracellular components also occur. These are not normally pathogenetic, although they may be diagnostically useful.
- **Transfusion reactions to erythrocytes** are produced by antibodies to blood group antigens, which may occur naturally or may have been induced by previous contact with incompatible tissue or blood following transplantation, transfusion or during pregnancy.
- **The antibodies** damage cells and tissues by activating complement, and by binding and activating effector cells carrying Fcγ receptors.
- **Haemolytic disease of the newborn** occurs when maternal antibodies to fetal blood group antigens cross the placenta and destroy the fetal erythrocytes.
- **Damage to tissues** may be produced by antibody to basement membranes, to intercellular adhesion molecules or to receptors. Examples include myasthenia gravis, pemphigus and Goodpasture's syndrome.

Type II hypersensitivity reactions are mediated by IgG and IgM antibodies binding to specific cells or tissues. The damage caused is thus restricted to the specific cells or tissues bearing the antigens. In general, those antibodies which are directed against cell surface antigens are usually pathogenic, while those against internal antigens usually are not so. The Type II reactions therefore differ from Type III reactions which involve antibodies directed against soluble antigens in the serum, leading to the formation of circulating antigen–antibody complexes. Damage occurs when the complexes are deposited non-specifically onto tissues and/or organs (see Chapter 23).

MECHANISMS OF DAMAGE

Cells engage their targets using Fc and C3 receptors

In Type II hypersensitivity, antibody directed against cell surface or tissue antigens interacts with complement and a variety of effector cells to bring about damage to the target cells (*Fig. 22.1*).

Once the antibody has attached itself to the surface of the cell or tissue, it can bind and activate complement component C1, with the following consequences:

- Complement fragments (C3a and C5a) generated by activation of complement attract macrophages and polymorphs to the site, and also stimulate mast cells and basophils to produce chemokines that attract and activate other effector cells.
- The classical complement pathway and activation loop lead to the deposition of C3b, C3bi and C3d on the target cell membrane.
- The classical complement pathway and lytic pathway result in the production of the C5b–9 membrane attack complex and insertion of the complex into the target cell membrane.

Effector cells – in this case macrophages, neutrophils, eosinophils and K (killer) cells – bind either to the complexed antibody, via their Fc receptors, or to the membrane-bound C3b, C3bi and C3d, via their C3 receptors (CR1, CR3, CR4).

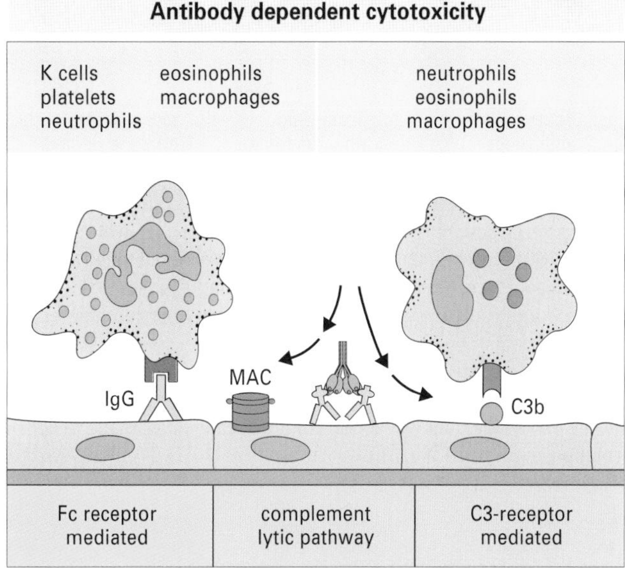

Fig. 22.1 Effector cells – K cells, platelets, neutrophils, eosinophils, and cells of the mononuclear phagocyte series – all have receptors for Fc, which they use to engage antibody bound to target tissues. Activation of complement C3 can generate complement-mediated lytic damage to target cells directly, and also allows phagocytic cells to bind to their targets via C3b, C3bi or C3d, which also activate the cells. (MAC = Membrane attack complex.)

Cells damage targets by exocytosis of their normal immune effector molecules

The mechanisms by which neutrophils and macrophages damage target cells in Type II hypersensitivity reactions reflect their normal methods of dealing with infectious pathogens (*Fig. 22.2*). Normally pathogens would be internalized and then subjected to a barrage of microbicidal systems including defensins, reactive oxygen and nitrogen metabolites, hypohalites, enzymes, altered pH and other agents that interfere with metabolism (see Chapter 9). But if the target is too large to be phagocytosed, the granule and lysosome contents are released in apposition to the

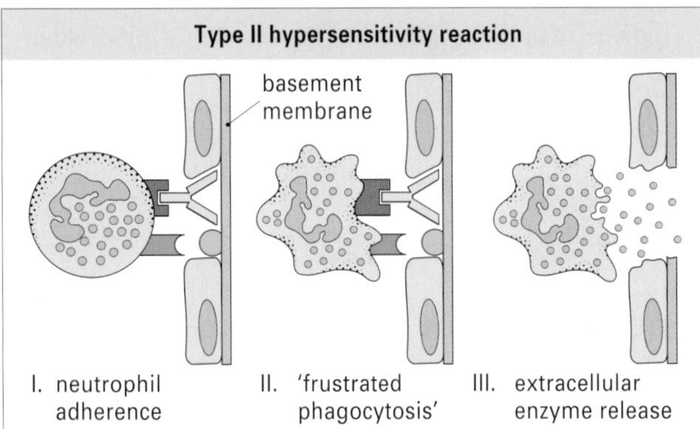

Fig. 22.2 Neutrophil-mediated damage is a reflection of normal antibacterial action. (**1**) Neutrophils engage microbes with their Fc and C3 receptors. (**2**) The microbe is then phagocytosed and destroyed as lysosomes fuse to form the phagolysosome (**3**). In Type II hypersensitivity reactions, individual host cells coated with antibody may be similarly phagocytosed, but where the target is large, for example a basement membrane (**I**), the neutrophils are frustrated in their attempt at phagocytosis (**II**). They exocytose their lysosomal contents, causing damage to cells in the vicinity (**III**).

sensitized target in a process referred to as exocytosis. Cross-linking of the Fc and C3 receptors during this process causes activation of the phagocyte with production of reactive oxygen intermediates, as well as activation of phospholipase A2 and the consequent synthesis of prostaglandins and leukotrienes. In some situations, such as the eosinophil reaction against schistosomes (see Chapter 16), exocytosis of granule contents is normal and beneficial; however, when the target is host tissue that has been sensitized by antibody, the result is damaging (*Fig. 22.3*). Antibodies may also mediate hypersensitivity by K cells. In this case, however, the nature of the target, and whether it can inhibit the K cells' cytotoxic actions, are as important as the presence of the sensitizing antibody.

The resistance of a target cell to damage varies. Susceptibility depends on the amount of antigen expressed on the target cell's surface, and on the inherent ability of different target cells to sustain damage. For example, an erythrocyte may be lysed by a single active C5 convertase site, whereas it takes many such sites to destroy most nucleated cells – their ion-pumping capacity and ability to maintain membrane integrity with anti-complementary defences is so much greater.

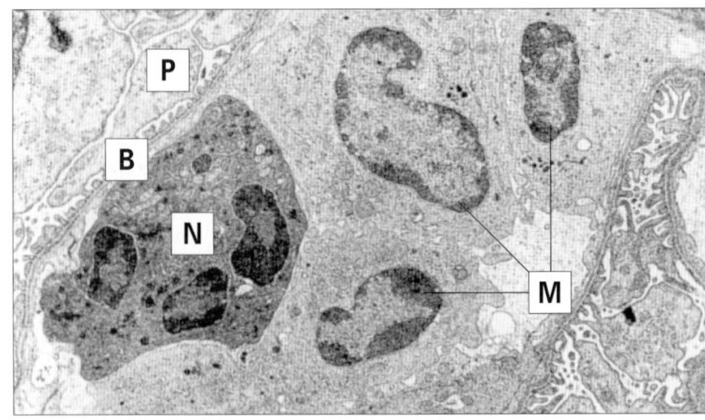

Fig. 22.3 Phagocytes attacking a basement membrane. This electronmicrograph shows a neutrophil (N) and three monocytes (M) binding to the capillary basement membrane (B) in the kidney of a rabbit containing anti-basement membrane antibody. P = podocyte. ×3500. (Courtesy of Professor G.A. Andres.)

The remainder of this chapter examines some of the instances where Type II hypersensitivity reactions are thought to be of prime importance in causing target cell destruction or immunopathological damage.

REACTIONS AGAINST BLOOD CELLS AND PLATELETS

Some of the most clear-cut examples of Type II reactions are seen in the responses to erythrocytes. Important examples are:

- Incompatible blood transfusions, where the recipient becomes sensitized to antigens on the surface of the donor's erythrocytes.
- Haemolytic disease of the newborn, where a pregnant woman has become sensitized to the fetal erythrocytes.
- Autoimmune haemolytic anaemias, where the patient becomes sensitized to his/her own erythrocytes.

Reactions to platelets can cause thrombocytopenia and reactions to neutrophils and lymphocytes have been associated with systemic lupus erythematosus.

Transfusion reactions occur when a recipient has antibodies that react against donor erythrocytes

More than 20 blood group systems, generating over 200 genetic variants of erythrocyte antigens, have been identified in man. A blood group system consists of a gene locus that specifies an antigen on the surface of blood cells (usually, but not always, erythrocytes). Within each system there may be two or more phenotypes. In the ABO system, for example, there are four phenotypes (A, B, AB and O), and thus four possible blood groups. An individual with a particular blood group can recognize erythrocytes carrying allogeneic (non-self) blood group antigens, and will produce antibodies against them. However, for some blood group antigens such antibodies can also be produced 'naturally', i.e. without prior sensitization by foreign erythrocytes (see below). Transfusion of allogeneic erythrocytes into an individual who already has antibodies against them

Five major blood group systems involved in transfusion reactions

system	gene loci	antigens	phenotype frequencies
ABO	1	A, B or O	A 42% B 8% AB 3% O 47%
Rhesus	2 closely linked loci: major antigen=RhD	C or c D or d E or e	RhD^+ 85% RhD^- 15%
Kell	1	K or k	K 9% k 91%
Duffy	1	Fy^a, Fy^b or Fy	Fy^aFy^b 46% Fy^a 20% Fy^b 34% Fy 0.1%
MN	1	M or N	MM 28% MN 50% NN 22%

Fig. 22.4 Not all blood groups are equally antigenic in transfusion reactions: thus, RhD evokes a stronger reaction in an incompatible recipient than the other Rhesus antigens; and Fy^a is stronger than Fy^b. Frequencies stated are for Caucasian populations – other races have different gene frequencies.

The ABO blood group antigens

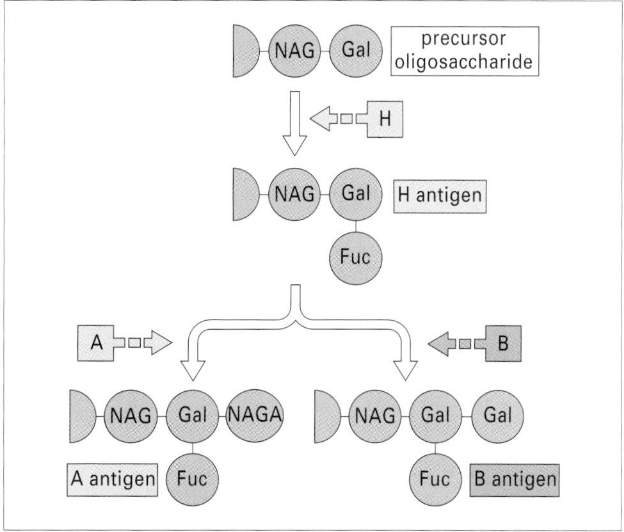

blood group (phenotype)	genotypes	antigens	antibodies to ABO in serum
A	AA, AO	A	anti-B
B	BB, BO	B	anti-A
AB	AB	A and B	none
O	OO	H	anti-A and anti-B

Fig. 22.5 The diagram shows how the ABO blood groups are constructed. The enzyme produced by the H gene attaches a fucose residue (Fuc) to the terminal galactose (Gal) of the precursor oligosaccharide. Individuals possessing the A gene now attach *N*-acetylgalactosamine (NAGA) to this galactose residue, while those with the B gene attach another galactose, producing A and B antigens, respectively. People with both genes make some of each. The table indicates the genotypes and antigens of the ABO system. Most people naturally make antibodies to the antigens they lack. NAG = *N*-acetylglucosamine.

may produce erythrocyte destruction and symptoms of a 'transfusion reaction'. Some blood group systems (e.g. ABO and Rhesus) are characterized by antigens that are relatively strong immunogens; such antigens are more likely to induce antibodies. When planning a blood transfusion, it is important to ensure that donor and recipient blood types are compatible with respect to these major blood groups, otherwise transfusion reactions will occur. Some major human blood groups are listed in *Figure 22.4*.

The ABO system – This blood group system is of primary importance. The epitopes concerned occur on many cell types in addition to erythrocytes and are located on the carbohydrate units of glycoproteins. The structure of these carbohydrates, and of those determining the related Lewis blood group system, is determined by genes coding for enzymes that transfer terminal sugars to a carbohydrate backbone (*Fig. 22.5*). Most individuals develop antibodies to allogeneic specificities of the ABO system without prior sensitization by foreign erythrocytes; this sensitization occurs through contact with identical epitopes, coincidentally and routinely expressed on a wide variety of microorganisms. Antibodies to ABO antigens are therefore extremely common, making it particularly important to match donor blood to the recipient for this system. However, all people are tolerant to the O antigen, and so O individuals are universal donors with respect to the ABO system.

The Rhesus system – This system is also of great importance, as it is a major cause of haemolytic disease of the newborn (HDNB). Rhesus antigens are associated with membrane proteins of 30 kDa which are expressed at moderate levels on the erythrocyte surface. The antigens are encoded by two closely linked loci, RhD and RhCcEe, with 92% homology. RhD is the most important clinically due to its high immunogenicity, but in RhD^- individuals the RhD locus is missing completely. The RhCcEe locus encodes a molecule which expresses the RhC/c and RhE/e epitopes.

Minor blood group systems – MN system epitopes are expressed on the N-terminal glycosylated region of glycophorin A, a glycoprotein present on the erythrocyte surface. Antigenicity is determined by polymorphisms at amino acids 1 and 5. The related Ss system antigens are carried on glycophorin B. Proteins expressed on erythrocytes which display allelic variation can also act as blood group antigens. Examples of these include the Kell antigen, a zinc endopeptidase, the Duffy antigen receptor for

Erythrocyte blood group antigens

erythrocyte surface glycoprotein	blood groups expressed	number of epitopes per cell
anion transport protein	ABO, Ii	10^6
glycophorin A	MN	10^6
glucose transporter	ABO, Ii	5×10^5
Mr 45 000–100 000	ABO	
Mr 30 000	ABO, Rh	1.2×10^5
glycophorin B	N, Ss	2.5×10^5
glycophorins C & D	Gerbich (Ge)	10^5
DAF (decay accelerating factor)	Cromer	<10 000
CD44 (80 kDa)	Ina/Inh	3000–6000
Zinc endopeptidase	Kell	3000–6000
DARC	Fy	12 000
Laminin-binding glycoprotein	lutheran	1500–4000

Fig. 22.6 Note that blood group epitopes based on carbohydrate moieties, such as ABO and Ii (expressed on the precursor of the ABO polysaccharide), can appear on many different proteins, including Rh antigens. Antigens such as Rhesus and Duffy are proteins, so the epitope only appears on one type of molecule. In general, the most important blood group antigens are present at high levels on the erythrocytes, thus providing plenty of targets for complement-mediated lysis or Fc receptor-mediated clearance.

chemokines (DARC) and variants of decay accelerating factor (DAF). The relationship of the blood groups to erythrocyte surface proteins is listed in *Figure 22.6*. Transfusion reactions caused by the minor blood groups are relatively rare, unless repeated transfusions are given. Again, the risks are greatly reduced by accurately cross-matching the donor blood to that of the recipient.

Cross-matching – The aim of cross-matching is to ensure that the blood of a recipient does not contain antibodies that will be able to react with and destroy transfused (donor) erythrocytes. For example, antibodies to ABO system antigens cause incompatible cells to agglutinate in a clearly visible reaction. Minor blood group systems cause weaker reactions that may only be detectable by an indirect Coombs' test (see *Fig. 22.10*). If the individual is transfused with whole blood, it is also necessary to check that the donor's serum does not contain antibodies against the recipient's erythrocytes. However, transfusion of whole blood is unusual – most blood donations are separated into cellular and serum fractions, to be used individually.

Transfusion reactions involve extensive destruction of donor blood cells

Transfusion of erythrocytes into a recipient who has antibodies to those cells produces an immediate reaction. The symptoms include fever, hypotension, nausea and vomiting, and pain in the back and chest. The severity of the reaction depends on the class and the amounts of antibodies involved.

Antibodies to ABO system antigens are usually IgM, and cause agglutination, complement activation and intravascular haemolysis. Other blood groups induce IgG antibodies, which cause less agglutination than IgM. The IgG-sensitized cells are usually taken up by phagocytes in the liver and spleen, although severe reactions may cause erythrocyte destruction by complement activation. This can cause circulatory shock, and the released contents of the erythrocytes can produce acute tubular necrosis of the kidneys. These acute transfusion reactions are often seen in previously unsensitized individuals, and develop over days or weeks as antibodies to the foreign cells are produced. This can result in anaemia or jaundice.

Transfusion reactions to other components of blood may also occur, though their consequences are not usually as severe as reactions to erythrocytes.

Hyperacute graft rejection is related to the transfusion reaction

Hyperacute graft rejection occurs when a graft recipient has preformed antibodies against the graft tissue. It is only seen in tissue that is revascularized directly after transplantation, in kidney grafts for example. The most severe reactions in this type of rejection are due to the ABO group antigens that are expressed on kidney cells. The damage is produced by antibody and complement activation in the blood vessels, with consequent recruitment and activation of neutrophils and platelets. However, donors and recipients are now always cross-matched for ABO antigens, and this reaction has become extremely rare. Antibodies to other graft antigens (e.g. MHC molecules) induced by previous grafting can also produce this type of reaction.

Haemolytic disease of the newborn is due to maternal IgG antibodies which react against the child's erythrocytes *in utero*

Haemolytic disease of the newborn (HDNB) occurs when the mother has been sensitized to antigens on the infant's erythrocytes and makes IgG antibodies to these antigens. These antibodies cross the placenta and react with the fetal erythrocytes, causing their destruction (*Figs 22.7* and *22.8*). Rhesus D (RhD) is the most commonly involved antigen.

A risk of HDNB arises when a Rh^+ sensitized Rh^- mother carries a second Rh^+ infant. Sensitization of the Rh^- mother to the Rh^+ erythrocytes usually occurs during birth of the first Rh^+ infant, when some fetal erythrocytes leak back across the placenta into the maternal circulation and are recognized by the maternal immune system. Thus the first incompatible child is usually unaffected, whereas subsequent children have an increasing risk of being affected, as the mother is resensitized with each successive pregnancy.

Reactions to other blood groups may also cause HDNB, the second most common being the Kell system K antigen. Reactions due to anti-K are much less common than reactions due to RhD because of the relatively low frequency (9%) and weaker antigenicity of the K antigen.

The risk of HDNB due to Rhesus incompatibility is known to be reduced if the father is of a different ABO group to the mother. This observation led to the idea that these Rh^- mothers were destroying Rh^+ cells more rapidly,

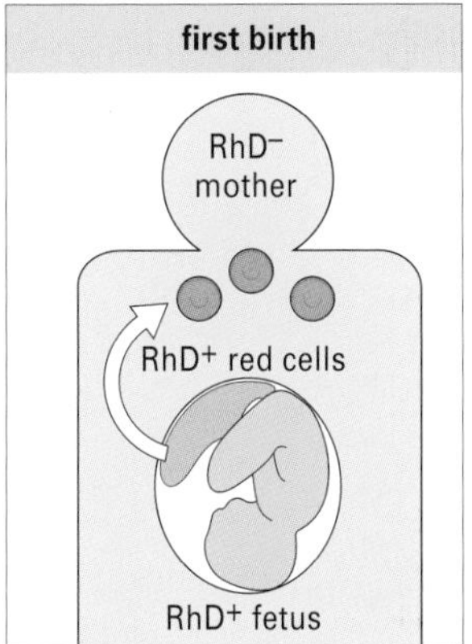

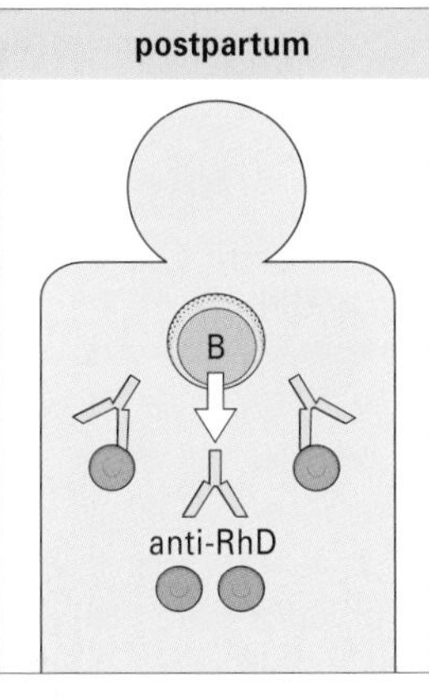

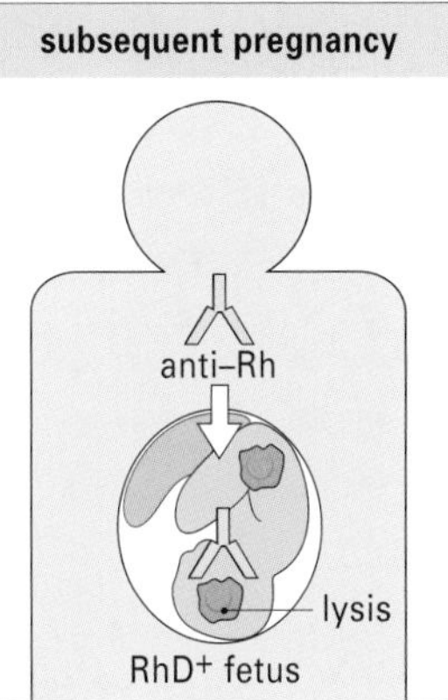

Fig. 22.7 Erythrocytes from RhD^+ fetus leak into the maternal circulation usually during birth. This stimulates the production of anti-Rh antibody of the IgG class postpartum. During subsequent pregnancies, IgG antibodies are transferred across the placenta into the fetal circulation (IgM cannot cross the placenta). If the fetus is again incompatible the antibodies cause erythrocyte destruction.

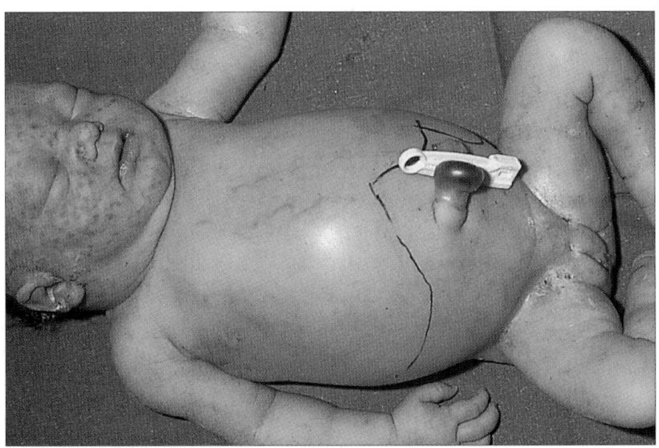

Fig. 22.8 A child suffering from HDNB. There is considerable enlargement of the liver and spleen associated with erythrocyte destruction caused by maternal anti-erythrocyte antibody in the fetal circulation. The child had elevated bilirubin (breakdown product of haemoglobin). The facial petechial haemorrhaging was due to impaired platelet function. The most commonly involved antigen is RhD. (Courtesy of Dr K. Sloper.)

because they were also ABO incompatible. Consequently, fetal Rh^+ erythrocytes would not be available to sensitize the maternal immune system to RhD antigen. This notion led to the development of Rhesus prophylaxis: preformed anti-RhD antibodies are given to Rh^- mothers immediately after delivery of Rh^+ infants, with the aim of destroying fetal Rh^+ erythrocytes before they can cause Rh^- sensitization. This practice has successfully reduced the incidence of HDNB due to Rhesus incompatibility (*Fig. 22.9*). Although the number of cases of HDNB has fallen dramatically and progressively, the proportion of cases caused by other blood groups, including Kell and the ABO system, has increased.

Autoimmune haemolytic anaemias arise spontaneously as autoimmune diseases, or may be induced as reactions to drugs

Reactions to blood group antigens also occur spontaneously in the autoimmune haemolytic anaemias, in which patients produce antibodies to their own erythrocytes. Autoimmune haemolytic anaemia is suspected if a patient gives a positive result on a direct antiglobulin test (*Fig. 22.10*), which identifies antibodies present on the

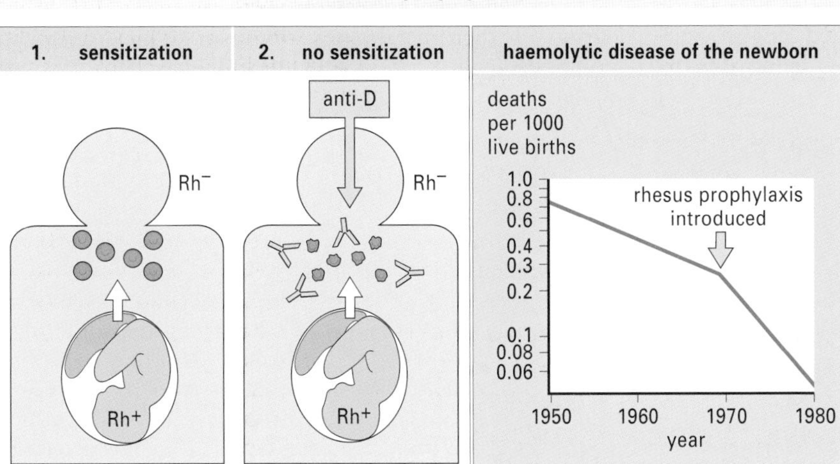

Fig. 22.9 (**1**) Without prophylaxis, Rh^+ erythrocytes leak into the circulation of a Rh^- mother and sensitize her to the Rh antigen(s). (**2**) If anti-Rh antibody (anti-D) is injected immediately postpartum it eliminates the Rh^+ erythrocytes and prevents sensitization. The incidence of deaths due to HDNB fell during the period 1950–66 with improved patient care. The decline in the disease was accelerated by the advent of Rhesus prophylaxis in 1969.

Direct antiglobulin test

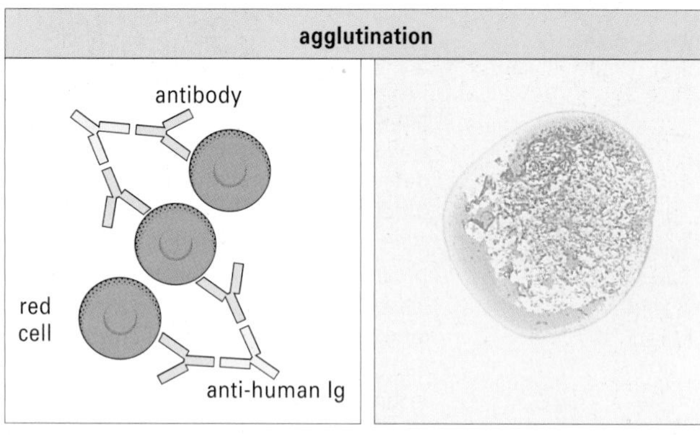

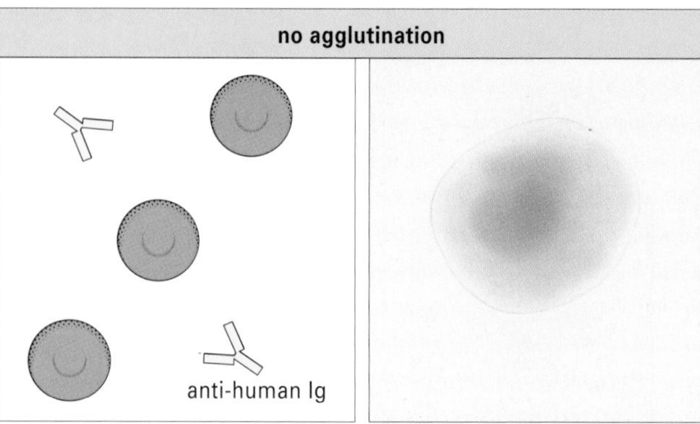

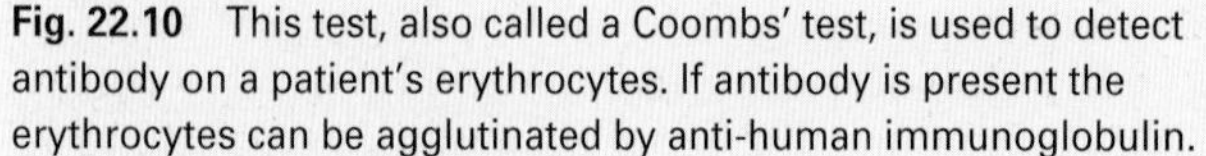

Fig. 22.10 This test, also called a Coombs' test, is used to detect antibody on a patient's erythrocytes. If antibody is present the erythrocytes can be agglutinated by anti-human immunoglobulin. If no antibody is present on the red cells, they are not agglutinated by anti-human immunoglobulin.

patient's erythrocytes. These are usually antibodies directed towards erythrocyte antigens, or immune complexes adsorbed onto the erythrocytes' surface. The direct antiglobulin test is also used to detect antibodies on red cells in mismatched transfusions, and in HDNB (see above). Autoimmune haemolytic anaemias can be divided into three types, depending upon whether they are due to:

- Warm-reactive autoantibodies, which react with the antigen at 37°C.
- Cold-reactive autoantibodies, which can only react with antigen at below 37°C.
- Antibodies provoked by allergic reactions to drugs.

Warm-reactive autoantibodies cause accelerated clearance of erythrocytes

Warm-reactive autoantibodies are frequently found against Rhesus system antigens, including determinants of the RhC and RhE loci as well as RhD. They differ from the antibodies responsible for transfusion reactions, in that they appear to react with different epitopes. Warm-reactive autoantibodies to other blood group antigens exist, but are relatively rare. Most of these haemolytic anaemias are of unknown cause, but some are associated with other autoimmune diseases. The anaemia appears to be a result of accelerated clearance of the sensitized erythrocytes by spleen macrophages more often than being due to complement-mediated lysis.

Cold-reactive autoantibodies cause erythrocyte lysis by complement fixation

Cold-reactive autoantibodies are often present in higher titres than the warm-reactive autoantibodies. The antibodies are primarily IgM and fix complement strongly. In most cases they are specific for the Ii blood group system. The I and i epitopes are expressed on the precursor polysaccharides that produce the ABO system epitopes, and are the result of incomplete glycosylation of the core polysaccharide.

The reaction of the antibody with the erythrocytes takes place in the peripheral circulation (particularly in winter), where the temperature in the capillary loops of exposed skin may fall below 30°C. In severe cases, peripheral necrosis may occur due to aggregation and microthrombosis of small vessels caused by complement-mediated destruction in the periphery. The severity of the anaemia is therefore directly related to the complement-fixing ability of the patient's serum. (Fc-mediated removal of sensitized cells in the spleen and liver is not involved, because these organs are too warm for the antibodies to bind.)

Most cold-reactive autoimmune haemolytic anaemias occur in older people. Their cause is unknown, but it is notable that the autoantibodies produced are usually of very limited clonality, indicating that a limited number of autoreactive clones are present. However, some cases may follow infection with *Mycoplasma pneumoniae*, and these are acute onset diseases of short duration with polyclonal autoantibodies. Such cases are thought to be due to cross-reacting antigens on the bacteria and the erythrocytes, producing a bypass of normal tolerance mechanisms (see Chapter 12).

Drug-induced reactions to blood components may be due either to antibodies binding to the drug adsorbed to cells, or to breakdown of self tolerance

Drugs (or their metabolites) can provoke hypersensitivity reactions against blood cells, including erythrocytes and platelets. This can occur in three different ways (*Fig. 22.11*):

- The drug binds to the blood cells, and antibodies are produced against the drug. In this case it is necessary for both the drug and the antibody to be present to produce the reaction. This phenomenon was first recorded by Ackroyd, who noted thrombocytopenic purpura (destruction of platelets leading to purpuric rash) following administration of the drug Sedormid. Haemolytic anaemias have been reported following the administration of a wide variety of drugs, including penicillin, quinine and sulphonamides. All these conditions are rare.
- Drug–antibody immune complexes are adsorbed on to the erythrocyte cell membrane. Damage occurs by complement-mediated lysis.

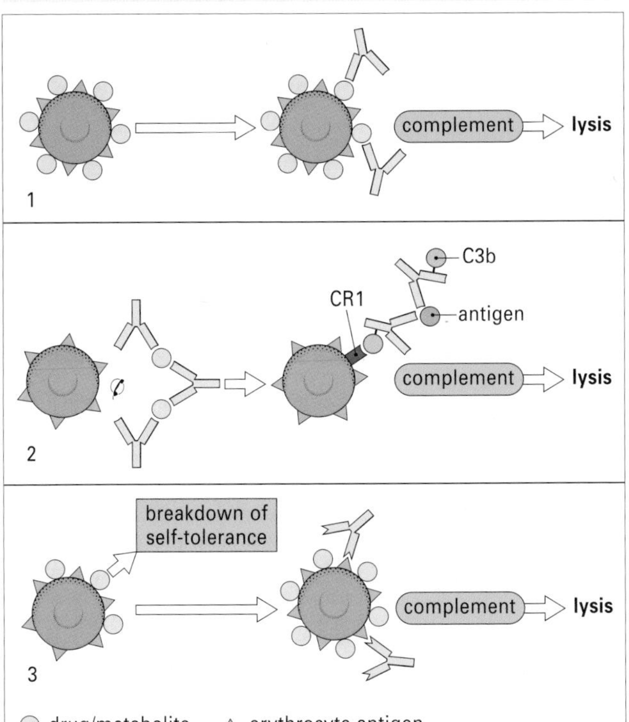

Fig. 22.11 Three ways that drug treatment can cause damage are illustrated.
(**1**) The drug adsorbs to cell membranes. Antibodies to the drug will bind to the cell and complement-mediated lysis will occur.
(**2**) Immune complexes of drugs and antibody become adsorbed to the red cell. This could be mediated by an Fc receptor, but is more probably via the C3b receptor CR1. Damage occurs by complement-mediated lysis.
(**3**) Drugs, presumably adsorbed onto cell membranes, induce a breakdown of self tolerance, possibly by stimulating T-helper (TH) cells. This leads to formation of antibodies to other blood group antigens on the cell surface.
Note that in examples 1 and 2, the drug must be present for cell damage to occur, whereas in 3 the cells are destroyed whether they carry absorbed drug or not.

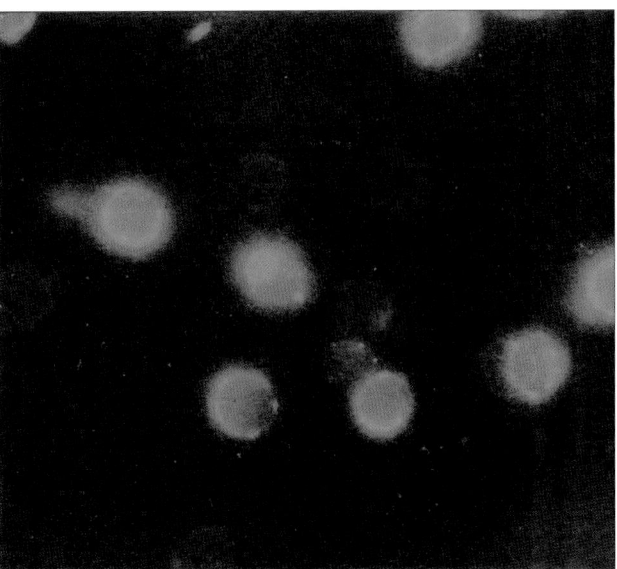

Fig. 22.12 Antibodies to neutrophils. Antibodies to neutrophils are demonstrated by immunofluorescence. In this instance, normal neutrophils were stained with antibodies from a neonate suffering from alloimmune neonatal neutropenia.

- The drug induces an allergic reaction, and autoantibodies are directed against the erythrocyte antigens themselves, as is the case with 0.3% of patients given α-methyldopa. The antibodies produced are similar to those in patients with warm-reactive antibody. However, the condition remits shortly after the cessation of drug treatment.

Reactions against other blood cells have been associated with systemic lupus erythematosus and with thrombocytopenia

Antibodies to neutrophils and lymphocytes – Autoantibodies to neutrophil cytoplasmic antigens (ANCAs) are associated with a number of diseases. For example, antibody to proteinase-3, a cytoplasmic antigen (C-ANCA), is associated with Wegener's granulomatosis, while antibodies to myeloperoxidase are seen more commonly in systemic lupus erythematosus (SLE), and are located in perinuclear granules (P-ANCA). Other granule components may also act as antigens in SLE but less commonly than myeloperoxidase. Such autoantigens are generally neutrophil specific and antibodies can be detected by immunofluorescent staining (*Fig. 22.12*). (By contrast, antibodies to MHC antigens also seen in SLE are highly non-tissue specific.) Antibodies to P-ANCAs are particularly characteristic of vasculitis and glomerulonephritis. Their contribution to disease pathogenesis appears to be relatively small, although they have some diagnostic use.

Antibodies to platelets – Autoantibodies to platelets are seen in up to 70% of cases of idiopathic thrombocytopenic purpura, a disorder in which there is accelerated removal of platelets from the circulation, mediated primarily by splenic macrophages. The mechanism of removal is via the immune adherence receptors on these cells. The condition most often develops after bacterial or viral infections, but may also be associated with autoimmune diseases including SLE. In SLE, antibodies to cardiolipin, which is present on platelets, can sometimes be detected. Autoantibodies to cardiolipin and other phospholipids can inhibit one aspect of blood clotting (lupus anticoagulant) and can be associated, in some cases, with venous thrombosis and recurrent abortions. Thrombocytopenia may also be induced by drugs, by similar mechanisms to those outlined in *Figure 22.11.*

REACTIONS AGAINST TISSUE ANTIGENS

A number of autoimmune conditions occur in which antibodies to tissue antigens cause immunopathological damage by activation of Type II hypersensitivity mechanisms. The antigens are extracellular, and may be expressed on structural proteins or on the surface of cells. Descriptions of such diseases – Goodpasture's syndrome, pemphigus and myasthenia gravis – are given below.

It is often possible to demonstrate autoantibodies to particular cell types, but in these cases the antigens are intracellular, and the importance of the Type II mechanisms is less well established. In these cases, recognition of autoantigen by T cells is probably more important pathologically, and the autoantibodies are of secondary importance.

Antibodies against basement membranes produce nephritis in Goodpasture's syndrome

A number of patients with nephritis are found to have antibodies to collagen type IV, which is a major component of basement membranes (see *Fig. 23.3*). Collagen Type IV undergoes alternate RNA splicing which produces a number of variant proteins (Goodpasture antigen), but the antibodies appear to bind just those forms which retain the characteristic N-terminus. The antibody is usually IgG and, in at least 50% of patients, it appears to fix complement. The condition usually results in severe necrosis of the glomerulus, with fibrin deposition. The association of this type of nephritis with lung haemorrhage was originally noticed by Goodpasture (hence Goodpasture's syndrome). Although the lung symptoms do not occur in all patients, the association of lung and kidney damage is due to cross-reactive autoantigens in the basement membranes of the two tissues.

A number of animal models for Goodpasture's syndrome have been developed. In nephrotoxic serum nephritis (Masugi glomerulonephritis), heterologous antibodies to glomerular basement membrane are injected into rats or rabbits. The injected antibody is deposited on to the basement membranes, and this is followed by further deposition of host antibodies to the injected antibody; this precipitates acute nephritis. Development of nephritis and proteinuria depends on the accumulation of neutrophils, which bind via complement-dependent and complement-independent mechanisms. Similar lesions can be induced by immunization with heterologous basement membrane (Steblay model).

Another animal model (Heymann nephritis), caused by raising autoantibodies to a protein present in the brush border of glomerular epithelial cells, resembles human membranous glomerulonephritis. In this model, the damage is mostly complement mediated: complement depletion of the animals alleviates the condition.

Pemphigus is caused by autoantibodies to an intercellular adhesion molecule

Pemphigus is a serious blistering disease of the skin and mucous membranes. Patients have autoantibodies against desmoglein-1 and desmoglein-3, components of desmosomes, which form junctions between epidermal cells (*Fig. 22.13*). The antibodies disrupt cellular adhesion, leading to breakdown of the epidermis. Clinical disease profiles can be related to the specificity of the antibodies. For example, patients with only anti-desmoglein-3 tend to show mucosal disease, while those with anti-desmoglein-1 and -3 have affected skin and mucosa. Disease has been correlated with the incidence of IgG4 antibodies against a different part of the molecule. Pemphigus is strongly linked to a rare haplotype of HLA-DR4 (DRB1*0402), and this molecule has been shown to present a peptide of desmoglein-3, which other DR4 subtypes cannot. This is therefore a clear example of an autoimmune disease producing pathology by Type II mechanisms.

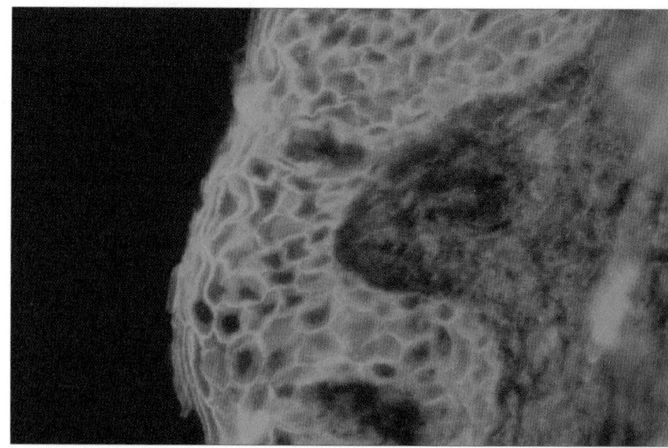

Fig. 22.13 Autoantibodies in pemphigus. The antibodies in pemphigus bind to components of the desmosome involved in cell adhesion. Desmoglein-1 and desmoglein-3 are most commonly involved, but other molecules, including the plakins and desmocollin, may also act as autoantigens. Immunofluorescence of human skin stained with anti-IgA. (Courtesy of Dr R. Mirakian and Mr P. Collins.)

Myasthenia gravis and Lambert–Eaton syndrome are caused by antibodies that reduce the availability of acetylcholine at motor endplates

Myasthenia gravis, a condition in which there is extreme muscular weakness, is associated with antibodies to the acetylcholine receptors present on the surface of muscle membranes. The acetylcholine receptors are located at the motor endplate where the neuron contacts the muscle. Transmission of impulses from the nerve to the muscle takes place by the release of acetylcholine from the nerve terminal and its diffusion across the gap to the muscle fibre.

It was noticed that immunization of experimental animals with purified acetylcholine receptors produced a condition of muscular weakness that closely resembled human myasthenia. This suggested a role for antibody to the acetylcholine receptor in the human disease. Analysis of the lesion in myasthenic muscles indicated that the disease was not due to an inability to synthesize acetylcholine, nor was there any problem in secreting it in response to a nerve impulse – the released acetylcholine was less effective at triggering depolarization of the muscle (*Fig. 22.14*).

Examination of neuromuscular endplates by immunochemical techniques has demonstrated IgG and the complement proteins, C3 and C9, on the postsynaptic folds of the muscle (*Fig. 22.15*). (Further evidence for a pathogenetic

Myasthenia gravis

normal nerve impulse
neuron
motor endplate
acetylcholine vesicles
postsynaptic folds
muscle fibre
acetylcholine receptor

myasthenic patient
anti-AChR antibody
acetylcholine
acetylcholine receptor

Fig. 22.14 Normally a nerve impulse passing down a neuron arrives at a motor endplate and causes the release of acetylcholine (ACh). This diffuses across the neuromuscular junction, binds ACh receptors on the muscle, and causes ion channels in the muscle membrane to open, which in turn triggers muscular contraction. In myasthenia gravis, antibodies to the receptor block binding of the ACh transmitter. The effect of the released vesicle is therefore reduced, and the muscle can become very weak. Antibody blocking receptors is only one of the factors operating in the disease.

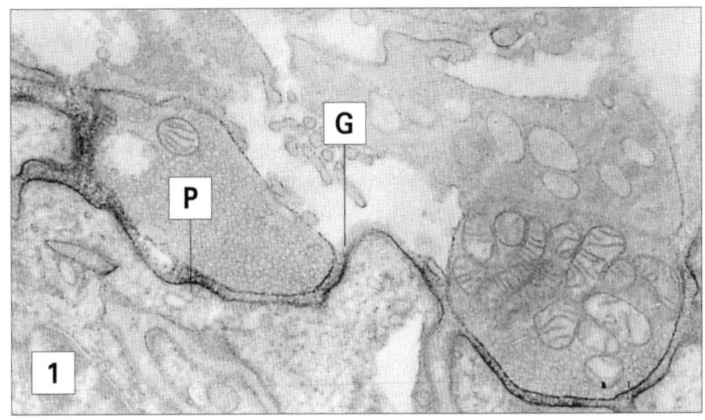

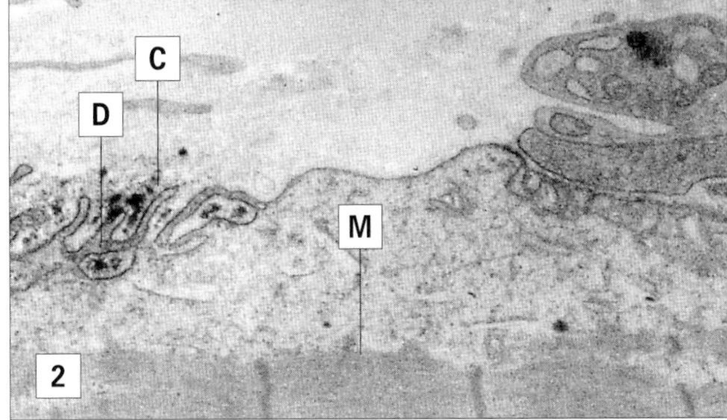

Fig. 22.15 Myasthenia gravis: motor endplate. (**1**) Electronmicrograph showing IgG deposits (G) in discrete patches on the postsynaptic membrane (P). ×13 000. (**2**) Electronmicrograph illustrating C9 (C) shows the postsynaptic region denuded of its nerve terminal: it consists of debris and degenerating folds (D). There is a strong reaction for C9 on this debris. M = muscle fibre. ×9000 (Courtesy of Dr A.G. Engel.)

role for IgG in this disease was furnished by the discovery of transient muscle weakness in babies born to myasthenic mothers. This is significant because it is known that IgG can and does cross the placenta, entering the bloodstream of the fetus.) IgG and complement are thought to act in two ways: by increasing the rate of turnover of the acetylcholine receptors, and by partial blocking of acetylcholine binding. Cellular infiltration of myasthenic endplates is rarely seen, so it is assumed that damage does not involve effector cells.

In a related condition, Lambert–Eaton syndrome, the muscular weakness is caused by defective release of acetylcholine from the neuron. If serum or IgG from patients with Lambert–Eaton syndrome is transfused into mice, the condition is also transferred, indicating the presence of autoantibody. The autoantibodies are directed against components of voltage-gated calcium channels or against the synaptic vesicle protein synaptotagmin. The different forms of the syndrome are thought to relate to the target antigen and the class and titre of antibodies involved. These two diseases exemplify conditions where autoantibodies to receptors block the normal function of the receptor. There are other diseases, however, where the autoantibody has an opposite effect; for example, in some forms of autoimmune thyroid disease antibodies to the TSH receptor mimic TSH (thyroid-stimulating hormone), thereby stimulating thyroid function (see Chapter 26).

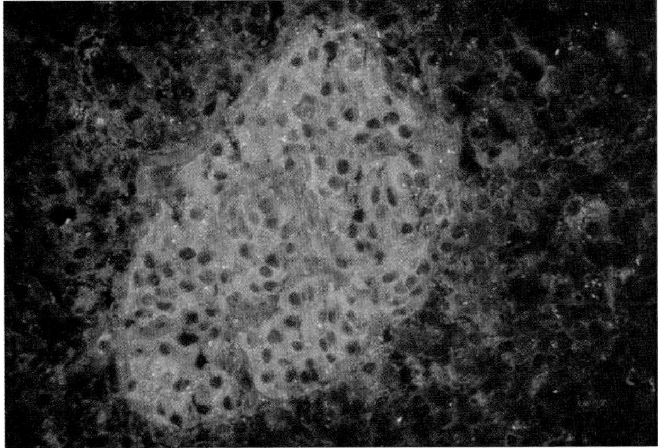

Fig. 22.16 Islet cell autoantibodies. Autoantibodies to the pancreas in diabetes mellitus may be demonstrated by immunofluorescence. The antibodies are diagnostically useful, and may contribute to the pathology. (Courtesy of Dr B. Dean.)

Autoantibodies to tissue antigens do not necessarily produce a Type II hypersensitivity reaction

Although a great number of autoantibodies react with tissue antigens, their significance in causing tissue damage and pathology *in vivo* is not always clear. For example, although autoantibodies to pancreatic islet cells can be detected *in vitro* using sera from some diabetic patients (*Fig. 22.16*), most of the immunopathological damage in autoimmune diabetes is thought to be caused by autoreactive T cells.

Until recently it was thought that autoantibodies against intracellular antigens would not usually cause immunopathology because they could not reach their antigen within a living cell. However, it now appears that antibodies such as anti-RNP and anti-DNA can reach the cell nucleus and modulate cell function – in some cases, they can induce apoptosis. Although the relative importance of antibody in causing cell damage is still debated, autoantibodies against internal antigens of cells often make excellent disease markers, as they are frequently detectable before immunopathological damage occurs.

CRITICAL THINKING • Blood groups and haemolytic disease of the newborn (Explanations on p. 461)

Mrs Chareston has the blood group O, Rhesus-negative, and her husband Mr Chareston is A, Rhesus-positive. They have had four children, of which two have been affected by haemolytic disease of the newborn, as follows:

First child	born 1968	unaffected.
Second child	born 1974	mildly affected.
Third child	born 1976	seriously affected, required intra-uterine blood transfusion.
Fourth child	born 1980	unaffected.

In both affected cases (second and third), the cause of the haemolytic disease was identified as antibodies to Rhesus-D binding to the child's red cells. Following the second, third and fourth deliveries, Mrs Chareston was given antibodies to the Rhesus-D blood group (Rhesus prophylaxis was introduced in the UK in 1972).

22.1 From this information, what can you deduce about the blood group of the first child?

22.2 Why does HDNB usually become more serious with succesive pregnancies?

22.3 What is the reason for giving anti-Rhesus D antibodies to the mother?

22.4 Why are the antibodies given postpartum and not earlier?

22.5 Give an explanation of why the Rhesus prophylaxis after the second delivery failed to prevent HDNB in the third child.

22.6 What explanation can be given to account for the fact that the fourth child is unaffected?

When the blood groups of the children are examined it is found that they are:

1. First child — O, Rh^+
2. Second child — B, Rh^+
3. Third child — A, Rh^+
4. Fourth child — A, Rh^-

22.7 As Mrs Chareston has antibodies to blood group A, why was the fourth child not affected by HDNB caused by these antibodies?

22.8 One of these children was definitely not fathered by Mr Chareston – which child?

FURTHER READING

Alarçon-Segovia D, Ruiz-Argüelles A, Llorente L. Broken dogma: penetration of autoantibodies into living cells. *Immunol Today* 1996;**17**:163–4.

Amagai M. Autoantibodies against desmosomal cadherins in pemphigus. *J Dermatol Sci* 1999;**20**:92–102.

Anstee DJ. Blood group active substances of the human red blood cell. *Vox Sang* 1990;**58**:1.

Bhol K, Natarajan K, Nagarwalla N, *et al.* Correlation of peptide specificity and IgG subclass with pathogenic and non-pathogenic autoantibodies in pemphigus vulgaris: a model for autoimmunity. *Proc Natl Acad Sci USA* 1995;**92**:5239–43.

Bloy C, Blanchard D, Lambin P, *et al.* Characterization of the D, C, E and G antigens of the Rh blood group system with human monoclonal antibodies. *Mol Immunol* 1988;**25**:926–30.

Druet P, Glotz D. Experimental autoimmune nephropathies: induction and regulation. *Adv Nephrol* 1984;**13**:115.

Le van Kim C, Mouro I, Cherif-Zahar B, *et al.* Molecular cloning and primary structure of the human blood group RhD polypeptide. *Proc Natl Acad Sci USA* 1992;**89**:10925–29.

King MJ. Blood group antigens on human erythrocytes – distribution, structure and possible functions. *Biochim Biophys Acta* 1994; **1197**:14–44.

Lang B, Newsom-Davis J. Immunopathology of the Lambert–Eaton myasthenic syndrome. *Springer Semin Immunopathol* 1995;**17**:3–15.

Lindstrom J. Immunobiology of myasthenia gravis, experimental autoimmune myasthenia gravis and Lambert–Eaton syndrome. *Annu Rev Immunol* 1985;**3**:109–31.

Mauro I, Colin Y, Chenif-Zahar B, *et al.* Molecular genetic basis of the human Rhesus blood group system. *Nature Genet* 1993;**5**:62–5.

Naparstek Y, Plotz PH. The role of autoantibodies in autoimmune disease. *Annu Rev Immunol* 1993;**11**:79–104.

Race R, Sanger R. *Blood Groups in Man,* 6th edn, Oxford: Blackwell Scientific Publications, 1975.

Russo D, Redman C, Lee S. Association of XK and Kell blood group proteins. *J Biol Chem* 1998; **273**:13960–6.

Schulz DR, Tozman EC. Anti-neutrophil cytoplasmic antibodies: major autoantigens, pathophysiology, and disease associations. *Semin Arthritis Rheum* 1995;**25**:143–59.

Yamamoto F–I, Clausen H, White T, *et al.* Molecular genetic basis of the histo-blood group ABO system. *Nature* 1990;**345**:229.

23 Hypersensitivity – Type III

- **Immune complexes are formed every time antibody meets antigen** and are removed by the mononuclear phagocyte system following complement activation.
- **Persistence of antigen** from continued infection or in autoimmune disease can lead to immune-complex disease.
- **Immune complexes** can form both in the circulation, leading to systemic disease, and at local sites such as the lung.
- **Complement** helps to disrupt antigen–antibody bonds and keeps immune complexes soluble.
- **Primate erythrocytes bear a receptor for C3b** and are important for transporting complement-containing immune complexes to the spleen for removal.
- **Complement deficiencies** lead to formation of large, relatively insoluble complexes which deposit in tissues.
- **Charged cationic antigens have tissue-binding properties**, particularly for the glomerulus, and help to localize complexes to the kidney.
- **Factors that tend to increase blood vessel permeability** enhance the deposition of immune complexes in tissues.

Immune complexes are formed every time antibody meets antigen, and generally they are removed effectively by the mononuclear phagocyte system, but occasionally they persist and eventually deposit in a range of tissues and organs. The complement and effector-cell-mediated damage that follows is known as a Type III hypersensitivity reaction, or immune-complex disease. The sites of immune complex deposition are partly determined by the localization of the antigen in the tissues and partly by how circulating complexes become deposited.

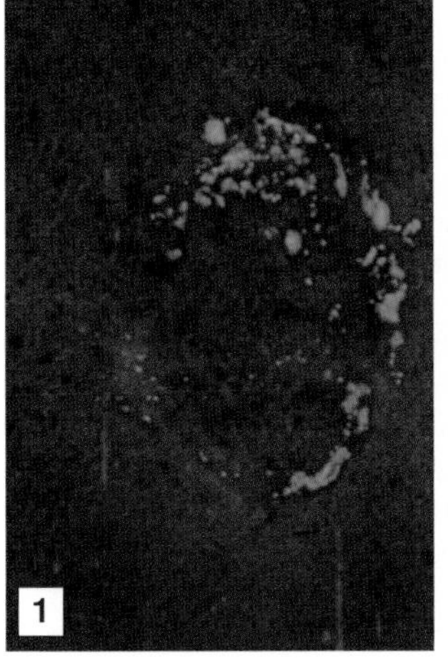

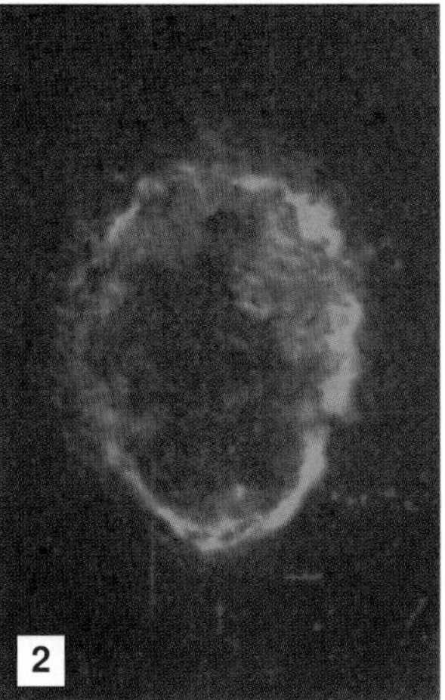

Fig. 23.2 Immunofluorescence study of immune complexes in infectious disease. These serial sections of the renal artery of a patient with chronic hepatitis B infection are stained with fluoresceinated anti-hepatitis B antigen (**1**) and rhodaminated anti-IgM (**2**). The presence of both antigen and antibody in the intima and media of the arterial wall indicates the deposition of complexes at this site. IgG and C3 deposits are also detectable with the same distribution. (Courtesy of Dr A. Nowoslawski.)

TYPES OF IMMUNE-COMPLEX DISEASE

Diseases resulting from immune-complex formation can be divided broadly into three groups: those due to persistent infection, those due to autoimmune disease, and those caused by inhalation of antigenic material (*Fig. 23.1*).

Persistent infection – The combined effects of a low-grade persistent infection and a weak antibody response lead to chronic immune-complex formation, and eventual deposition of complexes in the tissues (*Fig. 23.2*). Diseases with this aetiology include leprosy, malaria, dengue haemorrhagic fever, viral hepatitis and staphylococcal infective endocarditis.

Autoimmune disease – Immune-complex disease is a frequent complication of autoimmune disease, where the continued production of autoantibody to a self-antigen leads to prolonged immune complex formation. As the number of complexes in the blood increases, the systems that are responsible for the removal of complexes (mononuclear phagocyte, erythrocyte and complement) become overloaded, and complexes are deposited in the tissues (*Fig. 23.3*). Diseases with this aetiology include rheumatoid arthritis, systemic lupus erythematosus (SLE) and polymyositis.

Three categories of immune-complex disease

cause	antigen	site of complex deposition
persistent infection	microbial antigen	infected organ(s), kidney
autoimmunity	self antigen	kidney, joint, arteries, skin
inhaled antigen	mould, plant or animal antigen	lung

Fig. 23.1 This table indicates the source of the antigen and the organs most frequently affected.

Inhalation of antigenic material – Immune complexes may be formed at body surfaces following exposure to extrinsic antigens. Such reactions are seen in the lungs following repeated inhalation of antigenic materials from moulds, plants or animals. This is exemplified in Farmer's lung and

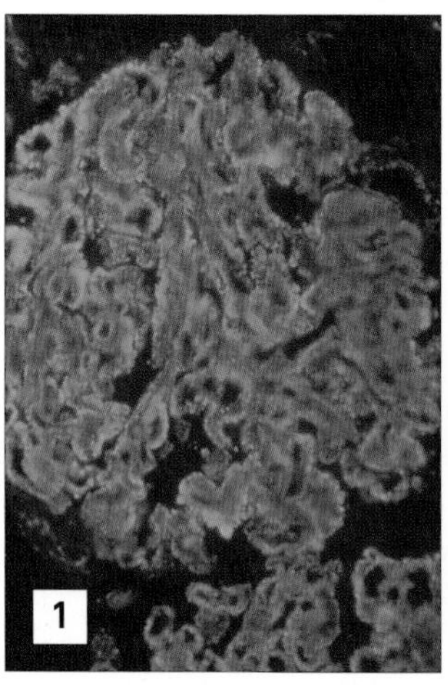
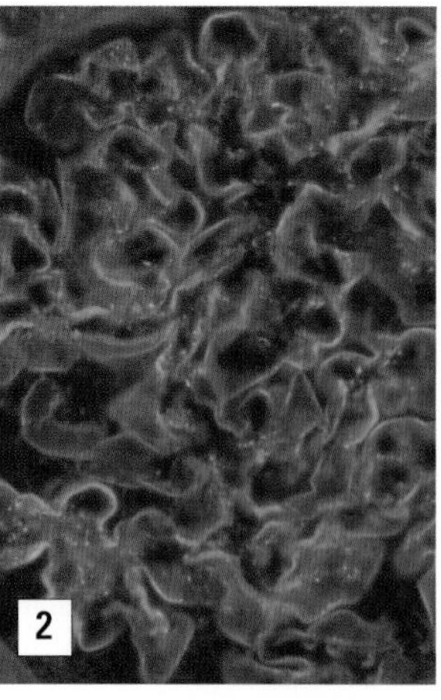

Fig. 23.3 Immunofluorescence study of immune complexes in autoimmune disease. These renal sections compare a patient with systemic lupus erythematosus (Type III hypersensitivity) (**1**) and one with Goodpasture's syndrome (Type II hypersensitivity) (**2**). In each case the antibody was detected with fluorescent anti-IgG. Complexes, formed in the blood and deposited in the kidney, form characteristic 'lumpy bumpy' deposits (**1**). The anti-basement membrane antibody in Goodpasture's syndrome forms an even layer on the glomerular basement membrane. (Courtesy of Dr S. Thiru.)

pigeon fancier's lung, where there are circulating antibodies to actinomycete fungi (found in mouldy hay) or to pigeon antigens. Both diseases are forms of extrinsic allergic alveolitis, and only occur after repeated exposure to the antigen. (Note that the antibodies induced by these antigens are primarily IgG, rather than the IgE seen in Type I hypersensitivity reactions.) When antigen again enters the body by inhalation, local immune complexes are formed in the alveoli leading to inflammation and fibrosis (*Fig. 23.4*). Precipitating antibodies to actinomycete antigens are found in the sera of 90% of patients with Farmer's lung. However, they are also found in some people with no disease, and are absent from some sufferers, so it seems that other factors are also involved in the disease process, including Type IV hypersensitivity reactions.

MECHANISMS IN TYPE III HYPERSENSITIVITY

Immune complexes are capable of triggering a wide variety of inflammatory processes:

- Complexes interact directly with basophils and platelets (via Fc receptors) to induce the release of vasoactive amines (*Fig. 23.5*).
- Macrophages are stimulated to release cytokines, particularly TNFα and IL-1, that are very important during inflammation.
- They interact with the complement system to generate C3a and C5a (anaphylatoxins). These complement fragments stimulate the release of vasoactive amines (including histamine and 5-hydroxytryptamine) and chemotactic factors from mast cells and basophils. C5a is also chemotactic for basophils, eosinophils and neutrophils.

Recent work with knockout mice indicates that complement has a less pro-inflammatory role than previously thought, whereas cells bearing Fc receptors for IgG and IgE appear to be critical for developing inflammation, with complement having a protective effect.

The vasoactive amines released by platelets, basophils and mast cells cause endothelial cell retraction and thus increase vascular permeability, allowing the deposition of immune complexes on the blood vessel wall (*Fig. 23.6*). The deposited complexes continue to generate C3a and C5a.

Platelets also aggregate on the exposed collagen of the vessel basement membrane, assisted by interactions with the Fc regions of deposited immune complexes, to form microthrombi. The aggregated platelets continue to pro-

Extrinsic allergic alveolitis

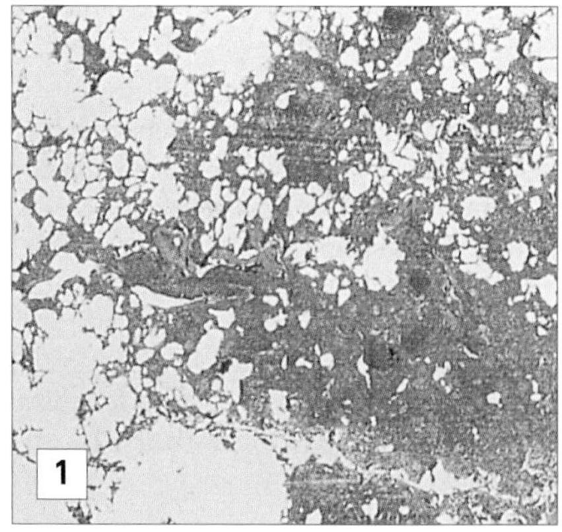
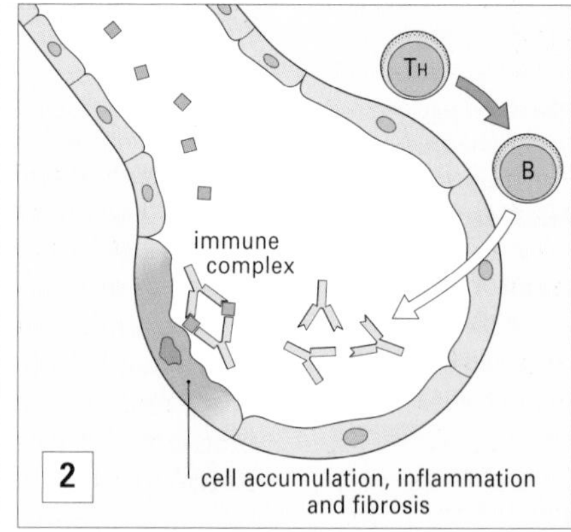

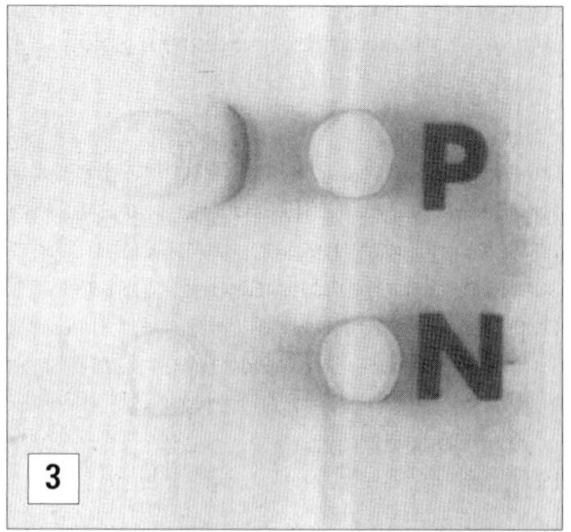

Fig. 23.4 When fungal antigen is inhaled into the lung of a sensitized individual, immune complexes are formed in the alveoli (**2**). Complement fixation leads to cell accumulation, inflammation and fibrosis. The histological appearance of the lung in extrinsic allergic alveolitis (**1**) shows consolidated areas due to cell accumulation. Precipitin antibody present in the serum of a patient with pigeon fancier's lung: P (**3**) is directed against the fungal antigen *Micropolyspora faeni*. Anormal serum (N) lacks antibodies to this fungus.

Immune complexes as a trigger for increasing vascular permeability

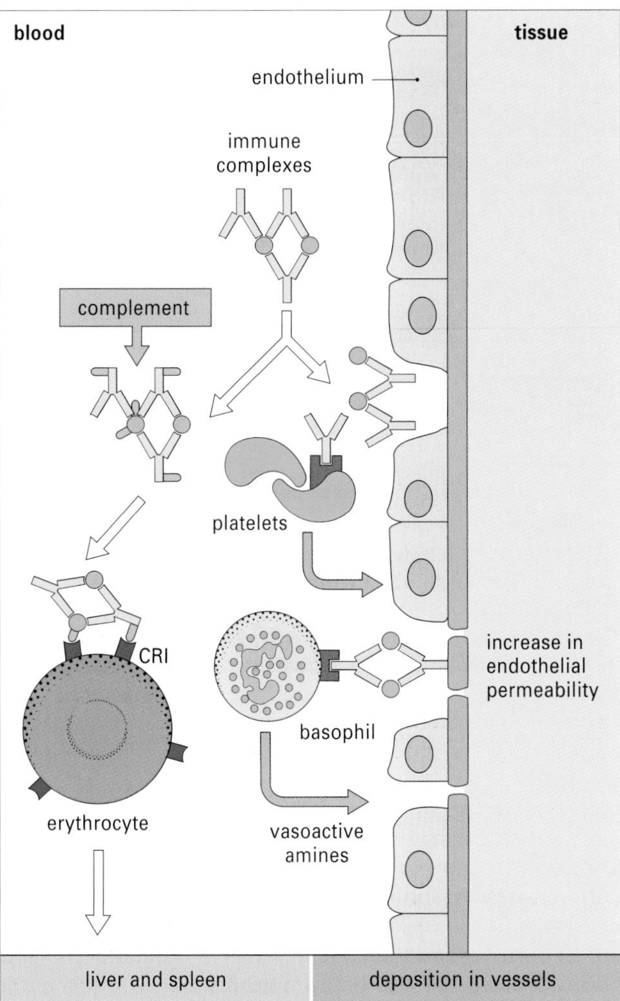

Fig. 23.5 Immune complexes normally bind complement and are removed to the liver and spleen after binding to CR1 on RBC. In inflammation, immune complexes act on basophils and platelets (in humans) to produce vasoactive amine release. The amines released (e.g. histamine, 5-hydroxytryptamine) cause endothelial cell retraction and thus increase vascular permeability.

Deposition of immune complexes in blood vessel walls

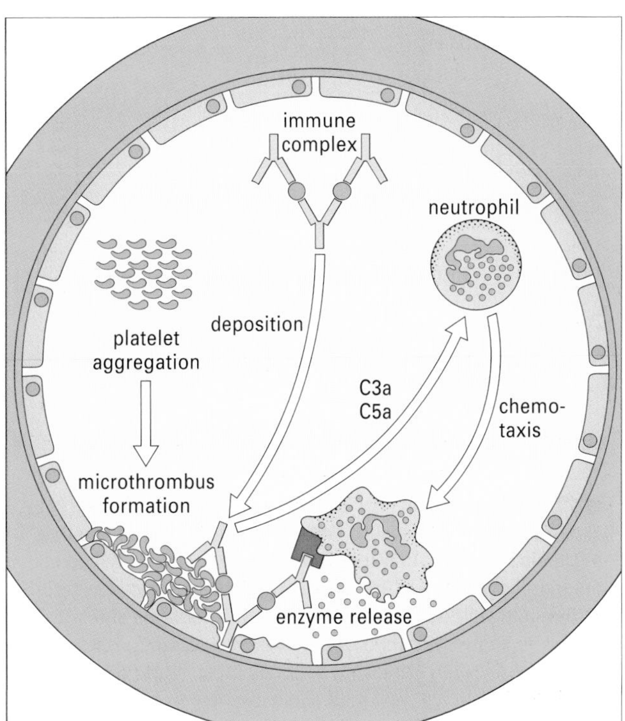

Fig. 23.6 Increased vascular permeability allows immune complexes to be deposited in the blood vessel wall. This induces platelet aggregation and complement activation. The aggregated platelets form microthrombi on the exposed collagen of the basement membrane of the endothelium. Neutrophils are attracted to the site by complement products, but cannot ingest the complexes. They therefore exocytose their lysosomal enzymes, causing further damage to the vessel wall.

duce vasoactive amines and to stimulate the production of C3a and C5a. (Platelets are also a rich source of growth factors – these may be involved in the cellular proliferation seen in immune-complex diseases such as glomerulonephritis and rheumatoid arthritis.)

Polymorphs are chemotactically attracted to the site by C5a. They attempt to engulf the deposited immune complexes, but are unable to do so because the complexes are bound to the vessel wall. They therefore exocytose their lysosomal enzymes onto the site of deposition (*Fig. 23.6*). If simply released into the blood or tissue fluids these lysosomal enzymes are unlikely to cause much inflammation, because they are rapidly neutralized by serum enzyme inhibitors. But if the phagocyte applies itself closely to the tissue-trapped complexes through Fc binding, then serum inhibitors are excluded and the enzymes may damage the underlying tissue.

EXPERIMENTAL MODELS OF IMMUNE-COMPLEX DISEASE

Experimental models are available for each of the three main types of immune-complex disease described above:

- Serum sickness, induced by injections of foreign antigen, mimics the effect of a persistent infection.
- The NZB/NZW mouse demonstrates autoimmunity.
- the Arthus reaction is an example of local damage by extrinsic antigen.

Care must be taken when interpreting animal experiments, as the erythrocytes of rodents and rabbits lack the receptor for C3b (known as CR1) which readily binds immune complexes that have fixed complement. This receptor is present on primate erythrocytes.

Serum sickness can be induced with large injections of foreign antigen

In serum sickness, circulating immune complexes deposit in the blood vessel walls and tissues, leading to increased

Time course of experimental serum sickness

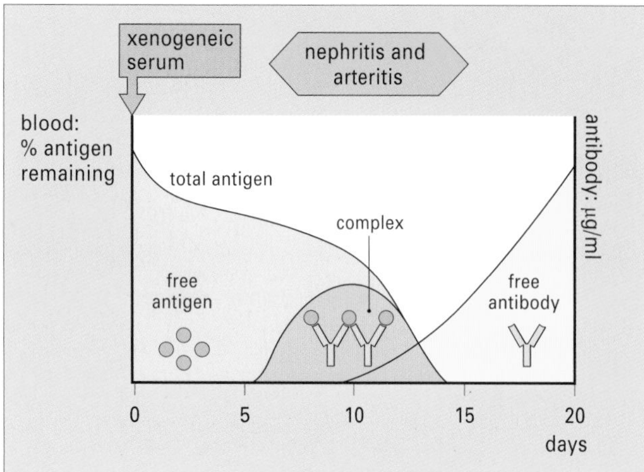

Fig. 23.7 Following an injection of xenogeneic serum there is a lag period of approximately 5 days, in which only free antigen is detectable in serum. After this time, antibodies are produced to the foreign proteins and immune complexes are formed in serum; it is during this period that the symptoms of nephritis and arteritis appear. To begin with, small soluble complexes are found in antigen excess; with increasing antibody titres, larger complexes are formed which are deposited and subsequently cleared. At this stage the symptoms disappear.

Autoimmune disease in NZB/NZW mice

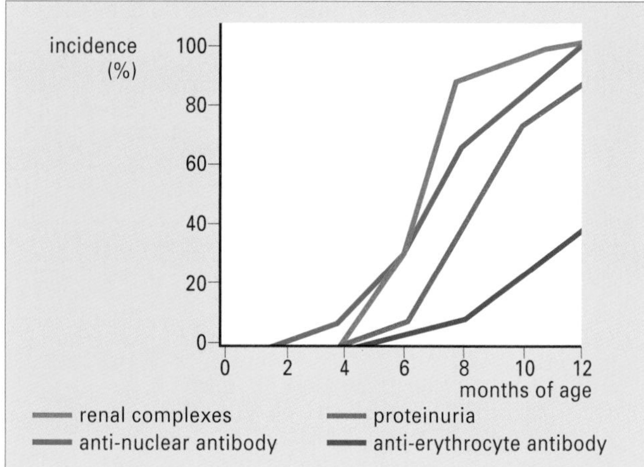

Fig. 23.8 The graph shows the onset of autoimmune disease in female NZB/NZW mice with advancing age. Incidence refers to the percentage of mice with the features identified. Immune complexes were detected by immunofluorescent staining of a kidney section. Anti-nuclear antibodies were detected in serum by indirect immunofluorescence. Proteinuria reflects kidney damage. Autoantibodies to erythrocytes develop later in the disease and so are less likely to relate to kidney pathology. Onset of autoimmune disease is delayed in male mice by approximately 3 months.

vascular permeability and thus to inflammatory diseases such as glomerulonephritis and arthritis.

In the pre-antibiotic era, serum sickness was a complication of serum therapy, in which massive doses of antibody were given for diseases such as diphtheria. Horse anti-diphtheria serum was usually used, and some individuals made antibodies against the horse proteins.

Serum sickness is now commonly studied in rabbits by giving them an intravenous injection of a foreign soluble protein such as bovine serum albumin (BSA). After about one week antibodies are formed which enter the circulation and complex with antigen. Because the reaction occurs in antigen excess, the immune complexes are small (*Fig. 23.7*). These small complexes are only removed slowly by the mononuclear phagocyte system and therefore persist in the circulation. The formation of complexes is followed by an abrupt fall in total haemolytic complement; the clinical signs of serum sickness that develop are due to granular deposits of antigen–antibody and C3 forming along the glomerular basement membrane (GBM) and in small vessels elsewhere. As more antibody is formed and the reaction moves into antibody excess, the size of the complexes increases and they are cleared more efficiently, so the animals recover. Chronic disease is induced by daily administration of antigen.

Autoimmunity causes immune-complex disease in the NZB/NZW mouse

The F_1 hybrid NZB/NZW mouse produces a range of autoantibodies (including anti-erythrocyte, anti-nuclear, anti-DNA and anti-*Sm*) and suffers from an immune-complex disease similar in many ways to SLE in humans. An NZB/NZW mouse is born clinically normal, but within 2–3 months shows sign of haemolytic anaemia. Tests for anti-erythrocyte antibody (the Coombs' test), anti-nuclear antibodies, lupus cells and circulating immune complexes are all positive, and there are deposits in the glomeruli and choroid plexus of the brain. The disease is much more marked in the females, who die within a few months of developing symptoms (*Fig. 23.8*).

Injection of antigen into the skin of presensitized animals produces the Arthus reaction

The Arthus reaction takes place at a local site in and around the walls of small blood vessels; it is most frequently demonstrated in the skin.

An animal is immunized repeatedly until it has appreciable levels of serum antibody (mainly IgG). Following subcutaneous or intradermal injection of the antigen a reaction develops at the injection site, sometimes with marked oedema and haemorrhage, depending on the amount of antigen injected. The reaction reaches a peak after 4–10 hours, then wanes and is usually minimal by 48 hours (*Fig. 23.9*). Immunofluorescence studies have shown that initial deposition of antigen, antibody and complement in the vessel wall is followed by neutrophil infiltration and intravascular clumping of platelets (*Fig. 23.10*). This platelet reaction can lead to vascular occlusion and necrosis in severe cases. After 24–48 hours the neutrophils are replaced by mononuclear cells and eventually some plasma cells appear.

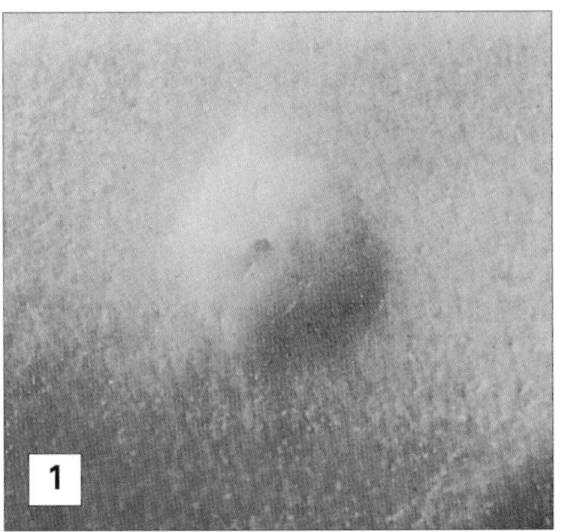

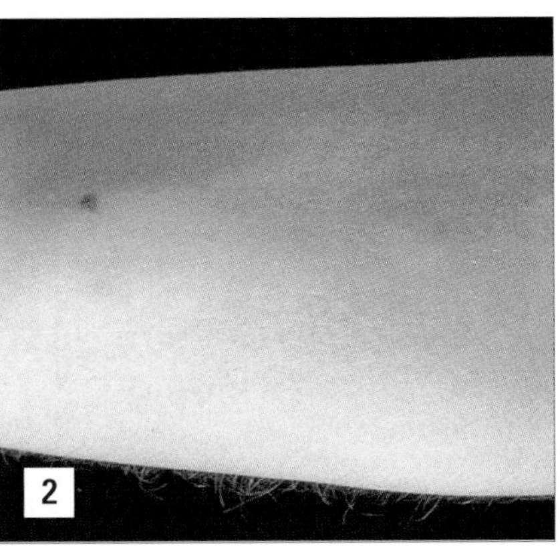

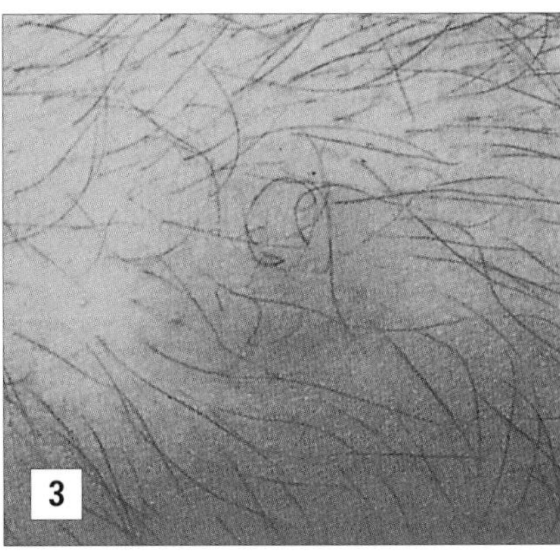

Fig. 23.9 The appearance of the three main skin test reactions. A type I hypersensitivity reaction (**1**) produces a raised wheal, 5–7 mm in diameter and with a well-defined edge after about 15 minutes. A Type III hypersensitivity Arthus reaction (**2**) produces a reaction after 5–12 hours that is larger (50 mm or more), and which has a less well defined edge. A Type IV (delayed) hypersensitivity reaction shows as a red indurated lesion, about 5 mm in diameter, at 24–48 hours (**3**).

The Arthus reaction

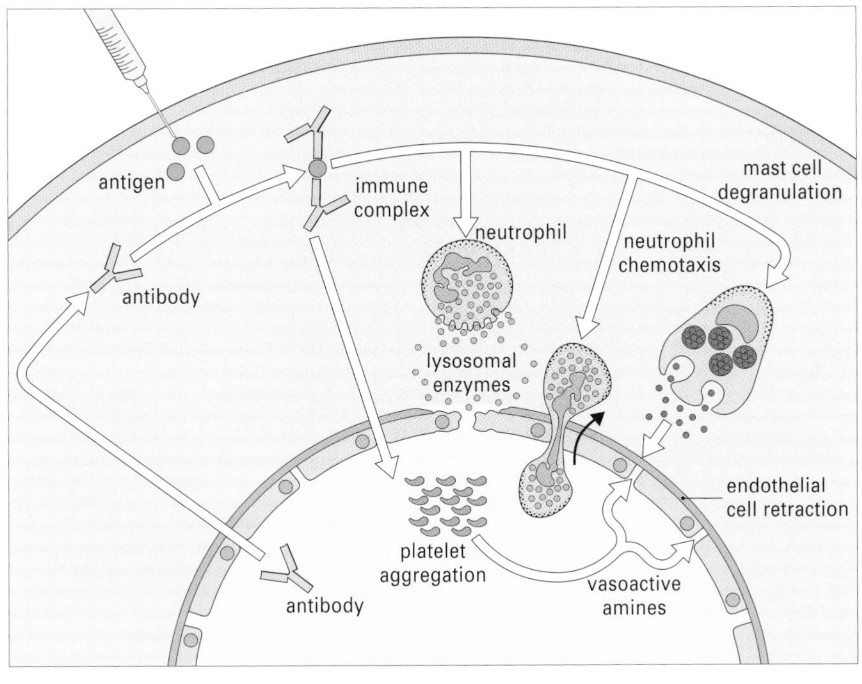

Fig. 23.10 Antigen injected intradermally combines with specific antibody from the blood to form immune complexes. The complexes act on platelets and mast cells, which release vasoactive amines. Immune complexes also induce macrophages to release TNF and IL-1 (not shown). Mast cell products, including histamine and leukotrienes, induce increased blood flow and capillary permeability. The inflammatory reaction is potentiated by lysosomal enzymes released from the polymorphs. The Arthus reaction can be seen in patients with precipitating antibodies, such as those with extrinsic allergic alveolitis associated with Farmer's lung disease.

Complement activation via either the classical or alternative pathways was thought to be essential for the Arthus reaction to develop. But C3, C4 or C5 deficient mice were able to mount a normal Arthus reaction. However, when mice were made deficient in FcγRI or FcγRIII they were unable to produce the reaction. Furthermore, when recombinant soluble FcγRII receptors were given they inhibited the development of the Arthus reaction.

TNFα enhances cell-mediated immune responses in various ways (see Chapter 9). Treatment with antibodies to TNF can reduce severity in the Arthus reaction and, interestingly, anti-TNF is useful in treating rheumatoid arthritis.

The ratio of antibody to antigen is directly related to the severity of the ensuing reaction. Complexes formed in either antigen or antibody excess are much less toxic than those formed at equivalence.

PERSISTENCE OF COMPLEXES

Immune complexes are normally removed by the mononuclear phagocyte system

Immune complexes are opsonized with C3b following complement activation, and removed by the mononuclear phagocyte system, particularly in the liver and spleen.

Removal is mediated by the complement C3b receptor, CR1. In primates, the bulk of CR1 in blood is found on erythrocytes. (Non-primates do not have erythrocyte CR1, and must therefore rely on platelet CR1.) There are about 700 receptors per erythrocyte, and their effectiveness is enhanced by the grouping of receptors in patches, allowing high-avidity binding to the large complexes. CR1 readily binds immune complexes that have fixed complement as has been shown by experiments with animals lacking complement (*Fig. 23.11*).

In normal primates the erythrocytes provide a buffer mechanism, binding complexes which have fixed complement and effectively removing them from the plasma. In small blood vessels 'streamline flow' allows the erythrocytes to travel in the centre of the vessel surrounded by the flowing plasma. Thus it is only the plasma that makes contact with the vessel wall. Only in the sinusoids of the liver and spleen, or at sites of turbulence, do the erythrocytes make contact with the lining of the vessels.

The complexes are transported to the liver and spleen, where they are removed by fixed tissue macrophages (*Fig. 23.12*). Most of the CR1 is also removed in the process so, in situations of continuous immune-complex formation, the number of active receptors falls rapidly, impairing the efficiency of immune complex handling. In patients with SLE, for example, the number of receptors may well be halved. With less complement receptors the complexes are cleared rapidly to the liver, but these complexes which have arrived directly rather than on red cells are later released into the circulation again and may then deposit in the tissues elsewhere and lead to inflammation.

Complexes can also be released from erythrocytes in the circulation by the enzymatic action of Factor I, which cleaves C3b leaving a small fragment (C3dg) attached to the CR1 on the cell membrane. These soluble complexes are then removed by phagocytic cells, particularly those in the liver, bearing receptors for IgG Fc (*Fig. 23.13*).

Effects of complement depletion on handling of immune complexes

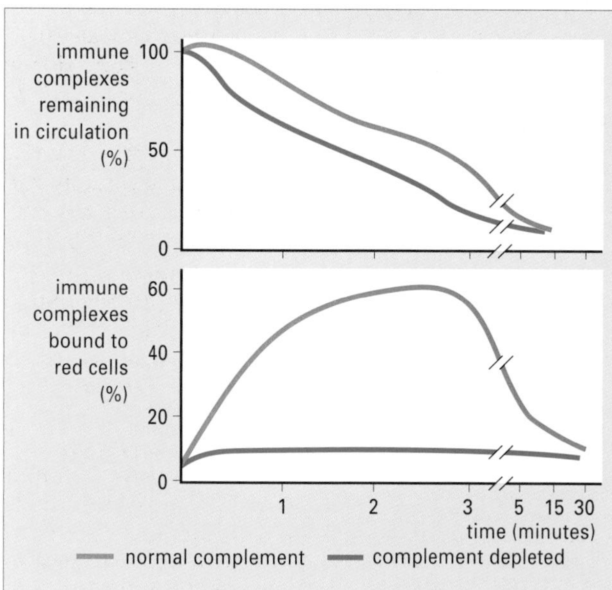

Fig. 23.11 A bolus of immune complexes was infused into the circulation of a primate. In animals with a normal complement system the complexes were bound quickly by the CR1 on erythrocytes. In animals whose complement had been depleted by treatment with cobra venom factor, the erythrocytes hardly bound immune complexes at all. Paradoxically, this results in slightly faster removal of complexes in the depleted animals, with the complexes being deposited in the tissues rather than being removed by the spleen. (Based on data from Waxman *et al. J Clin Invest* 1984;**74**:1329–40.)

Clearance of immune complexes in the liver

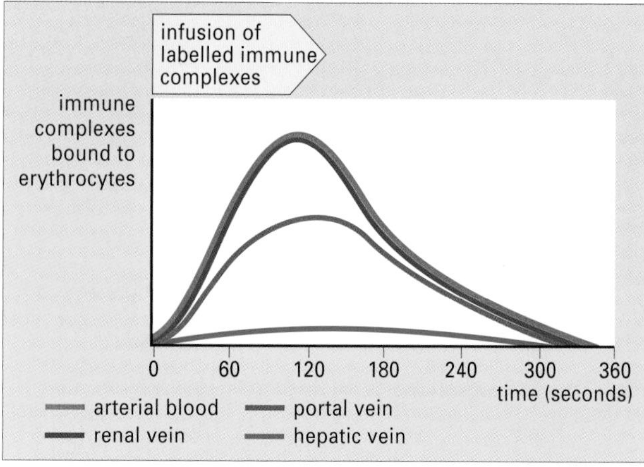

Fig. 23.12 ^{125}I-BSA/anti-BSA complexes were infused into a primate over a period of 120 seconds. Blood was sampled from renal, portal and hepatic veins, and the level of immune complexes bound to the erythrocytes was measured by radioactive counting. The levels of complexes in the renal and portal veins were similar to that in arterial blood. However, complexes were virtually absent from hepatic venous blood throughout, indicating that complexes bound to erythrocytes are removed during a single transit through the liver. (Based on data from Cornacoff *et al. J Clin Invest* 1983;**71**:236–47.)

Complement solubilization of immune complexes

It has been known since Heidelberger's work on the precipitin curve in the 1930s that complement delays precipitation of immune complexes, although this information was forgotten for a long time. The ability to keep immune complexes soluble is a function of the classical complement pathway. The complement components reduce the number of antigen epitopes that the antibodies can bind (i.e. they reduce the valency of the antigen) by intercalating into the lattice of the complex, resulting in smaller, soluble complexes. In primates these complement-bearing complexes are readily bound by the C3b receptor (CR1) on erythrocytes.

Complement can rapidly resolubilize precipitated complexes through the alternative pathway (*Fig. 23.14*). The solubilization appears to occur by the insertion of complement C3b and C3d fragments into the complexes.

Immune complex clearance

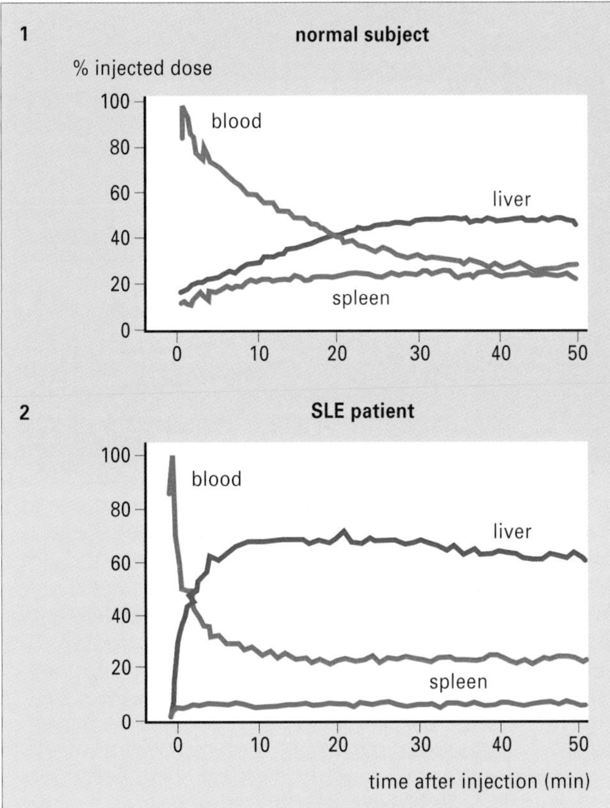

Fig. 23.13 (**1**) Immune complex clearance in healthy normal subject. (**2**) Immune complex clearance in patient with SLE. Radiolabelled soluble complexes were injected intravenously and immune complex localization monitored by dynamic imaging. In the normal subject complexes remained longer in the blood through binding to CR1 on red cells, followed by clearance to the liver and the spleen, where immune complexes take part in immunoregulation. In the hypocomplementaemic SLE patient there was little binding to red cells but rapid clearance to organs such as the liver, with little localizing to the spleen, leading to impaired immunoregulation which may be a factor in the persistence of autoimmunity.

It may be that complexes are continually being deposited in normal individuals, but are removed by solubilization. If this is the case, then the process will be inadequate in hypocomplementaemic patients and lead to prolonged complex deposition. Solubilization defects have indeed been observed in sera from patients with systemic immune-complex disease, but whether the defect is primary or secondary is not known.

Complement deficiency impairs clearance of complexes

In patients with low levels of classical pathway components there is poor binding of immune complexes to erythrocytes. The complement deficiency may be due to depletion, caused by immune-complex disease, or could be due to a hereditary disorder, as is the case in C2 deficiency. This might be expected to result in persistent immune complexes in the circulation but in fact the reverse occurs, with

Solubilization of immune complexes by complement

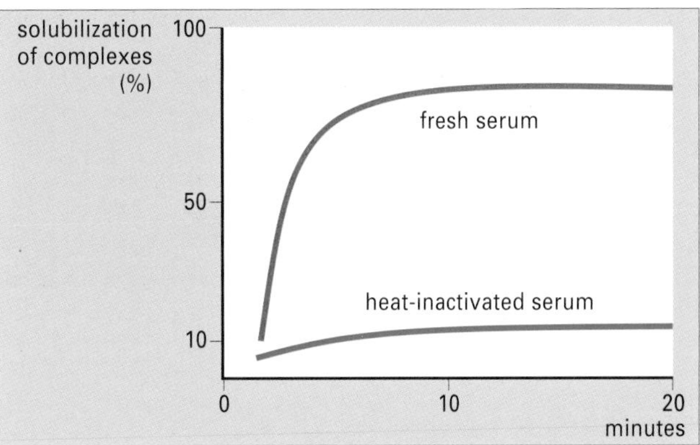

Fig. 23.14 Complement can solubilize precipitable complexes *in vitro*. Addition of fresh serum containing active complement to insoluble complexes induces solubilization over about 15 minutes at 37°C. Some of the complexes resist resolubilization. Heated serum (56°C for 30 minutes) lacks active complement and cannot resolubilize the complexes. Intercalation of complement components C3b and C3d into the complex causes their solubilization by disrupting antigen–antibody bonds. Complexes that have been artificially connected by covalent bonds cannot be solubilized by complement.

the complexes disappearing rapidly from the circulation. These non-erythrocyte-bound complexes are taken up rapidly by the liver (but not the spleen) and are then released to be deposited in tissues such as skin, kidney and muscle, where they can set up inflammatory reactions (*Fig. 23.15*).

Infusion of fresh plasma, containing complement, restores the clearance patterns to normal, illustrating the importance of complement in clearance of immune complexes. Failure to localize in the spleen not only results in immune-complex disease, but may also have important implications for the development of appropriate immune responses. This is because the spleen plays a vital role in antigen processing and induction of immune responses (see Chapter 2).

The size of immune complexes affects their deposition

In general, larger immune complexes are rapidly removed by the liver within a few minutes, whereas smaller complexes circulate for longer periods (*Fig. 23.16*). This is because larger complexes are more effective at binding to Fc receptors and at fixing complement so binding better to erythrocytes. Also, larger complexes are released more slowly from the erythrocytes by the action of Factor I. Anything that affects the size of complexes is therefore likely to influence clearance. It has been suggested that a genetic defect which favours produc-tion of low-affinity antibody could well lead to formation of smaller complexes, and so to immune-complex disease. Affinity maturation is dependent on efficient somatic mutation and selection of B cells within germinal centres following binding of antigen. This process is far more effective when B cells are stimulated by antigen or immune complexes coated with

Immune-complex transport and removal

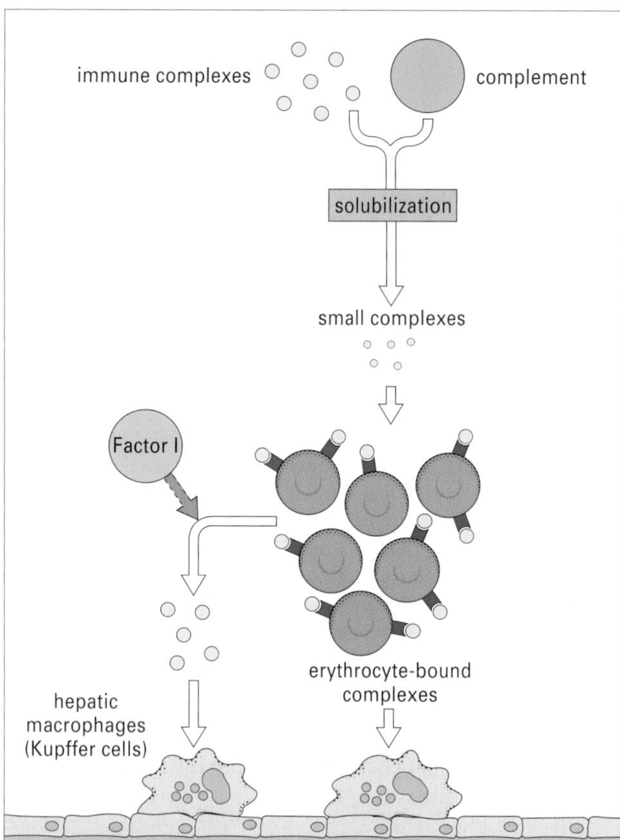

Fig. 23.15 In primates, complexes solubilized by complement are bound by CR1 on erythrocytes and transported to the liver where they are removed by hepatic macrophages. Complexes released from erythrocytes by Factor I are taken up by cells (including macrophages) bearing receptors for Fc and complement.

Complex clearance by mononuclear phagocytes

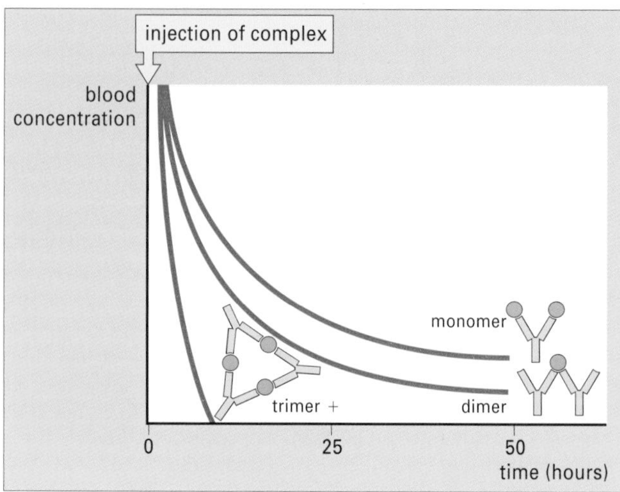

Fig. 23.16 Large immune complexes are cleared most quickly because they present an IgG–Fc lattice to mononuclear phagocytes cells with Fc receptors, permitting higher avidity binding to these cells. They also fix complement better than small complexes.

complement. Patients with complement deficiencies are particularly prone to develop immune complex disease and recent evidence indicates that one of the ways this is brought about is through poor targeting of antigen complexes to germinal centres so preventing affinity maturation. Antibodies to self antigens may have low affinity and recognize only a few epitopes. This results in small complexes and long clearance times, because the formation of large, cross-linked lattices is restricted.

Immunoglobulin classes affect the rate of immune-complex clearance

Striking differences have been observed in the clearance of complexes with different immunoglobulin classes. IgG complexes are bound by erythrocytes and are gradually removed from the circulation, whereas IgA complexes bind poorly to erythrocytes but disappear rapidly from the circulation, with increased deposition in the kidney, lung and brain.

Phagocyte defects allow complexes to persist

Opsonized immune complexes are normally removed by the mononuclear phagocyte system, mainly in the liver and spleen. However, when large amounts of complex are present, the mononuclear phagocyte system may become overloaded, leading to a rise in the level of circulating complex and increased deposition in the glomerulus and elsewhere. Defective mononuclear phagocytes have been observed in human immune-complex disease, but this may well be the result of overload rather than a primary defect.

Carbohydrate on antibodies affects complex clearance

Carbohydrate groups on immunoglobulin molecules have been shown to be important for the efficient removal of immune complexes by phagocytic cells. Abnormalities of these carbohydrates occur in immune-complex diseases such as rheumatoid arthritis, thus aggravating the disease process. IgGFc oligosaccharides lack the normally terminating galactose residue, enhancing rheumatoid-factor binding. Recently, mannan binding protein has been shown to bind agalactosyl IgG and subsequently activate complement.

DEPOSITION OF COMPLEXES IN TISSUES

Immune complexes may persist in the circulation for prolonged periods of time. However, simple persistence is not usually harmful in itself; the problems only start when complexes are deposited in the tissues.

Two questions are relevant to tissue deposition:

- Why are complexes deposited?
- Why do complexes show affinity for particular tissues in different diseases?

Effect of a vasoactive amine antagonist on immune-complex disease

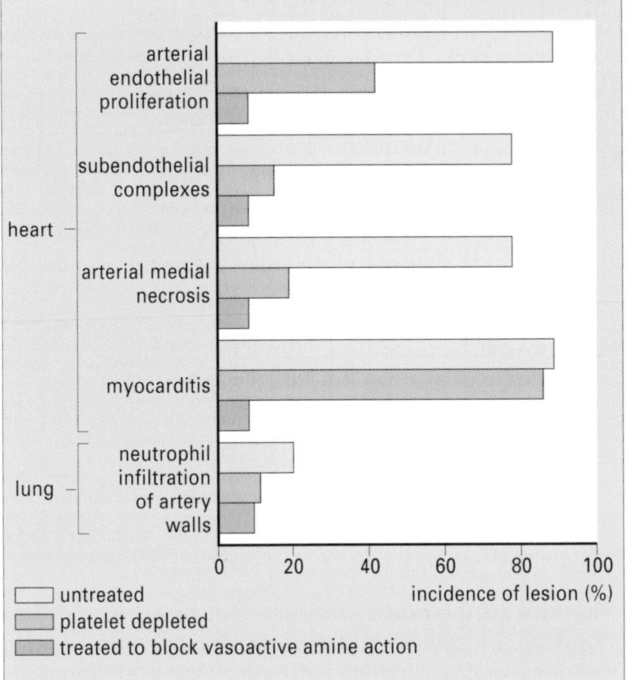

Fig. 23.17 Serum sickness was induced in rabbits with a single injection of bovine serum albumin. The animals were either untreated, platelet depleted or treated with drugs to block vasoactive amine action. The incidence of serum sickness lesions in the heart and lung was scored. Drug treatment considerably reduced the signs of disease by lowering vascular permeability and thus minimizing immune-complex deposition.

Effect of the vasoactive amine antagonist methysergide on kidney damage

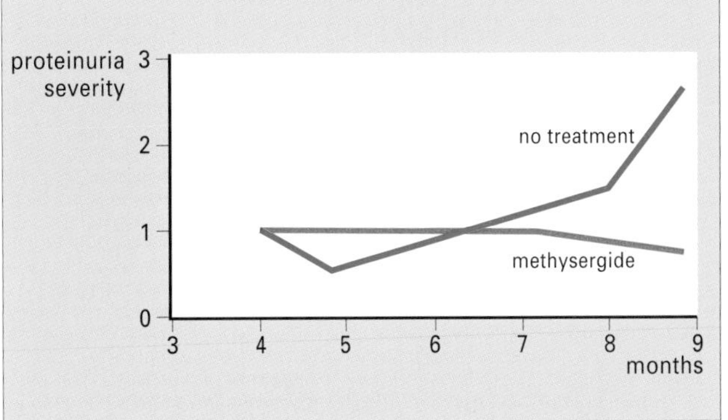

Fig. 23.18 Kidney damage, assessed by proteinuria, was measured in NZB/NZW mice over 5 months. Untreated animals developed severe proteinuria, while methysergide-treated animals did not. Methysergide blocks formation of the vasoactive amine, 5-HT, and thus blocks a variety of inflammatory events, e.g. deposition of complexes, neutrophil infiltration of capillary walls and endothelial proliferation, all of which produce the glomerular pathology.

The most important trigger for tissue deposition of immune complexes is probably an increase in vascular permeability

Animal experiments have shown that inert substances such as colloidal carbon will be deposited in vessel walls following administration of vasoactive substances, such as histamine or serotonin. Circulating immune complexes are deposited in a similar way following the infusion of agents that cause liberation of mast cell vasoactive amines (including histamine). Pretreatment with antihistamines blocks this effect.

In studies of experimental immune-complex disease in rabbits, long-term administration of vasoactive amine antagonists, such as chlorpheniramine and methysergide, has been shown considerably to reduce immune complex deposition (*Fig. 23.17*). More importantly (from the point of view of disease prevention), young NZB/NZW mice treated with methysergide show less renal pathology than controls (*Fig. 23.18*).

Increases in vascular permeability can be initiated by a range of mechanisms which vary in importance, depending on the diseases and species concerned. This variability makes interpretation of some of the animal models difficult. In general, however, complement, mast cells, basophils and platelets must all be considered as potential producers of vasoactive amines.

Haemodynamic factors affecting complex deposition

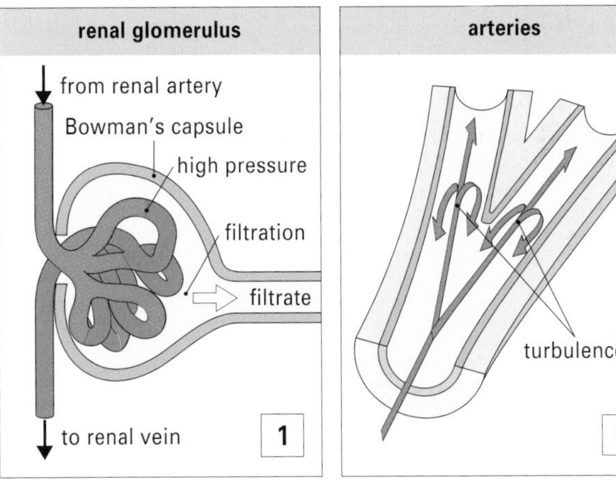

Fig. 23.19 Factors that affect complex deposition include filtration and high blood pressure, both of which occur in the formation of ultrafiltrate in the renal glomerulus (**1**). Turbulence at curves or bifurcations of arteries (**2**) also favours deposition of immune complexes.

Immune-complex deposition is most likely where there is high blood pressure and turbulence

Many macromolecules deposit in the glomerular capillaries, where the blood pressure is approximately four times that of most other capillaries (*Fig. 23.19*). If the glomerular blood pressure of a rabbit is reduced by partially constricting the renal artery or by ligating the ureter, deposition is also reduced. If the glomerular blood pressure is increased by experimentally induced hypertension, immune complex deposition is also enhanced as shown by the development of serum sickness. Elsewhere, the most severe lesions also occur at sites of turbulence. They occur at turns of bifurcations of arteries, and in vascular filters such as the choroid plexus, and the ciliary body of the eye.

Affinity of antigens for specific tissues can direct complexes to particular sites

Local high blood pressure explains the tendency for deposits to form in certain organs, but does not explain why complexes are deposited on specific organs in certain diseases. In SLE, the kidney is a particular target, whereas in rheumatoid arthritis, although circulating complexes are present, the kidney is usually spared and the joints are the principal target.

It is possible that the antigen in the complex provides the organ specificity, and a convincing model has been established to support this hypothesis. In the model, mice are given endotoxin causing cell damage and release of DNA, which then binds to healthy glomerular basement membrane. Anti-DNA is then produced by polyclonal activation of B cells, and is bound by the fixed DNA leading to local immune complex formation (*Fig. 23.20*). The production of rheumatoid factor IgM anti-IgG allows further immune-complex formation to occur *in situ*. It is possible that in other diseases antigens will be identified with affinity for particular organs.

The charge of the antigen and antibody may be important in some systems. For example, positively charged antigens and antibodies are more likely to be deposited in the negatively charged glomerular basement membrane. The degree of glycosylation also affects the fate of complexes containing glycoprotein antigens because certain clearance mechanisms are activated by recognition of sugar molecules, e.g. mannan binding protein.

In certain diseases the antibodies and antigens are both produced within the target organ. The extreme of this is reached in rheumatoid arthritis, where IgG anti-IgG rheumatoid factor is produced by plasma cells within the synovium; these antibodies then combine with each other (self-association), so setting up an inflammatory reaction.

Tissue binding of antigen with local immune-complex formation

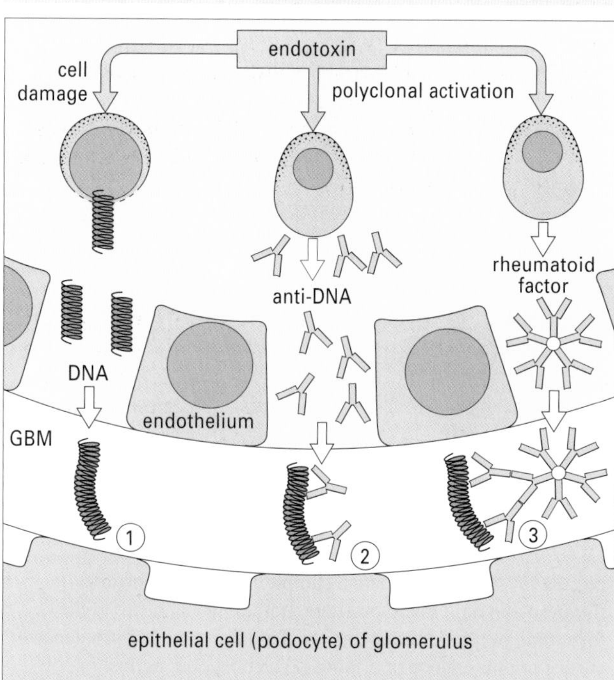

Fig. 23.20 Endotoxin, injected into mice, increases vascular permeability and induces cell damage and release of DNA. The DNA can then become deposited (**1**) on the collagen of the glomerular basement membrane (GBM) in the kidney. Endotoxin can also induce a polyclonal stimulation of B cells, some of which produce autoantibodies such as anti-DNA and anti-IgG – the latter are known as rheumatoid factors (RFs). Anti-DNA antibody can then bind to the deposited DNA forming a local immune complex (**2**). RFs have a low affinity for monomeric IgG, but bind with high avidity to the assembled DNA–anti-DNA complex (**3**). Thus further immune complex formation occurs *in situ*.

The site of immune-complex deposition depends partly on the size of the complex

This is exemplified in the kidney: small immune complexes can pass through the glomerular basement membrane,

Immune-complex deposition in the kidney

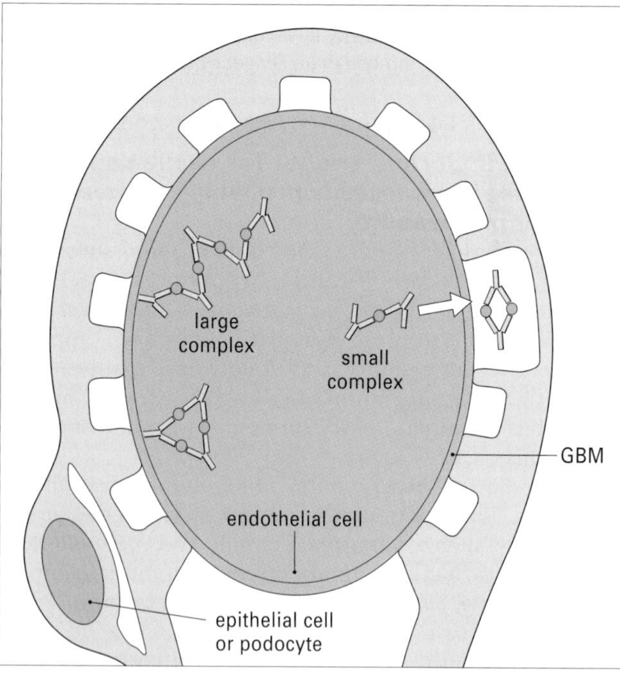

Fig. 23.21 The site of complex deposition in the kidney is dependent on the size of the complexes in the circulation. Large complexes become deposited on the glomerular basement membrane, while small complexes pass through the basement membrane and are seen on the epithelial side of the glomerulus.

and end up on the epithelial side of the membrane; large complexes are unable to cross the membrane and generally accumulate between the endothelium and the basement membrane or the mesangium (*Fig. 23.21*). The size of immune complexes depends on the valency of the antigen, and on the titre and affinity of the antibody.

The class of immunoglobulin in an immune complex can also influence its deposition

There are marked age- and sex-related variations in the class and subclass of anti-DNA antibodies seen in SLE. Similarly, as NZB/NZW mice grow older there is a class switch, from predominantly IgM to IgG2a. This occurs earlier in females than in males and coincides with the onset of renal disease, indicating the importance of antibody class in the tissue deposition of complexes (*Fig. 23.22*).

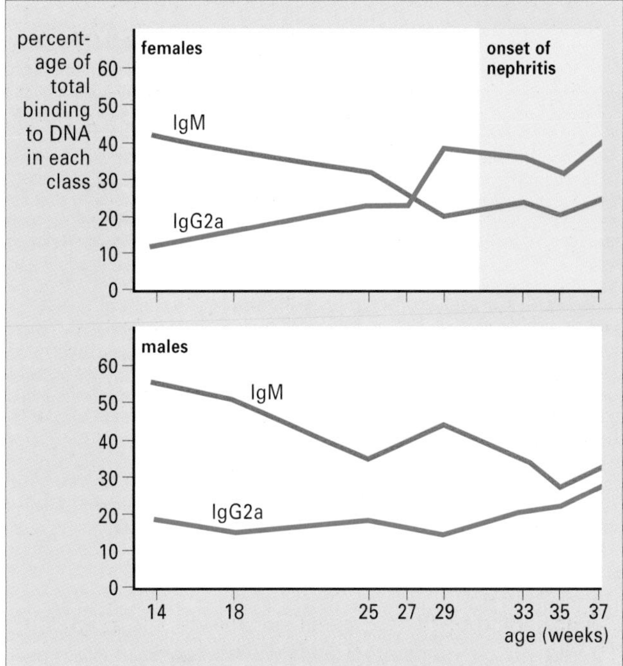

Fig. 23.22 Immune-complex disease is automatic in the NZB/NZW mouse and follows a class switch during early development, from IgM to IgG2a. The graphs show the proportions of anti-DNA antibodies of the IgM and IgG2a isotypes in females and males. Both the class switch and fatal renal disease occur earlier in the female mice of this strain.

DETECTION OF IMMUNE COMPLEXES

Deposited immune complexes can be visualized using immunofluorescence

The ideal place to look for complexes is in the affected organ. Tissue samples may be examined by immunofluorescence for the presence of immunoglobulin and complement. The composition, pattern and particular area of tissue affected all provide useful information on the severity and prognosis of the disease. For example, patients with the continuous, granular, subepithelial deposits of IgG found in membranous glomerulonephritis have a poor prognosis. In contrast, those whose complexes are localized in the mesangium have a good prognosis. Not all tissue-bound complexes give rise to an inflammatory response; for example in SLE, complexes are frequently found in skin biopsies from normal-looking skin, as well as from inflamed skin.

Assays for circulating immune complexes

Circulating complexes are found in two separate compartments: bound to erythrocytes and free in plasma. Erythrocyte-bound complexes are less likely to be damaging, so it is of more interest to determine the level of free complexes. Care is required when collecting the sample: bound complexes can easily be released during clotting by the action of Factor I. To obtain accurate assays of free complexes, the erythrocytes should be rapidly separated from the plasma to prevent the release of bound complexes.

CRITICAL THINKING • Drug allergy (Explanations on pp 461–462)

As a child, Yvonne had a number of sore throats for which the doctor had prescribed antibiotics, in particular penicillin. After a number of courses she developed a rash, was told that she had developed an allergy to penicillin and that she should not have it again. Fortunately, once she left school, she had very few further infections that needed antibiotic therapy.

Towards the end of a holiday abroad, at the age of 28, Yvonne developed acute cystitis with difficulty of micturition and some urinary frequency. When she got home she went to see her doctor, who gave her an antibiotic, trimethoprim, which she was to take for 8 days. She was, of course, not given penicillin.

She finished all the tablets and 3 days later developed a headache and some itchy lumps on her skin. The next day she had aching and swollen joints, mainly of the wrists and knees, although her hands were affected as well. She did not think that these symptoms had anything to do with the drug as she had already stopped taking it. She went to her doctor who confirmed that the rash was urticaria, but she also had a raised temperature and swollen glands in her neck. Examination of her urine showed evidence of protein.

The doctor asked for some further tests (see table below) but in the meantime gave her some antihistamines with the warning that if these were not helpful she would need a course of corticosteroids. He diagnosed a drug allergy.

Investigation	**Result** (normal range)
haemoglobin (g/dl)	14.1 (11.5–16.0)
white cell count ($\times 10^9$/l)	10.1 (4.0–11.0)
eosinophils ($\times 10^9$/l)	1.45 (0.4–0.44)
total lymphocytes ($\times 10^9$/l)	2.2 (1.6–3.5)
ESR	34 mm/h (0–20)
C3 (g/l)	0.41 (0.75–1.65)
C4 (g/l)	0.09 (0.20–0.65)
ANA	negative
rheumatoid factor	negative

Her symptoms did not improve and she was started on oral prednisone. A renal biopsy was considered but not done because all the symptoms cleared following a course of corticosteroids.

Three weeks later Yvonne went for a check up and all her tests had returned to normal.

23.1 What is the likely mechanism of the reaction she had whilst on holiday?

23.2 What non-immunological factors can lead to drug reactions?

23.3 Does a pre-existing drug allergy make the patient more likely to react to other drugs in the future?

23.4 What was the reason for asking for an autoantibody screen?

FURTHER READING

Agnello V. Immune complex assays in rheumatic diseases. *Hum Pathol* 1983;**14**:343–9.

Arthus M. Injections répétées de sérum de cheval chez le lapin. *C R Seances Soc Biol Filiales* 1903;**55**:817.

Birmingham DJ, Herbert LA, Cosio FG, *et al.* Immune complex erythrocyte complement receptor interactions *in vivo* during induction of glomerulonephritis in non-human primates. *J Lab Clin Med* 1990;**116**:242–52.

Boackle SA, Holer VM, Karp DR. CD21 augments antigen presentation in immune individuals. *Eur J Immunol* 1997;**27**:122–29.

Cornacoff JB, Hebert LA, Smead WL, Vanaman ME, Birmingham DJ, Waxman FJ. Primate erythrocyte immune complex clearing mechanism. *J Clin Invest* 1983;**71**:236–47.

Clynes R, Maizes JS, Guinamard R, Ono M, Takai T, Ravetch JV. Modulation of immune-complex-induced inflammation *in vivo* by the co-ordinate expression of activation and inhibitory Fc receptors. *J Exp Med* 1999;**189**:179–85.

Czop J, Nussenzweig V. Studies on the mechanism of solubilization of immune precipitates by serum. *J Exp Med* 1976;**143**:615–30.

Davies KA, Hird V, Stewart S, *et al.* A study of *in vivo* immune complex formation and clearing in man. *J Immunol* 1990;**144**:4613–20.

Davies KA, Peters AM, Beynon HLC, Walport MJ. Immune complex processing in patients with systemic lupus erythematosus – *in vivo* imaging and clearance studies. *J Clin Invest* 1992;**90**:2075–83.

Davies KA, Chapman PT, Norsworthy PJ, *et al.* Clearance pathway of soluble immune complexes in the pig. Insights into the adaptive nature of antigen clearance in humans. *J Immunol* 1995;**155**:5760–8.

Davies KA, Schifferli JA, Walport MJ. Complement deficiency and immune complex diseases. *Springer Seminars in Immunopathology* 1994;**15**:397–416.

Dixon FJ, Joseph D, Feldman JD, *et al.* Experimental glomerulonephritis: the pathogenesis of a laboratory model resembling the spectrum of human glomerulonephritis. *J Exp Med* 1961;**113**:899–919.

Dixon FJ, Vazquez JJ, Weigle WO, *et al.* Pathogenesis of serum sickness. *Arch Pathol* 1958;**65**:18–28.

Emlen W, Carl V, Burdick CG. Mechanism of transfer of immune complexes from red blood cell CR1 to monocytes. *Clin Exp Immunol* 1992;**89**:8–17.

Finbloom DS, Magilvary DB, Harford JB, *et al.* Influence of antigen on immune complex behaviour in mice. *J Clin Invest* 1981;**68**:214–24.

Heidelberger M. Quantitative chemical studies on complement or alexin. *J Exp Med* 1941;**73**:681–709.

Inman RD. Immune complexes in SLE. *Clin Rheum Dis* 1982;**8**:49–62.

Johnston A, Auda GR, Kerr MA, *et al.* Dissociation of primary antigen-antibody bonds is essential for complement mediated solubilization of immune complexes. *Mol Immunol* 1992;**29**:659–65.

Kijlstrea H, van Es LA, Daha MR. The role of complement in the binding and degradation of immunoglobulin aggregates by macrophages. *J Immunol* 1979;**123**:2488–93.

Lachmann PJ. Complement deficiency and the pathogenesis of autoimmune complex disease. *Chem Immunol* 1980;**49**:245–63.

Lucisano Valim M, Lachmann PJ. The effects of antibody isotype and antigenic epitope density on the complement-fixing activity of immune complexes: a systematic study using chimaeric anti-NIP antibodies with human Fc regions. *Clin Exp Immunol* 1991;**84**:1–8.

McKenzie SE, Taylor SM, Malladi P, *et al.* The role of the human Fc receptor FcγRIIA in the immune clearance of platelets: a transgene mouse model. *J Immunol* 1999;**162**:4311–18.

Miller GW, Nussenzweig V. A new complement function: solubilization of antigen-antibody aggregates. *Proc Natl Acad Sci* 1975;**72**:418–22.

Park SY, Ueda S, Ohno H, *et al.* Resistance of Fc receptor-deficient mice to fatal glomerulonephritis. *J Clin Invest* 1998;**102**:1229–38.

Qiao J-H, Castellani LW, Fishbein MC, *et al.* Immune-complex-mediated vasculitis increases coronary artery lipid accumulation in autoimmune-prone MRL mice. *Arteriosclerosis Thromb* 1993;**13**:932–43.

Ravetch JV. Fc receptors. *Curr Opin Immunol* 1997;**9**:121–5.

Schifferli JA, Ng YC, Peters DK. The role of complement and its receptor in the elimination of immune complexes. *N Engl J Med* 1986;**315**:488–95.

Sylvestre DL, Ravetch JV. A dominant role for mast cell Fc receptors in the Arthus reaction. *Immunity* 1996;**5**:387–90.

Takata Y, Tamura N, Fujita T. Interaction of C3 with antigen–antibody complexes in the process of solubilisation of immune precipitates. *J Immunol* 1984;**132**:2531–7.

Terino FL, Powell MS, McKenzie IF, Hogarth PM. Recombinant soluble human FcγRII: production, characterization, and inhibition of the Arthus reaction. *J Exp Med* 1993;**178**:1617–28.

Theofilopoulos AN, Dixon FJ. The biology and detection of immune complexes. *Adv Immunol* 1979;**28**:89–220.

Warren JS, Yabroff KR, Remick DG, *et al.* Tumour necrosis factor participates in the pathogenesis of acute immune complex alveolitis in the rat. *J Clin Invest* 1989; **84**:1873–82.

Waxman FJ, Hebert LE, Cornacoff JB, *et al.* Complement depletion accelerates the clearance of immune complexes from the circulation of primates. *J Clin Invest* 1984;**74**:1329–40.

Whaley K. Complement and immune complex diseases. In: Whaley K (ed). *Complement in Health and Disease.* Lancaster: MTP Press Ltd, 1987.

Williams RC. *Immune Complexes in Clinical and Experimental Medicine.* Massachusetts: Harvard University Press, 1980.

World Health Organization Scientific Group. *Technical Report 606. The Role of Immune Complexes in Disease.* Geneva: WHO, 1977.

24 Hypersensitivity – Type IV

- **There are three varieties of Type IV hypersensitivity:** contact, tuberculin, and granulomatous.
- **Langerhans' cells** internalize and process epicutaneously applied hapten and present it to antigen-specific T cells.
- **Cytokines produced by immune-competent skin cells** (e.g. keratinocytes, Langerhans' cells, T cells) recruit antigen-non-specific T cells and macrophages.
- **Tuberculin-type hypersensitivity** is useful as a diagnostic test for exposure to a number of infectious agents.
- **In granulomatous reactions** there is a balance between protective immunity and T-cell-mediated tissue damage to insoluble antigen. A good example of this is seen in tuberculoid leprosy.
- **Persistence of antigen** leads to differentiation of macrophages to epithelioid cells, and fusion to form giant cells. The whole pathological response is termed a granulomatous reaction and it results in tissue damage.
- **Granuloma formation** is driven by T-cell activation of macrophages, and is dependent on tumour necrosis factor (TNF).

According to the Coombs and Gel classification, Type IV or delayed hypersensitivity reactions take more than 12 hours to develop and involve cell-mediated immune reactions rather than antibody responses to antigens. They serve more widely as a model of T-cell-mediated inflammatory responses to either exogenous or autoantigens. When the exogenous antigen is applied to the epidermis or injected intradermally in a sensitized individual, antigen-specific T cells stimulate a local inflammatory response over 24–72 hours. If the antigen is an organ-specific self antigen, autoreactive T cells may produce localized cellular inflammation and autoimmune disease, such as Type I diabetes. Some hypersensitivity reactions may straddle this definition with a rapid antibody-mediated phase and a later cell-mediated phase. For example, the late phase IgE-mediated reaction may peak 12–24 hours after contact with an allergen, and cells, such as T-helper (TH) 2 cells and eosinophils, are involved as well as IgE.

Unlike other forms of hypersensitivity, Type IV hypersensitivity cannot be transferred from one animal to another by serum, but can be transferred by T cells, particularly CD4 TH1 cells in mice. Therefore it can occur in antibody-deficient humans, but is lost with the decline in CD4 T cells in HIV/AIDS. Type IV hypersensitivity reflects the presence of antigen-specific CD4 T cells and is associated with protective immunity against intracellular and other pathogens. However, there is not a complete correlation between Type IV hypersensitivity and protective immunity. The T cells responsible for the delayed response have been specifically sensitized by a previous encounter with the antigen, and act by recruiting macrophages and other lymphocytes to the site of the reaction.

Three variants of Type IV hypersensitivity reaction are recognized (*Fig. 24.1*). Contact hypersensitivity and tuberculin-type hypersensitivity both occur within 72 hours of antigen challenge. Granulomatous hypersensitivity reactions develop over a period of 21–28 days; the granulomas are formed by the aggregation and proliferation of macrophages, and may persist for weeks. In terms of its clinical consequences, this is by far the most serious type of Type IV hypersensitivity response. Note that more than one type of reaction may follow a single antigenic challenge, and that the reactions may overlap.

The variants of delayed hypersensitivity

delayed reaction	maximal reaction time
contact	48–72 hours
tuberculin	48–72 hours
granulomatous	21–28 days

Fig. 24.1 Contact and tuberculin-type hypersensitivity have a similar time course and are maximal at 48–72 hours. In certain circumstances (e.g. with insoluble antigen) granulomatous reactions also develop at 21–28 days (e.g. skin testing in leprosy).

The three types of delayed hypersensitivity were originally distinguished according to the reaction they produced when antigen was applied directly to the skin (epicutaneously) or injected intradermally. The degree of the response is usually assessed in animals by measuring thickening of the skin. The local response is also accompanied by a variety of systemic immune responses, such as T-cell proliferation and synthesis of cytokines including interferon-γ (IFNγ).

CONTACT HYPERSENSITIVITY

Contact hypersensitivity is characterized by an eczematous reaction at the point of contact with an allergen (*Fig. 24.2*). It is often seen following contact with agents such as nickel, chromate, rubber accelerators and pentadecacatechol (found in poison ivy). Contact with irritants that damage skin by toxic mechanisms not mediated by hypersensitivity can also produce eczema. Although the initial reactions are different, the inflammatory events following application of irritants and allergens show similarities.

The immunologically active portions of the agents listed above are called haptens. Haptens are too small to be antigenic by themselves, having a molecular weight often less than 1 kDa. They penetrate the epidermis and conjugate, most often covalently, to body proteins. The sensitizing

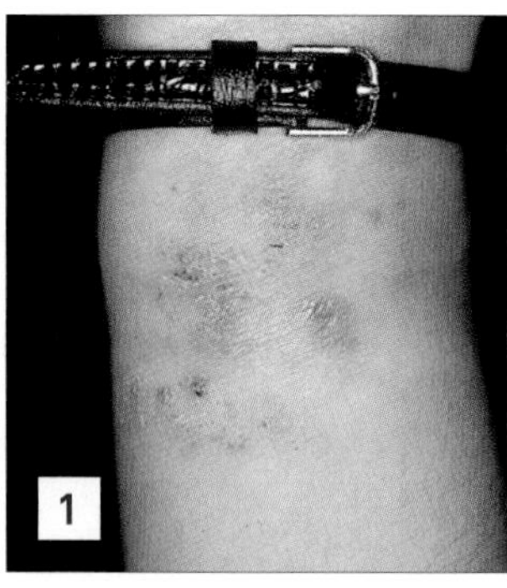

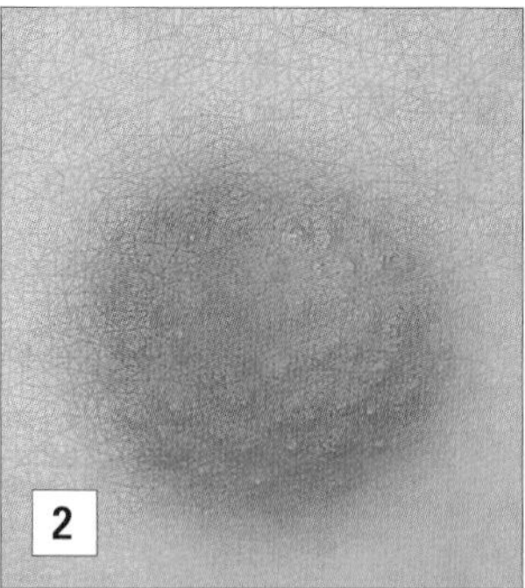

Fig. 24.2 Clinical and patch-test appearances of contact hypersensitivity. (**1**) The eczematous area at the wrist is due to sensitivity to nickel in the watch-strap buckle. (**2**) The suspected allergy may be confirmed by applying potential allergens, in the relevant concentrations and vehicles, to the patient's upper back (patch testing). A positive reaction causes a localized area of eczema at the site of the offending allergen, 2–4 days after application.

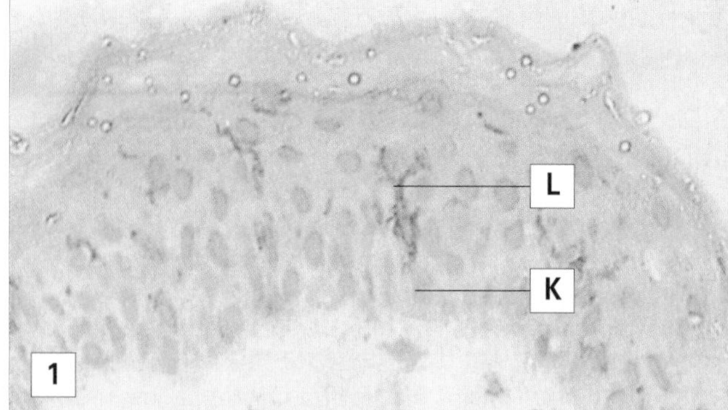

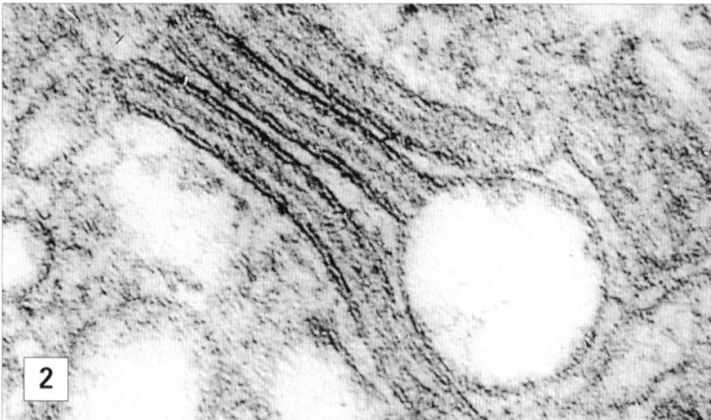

Fig. 24.3 The Langerhans' cell. (**1**) These dendritic cells constitute 3% of all cells in the epidermis. They express a variety of surface markers which allow them to be visualized. Here they have been revealed in a section of normal skin using a monoclonal antibody which reacts with the CD1 antigen (counterstained with Mayer's haemalum). L = Langerhans' cell; K = keratinocyte. ×312. (**2**) Electron micrograph of a Langerhans' cell showing the characteristic 'Birbeck granule'. This organelle is a plate-like structure with a distinct central striation and often has a bleb-like extension at one end. ×132 000.

potential of a hapten cannot reliably be predicted from its chemical structure, although there is some correlation with the number of haptens attached to the carrier and the ability of the molecule to penetrate the skin. Also, certain contact allergens have unsaturated carbon bonds and are easily oxidized. Some haptens, such as dinitrochlorobenzene (DNCB), sensitize nearly all individuals and can be used to assess cell-mediated immunity. Epicutaneously applied DNCB binds to epidermal proteins and to MHC-linked peptides through the -NH_2 groups of lysine.

Langerhans' cells and keratinocytes have key roles in contact hypersensitivity

The Langerhans' cell is the principal antigen-presenting cell

Contact hypersensitivity is primarily an epidermal reaction, and the dendritic Langerhans' cell, located in the suprabasal epidermis, is the principal antigen-presenting cell (APC) involved (*Fig. 24.3*). Langerhans' cells are derived from bone marrow and express CD1, MHC class II antigens and surface receptors for Fc and complement (see Chapter 2). Electron microscopy shows Birbeck granules, organelles derived from cell membrane and specific for the cell. Langerhans' cells are inactivated by ultraviolet B, which can thus prevent or alleviate the effects of contact hypersensitivity.

In vitro, Langerhans' cells act as APCs and are more potent in this regard than monocytes. Langerhans' cells take up hapten-modified proteins by micropinocytosis and under the influence of interleukin-1 (IL-1) and TNF from keratinocytes and other cells undergo maturation, increase the expression of MHC and co-stimulatory molecules and migrate to draining lymph nodes.

Keratinocytes produce a range of cytokines important to the contact hypersensitivity response

Keratinocytes provide the structural integrity of the epidermis and have a central role in epidermal immunology. They may express MHC class II molecules and intercellular adhesion molecule-1 (ICAM-1) in the cell membrane. They can also release cytokines including IL-1, IL-3, IL-6, IL-8, granulocyte- macrophage–colony-stimulating factor (GM–CSF), macrophage–colony-stimulating factor (M-CSF), TNFα, transforming growth factor-α (TGFα). IL-3 can activate Langerhans' cells, co-stimulate proliferative responses, recruit mast cells and induce the secretion of immunosuppressive cytokines (e.g. IL-10 and TGFβ). These latter dampen the immune response and induce clonal anergy (immunological unresponsiveness) in TH1 cells.

Keratinocytes can be activated by a number of stimuli, including allergens and irritants. Activated keratinocytes produce immunostimulatory cytokines such as TNFα and GM-CSF which activate Langerhans' cells. Some antigens, such as urushiol in poison ivy, may directly induce TNFα and IL-8.

A contact hypersensitivity reaction has two stages: sensitization and elicitation

Sensitization produces a population of memory T cells

Sensitization takes 10–14 days in humans. Once absorbed, the hapten combines with a protein and is internalized by epidermal Langerhans' cells, which leave the epidermis and

Sensitization phase of contact hypersensitivity

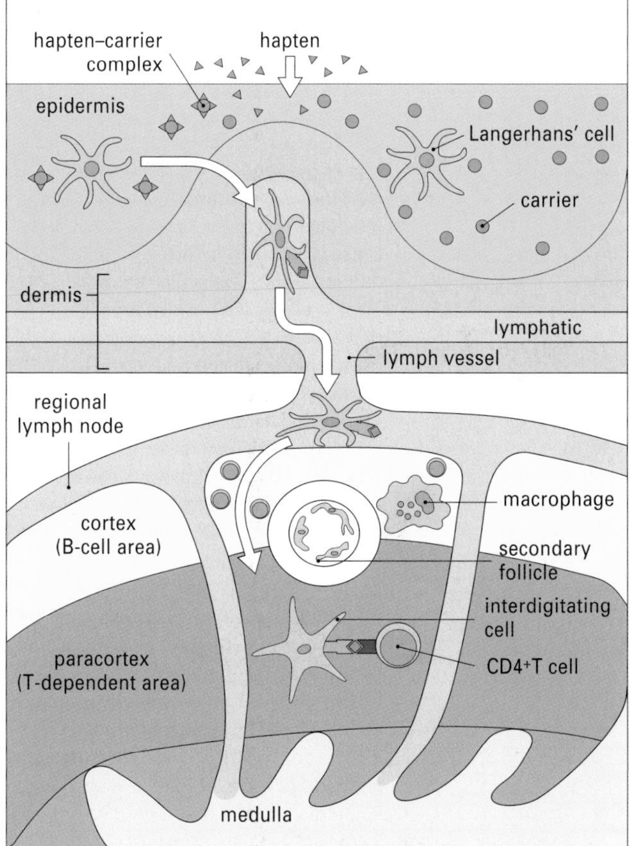

Fig. 24.4 The hapten forms a hapten–carrier complex in the epidermis. Langerhans' cells internalize the antigen, undergo maturation, and migrate via afferent lymphatics to the paracortical area of the regional lymph node where peptide/MHC complexes on the surface of the Langerhans' cell can also be directly haptenated. As interdigitating cells, they present antigen to $CD4^+$ T cells.

migrate as veiled cells through the afferent lymphatics to the paracortical areas of regional lymph nodes. Here they present processed hapten–protein conjugates (in association with MHC class II molecules) to $CD4^+$ lymphocytes, producing a population of memory $CD4^+$ T cells (*Fig. 24.4*). In addition to CD4 T cells, MHC class I-restricted CD8 T cells are important in contact hypersensitivity responses to some allergens in humans and mice. For example, lipid-soluble urushiol from poison ivy can enter the cytoplasm of APCs and the MHC class I processing pathway, leading to the activation of allergen-specific CD8 T-cell clones. These cause inflammation by direct cytolytic effect on epidermal cells or by the release of IFNγ.

Elicitation involves recruitment of $CD4^+$ lymphocytes and monocytes

The application of a contact allergen generally causes a modest decrease in Langerhans' cell numbers in the epidermis within hours of application. Antigen presentation by Langerhans' cells then occurs in skin and lymph nodes. TNFα and IL-1 from many cell types and from macrophages in particular, are potent inducers of endothelial cell adhesion molecules. These locally released cytokines produce a gradient signal for movement of mononuclear cells towards the dermo-epidermal junction and epidermis. For the elicitation phase of contact hypersensitivity, see *Figure 24.5*.

The earliest histological change, seen after 4–8 hours, is the appearance of mononuclear cells around adnexae and blood vessels, with subsequent epidermal infiltration. Macrophages invade the dermis and epidermis by 48 hours. The number of cells infiltrating the epidermis and dermis peaks at 48–72 hours (*Fig. 24.6*). Most infiltrating lymphocytes are $CD4^+$, with a few $CD8^+$. Less than 1% of infiltrating cells are antigen-specific memory $CD4^+$ TH1 cells. The later stages for T-cell recruitment are Ag independent. Askenase has shown that IgM antibodies to the hapten produced by B-1 cells are important for Ag localisation, to elicit the reaction. Experiments in gene-targeted mice show that selectins, ICAM-1 and the integrins, leucocyte functional antigen-1 (LFA-1) and very late antigen-4 (VLA-4), are all required for the elicitation of contact and delayed hypersensitivity.

The mechanisms of reactions to allergens and irritants share some features

TNFα, IFNγ and GM-CSF mRNA signals are induced in Langerhans' cells within 30 minutes of topical application of either an antigen or irritant, and a tenfold increase in mRNA expression is found in 2–4 hours. Certain changes in mRNA transcription occur only after application of a hapten. These include an increase in the IL-1β mRNA signal by Langerhans' cells at 15 minutes, and upregulation of transcription by keratinocytes of IL-1α, macrophage inflammatory protein 2 (MIP-2), and interferon-induced protein 10 (IP-10) (*Fig. 24.7*).

Chemical reagents applied to the epidermis can result in increased expression of ELAM-1 (endothelial leukocyte adhesion molecule) and VCAM-1 within 2 hours, and ICAM-1 within 8 hours, regardless of whether the individual is sensitive or not. ICAM-1 is more prominent than VCAM-1 or ELAM-1: it is the ligand for LFA-1, found on lymphoid and myeloid cells, and is important for localizing these cells to the skin. Chemotactic cytokines and the 'beacon effect' of in-transit Langerhans' cells attract TH1 cells. Memory T cells reside in dermal capillaries where they can trigger the reaction and recruit in a non-antigen-specific manner.

Suppression of the inflammatory reaction is mediated by a range of cytokines

The reaction wanes after 48–72 hours; macrophages and keratinocytes produce PGE, which inhibits IL-1 and IL-2 production; T cells bind to activated keratinocytes and the hapten conjugate undergoes enzymatic and cellular degradation. Downregulation is assisted by the following mechanisms:

- Migration-inhibitory lymphokines prevent spread of the inflammatory reaction.
- TGFβ, from dermal mast cells, activated keratinocytes and lymphocytes, inhibits inflammation and blocks the proliferative effects of IL-1 and IL-2.

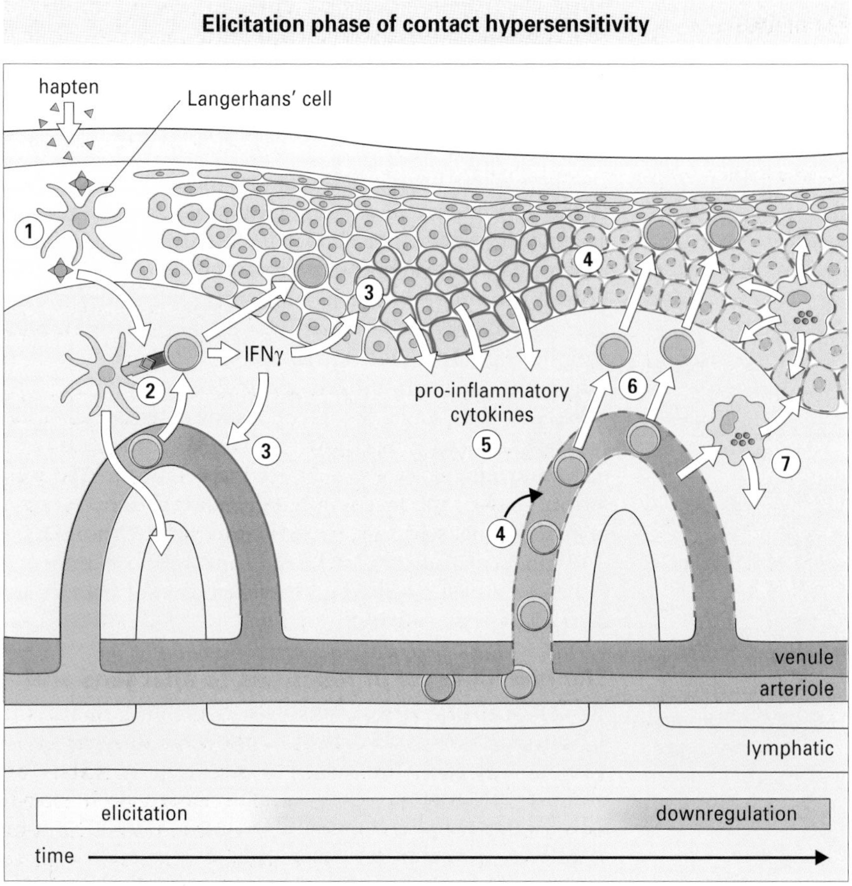

Elicitation phase of contact hypersensitivity

hapten
Langerhans' cell
IFNγ
pro-inflammatory cytokines
venule
arteriole
lymphatic
elicitation
downregulation
time

Fig. 24.5 Langerhans' cells carrying the hapten–carrier complex (**1**) move from the epidermis to the dermis, where they present the hapten–carrier complex to memory CD4⁺ T cells (**2**). Activated CD4⁺ T cells release IFNγ, which induces expression of ICAM-1 (**3**) and, later, MHC class II molecules (**4**) on the surface of keratinocytes and on endothelial cells of dermal capillaries and activates keratinocytes which release proinflammatory cytokines such as IL-1, IL-6 and GM–CSF (**5**). Non-antigen-specific CD4⁺ T cells are attracted to the site by cytokines (**6**) and may bind to keratinocytes via ICAM-1 and class II molecules. Activated macrophages are also attracted to the skin, but this occurs later. Thereafter the reaction starts to downregulate. This downregulation may be influenced by eicosanoids such as PGE, produced by activated keratinocytes and macrophages (**7**).

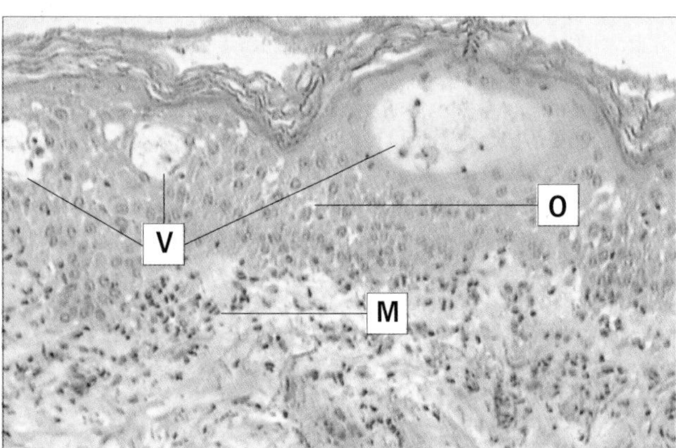

Fig. 24.6 Histological appearance of the lesion in contact hypersensitivity. Mononuclear cells (M) infiltrate both dermis and epidermis. The epidermis is pushed outwards and microvesicles (V) form within it due to oedema (O). H&E stain, ×130.

- IL-1, synthesized by keratinocytes following contact with allergens, inhibits oxidative metabolism in macrophages and depresses their production of pro-inflammatory mediators.
- IL-10 downregulates class II molecule expression, and suppresses cytokine production and antigen-specific proliferation by TH1 cells.
- External factors may also be involved: in mice UV light has been shown to induce a specific inhibitor of IL-1 activity.
- Keratinocytes expressing class II molecules without co-stimulatory molecules cannot act as prime lymphocytes but, when haptenated and incubated with TH1 cells, can induce clonal anergy.

TUBERCULIN-TYPE HYPERSENSITIVITY

This form of hypersensitivity was originally described by Koch. He observed that if patients with tuberculosis were injected subcutaneously with a tuberculin culture filtrate (antigens derived from the tubercle bacillus) they reacted with fever and generalized sickness. An area of hardening and swelling developed at the site of injection. Soluble antigens from a number of organisms, including *Mycobacterium tuberculosis*, *M. leprae* and *Leishmania tropica*, induce similar reactions in sensitive people. The skin reaction is frequently used to test for sensitivity to the organisms following previous exposure (*Fig. 24.8*). This form of hypersensitivity may also be induced by non-microbial antigens, such as beryllium and zirconium.

The tuberculin skin test reaction principally involves monocytes

The tuberculin skin test is an example of the recall response to soluble antigen previously encountered during infection. Following intradermal tuberculin challenge in a sensitized

Cytokines, prostaglandins and cellular interactions in contact hypersensitivity

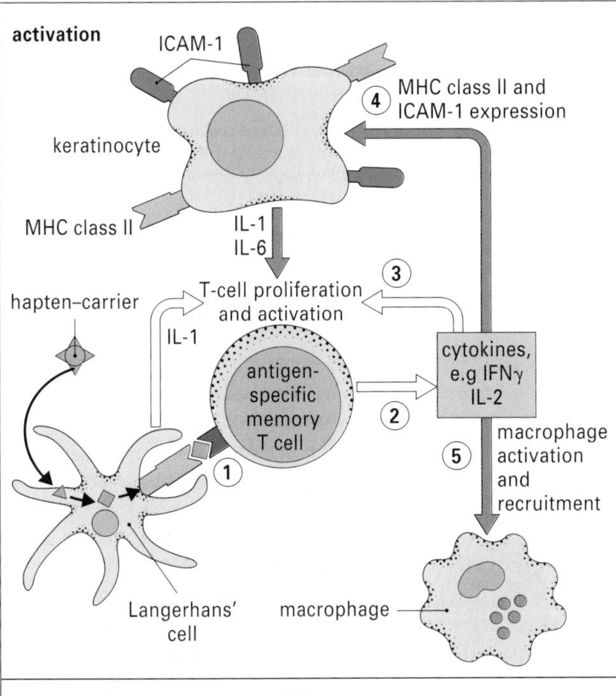

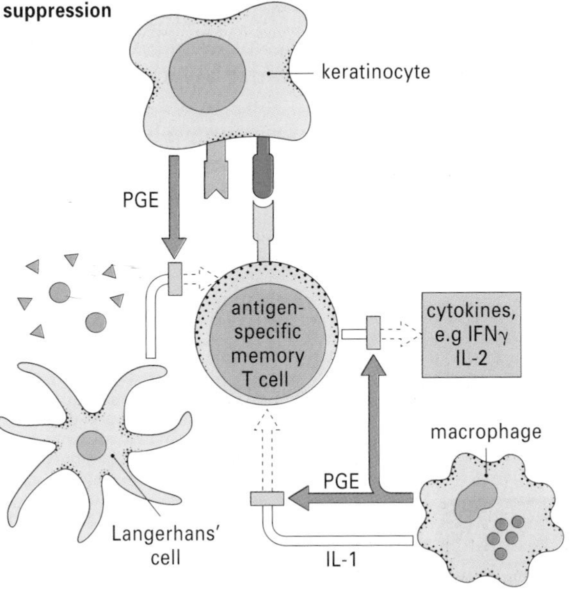

Fig. 24.7 Cytokines and prostaglandins are central to the complex interactions between Langerhans' cells, CD4⁺ T cells, keratinocytes, macrophages and endothelial cells in contact hypersensitivity. The act of antigen presentation (**1**) causes the release of a cascade of cytokines (**2**). This cascade initially results in the activation and proliferation of CD4⁺ T cells (**3**), the induction of expression of ICAM-1 and MHC class II molecules on keratinocytes and endothelial cells (**4**), and the attraction of further T cells and macrophages to the skin (**3, 5**). Subsequent PGE production by keratinocytes and macrophages may have an inhibitory effect on IL-1 and IL-2 production. Production of PGE, binding of activated T cells to keratinocytes and enzymatic and cellular degradation of the hapten– carrier complex all contribute to the downregulation of the reaction.

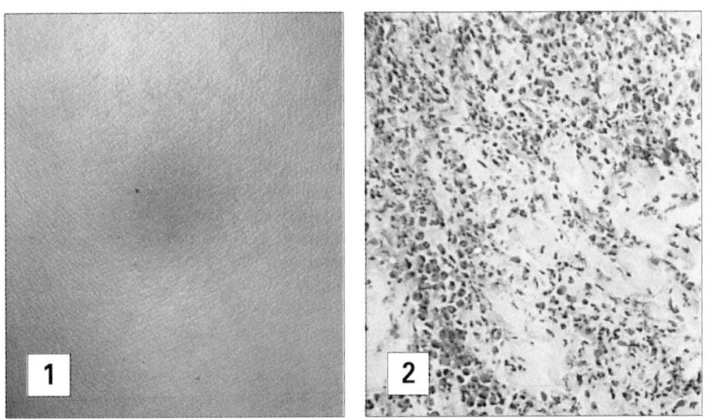

Fig. 24.8 Clinical and histological appearances of tuberculin-type sensitivity. The response to an injection of leprosy bacillus into a sensitized individual is known as the Fernandez reaction. The reaction is characterized by an area of firm red swelling of the skin and is maximal 48–72 hours after challenge (**1**). Histologically (**2**), there is a dense dermal infiltrate of leucocytes H&E stain, ×80.

individual, antigen-specific T cells are activated to secrete IFNγ which activates macrophages to produce TNFα and IL-1. These proinflammatory cytokines and chemokines from T cells and macrophages act on endothelial cells in dermal blood vessels to induce the sequential expression of the adhesion molecules E-selectin, ICAM-1 and VCAM-1. These molecules bind receptors on leucocytes and recruit them to the site of the reaction. The initial influx at four hours is of neutrophils, but this is replaced at 12 hours by monocytes and T cells. This infiltrate, which extends outwards and disrupts the collagen bundles of the dermis, increases to a peak at 48 hours. $CD4^+$ T cells outnumber $CD8^+$ cells by about 2 : 1. $CD1^+$ cells (Langerhans-like cells, but lacking Birbeck granules) are also found in the dermal infiltrate at 24 and 48 hours, and a few $CD4^+$ cells infiltrate the epidermis between 24 and 48 hours.

Monocytes constitute 80–90% of the total cellular infiltrate. Both infiltrating lymphocytes and macrophages express MHC class II molecules, and this increases the efficiency of activated macrophages as APCs. Overlying keratinocytes express HLA-DR molecules 48–96 hours after the appearance of the lymphocytic infiltrate. These events are summarized in *Figure 24.9*.

Macrophages are probably the main APCs in the tuberculin hypersensitivity reaction. However, there are $CD1^+$ cells in the dermal infiltrate, which suggests that Langerhans' cells or indeterminate dendritic cells may also participate. The circulation of immune cells to and from the regional lymph nodes is thought to be similar to that for contact hypersensitivity. The tuberculin lesion normally resolves within 5–7 days, but if there is persistence of antigen in the tissues it may develop into a granulomatous reaction.

Tuberculin-like delayed type hypersensitivity (DTH) reactions are used practically in two ways. First, reaction to soluble antigens from a pathogen demonstrates past infection with that pathogen. Thus, tuberculin reactivity confirms past infection with *M. tuberculosis*, but not necessarily active disease. Second, DTH responses to

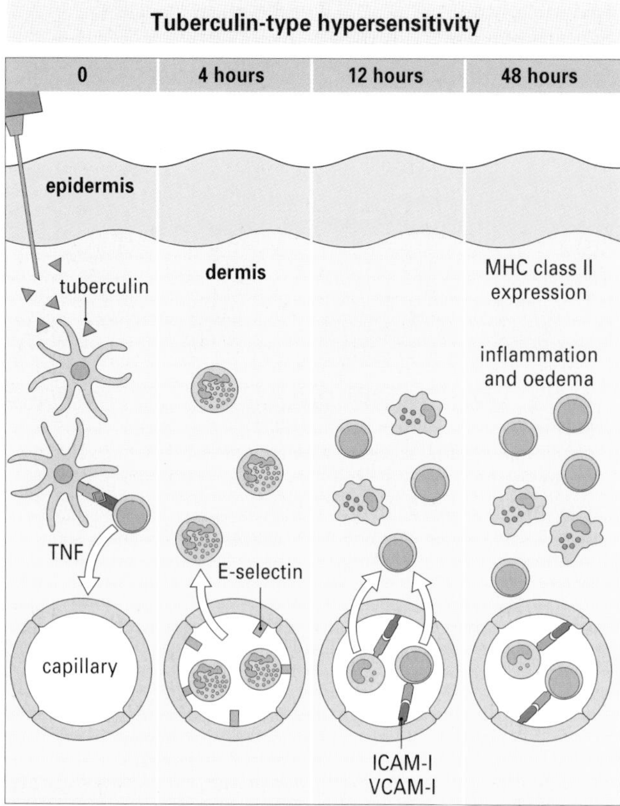

Fig. 24.9 This diagram illustrates cellular movements following intradermal injection of tuberculin. Within 1–2 hours there is expression of E-selectin on capillary endothelium leading to a brief influx of neutrophil leucocytes. By 12 hours ICAM-1 and VCAM-1 on endothelium bind the integrins LFA-1 and VLA-4 on monocytes and lymphocytes, leading to accumulation of both cell types in the dermis. This peaks at 48 hours and is followed by expression of the HLA class II molecules on keratinocytes. There is no oedema of the epidermis.

frequently encountered microbes are a general measure of cell-mediated immunity. This can be tested with intradermal injection of single antigens from common pathogens, or a multipuncture device which delivers seven common microbial antigens in a standardized fashion. Loss of recall responses to specific antigens occurs in a wide range of diseases and infections which impair T-cell function, and during therapy with corticosteroids or immunosuppressive agents.

GRANULOMATOUS HYPERSENSITIVITY

Granulomatous hypersensitivity is clinically the most important form of Type IV hypersensitivity, and causes many of the pathological effects in diseases that involve T-cell-mediated immunity. It usually results from the persistence within macrophages of intracellular microorganisms or other particles that the cell is unable to destroy. On occasion it may also be caused by persistent immune complexes, for example in allergic alveolitis. This process results in epithelioid cell granuloma formation.

The histological appearance of the granuloma reaction is quite different from that of the tuberculin-type reaction. However, they often result from sensitization to similar microbial antigens, for example the antigens of *M. tuberculosis* and *M. leprae* (*Fig. 24.10*). Immunological granuloma formation also occurs in the sensitivity reactions to zirconium and beryllium, and in sarcoidosis, although in the latter the antigen is unknown. Foreign-body granuloma formation occurs with talc, silica and a variety of other particulate agents. In this case macrophages are unable to digest the inorganic matter. These non-immunological granulomas may be distinguished by the absence of lymphocytes in the lesion.

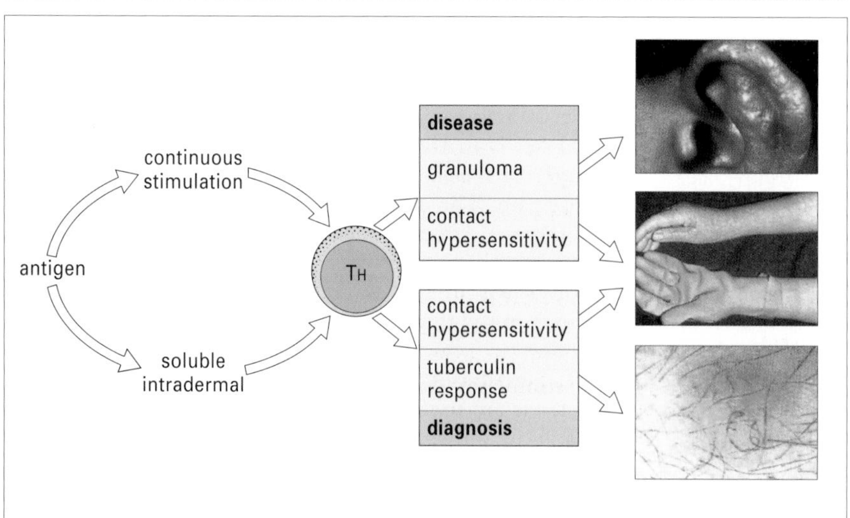

Fig. 24.10 The tuberculin skin reaction (lower: courtesy of Professor J. H. L. Playfair) is the classic diagnostic test for cell-mediated immunity in tuberculosis. If there is continuous antigenic stimulation instead of a single injection of soluble antigen, a granulomatous reaction (upper: courtesy of Dr A. du Vivier) or contact hypersensitivity (middle: courtesy Dr D. Sharvill) follows. This granulomatous reaction can also occur if the macrophages cannot destroy the antigen.

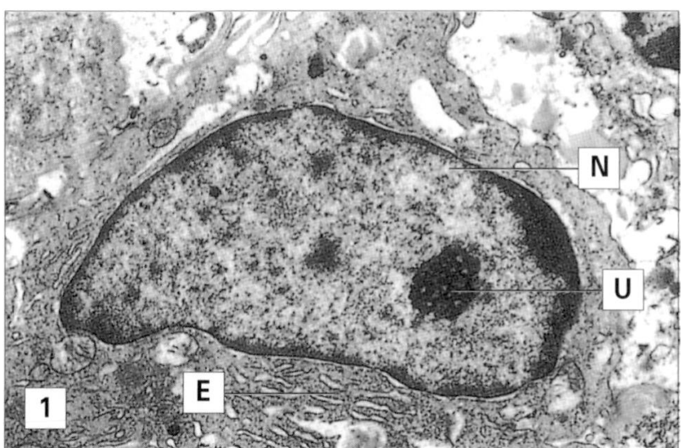

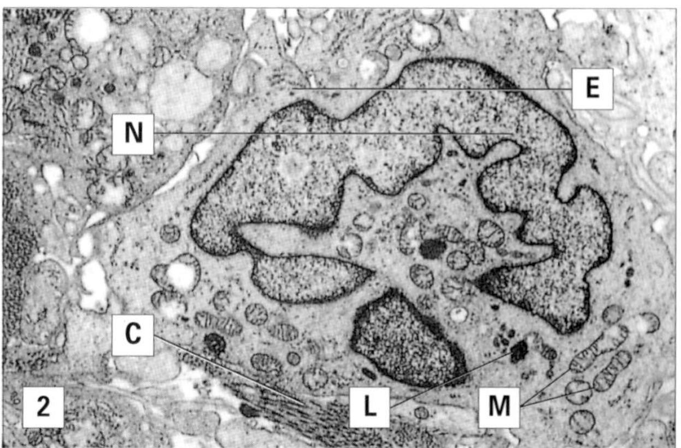

Fig. 24.11 Electron micrograph of an epithelioid cell. This is the characteristic cell of granulomatous hypersensitivity. Compare the extent of the endoplasmic reticulum (E) in the epithelioid cell (**1**) (×4800) with that of a tissue macrophage (**2**) (×4800). (Courtesy of M. J. Spencer.) U = nucleolus; N = nucleus; C = collagen; L = lysosome; M = mitochondria.

Epithelioid cells and giant cells are typical of granulomatous hypersensitivity

Epithelioid cells – These cells are large and flattened with increased endoplasmic reticulum (*Fig. 24.11*). They are derived from activated macrophages under the chronic stimulation of cytokines; they continue to secrete TNF and thus potentiate continuing inflammation.

Giant cells – Epithelioid cells may fuse to form multinucleate giant cells (*Fig. 24.12*), sometimes referred to as Langhans' giant cells (not to be confused with the Langerhans' cell discussed earlier). Giant cells have several nuclei, but these are not at the centre of the cell. There is little endoplasmic reticulum, and the mitochondria and lysosomes appear to be undergoing degeneration. The giant cell may therefore be a terminal differentiation stage of the monocyte/macrophage line.

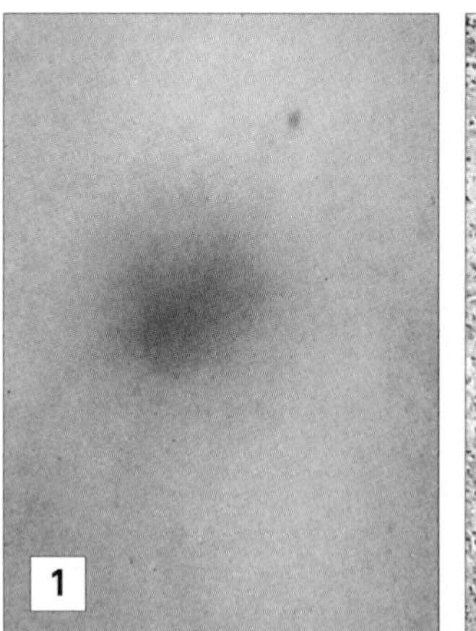

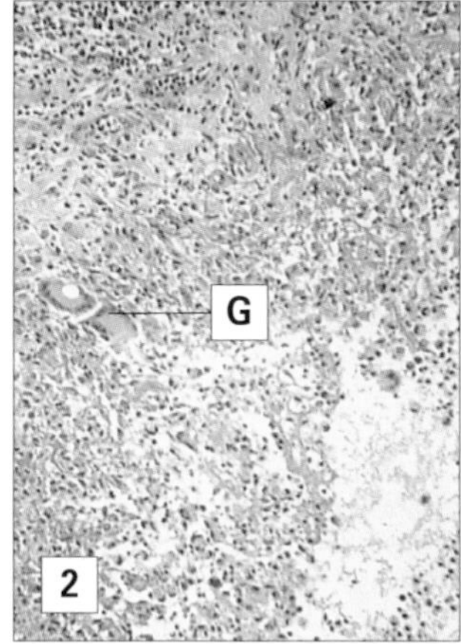

Fig. 24.12 Clinical and histological appearances of the Mitsuda reaction in leprosy seen at 28 days. (**1**) The resultant skin swelling (which may be ulcerated) is much harder and better defined than at 48 hours. (**2**) Histology shows a typical epithelioid-cell granuloma (H&E stain, ×60). Giant cells (G) are visible in the centre of the lesion, which is surrounded by a cuff of lymphocytes. This response is more akin to the pathological processes in delayed hypersensitivity diseases than the self-resolving tuberculin-type reaction. The reaction is due to the continued presence of mycobacterial antigen.

The granuloma contains epithelioid cells, macrophages and lymphocytes

An immunological granuloma typically has a core of epithelioid cells and macrophages, sometimes with giant cells. In some diseases, such as tuberculosis, this central area may have a zone of necrosis, with complete destruction of all cellular architecture. The macrophage/epithelioid core is surrounded by a cuff of lymphocytes, and there may also be considerable fibrosis (deposition of collagen fibres) caused by proliferation of fibroblasts and increased collagen synthesis. Examples of granulomatous reactions are the Mitsuda reaction to *M. leprae* antigens (see *Fig. 24.12*) or the Kveim test, where patients suffering from sarcoidosis react to (unknown) splenic antigens derived from other sarcoid patients. The three types of delayed hypersensitivity are summarized in *Figure 24.13*.

CELLULAR REACTIONS IN TYPE IV HYPERSENSITIVITY

Experiments with gene knock-out (gko) mice have confirmed that T cells bearing αβ TCR rather than γδ TCR are essential for initiating delayed hypersensitivity reactions in response to infection with intracellular bacteria. Sensitized αβ T cells, stimulated with the appropriate antigen and APCs, undergo lymphoblastoid transformation prior to cell division (*Fig. 24.14*). This forms the basis of the lymphocyte stimulation test (see Chapter 29). Lymphocyte stimulation is accompanied by DNA synthesis and this can be measured by assaying the uptake of radiolabelled thymidine, a nucleoside that is required for DNA synthesis. Lymphocytes from a patient are cultured with the suspect antigen to determine whether it induces transformation. It is important to stress that this is a test for T-cell memory

Delayed hypersensitivity reactions

type	reaction time	clinical appearance	histology	antigen
contact	48–72 hr	eczema	lymphocytes, later macrophages, oedema of epidermis	epidermal e.g. nickel, rubber, poison ivy
tuberculin	48–72 hr	local induration	lymphocytes, monocytes, macrophages	intradermal e.g. tuberculin
granuloma	21–28 days	hardening e.g. skin or lung	macrophages, epithelioid cells, giant cells, fibrosis	persistent Ag or Ag/Ab complexes or non-immunoglobin stimuli e.g. talc

Fig. 24.13 The characteristics of Type IV reactions comparing contact, tuberculin and granulomatous reactions.

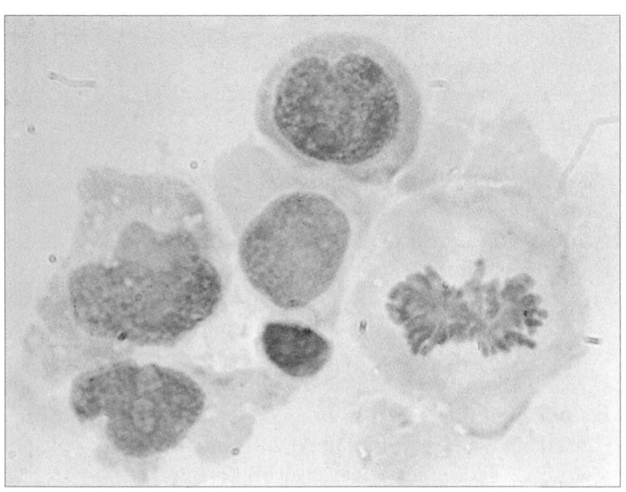

Fig. 24.14 **Transformed lymphocytes.** Following stimulation with appropriate antigen, T cells undergo lymphoblastoid transformation prior to cell division. Blast cells with expanded nuclei and cytoplasm (as well as one lymphocyte in the metaphase of cell division) are shown.

only, and does not necessarily imply the presence of protective immunity.

Following activation by APCs, T cells release a number of pro-inflammatory cytokines which attract and activate macrophages. These include IFNγ, lymphotoxin, IL-3 and GM–CSF. This TH1-like pattern of cytokines is enhanced by activation of the T cells in the presence of IL-12, which is released by macrophages on exposure to bacterial products. IL-12 suppresses the cytokine response of TH2 cells. The role of individual cytokines can be analysed in gko mice deficient for a single cytokine. For example, IFNγ gko mice are unable to activate macrophages and control infection with *M. tuberculosis* (*Fig. 24.15*). In granulomatous reactions the activated macrophages become a major source of TNF and the granulomas develop by auto-amplification, with differentiation of macrophages into

The importance of IFNγ in the activation of macrophages

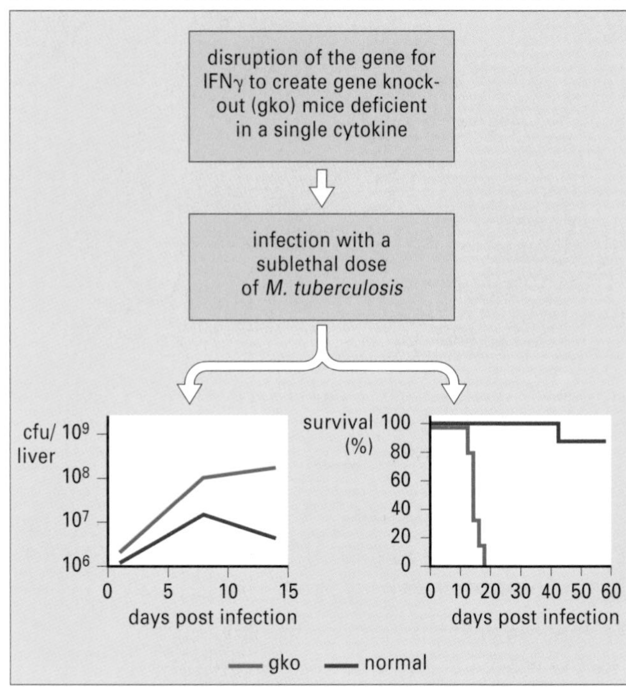

Fig. 24.15 Mice deficient in IFNγ (gko mice) are unable to activate macrophages in response to infection with an intracellular bacterium. Macrophages initially accumulate at the site of infection but do not form typical granulomas. Uncontrolled infection (graph, **left**) causes widespread tissue necrosis and death (graph, **right**). cfu: colony forming units of infectious agent in the liver.

epithelioid cells (*Figs 24.16* and *24.17*). These secrete more TNF, stimulating further epithelioid cell formation, with the fusion of epithelioid cells resulting in the formation of giant cells (*Fig. 24.18*). Granulomas fail to develop in the absence of TNF.

DISEASES MANIFESTING TYPE IV GRANULOMATOUS HYPERSENSITIVITY

There are many chronic diseases in man that manifest Type IV hypersensitivity. Most are due to infectious agents such as mycobacteria, protozoa and fungi, although in other granulomatous diseases such as sarcoidosis and Crohn's disease, no infectious agent has been established.

Important diseases in this respect include the following:

- Leprosy
- Tuberculosis
- Schistosomiasis
- Sarcoidosis
- Crohn's disease.

A common feature of these infections is that the pathogen presents a persistent, chronic antigenic stimulus. Activation of macrophages by lymphocytes may limit the infection, but continuing stimulation may lead to tissue damage through the release of macrophage products including reactive oxygen intermediates and hydrolases. Although

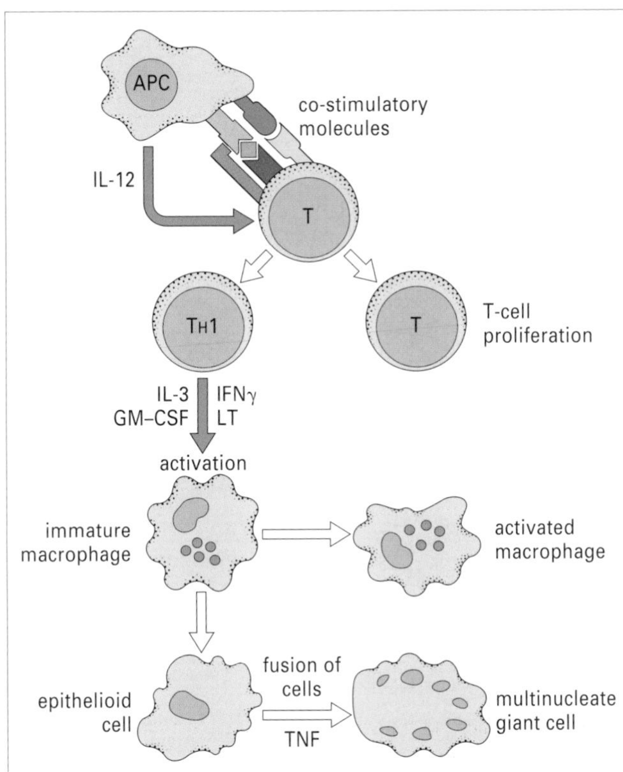

Fig. 24.16 Bacterial products stimulate macrophages to secrete IL-12. Activation of T cells in the presence of IL-12 leads to the release of IFNγ and other cytokines, lymphotoxin (LT), IL-3, and GM-CSF. These cytokines activate macrophages to kill intracellular parasites. Failure to eradicate the antigenic stimulus causes persistent cytokine release and promotes differentiation of macrophages into epithelioid cells which secrete large amounts of TNFα. Some fuse to form multinucleate giant cells.

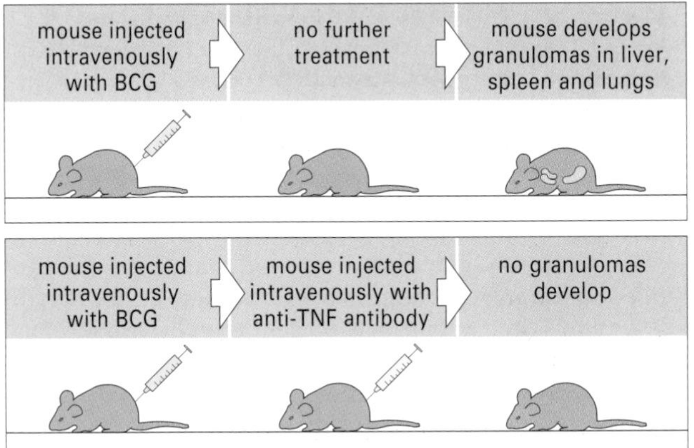

Fig. 24.17 TNF is essential for the development of epithelioid cell granulomas. If BCG-injected mice are injected with anti-TNFα antibodies, they do not develop granulomas.

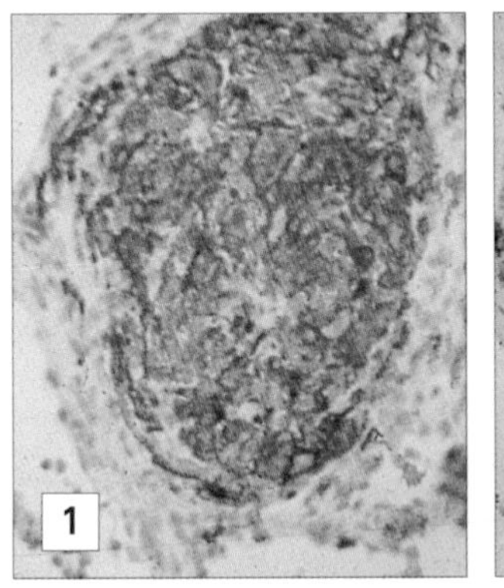

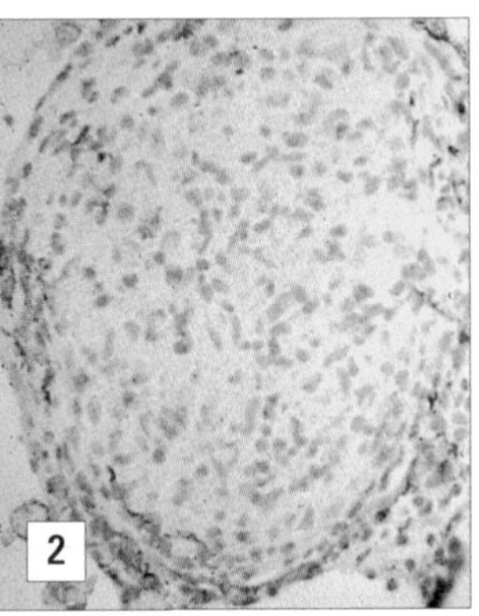

Fig. 24.18 Epithelioid cells in a granuloma from the lung of a patient with sarcoidosis. (**1**) The epithelioid cells and giant cells in the centre have been stained with the specific antibody RFD-9. (**2**) Mature tissue macrophages surrounding the granuloma are stained with the antibody RFD-7: the exact specificity of the antibody is not known. (Courtesy of C. S. Munro.)

delayed hypersensitivity is a measure of T-cell activation, the infection is not always controlled, with the result that protective immunity and delayed hypersensitivity do not necessarily coincide. Therefore some subjects showing delayed hypersensitivity may not be protected against disease in the future.

Leprosy – Leprosy is divided clinically into three main types: tuberculoid, borderline and lepromatous. In tuberculoid leprosy, the skin may have a few well-defined hypopigmented patches that show an intense lymphocytic and epithelioid infiltrate and no microorganisms. By contrast, the polar reaction of lepromatous leprosy shows multiple confluent skin lesions characterized by numerous bacilli, 'foamy' macrophages and a paucity of lymphocytes. Borderline leprosy has characteristics of both (*Fig. 24.19*). In leprosy, protective immunity is usually associated with cell-mediated immunity, but this declines across the leprosy spectrum towards the lepromatous pole with a rise in non-protective anti-*M. leprae* antibodies.

The borderline leprosy reaction is a dramatic example of delayed hypersensitivity. Borderline reactions occur either naturally or following drug treatment. In these reactions, hypopigmented skin lesions containing *M. leprae* become swollen and inflamed (*Fig. 24.20*), because the patient is now able to mount a delayed-type hypersensitivity reaction. The histological appearance shows a more tuberculoid pattern with an infiltrate of IFNγ-secreting lymphocytes. The process may occur in peripheral nerves, where Schwann cells contain *M. leprae*; this is the most important cause of nerve destruction in this disease. The lesion in borderline leprosy is typical of granulomatous hypersensitivity (*Fig. 24.20*). In patients with a tuberculoid type reaction, T-cell sensitization may be assessed *in vitro* by the lymphocyte stimulation test (see Chapter 27), using either whole or sonicated *M. leprae* as antigen (*Fig. 24.21*).

Tuberculosis – In tuberculosis there is a balance between the effects of activated macrophages controlling the

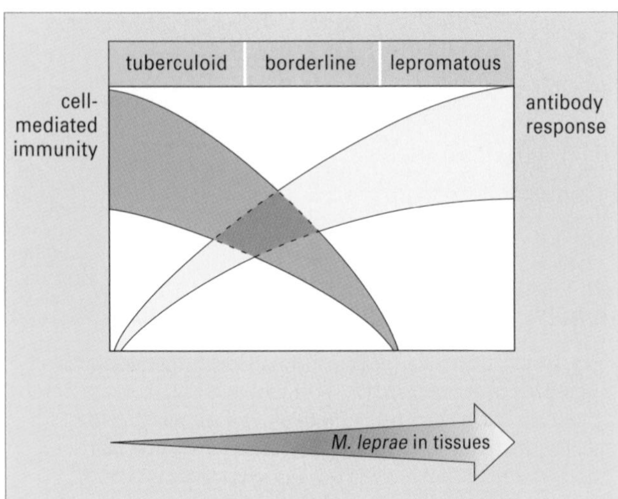

Fig. 24.19 The clinical spectrum of leprosy ranges from tuberculoid disease, with few lesions and bacteria, to lepromatous leprosy, with multiple lesions and uncontrolled bacterial proliferation. This range reflects host immunity as measured by specific cellular and antibody responses to *M. leprae*, and the tissue expression of cytokines.

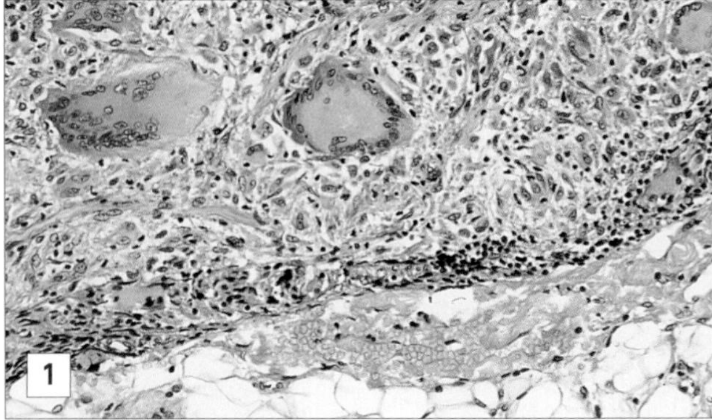

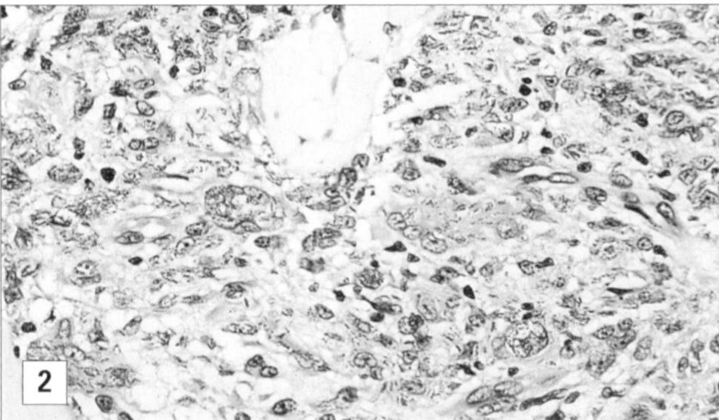

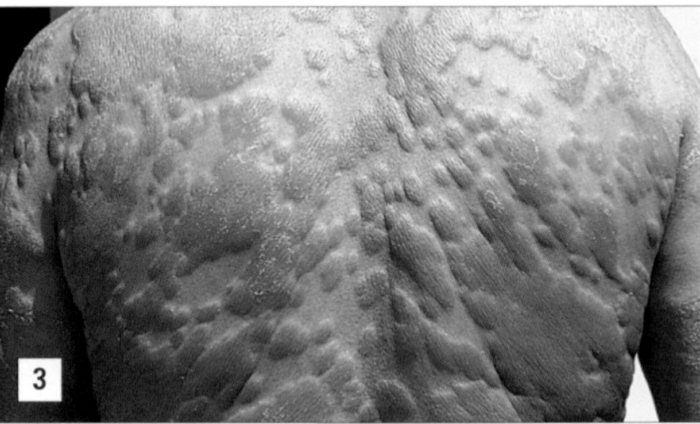

Fig. 24.20 A borderline leprosy reaction. (1) This small nerve is almost completely replaced by the granulomatous infiltrate. **(2)** Lepromatous leprosy. Large numbers of bacilli are present. (Courtesy of Dr Phillip McKee.) **(3)** Borderline lepromatous leprosy. There are gross infiltrated erythematous plaques with well-defined borders. (Courtesy of Dr S. Lucas.)

infection on the one hand, and causing tissue damage in infected organs on the other. In the lung, granulomatous reactions lead to cavitation and spread of bacteria. The reactions are frequently accompanied by extensive fibrosis and the lesions may be seen in the chest radiographs of affected patients (*Fig. 24.22*).

The histological appearance of the lesion is typical of a granulomatous reaction, with central caseous (cheesy) necrosis (*Fig. 24.23*). This is surrounded by an area of epithelioid cells, with a few giant cells. Mononuclear cell infiltration occurs around the edge.

Schistosomiasis – In schistosomiasis, caused by parasitic trematode worms (schistosomes), the host becomes sensitized to the ova of the worms, leading to a typical granulomatous reaction in the parasitized tissue mediated essentially by TH2 cells (*Fig. 24.24*; see also Chapter 16).

Sarcoidosis – Sarcoidosis is a chronic disease of unknown aetiology in which activated macrophages and granuloma accumulate in many tissues, frequently accompanied by fibrosis (*Fig. 24.25*). The disease particularly affects lymphoid tissue, and enlarged lymph nodes may be detected in chest radiographs of affected patients (*Fig. 24.26*). No infectious agent has been isolated, although mycobacteria have been implicated because of the similarities in the pathology.

One of the paradoxes of clinical immunology is that this disease is usually associated with depression of delayed hypersensitivity both *in vivo* and *in vitro*. Patients with sarcoidosis are anergic on testing with tuberculin; however, when cortisone is injected with tuberculin antigen the skin tests are positive, suggesting that cortisone-sensitive T-suppressor cells are responsible for the anergy. Cortisone would normally suppress delayed hypersensitivity.

In sarcoidosis, granulomas develop in a variety of organs, most commonly the lungs, lymph nodes, bone, nervous tissue and skin. Patients may present acutely with fever and malaise, although in the longer term those with pulmonary involvement develop shortness of breath caused by lung fibrosis. The diagnosis is often suggested by the clinical pattern and radiographic changes and confirmed by tissue biopsy. Angiotensin converting enzyme (ACE) and serum calcium are sometimes elevated, as activated macrophages are a source of both ACE and 1,25-dihydroxy-cholecalciferol (the active metabolite of vitamin D_3).

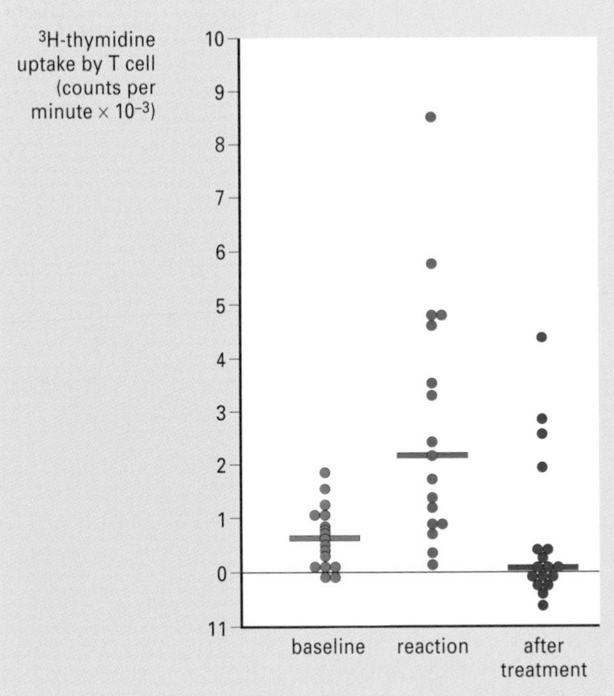

Fig. 24.21 During a borderline leprosy reaction, the lymphocyte stimulation response to *M. leprae* rises. There is a fall in response when the reaction is treated successfully with corticosteroids. The lymphocyte stimulation responses to sonicated *M. leprae* (measured by uptake of ^{3}H-thymidine) are shown for 17 patients who developed such reactions: (a) before starting treatment with anti-leprosy drugs (baseline); (b) during the reaction; and (c) following successful treatment with steroids. Medians are indicated by horizontal bars.

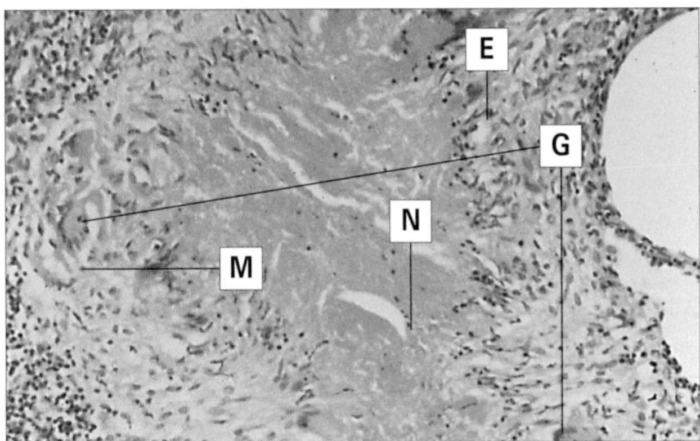

Fig. 24.23 Histological appearance of a tuberculous section of lung. This shows an epithelioid cell granuloma (E) with giant cells (G). Mononuclear cell infiltration can be seen (M). There is also marked caseation and necrosis (N) within the granuloma. H&E stain, ×75.

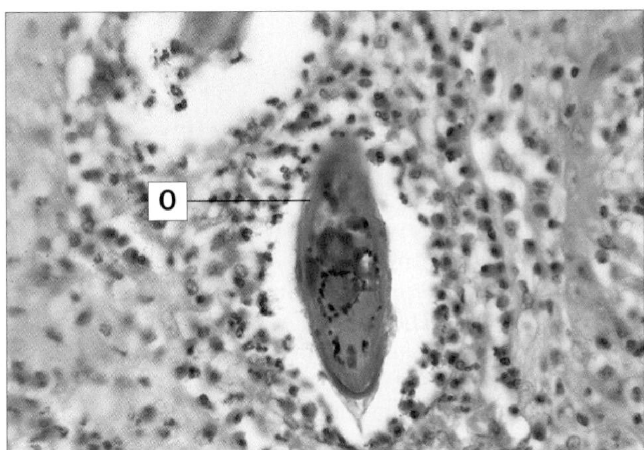

Fig. 24.24 Histological appearance of the liver in schistosomiasis. The epithelioid-cell granuloma surrounds the schistosome ovum (O). H&E stain, ×300. (Courtesy of Dr Phillip McKee.)

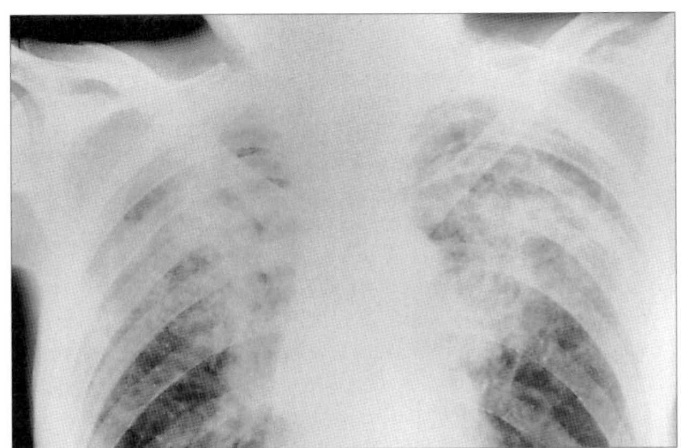

Fig. 24.22 Chest radiograph of a patient with pulmonary tuberculosis. There is extensive parenchymal streaking, predominantly in the upper fields of the lungs. These changes are typical of chronic bilateral pulmonary tuberculosis. Some enlargement of the heart is also evident.

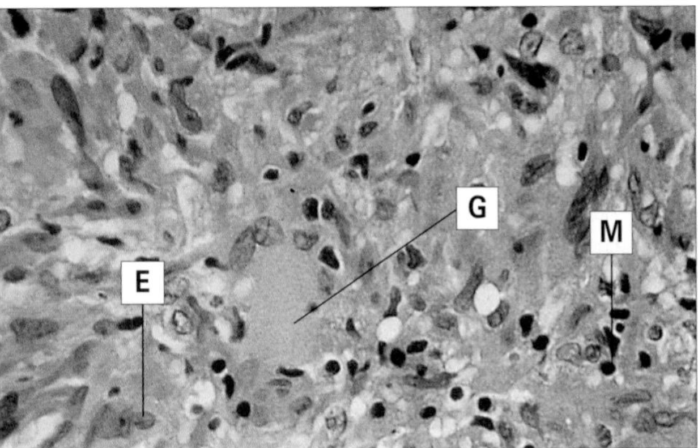

Fig. 24.25 Histological appearance of sarcoidosis in a lymph node biopsy. The granuloma of sarcoidosis is typically composed of epithelioid cells (E) and multinucleate giant cells (G), but without caseous necrosis. There is only a sparse mononuclear cell infiltrate (M) evident at the periphery of the granuloma. H&E stain, ×240.

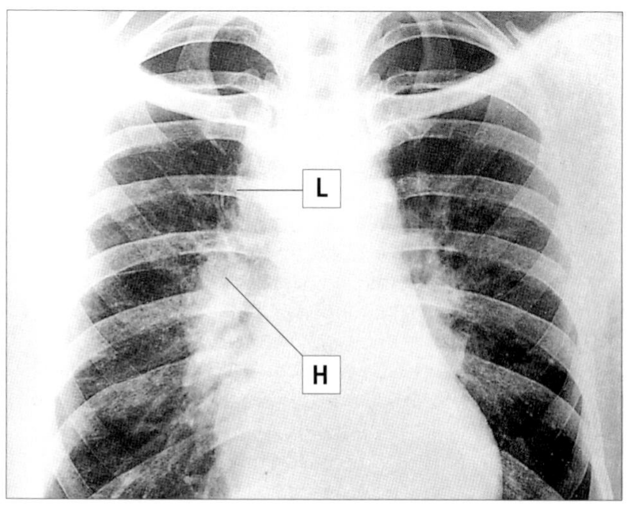

Fig. 24.26 The chest radiograph of a patient with sarcoidosis. There is enlargement of the lymph nodes adjacent to the hilar (H) and paratracheal (L) areas of the lungs, with diffuse pulmonary infiltration characteristic of the disease.

Crohn's disease – This is another non-infectious disease in which granulomas are prominent. In Crohn's disease, a chronic inflammatory disease of the ileum and colon, lymphocytes and macrophages accumulate in all layers of the bowel. The granulomatous reaction and fibrosis cause stricture of the bowel and penetrating fistulas into other organs. The natures of the antigens or infectious agents initiating and perpetuating this granulomatous reaction are unknown.

Activated T cells, showing restricted T-cell receptor repertoire and a TH1-like profile of cytokine production, are responsible for macrophage activation and the release of inflammatory cytokines, such as TNF, reactive oxygen metabolites and nitric oxide. These initiate and maintain the transmural intestinal inflammation. Inhibition of TNF activity with antibody reduces inflammation in patients with Crohn's disease.

CRITICAL THINKING • A hypersensitivity type IV reaction (Explanations on pp 462–463)

An 8-year-old boy with recent weight loss and mild fever is found to have an enlarged lymph node on the right side of the neck. He has no cough and his chest X-ray is normal. Surgical biopsy of the lymph node reveals a granulomatous infiltrate with no evident acid-fast bacilli. The result of microbiological culture for *Mycobacterium tuberculosis* is awaited. Intradermal skin testing with tuberculin causes swelling and erythema of 20 mm diameter after 48 hours.

24.1 What cell types make up the granulomas in the lymph node and what cytokines are involved in their formation?

24.2 What is the pathology at the site of the skin testing and how does it differ from that in the lymph node?

24.3 What type of lymphocyte is responsible for the skin test reactivity?

24.4 What other conditions cause granulomas in lymph nodes and how are they diagnosed?

24.5 When the family members are tested, the boy's 5-year-old brother is found to have a positive tuberculin reaction (18 mm at 48 hours), but he is well with a normal chest X-ray. What does this result indicate about his immune responses and what is its significance?

FURTHER READING

American Thoracic Society. Statement on sarcoidosis. *Am J Respir Crit Care Med* 1999;**160**:736–55.

Bean AGD, Roach DR, Briscoe H, *et al.* Structural deficiencies in granuloma formation in tumor necrosis factor gene-targeted mice underlie the heightened susceptibility to aerosol *Mycobacterium tuberculosis* infection which is not compensated for by lymphotoxin. *J Immunol* 1999;**162**:3504–11.

Bevilacqua MP. Endothelial-leukocyte adhesion molecules. *Annu Rev Immunol* 1993;**11**:767–804.

Bjune G, Barnetson RStC, Ridley DS, *et al.* Lymphocyte transformation test in leprosy; correlation of the response with inflammation of lesions. *Clin Exp Immunol* 1976;**25**:85–94.

Britton WJ. Immunology of leprosy. *Trans R Soc Trop Med Hyg* 1993;**87**:508–14.

Britton WJ, Garsia RJ. Mycobacterial infections. In: Bradley J, McCluskey J (eds). *Clinical Immunology*, vol. 38. London: Oxford University Press, 1997:483–98.

Daniel H, Present MD, Rutgeerts P, *et al.* Infliximab for the treatment of fistulas in patients with Crohn's disease. *N Engl J Med* 1999;**18**:1398–405.

Enk AH, Katz SI. Contact hypersensitivity as a model for T-cell activation in skin. *J Invest Dermatol* 1995;**105**:805–35.

Flynn JL, Chan J, Triebold KJ, *et al.* An essential role for interferon-γ in resistance to *Mycobacterium tuberculosis* infection. *J Exp Med* 1993;**178**:2249–54.

Gaspari AA. Advances in the understanding of contact hypersensitivity. *Am J Contact Derm* 1993;**4**:138–49.

Gawdrodger DJ, McVittie E, Carr MM, *et al.* Phenotypic characterisation of the early cellular responses in allergic and irritant contact dermatitis. *Clin Exp Immunol* 1986;**66**:590–8.

Gawkrodger DJ, McVittie E, Carr MM, *et al.* Keratinocyte expression of MHC class II antigens in allergic sensitisation and challenge reactions and in irritant contact dermatitis. *J Invest Dermatol* 1987;**88**:11–16.

Grabbe S, Schwarz, T. Immunoregulatory mechanisms involved in elicitation of allergic contact hypersensitivity. *Immunol Today* 1998;**19**:37–43.

Hoefakker S, Canbo M, van't Erre EHM, *et al. In vitro* cytokine profiles in allergic and irritant contact dermatitis. *Contact Dermatitis* 1995;**33**:258–66.

Kalish RS, Wood JA, LaPorte A. Processing of Urushiol (poison ivy) hapten by both endogenous and exogenous pathways for presentation to T cells *in vitro. J Clin Invest* 1994;**93**:2039–47.

Kindler V, Sappino A-P, Gran GE, *et al.* The inducing role of tumour necrosis factor in the development of bactericidal granulomas during BCG infection. *Cell* 1989;**56**:731–40.

Klimas N. Delayed hypersensitivity skin testing. In: *Manual of Clinical Laboratory Immunology*, 5th edn. Washington: ASM Press, 1997:276–80.

Romagnani P, Annunziato F, Baccari M, *et al.* T cells and cytokines in Crohn's disease. *Curr Opin Immunol* 1997;**9**:793–9.

Schaible U, Collins HL, Kaufmann S. Confrontation between intracellular bacteria and the immune system. *Adv Immunol* 1999;**71**:267–336.

Schwarzenberger K, Udey MC. Contact allergens and epidermal proinflammatory cytokines modulate Langerhans' cell E-cadherin expression *in situ. J Invest Dermatol* 1996;**106**:553–8.

Trinchieri G. Interleukin-12: a cytokine at the interface of inflammation and immunity. *Adv Immunol* 1998;**70**:133–95.

Yamamura M, Uyemura K, Deans RJ, *et al.* Defining protective immune responses to pathogens: cytokine profiles in leprosy lesions. *Science* 1991;**254**:277–9.

REFERENCE

A home page describing macrophage biology and the role of macrophages in the host response to infectious disease. http://www.path.ox.ac.uk/sg

25 Transplantation and rejection

- **Rejection of transplanted tissues** occurs because the immune system of the recipient recognizes and responds to foreign (tissue) histocompatibility antigens expressed on the graft.
- **The histocompatibility antigens** that are most important are those encoded by the major histocompatibility complex (MHC).
- **T lymphocytes** can directly recognize and respond to foreign MHC molecules.
- **Activated T-helper cells** make lymphokines which drive the activation of many different effector mechanisms of graft destruction.
- **Lymphokines** also act upon the graft to increase the expression of MHC molecules and adhesion molecules, making the graft more susceptible to rejection.
- **Graft rejection responses can be reduced** by matching of donor and recipient MHC molecules, especially for MHC class II molecules.
- **Non-specific immunosuppressive agents** can be used to block transplant rejection, but these may also reduce resistance to infections.
- **Specific immunosuppression** will be used in the future, inactivating only those lymphocyte clones which cause graft rejection.

The immunobiology of transplantation is important for many reasons, in terms of both its impact on our understanding of immunological processes and its application in the development of clinical transplantation. It was the study of mouse skin-graft rejection that led to the discovery of the major histocompatibility complex (MHC) molecules, which function in the presentation of antigens to T cells (see Chapter 5). T cells are pivotal in transplant rejection, and much of our knowledge of T-cell physiology and function, of self tolerance and autoimmunity, and of the role of the thymus in T-cell education, is derived from studies of transplantation. Last, but not least, transplantation of tissues is very important clinically. The need to prevent transplant rejection has led to the development and use of new immunomodulatory drugs and a search for ways to induce tolerance of the grafted tissues. These approaches also have a more general application in the treatment of various immune disorders, such as immune-mediated tissue damage in hypersensitivity and autoimmunity.

In clinical practice, organs are transplanted to make good a functional deficit (*Fig. 25.1*). Unless the donor and recipient are genetically identical, the graft antigens will elicit an immunological rejection response. Transplantation can stimulate all of the various active mechanisms of humoral and cellular immunity, both specific and non-specific. This is a consequence of the recognition by the recipient's T cells of large numbers of foreign and 'neo-self' peptides associated with the foreign MHC molecules on the grafted cells and of graft-derived peptides bound to self MHC (*Fig. 25.8*). Also, a transplant can activate all the regulatory mechanisms that control immune re-sponses (see Chapter 11), causing a state of unresponsiveness to the graft. Hence, transplantation immunobiology encompasses virtually all aspects of immune function.

Clinical transplantation

organ transplanted	examples of disease
kidney	end-stage renal failure
heart	terminal cardiac failure
lung or heart/lung	pulmonary hypertension, cystic fibrosis
liver	cirrhosis, cancer, biliary atresia
cornea	dystrophy, keratitis
pancreas or islets	diabetes
bone marrow	immunodeficiency, leukaemia
small bowel	cancer
skin	burns

Fig. 25.1 Organs and tissues are transplanted to treat various conditions. Each type of transplant has its own particular medical and surgical difficulties.

BARRIERS TO TRANSPLANTATION

Transplantation barriers can be described in terms of the genetic disparity between the donor and the recipient: grafts can be categorized as autografts, isografts, allografts or xenografts (*Fig. 25.2*). Autografts from one part of the body to another are not foreign and therefore do not elicit rejection. Similarly, isografts between isogeneic (genetically identical) individuals, such as monozygotic (identical) twins or mice of the same inbred strain, do not express antigens foreign to the recipient and so do not activate a rejection response. The allograft is the common clinical transplant, where one person donates an organ to a genetically different individual. In this case the graft is allogeneic (i.e. between members of the same species, having allelic variants of certain genes). The cells of the allograft will express alloantigens which are recognized as foreign by the recipient.

The maximal genetic disparity is between members of different species, and a xenograft across such a xenogeneic barrier is generally rapidly rejected, either by naturally occurring IgM antibodies in the recipient or by a rapid cell-mediated rejection (see below). If they are treated to reduce their immunogenicity, tissue xenografts that would

Genetic barriers to transplantation

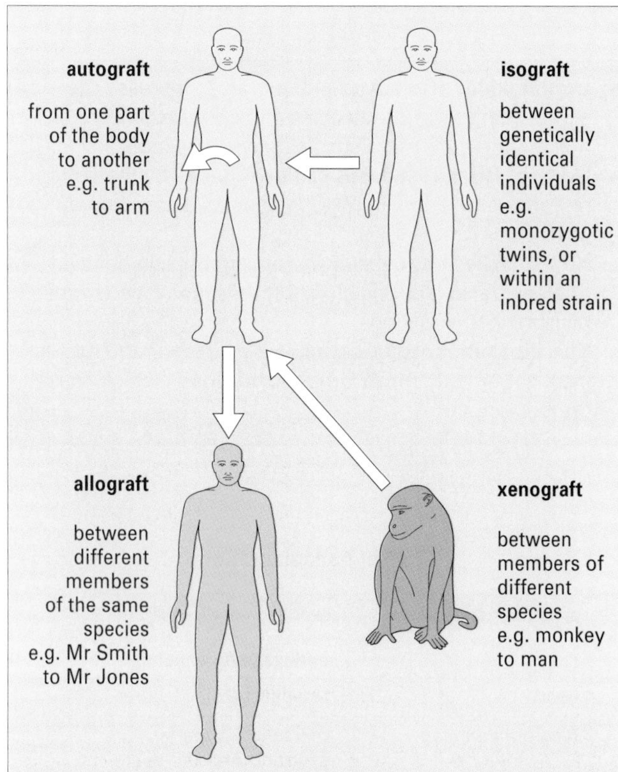

Fig. 25.2 The genetic relationship between the donor and recipient determines whether or not rejection will occur. Autografts or isografts are usually accepted, while allografts and xenografts are not.

otherwise be non-viable, such as pig skin, blood vessels or valves, can be grafted to man. Despite this, attempts to transplant whole organs from animal to man have been spectacularly unsuccessful, although some success has been achieved in xenografting between animal species. If the immunological problems of xenografting can be overcome, the use of animal donors could alleviate the worldwide shortage of human organs for transplantation. Nevertheless, various non-immunological problems remain, including donor organ size, physiological differences, transmission of animal diseases and the ethics of xenografting.

HISTOCOMPATIBILITY ANTIGENS

Histocompatibility antigens are the targets for rejection

The antigens primarily responsible for rejection of genetically different tissues are known as histocompatibility (i.e. tissue compatibility) antigens and the genes coding for these antigens are referred to as histocompatibility genes. There are more than 30 histocompatibility gene loci, and they cause rejection at different rates. Of these, alloantigens encoded by the genes of the MHC induce particularly strong reactions; these are the molecules that present

Mouse histocompatibility antigens and graft survival

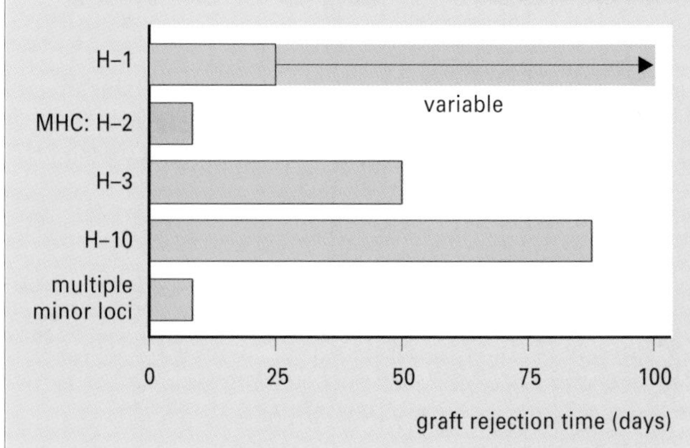

Fig. 25.3 This chart gives the rejection times for skin grafts between mice differing at the minor histocompatibility loci (red) or at the major histocompatibility H–2 locus (green). Grafts which differ at multiple minor loci are rejected as quickly as those that differ at H–2. (Data from Dr R. Graff and Dr D. Bailey.)

antigens in a form recognizable to T cells – all vertebrate species have an MHC. In mice the MHC is called H–2, while in man it is known as the human leucocyte antigen (HLA) system (see Chapter 5). The products of allelic variants of the other histocompatibility genes individually cause weaker rejection responses and are consequently known as minor histocompatibility antigens; these antigens are normal cellular constituents. None the less, combinations of several minor antigens can elicit strong rejection responses (*Fig. 25.3*).

MHC haplotypes are inherited from both parents and are co-dominantly expressed

The genes of the MHC are subject to simple Mendelian inheritance and are co-dominantly expressed. In other words, each individual has two 'half-sets' (haplotypes) of genes, one haplotype inherited from each parent (*Fig. 25.4*); both of these haplotypes are expressed equally, so that each cell in the offspring has both maternal and paternal MHC molecules on its surface (*Fig. 25.5*).

MHC molecules are expressed on transplanted tissues and induced by cytokines

MHC molecules are not equally distributed on all cells of the body. Class I molecules are normally expressed on most nucleated cells (and on erythrocytes and platelets in some species), while class II molecules are restricted to antigen-presenting cells (APCs, e.g. dendritic cells and activated macrophages), B cells and, in some species, activated T cells and vascular endothelial cells. The expression of MHC on cells is controlled by cytokines: interferon-γ (IFNγ) and tumour necrosis factor (TNF) are powerful inducers of MHC expression on many cell types which would otherwise express MHC molecules only weakly. As will be seen, this is important in graft rejection (see p. 389).

Haplotype inheritance of MHC antigens

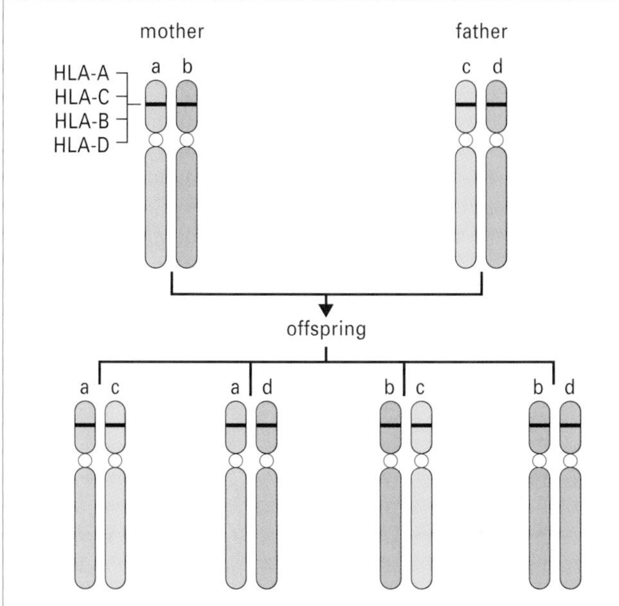

Fig. 25.4 The human MHC (HLA) is located on the short arm of chromosome 6. One set (haplotype) of the MHC class I (HLA-A, -B and -C) and class II (HLA-D) antigens are inherited en bloc from each parent according to simple mendelian inheritance.

Co-dominant expression of MHC antigens

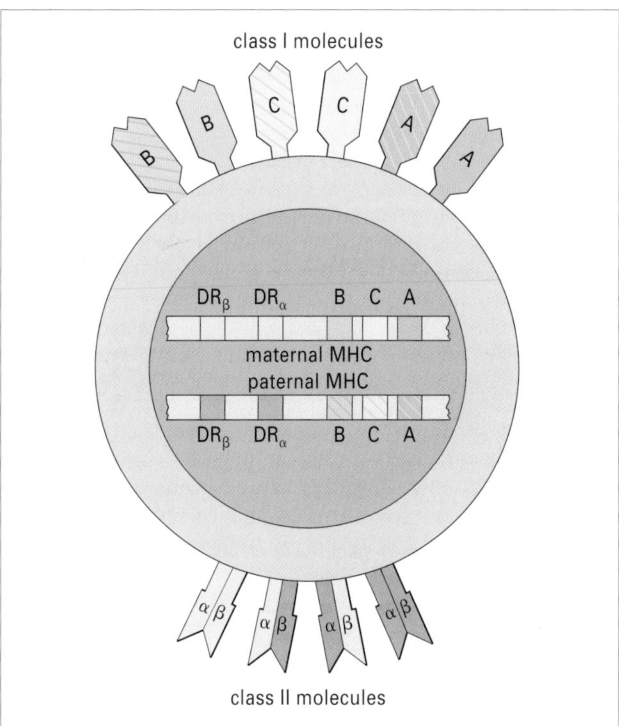

Fig. 25.5 Inherited MHC genes are all expressed on the cell surface. For each maternal and paternal class I gene there are class I molecules on the membrane. For each class II α and β gene there are α and β chains on the cell surface, but these can associate to form four different molecules. Note that there are other class II α and β genes coding for DP and DQ antigens as well. B cells have 23×10^5 class I molecules and the same number of class II molecules per cell.

THE LAWS OF TRANSPLANTATION

The transplant situation is unique in that foreign MHC molecules can directly activate T cells. Conventional T-cell responses against foreign proteins require that such antigens are processed into peptides and presented on the surface of the recipient's APCs in association with MHC molecules.

Host-versus-graft responses cause transplant rejection

The overriding consideration for organ allograft rejection is whether the graft carries any antigens that are not present in the recipient. This principle of host-versus-graft reactions is illustrated in *Figure 25.6*.

Graft-versus-host reactions result when donor lymphocytes attack the graft recipient

A special situation occurs in bone-marrow transplantation, in which graft-versus-host disease (GVHD) is induced by immunologically competent T cells being transplanted into allogeneic recipients which are unable to reject them. This inability may be due to the genetic differences between the donor and recipient, or because of a lack of immunocompetence (through immaturity or immunosuppression) of the recipient. In this situation, the immunocompetent T cells transplanted with the bone marrow can attack the recipient (*Fig. 25.7*). GVHD is a major complication of bone-marrow transplantation, causing severe damage, particularly to the skin and intestine, and is avoided by careful typing, removal of mature T cells from the graft and the use of immunosuppressive drugs.

THE ROLE OF T LYMPHOCYTES IN REJECTION

T cells are pivotal in graft rejection

Rodents born without a thymus (congenitally athymic or 'nude') have no mature T cells and cannot reject transplants. The same is true of normal rats or mice from which the thymus is removed in the neonatal period, before mature T cells are released to the periphery. Likewise, adult thymectomy (AT) of rats or mice (to stop the production of T cells), followed by irradiation (to remove existing mature T cells) and bone marrow (BM) transplantation (to restore haemopoiesis) produces 'ATx.BM recipients' which have no T cells and cannot reject grafts.

In any of these animals (nudes, neonatally thymectomized or ATx.BM), the ability to rejects grafts is restored by the injection of T cells from a normal animal of the same strain. Thus T cells are necessary for rejection. This does not imply that antibodies, B cells or other cells play no part. Indeed, antibodies cause graft damage and macrophages may be involved in inflammatory reactions in grafted tissue.

Host-versus-graft reactions

	donor	recipient	outcome
1	A	A	accepted
2	B	A	rejected
3	B	A X B	accepted
4	A X B	B	rejected

Fig. 25.6 Grafts between genetically identical animals are accepted. Grafts between genetically non-identical animals are rejected with a speed which is dependent on where the genetic differences lie. For example syngeneic animals, which are identical at the MHC locus, accept grafts from each other (**1**). Animals that differ at the MHC locus reject grafts from each other (**2**). The ability to accept a graft is dependent on the recipient sharing all the donor's histocompatibility genes: this is illustrated by the difference between grafting from parental to (A × B) F_1 animals (**3**) and *vice versa* (**4**). Animals that differ at loci other than the MHC reject graft from each other, but much more slowly.

Graft-versus-host disease

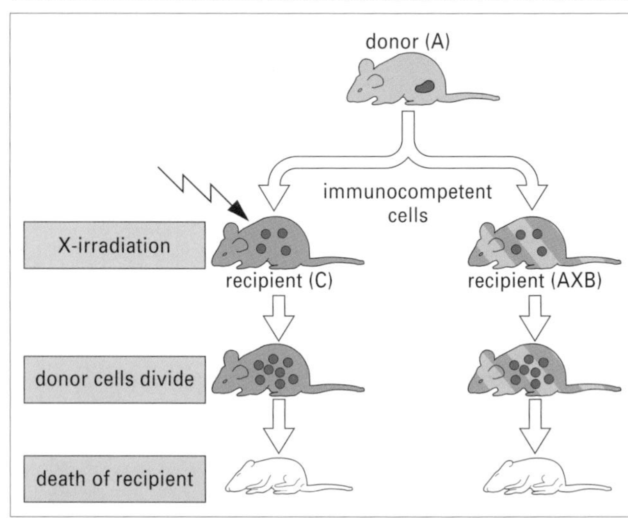

Fig. 25.7 Immunocompetent cells from a donor of Type A are injected into an immunosuppressed (X-irradiated) host of Type C, or a normal (A × B) F_1 recipient. The immunosuppressed individual is unable to reject the cells and the F_1 animal is fully tolerant to parental Type A cells. In both cases the donor cells recognize the foreign tissue Types B or C of the recipient. They divide and react against the recipient tissue cells and recruit large numbers of host cells to inflammatory sites. Very often the process leads to the death of the recipient.

Rejection responses have a molecular basis in the TCR–MHC interaction

Via their T-cell receptors (TCRs), the T cells involved in rejection recognize donor-derived peptides in association with the MHC antigens expressed on the graft. As we already know, the structure of the T-cell receptor (TCR) (see *Fig. 5.13*) is such that T cells can only 'see' peptide antigens when they are associated with MHC molecules, and this MHC restriction is imposed by positive selection in the thymus (see Chapters 2 and 12 and *Fig. 25.8*). So, to understand the involvement of T cells in rejection, we need to examine the differences between recipient and graft MHC molecules and how such differences affect the range of antigens presented to the recipient's TCR.

Different MHC molecules have similar structures but different peptide-binding grooves

The structures of different MHC molecules are almost identical, with the overall shape consisting of two α helices lying on a β-pleated sheet atop two immunoglobulin-like domains which sit on the cell membrane (see Chapter 5). Between the α helices is a deep groove into which peptides can be bound. The part of the MHC molecule that is important in T-cell recognition is the outer surface of these α helices, which is highly conserved between different MHC molecules.

The significant amino-acid sequence differences between two MHC molecules – comparing, for example, A2 and Aw68 allelic variants of the HLA-A antigen – lie deep in the groove between the α helices, not on the outer surface contacted by the TCR (see *Fig. 5.7*). Hence, for T-cell recognition, the principal difference between MHC molecules is in the shape and charge of the peptide-binding groove, and this governs which peptides can be bound and in what orientation they are presented to TCRs (see *Figs 5.11* and *5.12*).

Graft and host MHC molecules present different peptides

In the normal physiological situation, the MHC groove is occupied by peptides derived from normal cellular constituents by intracellular degradative pathways. Thymic tolerance mechanisms (clonal deletion of self-reactive T cell – see Chapter 12) ensure that T-cell recognition of these self peptide–self MHC complexes, which would lead to autoimmunity, does not occur. However, when cells are infected (with virus, for example), the normal cell-derived peptides are replaced by peptides of foreign origin, as is the case of 'professional' APCs. T cells then respond to these foreign peptides in association with self MHC molecules.

However in the case of a genetically distinct transplanted tissue a third situation arises. A different array of peptides is presented on the cell surface because of the different shape and charge of the peptide-binding sites of the graft MHC molecules. This allows binding, not only of peptides derived from the foreign MHC and minor allelic histocompatibility antigens, but also peptides of host molecules which do not bind to self MHC and which therefore have not induced tolerance (*Fig. 25.8*). This

Presentation of graft antigens

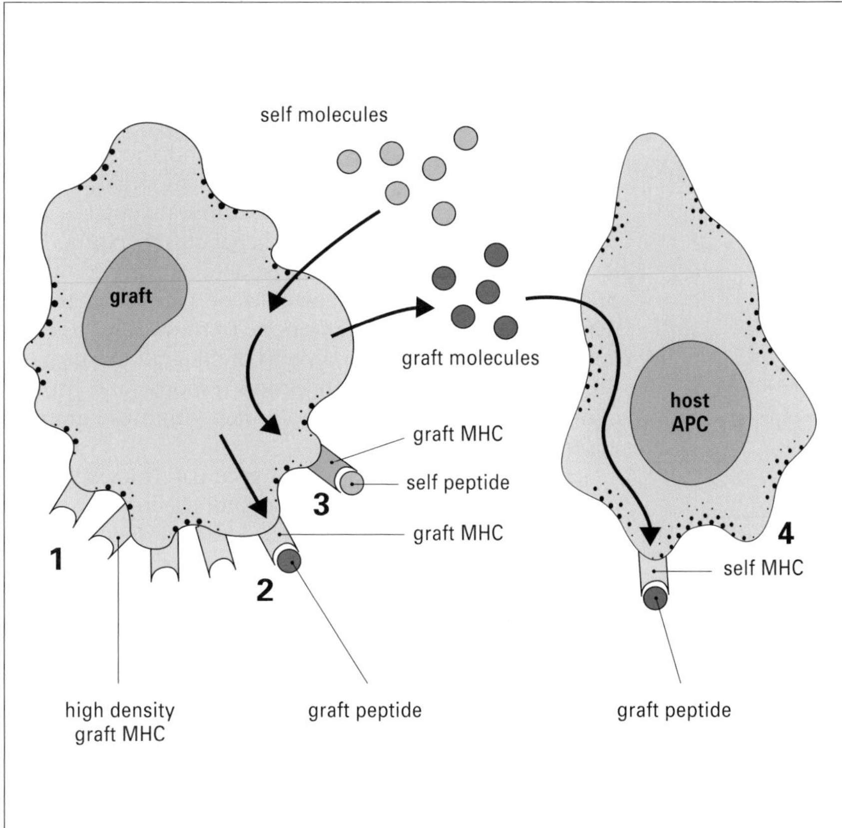

Fig. 25.8 There are several ways in which grafts and graft antigens can be recognised by T cells in the host. This may account for the relatively high proportion of host T cells which is capable of responding to engrafted tissue. **1.** A high density of graft MHC molecules, which individually react weakly with the TCR may generate a sufficient signal for T cell activation. **2.** Graft MHC molecules can present the graft's own peptides including molecules from both major and minor histocompatibility antigens. **3.** Graft MHC molecules can present processed antigens of host molecules. Because the graft MHC is different to self MHC it will present a different set of peptides to the host, and the host will not be tolerant of this MHC/antigen combination. **4.** Allotypically different graft molecules, including histocompatibility antigens can be taken up by host antigen presenting cells, and be processed and presented on self MHC molecules.

leads to the expression on transplanted APCs of a very large number of novel antigens which can be recognised by the recipient's T cells. This so-called 'direct' mode of antigen presentation is supplemented by the direct recognition of graft peptides bound by self MHC. It is not surprising therefore that up to 10% of an induvidual's T cells may respond to these antigens originating from the engrafted tissue.

T-helper (TH) cells and lymphokines are involved in rejection

The role of T-helper (TH) cells in rejection

Injecting T cells of the $CD4^+$ subpopulation (TH cells) into nude or ATx.BM recipients leads to acute skin-graft rejection. Naïve, unsensitized $CD8^+$ T cells (TC cells) are unable to do this, but when $CD8^+$ T cells are mixed with a very low number of $CD4^+$ T cells, or are presensitized to graft antigens (i.e. taken from animals which have already rejected a graft), rapid graft destruction is then seen. Treating recipients with monoclonal anti-$CD4^+$ antibodies (*Fig. 25.9*) confirms the importance of TH cells in rejection.

TH cells are activated by APCs derived from bone marrow and carrying MHC class II molecules. The APCs activating rejection can come from either the donor or the recipient. Those of donor origin are present in the graft as 'passenger leucocytes' (interstitial dendritic cells) and they cause 'direct' activation of the recipient's TH cells. Those of recipient origin are located in draining lymphoid tissues and acquire antigen that is shed from the transplant, and present it to the recipient's TH cells to cause 'indirect' activation. Direct activation is a more powerful stimulus to rejection than the so-called indirect route (*Fig. 25.10*). Thus passenger cells may have a strong influence on graft survival (*Fig. 25.11*).

The role of lymphokines in rejection

In addition to the role of $CD4^+$ TH cells, a multiplicity of immunological mechanisms including lymphokines are involved in the process of rejection. The overall picture is shown in *Figure 25.12*.

The most important lymphokines in cellular rejection are interleukin-2 (IL-2), which is required for activation of TC cells, and IFNγ, which induces MHC expression, increases APC activity, activates large granular lymphocytes and, in concert with lymphotoxin, activates macrophages. Macrophages, in turn, release TNFα, an important mediator of graft damage. (Note: the mixture of IFNγ and lymphotoxin was formerly known as macrophage activating factor or MAF.)

Lymphokines (IL-4, -5 and -6) are also required for B-cell activation, leading to the production of anti-graft antibodies. These antibodies fix complement and cause

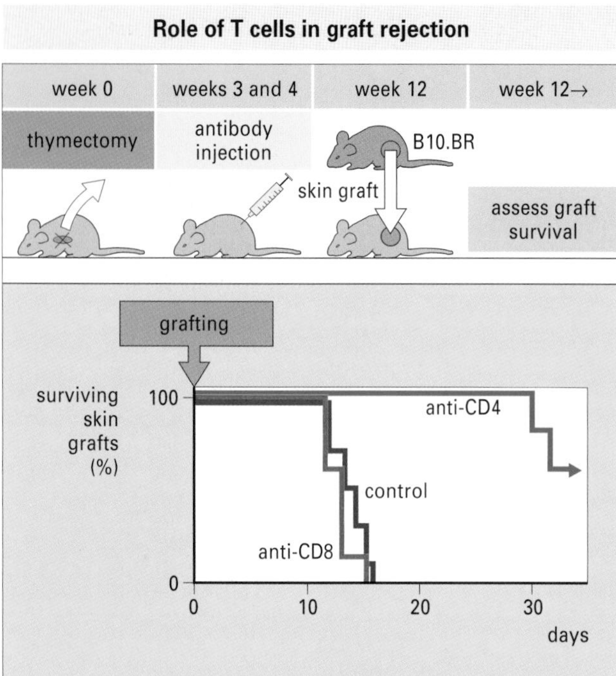

Fig. 25.9 Thymectomized CBA mice were treated with cytotoxic monoclonal antibodies to CD4 or CD8, to selectively deplete TH and Tc cell populations, respectively. They were then grafted with skin from B10.BR mice, which differ at minor histocompatibility loci. The survival of the grafts was assessed. Animals treated with anti-CD4 had greatly extended graft survival by comparison with untreated animals (control) or those treated with anti-CD8. This emphasizes the importance of the CD4+ (TH) population in graft rejection. (Based on data from Professor H. Waldman and Dr S. Cobbold.)

damage to the vascular endothelium, resulting in haemorrhage, platelet aggregation within the vessels, graft thrombosis, lytic damage to cells of the transplant, and the release of the pro-inflammatory complement components, C3a and C5a.

Not all parts of the graft need to be attacked for rejection to occur. The critical targets are the vascular endothelium of the microvasculature and the specialized parenchymal cells of the organ, such as renal tubules, pancreatic islets of Langerhans or cardiac myocytes.

IFNγ can cause vascular endothelial cells to express high levels of class II MHC molecules, and can induce the expression of class I and II molecules on parenchymal cells, which usually express little or none of these. This upregulation of MHC expression on cells of the graft can provoke greater stimulation of the rejection response and provide a greater number of target molecules within the graft for antibodies and activated cells.

Lymphotoxin and IFNγ also upregulate the expression of adhesion molecules on vascular endothelium. These are required for the adhesion of blood-borne leucocytes to the walls of blood vessels prior to their migration across the endothelium into the tissues.

THE TEMPO OF REJECTION

The rate of rejection depends in part on the underlying effector mechanisms (*Fig. 25.13*).

A comparison of direct and indirect antigen presentation

	Direct antigen presentation	**Indirect antigen presentation**
General comment	Abnormal situation restricted to recognition of transplanted tissues	Normal physiological route of antigen processing and presentation
Origin of antigen presenting cells	Donor	Recipient
Antigen recognised by recipient T cells	Donor MHC plus donor and 'neo-self' peptides	Recipient MHC plus donor peptide
Frequency of the activated T cells	1/1000 to 1/10 000	1/100 000 to 1/1000 000
Function of the activated T cells		
TH cells	Produce cytokines No cognate interaction with B cells	Produce cytokines Provide cognate help for B-cell activation and antibody formation
Tc cells	Can kill cells in the graft because they recognize donor MHC + peptide in the transplant	Cannot kill cells in the graft because they do not recognize antigens expressed on donor cells
Duration of stimulus	Donor APC (passenger leucocytes) are normally lost from the graft within days, therefore their influence is short-lived*	Continues for as long as the graft (source of donor peptide) survives, and can therefore stimulate chronic rejection

Fig. 25.10 Direct presentation of alloantigens stimulates a very powerful rejection response because of the large number of recipient T cells that may become activated. However, the T cells activated may act in different ways, and the stimulus through the direct route of alloantigen presentation is likely to be of limited duration. *Note there is evidence that donor-derived passenger leucocytes can remain in the recipient for a long time, a state known as chimerism. Some researchers suggest that the presence of chimerism is associated with graft acceptance, and may even play a role in maintaining unresponsiveness to the graft.

The role of passenger cells in graft destruction

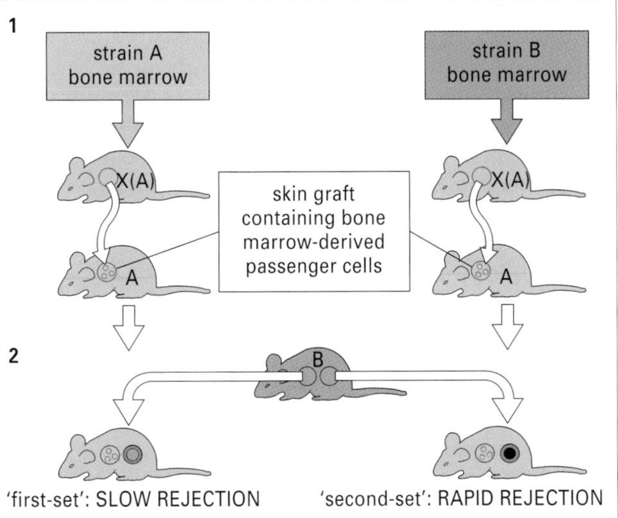

Fig. 25.11 Strain A mice were X-irradiated (X(A)) and then reconstituted with bone marrow cells of either strain A or strain B. Skin grafts from these mice were accepted by strain A mice (**1**). The recipients subsequently received strain B skin grafts. Animals whose first graft came from an animal reconstituted with strain A cells rejected the strain B graft more slowly than animals whose first graft came from a mouse reconstituted with strain B cells (**2**). This implies that strain B bone-marrow cells, carried as passengers in the first graft, primed the recipient to strain B alloantigen.

Hyperacute rejection – This occurs very rapidly in patients who already have antibodies against a graft. Anti-HLA antibodies are induced by prior blood transfusions, multiple pregnancies or the rejection of a previous transplant. In addition, antibodies against the ABO blood group system can cause hyperacute rejection. Preformed antibodies fix complement, damaging the endothelial cell lining of the blood vessels. This damage allows the leakage of cells and fluids and causes aggregation of platelets which then block the microvasculature, depriving the graft of a blood supply (*Fig. 25.14*). Hyperacute rejection can be avoided by ABO matching and by performing cross-matching, in which serum from a prospective recipient is tested for the presence of cytotoxic anti-donor antibodies.

Because humans have preformed IgM and IgG natural antibodies to animal cells, hyperacute rejection prevents transplantation of animal organs to man. Various approaches to overcoming this – by removing the antibodies, depleting complement or genetically engineering donor animals that have tissues less susceptible to hyperacute rejection – are under active investigation.

Immunological components of rejection

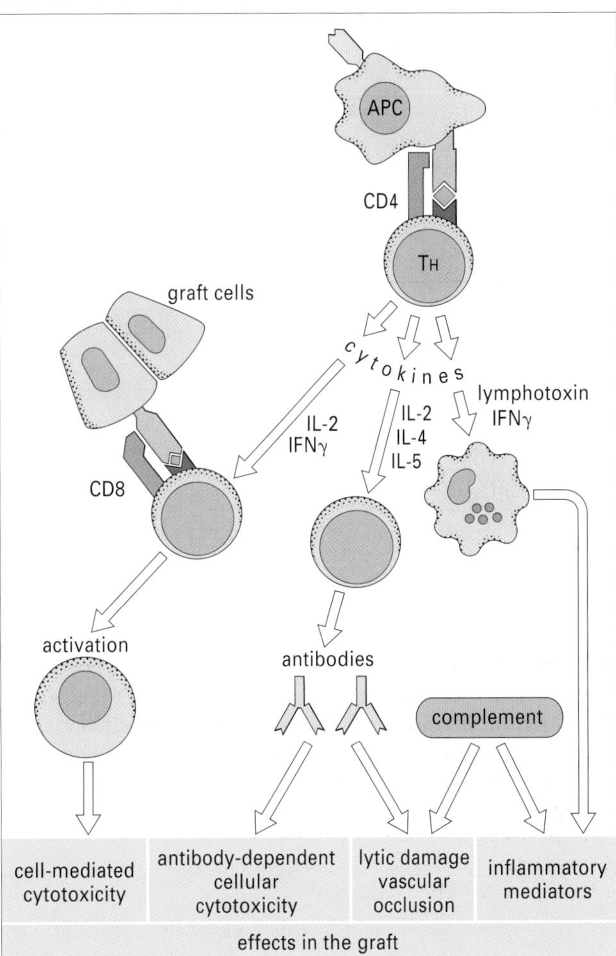

Fig. 25.12 TH cells are activated by APCs to release lymphokines. IL-2 and IFNγ are required for Tc-cell activation; IL-2, IL-4 and IL-5 are involved in B-cell activation; a mixture of lymphotoxin and IFNγ acts as macrophage-activating factor (MAF). These cells reject the graft by specific cell-mediated and antibody-mediated immune pathways, or by non-specific inflammatory reactions.

Tempo of rejection reactions

type of rejection	time taken	cause
hyperacute	minutes–hours	preformed anti-donor antibodies and complement
accelerated	days	reactivation of sensitized T cells
acute	days–weeks	primary activation of T cells
chronic	months–years	causes are unclear: antibodies, immune complexes, slow cellular reaction, recurrence of disease

Fig. 25.13 Much can be determined about the mechanisms of rejection by observing the speed of graft damage. Preformed antibodies and presensitized lymphocytes cause rapid rejection compared with primary and slowly evolving responses.

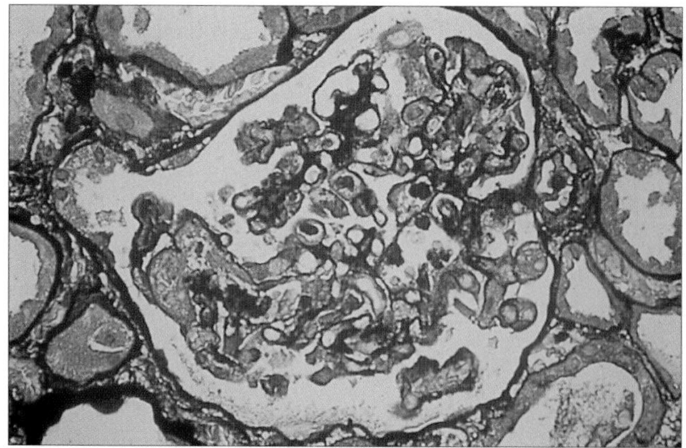

Fig. 25.14 Renal histology showing hyperacute graft rejection. There is extensive necrosis of the glomerular capillary associated with massive interstitial haemorrhage. This extensive necrosis is preceded by an intense polymorphonuclear infiltration which occurs within the first hour of the graft's revascularization. The changes shown here occurred 24–48 hours after this. H&E stain. ×200.

Acute rejection – This takes days or weeks to become manifest and is due to the primary activation of T cells and the consequent triggering of various effector mechanisms (*Figs 25.15–25.17*). If a transplant is given to someone who has been presensitized to antigens on the graft, a secondary reactivation of T cells occurs, leading to an accelerated cell-mediated rejection response. Accelerated or 'second-set' rejection of skin grafts is particularly dramatic – so-called 'white graft rejection' in which the graft is rejected before it has time to heal (*Fig. 25.18*).

Chronic rejection – Depending on the genetic disparity between donor and recipient and the use of immunosuppressive treatment, graft rejection can be a slow process taking months or years. The walls of the blood vessels in the graft thicken and eventually become blocked. This is called chronic rejection and may be due to several different causes, such as a low-grade cell-mediated rejection or the deposition of antibodies or antigen–antibody complexes in the grafted tissue, which damage or activate the endothelial cells lining the vessel and trigger inappropriate repair responses.

The cardinal features of chronic rejection are luminal obliteration (blocking of the blood vessels of the graft by proliferating smooth muscle cells which have migrated from the vessel wall and deposited matrix proteins) and interstitial fibrosis (formation of scar tissue throughout the grafted organ). These processes are controlled by various growth factors, such as TGFβ, released as a consequence of immune or other injury to the transplant (*Fig. 25.19*). The half-life of a kidney transplant is still only 7–8 years, and has not improved in the last 10 years despite the introduction of cyclosporin A to control acute rejection. This strongly suggests that we need to find new immunosuppressive drugs to control the chronic rejection process.

Grafts may also be damaged by the recurrence of the original disease process that necessitated the transplant.

GENETIC PREDISPOSITION TO GRAFT REJECTION

The amount of many of the cytokines that an individual makes is under genetic control. For example, a person may be a high or a low producer of IL-10. Indeed, there may be a ten-fold difference in the amount of IL-10 made by different people. This is related to small differences (polymorphisms) in the DNA sequences flanking the IL-10 gene, in the gene promoter region. Most other cytokine genes are polymorphic too, so that each individual inherits a pattern of higher and lower cytokine responses. By using simple genetic tests it is possible to determine whether someone is predisposed to make higher or lower amounts of each cytokine. A person who is genetically pre-programmed to be a high producer of TNFα (an inflammatory cytokine) and a low producer of IL-10 (an anti-inflammatory cytokine) is more susceptible to inflammatory conditions. Likewise, these inherited differences may contribute to susceptibility to infections, allergies and autoimmunity.

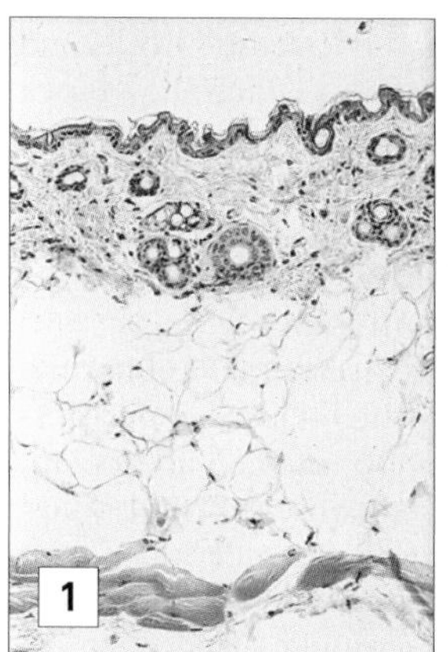

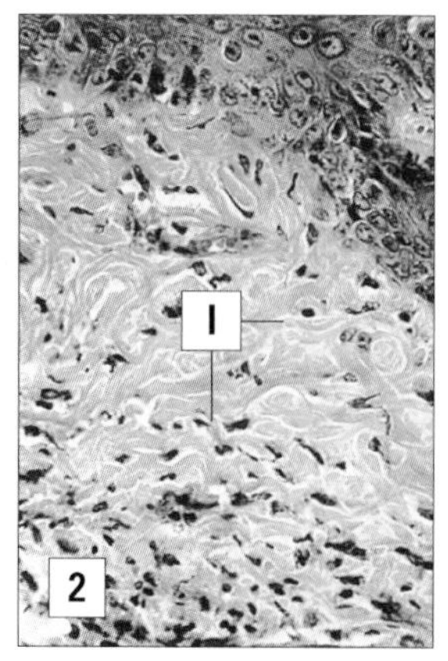

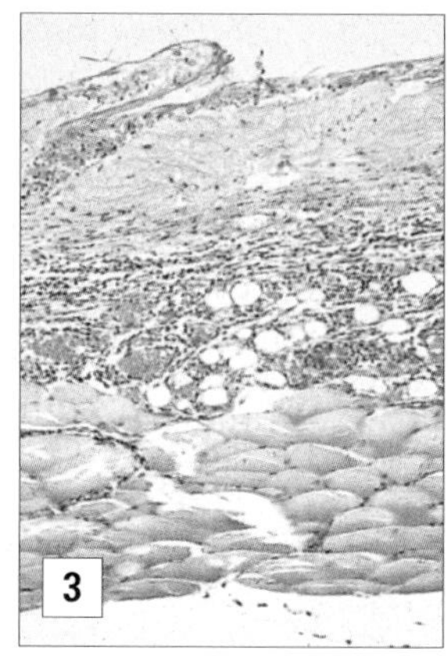

Fig. 25.15 Sections of strain A mouse skin showing the normal appearance (1) and the allograft 5 days (2) and 12 days (3) after transplantation to a mouse. At 5 days there is a substantial infiltration (I) of the allograft area by host mononuclear cells. At 12 days the epithelium has been totally destroyed and is lifting off the dermis, which is now free of cells; the infiltrating host cells have been destroyed by anoxia but there is still a brisk cellular traffic in the graft bed between the dermis and the panniculus carnosus. (Courtesy of Professor L. Brent.)

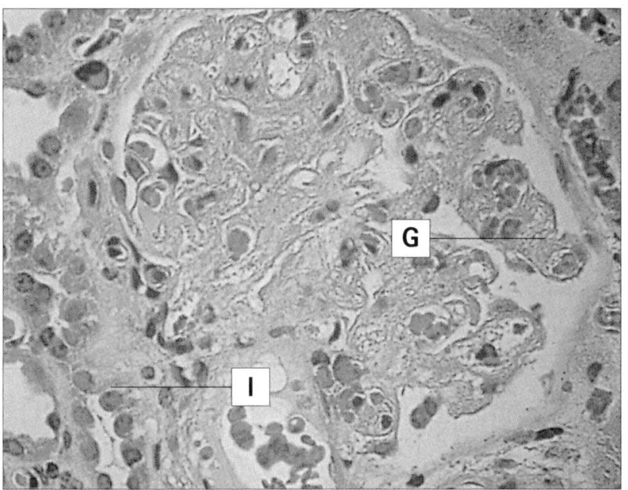

Fig. 25.16 Renal histology showing acute graft rejection – I. Small lymphocytes and other cells are accumulating in the interstitium of the graft. Such infiltration (I) is characteristic of acute rejection and occurs before the appearance of any clinical signs. G = glomerulus. H&E stain. ×200.

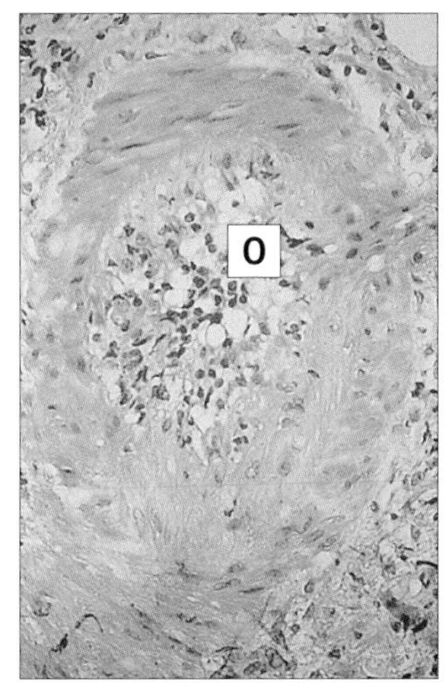

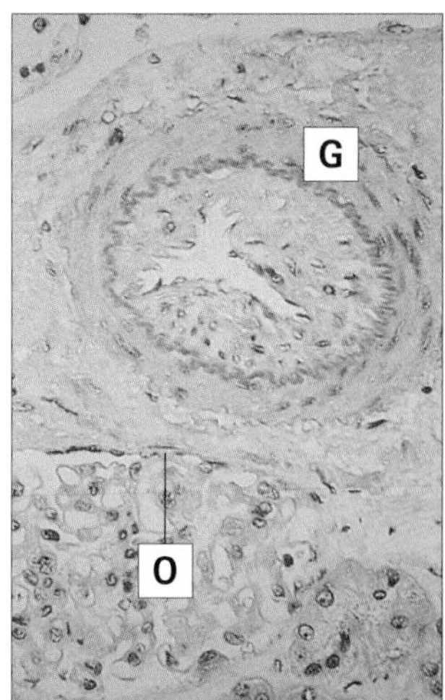

Fig. 25.17 Renal histology showing acute graft rejection – II. The section of acutely rejecting kidney on the left (H&E stain) shows vascular obstruction (O) and that on the right (van Gieson's stain) the end stage of this process. G = glomerulus. ×140.

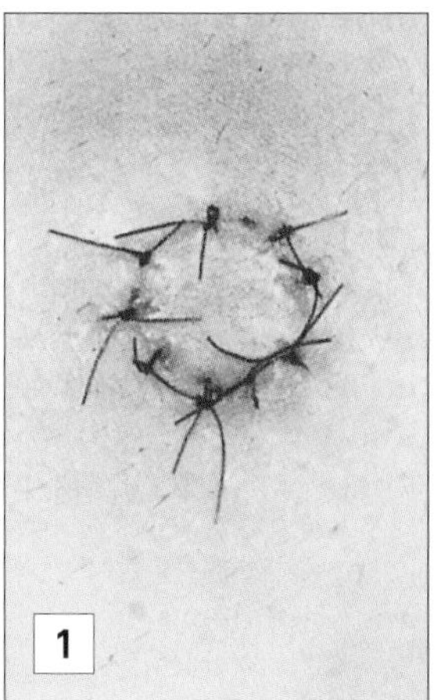

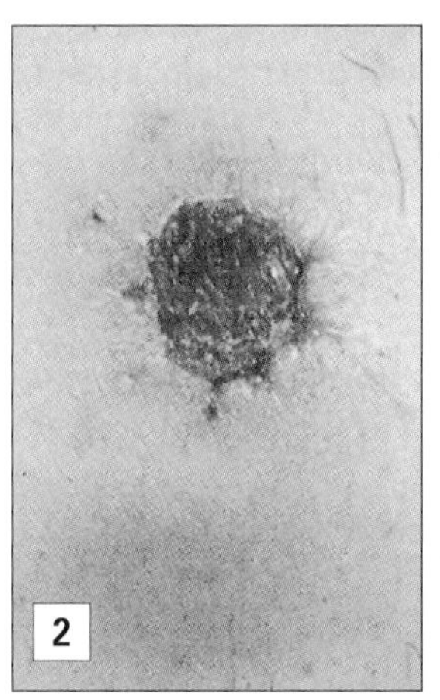

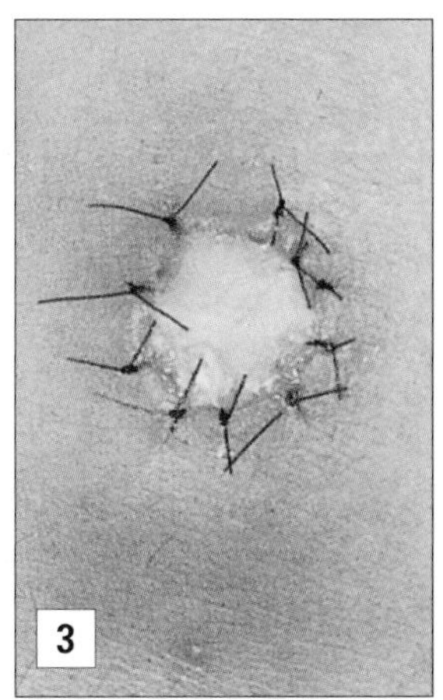

Fig. 25.18 Graft rejection displays immunological memory. A human skin allograft at day 5 (**1**) is fully vascularized and the cells are dividing, but by day 12 (**2**) it is totally destroyed. A second graft ('second-set' graft) from the same donor shown here on day 7 (**3**) does not become vascularized and is destroyed rapidly. This indicates that sensitization to the first graft produces immunological memory.

Cytokine gene polymorphisms have been shown to influence transplant rejection in humans. The high TNFα producer genotype is associated with the acute rejection of kidney, heart and liver transplants, so that 80% of recurrent acute rejection episodes occur in the 20% of recipients who are high TNFα producers. In addition, such people are more likely to suffer irreversible rejection, a fatal outcome in heart transplant recipients. Similarly, because TGFβ plays a major role in chronic rejection, recipients of high TGFβ producer genotype are more likely to suffer chronic rejection of heart and lung transplants.

This recent research will be important in many ways. For example, the drugs that are given to prevent rejection are toxic and can produce severe side-effects. Thus we would aim to give the lowest effective doses. Knowing that someone is unlikely to fiercely reject their graft may allow the use of minimal immunosuppression while, at the opposite extreme, closer monitoring for rejection and higher drug doses may be used. This is a concept called 'tailoring immunosuppression to the individual needs of the patient' and contrasts with giving the same treatment to everyone regardless of their requirement.

Another outcome of cytokine genotyping is that it identifies the cytokines that play a pivotal role in transplant rejection. The importance of TNFα in acute rejection suggests that giving an agent, either an anti-TNFα antibody or an engineered soluble TNFα receptor, that will neutralize TNFα in the patient may work to suppress acute rejection. Anti-TNFα antibody does suppress acute rejection in rats. Furthermore, anti-TNFα agents are already used clinically to treat patients with rheumatoid arthritis. At present there are no agents that can be used to reduce TGFβ production and influence chronic rejection.

Immunological mechanisms of chronic transplant rejection

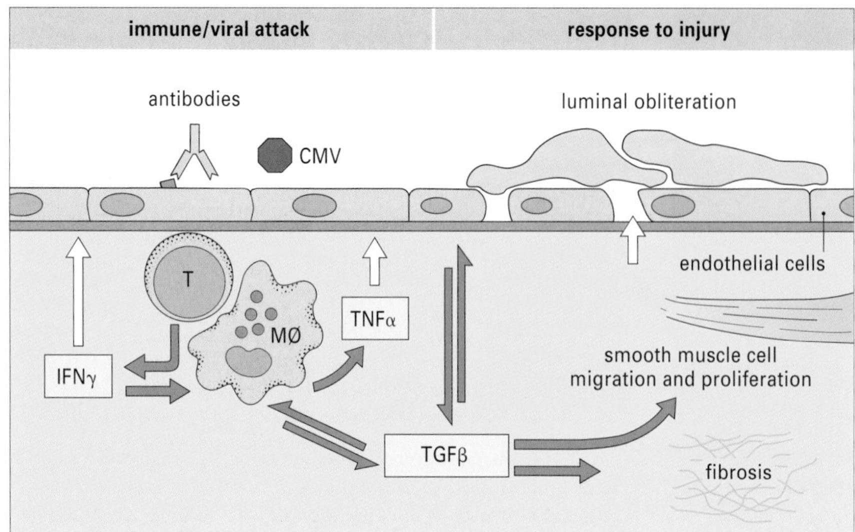

Fig. 25.19 Activation of endothelium by immune or viral attack stimulates the release of various growth factors. Of these, TGFβ is important because it causes fibrosis of the graft and contributes to arteriosclerosis. Obliteration of the lumen of the blood vessels supplying the graft occurs because smooth muscle cells from the intima migrate into the vessel wall, proliferate and deposit matrix components. The gradual loss of the blood supply to the graft tissues precipitates the fibrotic process, and this is seen as a steady loss of graft function.

PREVENTION OF REJECTION

The rejection response can be reduced by tissue matching

The perfectly matched donor and recipient would be isogeneic, for example monozygotic twins. However, this situation is rare, and in all other cases there will be major and/or minor histocompatibility differences between the donor and recipient. Only the major (MHC, i.e. HLA) antigens can be practicably matched. This can be done by serology (*Fig. 25.20*), which takes only a few hours and can therefore be performed while the donor organ is preserved on ice. Recently, sensitive and accurate typing has been achieved using the polymerase chain reaction (PCR) to identify HLA genes in the DNA of donors and recipients.

Matching for all known HLA antigens is practically impossible, but good organ graft survival is obtained when the donor and recipient share only the same MHC class II antigens, especially HLA-DR (*Fig. 25.21*), because these are the antigens that directly activate the recipient's TH cells.

The lists of known class I (HLA-A, HLA-B and HLA-C) and class II (HLA-DP, HLA-DQ and HLA-DR) antigens are long (see Appendix 2), and the chances of completely matching two individuals at random are extremely remote.

Serological tissue typing

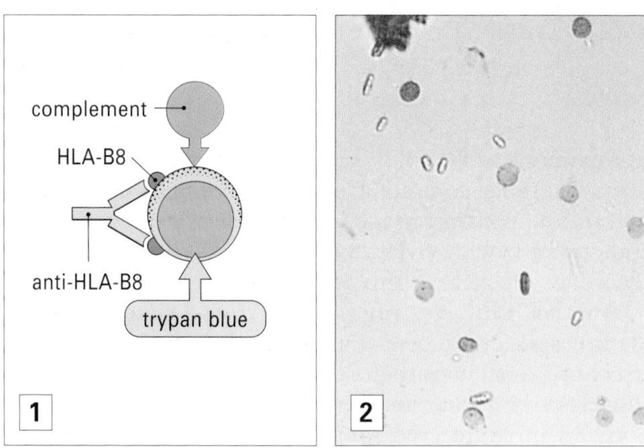

Fig. 25.20 (**1**) Tissue typing is performed serologically by adding typing antisera of defined specificity (e.g. anti-HLA-B8), complement and trypan blue stain to test cells on a microasssay plate. (**2**) Cell death, as assessed by trypan blue staining, confirms that the test cell carried the antigen in question (HLA-B8). Dead, trypan-blue-stained cells (dark staining) are shown on the right.

Kidney graft survival and HLA matching

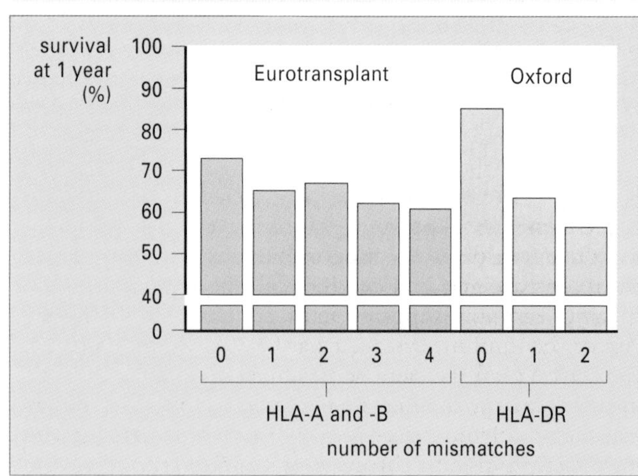

Fig. 25.21 The bar chart shows the percentage survival of cadaver kidney grafts at 1 year in humans in two separate studies. These studies were done before the use of cyclosporin; current outcomes of such engraftment are much improved. In the first study (Eurotransplant), donors were matched for HLA-A and -B (class I). In the second study (Oxford) donors were matched for HLA-DR (class II).

Tissue typing – mixed lymphocyte reaction

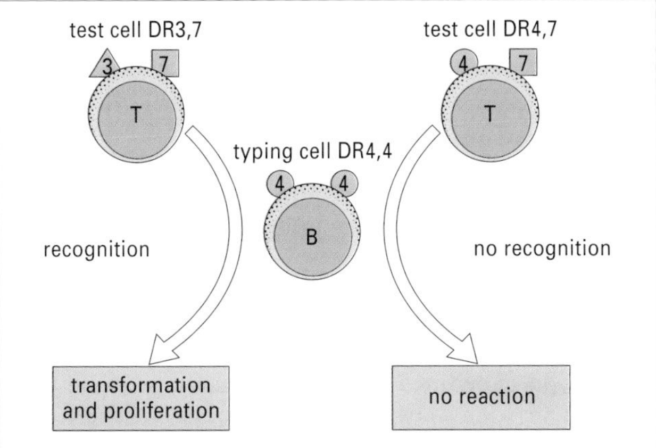

Fig. 25.22 In the mixed lymphocyte reaction, the cells being tested are incubated with 'typing' cells of known HLA specificity (DR4,4 in this case). The DR3,7 cells recognize the typing cell as foreign; this is revealed by the test cells transforming and proliferating (the typing cells are treated to stop them dividing in response to test cells). Conversely, DR4,7, which carries the typing cell's specificity (DR4), does not recognize the typing cell and so does not react to it.

Immunosuppression with drugs

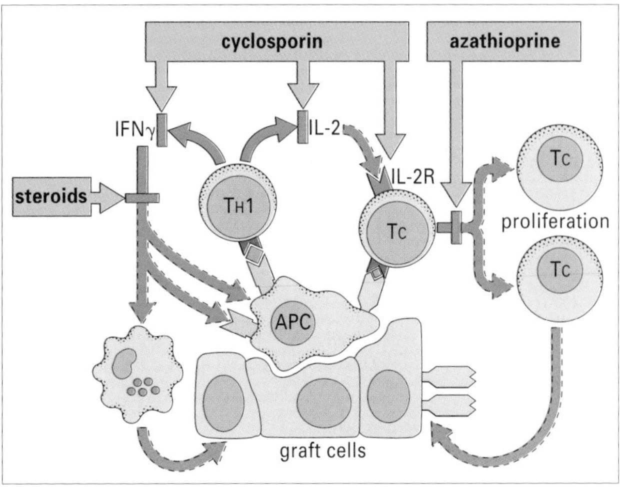

Fig. 25.23 The agents in common clinical use, steroids, cyclosporin and azathioprine, suppress the rejection response at different points. Steroids are anti-inflammatory and suppress activated macrophages, decrease APC function, and reduce MHC expression. Cyclosporin interferes with lymphokine production. Azathioprine prevents the proliferation of activated cells.

The mixed lymphocyte reaction (MLR) can also be used to test the responsiveness of recipient lymphocytes to antigens expressed on donor cells (*Fig. 25.22*). Low recipient anti-donor MLR responses are associated with excellent transplant survival. However, the 4–5 days required for the MLR test precludes its use in most clinical organ transplantation, because organs from dead or brain-dead donors cannot be preserved for more than 24–48 hours. In those for whom living donors (e.g. relatives) are to be used, MLR can be used. It is especially important in bone marrow transplantation, to assess whether the donor bone marrow cells can respond to recipient antigens and cause GVHD DNA typing has now largely superseded these older methods.

Non-specific immunosuppression can control rejection reactions

There are two main categories of immunosuppressive treatment: antigen-non-specific and antigen-specific. Non-specific immmunosuppression blunts or abolishes the activity of the immune system regardless of the antigen. This can leave a graft recipient very vulnerable to infections. For instance, a large dose of X-rays prevents rejection but also has many deleterious effects, as well as abolishing antimicrobial immunity. Most non-specific treatments used today are selective for the immune system, or are used in a way which creates some selectivity. The very best treatment would take this further and inactivate only those clones of lymphocytes with specificity for donor antigens, leaving other clones intact, so that the patient does not suffer infections or side-effects. Such highly specific immunosuppression remains the 'Holy Grail' of transplantation immunobiology and is described later.

The three non-specific agents that are most widely used in current clinical practice are steroids, cyclosporin and azathioprine (*Fig. 25.23*).

Steroids have anti-inflammatory properties and suppress activated macrophages, interfere with APC function and reduce the expression of MHC antigens. In effect, steroids reverse many of the actions of IFNγ on macrophages and transplanted tissues.

Cyclosporin is a fungal macrolide produced by soil organisms, and has interesting and potent immunosuppressive properties. Its principal action is to suppress lymphokine production by TH cells by interfering with the activation of lymphokine genes and, directly or indirectly, to reduce the expression of the receptors for IL-2 on lymphocytes undergoing activation. Other macrolides such as FK506 and rapamycin also have immunosuppressive properties. FK506 suppresses lymphokine production by TH cells in a way similar to cyclosporin. Rapamycin interferes with the intracellular signalling pathways of the IL-2 receptor and therefore prevents IL-2-dependent lymphocyte activation. The comparative structures of cyclosporin, FK506 and rapamycin are shown in *Figure 25.24*.

The rejection response involves the rapid division and differentiation – proliferation – of lymphocytes. Azathioprine is an antiproliferative drug, an analogue of 6-mercaptopurine. Its incorporation into the DNA of dividing cells prevents further proliferation. New antiproliferative drugs, such as mycophenolic acid derivatives, are under investigation.

These agents can be effective used alone, although high doses are usually required and the likelihood of adverse toxic effects is increased. Used together in various combinations, they work in synergy because they interfere with

The structure of immunosuppressive fungal macrolides

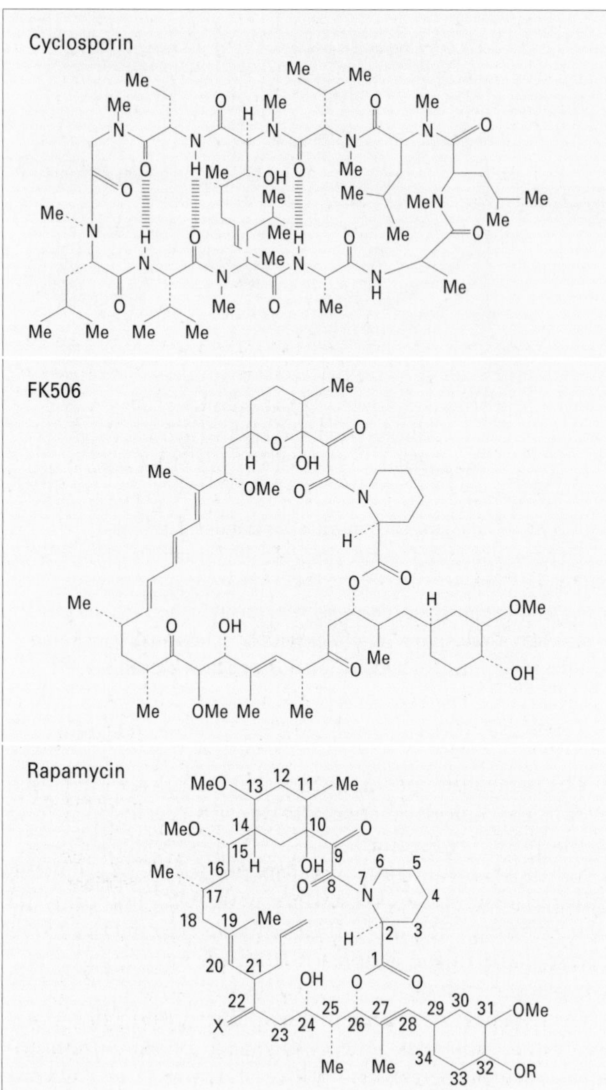

Fig. 25.24 The immunosuppressive fungal macrolides, cyclosporin, FK506 and rapamycin, have quite different structures. They act on lymphocytes in different ways, cyclosporin and FK506 affecting cytokine production and rapamycin interfering with signalling through the IL-2 receptor (IL-2R).

different stages of the same immune pathway. The doses of individual agents can thus be reduced and the adverse effects minimized. The clinical results obtained since the introduction of cyclosporin are very good (85–90% graft acceptance at 1 year for kidneys, hearts and livers). However, the expected half-life of a kidney transplant is 7–8 years because of the problem of chronic rejection, and long-term use of drugs is still associated with adverse effects. Further improvements might be obtained with the introduction of new drugs.

New non-specific but more selective agents are under development (*Fig. 25.25*). Monoclonal antibodies against lymphocyte surface molecules, especially CD3, CD4, CD8 and the IL-2 receptor, can be used to eliminate cells or to block their function. Cytotoxic drugs can be attached to these antibodies to increase their effectiveness. A related approach is to attach a toxin to IL-2 so that cells undergoing activation in response to graft antigens and expressing receptors for IL-2 take up the IL-2–toxin conjugate and are selectively poisoned.

Specific immunosuppression reduces anti-graft responses without increasing susceptibility to infection

The immune system is regulated by various feedback mechanisms that control the magnitude, type and specificity of immunological reactions (see Chapter 11). It is possible, in experimental models, to harness these feedback systems to prevent transplant rejection. There are three classical procedures which can be used: neonatally induced tolerance, active enhancement and passive enhancement.

Neonatal exposure to donor antigen can induce unresponsiveness to transplants in animals

Neonatal rodents (unlike humans) are born just before mature T cells are first exported from the thymus (the equivalent stage of human development is 16–20 weeks' gestation). If a persistent source of antigen, for instance viable cells with potential for growth or repeated injections of antigen, is given to the neonate rodents, the development of mature T cells that react with that antigen is suppressed. Classically, bone marrow cells from an (A × B) F_1 mouse are injected into a B-strain neonate. (The donor cells used are (A × B) F_1 to obviate the A-strain anti-B GVH reaction that occurs if A donor cells are used.) The bone marrow inoculum produces cells that provide a con-

Selective approaches to immunosuppression

	agent	target
heterologous antisera/ antibodies	anti-lymphocyte serum (ALS) anti-thymocyte globulin (ATG)	all lymphocytes selective for T cells
monoclonal antibodies	anti-CD3 anti-CD4 anti-CD25 (IL-2R)	mature T cells TH cells activated T cells
antibody–toxin conjugates	anti-CD5 coupled to the A chain of ricin toxin	activated ($CD5^+$) T cells
cytokine–toxin conjugates	IL-2 coupled to diphtheria toxin	activated T cells (which express IL-2R)
complement inactivating molecules	DAF/MCP CD59 transfected into donor cells (especially of xenografts)	complement-mediated damage via the classical and alternative pathways

Fig. 25.25 Antibodies and cytokines can be targeted to cells of the immune system. By contrast, drugs can have adverse effects on non-lymphoid tissue, e.g. nephrotoxicity and hepatotoxicity. The efficacy of biological agents can be increased by coupling drugs or toxins to them.

tinuous source of antigen. When the B-strain mouse grows to adulthood it is unresponsive to the A antigens to which it has been exposed neonatally and is tolerant of the A antigens on skin grafts and other tissues from A or (A × B) F_1 strain donors. Mechanisms to account for neonatal tolerance are detailed in Chapter 12.

Antigen may selectively activate certain subpopulations of lymphocytes. It is currently proposed that there are two major types of TH cell, known as TH1 and TH2 cells (see Chapter 7). Neonatally tolerized mice can have a deficit of donor-specific TH1 cells and an increased number of donor-specific TH2 cells. TH1 cells make IFNγ and IL-2 and are the TH cells illustrated in *Figure 25.23*, which are involved in rejection. By contrast, TH2 cells make other cytokines including IL-10 or cytokine synthesis inhibitory factor (CSIF), which interferes with the synthesis of lymphokines by TH1 cells. For neonatally tolerized mice, fewer donor-specific TH1 cells and more donor-specific TH2 cells mean a shift in the balance between rejection and acceptance, leading to tolerance of the graft. This form of tolerance is not strictly unresponsiveness *per se* but, rather, a deviated response. Interestingly, cyclosporin may have a preferential effect on TH1 cells and spare TH2 cells.

Finally, antigen can activate suppressor T cells (Ts cells). The precise identity of these T cells is still shrouded in mystery. What is known is that, when transferred to another animal, T cells from an animal tolerant of a graft from donor A can prevent rejection of a graft carrying A antigens. This is referred to as the adoptive transfer of suppression and the cells responsible can be TH or Ts cells. Much controversy still exists concerning Ts cells and their mode of action, but experimental data provide a clear indication that functional Ts cells do exist. They are resistant to cyclosporin and may contribute to this agent's mode of action and mediate tolerance by active suppression.

Equivalents in humans – A direct equivalent of neonatally induced tolerance is not possible in humans. However, procedures such as total lymphoid irradiation (TLI), in which mature lymphocytes are severely depleted by radiation while the bone marrow is shielded and therefore remains intact, may create in adults a situation analogous to that in the neonatal rodent. Indeed, TLI followed by antigen exposure induces profound tolerance. However, TLI is rather hazardous for routine clinical use. Antilymphocyte serum (ALS), made by immunizing animals with human lymphocytes, is widely used in heart transplant recipients to deplete circulating T cells. The use of monoclonal antibodies to mature T cells may achieve their depletion in a much safer but equally effective way, and anti-CD3 antibodies are in clinical use.

Unresponsiveness to transplants can be induced in humans by blood transfusions

In some cases, prior exposure to donor antigens can cause prolonged or indefinite graft survival (*Fig. 25.26*). This is, of course, contrary to expectation, as one might expect accelerated or hyperacute rejection. The phenomenon is called active enhancement of graft survival. The route of exposure of antigen is important, possibly because it

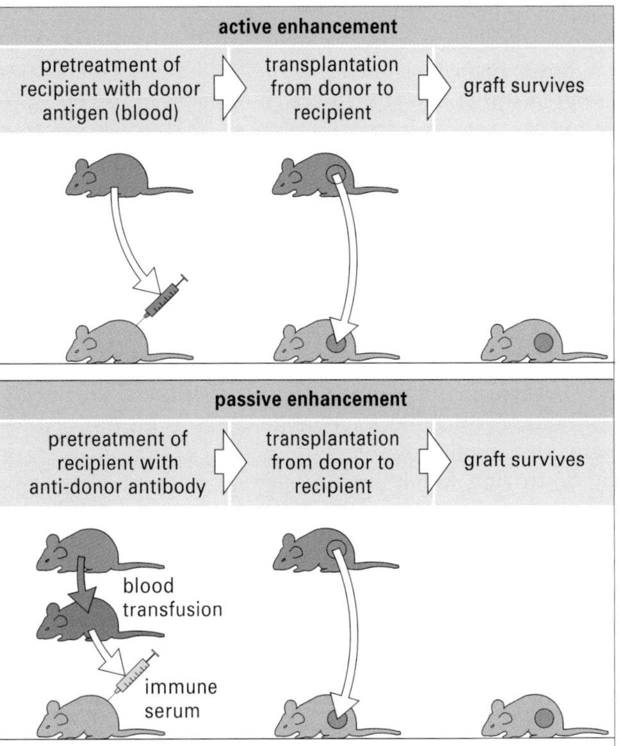

Fig. 25.26 Pretreatment of recipients with donor antigen given intravenously can prolong the survival of a subsequent allograft. This is known as active enhancement of graft survival because the effect requires an active response on the part of the recipient. (Note that the same blood, given by a different route, can result in rapid rejection.) Alternatively, anti-donor antibody given to the recipient at the time of transplantation can cause passive enhancement of graft survival. Both active and passive enhancement are immunologically specific, as only the response to the particular donor is suppressed and the survival of 'third-party' unrelated grafts is not enhanced.

impinges on particular lymphoid tissues. It has been shown in a rat kidney-graft model that a transfusion of donor blood given intravenously to the recipient 1 week before kidney transplantation leads to long-term organ-graft acceptance, while the same dose of blood given subcutaneously causes accelerated rejection. The effect is immunologically specific, so the blood donor and the kidney donor must share at least some antigens.

An active enhancement effect has been employed clinically using donor-specific transfusions (DST). For example, if a parent is about to donate a kidney to a child, the recipient can be treated with blood transfusions from the parent before transplantation. Unfortunately, about 20% of patients receiving DST develop anti-donor antibodies and cannot then receive the kidney as planned, for fear of hyperacute rejection. However, of the remaining 80% the transplant success rate is 95–100%.

The beneficial effect of pretransplant blood transfusion, known as the blood transfusion effect, has also been documented in patients receiving random transfusions, perhaps because of the chance exposure to antigens which happen to be on their transplant (*Fig. 25.27*). Indeed, the blood transfusion effect increases with the number of random transfusions, and for a time most transplant centres adopted the policy of deliberately transfusing prospective recipients. However, there is always a risk of sensitization of the patient, as well as the transmission of AIDS, and improvements in the availability and use of immunosuppressive drugs have largely made this practice redundant.

Active enhancement requires an active response by the recipient to the injected donor antigen. The mechanism could be induction of anergy, selective activation of TH2 cells, or activation of Ts cells by the blood transfusion, as described for neonatally induced tolerance. Alternatively, the mechanism might involve the production of 'enhancing antibodies' which block recognition of specific donor antigens, thus interfering with the graft rejection process, or by destroying highly immunogenic passenger leucocytes within the graft. Enhancing antibodies may also be formed to antigen receptors, thus eliminating donor reactive cells or affecting antigen presentation so that, for instance, TH2 and Ts cells are selectively activated after transplantation.

The effect of blood transfusion on kidney transplantation

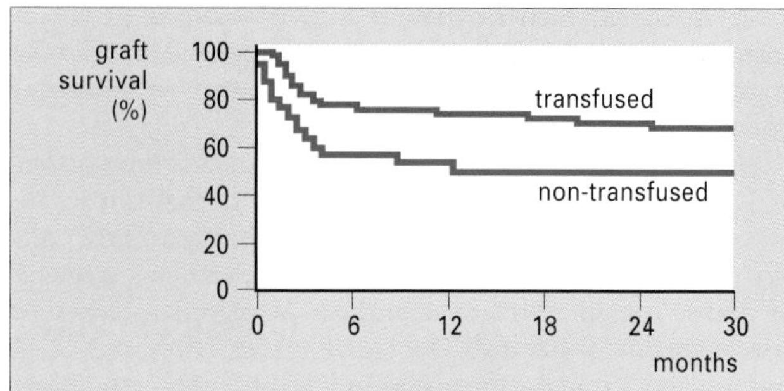

Fig. 25.27 Survival of kidney grafts is higher in transfused patients (102 patients) than in non-transfused patients (71 patients).

Antibody can have a feedback role in transplanted individuals. Injection of anti-donor antibody (passive enhancement) into a rat kidney-graft recipient at the time of grafting can cause long-term graft acceptance (*Fig. 25.26*).

CRITICAL THINKING • Kidney transplantation (Explanations on pp 463–464)

Mrs X had diabetes, and this caused severe damage to her kidneys. This complication is called diabetic nephropathy, and is one of the major indications for kidney transplantation. Mrs X was on dialysis treatment but this was not working well for her and she was advised that she would benefit from renal transplantation. However, it proved very difficult to find a suitable cadaveric donor for Mrs X and it was suggested that a family member might donate an organ. All of her immediate family, her husband, her five children and her two brothers, agreed to be considered as donors.

The HLA types and blood groups of the family members are shown in the table below. On the basis of these tests a donor was selected and the transplant was performed. Alas, despite successful surgery, the kidney soon turned dark and swelled. This started to happen within a few minutes of the restoration of blood flow through the transplant, and necessitated the immediate removal of the graft.

CRITICAL THINKING - *Continued*

Person	Age	Relationship to patient	HLA genotypes A	B	DR	Blood group genes phenotype
Mrs X	46	The patient	1 2	8 44	3 4	BODd BRh+
Mr X	52	Husband	2 3	14 7	8 2	AOdd ARh–
Anne	25	Daughter	2 3	44 7	4 2	AOdd ARh–
Bert	24	Son	1 2	8 14	3 8	ABDd ABRh+
Chas	21	Son	1 3	8 7	3 2	BOdd BRh–
Dave	15	Son	2 1	44 60	4 9	BODd BRh+
Edna	13	Daughter	1 2	8 14	3 8	AODd ARh+
Fred	48	Brother	1 2	8 44	3 4	ABDd ABRh+
Gary	56	Brother	2 2	44 14	4 15	BODD BRh+

Four years later Mrs X was still very ill on dialysis, no cadaveric donor was available and it was decided to try again with a living related transplant. Another member of the family was selected to donate a kidney and it functioned well from the onset. Mrs X was given triple immunosuppression. She had only one rejection episode at about 3 weeks after grafting, and this was treated successfully with anti-rejection therapy. There were no other problems.

The kidney continued to work for 8 years but its function gradually declined from the fourth year onwards. It seemed there was little the doctors could do to prevent this worsening situation, and Mrs X eventually had to return to dialysis.

25.1 What are the difficulties in finding a donor organ?

25.2 Comment on the HLA relationships between Mrs X and her brothers.

25.3 Comment on the relationships between the children of Mrs X.

25.4 Classify each member of the family in terms of their HLA relationship to Mrs X (HLA identical, HLA haplotype match, complete HLA mismatch).

25.5 In terms of HLA matching alone, who was the best donor for Mrs X?

25.6 Consider what effect the blood group antigens had on the choice of donor. From whom could kidneys have been transplanted, and who would not have been suitable?

25.7 Of those who had a compatible blood group, whom would you have chosen as the best donor? Explain your reasoning.

25.8 The outcome of the transplantation was a disaster! By what mechanism was the graft attacked?

25.9 Why was Mrs X at a greater risk of this untoward reaction?

25.10 What laboratory tests are used to avoid this rejection reaction, and what seems to have gone wrong on this occasion?

25.11 Four years after the first transplant it was decided to try again with a living related donor. Of all the family members, whom would you have chosen as the donor whose kidney was most likely to survive in Mrs X?

25.12 What is triple therapy immunosuppression?

25.13 What type of rejection occurred at 3 weeks after transplantation, and what immunological mechanisms were involved?

25.14 What is anti-rejection therapy?

25.15 There were no other problems with Mrs X. Can you think of some of the problems that might arise in a transplant recipient?

25.16 Why did the function of the transplant gradually decline, and why could the doctors not stop this process?

FURTHER READING

Alexandre GPJ, Latime D, Gianello P, *et al.* Preformed cytotoxic antibodies and ABO-incompatible grafts. *Clin Transplant* 1991;**5**:583.

Bach FH. Xenotransplantation: problems for consideration. *Clin Transplant* 1991;**5**:595.

Bjorkman PJ, Saper MA, Samaouri B, *et al.* The foreign antigen binding site and T cell recognition regions of class I histocompatibility antigens. *Nature* 1987;**329**:512.

Burdick JF. Chronic rejection. *Clin Transplant* 1991;**5**:489.

Concar D. The organ factory of the future? *New Scientist* 1994;**1930**:24–9.

Dallman MJ, Clark GJ. Cytokines and their receptors in transplantation. *Curr Opin Immunol* 1991;**3**:729.

Graff RJ, Bailey DW. The non-H-2 histocompatibility loci and their antigens. *Transplant Rev* 1973;**15**:26–49.

Hall BM, Dorsch S, Roser B. The cellular basis of allograft rejection *in vivo*. I. The cellular requirements for first set rejection of heart grafts. *J Exp Med* 1978;**148**:878.

Halloran PF, Broski AP, Batiuk TD, *et al.* The molecular immunology of acute rejection: an overview. *Transplant Immunol* 1993;**1**:3–27.

Hunt S, Billingham M. Long-term results of cardiac transplantation. *Ann Rev Med* 1991;**42**:437.

Hutchinson IV. Cellular mechanisms of allograft rejection. *Curr Opin Immunol* 1991;**3**:722.

Hutchinson IV, Pravica V, Hajeer AH, Sinnott PJ. Identification of high and low responders to allografts. *Rev Immunogenet* 1991;**1**:323–33.

Hutchinson IV, Turner DM, Sankaran D, *et al.* Cytokine genotypes in allograft rejection: guidelines for immunosuppression. *Transplant Proc* 1998;**30**:3991–2.

Lechler RI, Lombardi G, Batchelor JR, *et al.* The molecular basis of alloreactivity. *Immunol Today* 1990;**11**:83.

Mason DW, Morris PJ. Effector mechanisms in allograft rejection. *Annu Rev Immunol* 1986;**4**:119.

Masoor S, Schroeder TJ, Michler RE, *et al.* Monoclonal antibodies in organ transplantation: an overview. *Transplant Immunol* 1986;**4**:176–89.

Opelz G. Effect of HLA matching in heart transplantation. *Transplant Proc* 1989;**21**:794.

Platt JL, Bach FH. The barrier to xenotransplantation. *Transplantation* 1991;**52**:937.

Sablinski T, Hancock WW, Tilney NL, *et al.* CD4 monoclonal antibodies in organ transplantation. A review of progress. *Transplantation* 1991;**52**:579.

Sachs DH, Bach FH. Immunology of xenograft rejection. *Human Immunol* 1990;**28**:245.

Steinmuller D. Which T cells mediate allograft rejection? *Transplantation* 1985;**40**:229.

Thomson AW. Immunosuppressive drugs and the induction of transplantation tolerance. *Transplant Immunol* 1994;**2**:263–70.

Waldman H, Cobbold S. The use of monoclonal antibodies to achieve immunological tolerance. *Immunol Today* 1993;**14**:247–51.

Waldmann H. Manipulation of T-cell responses with monoclonal antibodies. *Annu Rev Immunol* 1989;**7**:407.

Wood KJ. Transplantation tolerance. *Curr Opin Immunol* 1991;**3**:710.

26 Autoimmunity and autoimmune disease

- **Autoimmune mechanisms** underlie many diseases, some organ-specific, others systemic in distribution.
- **Autoimmune disorders can overlap:** an individual may have more than one organ-specific disorder; or more than one systemic disease.
- **Genetic factors** such as HLA type are important in autoimmune disease, and it is probable that each disease involves several factors.
- **Autoimmune mechanisms** are pathogenic in experimental and spontaneous animal models associated with the development of autoimmunity.
- **Human autoantibodies** can be directly pathogenic.
- **Immune complexes** are often associated with systemic autoimmune disease.
- **Autoreactive B and T cells** persist in normal subjects but in disease are selected by autoantigen in the production of autoimmune responses.
- **Microbial cross-reacting antigens and cytokine** dysregulation can lead to autoimmunity.
- **Autoantibody tests** are valuable for diagnosis and sometimes for prognosis.
- **Treatment of organ-specific diseases** usually involves metabolic control.
- **Treatment of systemic diseases** includes the use of anti-inflammatory and immunosuppressive drugs.
- **Future treatment** will probably focus on manipulation of the pivotal autoreactive T cells by antigens or peptides, by anti CD4 and possibly T-cell vaccination.

THE ASSOCIATION OF AUTOIMMUNITY WITH DISEASE

The immune system has tremendous diversity and because the repertoire of specificities expressed by the B- and T-cell populations is generated randomly, it is bound to include many which are specific for self components. Thus, the body must establish self-tolerance mechanisms, to distinguish between self and non-self determinants, so as to avoid autoreactivity (see Chapter 7). However, all mechanisms have a risk of breakdown. The self-recognition mechanisms are no exception, and a number of diseases have been identified in which there is autoimmunity, due to copious production of autoantibodies and autoreactive T cells.

One of the earliest examples in which the production of autoantibodies was associated with disease in a given organ is Hashimoto's thyroiditis. Among the autoimmune diseases, thyroiditis has been particularly well-studied, and many of the aspects discussed in this chapter will draw upon our knowledge of it. It is a disease of the thyroid which is most common in middle-aged women and often leads to formation of a goitre and hypothyroidism. The gland is infiltrated, sometimes to an extraordinary extent, with inflammatory lymphoid cells. These are predominantly mononuclear phagocytes, lymphocytes and plasma cells, and secondary lymphoid follicles are common (*Fig. 26.1*). In Hashimoto's disease, the gland often shows regenerating thyroid follicles but this is not a feature of the thyroid in the related condition, primary myxoedema, in which comparable immunological features are seen and where the gland undergoes almost complete destruction and shrinks.

The serum of patients with Hashimoto's disease usually contains antibodies to thyroglobulin. These antibodies are demonstrable by agglutination and by precipitin reactions when present in high titre. Most patients also have antibodies directed against a cytoplasmic or microsomal antigen, also present on the apical surface of the follicular epithelial cells (*Fig. 26.2*), and now known to be thyroid peroxidase, the enzyme which iodinates thyroglobulin.

THE SPECTRUM OF AUTOIMMUNE DISEASES

The antibodies associated with Hashimoto's thyroiditis and primary myxoedema react only with the thyroid, so the resulting lesion is highly localized. By contrast, the serum from patients with diseases such as systemic lupus erythematosus (SLE) reacts with many, if not all, of the tissues in the body. In SLE, one of the dominant antibodies is directed against the cell nucleus (*Fig. 26.2*). These two diseases represent the extremes of the autoimmune spectrum (*Fig. 26.3*).

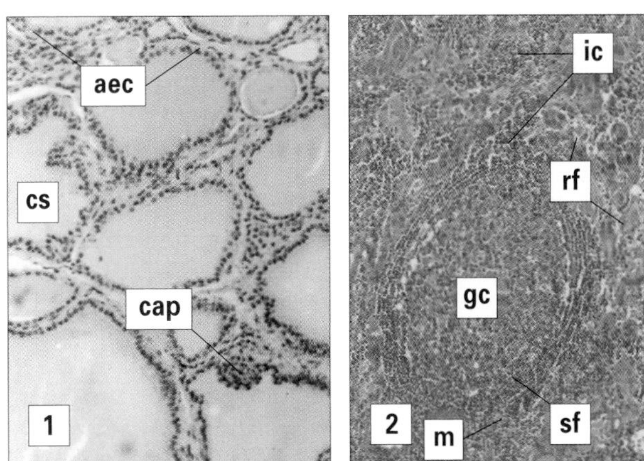

Fig. 26.1 Histological changes in Hashimoto's thyroiditis. In the normal thyroid gland (**1**), the acinar epithelial cells (aec) line the colloid space (cs) into which they secrete thyroglobulin, which is broken down on demand to provide thyroid hormones (cap = capillaries containing red blood cells). In the Hashimoto gland (**2**), the normal architecture is virtually destroyed and replaced by invading cells (ic), which consist essentially of lymphocytes, macrophages and plasma cells. A secondary lymphoid follicle (sf), with a germinal centre (gc) and a mantle of small lymphocytes (m), and small regenerating thyroid follicles (rf) are present. H&E stain. ×80.

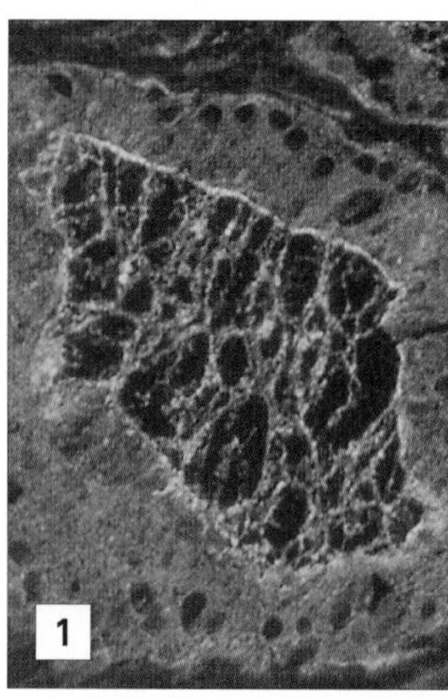

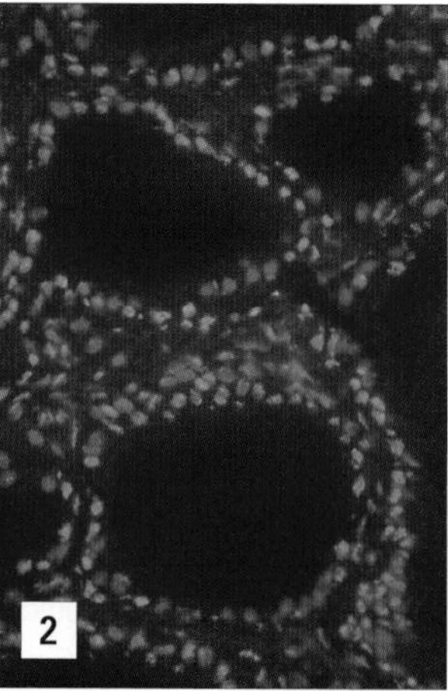

Fig. 26.2 Autoantibodies to thyroid. Healthy, unfixed human thyroid sections were treated with patients' serum, and then with fluoresceinated rabbit anti-human Ig. Some residual thyroglobulin in the colloid and the acinar epithelial cells of the follicles are stained by antibodies from a patient with Hashimoto's disease, which react with the cells' cytoplasm but not the nuclei (**1**). In contrast, serum from a patient with SLE (**2**) contains antibodies which react only with the nuclei of acinar epithelial cells and leave the cytoplasm unstained (**2**). (Courtesy of Mr G. Swana.)

The spectrum of autoimmune diseases

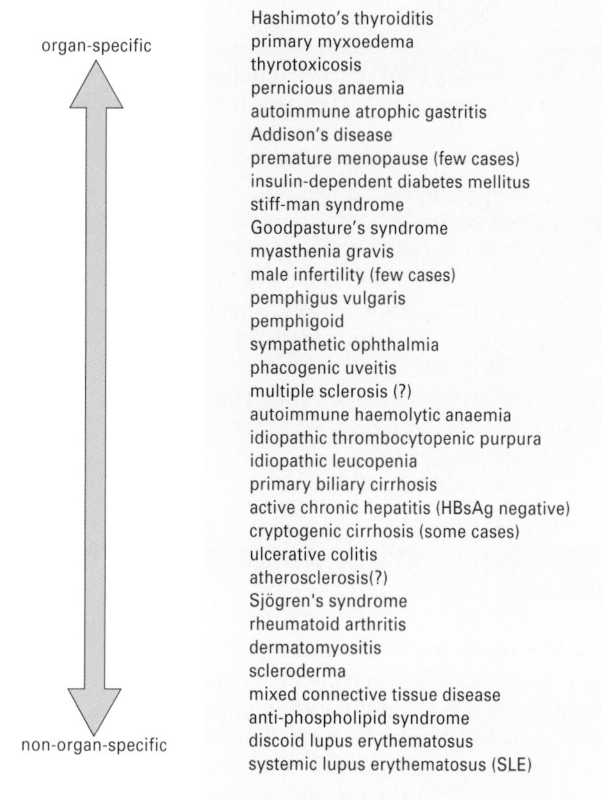

Fig. 26.3 Autoimmune diseases may be classified as organ-specific or non-organ-specific depending on whether the response is primarily against antigens localized to particular organs, or against widespread antigens.

The common target organs in organ-specific disease include the thyroid, adrenals, stomach and pancreas. The non-organ-specific diseases, which include the rheumatological disorders, characteristically involve the skin, kidney, joints and muscle (*Fig. 26.4*).

An individual may have more than one autoimmune disease

Interestingly, there are remarkable overlaps at each end of the spectrum. Thyroid antibodies occur with a high frequency in pernicious anaemia patients who have gastric autoimmunity, and these patients have a higher incidence of thyroid autoimmune disease than the normal population. Similarly, patients with thyroid autoimmunity have a high incidence of stomach autoantibodies and, to a lesser extent, the clinical disease itself, namely pernicious anaemia.

The cluster of rheumatological disorders at the other end of the spectrum also shows considerable overlap. Features of rheumatoid arthritis, for example, are often associated with the clinical picture of SLE. In these diseases immune complexes are deposited systemically, particularly in the kidney, joints and skin, giving rise to widespread lesions. By contrast, overlap of diseases from the two ends of the spectrum is relatively rare.

The mechanisms of immunopathological damage vary depending on where the disease lies in the spectrum. Where the antigen is localized in a particular organ, Type II hypersensitivity and cell-mediated reactions are most important (see Chapters 22 and 24). In non-organ-specific autoimmunity, immune complex deposition leads to inflammation through a variety of mechanisms, including complement activation and phagocyte recruitment (see Chapter 23).

GENETIC FACTORS

Autoimmune disease can occur in families

There is an undoubted familial incidence of autoimmunity. This is largely genetic rather than environmental, as may be seen from studies of identical and non-identical twins, and from the association of thyroid autoantibodies with abnormalities of the X-chromosome.

Within the families of patients with organ-specific autoimmunity, not only is there a general predisposition to develop organ-specific antibodies, it is also clear that other genetically controlled factors tend to select the organ that is mainly affected. Thus, although relatives of Hashimoto patients and families of pernicious anaemia patients both have higher than normal incidence and titre of thyroid autoantibodies, the relatives of pernicious anaemia patients have a far higher frequency of gastric autoantibodies, indicating that there are genetic factors which differentially select the stomach as the target within these families.

Certain HLA haplotypes predispose to autoimmunity

Further evidence for the operation of genetic factors in autoimmune disease comes from their tendency to be asso-

Two types of autoimmune disease

organ-specific	non-organ-specific
brain multiple sclerosis(?)	**muscle** dermatomyositis
thyroid Hashimoto's thyroiditis, primary myxoedema, thyrotoxicosis	**kidney** SLE
stomach pernicious anaemia	**skin** scleroderma, SLE
adrenal Addison's disease	**joints** rheumatoid arthritis
pancreas insulin-dependent diabetes mellitus	

Fig. 26.4 Although the non-organ-specific diseases characteristically produce symptoms in the skin, joints, kidney and muscle, individual organs are more markedly affected by particular diseases, for example the kidney in systemic lupus erythematosus (SLE) and the joints in rheumatoid arthritis.

HLA associations in autoimmune disease

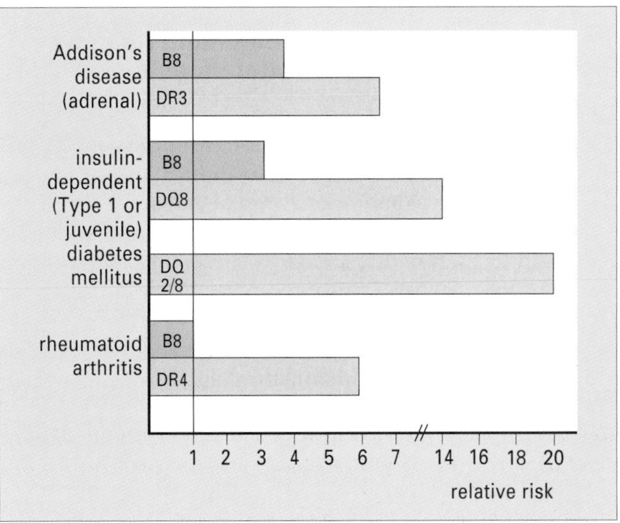

Fig. 26.5 The relative risk is a measure of the increased chance of contracting the disease for individuals bearing the HLA antigen, relative to those lacking it. Virtually all autoimmune diseases studied have shown an association with some HLA specificity. The greater relative risk for Addison's disease associated with HLA-DR3, as compared with HLA-B8, suggests that DR3 is closely linked to or even identical with the 'disease susceptibility gene'. In this case it is not surprising that B8 has a relative risk greater than 1, because it is known to occur with DR3 more often than expected by chance in the general population, a phenomenon termed linkage disequilibrium. Both DQ2 and DQ8 are associated with Type 1 diabetes mellitus, and when a gene for both is present, in the DQ2/8 heterozygote, there is a greatly increased risk, supporting the concept of multiple, additive genetic factors. Rheumatoid arthritis is linked to a pentamer sequence in DR1 and certain subtypes of DR4 but not to any HLA-A or HLA-B alleles.

ciated with particular HLA specificities (*Fig. 26.5*). Rheumatoid arthritis shows no associations with the HLA-A and -B loci haplotypes, but is associated with a nucleotide sequence (encoding amino acids 70–74 in the DRβ chain) that is common to DR1 and major subtypes of DR4. This sequence is also present in the dnaJ heat-shock proteins of various bacilli and EBV gp110 proteins, presenting an interesting possibility for the induction of autoimmunity by a microbial cross-reacting epitope (see below). The plot gets even deeper, though, with the realization that HLA-DR molecules bearing this sequence can bind to another bacterial heat shock protein, dnaK, and to the human analogue, namely hsp73, which targets selected proteins to lysosomes for antigen processing. The haplotype B8, DR3 is particularly common in the organ-specific diseases, although Hashimoto's thyroiditis tends to be associated more with DR5. It is notable that for insulin-dependent (type 1) diabetes mellitus, DQ2/8 heterozygotes have a greatly increased risk of developing the disease (*Fig. 26.5*). Although HLA risk factors tend to dominate, these disorders are genetically complex and genome-wide searches for mapping the genetic intervals containing genes for predisposition to disease by linkage to microsatellite markers (polymorphic variable numbers of tandem repeats, VNTR) reveal a plethora of genes affecting loss of tolerance, sustained inflammatory responses and end-organ targeting.

PATHOGENESIS

Autoimmune processes are often pathogenic. When autoantibodies are found in association with a particular disease there are three possible inferences:

- The autoimmunity is responsible for producing the lesions of the disease.
- There is a disease process which, through the production of tissue damage, leads to the development of autoantibodies.
- There is a factor which produces both the lesions and the autoimmunity.

Autoantibodies secondary to a lesion (the second possibility) are sometimes found. For example, cardiac autoantibodies may develop after myocardial infarction. However, sustained production of autoantibodies rarely follows the release of autoantigens by simple trauma. In most diseases associated with autoimmunity, the evidence supports the first possibility, that the autoimmune process produces the lesions.

The pathogenic role of autoimmunity can be demonstrated in experimental models

Examples of induced autoimmunity

The most direct test of whether autoimmunity is responsible for the lesions of disease is to induce autoimmunity deliberately in an experimental animal and see if this leads to the production of the lesions. Autoimmunity can be induced in experimental animals by injecting autoantigen (self antigen) together with complete Freund's adjuvant (see Chapter 15), and this does indeed produce organ-specific disease in certain organs. For example, thyroglobulin injection can induce an inflammatory disease of the thyroid while myelin basic protein can cause encephalomyelitis. In the case of thyroglobulin-injected animals, not only are thyroid autoantibodies produced, but the gland becomes infiltrated with mononuclear cells and the acinar architecture crumbles, closely resembling the histology of Hashimoto's thyroiditis.

The ability to induce experimental autoimmune disease depends on the strain of animal used. For example, it is found that the susceptibility of rats and mice to myelin basic protein-induced encephalomyelitis depends on a small number of gene loci, of which the most important are the MHC class II genes. The disease can be induced in susceptible strains by injecting T cells specific for myelin basic protein. These pathogenic T cells belong to the CD4/TH1 subset and it has been found that induction of disease can be prevented by treating the recipients with antibody to CD4 just before the expected time of disease onset, blocking the interaction of the TH cells' CD4 with the class II MHC of antigen-presenting target cells (see Chapter 5). The results indicate the importance of class II restricted autoreactive TH cells in the development of these conditions, and emphasize the prominent role of the MHC.

Examples of spontaneous autoimmunity

It has proved possible to breed strains of animals which are genetically programmed to develop autoimmune diseases closely resembling their human counterparts. One well-established example is the Obese strain (OS) chicken (*Fig. 26.6*) which parallels human autoimmune thyroid disease in terms of the lesion in the gland, the production of antibodies to different components in the thyroid, and the overlap with gastric autoimmunity. So it is of interest that when the immunological status of these animals is altered, quite dramatic effects on the outcome of the disease are seen. For example, removal of the thymus at birth appears to exacerbate the thyroiditis, suggesting that the thymus exerts a controlling effect on the disease, but if the entire T-cell population is abrogated by combining thymectomy with massive injections of anti-chick T-cell serum, both autoantibody production and the attack on thyroid are completely inhibited. Thus, T cells play a variety of pivotal roles as mediators and regulators of this disease. The non-obese diabetic (NOD) mouse provides an excellent model for human insulin-dependent diabetes mellitus (IDDM; type 1 diabetes) where the insulin-producing β cells of the pancreatic islets of Langerhans are under attack from a chronic leucocytic infiltrate of T cells and macrophages (*Fig. 26.7*). The role of the T cells in mediating this attack is evident from the amelioration and prevention of disease by treatment of the mice with a non-depleting anti-CD4 monoclonal antibody, which in the presence of the pancreatic autoantigens, insulin and glutamic acid decarboxylase (GAD) induces specific T-cell anergy.

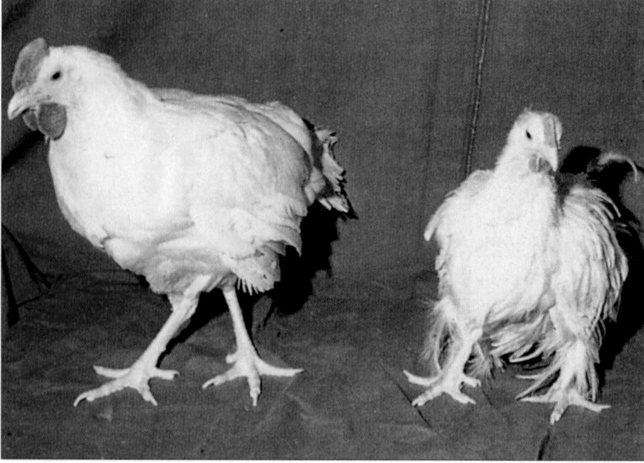

Fig. 26.6 Obese strain (OS) chicken. Chickens of this strain are affected with a spontaneously occurring autoimmune Hashimoto-like thyroiditis. They are much smaller (right) than age-matched normal controls and also show additional symptoms of hypothyroidism, such as cold sensitivity (ruffled feathers), skin abnormalities (long silky feathers), poor reproduction, subcutaneous and abdominal fat deposits (hence the name), high lipid serum, etc. These symptoms can be prevented by early thyroxine supplementation. (Courtesy of Professor G. Wick.)

The dependence of yet another spontaneous model, the F1 hybrid of New Zealand Black and White strains (NZB × W/F1), on the operation of immunological processes is aptly revealed by the suppression of the murine SLE which characterizes this strain, by treatment with anti-CD4 (*Fig. 26.8*).

Human autoantibodies can be directly pathogenic

When investigating human autoimmunity directly, rather than using animal models, it is of course more difficult to carry out experiments. Nevertheless, there is much evidence to suggest that autoantibodies may be important in pathogenesis, and we will discuss the major examples here.

Thyroid autoimmune disease – A number of diseases have been recognized in which autoantibodies to hormone receptors may actually mimic the function of the normal hormone concerned and produce disease. Graves' disease (thyrotoxicosis) was the first disorder in which such anti-receptor antibodies were clearly recognized. The phenomenon of neonatal thyrotoxicosis provides us with a natural 'passive transfer' study, because the IgG antibodies from the thyrotoxic mother cross the placenta and react

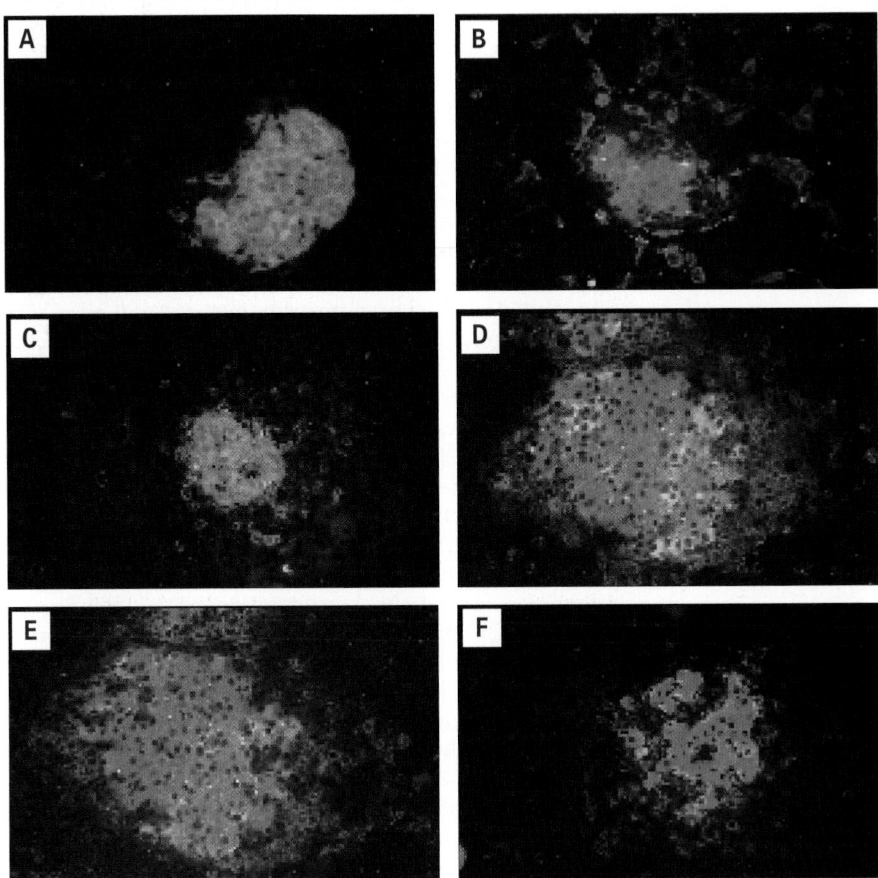

Fig. 26.7 NOD neonates were injected with the diabetogenic CD4$^+$ T-cell clone, BDC2.5. The cells infiltrated the pancreas and there was recruitment of other NOD cells. Eighty per cent of neonates that receive this clone become diabetic within 20 days. Snap-frozen pancreas sections taken from representative neonates killed 10 days after transfer of BDC2.5, before the onset of overt diabetes, were stained for insulin (red fluorescence) and infiltrating cells (green fluorescence). (**A**) is a section from a normal NOD neonate showing an islet, but no infiltration of CD3$^+$ T cells. Other sections show islets infiltrated with (**B**) macrophages (F4/80$^+$), (**C**) B cells (B220$^+$), (**D**) CD3$^+$ T cells, (**E**) CD4$^+$ T cells and (**F**) CD8$^+$ T cells, this section showing serious loss of insulin producing cells. ×400. (Figures generously provided by Drs Jenny Phillips and Anne Cooke.)

directly with the thyroid stimulating hormone (TSH) receptor on the neonatal thyroid. Many babies born to thyrotoxic mothers and showing thyroid hyperactivity have been reported, but the problem spontaneously resolves as the antibodies derived from the mother are catabolized in the baby over several weeks.

Whereas autoantibodies to the TSH receptor may stimulate cell division and/or increase the production of thyroid hormones, others can bring about the opposite effect by inhibiting these functions, a phenomenon frequently observed in receptor responses to ligands which act as agonists or antagonists. Different combinations of the various manifestations of thyroid autoimmune disease, chronic inflammatory cell destruction and stimulation or inhibition of growth and thyroid hormone synthesis, can give rise to a wide spectrum of clinical thyroid dysfunction (*Fig. 26.9*).

Myasthenia gravis – A parallel with neonatal hyperthyroidism has been observed with mothers suffering from myasthenia gravis, where antibodies to acetylcholine receptors cross the placenta into the fetus and may cause transient muscle weakness in the newborn baby.

Other receptor diseases – Somewhat rarely, autoantibodies to insulin receptors and to β-adrenergic receptors can be found, the latter associated with bronchial asthma. Neuromuscular defects can be elicited in mice injected with serum from patients with the Lambert–Eaton syndrome containing antibodies to presynaptic calcium channels, while sodium channel autoantibodies have been identified in the Guillain–Barré syndrome.

Male infertility – Yet another example of autoimmune disease is seen in rare cases of male infertility where antibodies to spermatozoa lead to clumping of spermatozoa, either by their heads or by their tails, in the semen.

Pernicious anaemia – In this disease an autoantibody interferes with the normal uptake of vitamin B_{12}. Vitamin B_{12} is not absorbed directly, but must first associate with a protein called intrinsic factor; the vitamin–protein complex is then transported across the intestinal mucosa. Early passive transfer studies demonstrated that serum from a patient with pernicious anaemia, if fed to a healthy individual together with intrinsic factor–B_{12} complex, inhibited uptake of the vitamin. Subsequently, the factor in the serum which blocked vitamin uptake was identified as antibody against intrinsic factor. It is now known that plasma cells in the gastric mucosa of patients with pernicious anaemia secrete this antibody into the lumen of the stomach (*Fig. 26.10*).

Suppression of autoimmune disease

NZW (New Zealand White) | NZB (New Zealand Black)

F_1(NZB/NZW)
DNA autoantibodies, immune-complex glomerulonephritis

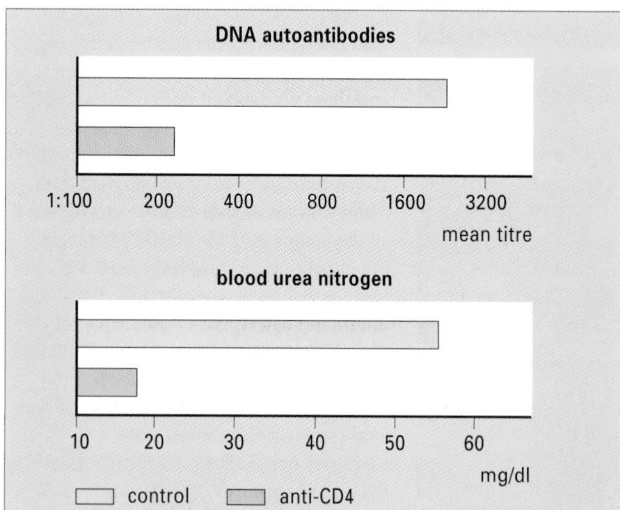

Fig. 26.8 The New Zealand Black mouse spontaneously develops autoimmune haemolytic anaemia. The hybrid between this and the New Zealand White strain develops DNA autoantibodies and immune-complex glomerulonephritis, as in patients with SLE. Immunosuppression with monoclonal antibodies to the TH cell marker CD4 considerably reduced the severity of the glomerulonephritis and the titre of double-stranded DNA autoantibodies at 8 months of age, showing the relevance of the immune processes to the generation of the disease. (Based on data from Wofsy *et al.*, *J Exp Med* 1985;**161**:378.)

Goodpasture's syndrome – In Goodpasture's syndrome, antibodies to the glomerular capillary basement membrane bind to the kidney *in vivo* (see *Fig. 23.3*). To demonstrate that the antibodies can have a pathological effect, a passive transfer experiment was performed. The antibodies were eluted from the kidney of a patient who had died with this disease, and injected into primates whose kidney antigens were sufficiently similar for the injected antibodies to localize on the glomerular basement membrane. The injected monkeys subsequently died with glomerulonephritis.

Blood and vascular disorders – Autoimmune haemolytic anaemia and idiopathic thrombocytopenic purpura result from the synthesis of autoantibodies to red cells and platelets, respectively. The primary antiphospholipid syndrome characterized by recurrent thromboembolic phenomena and fetal loss is triggered by the reaction of autoantibodies with a complex of β_2-glycoprotein 1 and cardiolipin. The β_2-glycoprotein turns up again as an abundant component of atherosclerotic plaques and there is increasing attention to the idea that autoimmunity may initiate or exacerbate the process of lipid deposition and plaque formation in this disease, the two lead candidate antigens being heat-shock protein 60 and the low-density lipoprotein, apoprotein B. The necrotizing granulomatous vasculitis which characterizes Wegener's granulomatosis is associated with antibodies to neutrophil cytoplasmic proteinase III (cANCA) but their role in pathogenesis of the vasculitis is ill defined.

Immune complexes appear to be pathogenic in systemic autoimmunity

In the case of SLE, it can be shown that complement-fixing complexes of antibody with DNA and other nucleosome components such as histones are deposited in the kidney (see *Fig. 23.3*), skin, joints and choroid plexus of patients, and must be presumed to produce Type III hypersensitivity reactions as outlined in Chapter 23. Cationic anti-DNA antibodies and histones facilitate the

The spectrum of autoimmune thyroid disease

thyroid disease	thyroid destruction	cell division		thyroid hormone synthesis	
		stimulation	inhibition	stimulation	inhibition
Hashimoto's thyroiditis	■				
Hashimoto's persistent goitre	■	■			
autoimmune colloid goitre		■			
Graves' disease		■		■	
non-goitrous hyperthyroidism				■	
'Hashitoxicosis'	■			■	
primary myxoedema	■		■		■

Fig. 26.9 Responses involving thyroglobulin and the thyroid peroxidase (microsomal) surface microvillous antigen lead to tissue destruction, whereas autoantibodies to TSH (and other?) receptors can stimulate or block metabolic activity or thyroid cell division. 'Hashitoxicosis' is an unconventional term which describes a gland showing Hashimoto's thyroiditis and Graves' disease simultaneously.

Failure of vitamin B_{12} absorption in pernicious anaemia

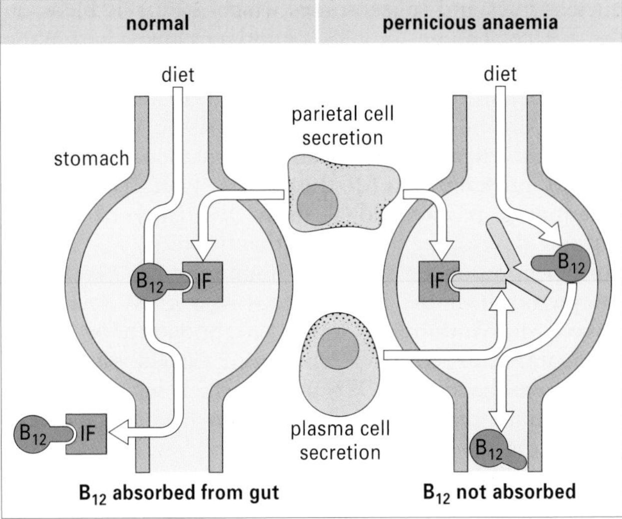

Fig. 26.10 Normally, dietary vitamin B_{12} is absorbed by the small intestine as a complex with intrinsic factor (IF), which is synthesized by parietal cells in gastric mucosa. In pernicious anaemia, locally synthesized autoantibodies, specific for intrinsic factor, combine with intrinsic factor to inhibit its role as a carrier for vitamin B_{12}.

Self-associated IgG rheumatoid factors forming immune complexes

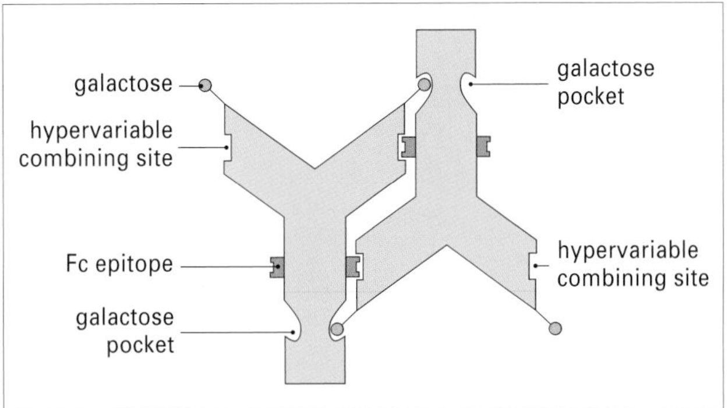

Fig. 26.11 The binding between the Fab on one IgG rheumatoid factor and the Fc of another involves the hypervariable region of the combining site. Since it has been established that the Fab oligosaccharides which occur on approximately one in three different immunoglobulin molecules are not defective with respect to glycosylation in rheumatoid arthritis, a Fab galactose residue could become inserted in the Fc pocket left vacant by a galactose-deficient $C\gamma2$ oligosaccharide, so increasing the strength of intermolecular binding. The stability and inflammatory potency of these complexes is increased by binding IgM rheumatoid factor and Clq.

binding to heparin sulphate in the connective tissue structures. Individuals with genetic deficiency of the early classical pathway complement components clear circulating immune complexes very poorly and are unduly susceptible to the development of SLE.

Turning to the experimental models, we have already mentioned the (NZB × W) F1 which spontaneously develops murine SLE associated with immune-complex glomerulonephritis and anti-DNA autoantibodies as major features. The fact that measures which suppress the immune response in these animals (e.g. treatment with azathioprine or anti-CD4) also suppress the disease and prolong survival, adds to the evidence for autoimmune reactions causing such disease (*Fig. 26.8*).

The erosions of cartilage and bone in rheumatoid arthritis are mediated by macrophages and fibroblasts which become stimulated by cytokines from activated T cells and immune complexes generated by a vigorous immunological reaction within the synovial tissue. The complexes can arise through the self-association of IgG rheumatoid factors specific for the Fcγ domains, a process facilitated by the striking deficiency of terminal galactose on the biantennary *N*-linked Fc oligosaccharides (*Fig. 26.11*). This agalacto glycoform of IgG in complexes can exacerbate inflammatory reactions through reaction with mannose-binding lectin and production of TNF.

Evidence for directly pathogenic T cells in human autoimmune disease is hard to get

Adoptive transfer studies have shown that TH1 cells are responsible for directly initiating the lesions in experimental models of organ-specific autoimmunity. In the human, the production of high affinity, somatically mutated IgG autoantibodies characteristic of T-dependent responses, the isolation of thyroid-specific T-cell clones from the glands of Graves' disease patients, the beneficial effect of cyclosporin in prediabetic individuals and the close associations with certain HLA haplotypes, make it abundantly clear that T cells are utterly pivotal for the development of autoimmune disease. However, it is difficult to identify a role for the T cell as a pathogenic agent as distinct from a T-helper function in the organ-specific disorders. Indirect evidence from circumstances showing that antibodies themselves do not cause disease, such as in babies born to mothers with insulin-dependent diabetes (IDDM), may be indicative.

AETIOLOGY

Self-reactive B and T cells persist even in normal subjects

Despite the complex selection mechanisms operating to establish self tolerance during lymphocyte development, the body contains large numbers of lymphocytes which are potentially autoreactive. This is particularly true of developing thymic T cells (thymocytes) that fail to be eliminated by a subset of self peptides (self epitopes). Normally, thymic APCs carrying self epitope deliver the negative selection that prompts the death of autoreactive T cells. But cryptic self epitopes are present in relatively low concentrations on APCs, because of either inefficient processing or low affinity for the MHC groove, or both, and are therefore unable to tolerize the autoreactive T cells which exit to the periphery (*Fig. 26.12*).

Cryptic self epitopes do not induce T-cell tolerance

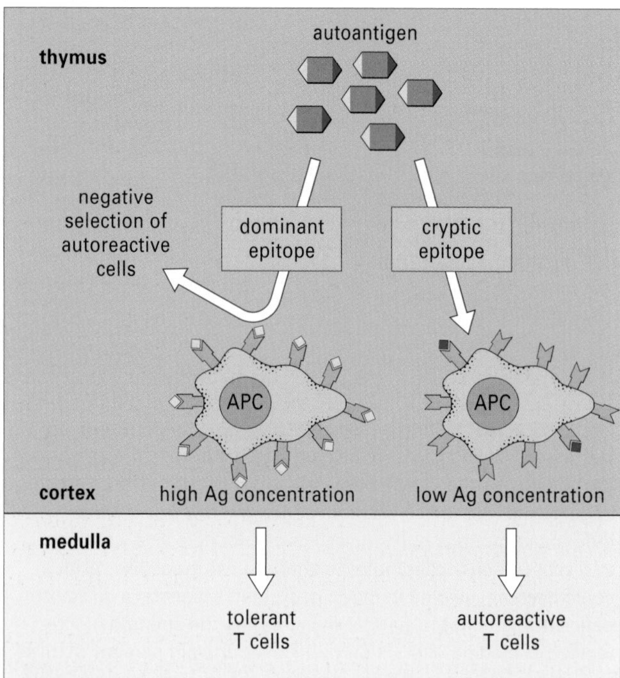

Fig. 26.12 Self epitopes which, after processing, appear in a high concentration on the surface of APCs in association with MHC are called dominant epitopes and are powerful stimulants which will delete or anergize developing autoreactive T cells, so that only tolerant T cells leave the thymus. By contrast, self epitopes which appear in a very low concentration on the APC are termed cryptic in the sense that they do not delete autoreactive T cells, which can then join the peripheral adult T-cell repertoire.

Many autoantigens, when injected with adjuvants, make autoantibodies in normal animals, demonstrating the presence of autoreactive B cells, and it is possible to identify a small number of autoreactive B cells (e.g. anti-thyroglobulin) in the normal population. Autoreactive T cells are also present in normal individuals, as shown by the fact that it is possible to produce autoimmune lines of T cells by stimulation of normal circulating T cells with the appropriate autoantigen (e.g. myelin basic protein) and IL-2.

Autoimmunity is antigen driven

Given that autoreactive B cells exist, the question remains whether they are stimulated to proliferate and produce autoantibodies by interaction with autoantigens or by some other means, such as non-specific polyclonal activators or idiotypic interactions (see *Fig. 26.14*). Evidence that B cells are selected by antigen comes from the existence of high affinity autoantibodies which arise through somatic mutation, a process which requires both T cells and autoantigen. Additionally, autoantibodies to epitope clusters occur on the same autoantigenic molecule. Apart from the presence of autoantigen itself, it is very difficult to envisage a mechanism that could account for the co-existence of antibody responses to different epitopes on the same molecule. A similar argument applies to the induction, in a single individual, of autoantibodies to organelles (e.g. nucleosomes and spliceosomes which appear as blebs on the surface of apoptotic cells) or antigens linked within the same organ (e.g. thyroglobulin and thyroid peroxidase).

The most direct evidence for autoimmunity being antigen driven comes from studies of the Obese strain chicken which, as described earlier, spontaneously develops thyroid autoimmunity. If the thyroid gland (the source of antigen) is removed at birth, the chickens mature without developing thyroid autoantibodies (*Fig. 26.13*). Furthermore, once thyroid autoimmunity has developed, later removal of the thyroid leads to a gross decline of thyroid autoantibodies, usually to undetectable levels. Comparable experiments have been carried out in the non-obese diabetic (NOD) mouse which models human autoimmune diabetes; chemical destruction of the β cells leads to decline in pancreatic autoantibodies. DNase treatment of lupus mice ameliorates the disease, presumably by destroying potentially pathogenic immune complexes.

In organ-specific disorders, there is ample evidence for T cells responding to antigens present in the organs under attack. But in non-organ-specific autoimmunity, identification of the antigens recognized by T cells is often inadequate. True, histone-specific T cells are generated in SLE patients and histone could play a 'piggy back' role in the formation of anti-DNA antibodies by substituting for natural antibody in the mechanism outlined in *Figure 26.14*. Another possibility is that the T cells do not see conventional peptide antigen (possibly true of anti-DNA responses) but instead recognize an antibody's idiotype (an antigenic determinant on the V region of antibody). In this view SLE, for example, might sometimes be initiated as an 'idiotype disease', like the model presented in *Figure 26.14*. In this scheme, autoantibodies are produced normally at low levels by B cells using germline genes. If these then form complexes with the autoantigen, the complexes can be taken up by APCs (including B cells) and components

Effect of neonatal thyroidectomy on Obese chickens

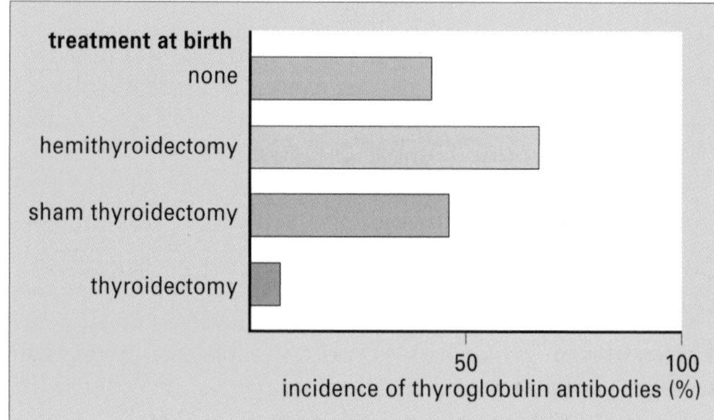

Fig. 26.13 Because removal of the thyroid at birth prevents the development of thyroid autoantibodies, it would appear that the autoimmune process is driven by the autoantigen in the thyroid gland. (Based on data from de Carvalho *et al., J Exp Med* 1982;**155**:1255.)

Model of T-cell help via processing of intermolecular complexes in the induction of autoimmunity

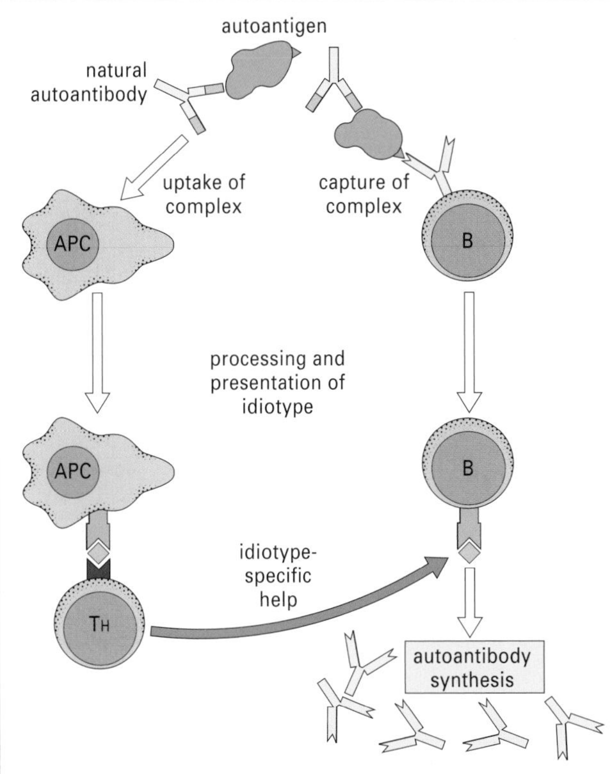

Fig. 26.14 An immune complex consisting of autoantigen (e.g. DNA) and a naturally occurring (germ-line) autoantibody is taken up by an antigen-presenting cell (APC), and peptides derived by processing of the idiotypic segment of the antibody (Id) are presented to TH cells. B cells that express the 'pathogenic' autoantibody can capture the complex and so can receive T-cell help via presentation of the processed Id to the TH cell. Similarly, an anti-DNA specific B cell which had endocytosed a histone/DNA complex, could be stimulated to autoantibody production by histone specific T-helpers.

of the complex, including the antibody idiotype, presented to T cells. Idiotype-specific T cells would then help the autoantibody-producing B cells. Evidence for the induction of anti-DNA and glomerulonephritis by immunization of mice with the idiotype of germline 'natural' anti-DNA autoantibody lends credence to this hypothesis.

Controls on the development of autoimmunity can be bypassed in a number of ways

Molecular mimicry by cross-reactive microbial antigens can stimulate autoreactive B and T cells

Normally, naïve autoreactive T cells recognizing cryptic self epitopes are not switched on because the antigen is only presented at low concentrations on 'professional' APCs or it may be presented on 'non-professional' APCs such as pancreatic β-islet cells or thyroid epithelial cells, which lack B7 or other co-stimulator molecules. However, infection with a microbe bearing antigens that cross-react with the cryptic self epitopes (i.e. have shared epitopes) will load the professional APCs with levels of processed peptides that are sufficient to activate the naïve autoreative T cells. Once primed, these T cells are able to recognize and react with the self epitope on the non-professional APCs since they no longer require a co-stimulatory signal and have a higher avidity for the target, due to upregulation of accessory adhesion molecules (*Fig. 26.15*).

Cross-reactive antigens which share B-cell epitopes with self molecules can also break tolerance but by a different mechanism. Many autoreactive B cells cannot be activated because the $CD4^+$ helper T cells which they need are unresponsive either because these helper T cells are tolerized at lower concentrations of autoantigens than the B cells or because they only recognize cryptic epitopes. However, these 'helpless' B cells can be stimulated if the cross-reacting antigen bears a 'foreign' carrier epitope to which the T cells have not been tolerized (*Fig. 26.16*). The autoimmune process may persist after clearance of the foreign antigen if the activated B cells now focus the autoantigen on their surface receptors and present it to normally resting autoreactive T cells which will then proliferate and act as helpers for fresh B-cell stimulation.

A disease in which such molecular mimicry operates is rheumatic fever, in which autoantibodies to heart valve antigens can be detected. These develop in a small proportion of individuals several weeks after a streptococcal infection of the throat. Carbohydrate antigens on the streptococci cross-react with an antigen on heart valves, so the infection may bypass T-cell self tolerance to heart valve antigens. Shared B-cell epitopes between *Yersinia*

Cross-reactive antigens induce autoimmune TH cells

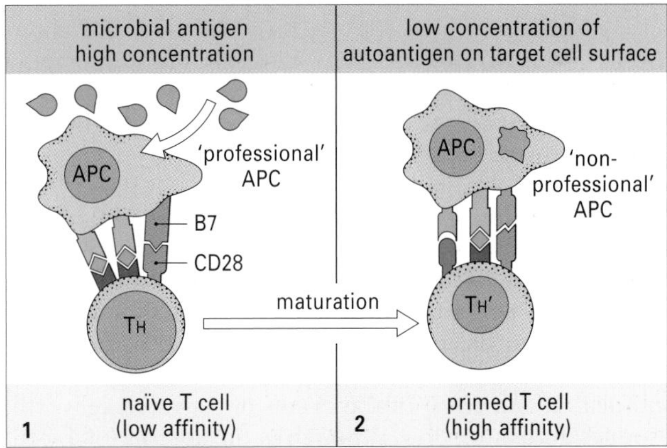

Fig. 26.15 The inability of naïve TH cells to recognize autoantigen on a tissue cell, whether because of low concentration or low affinity, can be circumvented by a cross-reacting microbial antigen at higher concentration or with higher innate affinity, together with a co-stimulator such as B7 on a 'professional' APC; this primes the TH cells (**1**). Due to increased expression of accessory molecules (e.g. LFA-1 and CD2) the primed TH cells now have high affinity and because they do not require a co-stimulatory signal, they can interact with autoantigen on 'non-professional' APCs such as organ-specific epithelial cells to produce autoimmune disease (**2**).

Induction of autoantibodies by cross-reactive antigens

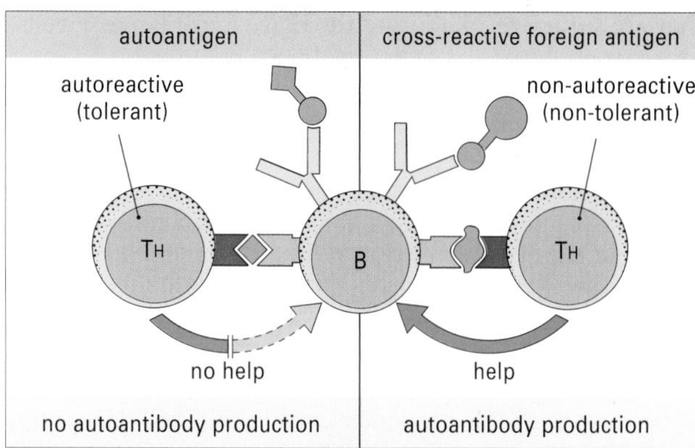

Fig. 26.16 The B cell recognizes an epitope present on autoantigen, but coincidentally present also on a foreign antigen. Normally the B cell presents the autoantigen but receives no help from autoreactive TH cells, which are functionally deleted. If a cross-reacting foreign antigen is encountered, the B cell can present peptides of this molecule to non-autoreactive T cells and thus be driven to proliferate, differentiate and secrete autoantibodies.

Autoimmunity due to cytokine dysregulation

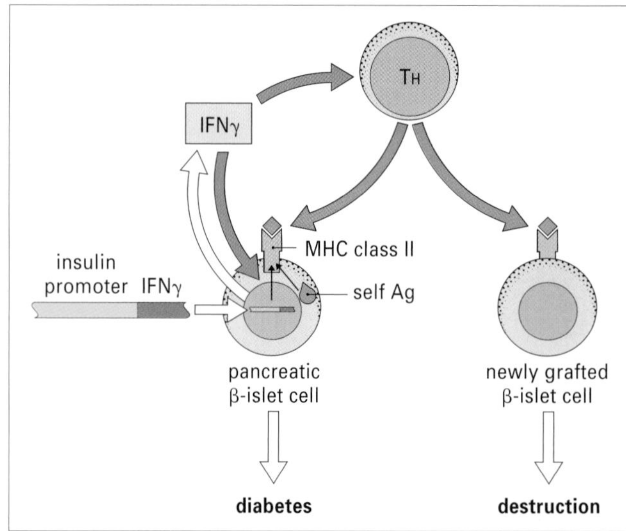

Fig. 26.17 Introduction of a transgene comprising IFNγ on an insulin promoter leads to copious pancreatic expression and secretion of IFNγ. This leads to upregulation of surface MHC class II and activation of autoreactive T cells by an as yet unexplained mechanism but probably mediated through uptake of autoantigen by cytokine-activated 'professional' APCs. The primed T cells now initiate autoimmune destruction of the β cells. That this is a true autoagression is shown by the prompt destruction of newly grafted normal syngeneic islet cells (genetically identical cells lacking the transgene).

enterolytica and the extracellular domain of the TSH receptor have recently been described. There may also be cross-reactivity between HLA-B27 and certain strains of *Klebsiella* in connection with ankylosing spondylitis, and cross-reactivity between bacterial heat-shock proteins and DR4 in relationship to rheumatoid arthritis.

In this connection, it has been suggested that because processed MHC molecules may represent a major fraction of the peptide epitopes presented to differentiating T cells within the thymus, a significant proportion of positively selected cells which escape negative selection and enter the periphery will be specific for weakly binding cryptic MHC epitopes. One might therefore expect autoimmune responses to arise not infrequently through activation of these cells by molecular mimicry.

In some cases foreign antigen can directly stimulate autoreactive cells

Another mechanism to bypass the tolerant autoreactive TH cell is where antigen or another stimulator directly triggers the autoreactive effector cells. For example, lipopolysaccharide or Epstein–Barr virus causes direct B-cell stimulation and some of the clones of activated cells will produce autoantibodies, although in the absence of T-cell help these are normally of low titre and affinity. However, it is conceivable that an activated B cell might pick up and process its cognate autoantigen and present it to a naïve autoreactive T cell.

Cytokine dysregulation, inappropriate MHC expression and failure of suppression may induce autoimmunity

It appears that dysregulation of the cytokine network can also lead to activation of autoreactive T cells. One experimental demonstration of this is the introduction of a transgene for interferon-γ (IFNγ) into pancreatic β-islet cells. If the transgene for IFNγ is fully expressed in the cells, MHC class II genes are upregulated and autoimmune destruction of the islet cells results (*Fig. 26.17*). This is not simply a result of a non-specific chaotic IFNγ-induced local inflammatory milieu since normal islets grafted at a separate site are rejected, implying clearly that T-cell autoreactivity to the pancreas has been established.

The surface expression of MHC class II in itself is not sufficient to activate the naïve autoreactive T cells but it may be necessary to allow a cell to act as a target for the primed autoreactive TH cells, and it was therefore most exciting when cells taken from the glands of patients with Graves' disease were found to be actively synthesizing class II MHC molecules (*Fig. 26.18*) and so were able to be recognized by CD4$^+$ T cells. In this context it is interesting that isolated cells from several animal strains that are susceptible to autoimmunity are also more readily induced by IFNγ to express MHC class II than are cells from non-susceptible strains.

The argument that imbalanced cytokine production may also contribute to autoimmunity receives further support from the unexpected finding that tumour necrosis factor (introduced by means of a TNF transgene) ameliorates autoimmune disease in NZB × NZW hybrid mice.

Aside from the normal 'ignorance' of cryptic self epitopes, other factors which normally restrain potentially autoreactive cells may include regulatory T cells, hormones (e.g. steroids), cytokines (e.g. TGFβ) and products of macrophages (*Fig. 26.19*). Deficiencies in any of them may

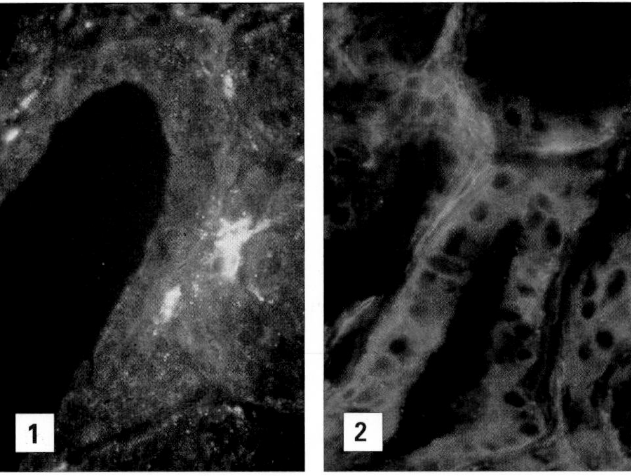

Fig. 26.18 Human thyroid sections stained for MHC class II. (**1**) Normal thyroid with unstained follicular cells, and an isolated dendritic cell that is strongly positive for MHC class II. (**2**) Thyrotoxic (Graves' disease) thyroid with abundant MHC class II molecules in the cytoplasm, indicating that rapid synthesis of MHC class II is occurring.

Regulatory mechanisms controlling autoimmunity

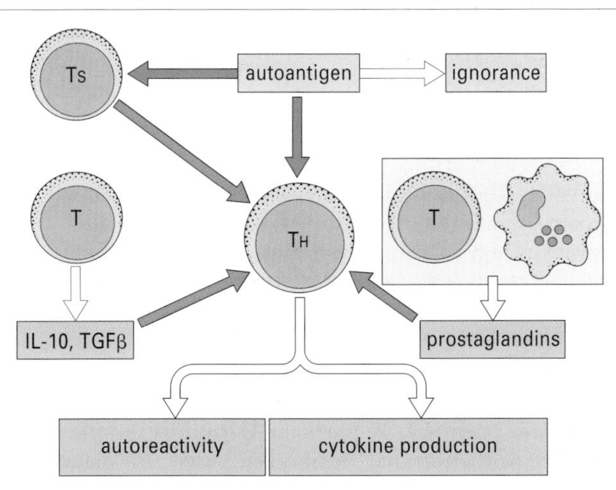

Fig. 26.19 Autoreactive TH cells are not normally stimulated by cryptic epitopes ('ignorance') but should they become activated, they would usually be held in check by a network of suppressive signals including antigen-specific suppression by T cells, which may be mediated directly or via suppressive cytokines such as IL-10 and TGFβ. Non-specific suppression (e.g. mediated by prostaglandins) also limits the capacity of the TH cell to respond. Should the TH cell show an enhanced capacity to respond, e.g. increased levels of IL-2 receptor, or the suppressive influences fail, the balance would be shifted towards autoimmune disease.

increase susceptibility to autoimmunity. The feedback loop on T-helpers and macrophages through the pituitary–adrenal axis is particularly interesting, as defects at different stages in the loop turn up in a variety of autoimmune disorders (*Fig. 26.20*). For example, patients with rheumatoid arthritis have low circulating corticosteroid levels

Defects in the cytokine/hypothalamic–pituitary–adrenal feedback loop in autoimmunity

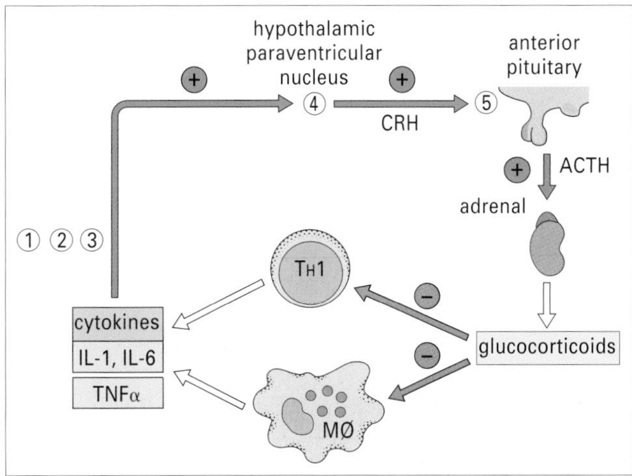

Fig. 26.20 Production of IL-1 is defective in the non-obese (NOD) mouse (**1**) and diabetes-prone BB rat (**2**); the disease can be corrected by injection of the cytokine. The same is true for the production of TNFα by the NZB × W lupus mouse (**3**). Rheumatoid arthritis patients have a poor hypothalamic response to IL-1 and IL-6 (**4**). The hypothalamic–pituitary axis is defective in the Obese strain chicken and in the Lewis rat which is prone to the development of Freund's adjuvant-mediated experimental autoimmune disease (**5**). CRH = corticotrophin releasing hormone; MØ = macrophage.

compared with controls, and after surgery, although they produce copious amounts of IL-1 and IL-6, a defect in the hypothalamic paraventricular nucleus prevents the expected increase in ACTH and adrenal steroid output. A subset of CD4 regulatory cells present in young healthy mice of the NOD strain can prevent the transfer of disease by spleen cells of diabetic animals to NOD mice congenic for the severe combined immunodeficiency trait; this regulatory subset is lost in older mice.

Pre-existing defects in the target organ may increase susceptibility to autoimmunity

We have already alluded to the undue sensitivity of target cells to upregulation of MHC class II by IFNγ in animals susceptible to certain autoimmune diseases. Other evidence also favours the view that there may be a pre-existing defect in the target organ. In the Obese strain chicken model of spontaneous thyroid autoimmunity (see p. 404), not only is there a low threshold of IFNγ induction of MHC class II expression by thyrocytes but it has also been shown that, when endogenous TSH is suppressed by thyroxine treatment, the uptake of iodine into the thyroid glands is far higher in the Obese strain than in a variety of normal strains. Furthermore, this is not due to any stimulating effect of the autoimmunity, because immunosuppressed animals show even higher uptakes of iodine (*Fig. 26.21*). Interestingly, the Cornell strain (from which the Obese strain was derived by breeding) shows even higher uptakes of iodine, yet these animals do not develop spontaneous thyroiditis. This could be indicative of a type

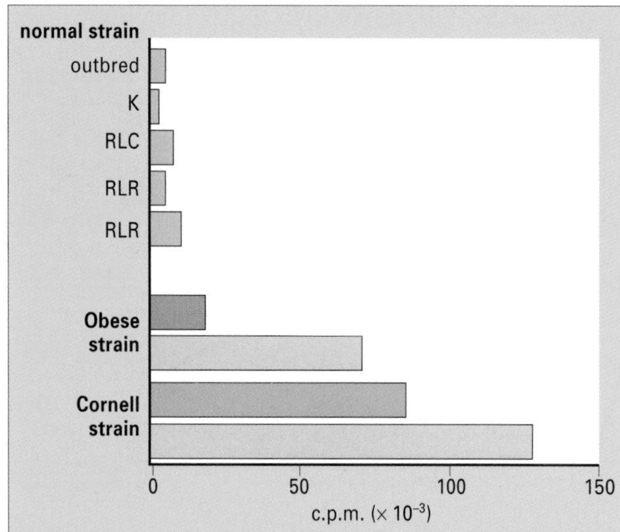

Fig. 26.21 Thyroid ^{131}I uptake in Obese strain chickens and in the related Cornell strain is abnormally high compared with normal strains. Endogenous TSH production was suppressed by administration of thyroxine; therefore the experiment measured TSH-independent ^{131}I uptake. Values were far higher than normal in Obese strain chickens, which spontaneously develop thyroid autoimmunity, and even higher in the non-autoimmune Cornell strain from which the Obese strain was bred. That this abnormality was not due to immune mechanisms was shown by the finding that immunosuppression (blue bars) actually increased ^{131}I uptake into the thyroid gland.

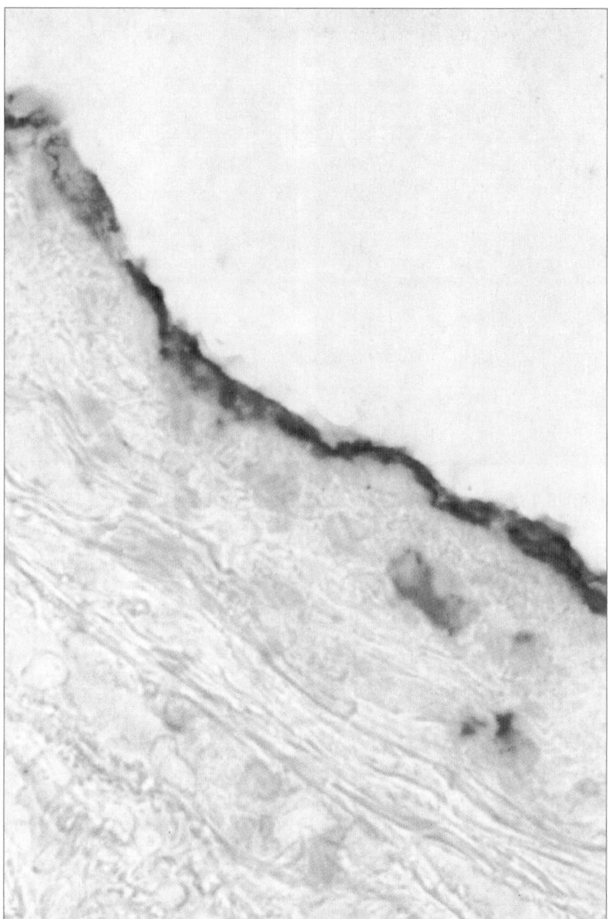

Fig. 26.22 Upregulation of heat-shock protein 60 (hsp60) in endothelial cells at a site of haemodynamic stress. Hsp60 expression (red) co-localized with ICAM-1 expression (black) by endothelial cells and cells in the intima (macrophages) at the bifurcation of the carotid artery of a 5-month-old child. ×240. (Photograph kindly provided by Professor G. Wick.)

of abnormal thyroid behaviour which in itself is insufficient to induce autoimmune disease but does contribute to susceptibility in the Obese strain. Other situations in which the production of autoantigen is affected are diabetes, in which one of the genetic risk factors is associated with a microsatellite marker lying within a transcription factor controlling the rate of insulin production, and rheumatoid arthritis, in which the agalacto IgG glycoform is abnormally abundant. The intriguing observations that immunization with mycobacterial heat-shock protein 65 (hsp65) elicits atherosclerotic lesions at classical predilection sites subject to major haemodynamic stress and that patients with atherosclerosis produce antibodies to human hsp60 which react with heat or TNFα-stressed endothelial cells, hints strongly at an autoimmune contribution to the pathology of the disease. Particularly relevant to the present discussion is the finding of upregulated hsp60 expression at such critical sites even in a 5-month-old child (*Fig. 26.22*). Again, one must re-emphasize the considerable importance of multiple factors in the establishment of prolonged autoimmunity.

DIAGNOSTIC AND PROGNOSTIC VALUE OF AUTOANTIBODIES

Whatever the relationship of autoantibodies to the disease process, they frequently provide valuable markers for diagnostic purposes. A particularly good example is the test for mitochondrial antibodies, used in diagnosing primary biliary cirrhosis (*Fig. 26.23*). Exploratory laparotomy was previously needed to obtain this diagnosis, and was often hazardous because of the age and condition of the patients concerned.

Autoantibodies often have predictive value. For instance, individuals testing positively for antibodies to both insulin and glutamic acid decarboxylase have a high risk of developing insulin-dependent diabetes.

TREATMENT

Often, in organ-specific autoimmune disorders, the symptoms can be corrected by metabolic control. For example, hypothyroidism can be controlled by administration of thyroxine, and thyrotoxicosis by antithyroid drugs. In pernicious anaemia, metabolic correction is achieved by injection of vitamin B_{12}, and in myasthenia gravis by administration of cholinesterase inhibitors. If the target

Diagnostic value of anti-mitochondrial antibodies

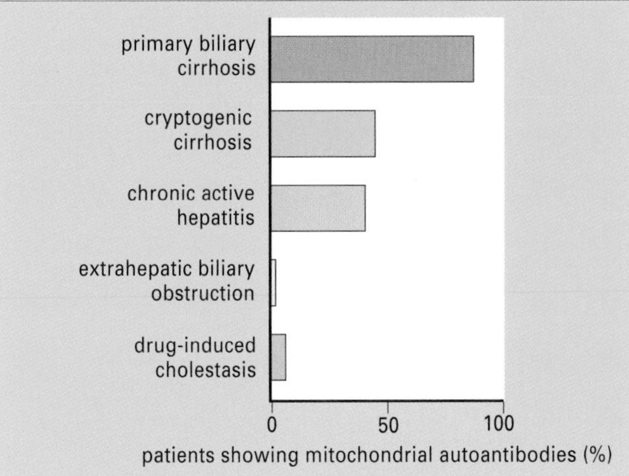

Fig. 26.23 Mitochondrial antibody tests using indirect immunofluorescence, together with percutaneous liver biopsy, can be used to assist in the differential diagnosis of these diseases. A large proportion of patients with primary biliary cirrhosis but less than half of patients with cryptogenic cirrhosis or chronic active hepatitis have anti-mitochondrial antibodies; the antibodies are rare in the other diseases.

organ is not completely destroyed, it may be possible to protect the surviving cells by transfection with *FasL* or *TGFβ* genes. Where function is completely lost and cannot be substituted by hormones, as may occur in lupus nephritis or chronic rheumatoid arthritis, tissue grafts or mechanical substitutes may be appropriate. In the case of tissue grafts, protection from the immunological processes which necessitated the transplant may be required.

Conventional immunosuppressive therapy with anti-mitotic drugs at high doses can be used to damp down the immune response but, because of the dangers involved, tends to be used only in life-threatening disorders such as SLE and dermatomyositis. The potential of cyclosporin and related drugs such as rapamycin has yet to be fully realized, but quite dramatic results have been reported in the treatment of type 1 diabetes mellitus. Anti-inflammatory drugs are, of course, prescribed for rheumatoid diseases with the introduction of selective cyclo-oxygenase-2 (COX-2) inhibitors representing a welcome development. Encouraging results are being obtained by treatment of rheumatoid arthritis patients with low steroid doses at an early stage to correct the apparently defective production of these corticosteroids by the adrenal feedback loop, and for those with more established disease, attention is now focused on the striking remissions achieved by synergistic treatment with anti-TNFα monoclonals plus methotrexate.

As we understand more about the precise defects, and learn how to manipulate the immunological status of the patient, some less well-established approaches may become practicable (*Fig. 26.24*). Several centres are trying out autologous stem-cell transplantation following haemato-immunoablation with cytotoxic drugs in severe cases of SLE, scleroderma and rheumatoid arthritis. Draconian reduction in the T cells in multiple sclerosis by Campath-1H (anti-CD52) and of the B-cell population with anti-CD20 in rheumatoid arthritis are both under scrutiny. Treatment with Campath-1H followed by a non-depleting

Current and potential treatment of autoimmune disease

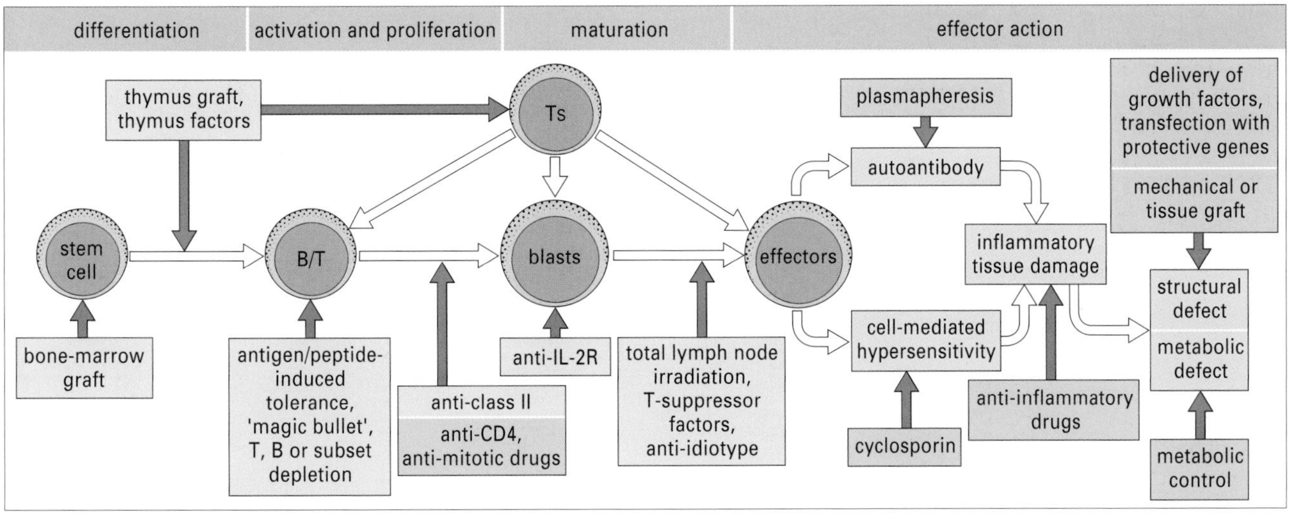

differentiation
activation and proliferation
maturation
effector action
thymus graft, thymus factors
Ts
plasmapheresis
delivery of growth factors, transfection with protective genes
mechanical or tissue graft
autoantibody
stem cell
B/T
blasts
effectors
inflammatory tissue damage
structural defect
metabolic defect
cell-mediated hypersensitivity
bone-marrow graft
antigen/peptide-induced tolerance, 'magic bullet', T, B or subset depletion
anti-class II
anti-CD4, anti-mitotic drugs
anti-IL-2R
total lymph node irradiation, T-suppressor factors, anti-idiotype
cyclosporin
anti-inflammatory drugs
metabolic control

Fig. 26.24 Current treatments for arresting the pathological developments in autoimmune disease are given in blue boxes, and those that may become practicable in green boxes. Anti-mitotic drugs are given in severe cases of SLE or chronic active hepatitis, and anti-inflammatory drugs are widely prescribed in rheumatoid arthritis. Organ-specific disorders (e.g. primary myxoedema) can be treated by supplying the defective component (e.g. thyroid hormone). When a live graft is necessary, immunosuppressive therapy can protect the tissue from damage.

anti-CD4 has produced excellent remissions in patients with Wegener's granulomatosis who were refractory to normal treatment. In an attempt to establish antigen-specific suppression, considerable clinical improvement has been achieved in exacerbating-remitting multiple sclerosis by repeated injection of Cop 1, a random copolymer of alanine, glutamic acid, lysine and tyrosine meant to simulate the postulated 'guilty' autoantigen, myelin basic protein. Some experimental autoimmune diseases have been treated successfully by feeding antigen to induce oral tolerance, by the inhalation of autoantigenic peptides and their analogues (*Fig. 26.25*), and by 'vaccination' with peptides from heat-shock protein 70 or the antigen-specific receptor of autoreactive T cells. This suggests that stimulating normally suppressive functions, including the idiotype network, could be promising.

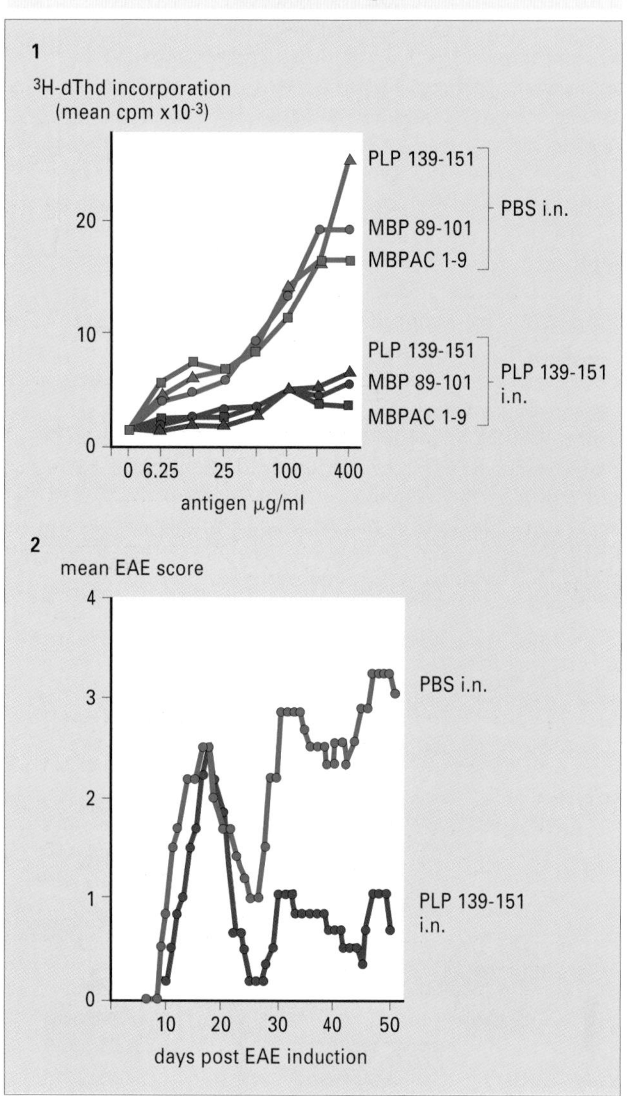

Fig. 26.25 (**1**) Proteolipid protein (PLP) peptide 139–151, administered intranasally prior to immunization with myelin, suppresses the proliferative responses to itself and to T-cell epitopes on another myelin antigen, myelin basic protein (MBP). This is bystander suppression. (**2**) PLP139–151 administered intranasally several days *after* induction of experimental allergic encephalitis by myelin in complete Freund's adjuvant, reduces disease severity. (Data reproduced from Anderton SM, Wraith DC. *Eur J Immunol* 1998;**28**:1251 with permission.)

CRITICAL THINKING • Autoimmunity and autoimmune disease (Explanations on p. 464)

Miss Jacob, a 30-year-old Caribbean lady, was seen in a rheumatology clinic with stiff painful joints in her hands, which were worse first thing in the morning. Other symptoms included fatigue, a low-grade fever, a weight loss of 2 kg, and some mild chest pain. Miss Jacob had recently returned to the UK from a holiday in Jamaica and was also noted to be taking the combined oral contraceptive pill. Past medical history of note was a mild autoimmune haemolytic anaemia 2 years previously.

On examination Miss Jacob had a non-specific maculopapular rash on her face and chest and patchy alopecia (hair loss) over her scalp. Her mouth was tender and examination revealed an ulcer on the soft palate. She had moderately swollen and tender proximal interphalangeal joints. Her other joints were unaffected, but she had generalized muscle aches. The results of investigations are shown in *Figure 26.26*.

Investigation	Result
Radiograph of hands	Soft-tissue swelling, but no bone erosions
Chest radiograph	A small pleural effusion at the right lung base
Full blood count	A mild normocytic, normochromic anaemia and mild lymphocytopenia
C-reactive protein levels	Normal
Erythrocyte sedimentation rate	Raised
Rheumatoid factor	Negative
Serum IgG levels	Elevated
Anti-nuclear antibodies (ANA)	Positive by immunofluorescence
Anti-double stranded DNA, anti-RNA, and anti-histone antibodies	Positive by ELISA
Complement (C3 and C4) levels	Low
Skin biopsy from an area unaffected by the rash	Deposition of IgG and complement components at the junction between dermis and epidermis (lupus 'band' test)

Fig. 26.26 Results of investigations.

A diagnosis of systemic lupus erythematosus (SLE) was made. Miss Jacob was treated with chloroquine, an antimalarial, for the rash on her face and chest.

At a follow-up appointment urinalysis showed protein and red cells. Serum creatinine was mildly elevated as was her blood pressure. A renal biopsy showed membranous lupus nephritis. She was prescribed oral corticosteroids and an antihypertensive agent, which improved her renal function. Her physician also gave advice regarding birth control and pregnancy, and regular check-ups were arranged.

26.1 What is the immunological mechanism leading to the glomerulonephritis?

26.2 Are immune complexes the main mediator of systemic damage?

26.3 What is the mechanism for the vasculitis seen in SLE?

26.4 Are anti-double-stranded DNA antibodies pathognomonic of SLE?

FURTHER READING

Albani S, Keystone EC, Nelson JL, *et al.* Positive selection in autoimmunity: abnormal immune responses to bacterial dnaJ antigenic determinant in patients with early rheumatoid arthritis. *Nat Med* 1995;**1**:448–52.

Alt F, Marrack P (eds). *Curr Opin Immunol* 1999;**11**: issue 6 (several critical essays in each annual volume).

Brostoff J, Scadding GK, Male D, *et al. Clinical Immunology.* London: Gower Medical Publishing, 1991.

Chapel H, Haeney M, Misbah S, Snowden N. *Essentials of Clinical Immunology,* 4th edn. Oxford: Blackwell Science, 1999.

Peter JB, Shoenfeld Y (eds). *Autoantibodies.* Amsterdam: Elsevier, 1996.

27 Immunological techniques

- **Antigen–antibody interactions** underlie many immunological techniques, in which the high specificity of the antibody is used to identify, isolate or quantify a particular antigen.
- **Cell populations can be identified** and characterized by their surface markers, using the techniques of immunofluorescence or immunohistochemistry.
- **Cell populations can be isolated** according to their surface markers, by techniques which include fluorescence-activated cell sorting (FACS), panning and density-dependent centrifugations.
- **The principal assays for lymphocyte function** are by antibody or cytokine production, by proliferation in response to antigen, or by cytotoxicity.

Immunologists employ a number of techniques which are common to other biological sciences. For example, the methods used to isolate antigens and antibodies are those of biochemistry and protein fractionation, while the gene sequences of immunologically important molecules have been elucidated by the standard techniques of molecular genetics. Immunology has, however, developed a number of its own techniques, particularly those based on the antigen–antibody interaction. These have found many uses in other biological sciences. For example, any molecule that acts as antigen can be identified in tissues by immunocytochemical methods. Very low concentrations of such molecules can be quantified by radioimmunoassay (RIA) and enzyme-linked immunosorbent assay (ELISA). There are hundreds of different immunological methods now being used, and some of the most common are outlined in this chapter.

ANTIGEN–ANTIBODY INTERACTIONS

Precipitation reactions

One of the first observations of antigen–antibody reactions was their ability to precipitate when combined in proportions at or near equivalence. This is seen in the classic precipitin reaction, where antigen and antibody are mixed in solution (*Fig. 27.1*). By performing these reactions in agar gels it is possible to distinguish separate antigen–antibody reactions produced by different populations of antibody which are present in a serum – the immunodouble-diffusion technique. This technique has been extended to the examination of the relationship between different antigens (*Fig. 27.2*).

Some antigen mixtures, however, are too complex to be resolved by simple diffusion and precipitation and so the technique of immunoelectrophoresis was developed – antigens are separated on the basis of their charge before being visualized by precipitation (*Fig. 27.3*).

These gel techniques only identify antigens and antibodies qualitatively, but by further modification, using the technique of single radial immunodiffusion, they can be made quantitative (*Fig. 27.4*).

By applying a voltage across the gels to move the antigens and antibodies together, immunodiffusion becomes counter-current electrophoresis, and single radial immunodiffusion becomes rocket electrophoresis (*Fig. 27.5*).

The precipitin reaction

free antibody	+	–	–
free antigen	–	–	+

immune complex precipitated

antibody excess zone

equivalence zone

antigen excess zone

antigen added →

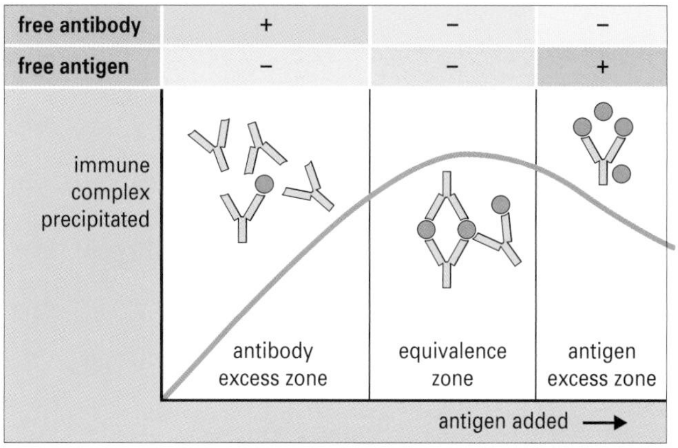

Fig. 27.1 The classical illustration of the antigen–antibody reaction *in vitro* is the precipitin reaction. As increasing concentrations of antigen are added to a constant amount of antibody, the amount of immune complex precipitated rises and then falls. The precipitin curve generated in this way has three zones:

Antibody excess zone: the amount of antigen is insufficient to react with and precipitate all the antibody present; thus free antibody can be detected in the supernatant.

Equivalence zone: the added antigen is sufficient to combine with and precipitate all the antibody present and neither free antigen nor antibody can be detected in the supernatant.

Antigen excess zone: the amount of antigen exceeds that required to bind all the antibody, and this leads to a reduction in the amount of antibody precipitated. This fall is due to the formation of soluble antigen–antibody complexes by the excess antigen. The extent to which this phenomenon occurs varies with different antibodies and with the species from which the antibody is derived.

These techniques operate in the range of 20 μg/ml to 2 mg/ml of antigen or antibody.

Haemagglutination and complement fixation

Antibody may be detected and measured by haemagglutination at lower concentrations than those detectable by countercurrent electrophoresis and rocket electrophoresis. This relies on the ability of antibody to cross-link

Precipitin reactions in gels: immuno-double-diffusion

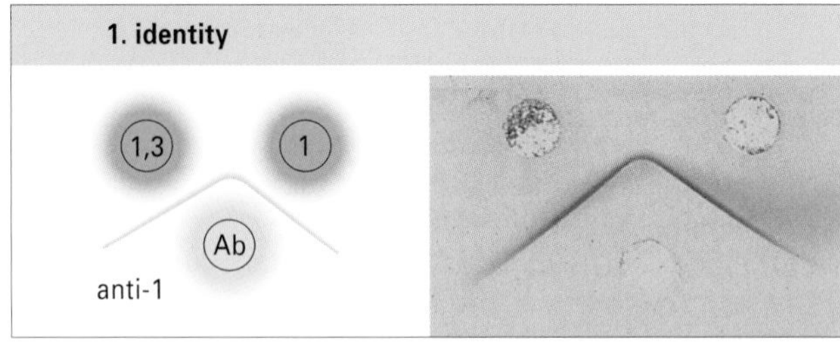

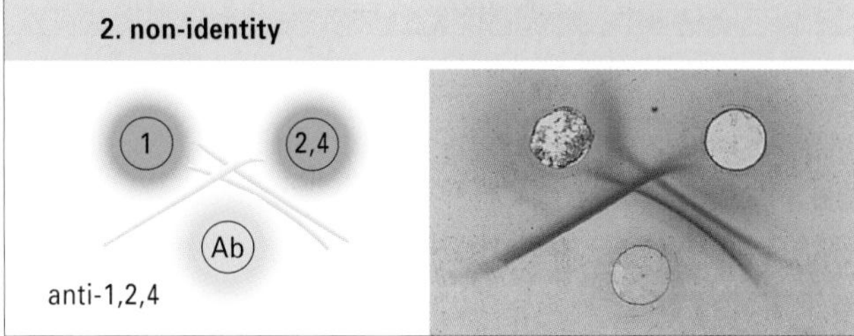

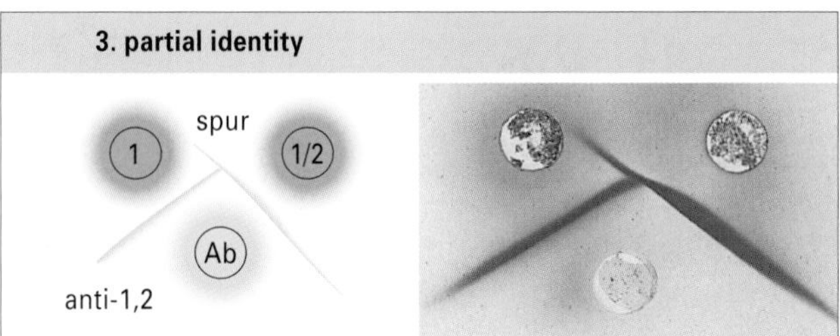

Fig. 27.2 In immuno-double-diffusion, agar gels are poured onto slides and allowed to set; wells are then punched in the gel and the test solutions of antigen (Ag) and antibody (Ab) are added. The solutions diffuse out and where Ag and Ab meet they bind to each other, cross-link and precipitate, leaving a line of precipitation. The precipitin bands can be visualized by washing the gel to remove soluble proteins and then staining the precipitin arcs with a protein stain such as Coomassie blue. This technique may be used to determine the relationship between antigens (blue) and a particular test antibody (yellow). Three basic patterns appear. The numbers in the blue wells refer to the epitopes present on the test antigen. In reaction (**1**) the precipitin arcs formed between the antibody and the two test antigens fuse, indicating that the antibody is precipitating identical epitopes in each preparation (epitope 1). This does not mean that the antigens are necessarily identical; they are only identical in as far as the antibody cannot distinguish a difference. In reaction (**2**) the antibody preparation distinguishes the three different antigens, which form independent precipitin arcs. In reaction (**3**) the antigens share epitope 1 but one antigen also has epitope 2. This is the same situation as in (1), but in this case the antibody can distinguish them, by virture of being able to react against both epitopes. A line of identity forms with anti-epitope 1, with the addition of a 'spur' where the anti-epitope 2 has reacted with the second epitope, thus indicating partial rather than total identity between the antigen preparations.

Immunoelectrophoresis

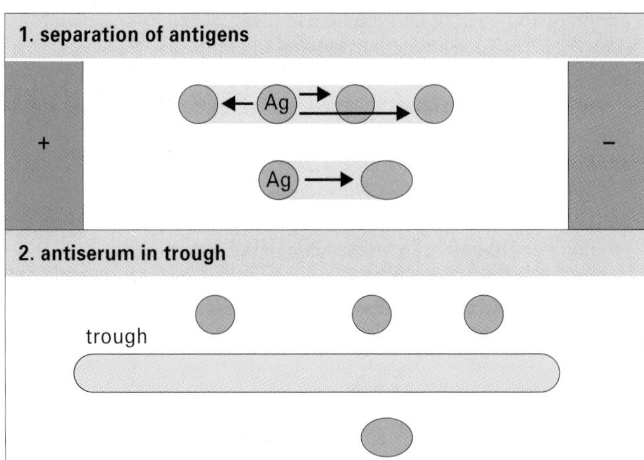

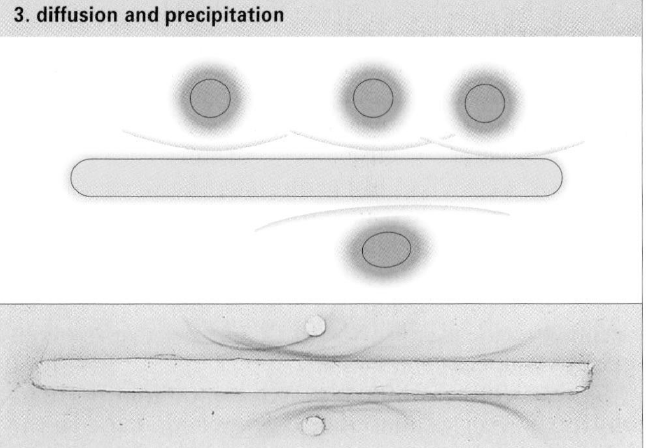

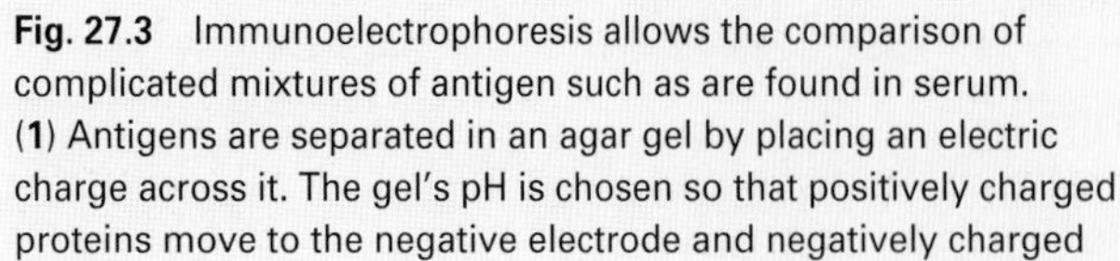

Fig. 27.3 Immunoelectrophoresis allows the comparison of complicated mixtures of antigen such as are found in serum. (**1**) Antigens are separated in an agar gel by placing an electric charge across it. The gel's pH is chosen so that positively charged proteins move to the negative electrode and negatively charged proteins to the positive. (**2**) A trough is then cut between the wells and filled with the antibody, which is left to diffuse. (**3**) The antigens and antibody form precipitin arcs. The lower Figure shows the complex patterns which result when different sera are analyzed by electrophoresis.

Single radial immunodiffusion

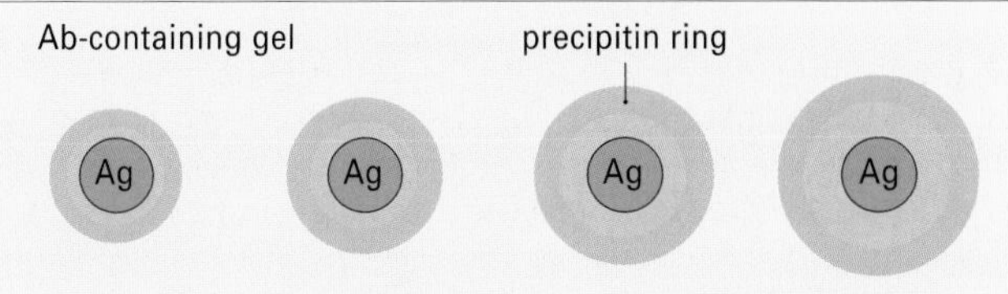

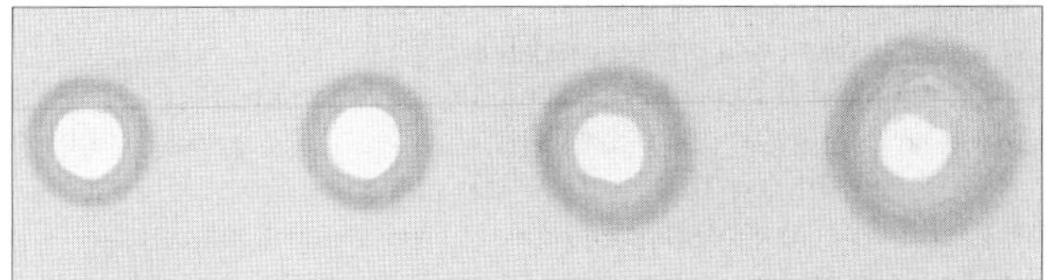

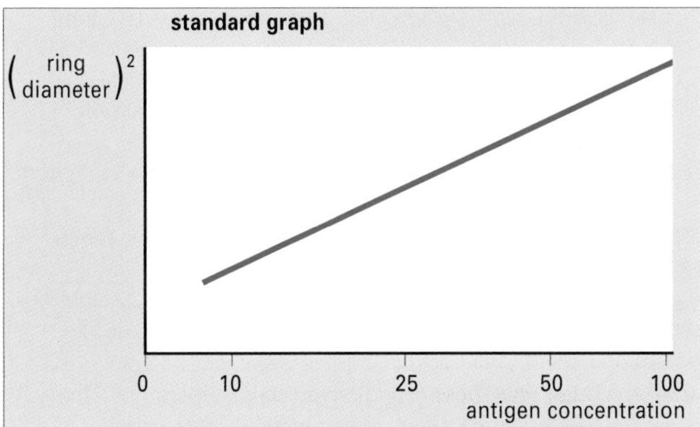

Fig. 27.4 Single radial immunodiffusion allows quantitation of antigens. Antibody is added to the agar gel which is then poured onto slides and allowed to set. Wells are punched in the agar and standard volumes of test antigen of different concentration are put in the wells. The plates are left for at least 24 hours, during which time the antigen diffuses out of the wells to form soluble complexes (in antigen excess) with the antibody. These continue to diffuse outwards, binding more antibody until an equivalence point is reached and the complexes precipitate in a ring. The area within the precipitin ring, measured as ring diameter squared, is proportional to the antigen concentration. Unknowns are derived by interpolation from the standard curve (graph). The whole process may be reversed using an antigen-containing gel to determine unknown concentrations of antibody.

Countercurrent electrophoresis and rocket electrophoresis

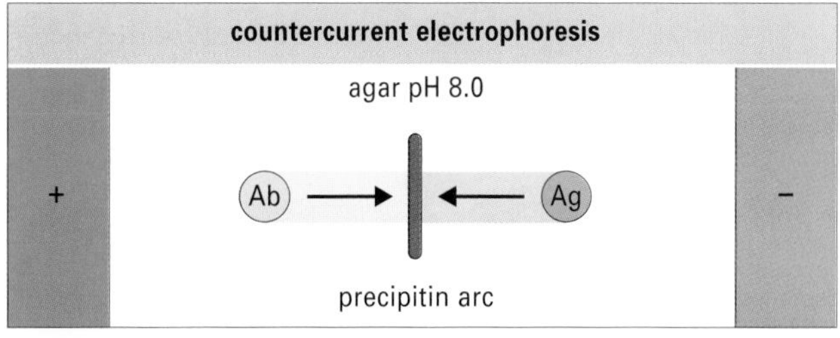

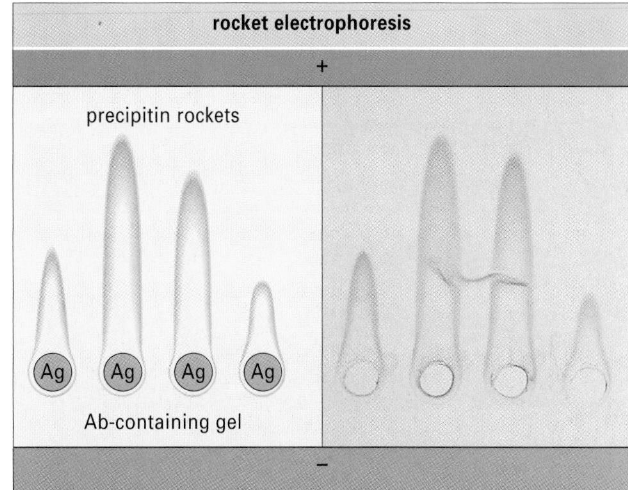

Fig. 27.5 Countercurrent electrophoresis is performed in agar gels where the pH is chosen so that the antibody is positively charged and the antigen being tested is negatively charged. By applying a voltage across the gel the antigen and antibody move towards each other and precipitate. The principle is the same as for immuno-double-diffusion but the sensitivity is increased 10–20-fold. Antigens may be quantitated by electrophoresing them into an antibody-containing gel in the technique termed rocket electrophoresis. The pH of the gel is chosen so that the antibodies are immobile and the antigen is negatively charged. Precipitin rockets form; the height of the rocket is proportional to antigen concentration, and unknowns are determined by interpolation from standards. The appearance of stained rockets is shown on the right. Both techniques rely on the antigen and antibody having different charges at the selected pH; this is true for most antigens since antibodies have a relatively high isoelectric point (i.e. they are neutrally charged at a more alkaline pH than most antigens). If the charges on the antigen and antibody do not differ sufficiently, the antibody or antigen can be chemically modified to alter its isoelectric point. Rocket electrophoresis can be reversed to estimate antibody concentration if a suitable pH gel can be found to immobilize the antigen, without damaging it or preventing the antigen–antibody reaction.

red blood cells by interacting with the antigens on their surface (*Fig. 27.6*).

Antigen–antibody reactions lead to immune complex formation which produces complement fixation via the classical pathway, and this may be exploited to determine the amount of antigen or antibody present (*Fig. 27.7*). Haemagglutination and complement fixation can detect antibody at levels of less than 1 μg/ml.

Direct and indirect immunofluorescence

Immunofluorescence is used extensively to detect autoantibodies and antibodies to tissue and cellular antigens (*Fig. 27.8*). Although these techniques are more cumbersome than those described earlier if a quantitative measure of antibody concentration is required, they do have advantages. By using tissue sections (which contain a large number of antigens), antibodies to several different antigens can be identified on a single slide according to their distribution between cells or in different subcellular compartments.

Furthermore, the immunofluorescence test can be used to identify particular cells in suspension, that is, to identify

Haemagglutination

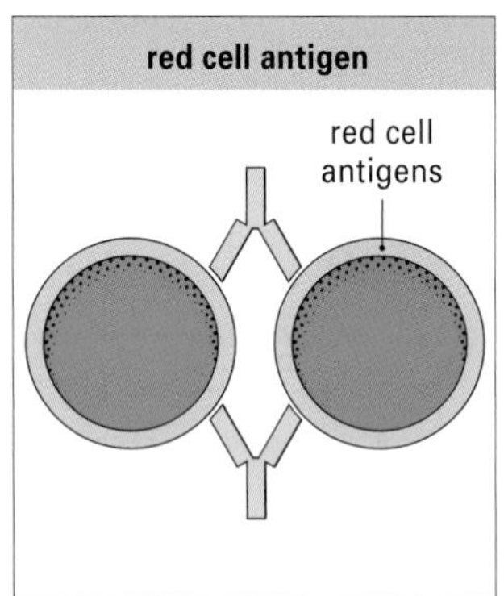

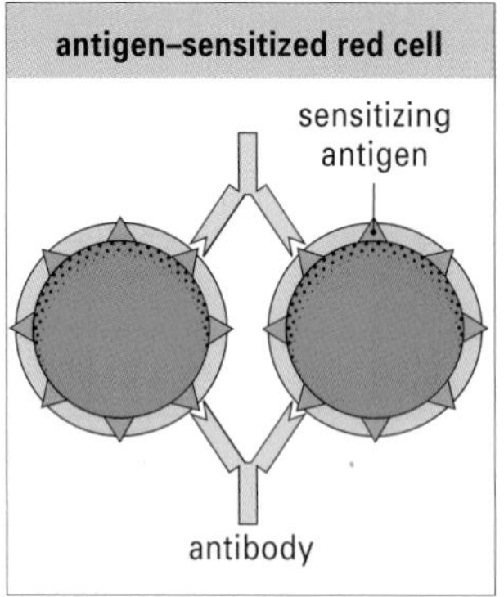

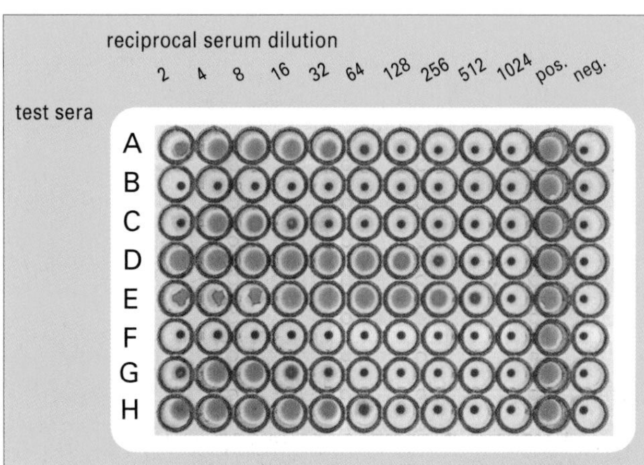

Fig. 27.6 The active haemagglutination test (upper panel, left) detects antibodies to red blood-cell antigens. The antibody is serially diluted (usually in doubling dilutions) in physiological saline and placed in the wells (columns 1–10, lower panel read left to right) of the haemagglutination plate. Positive controls (column 11) and negative controls (column 12) are included. In this example, eight different antisera (rows A–H) are being tested. A suspension of red cells (containing a protein to prevent the red cells agglutinating non-specifically) is added to each well to give a final concentration of about 1% cells. If sufficient antibody is present to agglutinate (cross-link) the cells, they sink as a mat to the bottom of the well. If insufficient antibody is present, the cells roll down the sloping sides of the plate to form a red pellet at the bottom. Some antibodies do not agglutinate red cells very effectively and may be detected in the indirect agglutination test by the addition of a second antibody which binds to the non-agglutinating antibody already bound on the red cell. By binding different antigens onto the red-cell surface, covalently or non-covalently, the test can be extended to detect antibodies to antigens other than those found on red cells (upper right panel). Chromic chloride, tannic acid, glutaraldehyde and a number of other chemicals are used to cross-link the antigen to the cells.

Complement fixation

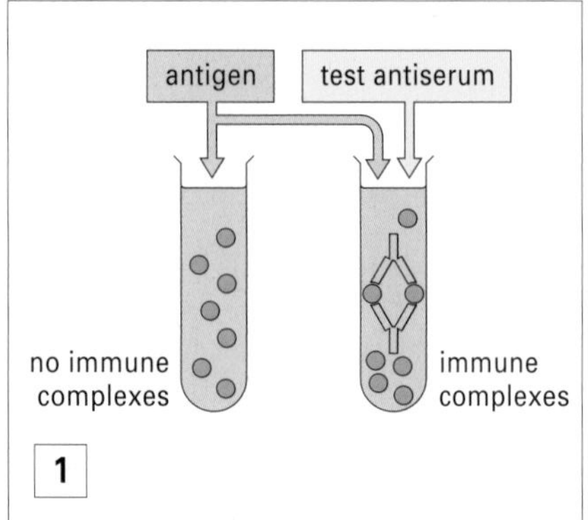

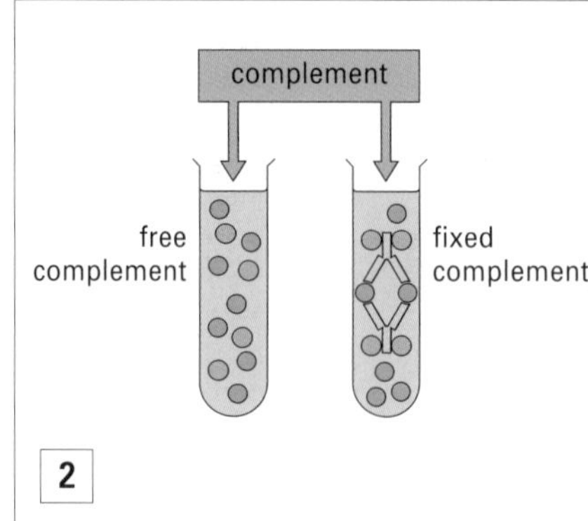

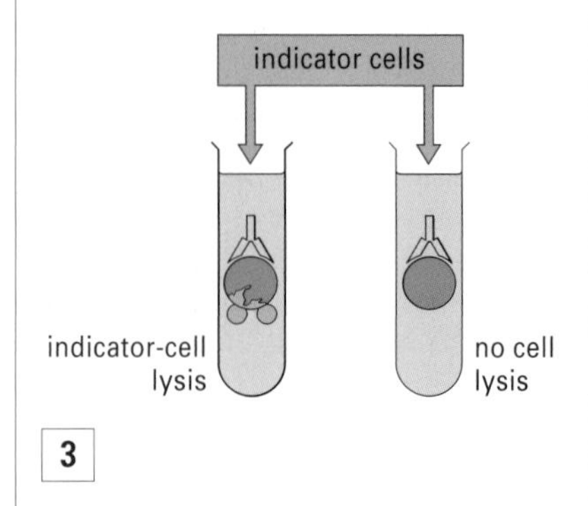

Fig. 27.7 The complement fixation test detects antibody. (**1**) A test antiserum is titred in doubling dilutions and a fixed amount of antigen is added to each tube or well. If antibody is present in the test serum, immune complexes will form. (**2**) Complement is then added to the mixture. If complexes are present, they will fix complement and 'consume' it. (**3**) In the final step, indicator cells (red cells) together with a subagglutinating amount of antibody (erythrocyte antibody) are added to the mixture. If there is any complement remaining these cells will be lysed; if it was consumed by immune complexes in stage 2, there will be insufficient to lyse the red cells. A quantity of complement is used that is just enough to lyse the indicator cells if none is consumed by the complexes. The assay is often performed on plastic plates. By using constant amounts of antibody and titrations of antigen, the assay can be applied to testing for antigens. Appropriate controls are most important in this assay because some antibody preparations consume complement without the addition of antigen, for example if the antibody preparation is serum that already contains immune complexes. Some antigens can also have anti-complement activity. The controls should therefore include antibody alone and antigen alone to check that neither fix complement by themselves.

Direct and indirect immunofluorescence

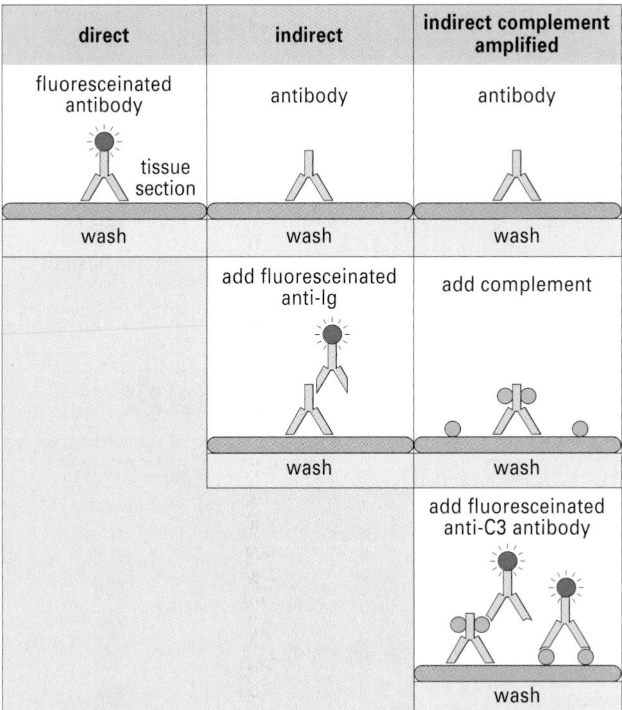

Fig. 27.8 Immunofluorescence detects antigen *in situ*. A section is cut on a cryostat from a deep-frozen tissue block. This ensures that labile antigens are not damaged by fixatives.

Direct: the test solution of fluoresceinated antibody is applied to the section in a drop, incubated and washed off. Any bound antibody is then revealed under the microscope; UV light is directed onto the section through the objective, thus the field is dark and areas with bound fluorescent antibody fluoresce green. The pattern of fluorescence is characteristic for each tissue antigen.

Indirect: antibody applied to the section as a solution is visualized using fluoresceinated anti-immunoglobulin.

Indirect complement amplified: this is an elaboration of the indirect method for the detection of complement-fixing antibody (see *Fig. 27.7*). In the second step fresh complement is added which becomes fixed around the site of antibody binding. Due to the amplification steps in the classical complement pathway (see Chapter 3) one antibody molecule can cause many C3b molecules to bind to the section; these are then visualized with fluoresceinated anti-C3.

Fluorescence-activated cell sorter (FACS)

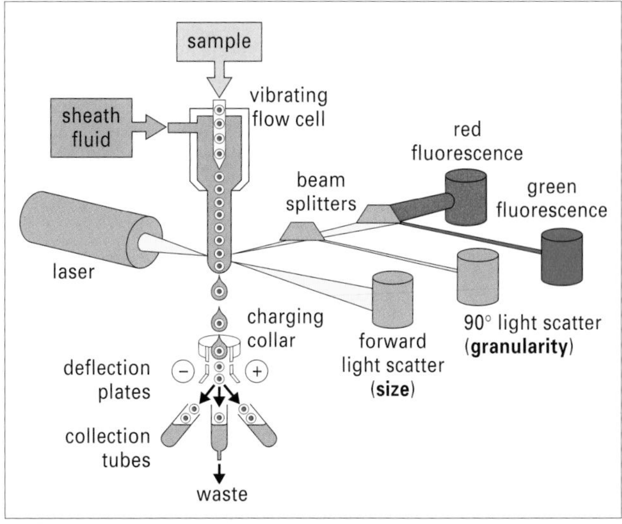

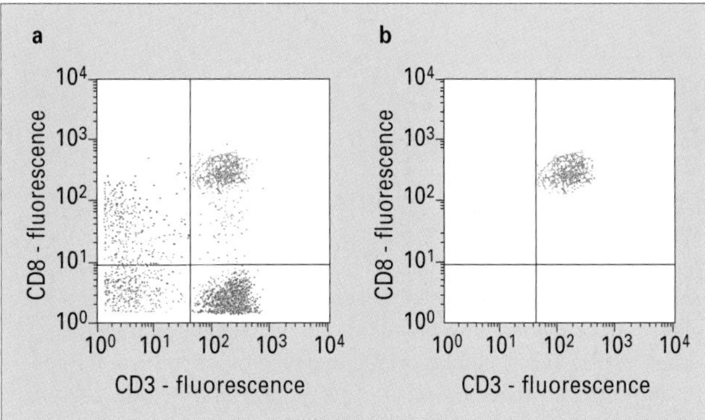

Fig. 27.9 (**1**) Cells in the sample are stained with specific fluorescent reagents to detect surface molecules and are then introduced into the vibrating flow chamber of the FACS. The cell stream passing out of the chamber is encased in a sheath of buffer fluid. The stream is illuminated by laser light and each cell is measured for size (forward light scatter) and granularity (90° light scatter), as well as for red and green fluorescence, to detect two different surface markers. The vibration in the cell stream causes it to break into droplets which are charged and may then be steered by deflection plates under computer control to collect different cell populations according to the parameters measured. The plots shown represent (**a**) peripheral blood mononuclear cells double stained with FITC-conjugated anti-CD3 antibody (x axis) and PE-labelled anti-CD8 antibody (y axis). Four populations can be seen, and the CD8 cells appear in the upper right quadrant. These are then selected (gated) and the isolated CD8 population is shown in (**b**).

antigens on live cells. When a live stained-cell suspension is put through a fluorescence-activated cell sorter (FACS), the machine measures the fluorescence intensity of each cell and then the cells are separated according to their particular fluorescent brightness. This technique permits the isolation of different cell populations with different surface antigens stained with different fluorescent antibodies (*Fig. 27.9*).

Immunoasssay

The techniques of immunoassay using labelled reagents for detecting antigens and antibodies are exquisitely sensitive and extremely economical in the use of reagents (*Fig. 27.10*). Solid-phase assays for antibodies employing ligands labelled with radioisotopes or enzymes (enzyme-linked immunosorbent test; ELISA, *Fig. 27.11*) are probably the most widely used of all immunological assays because large numbers can be performed in a relatively short time, although fluorescent or chemiluminescent markers are tending to replace radioisotopes for labelling. Antigen may

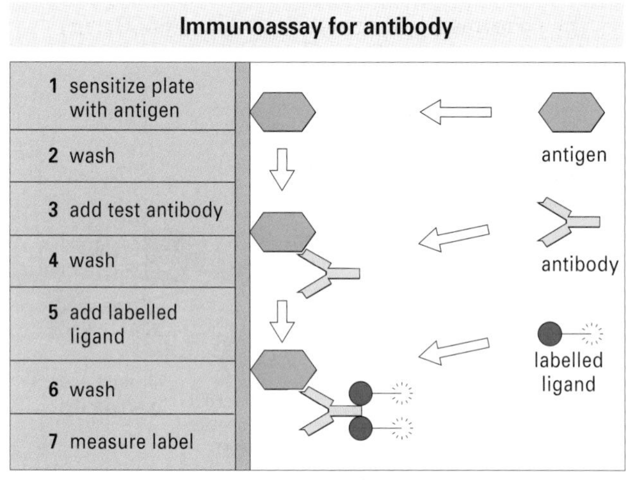

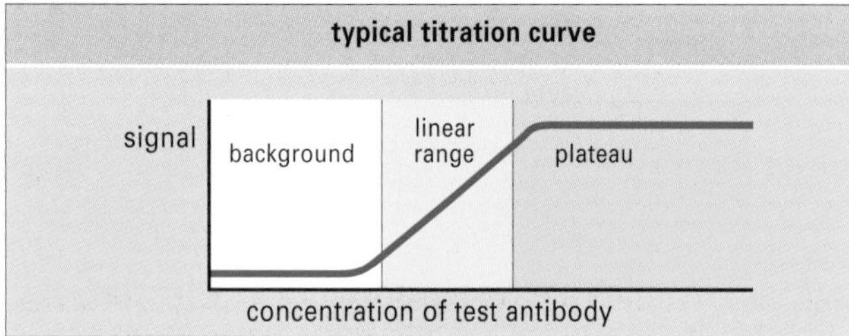

Fig. 27.10 Immunoassay for antibody. (**1**) Antigen in saline is incubated on a plastic plate or tube, and small quantities become absorbed onto the plastic surface. (**2**) Free antigen is washed away. (The plate may then be blocked with excess of an irrelevant protein to prevent any subsequent non-specific binding of proteins.) (**3**) Test antibody is added, which binds to the antigen. (**4**) Unbound proteins are washed away. (**5**) The antibody is detected by a labelled ligand. The ligand may be a molecule such as staphylococcal protein A which binds to the Fc region of IgG – more often it is another antibody specific for the test antibody. By using a ligand which binds to particular classes or subclasses of test antibody it is possible to distinguish isotypes. (**6**) Unbound ligand is washed away. (**7**) The label bound to the plate is measured. A typical titration curve is shown in the graph above. With increasing amounts of test antibody the signal rises from a background level through a linear range to a plateau. Antibody titres can only be detected correctly within the linear range. Typically the plateau binding is 20–100 times the background. The sensitivity of the technique is usually about 1–50 ng/ml of specific antibody. Specificity of the assay may be checked by adding increasing concentrations of free test antigen to the test antibody at step 3; this binds to the antibody and blocks it from binding to the antigen on the plate. Addition of increasing amounts of free antigen reduces the signal.

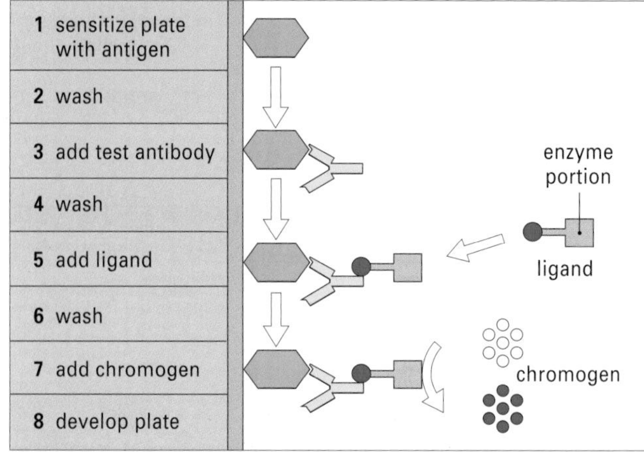

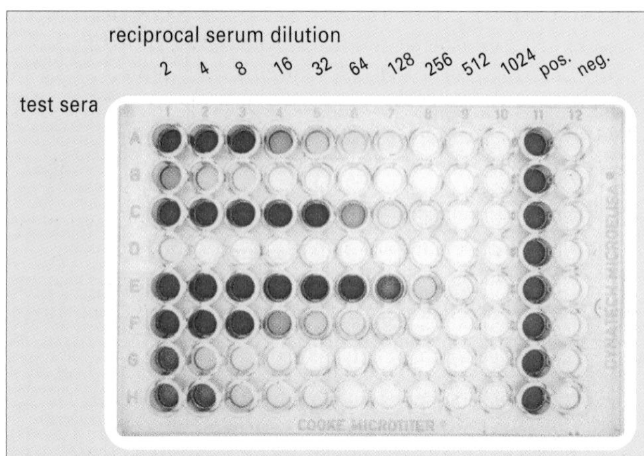

Fig. 27.11 The ELISA plate is prepared in the same way as the assay in *Figure 27.10* up to step **4**. In this system, ligand is a molecule which can detect the antibody and is covalently coupled to an enzyme such as peroxidase. This binds the test antibody and after free ligand is washed away (**6**) the bound ligand is visualized by the addition of chromogen (**7**) – a colourless substrate which is acted on by the enzyme portion of the ligand to produce a coloured end-product. A developed plate is shown in the lower panel (**8**). The amount of test antibody is measured by assessing the amount of coloured end-product by optical density scanning of the plate.

be measured by either the two-site capture assay or the competitive assay, which may be carried out using any of the labels for detection (*Fig. 27.12*).

Biosensor assay of intermolecular reactions

The measurement in real time of interactions between antibodies and antigens, ligands and receptors, and membrane reactions between cells is becoming increasingly important in biology. The rapid and simple measurement of the kinetics of such biomolecular reactions has been made possible by the development of optical biosensors such as the IAsys and BIAcore instruments.

The intensity and wavelength of light reflected off a sensing surface with a film of solution on it is affected by the concentrations of the components at the liquid–surface interface. When molecules in the liquid phase interact with molecules attached to the solid phase the concentrations are altered and this results in a change in the intensity of the reflected light at a particular angle caused by surface plasmon resonance. Biosensors measure these changes (*Fig. 27.13*), and the progress of the reaction is monitored as a sensorgram (*Fig. 27.14, p. 424*). In a BIAcore biosensor, antibody is immobilized on a gold-film-coated

Assay of antigen

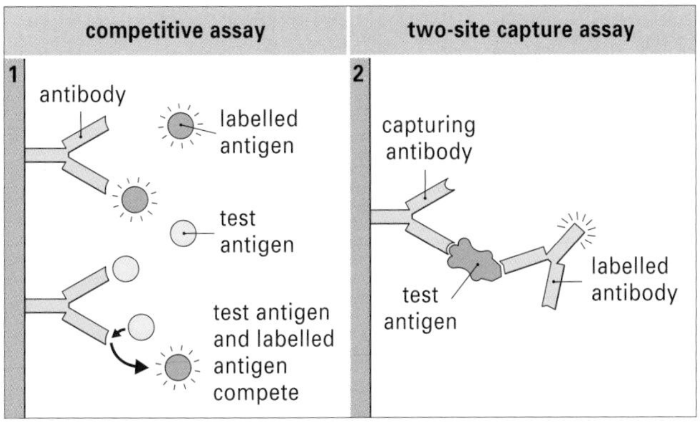

Fig. 27.12 (**1**) Competitive assay. The test antigen is placed together with labelled antigen onto a plate coated with specific antibody. The more test antigen is present, the less of the labelled standard antigen binds. This type of assay is often used to measure antigens at relatively high concentrations or hormones which only have a single site available for combination with antibody. (**2**) Two-site capture assay. The assay plate is coated with specific antibody, the test solution then applied and any antigen present captured by the bound antibody. After washing away unbound material, the captured antigen is detected using a labelled antibody against another epitope on the antigen. Since the antigen is detected by two different antibodies, the second in excess, such assays are both highly specific and sensitive.

chip. A solution containing antigen flows over the chip. The binding of antigen to the antibody is detected by illuminating the chip with polarized light. When antigen binds it alters the reflective properties of the chip, which can be detected photometrically.

Immunoblotting and immunoprecipitation

The methods described so far are particularly useful for measuring levels of certain known antigens or antibodies, but often it is necessary to identify and characterize previously unknown antigens from a complex mixture, in which case immunoblotting is very useful.

In immunoblotting, complex mixtures are resolved in analytical separation gels and then the molecules are transferred to membranes (blots) for the identification of individual antigens by specific antisera. By using sodium dodecyl sulphate (SDS) gels, isoelectric focusing gels or peptide mapping gels in the initial separation, it is possible to obtain data on the size, isoelectric point and molecular relationships of the antigens which are under investigation (*Fig. 27.15*).

In some cases an antigen becomes so denatured by the gel separations and blotting procedures that some of its epitopes are destroyed and it can no longer bind to particular antibodies. In this case it is necessary to use immunoprecipitation instead to identify which antigen an antibody binds to. The technique can be used either with soluble antigens or with cell-surface antigens (*Fig. 27.16*).

Flow cell and optical system of BIAcore biosensor

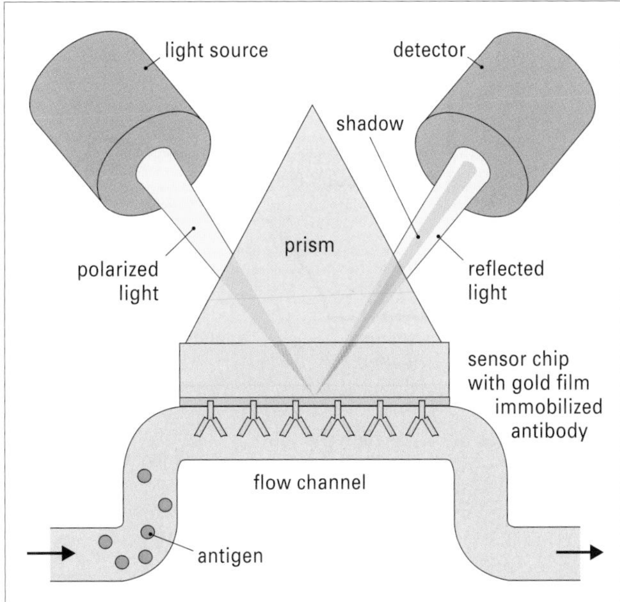

Fig. 27.13 Antibody is immobilized onto the sensing surface and the test antigen solution is passed over the surface. A wedge-shaped beam of polarized light is focused onto the gold film which is part of the sensing surface and is reflected. At one angle, the intensity of light reflected is reduced and a shadow is produced. This reduction in light intensity is caused by surface plasmon resonance. The angle at which the surface plasmon resonance occurs is dependent upon the refractive index of the fluid layer next to the gold surface and is affected by the association or dissociation of the antigen from the immobilized antibody. Measurement of the angle or wavelength at which the light intensity falls can be used to assess the amount of binding to the surface.

ISOLATION OF PURE ANTIBODIES

Immunologists often need to isolate pure antibodies, which may be either antigen-specific or non-specific immunoglobulin. Isolation of non-specific immunoglobulin from serum is usually carried out by sequential protein fractionation steps which may include:

- **Precipitation of the gammaglobulins** in 30–50% ammonium sulphate.
- **Gel filtration** to obtain molecules of the correct size.
- **Ion exchange chromatography** to isolate molecules which are positively charged at neutral pH.
- **Affinity chromatography** on natural ligands for immunoglobulin, such as protein A (protein A is a component of staphylococcal cell walls which binds to a region in Cγ2 and Cγ3 of most IgG subclasses, i.e. IgG1, IgG2 and IgG4).

Isolation of antigen-specific immunoglobulin is carried out by affinity chromatography using antigen coupled to Sepharose: pure antibody is eluted from the immunoabsorbent with chaotropic agents such as sodium thiocyanate, or glycine–HCl buffer, or diethylamine buffer.

Interaction of antigen with immobilized antibody monitored as a sensorgram

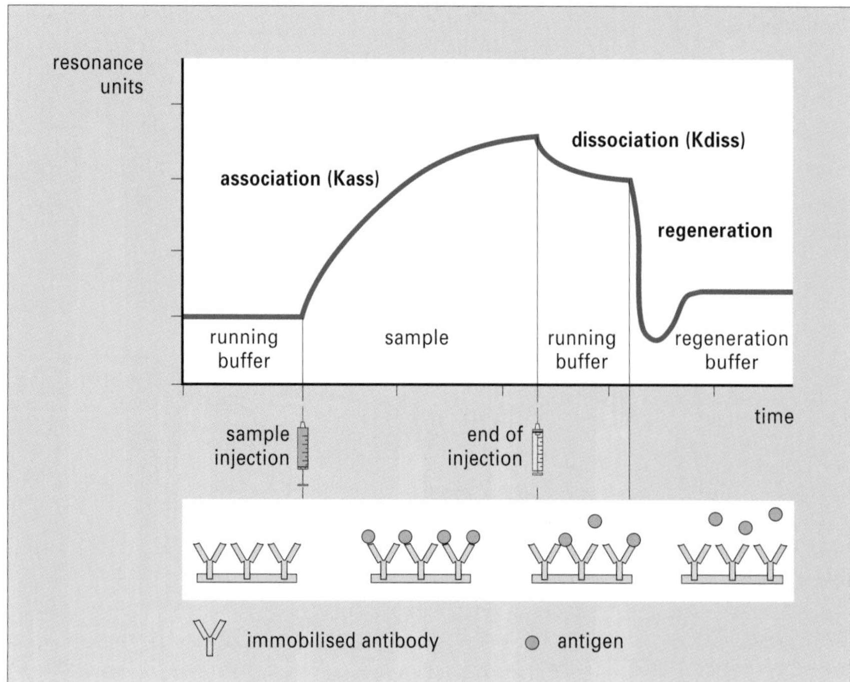

Fig. 27.14 In the case of an antibody : antigen reaction, the antigen binds to the surface-bound antibody during the injection period resulting in an increase in the resonance signal and k_{ass} can be determined. After injection, the sample is replaced by running buffer and a decrease in the signal is observed reflecting the dissociation of antigen from the antibody (k_{diss}).
These data can be used to determine the kinetics and affinity Ka of the reaction, because $Ka = k_{ass}/k_{diss}$.

Immunoblotting

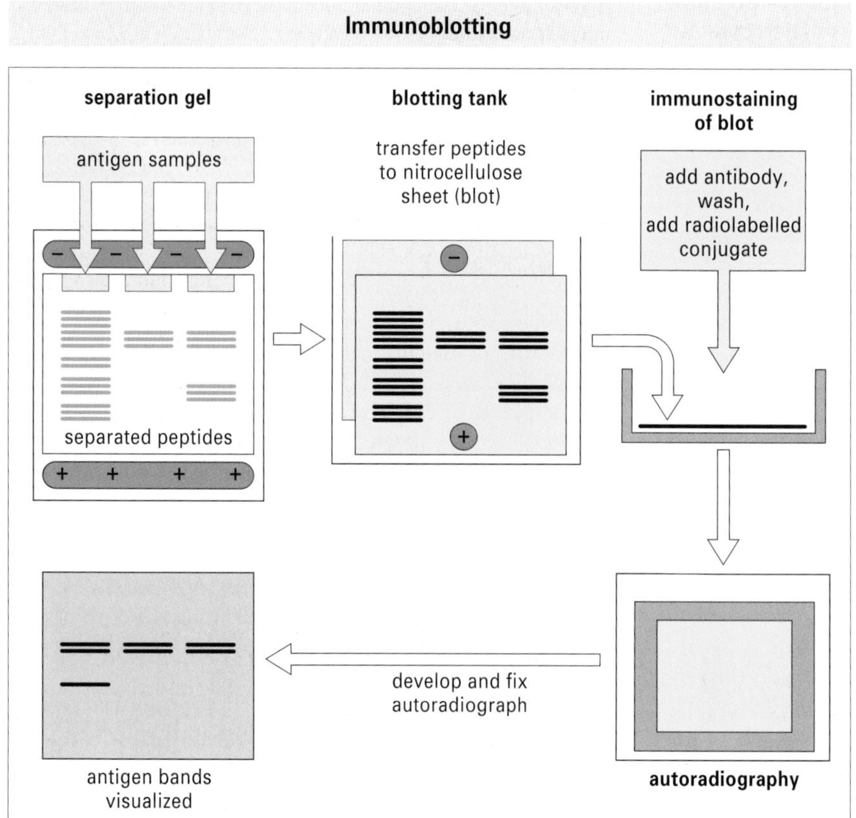

Fig. 27.15 In immunoblotting, antigen samples are first separated in an analytical gel, for example an SDS polyacrylamide gel or an isoelectric focusing gel. The resolved molecules are transferred electrophoretically to a nitrocellulose membrane in a blotting tank. The blot is then treated with antibody to the specific antigen, washed, and a radiolabelled conjugate to detect antibodies is bound to the blot. The principle is similar to that of a RIA or ELISA. After washing again, the blot is placed in contact with X-ray film in a cassette; the autoradiograph is developed and the antigen bands which have bound the antibody are visible. The technique can be modified for use with a chemiluminescent label or an enzyme-coupled conjugate (as in ELISA), where the bound material can be detected by treatment with a chromogen which deposits an insoluble reagent directly onto the blot.

Immunoprecipitation

add specific antibody
add co-precipitating reagents
spin down precipitate
labelled antigen mixture
complexed antigen
resolubilize
autoradiograph
SDS gel sample
separated proteins of the immune complex

Fig. 27.16 In immunoprecipitation the antigens being tested are labelled with ^{125}I, and antibody is added, which binds only to its specific antigen. The complexes are precipitated by the addition of co-precipitating agents, such as anti-immunoglobulin antibodies or staphylococcal protein A. The insoluble complexes are spun down and washed to remove any unbound labelled antigens. Then the precipitate is resolubilized, for example in SDS, and the components separated on analytical gels. After running, the fixed gels are autoradiographed, to show the position of the specific labelled antigen. Frequently the antigens are derived from the surface of radiolabelled cells, which are solubilized with detergents before the immunoprecipitation. It is also possible to label the antigens with biotin, and detect them at the end chromatographically using streptavidin (binds biotin) coupled to an enzyme such as peroxidase (cf. ELISA technique).

Affinity chromatography

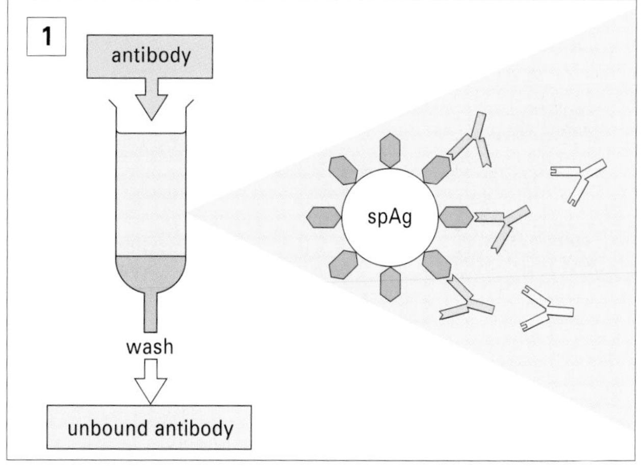

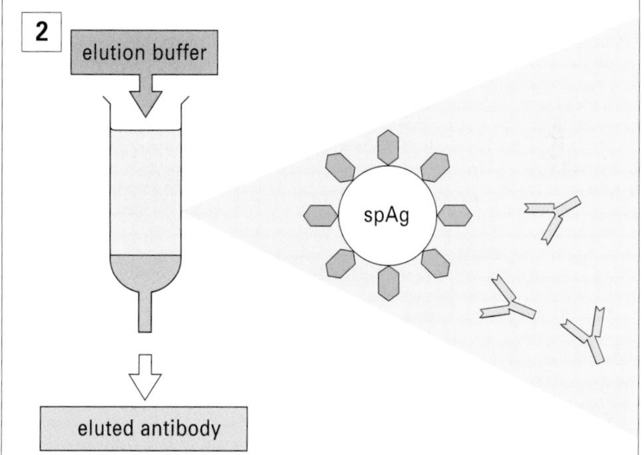

Fig. 27.17 By using affinity chromatography a pure population of antibodies may be isolated. (**1**) A solid-phase immunoabsorbent is prepared (spAg); this is an antigen covalently coupled to an inert support (e.g. cross-linked dextran beads). The immunoabsorbent is placed in a column and the antibody mixture is run in under physiological conditions. Antibody to the antigen binds to the column while unbound antibody washes through. (**2**) In the second step the column is eluted to obtain the bound antibody using elution buffer (e.g. acetate pH 3.0, diethylamine pH 11.5, 3 M guanidine HCl), which dissociates the antigen–antibody bond. By placing antibody on the column the process can be reversed to obtain pure antigen. The technique can also be used to obtain other types of molecule. For example, a lectin column will absorb all molecules with particular sugar residues and these can be eluted in buffer containing the free sugar molecules, which competes with the bound protein for the attachment site on the lectin.

Affinity chromatography is the technique used where the isolation of pure antibody or pure antigen is the objective (*Fig. 27.17*).

Monoclonal antibody production

Another way of obtaining pure antibody of a defined specificity is to produce monoclonal antibodies from cells in culture. By creating an immortal clone of cells which manufacture a single antibody of defined specificity, production can be maintained indefinitely (*Fig. 27.18*), obviating the vagaries of antiserum production (lack of uniformity). Monoclonal antibodies have found widespread use in many biological sciences, where the antibody is used as a highly specific probe.

Since any particular B cell is effectively producing a monoclonal antibody, the requirement is to immortalize and propagate individual B cells. Most monoclonal antibodies are generated by the fusion of mouse splenocytes with a B-cell myeloma from the same strain which does not secrete its own antibody. It is also possible to produce interstrain or even interspecies hybrids, but these are often unstable. An alternative method is to transform B cells; for example, human B cells may be immortalized for

Monoclonal antibody production

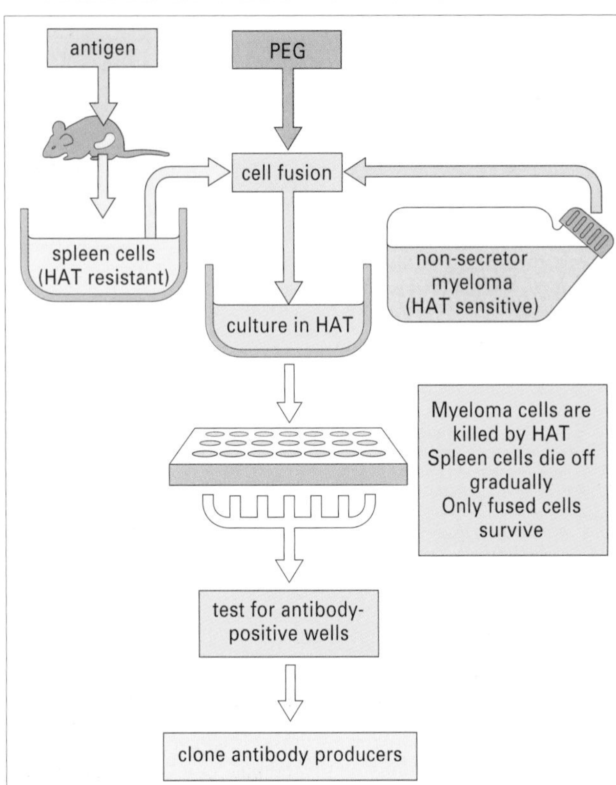

Fig. 27.18 Animals (usually mice or rats) are immunized with antigen. Once the animals are making a good antibody response their spleens are removed and a cell suspension is prepared (lymph node cells may also be used). These cells are fused with a myeloma cell line by the addition of polyethylene glycol (PEG) which promotes membrane fusion. Only a small proportion of the cells fuse successfully. The fusion mixture is then set up in culture with medium containing 'HAT'. HAT is a mixture of hypoxanthine, aminopterin and thymidine. Aminopterin is a powerful toxin which blocks a metabolic pathway. This pathway can be bypassed if the cell is provided with the intermediate metabolites hypoxanthine and thymidine. Thus spleen cells can grow in HAT medium, but the myeloma cells die in HAT medium because they have a metabolic defect and cannot use the bypass pathway. When the culture is set up in HAT medium it contains spleen cells, myeloma cells and fused cells. The spleen cells die in culture naturally after 1–2 weeks and the myeloma cells are killed by the HAT. Fused cells survive however, as they have the immortality of the myeloma and the metabolic bypass of the spleen cells. Some of them will also have the antibody producing capacity of the spleen cells. Any wells containing growing cells are tested for the production of the desired antibody (often by solid-phase immunoassay) and if positive the cultures are cloned by plating out so that there is only one cell in each well. This produces a clone of cells derived from a single progenitor, which is both immortal and a producer of monoclonal antibody.

monoclonal antibody production by infecting them with Epstein–Barr virus.

A new way of generating antibodies is by phage display. In this exciting technique it is possible to express antibody-

Production of Fv antibodies by phage display

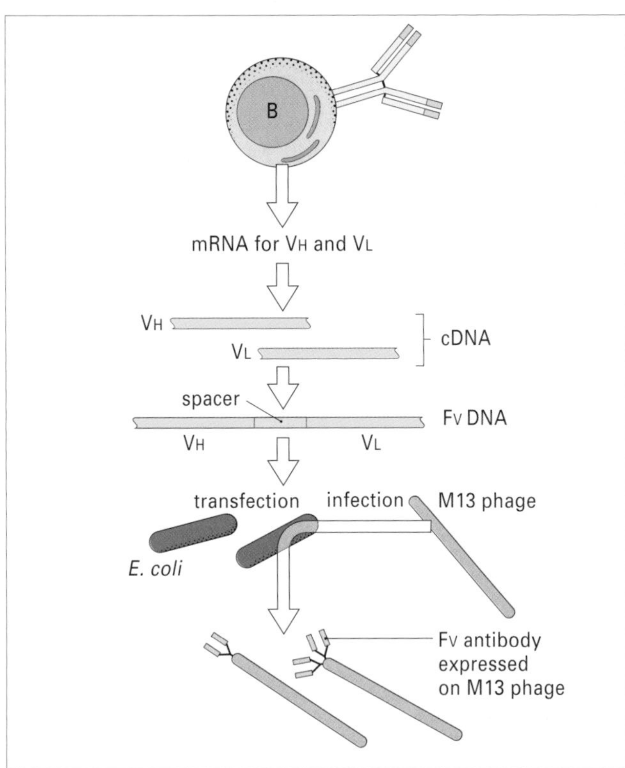

Fig. 27.19 To produce Fv antibodies by phage display, antibody VH and VL genes are first amplified from B-cell mRNA by the polymerase chain reaction. The genes are joined together with a spacer to give a gene for an Fv fragment. Bacteria are then transfected with the gene in a phagemid vector containing a leader sequence, a fragment of the gene expressing phage coat protein 3 and an M13 origin of replication and then infected with M13 phage. The phages replicate and express the Fv on their tips. Phages displaying the right specificity are isolated by panning on antigen-coated plates and amplified. The antigen-specific phage can be used to infect strains of bacteria which allow the secretion of the Fv protein into the culture medium.

variable regions (VH and VL) as part-molecules (Fv) of defined antigen-binding specificity and affinity on the surface of M13 filamentous phage so that they can be selected by antigen. In addition, if the phages are used to infect certain bacteria, the Fv protein is secreted in large amounts into the culture medium. This approach does not necessarily require the deliberate immunization of animals or humans (*Fig. 27.19*).

Although a monoclonal antibody is a well-defined reagent it does not have a greater specificity than a polyclonal antiserum which recognizes the antigen by means of a number of different epitopes.

ASSAYS FOR COMPLEMENT

The simplest measurement of complement activity is to determine the concentration of serum which will cause lysis of 50% of a standardized preparation of antibody-sensitized erythrocytes (EA). This is carried out in tubes or microwells. A simpler system, which provides a crude measure of complement activity, is single-radial haemolysis. The technique is similar to that of single-radial immunodiffusion (see *Fig. 27.4*) except that the wells contain the test serum and the gel contains EA. A zone of haemolysis develops around wells containing active complement, and the size of the zone is proportional to the amount of complement in the well. This technique measures the total activity of the classical and lytic pathways (C1–C9), but if a serum is deficient in complement activity it cannot identify which complement protein is lacking.

Individual components may be measured separately to determine either their total level or their functional level. This is an important distinction, since a component may be present in normal quantities but be functionally inactive. Total levels of individual complement proteins are usually measured by RIA or by ELISA using antibody specific for the protein under investigation. Functional levels are measured in assays tailored to detect each individual complement protein by providing a cocktail of sensitized red cells plus all the components required for lysis, except the one under investigation (*Fig. 27.20*).

Assays for complement components

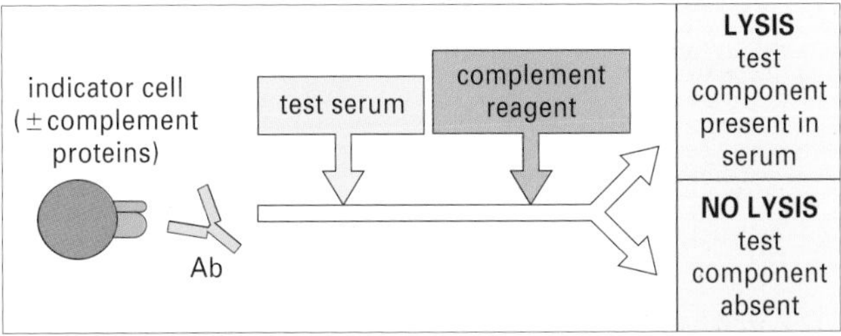

test	indicator	complement reagent
C1	EAC 4 (guinea-pig)	C1 reagent
C4	EA	C4-deficient guinea-pig serum
C2	EAC 4 (human) (antrypol)	C2 reagent
C3	EAC 142 (guinea-pig)	C5–9 (NH_3 treated guinea-pig serum)
C5	EAC 14 oxy 23	C5-deficient mouse serum
C6	EAC 143 (human) (antrypol)	C6-deficient rabbit serum
FB	EA+EGTA+Mg^{2+}	B-deficient serum (50°C treated)
FD	EA+EGTA+Mg^{2+}	D-deficient serum (Sephadex G75 exclusion peak)

Fig. 27.20 These assays detect specific complement components in a test serum. The principle of the assay is to mix sensitized red cells with a 'complement reagent' so that the sensitized cells plus the reagent contain all the complement components needed to lyse the red cells except for the component being tested. For example, to test for C4, erythrocytes sensitized with antibody (EA) are placed with C4-deficient guinea-pig serum. The cells will be lysed if there is C4 in the test serum, but not if none is present. The table lists the combinations of reagents used for each test component. The red cells are prepared by blocking the reactions of EA with complement at a specific point. The complement reagents may be sera thought to be deficient in one component or sera treated physicochemically to remove or inactivate one component. In practice the assay would be performed quantitatively, for example, by single-radial haemolysis, or in tubes to determine the point at which 50% of the red cells are lysed.

ASSAYS FOR CIRCULATING IMMUNE COMPLEXES

Circulating immune complexes are found in two compartments: free in plasma and bound to erythrocytes. Red cell bound complexes are less likely to be damaging, thus the estimate of free immune complexes may be more relevant.

C1q binding assays – Circulating complexes are often identified by their affinity for complement C1q, using either radiolabelled C1q or solid phase C1q (C1q linked to a solid support) (*Fig. 27.21*).

Precipitation of immune complexes – Precipitation of the immune complex with polyethylene glycol (PEG) and estimation of the precipitated IgG is frequently used to identify high molecular weight IgG, and forms the basis for one of the commercial assays (*Fig. 27.22*).

Immune complexes in autoimmune disease – However, care must be taken when determining complexes from patients with autoimmune diseases; these patients may have autoantibodies to components of the test system itself. In SLE, for example, patients produce anti-lymphocyte and anti-DNA antibodies that bind to the RAJI cells used in the assay, giving a false positive for immune complexes. Similarly, anti-C1q antibodies have been found in a number of connective tissue diseases (C1q has a structure similar to collagen), raising the possibility of false-positive results in C1q-based assays.

Interpretation of results – In all these assays, it is important to check that what is thought to be an immune complex is actually of higher molecular weight than monomeric IgG. Finally, note that evaluation of the importance of circulating complexes requires even more care than the interpretation of tissue complexes. Many circulating complexes will not in themselves be harmful. Damage only occurs if they are deposited in the tissue.

ISOLATION OF LYMPHOCYTE POPULATIONS

Many of the experiments performed by immunologists use populations of lymphocytes for work either *in vivo* or *in vitro*. The main sources of lymphocytes from experimental animals are the thymus, the spleen or the peripheral lymph nodes. Specialized studies may require isolation of cells from other areas such as Peyer's patches. Recirculating

An assay for immune complexes based on polyethylene glycol (PEG)

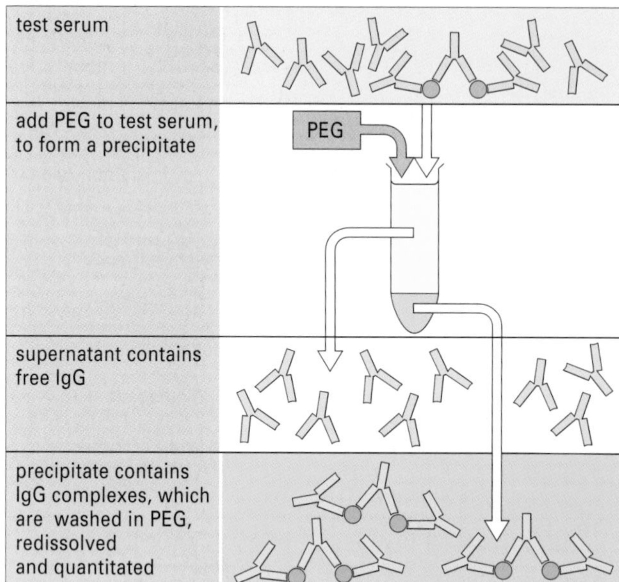

Fig. 27.21 Polyethylene glycol (PEG) is added to the test serum containing IgG complexes and IgG monomer. When the concentration of PEG reaches 2%, complexes are selectively precipitated; the free antibody remains in solution. The test tube is then centrifuged and the complexes form a pellet at the bottom. The supernatant containing free antibody is removed. The precipitate is washed and redissolved so that the amount of complexed IgG can be measured (e.g. by single radial immunodiffusion, nephelometry or radioimmunoassay).

Radioimmunoassay for immune complexes

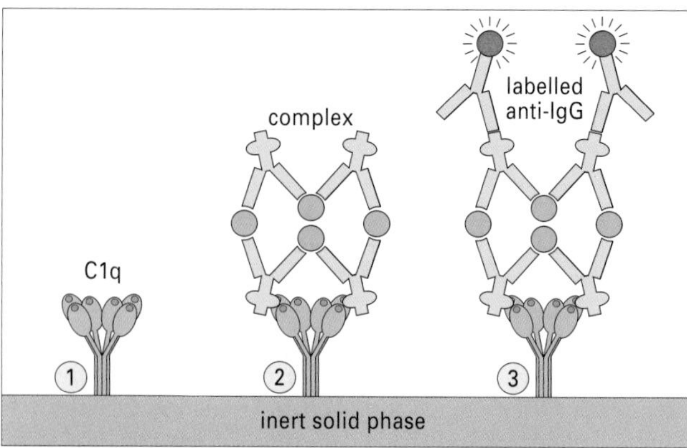

Fig. 27.22 A three-layer radioimmunoassay for immune complexes based on the use of C1q.
(1) C1q is linked to an inert solid phase support, usually a polystyrene tube or plate.
(2) Serum containing complexes is added. The complexes bind to the solid phase C1q by means of the array of Fc regions presented to the C1q.
(3) Radiolabelled anti-IgG antibody is added. The amount of radioactivity remaining on the solid phase after washing is measured in a gamma-counter, and is used to calculate the amount of complex bound to the C1q.

Density-gradient separation of lymphocytes on Ficoll Isopaque

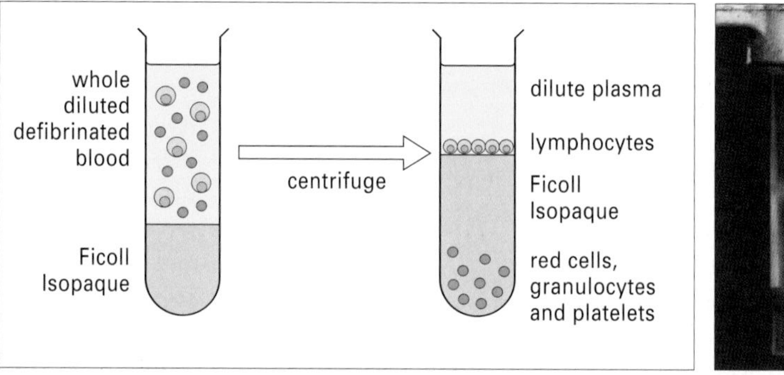

Fig. 27.23 Lymphocytes can be separated from whole blood using a density gradient. Whole blood is defibrinated by shaking with glass beads and the resulting clot removed. The blood is then diluted in tissue culture medium and layered on top of a tube half full of Ficoll. Ficoll has a density greater than that of lymphocytes but less than that of red cells and granulocytes (e.g. neutrophils). After centrifugation the red cells and polymorphonuclear neutrophils (PMNs) pass down through the Ficoll to form a pellet at the bottom of the tube while lymphocytes settle at the interface of the medium and Ficoll. The lymphocyte preparation can be further depleted of macrophages and residual PMNs by the addition of iron filings; these are taken up by phagocytes which can then be drawn away with a strong magnet. Macrophages can also be removed by leaving the cell suspension to settle on a plastic dish. Macrophages adhere to plastic, whereas the lymphocytes can be washed off.

Isolation of lymphocyte subpopulations – rosetting

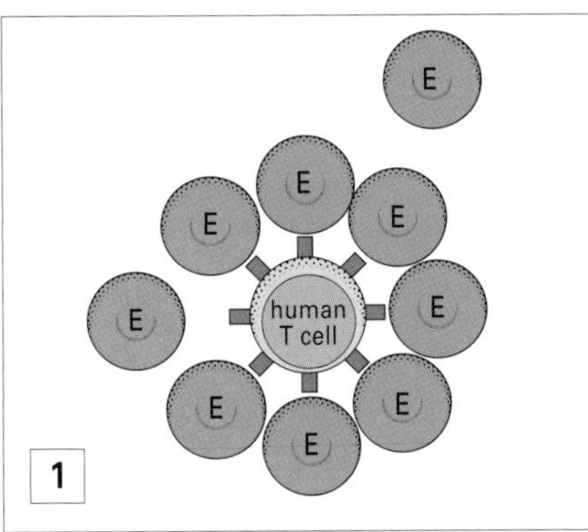

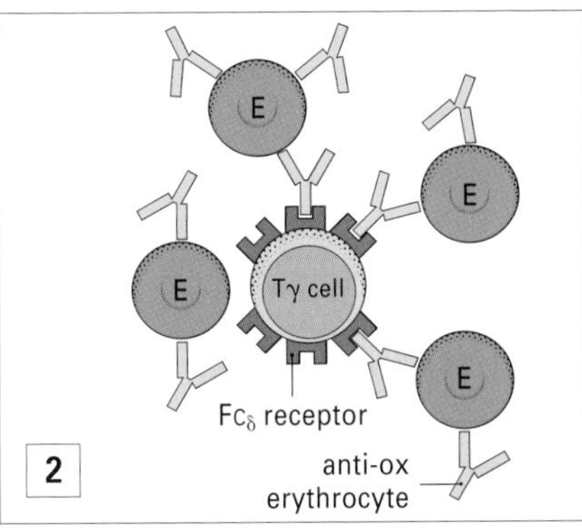

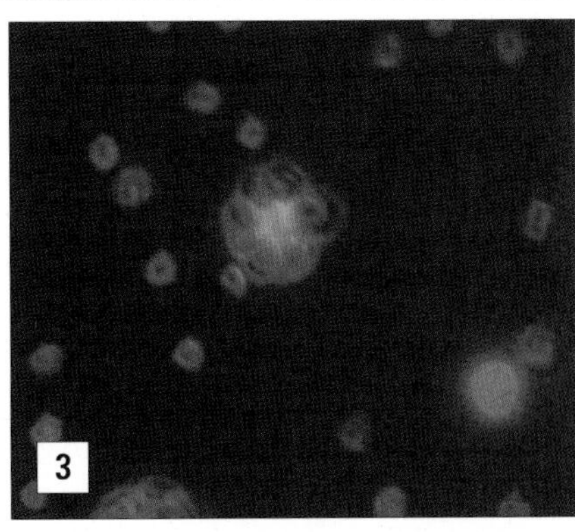

Fig. 27.24 Rosetting relies on the fact that some lymphocyte populations have receptors for erythrocytes. Human T cells have receptors for sheep erythrocytes (E); these are CD2 molecules (**1**). They are not present on mouse T cells in sufficient quantities, so mouse T cells cannot be isolated by this approach. When mixed together the T cells form rosettes with the erythrocytes and may be separated from non-rosetting B cells on Ficoll gradients. A modification of this technique to isolate cells with other receptors is also shown (**2**). For example, some T cells (Tγ cells) have a receptor for the Fc of IgG (Fcγ). These cells may be identified and isolated by rosetting with ox erythrocytes sensitized with a subagglutinating amount of anti-ox erythrocyte. A rosetted lymphocyte is shown (**3**). (Courtesy of Dr P.M. Lydyard.)

cells may be obtained by cannulating the thoracic duct and collecting the draining lymphocytes over a number of hours. In studies on humans, peripheral blood lymphocytes are the most readily available source of cells, but spleen, tonsil or lymph nodes may become available following surgical resection. However, problems can arise with surgical material due to the presence of infectious agents or tumour cells, depending on the circumstances that led to surgery. It should be emphasized that the cell populations derived from each of these tissues is quite distinct, with respect to the maturity of the lymphocytes and the proportions of different cell populations. The thymus is a source of fairly pure T cells but these are at varying stages of maturity. When working on lymphocytes from other sources, it is often desirable to separate the different cell populations so as to distinguish their effects.

Reference has already been made to the use of the fluorescence-activated cell sorter (FACS) for the isolation of lymphocyte populations, based on their surface markers. The number of cells isolated is, however, limited by the flow-through rate, which is slow because each cell is individually sorted. A number of bulk methods are also available for separating lymphocytes and the specific subpopulations. These include density-gradient separation, rosetting, panning and magnetic separations.

Density-gradient separation relies on lymphocytes being less dense than erythrocytes and granulocytes (*Fig. 27.23*), and is used to isolate the majority of blood lymphocytes. Rosetting and panning (or plating) are used to isolate subpopulations (*Figs 27.24* and *27.25*).

A simple and rapid way of separating lymphocyte populations, which does not require the use of expensive cell sorting equipment, is the technique of biomagnetic separation. This technique exploits the exquisite specificity of monoclonal antibodies and polymer particles containing magnetic material.

The beads are coated with a single monoclonal antibody to cellular antigens (such as CD3, CD4, CD8, CD19, etc.) as the primary antibody, or with a monoclonal antibody to immunoglobulin (of the appropriate species) or an antifluorochrome as the secondary antibody.

Two methods are available for cell separation using these beads (*Fig. 27.26*). These techniques can be used for the isolation of a wide range of cell types expressing antigens for which specific monoclonal antibodies are available and are most efficient when the antigens are expressed at a high level. The cells thus selected are pure and, most importantly, viable.

Another useful method for removing unwanted cell populations relies on antibody and complement. When a specific antibody (e.g. anti-CD8) is added to a mixture of cells, followed by complement, that subpopulation of cells will be lysed. Naturally this will only work with antibodies that fix complement, and where the target population of cells has sufficient surface antigens to fix a lytic dose of complement.

Another approach to the preparation of lymphocytes is to generate antigen-specific lines of T cells, and propagate them for an extended period (*Fig. 27.27*). This obviates the need for frequent isolation of primary cultures from animals.

EFFECTOR-CELL ASSAYS

Various methods have been developed for assaying lymphocyte-effector functions, including antibody production, cytotoxicity, and T-cell-mediated help and suppression.

Antibody-forming cells are measured by plaque-forming cell assay (*Fig. 27.28*), which can detect IgG- or IgM-producing cells. Another way of detecting antibody-producing cells is by the ELISPOT enzymatic test assay

Isolation of lymphocyte subpopulations – panning

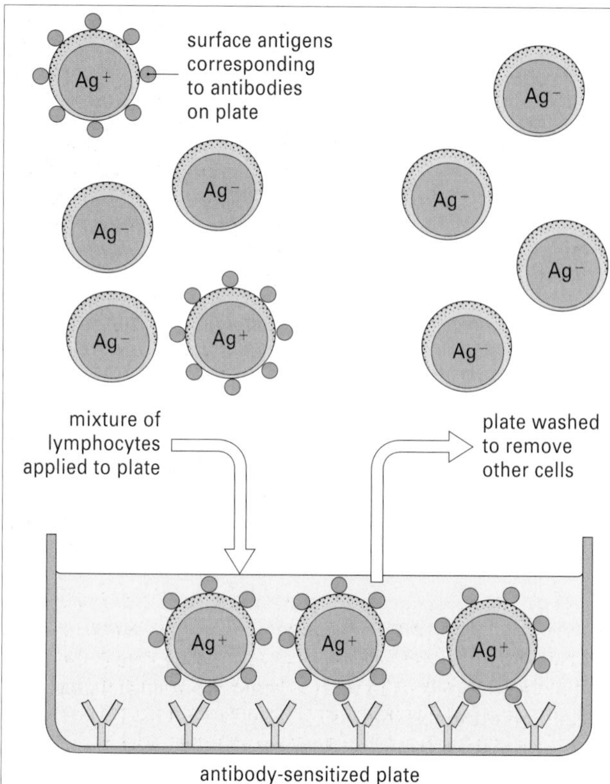

Fig. 27.25 Cell populations can be separated on antibody-sensitized plates. Antibody binds non-covalently to the plastic plate (as for solid-phase immunoassay) and the cell mixture is applied to the plate. Antigen-positive cells (Ag^+) bind to the antibody and the antigen-negative cells (Ag^-) can be carefully washed off. By changing the culture conditions or by enzyme-digestion of the cells on the plate it is sometimes possible to recover the cells bound to the plate. Often the cells that have bound to the plate are altered by their binding; for example, binding to the plate cross-links the antigen which can cause cell activation. Thus, the method is most satisfactory for removing a subpopulation from the population, rather than isolating it. Examples of the application of this method include separating TH and Tc cell populations using antibodies to CD4 or CD8, and separating T cells from B cells using anti-Ig (which binds to the surface antibody of the B cell). In reverse, by sensitizing the plate with antigen, antigen-binding cells can be separated from non-binding cells.

Cell separation by immunomagnetic beads

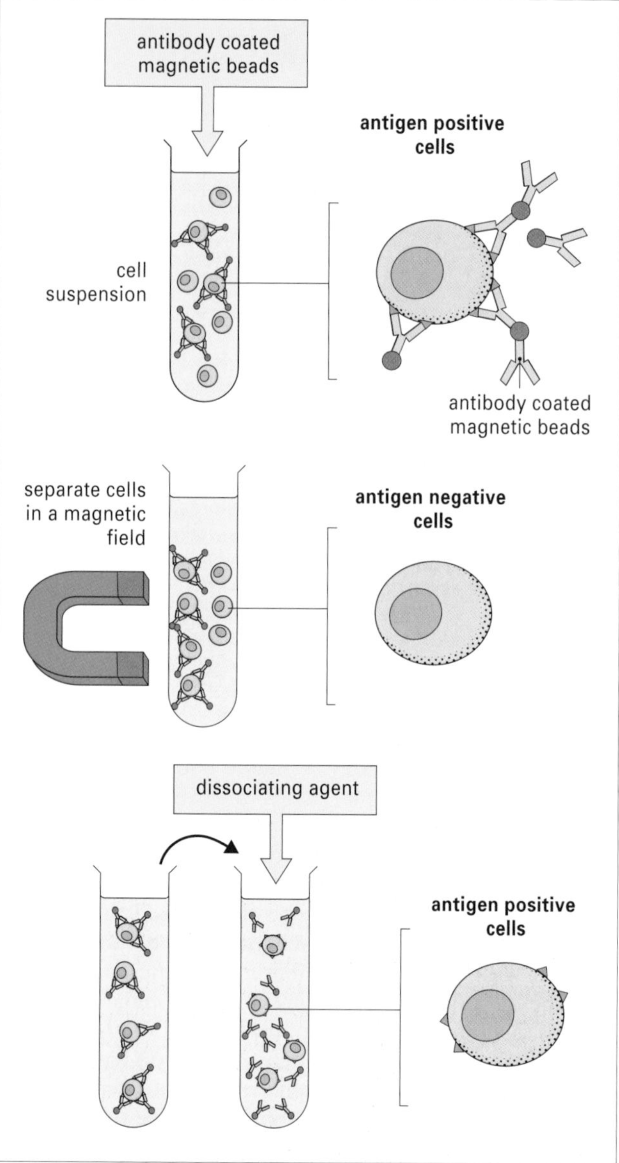

Fig. 27.26 In the **direct** method (illustrated), the beads are coated with a monoclonal antibody to the cellular antigen of interest, either by direct binding to the bead or by binding the primary antibody to secondary antibody-coated beads. The coated beads are then incubated with the cell suspension (or even whole blood) and the cells bound by the antibody on the beads (positively selected cells) are immobilized by applying a magnetic field to the tube. The non-immobilized cells (negatively selected) are removed from the tube and the positively selected cells are recovered following washing and dissociation from the antibody-coated beads.

In the **indirect** method, the monoclonal antibody to the target cellular antigen is first added to the cell suspension. Following incubation with the antibody, the cells are washed and mixed with beads coated with the appropriate secondary anti-Ig antibody. Cells bound to the magnetic beads (positively selected) are then immobilized with a magnetic field and the non-immobilized cells (negatively selected) removed. The positively selected cells are then washed and dissociated from the beads.

(*Fig. 27.29*). A development of this assay allows the detection of functional T cells according to the soluble mediators they release, i.e. cytokines. In this assay the plate is sensitized with an antibody to the specific cytokine (e.g. anti-IFN). This captures the specific cytokine released in a spot around the active T cell.

Antigen-specific T cells are often detected by the lymphocyte stimulation test, which measures their response to antigen as shown by their entering the cell cycle and incorporating precursors of DNA synthesis (*Fig. 27.30*). The cytotoxic activity of cell populations is usually

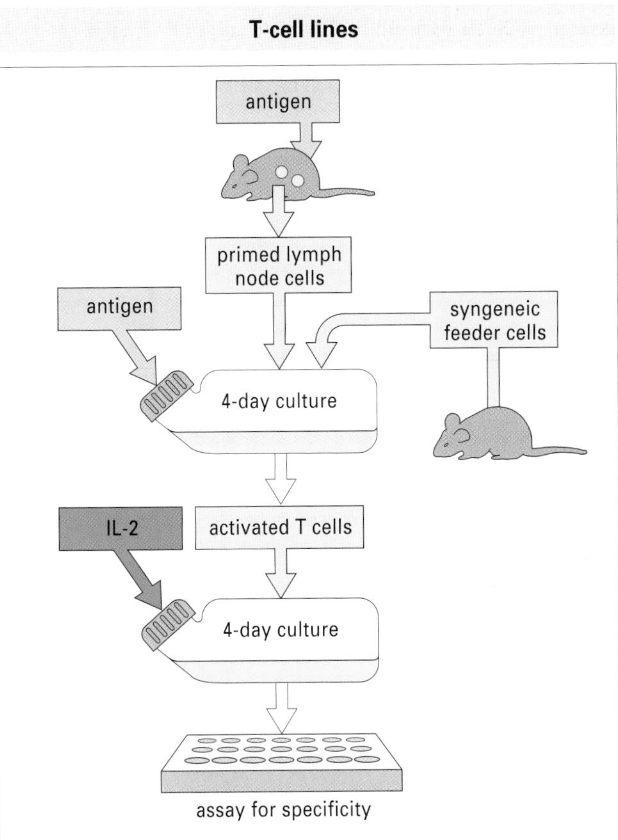

Fig. 27.27 The figure illustrates one protocol for the preparation of T-cell lines, although many other protocols are used. Mice are primed with antigen (usually subcutaneously in the rear foot pad), and the draining lymph nodes (in this case the popliteal and inguinal) are removed 1 week later and set up in co-culture with the antigen and with syngeneic feeder cells, i.e. cells from mice of the same inbred line (e.g. normal thymocytes or splenocytes). After 4 days the lymphoblasts are isolated and induced to proliferate with interleukin-2 (IL-2). When the population of cells has expanded sufficiently they are checked for antigen and MHC specificity in a lymphocyte transformation test, and are maintained by alternate cycles of culture on antigen-treated feeder cells and culture in IL-2-containing medium.

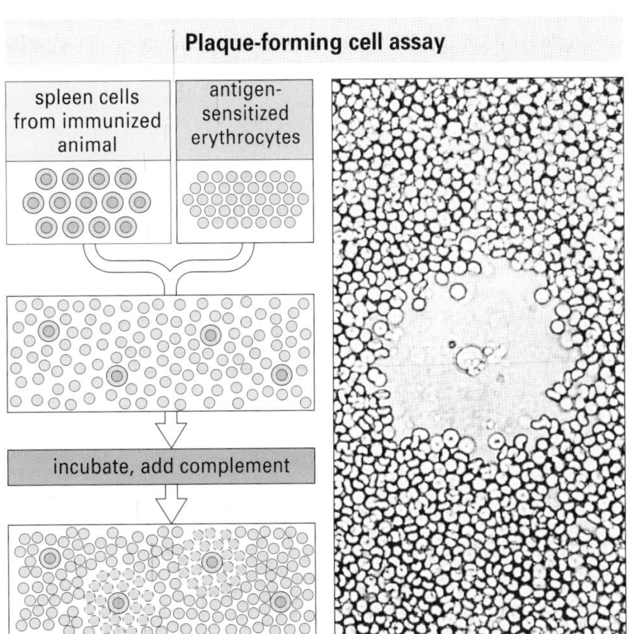

Fig. 27.28 Antibody-forming cells are measured by mixing the test population with antigen-sensitized red cells. Following incubation, the red cells surrounding the cells secreting specific antibody become coated with the antibody and so may be lysed by complement. The appearance of a plaque with a B cell in the centre is shown on the right. Two types of plaque can be identified:

Direct plaques: antigen-specific IgM antibodies produced by antibody-forming cells are able to directly cause complement-mediated lysis of antigen-sensitized red cells, because of their excellent complement-fixing ability.

Indirect plaques: antigen-specific IgG antibodies do not fix complement so efficiently and so anti-IgG antibodies must be added to enhance the ability of IgG-producing cells to lyse the target red cells.

By carrying out the assay with or without the anti-IgG step, it is possible to distinguish the number of IgM-producing B cells from the IgG-producing B cells.

detected by their ability to lyse target cells (e.g. virally infected cells, tumour cells, allogeneic tissue cells). Target-cell lysis is determined in the chromium-release assay (*Fig. 27.31*). This assay is insensitive with a cut off for detection of around 2000 activated antigen-specific CTL. *In vitro* stimulation of *ex vivo* cells is necessary to expand them and induce the formation of CTL precursors. The limiting dilution assay used to determine the frequency of CTL precursors is also insensitive.

The MHC tetramer assay allows the detection of antigen-specific CTL in *ex vivo* cell preparations without the need for *in vitro* expansion. The basis of this technique is to directly stain antigen-specific T cells with the MHC–peptide complex that they recognize via their T-cell receptors (TCRs). However, since the affinity of the TCR for the peptide–MHC complex is low, direct staining is not possible because of rapid dissociation. The formation of an MHC tetramer with four copies of the peptide–MHC complex results in a very enhanced avidity for the TCR (*Fig. 27.32*). MHC molecules of the appropriate haplotype are fused to a peptide (BSP) which acts as a substrate for biotinylation. MHC–BSP and beta$_2$ microglobulin are expressed in *E. coli*, mixed with the specific CTL epitopic peptide under folding conditions and the MHC–peptide complexes thus formed are purified. The complexes are biotinylated and mixed at a ratio of 4 : 1 with fluorescence-labelled streptavidin to produce the tetramers. The binding of these labelled tetramers by antigen-specific CTL can then be analysed by FACs.

Lymphocyte migration

Experiments for the detection of lymphocyte migration *in vivo* usually involve tracking of labelled lymphocytes to particular tissues after intravenous infusion. The cells may

ELISPOT assays

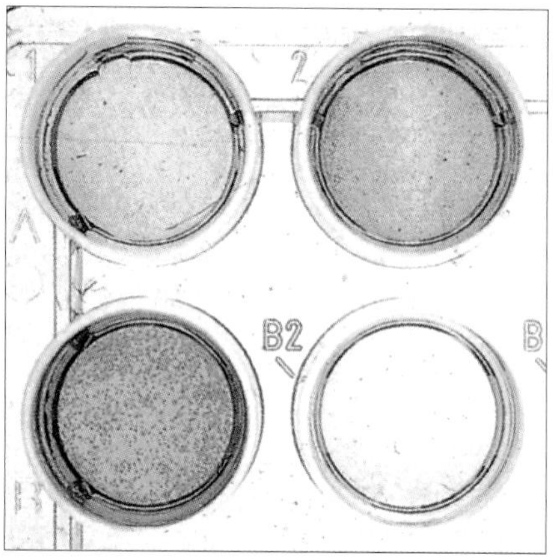

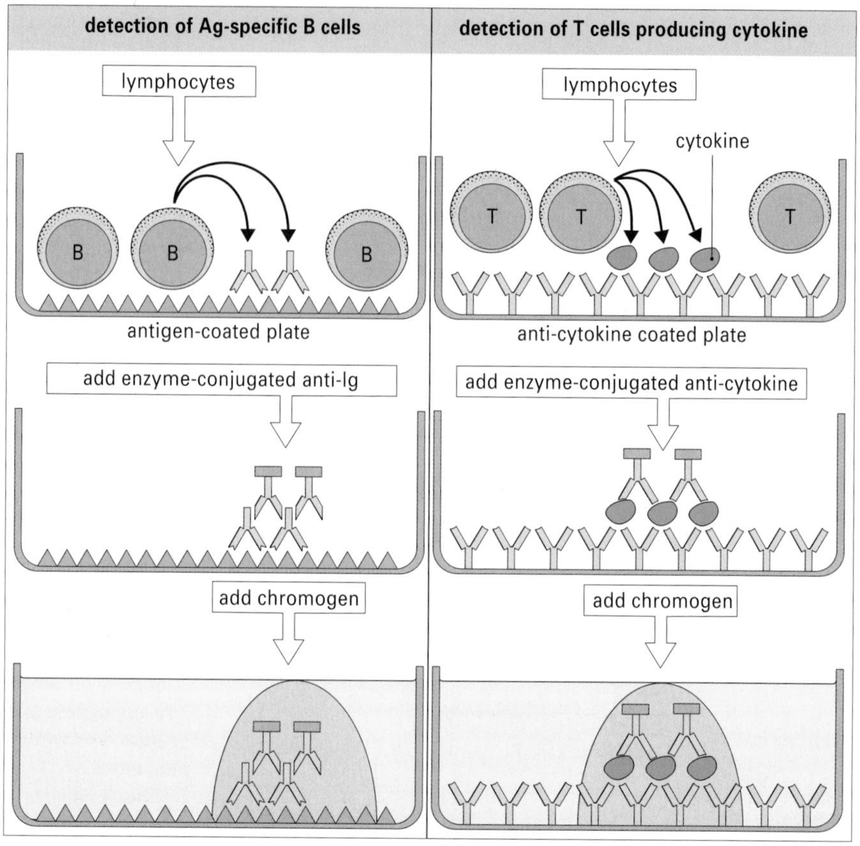

detection of Ag-specific B cells

lymphocytes

B B B

antigen-coated plate

add enzyme-conjugated anti-Ig

add chromogen

detection of T cells producing cytokine

lymphocytes

cytokine

T T T

anti-cytokine coated plate

add enzyme-conjugated anti-cytokine

add chromogen

Fig. 27.29 Individual B cells producing specific antibody or individual T cells secreting particular cytokines may be detected by ELISPOT assay. For detection of antibody-producing cells, the lymphocytes are plated onto an antigen-sensitized plate. Secreted antibody binds antigen in the immediate vicinity of cells producing the specific antibody. The spots of bound antibody are then detected chromatographically using enzyme coupled to anti-immunoglobulin and a chromogen. For detection of cytokine-producing cells the plates are coated with anti-cytokine and the captured cytokine is detected with enzyme-coupled antibody to a different epitope on the cytokine. The appearance of a developed plate is shown top left. (Photograph courtesy of P. Hutchings and Blackwell Scientific Publications.)

The lymphocyte stimulation test

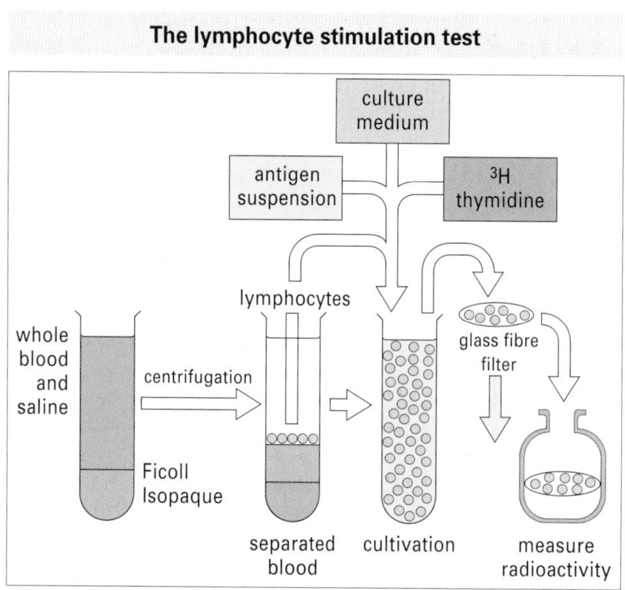

Fig. 27.30 In the lymphocyte stimulation test whole blood in saline solution is first layered on Ficoll Isopaque (which has a density between, and therefore separates, white cells and red cells) and centrifuged (400 × G). This separates the lymphocytes from the other cell and serum constituents (see *Fig. 27.23*). The cells are washed (to remove contaminants such as antigen) and then put into test tubes with a suspension of antigen and culture medium. Tritiated thymidine (^{3}H-thymidine) is added 16 hours before the cells are harvested. The cells are harvested on a glass-fibre filter disc and their radioactivity measured by placing the disc in a liquid scintillation counter. A high count indicates that the lymphocytes have undergone transformation and confirms their responsiveness to the antigen. This test can also be used for cells from lymphoid tissue.

Cytotoxicity assay by chromium release

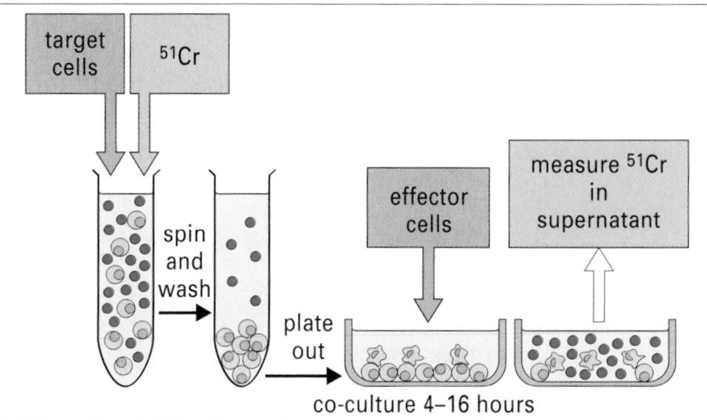

Fig. 27.31 To assay the cytotoxicity of effector cells, target cells are incubated with ^{51}Cr, which is taken up into the cells and binds to protein. After incubation the free ^{51}Cr is washed away and the target cells are plated out. They are then co-cultured with the effector cells for 4–16 hours and the supernatant is removed and counted to detect chromium released from target cells lysed by the effector cells.

A class I MHC tetramer

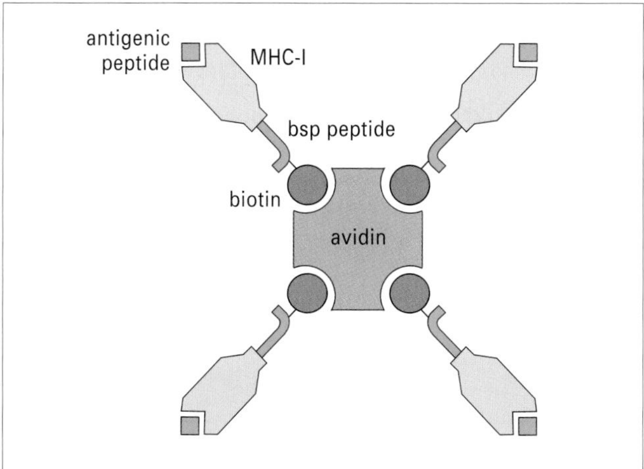

Fig. 27.32 A tetrameric MHC peptide is produced by biotinylating the MHC molecules, via a linking peptide (bsp), and allowing them to bind to the tetravalent molecule avidin – a natural receptor for biotin.

be radiolabelled or marked with stable fluorescent dyes. Radiolabelled cells are used for quantitative measurements of cell migration. Localization patterns within organs can be seen by autoradiography of labelled cells, or by direct visualization of fluorescent cells by microscopy under ultraviolet illumination.

Analysis of the adhesion molecules involved in lymphocyte migration has mostly been carried out *in vitro*. In the Stamper–Woodroofe assay, the direct binding of lymphocytes to high endothelial venules is measured by allowing the lymphocytes to adhere to tissue sections of lymph node, Peyer's patch or other tissues containing high endothelial venules. Adherent cells are counted under the microscope. Antibodies to intercellular adhesion molecules will reduce the level of binding, provided that the antibodies attach to the adhesion molecules near their active sites. The adhesion of lymphocytes to endothelial-cell monolayers can also be blocked *in vitro*. The identity of the adhesion molecules may then be confirmed by labelling the lymphocytes or endothelial cells and using the antibodies which block adhesion, to immunoprecipitate the specific adhesion molecules.

GENE TARGETING AND TRANSGENIC ANIMALS

Transgenic animals

One way of investigating the function of a particular molecule is to produce a transgenic animal in which the gene for that molecule is deleted, over-expressed, or expressed in a mutated form. The original way of producing transgenic mice was to inject about 100 copies of the gene in question directly into the pronucleus of a fertilized oocyte. This is then transferred to the oviduct of a pseudopregnant

Gene targeting by homologous recombination

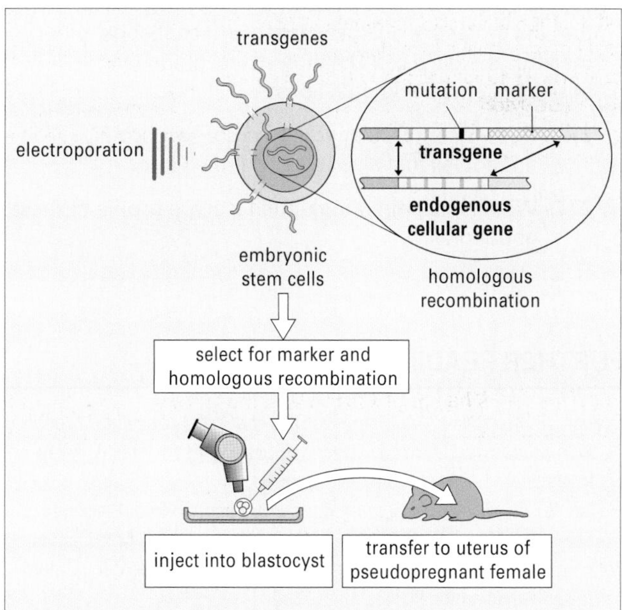

Fig. 27.33 Transgenic animals can be produced by gene targeting by homologous recombination. A gene segment is used which contains a sequence homologous to a cellular gene but with a mutation, for example, and with a ligated marker gene. These are electroporated into embryonic stem cells, which are then selected, using the marker gene, for cells which have taken up the exogenous gene. The cells are further selected for those which have recombined the exogenous gene with the endogenous gene. These cells are now injected into blastocysts, which are implanted into the uteri of pseudopregnant mice. The transgenic embryos are then left to develop and to be born normally.

female mouse, and the embryo left to develop. A variety of animals develop from such implantations. In a minority of embryos, one or more copies of the gene become incorporated into one of the chromosomes, before the first cell division occurs; these animals are heterozygous for the transgene. In another minority of the animals, the transgene becomes incorporated after the first division, and these are chimeras of normal cells and cells containing the transgene. In the majority of animals, no genes are incorporated. The status of each animal is established by taking some cells and establishing whether the gene is present by Southern blotting. Once heterozygous transgenics have been identified, these can be used in a programme of inbreeding to create a homozygous transgenic line.

Usually the transgenes become incorporated into a chromosome at random as a block. The number of transgenes incorporated is referred to as the copy number. It is important that this block does not disrupt another essential gene. How the transgenes are expressed depends on a number of factors. Sometimes the genes will be under the control of general promotors, and will be expressed in most tissues. Sometimes they will be linked with tissue-specific promotors so that they will only be expressed in some tissues (e.g. only in lymphocytes) or at particular stages of development. Care must be taken when interpreting the phenotype of transgenic animals, since it is unphysiological to express high quantities of transgenes in the wrong tissue.

Gene targeting

A more subtle approach is to use gene targeting. In this technique, a gene is transferred which interacts or recombines with the endogenous gene causing it to be altered in some way. For example the endogenous gene could be deleted (so-called 'knockout mice') or point mutated, or an exon could be removed. The altered gene in this case is injected into a pluripotent embryonic stem cell, where it recombines with the endogenous gene. The stem cell is then injected into a blastocyst and implanted as above (*Fig. 27.33*).

CRITICAL THINKING • Immunological techniques (Explanations on p. 464)

You have identified a protein fragment from an important viral pathogen which, when injected into experimental animals, induces immune responses that are protective against subsequent challenge with the virus. Select a combination of techniques to answer the following questions:

27.1 Does the molecule induce serum anti-protein antibodies that also react with the virus?

27.2 What is the immunoglobulin isotype profile of these antibodies?

27.3 How would you determine whether or not these antibodies show affinity maturation?

27.4 Does the molecule induce proliferative lymphocyte responses and/or cytotoxic lymphocyte responses?

27.5 How would you identify the lymphocyte subset (i.e. either $CD4^+$ or $CD8^+$) of the cells responsible for the proliferative responses and the cells responsible for the cytotoxic responses?

FURTHER READING

Coligan JE, Kruisbeck AM, Margulies DH, *et al.* (eds). *Current Protocols in Immunology*, New York: Greene Publishing Associates & Wiley-Interscience, 1991 – continually updated.

Hudson L, Hay FC. *Practical Immunology.* 3rd edn. Oxford: Blackwell Scientific Publications, 1989.

Johnstone A, Thorpe R. *Immunochemistry in Practice.* 2nd edn. Oxford: Blackwell Scientific Publications, 1987.

Rose NR *et al.* (eds). *Manual of Clinical Laboratory Immunology.* 4th edn. Washington: American Society of Microbiology, 1992.

Weir DM. *Handbook of Experimental Immunology.* Vols I & II. 4th edn. Oxford: Blackwell Scientific Publications, 1986.

Winter G, Griffith AD, Hawkins RE, *et al.* Making antibodies by phage display technology. *Annu Rev Immunol*; 1994;**12**:433–55.

Appendices

Appendix 1: Major histocompatibility complex

The Major Histocompatibility Complex is the most polymorphic gene locus known in man. Originally the MHC class I and class II molecules from the principal loci (HLA-A, -B, -C and -D) were distinguished using specific antibodies, which could recognize polymorphic variants at these loci. For example HLA-A2 identifies a particular variant at the HLA-A locus. These are termed serological HLA specificities. Later it became clear that the HLA-D region contained several class II loci (HLA-DP, -DQ and -DR), and that some serological specificities were specific for variants at these loci.

As serological analysis became more refined, it was found that some specificities could be subdivided into two or more types, using newer antibodies. For example, HLA-A9 is made up of two subgroups, HLA-A23 and HLA-A24.

In some cases the designation of the serologically defined MHC molecules was not fully certain, so they were given provisional or workshop designations 'w'. HLA-DPw1 is an example of such.

Later, sequence analysis of MHC genes was undertaken and the sequences could be related to the serological specificities. For example the sequences termed HLA-B*1301, B*1302, B*1303, B*1304, B*1305 and B*1306 are six different sequences, all of which encode HLA-B molecules which can be serologically defined by anti-HLA-B13 antibody. Following the '*', the first two digits indicate the serological specificity, and the subsequent digits the sequence number associated with that specificity. Hence several genetic variants can have the same serological specificity. The table below lists the full set of serological specificities.

Listing of all recognized serological and cellular HLA specificities. (Based on data at *http://anthonynolan.com/HIG/lists/specs.html*)

A	B	C	D	DR	DQ	DP
A1	B5	Cw1	Dw1	DR1	DQ1	DPw1
A2	B7	Cw2	Dw2	DR103	DQ2	DPw2
A203	B703	Cw3	Dw3	DR2	DQ3	DPw3
A210	B8	Cw4	Dw4	DR3	DQ4	DPw4
A3	B12	Cw5	Dw5	DR4	DQ5(1)	DPw5
A9	B13	Cw6	Dw6	DR5	DQ6(1)	DPw6
A10	B14	Cw7	Dw7	DR6	DQ7(3)	
A11	B15	Cw8	Dw8	DR7	DQ8(3)	
A19	B16	Cw9(w3)	Dw9	DR8	DQ9(3)	
A23(9)	B17	Cw10(w3)	Dw10	DR9		
A24(9)	B18		Dw11(w7)	DR10		
A2403	B21		Dw12	DR11(5)		
A25(10)	B22		Dw13	DR12(5)		
A26(10)	B27		Dw14	DR13(6)		
A28	B2708		Dw15	DR14(6)		
A29(19)	B35		Dw16	DR1403		
A30(19)	B37		Dw17(w7)	DR1404		
A31(19)	B38(16)		Dw18(w6)	DR15(2)		
A32(19)	B39(16)		Dw19(w6)	DR16(2)		
A33(19)	B3901		Dw20	DR17(3)		
A34(10)	B3902		Dw21	DR18(3)		
A36	B40		Dw22			
A43	B4005		Dw23	DR51		
A66(10)	B41		Dw24	DR52		
A68(28)	B42		Dw25	DR53		
A69(28)	B44(12)		Dw26			
A74(19)	B45(12)					
A80	B46					
	B47					
	B48					
	B49(21)					
	B50(12)					
	B51(5)					
	B5102					
	B5103					
	B52(5)					
	B53					
	B54(22)					
	B55(22)					

Appendix 1: Major histocompatibility complex (*contd.*)

A	B	C	D	DR	DQ	DP
	B56(22) B57(17) B58(17) B59 B60(40) B61(40) B62(15) B63(15) B64(14) B65(14) B67 B70 B71(70) B72(70) B73 B75(15) B76(15) B77(15) B78 B81 Bw4 Bw6					

The number of genetic variants is very large, and the current list (July 2000) can be viewed at *http://www.anthonynolan.com/HIG/lists/*.

Locus:	**Number of variants:**
HLA-A	206
HLA-B	403
HLA-C	92
HLA-E	5
HLA-F	1
HLA-G	14
HLA-DRA	2
HLA-DRB1	254
HLA-DRB2-9	63
HLA-DQA1	20
HLA-DQB1	45
HLA-DPA1	19
HLA-DPB1	89
TAP1	6
TAP2	4

Appendix 2: CD markers

CD	identity/function	family	mol. wt kDa	T cell	B cell	NK cell	monocyte/ macrophage	granulocyte	platelet	dendritic cell	other
CD1a	Presentation of lipids/glycolipids	IgSF	49	Thy						LC	
CD1b	Presentation of lipids/glycolipids	IgSF	45	Thy						LC	
CD1c	Presentation of lipids/glycolipids	IgSF	43	Thy						DC	
CD1d	Presentation of lipids/glycolipids	IgSF	55	Thy							
CD1e	Presentation of lipids/glycolipids	IgSF	50								
CD2	LFA-3 receptor (adhesion)	IgSF	50								
CD3	TCR signalling complex ($\gamma,\delta,\varepsilon$) ($\zeta,\upsilon$)	IgSF IgSF	25,20,19, 16,22								
CD4	MHC class II receptor	IgSF	55								
CD5	co-stimulator (activation)	Scav	67								
CD6	co-stimulator (activation)	Scav	105								
CD7	signal transduction	IgSF	40								LSC
CD8	MHC class I receptor	IgSF	36,32								
CD9	platelet activation	TM4	24		p			Eo B			
CD10	neutral endopeptidase	ZnMP	100	p	p						
CD11a	LFA-1	Intα	180								
CD11b	CR3	Intα	165								
CD11c	CR4	Intα	150								
CDw12		P-prot	120					Eo N			
CD13	Aminopeptidase N	ZnMP	150								End
CD14	LPS-binding protein receptor		53–55								
CD15	sialyl Lewis	Carb									
CD16	FcγRIIIA/FcγRIIIB	IgSF	50–65								
CD16b	FcγRIIIB	IgSF	48								
CDw17	Lactosyl ceramide	Carb	120								
CD18	LFA-1/CR3/CR4	Intβ	95								
CD19	B-cell co-receptor subunit	IgSF	95								FDC
CD20	Ca^{++} channel	TM4	33–37								
CD21	CR2 B-cell co-receptor subunit	CCP	140								FDC
CD22	adhesion moleculle	IgSF	130–140								
CD23	FcεRII	Clec	45		★		★	Eo			
CD24	co-stimulator (activation)		41,38								
CD25	IL-2R	CytR	55	★	★						
CD26	Dipeptidyl peptidase IV		120	★	★						
CD27	binds CD70	TNFR	55								
CD28	binds CD80, CD86	IgSF	44		★						
CD29	VLA-1–VLA-6	Intβ	130								
CD30	signal transduction (apoptosis)	TNFR	120	★	★	★					
CD31	PECAM-1	IgSF	140								End
CD32	FcγRII	IgSF	40								
CD33		IgSF	67								MSC
CD34	binds L-selectin	Muc	105–120								End MSC
CD35	CR1	CCP	160–260					Eo N			FDC
CD36	adhesion molecule	Scav	88								End
CD37	signal transduction (activation)	TM4	40–52								
CD38	ribosyl cyclase	Ect	45	★	PC						LSC
CD39	ecto-apyrose	Ect	70–100		★	★					FDC
CD40	binds CD154, co-stimulatory	TNFR	48								FDC
CD41	GPIIb adhesion to matrix	Intα	120,25								
CD42a	GPIX adhesion		23								
CD42b	GPIbα adhesion		135,23								
CD42c	GPIbβ adhesion		22								
CD42d	GPV adhesion		85								

Appendix 2: CD markers *(contd.)*

CD	identity/function	family	mol. wt kDa	T cell	B cell	NK cell	monocyte/ macrophage	granulocyte	platelet	dendritic cell	other
CD43	Leukosialin (anti-adhesive)	Muc	95								
CD44	Pgp-1 adhesion to matrix		80–95								
CD45	Leucocyte common antigen (LCA)		200								
CD45RA	Restricted LCA		220								
CD45RB	Restricted LCA		190,205								
CD45RO	Restricted LCA		190								
CD46	MCP (membrane cofactor protein)	CCP	66,56								
CD47		IgSF	47–52								
CD48	binds CD2 (rodents)	IgSF	41								
CD49a	VLA-1 adhesion to matrix	Intα	210	★							
CD49b	VLA-2 adhesion to matrix	Intα	160								
CD49c	VLA-3 adhesion to matrix	Intα	125								
CD49d	VLA-4 adhesion	Intα	150,80,70							LC	
CD49e	VLA-5 adhesion to matrix	Intα	135,25								
CD49f	VLA-6 adhesion to matrix	Intα	120,25								
CD50	ICAM-3	IgSF	124							LC	
CD51	Vitronectin receptor α	Intα	120,24								
CD52	Campath-1		21–28								
CD53	Signal transduction	TM4	32–40								
CD54	ICAM-1	IgSF	75–115								
CD55	DAF (decay accelerating factor)	CCP	70								
CD56	NCAM (neural cell adhesion molecule)	IgSF	220,135								
CD57	HNK-1	Carb	110								
CD58	LFA-3 binds CD2	IgSF	40–65								
CD59	Protectin inhibits MAC		19								
CDw60	NeuAc-NeuAc-Gal	Carb									
CD61	Vitronectin receptor subunit	Intβ	105								End
CD62E	E-selectin	Clec	115								★End
CD62L	L-selectin	Clec	75–80								
CD62P	P-selectin	Clec	150								★End
CD63	Adaptor	TM4	53					★	★		End
CD64	FcγRI	IgSF	70								
CD65	Ceramide dodecasaccharide	Carb									
CD66a	BGB-1 adhesion	IgSF	180–200								
CD66b	was CD67 adhesion	IgSF	95–100								
CD66c	NCA adhesion	IgSF	90–95								
CD66d	CGMI	IgSG	30								
CD66e	CEA (carcinoembryonic antigen)	IgSF	180–200								
CD66f	Pregnancy specific glycoprotein	IgSF	54–72								
CD68	Macrosialin	Scav	110					N B			MC Sav
CD69	activation induction	Clec	32,28	★	★	★	★				Thy
CD70	binds CD27	TNF	175,95,75	★	★		★				
CD71	Transferrin receptor		95	★	★	★	★				★
CD72		Clec	43,39								
CD73	Ecto-5′-nucleotidase	Ect	69								End FDC
CD74	Ii (MHC class II invariant chain)		41,35,33								
CDw75	α-2,6 sialyl transferase, binds CD22	Sial	53								
CDw76	NeuAc α-2,6(Galβ1,4GlcNac)n	Carb									End
CD77	Globotriaosylceramide	Carb									
CD79a	Igα	IgSF	33								
CD79b	Igβ	IgSF	39								
CD80	B7-1, binds CD28 and CD152	IgSF	60	★	★						
CD81	TAPA B-cell co-receptor unit	TM4	26								End

Appendix 2: CD markers *(contd.)*

CD markers											
CD	identity/function	family	mol. wt kDa	T cell	B cell	NK cell	monocyte/ macrophage	granulocyte	platelet	dendritic cell	other
CD82	Signal transduction	TM4	60								
CD83	? antigen presentation	IgSF	43								
CD84	? co-stimulation	IgSF	74								
CD85											
CD86	B7-2 binds CD28 and CD152	IgSF	80		★						
CD87	Urokinase plasminogen activator		35–39								
CD88	C5αR	TM7	43								MC
CD89	FcαR	IgSF	50–70								
CD90	Thy-1	IgSF	25–35	Thy							
CD91	α2-macroglobulin receptor	LDLR	515,85								
CDw92			70					N			End
CDw93			120					N			End
CD94	binds MHC class I	Clec	70								
CD95	FAS signal transduction (apoptosis)	TNFR	43	★	★						
CD96		IgSF	160	★							
CD97	binds CD55	EGFR	75–85	★	★						
CD98	modulates intracellular Ca^{++}		80,45								
CD99		Muc	32								
CD100	? proliferation	IgSF	150								
CD101		IgSF	120	★							
CD102	ICAM-2 binds LFA-1	IgSF	55,65								End
CD103	αEβ7 integrin	Intα	150,25								
CD104	β4 integrins	Intβ	220								End
CD105	Endoglin binds TGFβ		90				★				End
CD106	VCAM-1 binds VLA-4	IgSF	90–110								★End
CD107a	LAMP-1		110	★				★	★		★End
CD107b	LAMP-2		120	★				★	★		★End
CDw108	? adhesion		80								
CD109	Platelet activation factor		170	★					★		End
CD114	G-CSFR		110–130					N			
CD115	M-CSFR	IgSF	150–130								
CD116	GM-CSFR α chain	CytR	60					N Eo			
CD117	c-kit stem cell factor receptor	IgSF	145	Thy							SC
CD118	IFNα/β receptor										
CD119	IFNγ receptor		90–100								
CD120a	TNFR-I	TNFR	60								
CD120b	TNFR-II	TNFR	75–85								
CD121a	IL-1R type I	IgSF	80								End
CDw121b	IL-1R type II	IgSF	60–70								
CD122	IL-2R β chain	CytR	75								
CD123	IL-3R	CytR	70								SC
CD124	IL-4R	CytR	130–150								
CD125	IL-5R	CytR	55–60		★			Eo B			
CD126	IL-6R	IgSF	80		★						End
CD127	IL-7R		68–80		Pre B						LSC
CD128	IL-8R chemokine receptor CXCR1	TM7	58								
CD130	IL-6R, IL-11R common subunit	IgSF	130		★						
CDw131	IL-3R, IL-5R common subunit	CytR	140								SC
CD132	IL-2R, -4R, -7R, -4R, -15R common subunit	CytR	64								
CD134	? adhesion molecule	TNFR	50	★							
CD135	growth factor receptor		155,130		p		p				SC
CDw136	Macrophage-stimulating protein receptor		180								

Appendix 2: CD markers *(contd.)*

CD	identity/function	family	mol. wt kDa	T cell	B cell	NK cell	monocyte/ macrophage	granulocyte	platelet	dendritic cell	other
CDw137	co-stimulatory (activation)	TNFR	30								
CD138	Syndecan binds type I collagen										
CD139			228,209								FDC
CD140	PDGF receptor		180,180								End
CD141	Thrombomodulin	Clec	105					N			End
CD142	Tissue factor procoagulant		46								
CD143	ACE (angiotensin converting enzyme)	ZnMP	170–180	★		★					End
CD144	VE-cadherin adhesion		135								End
CDw145			110,90,25								End
CD146	? adhesion	IgSF	130	★							End
CD147	Neurothelin, basigin ? adhesion	IgSF	55–65								End
CD148	contact inhibition		250								
CDw149	≡ CD47	IgSF	47–52								
CDw150	SLAM ? costimulation		75–95	Thy							End
CD151	PETA3 ? signalling (adhesion)	TM4	32								End
CD152	CTLA-4 binds CD80 and CD86	IgSF	33	★							
CD153	CD30L binds CD30	TNF	38–40	★			★				
CD154	CD40L binds CD40	TNF	32–39	★							
CD155	Polio virus receptor	IgSF	80–90	Thy							
CD156	ADAM8	ZnMP	60–70					N			
CD157	ADP-ribosyl cyclase	Ect	42–50		p						FDC End
CD158a	p58.1,p50.1 binds MHC class I(KIR)	IgSF	58,50								
CD158b	p58.2,p50.2 binds MHC class I(KIR)	IgSF	58,50								
CD158c	p58.3,p50.3 activation(cytotoxicity)	IgSF	58,50								
CD161	NKRP-1 modulates cytotoxicity	Clec	44								
CD162	PSGL-1 binds selectins	Muc	240								
CD163	M130	Scav	130								
CD164	MGC-24 adhesion to stromal cells	Muc	80								SC
CD165	AD2 adhesion to thymic epithelium		37	Thy							
CD166	ALCAM binds CD6	IgSF	100	★			★				

This table shows the recognized CD markers of haemopoietic cells and their distribution:

Filled box = Molecule is expressed
Open box = Molecule not expressed or not determined yet
Half-filled box = Subpopulation only
★ = Activated cells only

B = Basophil
B = B cell
Carb = Carbohydrate
CCP = Complement control protein domains
Clec = C-type lectin
CytR = Haemopoietic cytokine receptor family
DC = Dendritic cell
Ect = Ectoenzyme
End = Endothelium
Eo = Eosinophil
FDC = Follicular dendritic cell
G = Granulocyte
IgSF = Immunoglobulin supergene family
Intα = Integrin alpha chain
Intβ = Integrin beta chain
LC = Langerhans' cell
LSC = Lymphoid stem cell
M = Mononuclear phagocyte lineage
MC = Mast cell
MSC = Myeloid stem cell
Muc = Mucin
N = Neutrophil
NK = Natural killer cell
P = Platelet
p = Precursor
PC = Plasma cell
P-prot = Phosphoprotein
SC = Stem cell
Scav = Scavenger receptors
Sial = Sialoglycan
T = T cell
Thy = Thymocyte
TM4 = Tetramembrane pass family
TM7 = 7 transmembrane pass G-protein coupled receptor
TNF = TNF-like
TNFR = TNF receptor/NGF receptor family
ZnMP = Zinc metalloproteinase

This gives principle family relationships only. Some molecules are composite.
The designation 'w' (workshop) indicates a provisional assignment only.
Detailed information on many of the CD molecules is distributed as 'CD guides' from http://www.ncbi.nlm.nih.gov/prow.
A further set of CD numbers were assigned at the 7th International Workshop in June 2000 numbered CD167–CD247. Minor refinements and corrections were also made to existing designations. The new designations can be seen at http://gryphon.jr2.ox.ac.uk/.

Appendix 3: The major cytokines

cytokine	immune system source	other cells	principal targets	principal effects
IL-1α IL-1β	macrophages, LGLs, B cells	endothelium, fibroblasts, astrocytes, etc.	T cells, B cells, macrophages, endothelium, tissue cells	lymphocyte activation, macrophage stimulation, ↑ leucocyte/endothelial adhesion, pyrexia, acute phase proteins
IL-2	T cells		T cells	T-cell proliferation and differentiation, activation of cytotoxic lymphocytes and macrophages
IL-3	T cells	stem cells		multilineage colony stimulating factor
IL-4	T cells		B cells, T cells	B-cell growth factor, isotype selection, IgE, IgG1
IL-5	T cells		B cells	B-cell growth and differentiation, IgA selection
IL-6	T cells, B cells	fibroblasts, macrophages	B cells, hepatocytes	B-cell differentiation, induces acute phase proteins
IL-7		bone marrow stromal cells	pre-B cells, T cells	B-cell and T-cell proliferation
IL-8	monocytes	fibroblasts	neutrophils, basophils, T cells, keratinocytes	chemotaxis, angiogenesis, superoxide release, granule release
IL-9	T cells			enhances T-cell survival, mast cell activation, synergy with erythropoietin
IL-10	T cells		TH1 cells	inhibition of cytokine synthesis
IL-11		bone marrow stromal cells, fibroblasts	haemopoietic progenitors osteoclasts	osteoclast formation, colony stimulating factor, elevates platelet count *in vivo*, inhibits pro-inflammatory cytokine production
IL-12	monocytes		T cells	induction of TH1 cells
IL-13	activated T cells		monocytes, B cells	B-cell growth and differentiation, inhibits pro-inflammatory cytokine production
IL-14	T cells			stimulates proliferation of activated B cells, inhibits Ig secretion
IL-15	monocytes	epithelium, muscle	T cells, activated B cells	proliferation
IL-16	eosinophils, $CD8^+$ T cells		$CD4^+$ T cells	chemoattraction of $CD4^+$ cells
IL-17	$CD4^+$ T lymphocytes		epithelium, fibroblasts, endothelium	release of IL-6, IL-8, G–CSF, PGE2, enhances ICAM-1, stimulates fibroblasts to sustain $CD34^+$ progenitors
IL-18	macrophages	hepatocytes, keratinocytes	PBMC, co-factor in TH1 induction	induces IFNγ production, enhances NK activity
IL-21	T cells, mast cells		T cells, B cells, mast cells, eosinophils, hepatocytes	induces acute phase reactants, levels raised after LPS
IL-22	activated T cells		TH2 cells	inhibits IL-4 production
TGFβ1			most cell types	downregulates inflammatory cytokine production, promotes wound healing responses and scar tissue, growth inhibition
TNFα	macrophages, mast cells, lymphocytes		macrophages, granulocytes, tissue cells	activation of macrophages, granulocytes and cytotoxic cells, leucocyte/endothelial cell adhesion, cachexia, pyrexia, induction of acute phase protein, stimulation of angiogenesis, enhanced MHC class I production
TNFβ (LT)	lymphocytes			as for TNFα

Appendix 3: The major cytokines *(contd.)*

cytokine	immune system source	other cells	principal targets	principal effects
IFNα	leucocytes	epithelia, fibroblasts	tissue cells	MHC class I induction, antiviral state, stimulation of NK cells, anti-proliferative, stimulates IL-12 production and TH1 cells
IFNβ		fibroblasts, epithelia	tissue cells, leucocytes	MHC class I induction, antiviral state, anti-proliferative
IFNγ	T cells, NK cells	epithelia, fibroblasts	leucocytes, tissue cells, TH2 cells	MHC class I and II induction, macrophage activation, ↑ endothelial cell/lymphocyte adhesion, MØ cytokine synthesis, antiviral state, anti-proliferative (TH1 cells)
M–CSF	monocytes	endothelium, fibroblasts		proliferation of macrophage precursors
G–CSF	macrophages	fibroblasts	stem cells	stimulates division and differentiation
GM–CSF	T cells, macrophages	endothelium, fibroblasts		proliferation of granulocyte and macrophage precursors and activators
MIF	T cells, macrophages		macrophages	migration inhibition, macrophage activation, enhances T-cell activation

Appendix 4: Chemokine receptors and chemokines

The table below lists the chemokine receptors, their principal ligands and the cells which express the receptors. This list is not complete (May 2000): additional chemokines and receptors are under investigation. Not all chemokines have been tested on all cell types, therefore entries in the table indicate only those chemokines which have been tested and show positive chemotaxis or activation. A new nomenclature is under development, in which each chemokine is given a designation according to the group of receptors it binds to and a number. For example: MCP-1 = CCL2; MIP-1α = CCL3; SDF-1 = CXCL12.

Cells: * = activated cells only; +/– = subpopulation; Endoth. = endothelium; DC = dendritic cells; B = basophil; E = eosinophil; N = neutrophil; Monocyte = mononuclear phagocytes; Imm. = immature; Mat. = mature; M = memory; TH1 = type 1 T helper cells; TH2 = type 2 T helper cells.

Chemokines: BCA = B-cell attracting chemokine; GCP = granulocyte chemotactic protein; Gro = growth-related oncogene; I309 = inducible-309; IL-8 = interleukin-8; IP-10 = interferon-inducible protein-10, I-TAC = interferon-inducible T-cell α chemoattractant; LARC = liver and activation regulated chemokine; MCP = monocyte chemotactic protein; MDC = macrophage-derived chemokine; Mig = monokine induced by interferon-γ; MIP = macrophage inflammatory protein; NAP = neutrophil-activating peptide; RANTES = regulated on activation normal T cell expressed and secreted; SDF = stromal cell-derived factor; SLC = secondary lymphoid tissue chemokine; TARC = thymus and activation regulated chemokine; TECK = thymus-expressed chemokine.

REFERENCE

Murphy PM *et al.* International Union of Pharmacology XXII. Nomenclature for chemokine receptors. *Pharmacol Rev* 2000;**52**:145–76. Available from http://www.pharmrev.org

Receptor	Ligands	T cell	B cell	NK cell	Monocyte	Granulocyte	Other
CCR1	RANTES, MCP-2, MCP-3, MIP-1α, MIP-3, MIP-5	+		+	+	E,B,N	Imm.DC
CCR2	MCP-1, MCP-2, MCP-3, MCP-4, MCP-5	*	+	*	+		
CCR3	RANTES, MCP-2, MCP-3, MCP-4, MIP-5, Eotaxins-1-3	TH2			+	E,B	
CCR4	MDC, TARC, MIP-1α	TH2		+			Imm.DC
CCR5	RANTES, MCP-2, MIP-1α, MIP-1β	TH1	+		+		Imm.DC
CCR6	MIP-3α	+	+				Imm.DC
CCR7	SLC, MIP-3β	Naïve	+				Mat.DC
CCR8	TARC, MIP-1β, I309	TH2*				E,B	
CCR9	TECK	+			*		DC
CCR10	RANTES, MCPs-1-5, MIP-1β, Eotaxin-1, skinkine	M			+		
CCR11	MCP-1, MCP-2, MCP-4						
CXC1	IL-8, GCP-2	*				N	Endoth.
CXCR2	IL-8, Gro-α, Gro-β, Gro-γ, NAP-2	*	+			N	Endoth.
CXCR3	IP-10, Mig, I-TAC	TH1					Endoth.
CXCR4	SDF-1	Naïve	+		+		Many cells
CXCR5	BCA-1	+/–	+				
XCR1	Lymphotactin	+					
CX3CR1	Fractalkine	*		+	+		

Glossary

Acquired immune deficiency syndrome (AIDS). A progressive immune deficiency caused by infection of CD4 T cells with the human retrovirus HIV.
Acute phase proteins. Serum proteins whose levels increase during infection or inflammatory reactions.
ADCC (antibody-dependent cell-mediated cytotoxicity). A cytotoxic reaction in which Fc receptor-bearing killer cells recognize target cells via specific antibodies.
Adhesion molecules. Cell surface molecules involved in the binding of cells to extracellular matrix or to neighbouring cells, where the principal function is adhesion, rather than cell activation, e.g. integrins and selectins.
Adjuvant. A substance that non-specifically enhances the immune response to an antigen.
AFCs (antibody-forming cells). Functionally equivalent to plasma cells.
Affinity. A measure of the binding strength between an antigenic determinant (epitope) and an antibody-combining site.
Affinity maturation. The increase in average antibody affinity frequently seen during a secondary immune response.
Allelic exclusion. Occurs when the use of a gene from the maternal or paternal chromosome prevents the use of the other. This is seen with antibody and T-cell receptor genes.
Allergen. An agent, e.g. pollen, dust, animal dander, that causes IgE-mediated hypersensitivity reactions.
Allergy. Originally defined as altered reactivity on second contact with antigen; now usually refers to a Type I hypersensitivity reaction.
Allotype. The protein of an allele which may be detectable as an antigen by another member of the same species.
Alternative pathway. The activation pathways of the complement system involving C3 and factors B, D, P, H and I, which interact in the vicinity of an activator surface to form an alternative pathway C3 convertase.
Amplification loop. The alternative complement activation pathway, which acts as a positive feedback loop when C3 is split in the presence of an activator surface.
Anaphylatoxins. Complement peptides (C3a and C5a) which cause mast cell degranulation and smooth muscle contraction.
Anaphylaxis. An antigen-specific immune reaction mediated primarily by IgE which results in vasodilation and constriction of smooth muscle, including those of the bronchus, and which may result in death.
Anchor residues. Certain amino acid residues of antigenic peptides are required for interaction with sites in the binding pocket of MHC molecules.
Anergy. Failure to make an immune response following stimulation with a potential antigen.
Antagonist peptides. Analogues of antigenic peptides which bind to MHC molecules and prevent stimulation of specific clones of T cells.
Antibody. A molecule produced by animals in response to antigen which has the particular property of combining specifically with the antigen which induced its formation.
Antigen. A molecule which reacts with preformed antibody and the specific receptors on T and B cells.
Antigen receptors. The lymphocyte receptors for antigens including the T-cell receptor (TCR) and surface immunoglobulin on B cells which acts as the B cell's antigen receptor (BCR).
Antigenic determinants. See epitopes.
Antigenic peptides. Peptide fragments of proteins which bind to MHC molecules and induce T-cell activation.
Antigen presentation. The process by which certain cells in the body (antigen-presenting cells) express antigen on their cell surface in a form recognizable by lymphocytes.
Antigen processing. The conversion of an antigen into a form in which it can be recognized by lymphocytes.
Antiviral proteins. Proteins whose synthesis is induced by interferons. They become activated if the cell is infected by virus and limit viral replication.
APCs (antigen-presenting cells). A variety of cell types which carry antigen in a form that can stimulate lymphocytes.
Apoptosis. Programmed cell death, which involves nuclear fragmentation and condensation of cytoplasm, plasma membranes and organelles into apoptotic bodies.
ARAMs (antigen receptor activation motifs). Target amino acid sequences on the intracellular domains of CD79 and CD3, which may become phosphorylated when a lymphocyte is activated via its antigen receptor.
Arthus reaction. Inflammation seen in the skin some hours following injection of antigen. It is a manifestation of a type III hypersensitivity reaction.
Atopy. The clinical manifestation of Type I hypersensitivity reactions including eczema, asthma, rhinitis and food allergy.
Autocrine. This refers to the ability of a cytokine to act on the cell that produced it.
Autoimmunity. Immune recognition and reaction against the individual's own tissue.
Avidity. The functional combining strength of an antibody with its antigen which is related to both the affinity of the reaction between the epitopes and paratopes, and the valencies of the antibody and antigen.
β_2-microglobulin. A polypeptide which constitutes part of some membrane proteins including the Class I MHC molecules.
B7-1 (CD80) and B7-2 (CD86). Two molecules which are present on antigen-presenting cells. They ligate CD28 on T cells and act as powerful co-stimulatory signals.
B cells. Lymphocytes which develop in the bone marrow in adults and produce antibody. They can be subdivided into two groups, B1 and B2. B1 cells use minimally mutated receptors which are close to the germline

immunoglobulin sequences, whereas B2 cells are the major responding population in conventional immune responses to protein antigens.

B-cell–co-receptor complex. A group of cell surface molecules consisting of complement receptor type 2 (CD21), CD81 and CD19, which act as a co-stimulatory receptor on mature B cells.

B-cell–receptor complex (BCR). B-cell surface immunoglobulin and its associated signalling molecules, CD79a and CD79b.

Basophil. A population of polymorphonuclear leucocytes which stain with basic dyes and which have important roles in the control of inflammation.

BCG (Bacille Calmette Guérin). An attenuated strain of *Mycobacterium tuberculosis* used as a vaccine, an adjuvant or a biological response modifier in different circumstances.

Bcl-2. A molecule expressed transiently on activated B cells which have been rescued from apoptosis.

Biozzi mice. Lines of mice bidirectionally bred to produce low or high antibody responses to a variety of antigens (originally sheep erythrocytes).

Blood groups. Sets of allelically variable molecules expressed on red cells, and sometimes other tissues, which may be the target of transfusion reactions.

Bradykinin. A vasoactive nonapeptide which is the most important mediator generated by the kinin system.

Bursa of Fabricius. A lymphoepithelial organ found at the junction of the hind gut and cloaca in birds which is the site of B-cell maturation.

Bystander lysis. Complement-mediated lysis of cells in the immediate vicinity of a complement activation site, which are not themselves responsible for the activation.

C domains. The constant domains of antibody and the T-cell receptor. These domains do not contribute to the antigen-binding site and show relatively little variability between receptor molecules.

C genes. The gene segments which encode the constant portion of the immunoglobulin heavy and light chains and the α, β, γ and δ chains of the T-cell antigen receptor.

c-Kit (CD117). A receptor for stem cell factor, required for the early development of leucocytes.

C1–C9. The components of the complement classical and lytic pathways which are responsible for mediating inflammatory reactions, opsonization of particles and lysis of cell membranes.

C3 convertases. The enzyme complexes $C\overline{3b,3b}$ and $\overline{C4b2a}$ that cleave complement C3.

Capping. A process by which cell surface molecules are caused to aggregate (usually using antibody) on the cell membrane.

Carrier. An immunogenic molecule, or part of a molecule that is recognized by T cells in an antibody response.

Caspases. A group of enzymes which are particularly involved in the transduction of signals for apoptosis.

CD markers. Cell surface molecules of leucocytes and platelets that are distinguishable with monoclonal antibodies and may be used to differentiate different cell populations.

CDRs (complementary-determining regions). The sections of an antibody or T-cell receptor V region responsible for antigen or antigen–MHC binding.

Cell adhesion molecules (CAMs). A group of proteins of the immunoglobulin supergene family involved in intercellular adhesion, including ICAM-1, ICAM-2, ICAM-3, VCAM-1, MAdCAM-1 and PECAM.

Central tolerance. Tolerance of T cells or B cells induced during their development in the thymus or bone marrow.

Chemokines. A large group of cytokines, falling into four separate families. The main families are the CC group and the CXC group. They include IL-8, MCP-1, RANTES, MIP-1α, MIP-1β, IP-10 and many others. They act on 7 transmembrane pass receptors and have a variety of chemotactic and cell-activating properties, acting on selected populations of target cells.

Chemokinesis. Increased random migratory activity of cells.

Chemotaxis. Increased directional migration of cells particularly in response to concentration gradients of certain chemotactic factors.

Chimerism. The situation in which cells from genetically different individuals coexist in one body.

Class I/II/III MHC molecules. Three major classes of molecule are coded within the MHC. Class I molecules have one MHC-encoded peptide complexed with β_2-microglobulin, class II molecules have two MHC-encoded peptides which are non-covalently associated, and class III molecules are other molecules including complement components.

Class I/II restriction. The observation that immunologically active cells will only cooperate effectively when they share MHC haplotypes at either the class I or class II loci.

Classical pathway. The pathway by which antigen–antibody complexes can activate the complement system, involving components C1, C2 and C4, and generating a classical pathway C3 convertase.

Class switching. The process by which an individual B cell can link immunoglobulin heavy chain C genes to its recombined V gene to produce a different class of antibody with the same specificity. This process is also reflected in the overall class switch seen during the maturation of an immune response.

Clonal selection. The fundamental basis of lymphocyte activation in which antigen selectively causes activation, division and differentiation only in those cells which express receptors with which it can combine.

CMI (cell-mediated immunity). A term used to refer to immune reactions that are mediated by cells rather than by antibody or other humoral factors.

Collectins. A group of large polymeric proteins, including conglutinin and mannan-binding lectin (MBL), that can opsonize microbial pathogens.

Complement. A group of serum proteins involved in the control of inflammation, the activation of phagocytes and the lytic attack on cell membranes. The system can be activated by interaction with the antibodies of the immune system (classical pathway).

Complement control protein (CCP) domains (also called short consensus repeats). A domain structure

found in many proteins of the complement classical and alternative pathways and in some complement receptors and control proteins.
Complement receptors (CR1–CR4 and C1qR). A set of four cell surface receptors for fragments of complement C3. CR1 and CR2 have numerous CCP domains, while CR3 and CR4 are integrins. C1qR binds C1q.
ConA (concanavalin A). A mitogen for T cells.
Congenic. Animals which are genetically constructed to differ at one particular locus.
Conjugate. A reagent which is formed by covalently coupling two molecules together, such as fluorescein coupled to an immunoglobulin molecule.
Constant regions. The relatively invariant parts of immunoglobulin heavy and light chains, and the α, β, γ and δ chains of the T-cell receptor.
Contact hypersensitivity. A delayed inflammatory reaction on the skin seen in type IV hypersensitivity.
Co-stimulation. The signals required for the activation of a lymphocyte, in addition to the antigen-specific signal delivered via their antigen receptors. CD28 is an important co-stimulatory molecule for T cells and CD40 for B cells.
Cross reaction. The sharing of antigenic determinants by two different antigens.
CSFs (colony stimulating factors). A group of cytokines which control the differentiation of haemopoietic stem cells.
CTLA-4 (CD152). A downregulatory signalling molecule of T cells that competes with CD28 for ligation by B7 on antigen-presenting cells.
Cyclophosphamide. A cytotoxic drug frequently used as an immunosuppressive.
Cyclosporin. A T-cell suppressive drug that is particularly useful in suppression of graft rejection.
Cytokines. A generic term for soluble molecules which mediate interactions between cells.
Cytotoxic T cells. Cells which can kill virally infected targets expressing antigenic peptides presented by MHC class I molecules.
D genes. Sets of gene segments lying between the V and J genes in the immunoglobulin heavy chain genes, and in the T-cell receptor β and δ chain genes which are recombined with V and J genes during ontogeny.
Decay accelerating factor (DAF). A cell surface molecule on mammalian cells which limits activation and deposition of complement C3b.
Defensins. A group of small antibacterial proteins produced by neutrophils.
Degranulation. Exocytosis of granules from cells such as mast cells and basophils.
Dendritic cells. A set of cells present in tissues, which capture antigens and migrate to the lymph nodes and spleen, where they are particularly active in presenting the processed antigen to T cells. Dendritic cells can be derived from either the lymphoid or mononuclear phagocyte lineages.
DM molecules. Molecules related to MHC class II molecules, that are required for loading antigenic peptides onto class II molecules.
Domain. A region of a peptide having a coherent tertiary structure. Both immunoglobulins and MHC class I and II molecules have immunoglobulin supergene family domains.
Dominant idiotypes. Individual idiotypes which are present on a large proportion of the antibodies generated by a particular antigen.
DTH (delayed type hypersensitivity). This term includes the delayed skin reactions associated with Type IV hypersensitivity.
Education of T cells. The process by which developing thymocytes are selected for those that recognize peptides on self MHC molecules, but not for those that recognize self antigenic peptides.
Effector cells. A functional concept, which in context means those lymphocytes or phagocytes that produce an end effect.
Eicosanoids. Products of arachidonic acid metabolism including prostaglandins, leukotrienes and thromboxanes.
Endocytosis. Internalization of material by a cell, by phagocytosis or pinocytosis.
Endothelium. Cells lining blood vessels and lymphatics.
Endotoxin. Lipolysaccharide produced by Gram-negative bacteria, which activates B cells and macrophages.
Enhancement. Prolongation of graft survival by treatment with antibodies directed towards the graft alloantigens.
Eosinophils. A population of polymorphonuclear granulocytes which stain with acidic dyes and which are particularly involved in reactions against parasitic worms and in some hypersensitivity reactions.
Epithelioid cells. A population of activated mononuclear phagocytes, present in granulomatous reactions.
Epitopes. The parts of an antigen which contact the antigen-binding sites of an antibody or the T-cell receptor.
Epstein–Barr virus (EBV). Causal agent of Burkitt's lymphoma and infectious mononucleosis, which has the ability to transform human B cells into stable cell lines.
Exon. Gene segment encoding protein.
Fab. The part of an antibody molecule which contains the antigen-combining site, consisting of a light chain and part of the heavy chain; it is produced by enzymatic digestion.
Factors B, P, D, H and I. Components of the alternative complement pathway.
Fas (CD95) A molecule expressed on a variety of cells, which acts as a target for ligation by FasL on the surface of cytotoxic lymphocytes.
Fc. The portion of an antibody that is responsible for binding to antibody receptors on cells and the C1q component of complement.
Fc receptors. Surface molecules on a variety of cells that bind to the Fc regions of immunoglobulins. They are antibody class specific and isotype selective.
Flow cytometry. Analysis of cell populations in suspension according to each individual cell's expression of selected surface markers.

Fluorescence activated cell sorter (FACS). A machine that analyses cells by flow cytometry and then allows them to be sorted into different populations and collected separately.
Follicular dendritic cells (FDCs). Antigen-presenting cells present in the B-cell areas of lymphoid tissues which retain stores of antigen.
Formyl-methionyl peptides. Prokaryotes initiate protein synthesis with f-Met. Peptides such as f-Met-Leu-Phe are highly chemotactic for mononuclear phagocytes and neutrophils.
Framework segments (FR). Sections of antibody V regions which lie between the hypervariable regions.
Freund's adjuvant. An emulsion of aqueous antigen in oil. Complete Freund's adjuvant contains killed *Mycobacterium tuberculosis,* while incomplete Freund's adjuvant does not.
Frustrated phagocytosis. A term to describe the events which occur when a phagocyte attempts to internalize an antigen or antigenic particle, but is unable to do so, e.g. because of its size.
γδ **T cells.** The minor subset of T cells which express the γδ form of the T-cell receptor.
GALT (gut-associated lymphoid tissue). Refers to the accumulations of lymphoid tissue associated with the gastrointestinal tract.
Genetic association. A term used to describe the condition where particular genotypes are associated with other phenomena, such as particular diseases.
Genetic restriction. The term used to describe the observation that lymphocytes and antigen-presenting cells cooperate most effectively when they share particular MHC haplotypes.
Genome. The total genetic material contained within the cell.
Genotype. The genetic material inherited from parents; not all of it is necessarily expressed in the individual.
Germ line. The genetic material which is passed down through the gametes before it is modified by somatic recombination or maturation.
Germinal centres. Areas of secondary lymphoid tissue in which B-cell differentiation and antibody class-switching occurs.
Giant cells. Large multinucleated cells sometimes seen in granulomatous reactions and thought to result from the fusion of macrophages.
Granulocytes. Neutrophils, eosinophils and basophils.
Granulomatous reactions. Chronic inflammatory reactions (often a manifestation of type IV hypersensitivity) caused by a failure to clear antigen.
Granzymes. Granule-associated enzymes of cytotoxic T cells and large granular lymphocytes.
GVH (graft versus host) disease. A condition caused by allogeneic donor lymphocytes reacting against host tissue in an immunologically compromised recipient.
H–2. The mouse major histocompatibility complex.
Haemagglutination. Clumping of erythrocytes, caused by antibody. This forms the basis of a number of immunoassays and blood group typing.
Haplotype. A set of genetic determinants located on a single chromosome.
Hapten. A small molecule which can act as an epitope but is incapable by itself of eliciting an antibody response.
Helper (TH) cells. A functional subclass of T cells which can help to generate cytotoxic T cells and cooperate with B cells in the production of antibody responses. Helper cells recognize antigen in association with class II MHC molecules.
Heterologous. Refers to interspecies antigenic differences.
HEV (high endothelial venule). An area of venule from which lymphocytes migrate into lymph nodes.
Hinge. The portion of an immunoglobulin heavy chain between the Fc and Fab regions which permits flexibility within the molecule and allows the two combining sites to operate independently. The hinge region is usually encoded by a separate exon.
Histamine. A major vasoactive amine released from mast cell and basophil granules.
Histocompatibility. The ability to accept grafts between individuals.
HIV (human immunodeficiency virus). The causative agent of acquired immune deficiency syndrome (AIDS).
HLA. The human major histocompatibility complex.
hnRNA (heteronuclear RNA). The fraction of nuclear RNA which contains primary transcripts of the DNA prior to processing to form messenger RNA.
Homologous restriction factors. Complement components that restrict the action of the membrane attack complex on cells of the host.
Humoral. Pertaining to the extracellular fluids, including the serum and lymph.
Hybridoma. Cell line created *in vitro* by fusing two different cell types, usually lymphocytes, one of which is a tumour cell.
5-Hydroxytryptamine. A vasoactive amine present in platelets and a major mediator of inflammation in rodents.
Hypersensitivity. An inordinately strong immune response, which causes more damage than the antigen or pathogen which induced the response.
Hypervariable region. The most variable areas (3) of the V domains of immunoglobulin and T-cell receptor chains. These regions are clustered at the distal portion of the V domain and contribute to the antigen-binding site.
ICAM-1 (CD54), ICAM-2 (CD102) and ICAM-3 (CD50) (intercellular adhesion molecules). Cell surface molecules found on a variety of leucocytes and non-haematogenous cells which interact with LFA-1.
Iccosomes. Immune complexes in the form of small inclusion bodies found in follicular dendritic cells.
Idiotope. A single antigenic determinant on an antibody V region.
Idiotype. The antigenic characteristic of the V region of an antibody.
IELs (intraepithelial lymphocytes). A population of lymphocytes defined according to location, in which γδ T cells are strongly represented.
Immune-complex. The product of an antigen–antibody reaction which may also contain components of the complement system.

Immune response (Ir) genes. Genes that affect the level of immune responses. MHC class II genes are very important in controlling responses to specific antigens.
Immunoblotting (Western blotting). A technique for identifying and characterizing proteins using antibodies.
Immunofluorescence. A technique used to identify particular antigens microscopically in tissues or on cells by the binding of a fluorescent antibody conjugate.
Immunogenic. Having the ability to evoke B- and/or T-cell mediated immune reactions.
Immunoglobulins. The serum antibodies, including IgG, IgM, IgA, IgE and IgD.
Immunoglobulin supergene family (IgSF). Molecules which have domains homologous to those seen in immunoglobulins, including MHC class I and II molecules, the T-cell receptor, CD2, CD3, CD4, CD8, ICAMs, VCAM and some of the Fc receptors.
Induced fit. A description of the way in which an antigen can alter the normal tertiary structure of the binding site on a receptor following binding, by displacing amino acids.
Inflammation. A series of reactions, which bring cells and molecules of the immune system to sites of infection or damage. This appears as an increase in blood supply, increased vascular permeability and increased transendothelial migration of leucocytes.
Integrins. A large family of cell surface adhesion molecules, some of which interact with CAMs, others with complement fragments, and others with components of the extracellular matrix.
Interferons (IFNs). A group of molecules involved in signalling between cells of the immune system, and in protection against viral infections.
Interleukins (IL-1–IL-22). A group of molecules involved in signalling between cells of the immune system.
Intron. Gene segment between exons, not encoding protein.
Ir gene. A group of immune response (Ir) genes determining the level of an immune response to a particular antigen or foreign stimulus. A number of them are found in the major histocompatibility complex.
Isotype. Refers to genetic variation within a family of proteins or peptides such that every member of the species will have each isotype of the family represented in its genome (e.g. immunoglobulin classes).
ITAMs and ITIMs. Immunoreceptor activation motifs and immunoreceptor inhibitory motifs respectively. These are target sequences for phosphorylation by kinases involved in cell activation or inhibition.
JAKs (Janus kinases). These are a group of enzymes with two catalytic domains. They activate by cross-phosphorylation and are particularly involved in signalling from types I and II cytokine receptors.
J chain. A monomorphic polypeptide present in polymeric IgA and IgM, and essential to their formation.
J genes. Sets of gene segments in the immunoglobulin heavy and light chain genes, and in the genes for the chains of the T-cell receptor, which are recombined during lymphocyte ontogeny and contribute towards the genes for variable domains.
K cells. A group of lymphocytes which are able to destroy their target by antibody-dependent cell-mediated cytotoxicity. They have Fc receptors.
κ (kappa) chains. One of the immunoglobulin light chain isotypes.
Karyotype. The chromosomal constitution of a cell which may vary between individuals of a single species, depending on the presence or absence of particular sex chromosomes or on the incidence of translocations between sections of different chromosomes.
Killer inhibitory receptors (KIRs). Receptors on natural killer cells, belonging to the Ig superfamily or the C-type lectin family, which when ligated by MHC molecules, inhibit cytotoxicity.
Kinins. A group of vasoactive mediators produced following tissue injury.
Knockout. An animal whose endogenous gene for a particular protein has been deleted or mutated to be non-functional.
Kupffer cells. Phagocytic cells which line the liver sinusoids.
λ (lambda) chains. One of the immunoglobulin light chain isotypes.
Langerhans' cells. Antigen-presenting cells of the skin which emigrate to local lymph nodes to become dendritic cells; they are very active in presenting antigen to T cells.
Large granular lymphocytes (LGLs). A group of morphologically defined lymphocytes containing the majority of K-cell and NK-cell activity. They have both lymphocyte and monocyte/macrophage markers.
Lectin pathway. A pathway of complement activation, initiated by mannan-binding lectin (MBL), which intersects the classical pathway.
Leukotrienes. A collection of metabolites of arachidonic acid which have powerful pharmacological effects.
LFAs (leucocyte functional antigens). A group of three molecules which mediate intercellular adhesion between leucocytes and other cells in an antigen non-specific fashion. LFA-1 is CD11a/CD18, LFA-2 is CD2 and LFA-3 is CD58.
Ligand. A linking (or binding) molecule.
Line. A collection of cells produced by continuously growing a particular cell culture *in vitro*. Such a cell line will usually contain a number of individual clones.
Linkage. The condition where two genes are both present in close proximity on a single chromosome and are usually inherited together.
Linkage disequilibrium. A condition where two genes are found together in a population at a greater frequency than that predicted simply by the product of their individual gene frequencies.
LPS (lipopolysaccharide). A product of some Gram-negative bacterial cell walls which can act as a B-cell mitogen.
Lymphokines. A generic term for molecules other than antibodies which are involved in signalling between cells of the immune system and are produced by lymphocytes (cf. interleukins).
Lymphokine activated killer cells (LAKs). Cytotoxic cells generated *ex vivo*, by stimulation with IL-2, and possibly other cytokines.

Ly antigens. A group of cell surface markers found on murine T cells which relate to the differentiation of T-cell subpopulations. Many are now assigned to the CD system.
Lysosomes. Intracellular vesicles containing stored enzymes/adhesion molecules/toxic molecules depending on the cell type.
Lytic pathway. The complement pathway effected by components C5–C9 that is responsible for lysis of sensitized cell plasma membranes.
MALT (mucosa-associated lymphoid tissue). Generic term for lymphoid tissue associated with the gastrointestinal tract, bronchial tree and other mucosa.
MAP kinases. A group of intracellular enzymes involved in signalling cascades which lead to the activation of transcription factors.
Marginal zone. An area surrounding the splenic white pulp which separates the lymphoid areas from the surrounding red pulp.
Mast cells. Cells found distributed near blood vessels in most tissues. These cells are full of granules containing inflammatory mediators.
MCPs (macrophage chemotactic proteins). A group of chemokines.
Membrane attack complex (MAC). The assembled terminal complement components C5b–C9 of the lytic pathway which becomes inserted into cell membranes.
Memory cells. Long-lived lymphocytes which have already been primed with their antigen, but have not undergone terminal differentiation into effector cells. They react more readily than naïve lymphocytes when restimulated with the same antigen.
MHC (major histocompatibility complex). A genetic region found in all mammals whose products are primarily responsible for the rapid rejection of grafts between individuals, and function in signalling between lymphocytes and cells expressing antigen.
Microglia. Mononuclear phagocytes resident in the brain and spinal cord. Microglial precursors colonize the human CNS early in gestation.
MHC restriction. A characteristic of many immune reactions in which cells cooperate most effectively with other cells that share an MHC haplotype.
MIF (migration inhibition factor). A group of peptides produced by lymphocytes which are capable of inhibiting macrophage migration.
MIIC compartment. An endosomal compartment where MHC class II molecules are loaded with antigenic peptides.
MIPs (macrophage inflammatory proteins). A group of chemokines.
Mitogens. Substances which cause cells, particularly lymphocytes, to undergo cell division.
MLR/MLC (mixed lymphocyte reaction/mixed lymphocyte culture). Assay system for T-cell recognition of allogenic cells in which response is measured by proliferation in the presence of the stimulating cells.
Mononuclear phagocyte system. The lineage of fixed and mobile long-lived phagocytic cells, related to blood monocytes and tissue macrophages.
Myeloid cells. The lineages of bone marrow-derived phagocytes, including neutrophils, eosinophils and monocytes.
Myeloma. A lymphoma produced from cells of the B-cell lineage which can invade bone.
N regions. Gene segments present in recombined antigen receptor genes which are not present in the germline DNA.
Neoplasm. A synonym for cancerous tissue.
Neutrophils. Polymorphonuclear granulocytes, which form the major population of blood leucocytes.
NFκB. A transcription factor which is widely used by different leucocyte populations to signal activation – sometimes called the master-switch of the immune system.
NK (natural killer) cells. A group of lymphocytes which have the intrinsic ability to recognize and destroy some virally infected cells and some tumour cells.
Nude mouse. A genetically athymic mouse which lacks a transcription factor which is also required for hair production.
Opsonization. A process by which phagocytosis is facilitated by the deposition of opsonins (e.g. antibody and C3b) on the antigen.
PAF (platelet activating factor). A factor released by basophils which causes platelets to aggregate.
PALS (periarteriolar lymphatic sheath). The accumulations of lymphoid tissue constituting the white pulp of the spleen.
Paracrine. The action of a cytokine on a cell distinct from that which produced it.
Passenger cells. Donor leucocytes present in a tissue graft that may sensitize the recipient to the graft.
Patch test. Application of antigen to skin on a patch to test for type IV hypersensitivity reactions.
Pathogen. An organism which causes disease.
PC (phosphorylcholine). A commonly used hapten which is also found on the surface of a number of microorganisms.
PCA (passive cutaneous anaphylaxis). The technique used to detect antigen-specific IgE, in which the test animal is injected intravenously with the antigen and dye, the skin having previously been sensitized with IgE antibody.
Perforin. A granule-associated molecule of cytotoxic cells, homologous to complement C9. It can form pores on the membrane of a target cell.
Peyer's patches. Collections of lymphoid cells in the wall of the gut which form a secondary lymphoid tissue.
PFC (plaque forming cell). An antibody-producing cell detected *in vitro* by its ability to lyse antigen-sensitized erythrocytes in the presence of complement.
PHA (phytohaemagglutin). A mitogen for T cells.
Phagocytosis. The process by which cells engulf material and enclose it within a vacuole (phagosome) in the cytoplasm.
Phenotype. The expressed characteristics of an individual (cf. genotype).
Plasma cell. An antibody-producing B cell which has reached the end of its differentiation pathway.
Pokeweed mitogen. A mitogen for B and T cells.

Polymorphs. A common acronym for polymorphonuclear leucocytes, including basophils, neutrophils and eosinophils.
Prick test. Introduction of minute quantities of antigen into the skin, to test for type I hypersensitivity.
Primary lymphoid tissues. Lymphoid organs in which lymphocytes complete their initial maturation steps; they include the fetal liver, adult bone marrow and thymus, and bursa of Fabricius in birds.
Primary response. The immune response (cellular or humoral) following an initial encounter with a particular antigen.
Prime. To induce an initial sensitization to antigen.
Privileged tissues/sites. In the context of transplantation these are tissues which induce weak immune responses, or sites of the body which are partly shielded from graft rejection reactions.
Prostaglandins. Pharmacologically active derivatives of arachidonic acid. Different prostaglandins are capable of modulating cell mobility and immune responses.
Proteasomes. Organelles which degrade cellular proteins that have been tagged for breakdown by ubiquitination.
Protein A and Protein G. Components of the cell wall of some strains of staphylococcus, which bind to Fc of most IgG isotypes.
Pseudoalleles. Tandem variants of a gene: they do not occupy a homologous position on the chromosome (e.g. C4).
Pseudogenes. Genes which have homologous structures to other genes but which are incapable of being expressed, e.g. *Jk3* in the mouse.
Radioimmunoassay (RIA). A number of different, sensitive techniques for measuring antigen or antibody titres, using radiolabelled reagents.
RAG-1 and RAG-2. Recombination activating genes, required for recombination of V, D and J gene segments during generation of functional antigen receptor genes.
Reactive oxygen/nitrogen intermediates (ROIs/RNIs). Bactericidal metabolites produced by phagocytic cells, including hydrogen peroxide, hypohalites and nitric oxide.
Receptor. A cell surface molecule which binds specifically to particular extracellular molecules.
Recombination. A process by which genetic information is rearranged during meiosis. This process also occurs during the somatic rearrangements of DNA which occur in the formation of genes encoding antibody molecules and T-cell antigen receptors.
Recurrent idiotype. An idiotype present in the immune response of different animals or strains to a particular antigen.
Relative risk. A number which expresses how much more likely (>1) or less likely (<1) an individual is to develop a particular disease, if they possess a particular genotype.
Respiratory burst. Increase in oxidative metabolism of phagocytes following uptake of opsonized particles.
Reticuloendothelial system. A diffuse system of phagocytic cells derived from the bone marrow stem cells which are associated with the connective tissue framework of the liver, spleen, lymph nodes and other serous cavities. An old-fashioned term, rarely used, mononuclear phagocyte system being preferred.
Rosetting. A technique for identifying or isolating cells by mixing them with particles or cells to which they bind (e.g. sheep erythrocytes to human T cells). The rosettes consist of a central cell surrounded by bound cells.
SCID (severe combined immunodeficiency). A group of genetic conditions leading to major deficiencies or absence of both B cells and T cells.
Secondary response. The immune response which follows a second or subsequent encounter with a particular antigen.
Secretory component. A polypeptide produced by cells of some secretory epithelia which is involved in transporting secreted polymeric IgA across the cell and protecting it from digestion in the gastrointestinal tract.
Selectins. Three adhesion molecules, P-selectin (CD62P), E-selectin (CD62E) and L-selectin (CD62L), involved in slowing leucocytes during their transit through venules.
Serotonin. 5-Hydroxytryptamine
SLE (systemic lupus erythematosus). An autoimmune disease (non-organ specific) of humans usually involving anti-nuclear antibodies.
Spleen. A major secondary lymphoid organ lying in the peritoneal cavity next to the stomach.
Somatic mutation. A process occurring during B-cell maturation and affecting the antibody gene region, which permits refinement of antibody specificity.
STATs. A group of proteins which form components of transcription factors following activation by kinases.
Stem cell factor (SCF). Also called Steel factor. A cytokine required for the earliest stages of leucocyte development in bone marrow.
Superantigens. Antigens which stimulate clones of T cells which have different antigen specificity, but which use the same TCR V genes.
Suppressor (Ts) cell. Functionally defined populations of T cells which reduce the immune responses of other T cells or B cells, or switch the response into a different pathway to that under investigation.
Surface plasmon resonance. A biophysical phenomenon, which can be used to measure the association and binding constants of proteins in solution interacting with bound ligands.
Synergism. Cooperative interaction.
Syngeneic. Strains of animals produced by repeated inbreeding so that each pair of autosomes within an individual is identical.
T cells. Lymphocytes that differentiate primarily in the thymus and are central to the control and development of immune responses. The principal subgroups are cytotoxic T cells (TC) and T-helper cells (TH0, TH1 and TH2).
T15. An idiotype associated with anti-phosphorylcholine antibodies, named after the TEPC15 myeloma prototype sequence.
TAP transporters. A group of molecules which transport proteins and peptides between intracellular compartments.
T-cell receptor (TCR). The T-cell antigen receptor

consisting of either an $\alpha\beta$ dimer (TCR-2) or a $\gamma\delta$ dimer (TCR-1) associated with the CD3 molecular complex.
T-dependent/T-independent antigens. T-dependent antigens require immune recognition by both T and B cells to produce an immune response. T-independent antigens can directly stimulate B cells to produce specific antibody.
Thoracic duct. The thoracic ducts drain efferent lymph into the venous system.
Thromboxanes. Products of arachidonic acid metabolism, some of which are involved in inflammation.
Thymus. A primary lymphoid organ lying in the thoracic cavity over the heart.
Tissue typing. Determination of an individual's allotypic variants of MHC molecules.
TNF (tumour necrosis factor). A cytokine released by activated macrophages that is structurally related to lymphotoxin released by activated T cells.
Tolerance. A state of specific immunological unresponsiveness.
Toll receptors. A group of evolutionarily ancient cell surface molecules (e.g. the IL-1 receptor), some of which are involved in transducing signals for inflammation.
Tonsils. Paired lymphoid organs situated in the throat which form part of the MALT.
Transformation. Morphological changes in a lymphocyte associated with the onset of division. Also used to denote the change to the autonomously dividing state of a cancer cell.
Transforming growth factors (TGFs). A group of cytokines identified by their ability to promote fibroblast growth, that are also generally immunosuppressive.
Transgenic animal. An animal in which one or more new genes have been incorporated. These are often placed under specific promotors so that they are only expressed in particular tissues for limited periods.
Tumour necrosis factors (TNFs). A group of proinflammatory cytokines encoded within the MHC.
V domains. The N-terminal domains of antibody heavy and light chains and the α, β, γ and δ chains of the T-cell receptor, and which become recombined with appropriate sets of D and J genes during lymphocyte ontogeny.
Vaccination. A general term for immunization against infectious disease, orginally derived from immunization against smallpox which uses the Vaccinia virus.
Vasoactive amines. Products such as histamine and 5-hydroxytryptamine released by basophils, mast cells and platelets which act on the endothelium and smooth muscle of the local vasculature.
Veiled cells. Cells of the dendritic cell lineage as seen in afferent lymph. They may be derived from Langerhans' cells or other dendritic cell types.
Very late antigens (VLA-1–VLA-6). The set of integrins which share a common $\beta 1$ chain (CD29).
Waldeyer's ring. The secondary lymphoid tissues of the nasopharynx, which include the tonsils and adenoids.
Western blotting. Synonymous with immunoblotting – see immunoblotting.
White pulp. The lymphoid component of spleen, consisting of periarteriolar sheaths of lymphocytes and antigen-presenting cells.
Xenogeneic. Referring to interspecies antigenic differences.

Explanations

1. SPECIFICITY AND MEMORY IN IMMUNE RESPONSES

1.1 The immunological 'memory' induced by vaccination does not depend just on the antibodies. Memory is due to long-lived memory lymphocytes, which persist in the lymphoid tissues for many years. They will be re-activated if the individual encounters the toxin or the vaccine on a later occasion.

1.2 The tetanus toxoid is a stable molecule – it does not change or mutate, so antibodies and lymphocytes which recognize it continue to be effective. By contrast, influenza-A mutates every year. Last year's antibodies may be marginally effective or ineffective against this year's virus. Researchers must identify newly emerging virus strains and prepare vaccine from those strains which they think will produce new epidemics. Often they get it right, but not always.

1.3 This is a question of practicality. It is impossible to prepare sufficient vaccine each year to immunize everyone against influenza. There is not enough time to do it and not enough laboratory resources available. So the highest risk groups are targetted – health workers because they will likely be in contact with the disease and old people because the disease can lead to serious complications.

2. DEVELOPMENT OF THE IMMUNE SYSTEM

2.1 The total numbers of blood lymphocytes are drastically reduced, with T cells being virtually absent and B cells significantly reduced – B cells require T cells to complete their own development. The lymph nodes are much reduced in size and this particularly affects the paracortex (T-cell areas). Compare this with diGeorge syndrome. The animals have a reduced ability to fight infections, but this is selective, affecting particularly some viruses and parasites – possibly because there is still good NK cell activity, and macrophage-mediated anti-bacterial defences.

2.2 Adult thymectomy has very little effect on the individual's ability to fight infection. By this stage of life, there is a large pool of peripheral T cells which may to some extent self renew. The thymus progressively involutes and becomes less important as a site of T-cell development in the adult.

2.3 As the lymphocyte precursors fail to make productive rearrangements of their antigen receptor genes, they die by apoptosis during development. This leads to a profound immune deficiency of all lymphocytes, which is analagous to severe combined immunodeficiency (SCID) in man.

2.4 Interleukin-7 is required for lymphocyte development in primary lymphoid organs. There is a profound reduction in thymocytes and peripheral lymphocytes and a total absence of gd T cells.

2.5 The $\alpha_4\beta_7$-integrin is required for binding of cells to adhesion molecules on the HEV of gut-associated lymphoid tissue (GALT), so this knockout results in drastically reduced lymphocyte numbers in these tissues.

3. A COMPLEMENT DEFICIENCY

3.1 Deficiencies of components of the classical or alternative pathways, particularly of C3, produce a reduced ability to opsonize bacteria, resulting in impaired phagocytosis by macrophages and neutrophils. Patients suffer from repeated bacterial infections from Gram-positive bacteria – staphylococci, streptococci, etc. These children are unable to clear bacterial infections because their phagocytes do not take up bacteria efficiently. (Deficiencies in the lytic pathway components (C5–C9) can render patients more susceptible to neisserial infections because the lytic pathway can damage the outer membrane of Gram-negative bacteria such as Neisseria.)

3.2 There is a clear deficiency in C3 and components of the alternative pathway. Components of the classical pathway are on the lower end of normal. At first this looks surprising, because the initial assay for lytic complement required the activity of the classical and lytic pathways. However the bacterial infections and the lack of total haemolytic complement can both be explained by the very low levels of C3. Note that the genes for C3, factor B, factor I and factor H are not genetically linked, so this apparent multiple deficiency of alternative pathway components cannot be explained by some multiple gene deletion. The explanation lies in the alternative pathway amplification loop. Because the children lack factor I, they cannot break down the alternative pathway C3 convertase $\overline{C3bBb}$. Thus C3 is continuously activated and binds both factor B and factor H. All the factor B is consumed, most of the free C3 and factor H is consumed. Hence the genetic deficiency of factor I leads to secondary deficiencies in the components of the alternative pathway and this then affects C3 and the function of the classical and lytic pathways.

3.3 The children have a homozygous factor I deficiency – both copies of the gene are missing. Replacing factor I, either by an infusion of normal serum, or by providing pure factor I restores all the other components to normal levels and allows the children to clear bacterial infections.

4. THE SPECIFICITY OF ANTIBODIES

4.1 In the presence of the antibodies mutated variants of the virus are selected which do not bind those antibodies. By detecting which of the virus proteins are mutated, one can infer that these are the proteins which normally would bind to the antibody. Neutralizing antibodies against viruses are generally directed against proteins in the capsid of the virus, particularly against the proteins which the virus uses to attach to the surface of its target cell. Antibodies cannot gain access to the inside of the virus, so neutralizing antibodies do not bind the core protein VP4.

4.2 The antibody VP1-a binds to an epitope which includes two closely spaced residues (91 and 95). This is a 'continuous epitope' and is located on a single external loop of polypeptide. By contrast, the epitope recognized by VP1-b is located in at least two distinct areas of the polypeptide chain (83–85 and 138–139). This is a 'discontinuous epitope': examination of the VP1 antigen shows that these residues are located on two adjacent areas of beta-pleated sheet.

4.3 A mutation of residue 138 does not affect the epitope recognized by antibody VP1-a, so it continues to bind with high affinity to the antigen. This confirms that the epitopes recognized by VP1-a and VP1-b are physically separate. The mutant with Gly at position 95 still binds the VP1-a antibody weakly. Glycine is a smaller amino acid than aspartate, which is present in the wild type, hence the antibody can still bind to the epitope, although the 'fit' is less good, so the affinity of binding is lower. By contrast, Lysine (Lys) is a larger residue than Aspartate. It protrudes further out into the antibody's binding site and completely disrupts the antigen–antibody bond.

5. THE SPECIFICITY OF T CELLS

5.1 This is an example of genetic restriction in antigen presentation. The SM/J T cells are primed with antigen on MHC molecules of the SM/J haplotype and will only respond to this combination of antigen–MHC. They do not recognize the same antigen presented by other MHC molecules. Because MHC molecules are co-dominantly expressed, the H–2^v MHC molecules are present on the APCs from the F1 animal and so they too stimulate the T cells.

5.2 The minimum peptide needed to activate the T cells appears to be 80–94, which is 15 residues long and therefore corresponds well to the expected size of antigen peptides which can fit into the MHC class II binding site. This peptide is included within peptide 80–102, which also stimulates strongly. Peptides 84–98 and 73–88 lack the N- and C-termini of the antigenic peptide respectively, and therefore lack some of the anchor residues need to hold them in the MHC peptide binding groove.

5.3 This is called a superagonist or a strong agonist peptide. Typically such a peptide will have a stronger binding affinity for the MHC molecule and/or the TCR.

6. ANTIGEN PROCESSING AND PRESENTATION

6.1 Macrophages express both MHC class I and class II molecules, and can therefore present antigen to either of the clones. Fibroblasts do not generally express class II molecules and one would not expect them to stimulate the class II-restricted clone.

6.2 Live flu virus infects the macrophages and flu virus polypeptides are synthesized in the cytoplasm of the cell. So the viral antigens are presented by the internal (class I) pathway as well as the external (class II) pathway. Inactivated virus is taken up by the macrophage, processed and presented via the class II pathway only – as there is no viral protein synthesis there is no presentation via the class I pathway.

6.3 Emetine blocks protein synthesis, so no protein fragments are fed into the class I pathway by the proteasomes. Chloroquine prevents phagosome/lysosome fusion so that endocytosed virus cannot be broken down into peptides. Consequently no peptides are available for the class II pathway.

6.4 The class I-restricted T cells express CD8 and the class II-restricted cells CD4, because CD8 and CD4 are co-receptors for class I and class II respectively.

7. CYTOKINE PRODUCTION

7.1 Some of the variability may be due to functional polymorphisms of cytokine genes, not only in the TNF and IL-6 genes but possibly in genes of other cytokines that may induce TNF and IL-6. Cytokine production can also be influenced by medication, or underlying disease, but genetic variability is the most likely cause.

7.2 There appears to be a correlation between TNF and IL-6 production in most cases. This could mean that TNF induces IL-6 or vice versa, or they may be co-induced independently.

7.3 As only TNF is found after 2 hours' culture, this suggests that TNF induces IL-6. It is possible to test this hypothesis by including antibody to TNF in the culture medium to determine if blocking TNF production causes a consequent block in IL-6 production.

8. DEVELOPMENT OF THE ANTIBODY RESPONSE

8.1 In a developing immune response to a T-dependent antigen, B cells will switch from IgM production to IgG. Because the antigen is continuously present as a depot, by day 14 the response has the characteristics of a secondary response – IgG antibody titres are climbing rapidly.

8.2 Perhaps the two mice have already been infected by mouse hepatitis virus. By day 5 they are already making a secondary IgG response. This could be a problem in the colony, although usually all animals housed together would become infected. If these mice have been naturally infected it would be through the gut (unlike the vaccine) and one would therefore expect a stronger IgA response.

8.3 IgA-producing clones tend to be located in the mucosa-associated lymphoid tissues, and it is not surprising that no IgA-producing clones were generated from the spleen.

8.4 IgG-producing clones at day 14 are likely to be of higher affinity than IgM producers.

9. MONONUCLEAR PHAGOCYTES IN IMMUNE DEFENCE

Problem 1

9.1 TNFα, IL-1, IL-6, IL-10.

9.2 Lack of activity, ruffling of fur, respiratory distress, possibly leading to death within 24 hours.

9.3 BCG activates macrophages via infection of antigen-presenting cells (APC) and induction of IFNγ by NK and CD4 T cells, which primes macrophages. LPS delivers stimulus via LPS binding protein, CD14, Toll-like receptor and NFκB activation, to enhance pro-inflammatory cytokine release. TNFα and IL-1, especially, act locally and systemically on vascular endothelium, neutrophils and central nervous centres, causing hypotension and circulatory collapse.

9.4 CD14 knockout mice are extremely resistant to septic shock. SR-A knockout mice are more susceptible to septic shock. IFNγ knockout mice are relatively resistant to septic shock.

9.5 CD14 is central to the LPS recognition and signalling pathway. SR-A clears LPS from circulation to protect host. IFNγ is needed to prime macrophages.

9.6 Evaluate the kinetics of pro- and anti-inflammatory cytokine production to establish endogenous regulation of macrophage activation.
Use blocking antibodies for TNFα and other cytokines, and receptor knockout mice to establish the roles of each. Evaluate cytokine production by peritoneal macrophages taken from BCG-primed mice after LPS challenge *in vitro*.

9.7 Septic shock is a major complication of Gram-negative (e.g. *Neisseria meningitidis*) infection. Therapeutic approaches include circulatory support, antibiotics and possibly combinations of cytokine and receptor antagonists (blocking antibodies, inhibitors of TNFα cleavage, soluble receptors).

For further reading see:

Haworth R, Platt N, Keshav S, *et al.* The macrophage scavenger receptor type A (SR-A) is expressed by activated macrophages and protects the host against lethal endotoxic shock. *J Exp Med* 1997;**186**:1431–9.

Haziot A, Ferrero E, Kontgen F, *et al.* Resistance to endotoxin shock and reduced dissemination of gram-negative bacteria in CD14 deficient mice. *Immunity* 1998;**4**:407–14.

Problem 2

9.8 Use blocking antibodies for phagocytic receptors, e.g. vitronectin receptors, or cells from knockout mice, if available.

9.9 Ligation and cross-linking of phagocytic receptors by apoptotic cells induce signalling pathways resulting in the suppression of inflammatory and anti-microbial responses.

9.10 Use antibodies and antagonists to receptors to study candidate inhibitory responses such as production of prostaglandin E_2 and TGFβ.

9.11 Pathogens can exploit and induce the downregulation of inflammation by apoptotic cells to evade killing by host cells. This may be counteracted by use of drugs to prevent inhibitory pathways, even *in vivo*.

For further reading see:

Freire-de-Lima CG, Nascimento DO, Soares MBP, *et al.* Uptake of apoptotic cells drives the growth of a pathogenic trypanosome in macrophages. *Nature* 2000;**403**:199–203.

Stein M, Keshav S, Harris N, Gordon S. IL-4 potently enhances murine macrophage mannose receptor activity; a marker of alternative immunologic macrophage activation. *J Exp Med* 1992;**176**:287–92.

Problem 3

9.12 Macrophage activation involves a complex pattern of altered gene expression, covering a spectrum of activities and not just polar opposites between activation (TH1, IFNγ) and deactivation (TH2, IL-10). IL-4 and IL-13, TH2 cytokines, utilize common receptor chains to induce an alternate pathway of macrophage activation, involved in humoral immunity and possibly repair (enhanced APC function via MHC class II expression and MR, as well as other effects on B-cell production of antibody). IFNγ and IL-10 regulate cellular immune effector functions.

9.13 Broaden the range of macrophage markers examined, ultimately by DNA gene chip analysis, and look for consistency and reproducibility of similar patterns of altered gene expression by the cytokines above. Analyse macrophage functions in mice with knockouts of cytokines or their receptors.

9.14 Find model antigens, e.g. parasites, which induce TH2 responses *in vivo*, and establish whether these are recognized by APC receptors which enhance IL-4/IL-13 or inhibit IFNγ production by appropriate cells.

10. MECHANISMS OF CYTOTOXICITY

10.1 Cytotoxic T cells kill their targets using both granule-associated mechanisms such as perforin, and by activating pathways of apoptosis, hence they produce both cell lysis and DNA fragmentation. The Tc cells recognize allogeneic MHC class I molecules on the targets – the effectors and targets come from different individuals. Note that there is always a low level of cell damage in the controls which contain no effector cells.

10.2 Tumour cells typically show reduced expression of MHC molecules by comparison with normal cells, and as they do, they become susceptible to damage mediated by NK cells. Because NK cells recognize several different types of MHC molecule, the fact that the targets are allogeneic is not so relevant. Antibody can crosslink the NK cells to their targets (K cell activity) via their Fc receptor (CD16). This moves the balance of activity towards activation of the NK cell. Note that antibody itself does not damage the targets in this type of assay, because the culture medium does not contain functional complement.

10.3 Purified perforin is extremely efficient at causing cell lysis, but does not activate the pathways of apoptosis, so there is no DNA fragmentation.

11. IMMUNE RESPONSE MODULATION BY EXPERIMENTAL TREATMENT

11.1 Anti-IgD will bind to IgD which is expressed primarily on the surface of B cells. Therefore the anti-IgD–peptide conjugate is directed towards B cells, and the peptide is preferentially presented by the B cells to TH2 cells. The peptide-specific immune response is therefore deviated towards antibody production and the pathogenic TH1 response which occurs in EAE is inhibited.

11.2 At first sight, it appears that the anti-IL-4 inhibits the TH2 response and thus promotes a TH1 type of response with a protective IFNγ/macrophage response. However, it cannot be this simple, since administration of exogenous IFNγ does not produce a cure, and neutralizing it does not prevent a cure. Therefore the anti-IL-4 may be inhibiting some other facet of the TH2 response. This could be by preventing the accumulation of TH2 cells at the site of infection (IL-4 induces eotaxin), reducing the production of suppressive cytokines (e.g. IL-10), or allowing the development of additional TH1 cells. (The paper did not investigate the precise mechanism.)

11.3 The anti-TNP antibody binds to TNP on the antigen and to the Fc receptor on the surface of the anti-SRBC B cells; it thereby delivers an inhibitory signal to those B cells. In this case, antibody to one antigenic determinant (TNP) is able to inhibit the response to other determinants (SRBC) because the antigen (SRBC–TNP) effectively cross-links the B cells' antigen receptor and Fc receptor. $F(ab')_2$ of the anti-TNP cannot do this, because it lacks Fc and therefore cannot bind the Fc receptor.

12. TOLERANCE

Lineage commitment in thymocyte development

12.1 The presence of a constitutively active Lck molecule in developing thymocytes. This is revealed in the OT-1/dLGF experimental mouse.

12.2 The presence of a catalytically inactive Lck causes a massive reduction in the number of CD4 SP cells that are selected in the AND mouse. There is a limited increase in the number of CD8 SP cells.

12.3 Yes the results are consistent. Overexpression of Lck promotes CD4 cells and reduced expression of CD8 cells, regardless of the MHC restriction of the majority population of T-cell receptors.

The molecular basis of activation-induced cell death (AICD)

12.4 AICD is mediated by signalling through the Fas pathway.

12.5 Activation of T cells with anti-CD3 fails to induce apoptosis in mice bearing defective Fas and FasL genes.

12.6 Despite having a defective FasL, the gld mouse has a normal Fas gene and ligation of this with the anti-Fas antibody is sufficient to cause apoptosis.

12.7 This is an important way of controlling immune homeostasis. If cells were to keep on proliferating after antigen encounter the lymph nodes would explode!

12.8 This is a good question! The answer is not yet known and obviously requires a lot more critical thinking.

The role of regulatory T cells in peripheral tolerance

12.9 This is because autoreactive lymphocytes exist as part of the normal T-cell repertoire. $CD25^+$ cells clearly suppress these cells and prevent them from causing disease. Precisely how the $CD25^+$ cells work is not yet known.

12.10 It seems likely that these cells arise in the thymus. Comparison of groups A–D shows that $CD25^-$ thymocytes can cause disease and that their activity is normally regulated by $CD25^+$ thymocytes.

12.11 It looks like tissues such as the adrenal gland are relatively resistant to disease. This could be:
(a) Because the antigenic targets for autoimmune disease are more sequestered in these tissues.
(b) Because mechanisms that create immunologically privileged sites operate in these tissues to some extent.

13. THE EVOLUTION OF IMMUNITY

13.1 The following list comprises a 'top 10' of major areas that need to be addressed in comparative immunology. This list was compiled on the basis of issues raised in a volume dedicated to current research on ectothermic vertebrate immune systems (Flajnik MF *Immunol Rev* 1998; **166**:5–14), but might have been constructed from points mentioned in this chapter on 'Evolution of immunity'.

1. Determine the functions of novel Ig isotypes identified in cartilaginous and teleost fish.
2. Examine the reasons why most ectothermic vertebrates lack affinity maturation during an antibody

response, despite the presence of somatic mutation of Ig genes.
3. Further investigate the functional significance (e.g. prevention of autoimmunity) of the turnover of lymphocytes that occurs during amphibian metamorphosis.
4. Probe the structure and function of the cells and receptors that delineate NK phenomena in diverse vertebrates.
5. Determine whether sharks, which have a 'cluster-type' organization of Ig genes, display B-cell clonal restriction.
6. Understand the nature of adaptive and non-adaptive immunity to natural pathogens in diverse organisms (e.g. in farmed fish).
7. Continue the search for the origins of TCR/MHC/Ig.
8. Understand the functional significance of various complement components identified in invertebrate and vertebrate organisms.
9. Isolate additional cytokines and their receptors.
10. Identify at least one gene relevant to the study of adaptive immunity in hagfish and lampreys!

14. VIRUS–IMMUNE SYSTEM INTERACTIONS

14.1 Antigenic variation as seen for example in HIV and influenza virus. Evasion of antibody and T-cell recognition by mutation arising in genes encoding major antigenic targets.

Production of 'decoy' molecules that interfere with host immune defences, in particular molecules targeting the interferon system, downregulating MHC class I expression, subverting the function of cytokines and chemokines, and the action of complement.

Establishment of virus latency, thereby avoiding detection by immune system, e.g. HSV-1 in sensory ganglia, EBV in B lymphocytes.

14.2 **i.** Non-neutralizing antibodies could function by mediating antibody-dependent complement-mediated lysis of infected cells, complement-mediated neutralization, antibody-dependent cellular cytotoxicity (ADCC) or antibody-enhanced phagocytosis by macrophages.

ii. Experiments to support the conclusions could involve:

a. examination *in vitro* of whether complement mediates neutralization of virus in the presence of non-neutralizing antibodies;
b. use of mice deficient in late complement components, i.e. C5-deficient mice;
c. analysis of whether IgG subclasses were able to mediate ADCC *in vitro* using virus-infected cells.

15. IMMUNO-ENDOCRINE INTERACTIONS IN THE RESPONSE TO INFECTION

15.1 The immune system cannot be understood in isolation from the rest of mammalian physiology. One of the many effects of stress is increased production of adrenocorticotrophic hormone (ACTH) from the pituitary. This in turn drives increased production of cortisol by the adrenal. The proof is that in the animal models mentioned, the stressor can be replaced by mimicking the stress-induced levels of cortisol (or the rodent equivalent, corticosterone) with implanted slow-release cortisol pellets. The cortisol downregulates cell-mediated immunity to tuberculosis; why does it?

15.2 These observations provide clues as to why increased cortisol levels can lead to reduced immunity to tuberculosis. Raised cortisol levels cause antigen-presenting cells to release more IL-10 and less IL-12, so that newly recruited T cells tend to develop a TH2 cytokine profile. Moreover, cortisol actually synergizes with some functions of TH2 cytokines, and enhances the ability of IL-4 to drive IgE production. It is interesting that BCG vaccination does not lead to protective immunity if the BCG is given to animals bearing cortisol pellets that mimic stress levels of cortisol. Cortisol also reduces the antimycobacterial functions of macrophages.

These points emphasize the need for a physiological approach to the understanding of infection. A narrowly immunological approach has solved some of the easy infections but global emergencies such as tuberculosis and HIV may require integrated physiological thinking as well as pure immunology.

16. IMMUNITY TO PROTOZOA AND HELMINTHS

16.1 Protozoa replicate within the host, so there is usually a balance between the effectiveness of the immune response and the virulence of the parasite. With certain parasites the infections may be short lived and indeed may kill the host, but this may not be a disadvantage to the parasite if it has already been transmitted to a new host. A good example is falciparum malaria which is potentially fatal, particularly in children in endemic areas who have not developed any immunity but are likely to have been bitten during the course of the infection by mosquitos which will ensure further transmission.

Helminths, by contrast, do not replicate within the host and are generally long-lived chronic infections. Transmission is by the release of eggs/larvae from an adult parasite which may be excreted or be taken up by a vector.

16.2 By adopting an intracellular mode of existence parasites may be able to 'hide' from the immune response. A good example is falciparum malaria which lives in mature red blood cells. As this cell type has no nucleus it is not possible to express MHC class I molecules on the surface of the cell, so that the parasite is invisible to $CD8^+$ cytotoxic T cells. Other parasites live in nucleated cells which will express class I MHC but experiments have shown this to be downregulated in cells infected with some parasites.

T. gondii avoids being killed by the macrophage by inhibiting the fusion of the lysosome with the phagosome; *T. cruzi* escape from the phagosome into the cytoplasm of the cell, and *Leishmania* spp. can resist the low pH of the phagolysosomes and are resistant to lysosomal enzymes.

16.3 Extracellular parasites can adopt a number of ways of avoiding immune attack. Parasites may *disguise* themselves, for example, by undergoing antigenic variation (African trypanosomes) or by adsorbing host molecules or undergoing molecular mimicry of the host (schistosomes). Parasites may *hide* from the host immune response by becoming cysts (*Entamoeba*) or by living in an immunoprivileged location (*Toxoplasma* in brain). They may *resist* attack by having a physical barrier (helminths) or by producing enzymes that resist the oxidative burst or disable antibodies. Many parasites are able to *modulate* the host immune response to their advantage.

17. VACCINATION

17.1 Successful attenuation results in an organism still capable of generating an immune response against the wild-type virulent organism but no longer capable of causing disease. This is a delicate balance to achieve. In some instances (e.g. hepatitis B and C viruses) the organisms cannot be cultured so that attenuation by repeated *in vitro* passage is impossible.

17.2 There is no reason to believe that a vaccine cannot improve on nature. Many organisms express gene products that interfere with immune responses. Removal of these from the vaccine may allow protective responses to be generated.

17.3 Although smallpox was eliminated because there was no animal reservoir or carrier state, this is also the case for some other microorganisms and it should be possible to eliminate them. For other organisms, elimination will be very difficult and maintenance of herd immunity will remain important.

17.4 Vaccines are unlikely ever to replace antibiotics completely. Microorganisms evolve very rapidly and vaccine production against complex organisms, such as mycobacteria, has proved very difficult. In addition, immunodeficient individuals and the elderly remain at risk even after vaccination.

17.5 BCG clearly has multiple effects. Specific immune responses to BCG antigens can be detected but cell wall and other components of the bacterium have potent immunomodulatory effects. The efficacy of BCG as a vaccine has been suggested to depend on cross-reactions of BCG with environmental mycobacteria as well as *Mycobacterium tuberculosis* itself.

17.6 Strong immune responses may cause tissue damage in individuals with parasites already present. However, a vaccine that prevented establishment of infection would be unlikely to be damaging.

17.7 Antigens that induce T-cell immunity may be useful vaccine antigens. Molecules that contribute to virulence such as toxins, may be the best targets for vaccines. Because the genomes of many pathogens have been or are being sequenced, searching homologous gene products may identify potential targets.

18. THE HOST IMMUNE RESPONSE TO TUMOURS

18.1 Several factors contribute to the progressive growth of tumours in the face of an immune response. Because tumours may not generate 'danger signals' until many tumour cells are present and tissue damage occurs, the immune response is a late event and may be unable to deal with the large burden of tumour. Tumour cells are poor antigen-presenting cells as they lack co-stimuli and may lose MHC expression, probably by immunoselection. Finally the tumour is often a hostile environment for leucocytes, as tumours produce a number of immunosuppressive factors that prevent an effective immune response.

18.2 Immunotherapy has failed because understanding of immune mechanisms has been poor and tumour antigens ill defined. Cloning of many tumour antigens is providing defined targets for immunotherapeutic vaccines, and better understanding of the need for co-stimulation and for the prevention of immunosuppression will allow more rational design of effective vaccines.

18.3 The parallels between tumours and infectious disease are many. Successful parasites employ many of the strategies of tumours for evading immune responses. They may downregulate MHC molecules or mutate their antigens to avoid the host response and they produce immunosuppressive or immunomodulatory substances to interfere with damaging host effector mechanisms.

18.4 Although there are grounds for cautious optimism about immunotherapy, tumour cells carry a very large amount of genetic information that allows them to deploy many evasion strategies. Prophylactic vaccination prevents this occurring and is cheap and effective. As microorganisms are being shown to play a role in the aetiology of an increasing number of tumours, this may provide the opportunity to vaccinate against the development of these types of cancer.

19. HYPER IGM IMMUNODEFICIENCY

19.1 Normal infants do not become infected with *Pneumocystis carinii*. The occurrence of this type of pneumonia suggests the presence of an immunodeficiency disorder. His immunoglobulin levels point to an elevated IgM level whereas the IgG, IgA and IgE levels are very low. These findings almost certainly rule out the diagnosis of X-linked agammaglobulinaemia because in that case the IgM would be undetectable. The normal white blood cell count probably rules out severe combined immunodeficiency (SCID) because an infant with SCID would have a very low lymphocyte count

(<3000/mm^3). Had the IgD level been measured it would probably also be high as is found in males with hyper IgM immunodeficiency.

19.2 A blood sample should be obtained to isolate the B lymphocytes. In the hyper IgM immunodeficiency the B cells would stain only with fluorescent anti-IgM and anti-IgD. In a normal infant B cells that stain with anti-IgA and anti-IgG would also be present in addition to IgM+ and IgD+ cells. Furthermore, the mononuclear cells from the blood sample should be stimulated with phytohaemagglutinin. After several hours of stimulation, the cells should be stained with fluorescent anti-CD40 ligand. 50% of normal T cells would stain positively whereas none would be positive in hyper IgM immunodeficiency.

19.3 The baby should be given intravenous gamma globulin at regular monthly intervals to protect him against pyogenic infections. Intravenous gamma globulin is virtually pure IgG. As this child is incapable of making IgG he will need lifelong infusions for passive protection. Intravenous gamma globulin does not protect against intracellular microorganisms such as *P. carinii.* These and other microorganisms that reside in macrophages are eliminated by activating macrophages. Macrophages, like B cells, express CD40 and require interaction with the CD40 ligand on activated T cells to become highly microbicidal. This baby therefore remains susceptible to recurrent *P. carinii* infection despite the gamma globulin therapy. If it recurs he would need treatment again with pentamidine.

19.4 Antibodies formed to tetanus toxoid immunization are of the IgG class. Because this baby is incapable of undergoing isotype switching he cannot make IgG antibodies. However, antibodies to the blood group substances are predominantly of the IgM class, which this infant can synthesize. Furthermore the isohaemagglutinins are so called T-independent antibodies; their formation does not require T-cell help. Isotype switching to IgG, IgA or IgE requires that the CD40 ligand on activated T cells engages CD40 on B cells. This is a critical first step in providing T-cell help to antibody formation by B cells. This infant with a genetic defect in the CD40 ligand cannot effect isotype switching.

19.5 A normal result. The mother would exhibit random inactivation of her X-chromosomes. In X-linked agammaglobulinaemia non-random inactivation of B lymphocytes is observed in females who carry this X-linked disorder because the B cells that have the mutated btk gene cannot clonally expand; only the B cells carrying the normal allele can. The same is true in X-linked severe combined immunodeficiency (SCID). The T cells of heterozygous females which have a mutation in the common gamma chain cannot clonally expand; only the T cells with the normal allele can. The CD40 ligand is not required for clonal expansion of T cells. This molecule is only expressed when T cells are activated. Thus females who must be heterozygous for hyper IgM immunodeficiency are immunologically normal and the clonal expansion of T cells bearing the wild-type allele and the mutated allele is normal.

19.6 It depends on the severity of the mutation in the child. If he has a missense mutation and expresses some mutated CD40 ligand on his activated T cell the prognosis is good if he continues to receive intravenous gamma globulin. However, if his mutation results in an inability to express any CD40 ligand, his future is uncertain because these affected males usually develop an extensive polyclonal expansion of IgM-producing B cells that invade the liver and other parts of the gastrointestinal tract and cause fatal complications (*Fig. 19.4*). In this case a bone marrow transplant from a histoidentical donor should be recommended as this would have a favourable outcome and would essentially be a cure of the disease.

20. SECONDARY IMMUNODEFICIENCY

20.1 Approximately 95% of HIV-positive individuals seroconvert within 3 months of infection. ELISAs for antibodies to gp41, an HIV surface glycoprotein, and p24, a core protein, are the most widely used to detect HIV infection. Confirmation is obtained by Western blot analysis to decrease the rate of false positive results. The Centre for Disease Control recommends that the blot should be positive for 2 of the p24, gp41 and gp120/160 markers (gp160 is the precursor form of gp41 and gp120, the envelope protein). ELISAs for p24 antigen can also be used although the false negative rate is higher.

The polymerase chain reaction (PCR) is a technique for amplifying specific sequences of DNA or RNA to produce quantities that are readily detectable. The test in the context of HIV is highly sensitive and specific but is more costly than ELISA techniques.

20.2 The mother's serological state should be tested by ELISA and confirmed by Western blot if positive.

Around 20–30% of infants born to HIV-positive mothers are infected with the virus. Transmission can occur *in utero* or very rarely by breast feeding. Diagnosis presents a problem because maternal IgG specific for HIV antigens crosses the placenta and can be detected in the infant even if it has not become infected.

The presence of HIV-specific antibodies of IgA and IgM classes in the infant should imply infection because they do not cross the placenta. Current tests lack sensitivity and remain in development. The method most widely used in the UK and USA is PCR which demonstrates the virus directly. Below the age of 1 month PCR may be negative in infected children. It has been shown that, in many children, HIV is sequestered into regional lymph nodes at this age. After establishng infection at these sites a viraemia follows.

20.3 *Figure 20.10* shows the change in a variety of indices of HIV infection over time. Acute seroconversion causes an infectious mononucleosis-like illness in up to 50% of those infected with HIV. Common symptoms are fever, lymphadenopathy, pharyngitis, rashes and myalgia. At

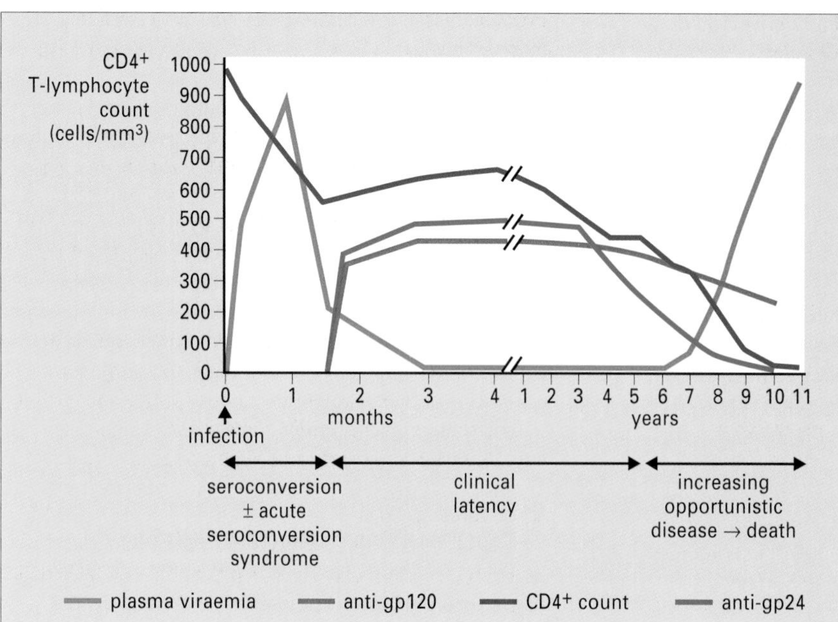

Fig. 20.10 A typical course of HIV infection.

this point there is drop in the CD4 (and also CD8) lymphocyte count and a rise in plasma viraemia and p24 antigen concentration. Antibodies to HIV surface glycoproteins gp120 and gp41 are produced from approximately 6 weeks after infection and are initially of the IgM class. IgG antibodies of the same specificities follow the IgM response and persist during the latent phase. Viraemia and p24 antigenaemia are generally low during this period. Disease progression is heralded by a declining CD4 lymphocyte count and a rise in plasma viraemia. Clinically, CD4 counts have become a widely used index of progression. Plasma viraemia is the most accurate measure of disease progression, and is becoming a more commonly used method.

21. SEVERE ANAPHYLACTIC SHOCK

21.1 Traditionally, the term anaphylaxis has been used to describe a systemic clinical syndrome caused by IgE-mediated degranulation of mast cells and basophils. Susceptible individuals exposed to a sensitizing antigen produce specific IgE antibodies which bind to high-affinity IgE receptors (FcεRI) found on mast cells and basophils. The receptor binds the Fc portion of the antibody-leaving the Fab binding sites available to interact with antigen. The avidity of this Fc binding reaction is high and therefore the dissociation of IgE from the receptors is slow, with a long half-life. On subsequent exposure, the antigen is bound by the IgE receptor complexes, which causes receptor-mediated activation of the cells with release of preformed and *de novo* synthesized mediators. Degranulation is rapid and is completed within 30 minutes. These mediators, released on a large scale, are responsible for the clinical manifestations of anaphylaxis.

The IgE-mediated mechanism of mast cell degranulation has been implicated in the pathogenesis of anaphylaxis triggered by a variety of agents. These include antibiotics (e.g. penicillins, cephalosporins), foods (e.g. milk, nuts, shellfish), foreign proteins (e.g. insulin, bee venom, latex) and pharmacological agents (e.g. streptokinase, vaccines). Patients who have anaphylaxis may or may not have a history of atopy. Natural exposure to common allergens such as pollen or dust mites is only very rarely a cause of anaphylaxis. However, when patients who also have asthma develop anaphylaxis due to venom, penicillin or food antigens, the reactions are more dangerous because they can include rapid onset of bronchospasm.

Mast cell degranulation can occur by IgE independent pathways. Prior exposure is not a prerequisite as specific IgE antibodies are not involved. Three putative mechanisms of anaphylactoid reactions are given below:

- Blood, blood products and immunoglobulins can cause an anaphylactoid reaction. The suggested mechanism is the formation of immune complexes with subsequent complement activation and production of C3a and C5a. Both of these complement components (anaphylatoxins) are capable of degranulating mast cells directly. In addition, both components increase vasopermeability and may induce hypotension.
- Certain therapeutic and diagnostic agents such as opiates, muscle relaxants and contrast media are also capable of directly causing mast cell degranulation and anaphylaxis.
- Five to ten per cent of asthmatic subjects produce a reaction to non-steroidal anti-inflammatory drugs (NSAIDs), such as aspirin or indomethacin. Symptoms commonly include bronchospasm, rhinorrhoea and, rarely, vascular collapse. The ability of these agents to cause anaphylaxis appears to correlate with their effectiveness in inhibiting prostaglandin synthesis. The mechanism of this sensitivity is unknown, but increased leukotriene production occurs which strongly suggests that triggering of mast cells is part of the reaction.

21.2 There is a great variation in the timing and nature of anaphylactic symptoms. The onset is usually within seconds or minutes of exposure although delays of an hour have been reported. The following are common presentations which may occur singly or in combination:

- Cutaneous: erythema, pruritus of hands, feet and abdomen, urticaria, angioedema.
- Respiratory: laryngeal oedema causing hoarseness which may progress to asphyxia, bronchoconstriction causing wheezing, rhinorrhoea.
- Cardiovascular: hypotension, arrhythmias, tachycardia, vascular collapse.
- Gastrointestinal: cramping abdominal pain, nausea, vomiting, diarrhoea.

The majority of cases of anaphylactic reactions are not fatal. It has been estimated that 1–2% of courses of penicillin therapy are complicated by systemic reactions but only 10% of these are serious. In the USA some 400–800 people die annually from penicillin anaphylaxis with a similar figure for contrast media. Seventy per cent of deaths result from respiratory complications (laryngeal oedema and/or bronchospasm) with 25% resulting from cardiovascular dysfunction.

Prompt treatment of anaphylaxis is essential as death may occur rapidly. The patient is placed in the recovery position, oxygen is given by mask and 0.5–1.0 ml of adrenaline is injected intramuscularly. This has the effect of raising the blood pressure, relaxing bronchial smooth muscle and preventing further mediator release. Intravenous antihistamines (e.g. 10 mg of chlorpheniramine) can be useful as histamine can cause vasodilation, cardiac arrhythmias and bronchospasm. Corticosteroids (e.g. 100 mg of hydrocortisone) intravenously may help to reduce any late phase response.

21.3 The first step is to obtain a thorough history of previous adverse reactions. The timing and nature of such reactions should be noted. Skin prick testing with insect venom is a fast and sensitive method of detecting anti-venom IgE. Radioallergosorbent tests can detect venom-specific IgE, but are positive in only 80% of those with significant reactions to venom skin prick tests.

Immunotherapy is best reserved for those with life-threatening systemic reactions to insect venom. The patient is given increasing subcutaneous dosages and is then given a monthly maintenance dose of 100 μg. The clinical protection rate is in the order of 98% for both adults and children.

22. BLOOD GROUPS AND HAEMOLYTIC DISEASE OF THE NEWBORN

22.1 Since Mrs Chareston has clearly becomed sensitized to Rhesus-D, it is most likely that the first child is RhD$^+$. The alternative explanation, that she has become sensitized by a blood transfusion, is highly unlikely, because of the routine matching of this blood group when carrying out transfusions.

22.2 The mother has become sensitized to the fetal red cells and successive sensitizations produce progressively stronger responses in the mother, and more serious disease in susceptible children.

22.3 The aim is to clear the fetal RhD$^+$ erythrocytes, before they have a chance to sensitize the mother's immune system.

22.4 If one gave them pre-partum, the antibodies would cross the placenta and produce or exacerbate HDNB in the fetus.

22.5 Rhesus prophylaxis is not always successful, but in this case, there was no treatment after the first pregnancy and Mrs Chareston was already sensitized to RhD. Preventing further responses in an individual who is already sensitized is less likely to succeed because of the nature of secondary immune responses – less antigen is required to trigger the response.

22.6 The most likely explanation is that the child is Rh$^-$. Indeed this turns out to be the case. A Rh$^-$ child must have received a Rh$^-$ gene from both parents. Assuming that Mr Chareston is the father of the fourth child, we can say that his genotype is RhD$^+$/RhD$^-$ (heterozygote), and that the child received RhD$^-$ genes from both parents.

22.7 Antigens of the ABO blood group are carbohydrates and tend to induce IgM antibodies which do not undergo affinity maturation or class-switching (see Chapter 8). IgM does not cross the placenta (see Chapter 4), and so does not produced HDNB.

22.8 The second child. Because ABO blood groups are co-dominately expressed, for a child to have the blood group 'B', one or both parents must have blood group 'B'. As neither Mr or Mrs Chareston have this blood group, the B gene must have come from someone else.

23. DRUG ALLERGY

23.1 The symptoms of rash, arthralgia and headache do have the hallmarks of an allergic drug response. However, the onset of the symptoms was after the drug had been discontinued, perhaps throwing doubt onto the causal relationship between drug intake and adverse response. Such a profile of symptoms is seen in the 'post-infection' syndrome and in that case is not caused by a drug reaction.

The delayed onset reflects the need for antigen to remain in the circulation for a prolonged period so that when sufficient antibody is synthesized, circulating antigen–antibody complexes are formed which 'precipitate' out into the various target tissues. Wherever the complexes are sited, complement can be fixed and local damage occur. This patient probably had damage to the glomeruli of the kidney as shown by the proteinuria as well as inflammation in the joints and skin. It is also possible that the urinary tract infection had not cleared and that was the origin of the proteinuria.

She also had abnormalities which showed that

complement was being consumed – low C4 and C3 – as well as an increase in breakdown products, namely C3a. Named anaphylatoxins, C3a and C5a can directly release histamine from mast cells. This can lead to a confusing picture of a Type III hypersensitivity reaction presenting clinically as anaphylactic shock.

Similar symptoms to Yvonne's were seen with old fashioned serum sickness reactions that followed foreign protein injections such as anti-tetanus serum (ATS) which was made in horses. ATS was given when there was a danger of tetanus to provide passive immunity to the patient whilst active immunization was being given. Blood products can also give a serum sickness syndrome.

23.2 A variety of drugs can cause reactions by activating effector pathways by non-immunological means. Some drugs, such as opiates, can cause the release of mediators from mast cells by direct action on the cell, without the involvement of IgE. Some compounds, such as X-ray contrast material given intravenously in order to visualize the excretion pattern of the kidney, activate the alternative pathway of complement and thereby produce anaphylatoxins, C3a and C5a. As mentioned above, this can lead to anaphylactic shock. Other drugs such as aspirin and non-steroidal anti-inflammatory drugs (NSAIDs) alter arachidonic acid pathways and can again produce anaphylactic shock. There is a well-described triad of asthma, nasal polyps and aspirin sensitivity. These patients are at risk of acute status asthmaticus if they take an aspirin or other NSAID.

Other reactions can be produced by overdose where the symptoms are predictable and due to the main action of the drug. This may not be deliberate but due to the poor excretion of the drug by the patient or its slow breakdown. Secondary effects are often seen and these represent actions of the drugs that are not the ones for which the drug is given. Examples of this are the alopecia, gut problems and bone marrow toxicity of many immunosuppressive compounds.

Other factors relate to the 'ecology' of the patient taking the drugs. Broad spectrum antibiotics change the bacterial flora in the gut and often lead to an overgrowth of candida in the mouth, gastrointestinal tract or vagina. Drug interactions can also lead to clinical problems. Probenecid given for gout interferes with penicillin excretion by the kidney. Phenytoin given for epilepsy interferes with folate metabolism. It has also been reported to lead to reduced levels of IgA if given long term.

Some drugs actually make the pre-existing disease worse. This is best seen in skin disease where lithium given for manic-depressive illnesses can exacerbate both acne and psoriasis.

23.3 If a patient has already had an allergic reaction to penicillin, they are 10 times more likely to react to other antibiotics. The reverse is also true in that if a patient has already reacted to other antimicrobials, he or she is more likely to react to penicillin. There are definable risk factors for drug allergy such as genetic background, metabolic status, concurrent drug therapy and the role of the illness itself, such as HIV infection or autoimmune disease, in altering the handling of drugs. This can be seen in patients taking aminophylline for asthma who have a virus infection. The virus reduces the degradation of aminophylline by the cytochrome P450 enzyme system, increases the half-life and can cause toxicity.

23.4 The patient presented with a rash, painful joints and evidence of renal damage as shown by proteinuria. A possible diagnosis was systemic lupus erythematosus (SLE). In this instance it could have been induced by drugs when the anti-nuclear antibody would have been positive. A number of drugs, especially hydralazine and procainamide, are capable of inducing anti-nuclear antibodies in a significant proportion of patients taking them – in the region of 60%. In most of the patients the antibodies are harmless and may remain at a high titre even when the drugs have been discontinued for years.

In a small percentage of patients, a clinical syndrome resembling SLE does develop. The main symptoms in these instances are pulmonary and polyserositis but there is a general lack of kidney or nervous system involvement. It would be unlikely on clinical grounds that Yvonne had drug-induced SLE and her anti-nuclear antibodies were negative. The mechanisms by which these drugs induce the autoantibodies is unknown. The lupus inducing drugs can be given to patients with pre-existing SLE without making the condition worse.

24. A HYPERSENSITIVITY TYPE IV REACTION

24.1 Granulomas are composed of lymphocytes, macrophages and epithelioid cells. The latter develop from macrophages following chronic antigenic stimulation and may fuse to form multinucleate giant cells, typical of granulomas. Cytokines involved in this process include T-cell-derived IFNγ and TNF, both for the activation of macrophages and the organization of the granuloma.

24.2 Histological examination at the site of a DTH reaction reveals odema of the dermis with an infiltrate of monocytes and lymphocytes. This resolves over 1–2 weeks. Granulomas do not form at the sites of DTH reactions if soluble antigen, such as tuberculin, are used. By contrast, in the lymph node a chronic granulomatous response develops as the mycobacteria survive within macrophages leading to persistent stimulation of T cells and chronic inflammation.

24.3 CD4 T lymphocytes are the major cells responsible for the recognition of soluble recall antigens and the stimulation of DTH reactions.

24.4 Other infections, such as cat scratch fever due to *Bartonella henselae*, histoplasmosis and tularaemia, may cause granulomas in lymph nodes. These are diagnosed by the clinical pattern and microbial cultures. Sarcoidosis causes non-caseating granulomas and is diagnosed by clinical features, histology and the absence of an infectious cause. Granulomas may also develop in response to foreign bodies, such as talc and silica, or exposure to beryllium.

24.5 The brother's DTH reaction is evidence of a strong T-cell response to soluble antigens from *M. tuberculosis*. This indicates that he has been infected with *M. tuberculosis*, but does not mean that he has active tuberculosis disease at present. Normally he would have investigations to exclude active tuberculosis, and if this is not present he would be considered for chemoprophylaxis to eradicate the infection and prevent progression to disease in later life.

25. KIDNEY TRANSPLANTATION

25.1 There is a great shortage of donor organs. The supply of cadaveric organs depends on the unfortunate deaths of healthy individuals and the willingness of their relatives to allow donation. In addition, the available organs are given to recipients with the best HLA tissue match. At random there is less than a 1 in 20 000 chance of finding a perfect match. In the case of kidney transplantation the blood group antigens must be taken into account. Mrs X is blood group B, which is uncommon (less than 10%), and will therefore have antibodies to tissues from blood group A donors. Blood group A is the most common blood group (about 45% of individuals).

25.2 Mrs X is HLA identical to her brother Fred and shares one HLA haplotype with her brother Gary. There is a 1 in 4 chance of siblings inheriting the same mendelian characteristics from their parents.

25.3 Like Mrs X and her brother Fred, Bert and Edna are HLA identical to each other. Of the five children of Mrs X, four have Mr X as their biological father. However, it is clear that Dave was fathered by a man other than Mr X! This is not uncommon. Approximately 5–10% of children may be like Dave!

25.4 HLA identical: Fred
HLA haplotype match: Anne, Bert, Chas, Dave, Gary
Complete HLA mismatch: Mr X.

25.5 If only HLA matching is considered, Fred would be the best donor because there would be no HLA mismatch between the donor and recipient.

25.6 Mrs X is blood group B, and therefore has antibodies to blood group A, thus excluding Mr X, Anne, Bert, Edna and Fred. Only Chas, Dave and Gary would be suitable. Because Mrs X is Rhesus positive (has antigen D) she will not have anti-Rh antibodies, so typing for this blood group can be ignored in this instance.

25.7 Chas is first choice. He is HLA haplotype matched, he is ABO compatible, and is a young man. In general, younger kidneys last for longer than older kidneys, and younger people respond better to surgery.

Gary might be considered. He too is haplotype identical and ABO compatible. In fact, in terms of his ABO blood group, being blood group O he is the 'universal donor', having no A or B blood group antigens on his tissues. However, he is older and therefore not an ideal donor.

Dave is like his brother Chas, HLA haplotype identical and ABO compatible with his mother. However, he is only 15 years of age and minors are generally excluded from this kind of surgery.

25.8 The organ from Chas suffered hyperacute rejection. This is mediated by preformed antibodies in the recipient binding to antigens in the graft. The antibodies fix complement and initiate the process of graft thrombosis. Platelet aggregation in the blood vessels blocks blood flow and the graft dies of lack of oxygen (ischaemia).

25.9 The main stimuli for antibodies that cause hyperacute rejection are rejection of a previous graft, blood transfusions and multiple pregnancies by the same partner. Mrs X has had four children by the same father, Mr X, and is likely to have become sensitized towards class I HLA antigens that Mr X has but Mrs X does not possess. In this case antibodies to either HLA-A3 or HLA-B7 could have been responsible for the hyperacute rejection.

25.10 Cross-match tests are used to detect anti-donor antibodies before transplantation. These tests are becoming more and more sensitive, but occasionally an antibody in low titre may go undetected. It appears that the cross-match test used at the time of the transplantation failed to detect an antibody to a HLA class I antigen. Fortunately this seldom happens nowadays and hyperacute rejection is now very rare indeed.

25.11 There were three family members who were originally suitable for donation, Chas, Dave and Gary.

The kidney from Chas was transplanted and rejected by Mrs X. Gary is now 60 and is less attractive as a donor. In any case he shares the HLA-B14 antigen with Mr X which, because Mrs X is sensitized to Mr X, may be a target for hyperacute rejection. The possibility that Mrs X has an antibody to HLA-B14 would have to be investigated very carefully! Dave has by now reached the age of majority and could be considered as a donor. He is HLA haplotype identical to his mother, and is ABO compatible. Furthermore, because he has a different father, Dave is less likely to express antigens that might be the target of hyperacute rejection. It seems that Dave would be the most suitable donor. You might like to consider the emotional pressure this puts on Dave, given the seriousness of his mother's condition and how his family are likely to react if he wants to change his mind about donation.

25.12 Triple immunosuppression is standard in most transplant centres. It consists of steroids plus either cyclosporin or FK506 and either azathioprine or mycophenolate. Some centres do add other agents such as anti-lymphocyte serum or a monoclonal antibody to T cells (OKT3).

25.13 About a third of all transplant recipients suffer an episode of acute rejection in the first few weeks. This is mainly a cell-mediated immune response.

25.14 The anti-rejection therapy often used is to give three large doses of steroids on three consecutive days (totalling 2–3 g of steroids). This causes apoptosis (programmed cell death) of activated lymphocytes and stops the rejection episode very effectively. Other anti-rejection therapies are used, such as giving OKT3 anti-T-cell monoclonal antibody.

25.15 Because of the immunosuppression, patients are more prone to infection. The immunosuppressive drugs used can be toxic, so a dose reduction or a change in medication may be required. In addition, transplant patients on high doses of immunosuppression may develop a post-transplant lymphoproliferative disorder caused by Epstein–Barr virus infection. Reduction of the dose usually helps. In the longer term transplant patients have a higher risk of cancer, because of depressed immune surveillance.

25.16 Mrs X finally lost her kidney transplant to chronic rejection. This may involve both immunological and non-immunological damage. The damage initiates a repair process involving the production of growth factors in the graft. None of the drugs in current use control this process very well so, although the doctors change drugs and doses, it is very difficult to control chronic rejection.

26. AUTOIMMUNITY AND AUTOIMMUNE DISEASE

26.1 It is thought that free DNA filtered in the kidney fixes to the glomerular basement membrane and can then bind anti-DNA antibodies, which then form an immune complex *in situ*. Complement is then fixed, resulting in local damage.

26.2 This is a vexed question. Although DNA–anti-DNA complexes are found in tissues, efforts to find these complexes in the serum have failed. In addition, immunizing lupus-prone animals with DNA does not produce clinical lupus. However, introduction of transgenes encoding anti-ds DNA in mice can produce lupus.

26.3 A possible explanation is that the mononuclear–phagocyte system becomes saturated and is therefore unable to clear the soluble complexes, which are thought to be most likely pathogenic. It is also possible that the reduction in the complement receptors on red cells (CRI) might also predispose to poor clearance of complexes.

26.4 Over 95% of patients with SLE have ANA as the major autoantibody. Antibodies to extractable nuclear antigens are also seen, but much less frequently. Anti-double-stranded DNA antibodies are the most specific to SLE because anti-single-stranded antibodies are found in a variety of other situations, such as other autoimmune disease, a variety of infections and inflammatory conditions.

27. IMMUNOLOGICAL TECHNIQUES

27.1–3 Immunise inbred animals with the protein and collect serum samples during the immunization regimen. Coat microtitre plates with either the protein or purified virus and perform ELISA using enzyme-labelled immunoglobulin class and subclass-specific antibodies. The affinity of the antibodies in the serum samples during the immune response can be assessed using biosensor assays in which the sensing surface has been coated with either protein or purified virus.

27.4 The proliferation of splenocytes from protein- or virus-immunized inbred mice can be assessed following *in vitro* culture with various concentrations of either protein or purified virus. Cytotoxic activity of the splenocytes can be assessed *in vitro* using chromium ^{51}-labelled virus-infected target cells of the same haplotype as the effectors.

27.5 FACS can be used to separate CD4$^+$ and CD8$^+$ cell populations from the splenocytes from protein- and virus-immunized mice and these purified sub-populations used *in vitro* proliferation and cytotoxicity assays.

Index

J

K

L

N